*Editors*
Berger, Engelhardt, Henß, Mertelsmann

Co-Editors
Andreeff, Koziner, Messner, Thatcher

# Concise Manual
# of Hematology and Oncology

*Editors*
D. P. Berger, M. Engelhardt, H. Henß, R. Mertelsmann

Co-Editors
M. Andreeff, B. Koziner, H. A. Messner, N. Thatcher

# Concise Manual of Hematology and Oncology

With 138 Figures and 474 Tables

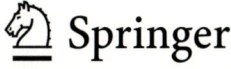 Springer

*Editors*

**Dietmar P. Berger**
University Medical Center
Department of Hematology and Oncology
Hugstetter Strasse 55
79106 Freiburg, Germany

**Monika Engelhardt**
University Medical Center
Department of Hematology and Oncology
Hugstetter Strasse 55
79106 Freiburg, Germany

**Hartmut Henß**
Tumorzentrum Ludwig-Heilmeyer
Comprehensive Cancer Center
University Medical Center
Hugstetter Strasse 55
79106 Freiburg, Germany

**Roland Mertelsmann**
University Medical Center
Department of Hematology and Oncology
Hugstetter Strasse 55
79106 Freiburg, Germany

*Co-Editors*

**Michael Andreeff**
MD Anderson Cancer Center
1515 Holcombe Boulevard 081
Houston, TX 77030-4095, USA

**Benjamin Koziner**
Unitad de Investigaciones
Oncohematologicas
Laboratorio 'Nelly Arrieta de Blaquier'
Agrelo 3038
Buenos Aires C.P. 1221, Argentinia

**Hans A. Messner**
Princess Margaret Hospital
5th Floor, Room 107
610 University Avenue
Toronto, ON M5G 2M9, Canada

**Nick Thatcher**
Department of Medical Oncology
Christie Hospital NHS Trust
Wilmslow Road
Manchester M20 4BX, United Kingdom

We would like to thank Dr. Milena Pantic and Dr. Ralph Wäsch for kindly providing the figures used for the cover.

Dietmar P. Berger is an employee of Amgen Inc., USA.

ISBN 978-3-540-73276-1 Springer Berlin Heidelberg New York

Library of Congress Control Number: 2007934266

Springer-Verlag is a part of Springer Science+Business Media
springer.com

© Springer-Verlag Berlin Heidelberg 2008

Editor: Ute Heilmann, Heidelberg, Germany
Desk Editor: Meike Stoeck, Heidelberg, Germany
Cover design: Frido Steinen-Broo, eStudio Calamar, Spain
Typesetting and Production: le-tex publishing oHG, Leipzig, Germany

Printed on acid-free paper 24/3180/YL 5 4 3 2 1 0

# Preface

## How Do We Treat?

Hematology and Oncology have seen rapid progress and advances during recent years. Increased knowledge of tumor biology, epidemiology, molecular genetics, growth regulation, and cellular functions has led to novel therapeutic paradigms. Targeted treatment approaches, antibodies, immunotherapy, and other new techniques complement classic chemotherapy, radiotherapy, and surgery. Patients are increasingly well educated as web-based information on diagnostic and therapeutic options as well as quality management and tumor outcome data are readily available.

In this dynamic and fast-paced environment, it is of central importance to base clinical decisions and medical practice on the best available evidence. Continuous quality management, with clinical process documentation, standardization, and evaluation, leads to improved patient care and long-term outcomes. For these reasons, we have started to systematically capture and evaluate data on diagnosis, treatment, and outcomes of patients with solid tumors and hematological neoplasms at the Freiburg University Medical Center. We have developed standard operating procedures, clinical pathways, and diagnostic and therapeutic processes, following the principles of "Good Clinical Practice." These processes (e.g., detailed protocols for chemotherapy application, treatment flowcharts, clinical pathways) are continuously tested and validated in clinical practice. National and international guidelines, new clinical study data, and international expert advice are incorporated into a framework of clinical standards. Based on this work, the Freiburg University Medical Center and the Comprehensive Cancer Center Freiburg have been recognized as one of the centers of excellence in hematology and oncology in Germany and Europe.

The *Concise Manual of Hematology and Oncology* is the result of this continuous process. It offers a specific view based on the daily practice at a large European academic medical center, and we welcome any comments and discussion. Several German language editions of the manual have been published since 1998, and we are thankful for all the positive feedback and constructive criticism we received. With the first English edition, we again want to support practicing physicians and healthcare providers in their daily interaction with patients in hematology and oncology. Treatment of patients with malignant diseases is always a challenge, in curative, supportive, and palliative settings, and each patient—in his or her unique situation—deserves the best available therapy and care.

The Editors
March 2008

# Contents

# Abbreviations

| | | | |
|---|---|---|---|
| **A.** | Arteria | **DDAVP** | Desamino-D-Arginin-Vasopressin (Desmopressin) |
| **Aa.** | Arteriae | | |
| **Ab** | Antibody | **Def** | Definition |
| **abs.** | absolute (ly) | **DFS** | Disease free survival |
| **Ad** | Adresses | **DFI** | Disease free interval |
| **Ag** | Antigen | **Dg** | Diagnostic |
| **AIDS** | Aquired Immune Deficiency Syndrome | **DIC** | Disseminated intravascular Coagulation |
| **AIHA** | Autoimmune Hemolytic Anemia | **dl** | Deciliter (100 ml) |
| **AJCC** | American Joint Committee on Cancer | **DNA** | Deoxyribonucleic Acid |
| | | **Dos** | Dosing |
| **ALL** | Acute lymphoblastic Leukemia | | |
| **AML** | Acute myeloid Leukemia | **EBV** | Epstein Barr Virus |
| **ANA** | Antinuclear Antibodies | **ECOG** | Eastern Cooperative Oncology Group (ECOG Performance Scale) |
| **a.o.** | among others | | |
| **ARDS** | Acute Respiratory Distress Syndrome | **ECG** | Elektrocardiogram |
| | | **e.g.** | for instance |
| **ATIII** | Antithrombin III | **EORTC** | European Organisation for Research and Treatment of Cancer |
| **ATTN** | Attention, be careful, | | |
| | | **Ep** | Epidemiology |
| **B** | Bolus injection | **ES** | Extrasystoles |
| **BC** | Blood Count | **ESR** | Erythrocyte Sedimentation Rate |
| **BCh** | Biochemistry | **Et** | Etiology |
| **BM** | Bone marrow | **etc.** | et cetera |
| **BW** | Body weight | | |
| **BSA** | Body surface area | **F** | Factor (Clotting factors FI to FXIII) |
| | | **FBC** | Full Blood Count |
| **°C** | Degree Celsius | **FIGO** | International Federation of Gynecology and Obstetrics |
| **Ca²⁺** | Calcium | | |
| **CD** | Cluster of Differentiation | **F/U** | Follow Up |
| **CFU** | Colony Forming Units | | |
| **Chap.** | Chapter | **g** | Gram |
| **Chem** | Chemistry | **GFR** | Glomerular Filtration Rate |
| **Ci.** | Contraindication | **GvHD** | Graft versus Host Disease |
| **c.i.v.** | continuous intravenous | **GvL** | Graft versus Leukemia |
| **Cl⁻** | Chloride | | |
| **Class** | Classifikation | **h** | hour(s) (hora) |
| **CLL** | Chronic lymphatic Leukemia | **HAV** | Hepatitis A Virus |
| **CML** | Chronische myeloid Leukemia | **Hb** | Hemoglobin |
| **CMV** | Cytomegalie Virus | **HBV** | Hepatitis B Virus |
| **CNS** | Central nervous system | **HCV** | Hepatitis C Virus |
| **Co** | Complications | **hd** | high dose |
| **CRP** | C-reactive Protein | **HIT** | Heparin-induced Thrombopenia |
| **CSF** | CerebroSpinal Fluid | **HIV** | Human Immunodeficiency Virus |
| **CT** | Computed tomography | **Hkt** | Hematocrit |
| **CVC** | Central Venous Catheter | **HSV** | Herpes Simplex Virus |
| **CVL** | Central Venous Line | **HUS** | Hemolytic-uremic Syndrome |
| **CVP** | Central Venous Pressure | | |
| | | **i.a.** | Intraarterial |
| **d** | day(s) (dies) | **i.m.** | Intramuscular |
| **DLCBL** | Diffuse Large B-Cell Lymphoma | **i.p.** | intraperitoneal |
| **Dd** | Differential diagnosis | **i.th.** | Intrathecal |
| **Ddi** | Drug drug interaction | **i.v.** | Intravenous |

| | |
|---|---|
| ICD-10 | International Classification of Diseases (10. edition) |
| Ig | Immunglobulin(e) |
| Ind | Indication |
| ITP | Idiopathic thrombocytopenic Purpura |
| IU | International Units |
| $K^+$ | Potassium |
| kDa | kilo Dalton |
| kg | Kilogramm |
| l | Liter |
| LDH | Lactate dehydrogenase |
| LFT | Liver Function Tests |
| Lit | Literature |
| LMWH | Low Molecular Weight Heparin |
| Ln | Lymph nodes |
| LPHD | Lymphocyte Predominant Hodgkin's Disease |
| M. | Morbus |
| MALT | mucosa associated lymphoid tissue |
| MDS | Myelodysplastic Syndrome(s) |
| Meth | Methods |
| mg | Milligram |
| µg | Microgram |
| $Mg^{2+}$ | Magnesium |
| MGUS | Monoclonal Gammopathy of Unknown Significance |
| min | Minute(s) |
| ml | Milliliter |
| µl | Microliter |
| MOA | Mechanism of Action |
| MPS | Myeloproliferative Syndrome(s) |
| MW | Molecular weight |
| $Na^+$ | Sodium |
| NCI | National Cancer Institute |
| NHL | Non-Hodgkin's Lymphoma |
| NMR | Nuclear Magnetic Resonance Tomography |
| Path | Pathology |
| PBCh | Pathobiochemistry |
| PBSCT | Peripheral Blood Stem Cell Transplantation |
| PCP | Pneumocystis Carinii Pneumonia |
| PCR | Polymerase Chain Reaction |
| PET | Positron Emission Tomography |
| Persp. | Perspective |
| Pg | Pathogenesis |

| | |
|---|---|
| Pharm | Pharmacology |
| Phys | Physiology |
| PKin | Pharmacokinetics |
| Phys | Physiology |
| PNH | Paroxysmal Nocturnal Hemoglobinuria |
| PPhys | Pathophysiology |
| PPSB | Prothrombin Complex Concentrate |
| Prg | Prognosis |
| PT | Prothrombin Time |
| PTT | Partial Prothromin Time |
| Px | Prophylaxis |
| ® | registered trade mark |
| RFA | Radio frequency ablation |
| RNA | Ribonucleic Acid |
| Ref | references |
| RT | Radiotherapy |
| s | seconds |
| s.c. | subcutaneous |
| SCC | Squamous Cell Cancer |
| Se | Side effects |
| SLE | Systemic Lupus erythematodes |
| SOP | Standard Operating Procedure |
| Stag | Staging |
| SVES | Supraventricular Extasystoles |
| Sy | Symptoms |
| $t\frac{1}{2}$ | Half life time |
| TBI | Total Body Irradiation |
| TBC | Tuberculosis |
| Th | Treatment, Therapy |
| TNM | TNM-System, Tumor classifikation (defines T = Tumor, N = Lymph nodes and M = Metastases) |
| TRALI | Transfusion Associated Lung Injury |
| TTP | Thrombotic-thrombozytopenic Purpura |
| U | Units |
| U&E | Urine and Electrolytes |
| UICC | Union Internationale Contre le Cancer |
| UFH | Unfractionated Heparin |
| V. | Vena |
| VES | Ventricular Extrasystoles |
| Vv. | Venae |
| VZV | Varicella Zoster Virus |
| WHO | World Health Organisation |
| Web | Internet adresses |

## Special symbols

| | |
|---|---|
| α | Alpha |
| β | Beta |
| γ | Gamma |
| δ | Delta |
| κ | Kappa |
| λ | Lambda |
| μ | Mu, Micro |
| → | leading to |
| ↑ | increased |
| ↓ | lowered, decreased |
| > | larger than, more frequent than |
| < | smaller than, less frequent as |
| ≥ | larger or equal |
| ≤ | smaller or equal |
| ≈ | about |
| ♀ | women, female |
| ♂ | men, male |
| ▶ | see (refers to other chapter) |
| ☎ | phone |

## Additional Abbreviations are explained in the respective chapters

# Contributors

**Adam, Gerhard**
Asklepios Klinik Triberg
Fachklinik f. Innere Medizin
Hematologie/Onkologie
Ludwigstrasse 1-2
78098 Triberg, Germany

**Allgaier, H.-P.**
Deaconness Hospital
Wirthstrasse 11
79110 Freiburg, Germany

**Andreeff, Michael**
MD Anderson Cancer Center
1515 Holcombe Boulevard 081
Houston, TX 77030-4095, USA

**Behringer, D.**
Augusta-Kranken-Anstalt
Hematology, Oncology
Bergstrasse 26
44791 Bochum, Germany

**Berger, Dietmar P.**
University Medical Center
Department of Hematology and Oncology
Hugstetter Strasse 55
79106 Freiburg, Germany

**Bertz, Hartmut**
University Medical Center
Department of Hematology and Oncology
Hugstetter Strasse 55
79106 Freiburg, Germany

**Blattmann, Ursula**
University Medical Center
Central Physiotherapy
Department of Internal Medicine
Hugstetter Strasse 55
79106 Freiburg, Germany

**Burger, Jan**
MD Anderson Cancer Center
PO Box 301402
Houston, TX 77230-1402, USA

**Burger, Meike**
University Medical Center
Department of Hematology and Oncology
Hugstetter Strasse 55
79106 Freiburg, Germany

**Daskalakis, Michael**
University Medical Center
Department of Hematology and Oncology
Hugstetter Strasse 55
79106 Freiburg, Germany

**Deschler, Barbara**
University Medical Center
Department of Hematology and Oncology
Hugstetter Strasse 55
79106 Freiburg, Germany

**Digel, Werner**
University Medical Center
Department of Hematology and Oncology
Hugstetter Strasse 55
79106 Freiburg, Germany

**Engelhardt, Andrea**
University Medical Center
Department of Hematology and Oncology
Hugstetter Strasse 55
79106 Freiburg, Germany

**Engelhardt, Monika**
University Medical Center
Department of Hematology and Oncology
Hugstetter Strasse 55
79106 Freiburg, Germany

**Engelhardt, Rupert**
University Medical Center
Department of Hematology and Oncology
Hugstetter Strasse 55
79106 Freiburg, Germany

**Fetscher, Sebastian**
Sana Kliniken Lübeck
Klinik für Hämatologie/Onkologie
Städt. Krankenhaus Süd
Kronsforder Allee 71/73
23560 Lübeck, Germany

**Finke, Jürgen**
University Medical Center
Department of Hematology and Oncology
Hugstetter Strasse 55
79106 Freiburg, Germany

**Frank, Uwe**
University Medical Center
Department of Environmental Medicine
and Hygiene
Hugstetter Strasse 55
79106 Freiburg, Germany

**Gärtner, Frank**
University Medical Center
Department of Hematology and Oncology
Hugstetter Strasse 55
79106 Freiburg, Germany

**Göbel, Alexandra**
University Medical Center
Hospital Pharmacy
Hugstetter Strasse 55
79106 Freiburg, Germany

**Gölz, Tanja**
University Medical Center
Department of Hematology and Oncology
Hugstetter Strasse 55
79106 Freiburg, Germany

**Grüllich, Carsten**
University Medical Center
Department of Hematology and Oncology
Hugstetter Strasse 55
79106 Freiburg, Germany

**Harder, Jan**
University Medical Center
Department of Gastroenterology
Hepatology, Endocrinology
and Infectious Diseases
Hugstetter Strasse 55
79106 Freiburg, Germany

**Heeskens, Katrin**
Blumhardtstrasse 17
75378 Bad Liebenzell, Germany

**Heining-Mikesch, Kristina**
University Medical Center
Department of Hematology and Oncology
Hugstetter Strasse 55
79106 Freiburg, Germany

**Heinz, Jürgen**
University Medical Center
Department of Hematology and Oncology
Hugstetter Strasse 55
79106 Freiburg, Germany

**Henne, Karl**
University Medical Center
Department of Radiation Therapy
Hugstetter Strasse 55
79106 Freiburg, Germany

**Henß, Hartmut**
Tumorzentrum Ludwig-Heilmeyer
Comprehensive Cancer Center
University Medical Center
Hugstetter Strasse 55
79106 Freiburg, Germany

**Houet, Leonora**
University Medical Center
Department of Hematology and Oncology
Hugstetter Strasse 55
79106 Freiburg, Germany

**Illerhaus, Gerald**
University Medical Center
Department of Hematology and Oncology
Hugstetter Strasse 55
79106 Freiburg, Germany

**Jüttner, Eva**
University Medical Center
Department of Pathology
Breisacher Strasse 115a
79106 Freiburg, Germany

**Kaskel, Anna-Katharina**
University Medical Center
Department of Hematology and Oncology
Hugstetter Strasse 55
79106 Freiburg, Germany

**Kiani, Alexander**
Medizinische Klinik und Poliklinik I
Universitätsklinikum Carl Gustav Carus
Technical University Dresden
Fetscherstrasse 74
01307 Dresden, Germany

**Koziner, Benjamin**
Unitad de Investigaciones
Oncohematologicas
Laboratorio 'Nelly Arrieta de Blaquier'
Agrelo 3038
Buenos Aires C.P. 1221, Argentinia

**Kunzmann, Regina**
University Medical Center
Department of Hematology and Oncology
Hugstetter Strasse 55
79106 Freiburg, Germany

**Leo, Albrecht**
Ruprecht-Karls University Heidelberg
Institute of Immunology, Serology
and Transfusion Medicine
Im Neuenheimer Feld 305
69120 Heidelberg, Germany

**Leo, Eugen**
Johnson & Johnson
Turnhoutseweg 30b
2340 Beerse, Belgium

**Lubrich, Beate**
University Medical Center
Hospital Pharmacy
Hugstetter Strasse 55
79106 Freiburg, Germany

**Luebbert, Michael**
University Medical Center
Department of Hematology and Oncology
Hugstetter Strasse 55
79106 Freiburg, Germany

**Maier-Lenz, Herbert**
University Medical Center
Center of Clinical Trials
Elsässer Strasse 2
79106 Freiburg, Germany

**Marks, Reinhard**
University Medical Center
Department of Hematology and Oncology
Hugstetter Strasse 55
79106 Freiburg, Germany

**Martens, Uwe**
University Medical Center
Department of Hematology and Oncology
Hugstetter Strasse 55
79106 Freiburg, Germany

**Messner, Hans A.**
Princess Margaret Hospital
5th Floor, Room 107
610 University Avenue
Toronto, ON M5G 2M9, Canada

**Mertelsmann, Roland**
University Medical Center
Department of Hematology and Oncology
Hugstetter Strasse 55
79106 Freiburg, Germany

**Mielke, Stephan**
Medizinische Klinik und Poliklinik I
Universitätsklinikum Carl Gustav Carus
Technical University Dresden
Fetscherstrasse 74
01307 Dresden, Germany

**Müller, Antonia**
University Medical Center
Department of Hematology and Oncology
Hugstetter Strasse 55
79106 Freiburg, Germany

**Müller, Claudia I.**
University Medical Center
Department of Hematology and Oncology
Hugstetter Strasse 55
79106 Freiburg, Germany

**Neumann, Hartmut**
University Medical Center
Department of Nephrology
Hugstetter Strasse 55
79106 Freiburg, Germany

**Otto, Florian**
University Medical Center
Department of Hematology and Oncology
Hugstetter Strasse 55
79106 Freiburg, Germany

**Potthoff, Karin**
National Center for Tumor Diseases
Heidelberg (NCT)
Department of Translational Oncology
German Cancer Research Center (DKFZ)
Im Neuenheimer Feld 350
69120 Heidelberg, Germany

**Reincke, Martin**
Klinikum der Universität München
Medizinische Klinik – Innenstadt
Ziemssenstrasse 1
80336 München, Germany

**Reinert, Elke**
Tumorzentrum Ludwig Heilmeyer
Comprehensive Cancer Center Freiburg
Hugstetter Strasse 55
79106 Freiburg, Germany

**Rosenthal, F. M.**
CellGenix Technologie Transfer GmbH
Am Flughafen 16
79108 Freiburg, Germany

**Runnebaum, Ingo**
Department of Gynecology
Jena University Medical Center
Bachstrasse 18
07743 Jena, Germany

**Rüter, Björn-Hans**
University Medical Center
Department of Hematology and Oncology
Hugstetter Strasse 55
79106 Freiburg, Germany

**Rüter, Simone**
University Medical Center
Department of Hematology and Oncology
Hugstetter Strasse 55
79106 Freiburg, Germany

**Scheele, Jürgen**
University Medical Center
Department of Hematology and Oncology
Hugstetter Strasse 55
79106 Freiburg, Germany

**Schmah, Oliver**
University Medical Center
Department of Hematology and Oncology
Hugstetter Strasse 55
79106 Freiburg, Germany

**Schmoor, Claudia**
University Medical Center
Center of Clinical Trials
Elsässer Strasse 2
79106 Freiburg, Germany

**Schultze-Seemann, Wolfgang**
University Medical Center
Department of Urology
Hugstetter Strasse 55
79106 Freiburg, Germany

**Schwabe, Michael**
University Medical Center
Department of Hematology and Oncology
Hugstetter Strasse 55
79106 Freiburg, Germany

**Seufert, Jochen**
University Medical Center
Department of Gastroenterology
Hepatology, Endocrinology
and Infectious Diseases
Hugstetter Strasse 55
79106 Freiburg, Germany

**Spyridonidis, Alexandros**
University Medical Center
Department of Hematology and Oncology
Hugstetter Strasse 55
79106 Freiburg, Germany

**Stockschläder, Marcus**
Institute of Hemostaseology
and Transfusion Medicine
Düsseldorf University Hospital
Moorenstrasse 5
40227 Düsseldorf, Germany

**Thatcher, Nick**
Department of Medical Oncology
Christie Hospital NHS Trust
Wilmslow Road
Manchester M20 4BX, United Kingdom

**Thierry, Veronique**
University Medical Center
Department of Hematology and Oncology
Hugstetter Strasse 55
79106 Freiburg, Germany

**Trepel, Martin**
University Medical Center
Department of Hematology and Oncology
Hugstetter Strasse 55
79106 Freiburg, Germany

**Veelken, Hendrik**
University Medical Center
Department of Hematology and Oncology
Hugstetter Strasse 55
79106 Freiburg, Germany

**Waesch, Ralph**
University Medical Center
Department of Hematology and Oncology
Hugstetter Strasse 55
79106 Freiburg, Germany

**Waller, Cornelius**
University Medical Center
Department of Hematology and Oncology
Hugstetter Strasse 55
79106 Freiburg, Germany

**Weissenberger, Christian**
University Medical Center
Department of Radiation Therapy
Hugstetter Strasse 55
79106 Freiburg, Germany

**Wetterauer, Ulrich**
University Medical Center
Department of Urology
Hugstetter Strasse 55
79106 Freiburg, Germany

**Wünsch, Alexander**
University Medical Center
Department of Hematology and Oncology
Hugstetter Strasse 55
79106 Freiburg, Germany

**Zahradnik, Hans-Peter**
University Medical Center
Department of Gynecology
Hugstetter Strasse 55
79106 Freiburg, Germany

**Zeller, Christoph**
Asklepios Klinik Triberg
Fachklinik für Innere Medizin
Hematologie/Oncologie
Ludwigstrasse 1–2
78098 Triberg, Germany

**Zürcher, Gudrun**
University Medical Center
Department of Hematology and Oncology
Hugstetter Strasse 55
79106 Freiburg, Germany

**1.1**　**Epidemiology**

**D.P. Berger, H. Henß**

**Def:**　Describes the frequency with which a disease occurs and examines possible links between disease occurrence and risk factors.

**Meth:**　*Terms*
- *Incidence:* total number of new cases of a given disease occurring in a population during a defined time interval (e.g., new cases per year)
- *Incidence Rate:* incidence within a given population (e.g., incidence per 100,000 people)
- *Prevalence:* total number of affected members of the population at a set point in time
- *Prevalence Rate:* prevalence within a given population (e.g., prevalence per 100,000 people)
- *Mortality:* total number of disease-related deaths occurring during a defined time interval (e.g., disease-related deaths per year)
- *Mortality Rate:* mortality within a given population (e.g., disease-related deaths per 100,000 people per year)

*Risk*
Describes the likelihood of an event occurring within a defined time interval, e.g., risk of developing a particular tumor (incidence risk) or risk of dying of a disease (mortality risk).

*Risk Factors*
Factors contributing to a specific risk. Risk factors for malignant diseases include demographical data (age, sex), geographical distribution, socio-economic factors, environmental factors, and biological parameters ("molecular epidemiology").

*Relative Risk (RR)*
Epidemiological term which compares the risk (e.g., of disease occurrence) within a specific sub-population ("high-risk group," e.g., smokers) with the average population. A factor > 1.0 represents an increased RR, factors < 1.0 constitute a reduced RR.

*Average Age at Which a Disease Occurs*
Maximum of the age-specific distribution of cases of a disease.

Incidence, age distribution, and gender distribution of each entity are shown in the disease-related chapters (▶ Chaps. 6.1–8.13). Recent research suggests that 70–80% of all malignant diseases are triggered by certain lifestyle habits or environmental carcinogens. In addition, hereditary factors are of particular importance (▶ Chap. 1.2).

**Development of mortality rates of female patients with solid tumors (USA, 1930–2003, age-adjusted mortality rate per 100,000)**

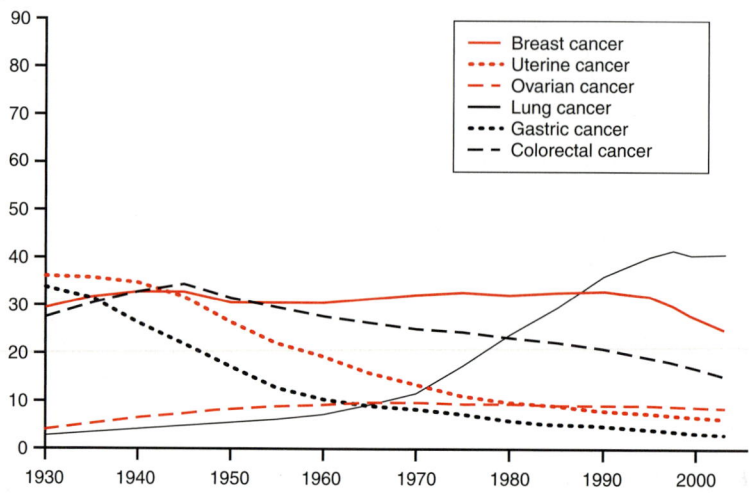

*Source:* American Cancer Society, Cancer Facts and Figures 2003

**Development of mortality rates of male patients with solid tumors (USA, 1930–2003, age-adjusted mortality rate per 100,000)**

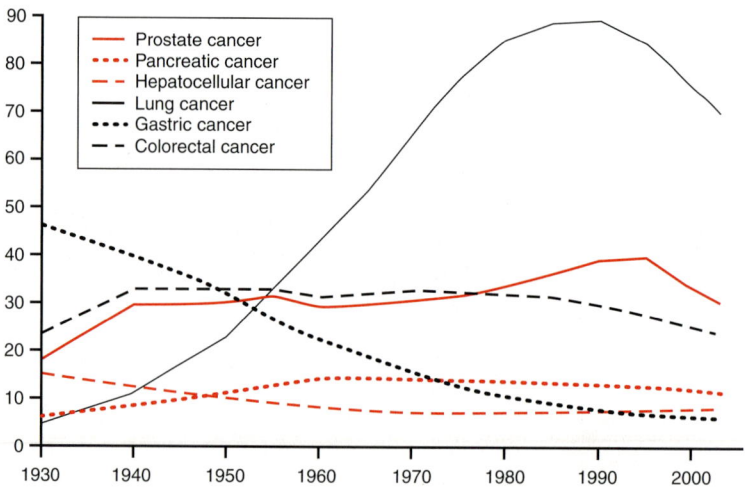

**Ref:**
1.  American Cancer Society. Cancer Facts and Figures 2003. Atlanta, GA, 2003
2.  Jemal A, Siegel R., Ward E et al. Cancer Statistics, 2007. CA Cancer J Clin 2007;57:43–66
3.  Lichtenstein P, Holm NV, Verkasalo PK et al. Environmental and heritable factors in the causation of cancer. N Engl J Med 2000;343:78–85
4.  Kamangar F, Dores GM, Anderson WF. Patterns of Cancer incidence, mortality, and prevalence across five continents. J Clin Oncol 2006;24:2137–50.

**Web:**
1.  http://www.cancer.org/              American Cancer Society
2.  http://www.iacr.com.fr/             Intl. Association of Cancer Registries
3.  http://seer.cancer.gov/             NCI SEER Database

## 1.2 Carcinogenesis, Molecular Tumor Biology

### D.P. Berger, U. Martens

**Def:** Development of malignant diseases is a result of multiple exogenic and endogenic factors. Of pivotal importance is the accumulation of genetic and epigenetic changes leading to the selection of a cell population with malignant phenotype. Characteristics are:
- Unlimited proliferation, immortalization
- Loss of antiproliferative feedback mechanisms, autonomous growth, not dependent on proliferation signals (e.g., autocrine stimulation)
- Loss of ability to induce apoptosis
- Neovascularization
- Metastatic and invasive properties

**Pg:** The development of a malignant tumor requires several steps (see model of multistep carcinogenesis). Point mutations (single nucleotide changes) or cytogenetic aberrations (e.g., translocation / inversion / deletion) lead to altered activity of genes (e.g., p53, pRB) impacting tumor growth regulation and biology of malignant cells. These can be hereditary ("germline mutation") or spontaneous ("somatic mutation") as a result of multiple factors ("carcinogens" or carcinogenic defects).

#### Exogenous Carcinogens:
- Chemicals, drugs
- Ionizing radiation
- Infections (viruses, bacteria, protozoa, particularly chronic infections)

#### Endogenous Carcinogens:
- Defective DNA repair mechanisms
- Defective regulation of epigenetic events
- Genetic instability

**Model of multistep carcinogenesis**

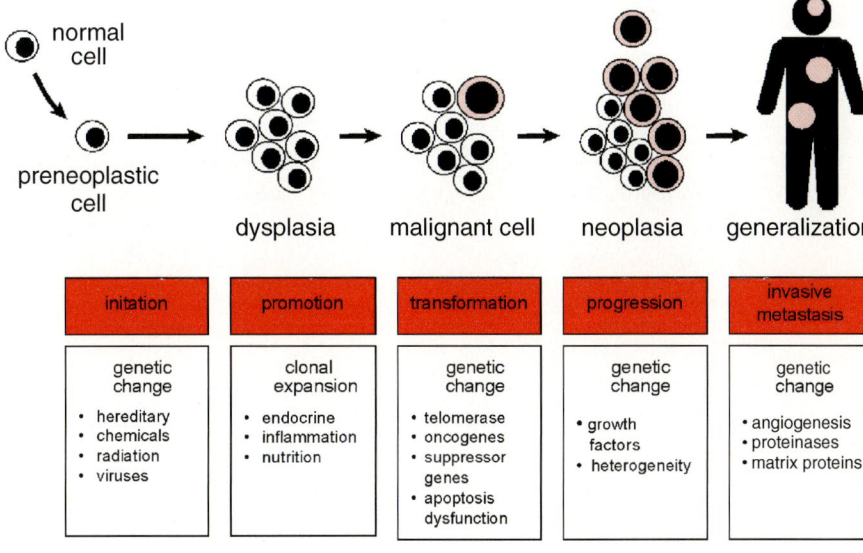

| initation | promotion | transformation | progression | invasive metastasis |
|---|---|---|---|---|
| genetic change | clonal expansion | genetic change | genetic change | genetic change |
| • hereditary<br>• chemicals<br>• radiation<br>• viruses | • endocrine<br>• inflammation<br>• nutrition | • telomerase<br>• oncogenes<br>• suppressor genes<br>• apoptosis dysfunction | • growth factors<br>• heterogeneity | • angiogenesis<br>• proteinases<br>• matrix proteins |

**Carcinogens and associated human neoplasias**

| Carcinogen / group | Associated diseases |
| --- | --- |
| *Alcohol / Tobacco:* | |
| Alcohol | Hepatic carcinoma, head and neck tumors, gastrointestinal tumors |
| Tobacco | Lung cancer, head and neck tumors, esophageal carcinoma, pancreatic carcinoma, renal cell carcinoma, carcinoma of renal pelvis, bladder carcinoma |
| *Industrial substances and environmental pollutants:* | |
| Aromatic amines | Bladder carcinoma, urinary tract tumors |
| Arsenic, arsenic compounds | Lung cancer, skin tumors |
| Asbestos | Lung cancer, mesothelioma |
| Benzol, styrol, benzene | Acute myeloid leukemia |
| Benzidine | Bladder carcinoma |
| Beryllium | Lung cancer |
| Chloromethyl ether | Lung cancer |
| Chromium, chromium compounds | Lung cancer, head and neck tumors |
| Halogenated hydrocarbons | Hepatic carcinoma, urinary tract tumors |
| Halogenated alkyl, aryl and alkylaryl oxides | Lung cancer, head and neck / gastrointestinal / urinary tract / skin tumors |
| Wood dust | Tumors of paranasal sinuses |
| Ionizing radiation | Various solid tumors, leukemias |
| Isopropanol production | Tumors of paranasal sinuses |
| Cadmium | Lung cancer |
| Crude coking plant gases | Lung cancer, head and neck tumors |
| Nickel and nickel compounds | Lung cancer, head and neck tumors |
| Nitrosamines | Esophageal carcinoma |
| Polycyclic hydrocarbons | Lung cancer, scrotal carcinoma, skin tumors |
| Radon and radon decay products | Lung cancer |
| Soot, tar, anthrazene | Skin tumors |
| Quartz dust (silicosis) | Lung cancer |
| Mustard gas | Lung cancer, head and neck tumors |
| Trichloroethylene | Renal cell carcinoma |
| Ultraviolet light (sunlight, UV-B) | Skin tumors, melanoma |
| Vinyl chloride | Hepatic angiosarcoma |

**Carcinogens and associated human neoplasias** *(continued)*

| Carcinogen / group | Associated diseases |
|---|---|
| *Drugs:* | |
| Alkylating agents | Acute myeloid leukemia, bladder carcinoma |
| Androgenic steroids | Hepatic carcinoma |
| Diethylstilbestrol (prenatal) | Vaginal adenocarcinoma |
| Epipodophyllotoxin derivates | Acute myeloid leukemia |
| Immunosuppressants (azathioprine, cyclosporine) | Non-Hodgkin's lymphomas, skin tumors, sarcomas |
| Phenacetine | Carcinoma of renal pelvis, bladder carcinoma |
| Synthetic estrogens | Endometrial carcinoma |
| *Bacteria, viruses, fungi:* | |
| Aflatoxins | Hepatic carcinoma |
| Chronic hepatitis B, C (HBV, HCV) | Hepatic carcinoma |
| Epstein-Barr virus (EBV) | Burkitt's lymphoma, nasopharyngeal carcinoma |
| Helicobacter pylori | Gastric cancer, MALT-lymphoma of the stomach |
| HIV | Lymphomas, Kaposi's sarcoma |
| HTLV-1 | Adult T-cell leukemia / lymphomas |
| Human papillomaviruses (HPV) | Cervical / vulvar / anal / penile carcinoma |
| KSHV / HHV-8 | Kaposi's sarcoma, multiple myeloma (?) |
| Schistosomiasis | Bladder carcinoma |

**Ref:**

1. Bergen AW, Caporaso N. Cigarette smoking. J Natl Cancer Inst 1999;91:1365–75
2. Berrington de Gonzales A, Darby S. Risk of cancer from diagnostic X-rays. Lancet 2004;363:345–51
3. Hahn WC, Weinberg RA. Rules for making tumor cells. N Eng J Med 2002;347:1593–603
4. Jordan CT, Guzman ML, Noble M. Cancer stem cell. N Engl J Med 2006;355:1253–61
5. Lichtenstein P, Holm NV, Verkasalo PK et al. Environmental and heritable factors in the causation of cancer. N Eng J Med 2000;343:78–85
6. Ponder BAJ. Cancer genetics. Nature 2001;411:336–41
7. Vogelstein B, Kinzler KW. Cancer genes and the pathways they control. Nat Med 2004;10:789-99
8. World Health Organisation IARC monographs on the evaluation of carcinogenic risks to humans, 1–74. Lyon, IARC, 1972-2000

**Web:**

1. http://www.iarc.fr — Intl. Agency for Research on Cancer
2. http://www.nlm.nih.gov/pubs/factsheets/ccrisfs.html — Chemical Carcinogen Information
3. http://ehp.niehs.nih.gov/roc/toc10.html — NIH Report on Carcinogens
4. http://potency.berkeley.edu/cpdb.html — Carcinogenic Potency Database
5. http://cancer.gov/cancerinfo/prevention-genetics-causes — Cancer Genetics, NIH
6. http://AtlasGeneticsOncology.org — Cytogenetics Atlas
7. http://www.carcinogenesis.com/home/ — Journal of Carcinogenesis
8. http://www.nature.com/nrc/poster/subpathways/index.html — A subway map to cancer

**Genetic variations and associated solid tumors**

| Hereditary syndrome | Gene | Locus | Primary tumor | Associated disease |
|---|---|---|---|---|
| Li-Fraumeni syndrome | TP53 | 17p13.1 | Breast cancer, sarcomas | CNS tumors, leukemias, lymphomas |
| Familial adenomatous polyposis (FAP, Gardner's syndrome) | APC,MYH | 5q21 | Colorectal cancer | Gastric cancer, pancreatic carcinoma, osteomas, medulloblastoma |
| Hereditary non-polyposis colorectal cancer (HNPCC, Lynch's syndrome) | MSH2,MLH1, PMS1, PMS2, MSH6 | 2p16, 3p21, 2q32, 7p22 | Colorectal cancer | Endometrial / ovarian / hepatic carcinoma, renal carcinoma, glioblastoma |
| Hereditary diffuse gastric carcinoma | CDH1 | 16q21-22 | Gastric cancer | Breast cancer, colorectal tumors? |
| Neurofibromatosis type 1 | NF1 | 17q11.2 | Neurofibromas | Neurofibrosarcoma, AML, CNS tumors |
| Neurofibromatosis type 2 | NF2 | 22q12.2 | Acoustic neurinoma, meningioma | Gliomas, ependymomas |
| Wilms' tumor | WT1, WT2 | 11p13, 11p15 | Wilms' tumor (nephroblastoma) | Aniridia, urogenital defects, mental retardation |
| Hereditary breast cancer type 1, 2 | BRCA1, BRCA2 | 17q21, 13q12 | Breast cancer | Ovarian carcinoma, pancreatic carcinoma |
| Bloom's syndrome | BLM | 15q26 | Leukemias, lymphomas | Diverse solid tumors, immunodeficiencies |
| von Hippel-Lindau's (VHL) syndrome | VHL | 3p12 | Hypernephroid carcinoma | Pheochromocytoma, retinal angiomas, cerebellar hemangiomas |
| Hereditary papillary renal carcinoma | MeT | 7q31 | Papillary renal carcinoma | Other solid tumors |
| Familial melanoma | CDKN2A(p16), CDK4 | 9p21, 12q13 | Melanoma | Pancreatic carcinoma, dysplastic moles |
| Multiple endocrine neoplasia 1 (MEN 1) | MEN 1 | 11q13 | Islet carcinoma | Parathyroid adenomas |
| Multiple endocrine neoplasia 2 (MEN 2) | MEN 2 (RET) | 10q11.2 | Medullary thyroid carcinoma | Pheochromocytomas, hamartomas, parathyroid adenomas |
| Cowden's syndrome | PTEN, MMAC1 | 10q23 | Breast cancer, follicular thyroid carcinoma | Hamartomas, intestinal polyps, cutaneous lesions |
| Ataxia telangiectasia (Louis-Bar) | ATM | 11q22 | Lymphomas | Ataxia, immunodeficiency, breast cancer |
| Xeroderma pigmentosum | XBD, XPD, XPA | Variable | Skin tumors | Abnormal pigmentation, hypogonadism |
| Fanconi's anemia | FACC, FACA | 9q22, 16q24 | AML | Pancytopenia, skeletal defects |
| Retinoblastoma | RB | 13q14 | Retinoblastoma | Osteosarcomas |
| Tuberous sclerosis | TSC1, TSC2 | 9q34, 16p13 | Cutaneous fibroadenomas | Astrocytomas, skin tumors |

# 1.3 Hematopoiesis and Development of Hematological Neoplasia

### C.I. Müller, D.P. Berger, M. Engelhardt

**Def:** Hematopoiesis is the formation of effector cells of the peripheral blood and bone marrow. In the bone marrow, approximately $1 \times 10^{12}$ cells are formed daily.
Differentiation:
- *Myelopoiesis:* formation of myeloid effector cells (granulocytes, monocytes, macrophages)
- *Lymphopoiesis:* formation of lymphocytic effector cells (T lymphocytes, B lymphocytes)
- *Erythropoiesis:* formation of erythrocytes
- *Thrombopoiesis:* formation of thrombocytes (platelets)
- *Granulopoiesis:* formation of granulocytes (eosinophils, basophils, neutrophils)

**Phys:** ## Location of Hematopoiesis
- Embryogenesis: hematopoiesis in liver → spleen → bone marrow
- Adulthood: bone marrow. In case of medullary insufficiency, liver and spleen can take over hematopoietic function ("extramedullary hematopoiesis")

## Regulation of Hematopoiesis
Proliferation and differentiation of stem cells, progenitor cells and effector cells are regulated by hematopoietic growth factors (HGF):
- Stem and progenitor cells: Flt-2 / flk-3 ligand, stem cell factor (SCF)
- Erythropoiesis: erythropoietin, SCF, interleukin-3 (IL-3)
- Thrombopoiesis: thrombopoietin, SCF, IL-3, IL-6, IL-11
- Granulopoiesis: IL-3, granulocyte colony-stimulating factor (G-CSF), GM-CSF
- Lymphopoiesis: Flt-2 / flk-3 ligand, SCF, IL-2, IL-6, IL-7

## Effector Cell Characteristics
- *Erythrocytes:* carry oxygen and hemoglobin, diameter 8 μm, biconcave, akaryotic, developmental period 7 days, life span 120 days
- *Thrombocytes:* "platelets," essential for coagulation, size 1–2 μm, granular, basophilic, developmental period 10–12 days, life span of circulating thrombocytes 7–8 days
- *Neutrophil granulocytes:* defense against infections (particularly bacterial infections), ≤ 5 nuclear segments connected by chromatin bridges ("segmented granulocyte"), developmental period 7–10 days, life span of mature neutrophil granulocyte 7–10 h, average production $10 \times 10^9$/h, in response to infection up to $500 \times 10^9$/h
- *Eosinophil granulocytes:* relevant in allergic and parasitic diseases, two nuclear segments connected by chromatin bridges, eosinophilic cytoplasm
- *Basophil granulocytes:* relevant in allergic and parasitic diseases, two nuclear segments connected by chromatin bridges, rough basophilic cytoplasmic granules
- *Monocytes:* resistance to infection and phagocytosis, nuclear sinuses and loosely structured chromatin, median life span in peripheral blood 20–40 days
- *B lymphocytes:* antibody-mediated immune response, plasmacytic precursors, diameter 7–12 μm, basophilic cytoplasm, central round nucleus with densely structured chromatin
- *T lymphocytes:* cellular immune response, diameter 7–12 μm, basophilic cytoplasm, central round nucleus with densely structured chromatin

**Phys:** ## Hematological Neoplasia
Hematologic neoplasms are formed by malignant transformation of cells of certain developmental stages → some characteristics of the neoplastic disease may be aligned with features of the corresponding stage of differentiation, e.g., proliferative activity, surface markers (CD antigens), molecular markers.

**Model of hematopoiesis**

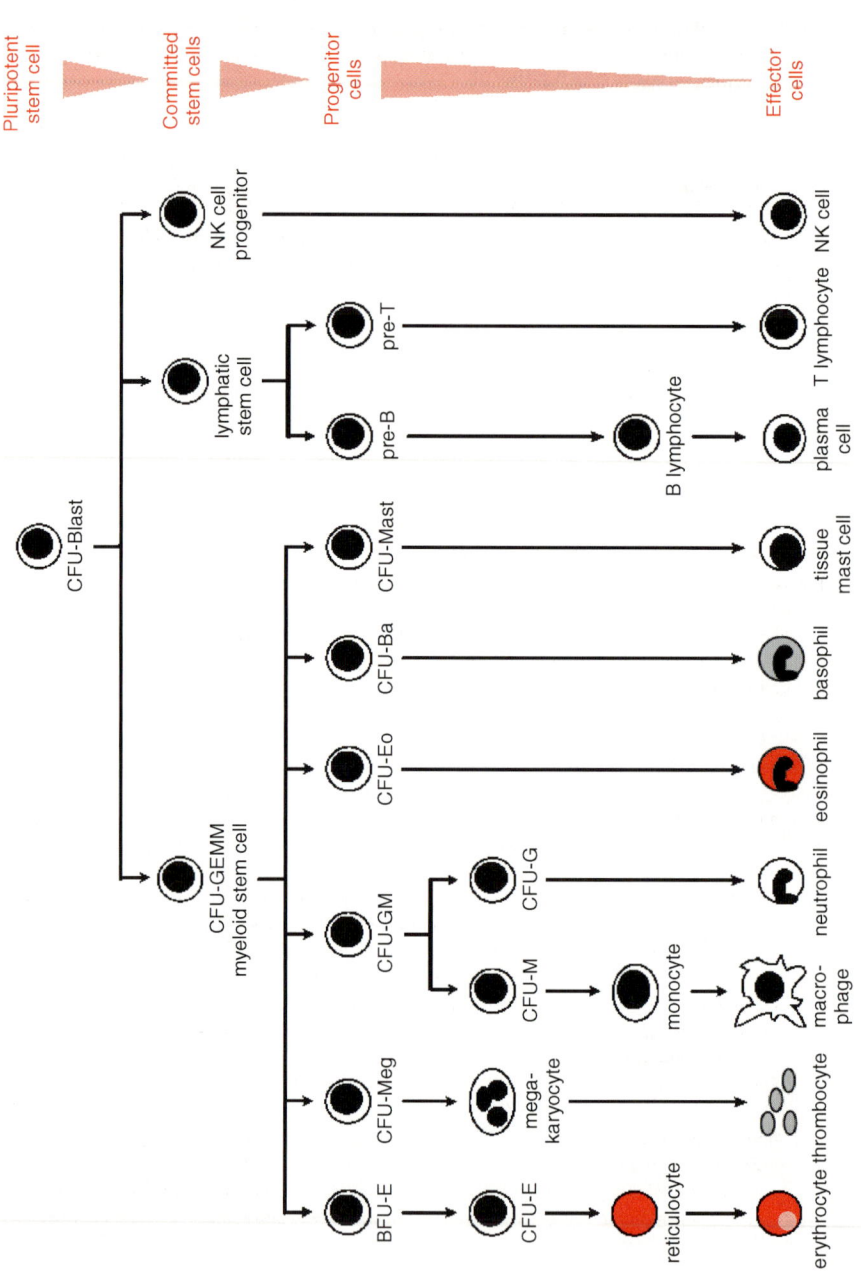

*BFU-E* burst-forming unit–erythroid, *CFU* colony-forming unit, *Ba* basophils, *E* erythrocytes, *Eo* eosinophils, *G* granulocytes, *M* monocytes or macrophages, *Meg* megakaryocytes, *NK* natural killer

**Example: B-cell development, differentiation, and expression of surface markers (CD antigens). Hematologic malignancies developing at a specific stage of differentiation will carry the given CD antigen expression pattern.**

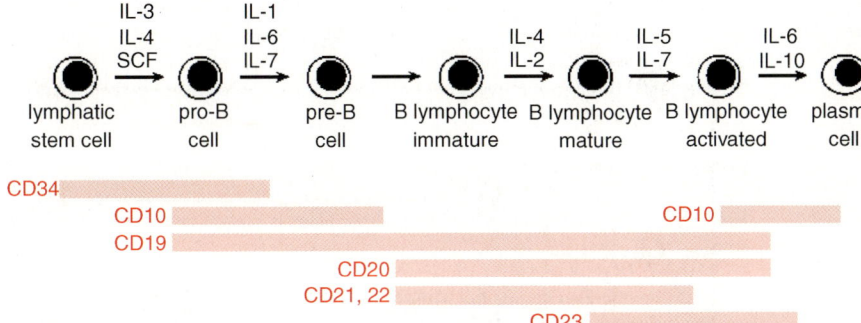

*IL* Interleukin, *SCF* Stem Cell Factor, *CD* Surface Marker (Cluster of Differentiation ►Chap. 2.5)

Formation of hematological neoplasias on the basis of:
- Erythropoiesis → erythroleukemias (AML M6) (► Chap. 7.1.2)
- Thrombopoiesis → megakaryoblastic leukemias (AML M7) (► Chap. 7.1.2)
- Granulopoiesis → acute myeloid leukemias (► Chap. 7.1.2)
- Lymphopoiesis → lymphomas, lymphatic leukemias (► Chaps. 7.1.1, 7.4, 7.5)

**Ref:**

1. Akashi K, Traver D, Kondo M et al. Lymphoid development from hematopoietic stem cells. Int J Hematol 1999;69:217–26
2. Baraldi-Junkins CA, Beck AC, Rothstein G. Hematopoiesis and cytokines. Hematol Oncol Clin North Am 2000;14:45–61
3. Broxmeyer HE, Kim CH. Regulation of hematopoiesis in a sea of chemokine family members with a plethora of redundant activities. Exp Hematol 1999;27:1113–23
4. Fey MF. Normal and malignant hematopoiesis. Ann Oncol 2007;18(suppl. 1):i9–i13
5. Gilliland DG, Griffin JD. The roles of FLT3 in hematopoiesis and leukemia. Blood 2002;100:1532–42
6. Hoang T. The origin of hematopoietic cell type diversity. Oncogene 2004;23:7188–98
7. Kondo M, Wagers AJ, Manz MG et al. Biology of hematopoietic stem cells and progenitors: implications for clinical application. Annu Rev Immunol 2003;21:759–806
8. Kyba M, Daley GQ. Hematopoiesis from embryonic stem cells: lessons from and for ontogeny. Exp Hematol 2003;31:994–1006
9. LeBien TW. Fates of human B-cell precursors. Blood 2000;96:9–23

**Web:**

1. http://www.hematology.org    American Society of Hematology (ASH)
2. http://www.bloodline.net/    Hematological Education and News
3. http://pathy.med.nagoya-u.ac.jp/atlas/doc/    Hematology Atlas of the University of Nagoya
4. http://www.hematologyatlas.com/    Hematology Atlas

## 1.4    Prevention and Screening

### H. Henß

**Def:**    Primary prevention = prevention of tumor development
Secondary prevention = tumor screening
Tertiary prevention = post-treatment follow-up and care to ensure early detection of relapse

### Primary Prevention

**Def:**    Successful primary prevention of all malignancies is currently unrealistic for the following reasons:
- Unresolved etiology and pathogenesis of malignant diseases
- Multiple oncogenetic mechanisms of malignant diseases
- Uncertain efficacy of the majority of primary preventive measures (chemoprevention, antioxidant therapy, etc.)

However, epidemiological research suggests that specific measures may reduce the risk of developing certain tumors. Activities with the potential for tumor prevention are:
- Sufficient physical exercise
- Adequate nutrition
- Avoidance of exogenous risk factors (e.g., smoking)

**Pg:**    Primary prevention focuses on definition, recognition, and avoidance of risk factors, which can be genetically determined and/or acquired. Once genetic risk factors have been identified, they can be used to define a high-risk population.

### Genetic Risk Factors: Examples (▶ Chap. 1.2)
- Familial adenomatous polyposis (FAP) and other familial colorectal tumors (HNPCC)
- Familial breast cancer and/or familial ovarian carcinoma (BRCA1, BRCA2)
- Xeroderma pigmentosum

In the presence of genetic risk factors, cancer screening, preventive therapy, and chemoprevention have to be considered.

### Acquired Risk Factors Associated with Certain Tumors (▶ Chap. 1.2)
- *Smoking:* lung cancer, squamous cell carcinoma of the head and neck, breast cancer, pancreatic carcinoma, bladder carcinoma, renal cell carcinoma
- *Alcohol:* squamous cell carcinoma of the head and neck, hepatocellular carcinoma, breast cancer, gastrointestinal tumors
- *Hazardous substances:* lung cancer (e.g., asbestos), nasopharyngeal carcinoma (hardwood dust), bladder carcinoma (tar, solvents)
- *Infections:* hepatocellular carcinoma (hepatitis B / C), cervical carcinoma (papilloma virus, HPV), gastric cancer (*Helicobacter pylori*)
- *Excess exposure to sunlight / UV light:* malignant melanoma, basal cell carcinoma
- *Obesity (esp. postmenopausal):* breast cancer, endometrial carcinoma, prostatic cancer, colorectal cancer

**Px:**    The "European Code Against Cancer" was developed as a source of information for patients. It contains general rules of conduct in order to prevent tumor development.

**European Code Against Cancer (2003)**

*Many aspects of general health can be improved, and certain cancers avoided, if you adopt a healthier life style*

1. Do not smoke. If you smoke, stop doing so. If you fail to stop, do not smoke in the presence of non-smokers

2. Avoid obesity

3. Undertake some brisk physical activity every day

4. Increase your daily intake and variety of vegetables and fruits: eat at least 5 servings daily. Limit your intake of foods containing fats from animal sources

5. If you drink alcohol, whether beer, wine, or spirits, moderate your consumption to two drinks per day if you are a man and one drink per day if you are a woman

6. Care must be taken to avoid excessive sun exposure. It is specifically important to protect children and adolescents. For individuals who have a tendency to burn in the sun, active protective measures must be taken throughout life

7. Apply strictly regulations aimed at preventing any exposure to known cancer-causing substances. Follow all health and safety instructions on substances which may cause cancer. Follow advice of national radiation protection offices

*There are public health programs that could prevent cancers developing or increase the probability that a cancer may be cured*

8. Women from 25 years of age should participate in cervical screening. This should be within programs with quality control procedures in compliance with European Guidelines for Quality Assurance in Cervical Screening

9. Women from 50 years of age should participate in breast screening. This should be within programs with quality control procedures in compliance with European Guidelines for Quality Assurance in Mammography Screening

10. Men and women from 50 years of age should participate in colorectal screening. This should be within programs with built-in quality assurance procedures

11. Participate in vaccination programs against hepatitis B virus infection

*Other measures*

12. See a doctor if you notice a lump, a persistent wound (including inside the mouth), changes in shape, color, or size of a mole, any abnormal bleeding

13. See a doctor if you have persistent symptoms such as a chronic cough or persistent hoarseness, a change in bowel habits / urination, or unexpected weight loss

## Chemoprevention

**Def:** Prevention of tumor development via prophylactic medication.

**Th:** *Colorectal Tumors*
- Retrospective studies demonstrate risk reduction through regular use of acetylsalicylic acid or non-steroidal antiinflammatory drugs (NSAIDs).
- Prospective studies showed decreased numbers of adenomas, but no significant influence on carcinoma-related mortality → General use of acetylsalicylic acid or NSAIDs for the prevention of colorectal tumors is presently not recommended due to the possible side effects.

### Breast Cancer

- Positive family history and/or identification of the BRCA-1 and BRCA-2 genes constitute a higher risk. However, the extent of this risk remains uncertain. Recent studies have shown that women carrying the genes have up to an 80% lifetime risk of developing the disease by the age of 80.
- Initial larger studies using tamoxifen in high-risk populations showed a positive influence on the disease risk. Consequently, the US National Cancer Institute (NCI) formulated a recommendation for the prophylactic use of tamoxifen in patients at risk of developing breast cancer. At present, this recommendation is judged controversial as other studies failed to reproduce the initial results or have even shown a negative influence of tamoxifen → *Outside of studies, tamoxifen use should be limited to clearly defined high-risk populations. Frequent follow-up is required due to the increased risk of endometrial carcinoma.*

### Cervical Carcinoma

Vaccination against human papillomavirus type 16 (HPV-16) prevents intraepithelial cervical neoplasias.

### Lung Cancer

Two large studies were conducted on the influence of protective substances in high-risk populations:

- ATBC study: administration of alpha-tocopherol (vitamin E) and β-carotene
- CARET study: administration of β-carotene and retinol

Neither study showed any benefit in relation to the occurrence of lung cancer. Instead, mortality was increased in the β-carotene group (higher incidence of bronchial carcinomas and myocardial infarction). Hence, further similar studies were discontinued.

### Head and Neck Tumors

Patients with successfully removed head and neck tumors show a reduced incidence of metachronous secondary tumors after prophylactic use of retinoids. However, retinoids appeared to have no influence on relapse frequency or metastasis of the primary tumor.

### Xeroderma Pigmentosum

The use of retinoids also had a positive effect in known cases of xeroderma pigmentosum.

### Selenium

Clinical studies do not conclusively verify the usefulness of selenium substitution. While substitution is useful in selenium deficient areas (e.g., China), it seems to have no protective effect in areas with sufficient selenium supply (e.g., Germany). Results of current clinical studies remain to be seen.

## Secondary Prevention (Cancer Screening)

**Def:** Cancer screening remains the main focus of prophylaxis. Its benefits are, however, still subject to debate.

- On the one hand, there is definite increase in cure rates and prolonged life expectancy in early stages of tumor development.
- On the other hand, there is lead time bias and diagnosis of asymptomatic tumors which have no influence on life expectancy ("over-diagnosis bias").
- Furthermore, false-positive screening results lead to increased technology-intensive and invasive diagnostic procedures with a higher risk of acute and chronic side effects (exposure to radiation, risk of invasive measures, etc.).

**Meth:** The following World Health Organization (WHO) criteria are adequate guidelines for screening measures.

**WHO criteria for sensible and effective cancer screening programs**

- The disease should be an important health problem
- There should be an accepted treatment
- There should be facilities for diagnosis and treatment of the disease
- The disease should have a detectable preclinical phase
- The natural history of the disease should be understood
- A suitable screening test should be available
- The test should be acceptable to the general public
- There should be a generally accepted strategy for determining whom to treat
- The costs generated should be acceptable
- The program should be designed to carry out screening continuously

**Px:**

## Cancer Screening Programs

Cancer screening programs are considered standard medical care for:
- Cervical and endometrial carcinoma → women from 20 years of age
- Breast cancer → women from 30 years of age
- Colorectal cancer → women and men from 45 years of age
- Prostate cancer → men from 45 years of age
- Malignant skin tumors → women from 30 years of age / men from 45 years of age.

International publications have firmly established the benefits of screening for:
- Colorectal cancer
- Breast cancer in postmenopausal women
- Cervical carcinoma

Up to now, the exact benefits of screening for prostate cancer have not been verified by published studies. There is a positive trend toward using mammography to screen for breast cancer in premenopausal women. Screening for malignant melanoma is also recommended, especially given the low costs involved and the importance of early treatment. There are no recommendations for lung cancer and ovarian carcinoma. In both cases, currently published studies do not show any correlation between detection by screening and decreased mortality.

**Ref:**

1. Boyle P, Autier P, Bartelink H et al. European Code Against Cancer and scientific justification: third version (2003). Ann Oncol 2003;14:973–1005
2. Chlebowski RT, Col N et al. ASCO Technology Assessment of Pharmacology Interventions for Breast Cancer Risk Reduction Including Tamoxifen, Raloxifen and Aromatase Inhibition. J Clin Oncol 2002;20:3328–43
3. Imperiale TF. Aspirin and the prevention of colorectal cancer. N Engl J Med 2003;348:879–80
4. Jordan VC. Chemoprevention of breast cancer with selective oestrogenreceptor modulators. Nat Rev Cancer 2007,7:46–53
5. Key TJ, Allen NE et al. The effect of diet on risk of cancer. Lancet 2002;360:861–68
6. Koutsky LA, Ault KA et al. A controlled trial of a human papillomavirus type 16 vaccine. N Engl J Med 2002;347:1645–51
7. Kushi LH, Byers T, Doyle C et al. ACS Guidelines on Nutrition and Physical Activity for Cancer Prevention: Reducing the Risk of Cancer With Healthy Food Choices and Physical Activity. CA Cancer J Clin 2006;56:254–81
8. Smith RA, Cokkinides V, Eyre HJ. Cancer screening in the US, 2007: A review of current guidelines, practies, and prospects. CA Cancer J Clin 2007;57:90–104

**Web:**

1. http://www.cancerprevention.org/ — Cancer Prevention Foundation
2. http://www.cancerprev.org/ — Cancer Detection and Prevention
3. http://www.cancerpreventionfund.com/ — National Cancer Prevention Fund
4. http://www.preventcancer.com/ — Cancer Prevention Coalition
5. http://www.prevention.cancer.gov — Division of Cancer Prevention (NCI)
6. http://www.cdc.gov/cancer/az/ — Center for Disease Control (CDC)

## 1.5     Classification of Diseases and ICD System

**D.P. Berger, H. Henß**

**Def:** Coded disease classifications using internationally standardized systems allow for world wide investigation of causes of morbidity and mortality. For the classification of diseases and causes of death, the World Health Organization (WHO) has established the "International Classification of Diseases" (ICD). In the case of malignant diseases, it focuses particularly on tumor location. Since 1993, the 10th revision of the ICD (ICD-10) has been in use.

In oncology, two codes are being distinguished: "the location code" (ICD-10) and the "ICD-O" which describes the morphology of a malignant disease ("morphology code"). A definite disease classification is only possible by combining ICD-10 and ICD-O.

**Meth:** *ICD-10*

ICD-10 describes 21 categories of diseases and causes of death which are coded using a combination of letters and numbers. Hematological and oncological diseases are classified between "C00" and "D90".

**General principles of the international classification of diseases, 10th revision (ICD-10)**

| Chapter | Blocks | Title |
|---|---|---|
| I | A00–B99 | Certain infectious and parasitic diseases |
| II | C00–D48 | Neoplasms |
| III | D50–D89 | Diseases of the blood and blood-forming organs and certain disorders involving the immune system |
| IV | E00–E90 | Endocrine, nutritional, and metabolic diseases |
| V | F00–F99 | Mental and behavioral disorders |
| VI | G00–G99 | Diseases of the nervous system |
| VII | H00–H59 | Diseases of the eye and adnexa |
| VIII | H60–H95 | Diseases of the ear and mastoid process |
| IX | I00–I99 | Diseases of the circulatory system |
| X | J00–J99 | Diseases of the respiratory system |
| XI | K00–K93 | Diseases of the digestive system |
| XII | L00–L99 | Diseases of the skin and subcutaneous tissue |
| XIII | M00–M99 | Diseases of the musculoskeletal system and connective tissue |
| XIV | N00–N99 | Diseases of the genitourinary system |
| XV | O00–O99 | Pregnancy, childbirth, and the puerperium |
| XVI | P00–P96 | Certain conditions originating in the perinatal period |
| XVII | Q00–Q99 | Congenital malformations, deformations, and chromosomal abnormalities |
| XVIII | R00–R99 | Symptoms, signs, and abnormal clinical and laboratory findings, not elsewhere classified |
| XIX | S00–T98 | Injury, poisoning, and certain other consequences of external causes |
| XX | V01–Y98 | External causes of morbidity and mortality |
| XXI | Z00–Z99 | Factors influencing health status and contact with health services |

**ICD-10 classification of malignant solid tumors**

| Code | Tumor location | Code | Tumor location |
|------|----------------|------|----------------|
| C00 | Lips | C46 | Kaposi's sarcoma |
| C01–02 | Tongue | C47 | Peripheral nervous system |
| C03–04 | Mouth, gum | C48 | Retroperitoneum, peritoneum |
| C05 | Palate | C49 | Connective and soft tissue |
| C06 | Cheek | C50 | Breast |
| C07–08 | Parotid gland, salivary glands | C51 | Vulva, labium |
| C09 | Tonsils | C52 | Vagina |
| C10–11 | Naso- / oropharynx | C53 | Cervix uteri |
| C13 | Hypopharynx | C54 | Corpus uteri |
| C14 | Other sites in lip / oral cavity / pharynx | C55 | Other uterine carcinomas |
| C15 | Esophagus | C56 | Ovaries |
| C16 | Stomach | C57 | Other genital organs, ♀ |
| C17 | Small intestine | C58 | Placenta |
| C18 | Colon | C60 | Penis |
| C19 | Rectosigmoid junction | C61 | Prostate |
| C20 | Rectum | C62 | Testis |
| C21 | Anus, anal canal | C63 | Other genital organs, ♂ |
| C22 | Liver | C64–65 | Kidney, renal pelvis |
| C23–24 | Gallbladder, biliary tract | C66 | Ureter |
| C25 | Pancreas | C67–68 | Bladder, urethra |
| C26 | Other digestive organs | C69 | Eye |
| C30 | Nasal cavity, middle ear | C70 | Meninges |
| C31 | Accessory sinuses | C71 | Brain |
| C32 | Larynx | C72 | Spinal cord, cranial nerves |
| C33 | Trachea | C73 | Thyroid gland |
| C34 | Bronchus, lung | C74 | Adrenal gland |
| C37 | Thymus | C75 | Other endocrine glands |
| C38 | Heart, mediastinum, pleura | C76 | Ill-defined primary sites |
| C39 | Other intrathoracic tumors | C77 | Lymph node metastasis |
| C40–41 | Bone, articular cartilage | C78 | Thoracic / abdominal metastasis |
| C43 | Melanoma | C79 | CNS / skeletal metastasis |
| C44 | Other malignant neoplasms of skin | C80 | Disseminated metastasis |
| C45 | Mesothelioma | C97 | Multiple primary tumors |

## ICD-10 classification of hematological neoplasms

| Code | Tumor location |
| --- | --- |
| C81 | Hodgkin's disease |
| C82 | Follicular non-Hodgkin's lymphoma |
| C83 | Diffuse non-Hodgkin's lymphoma |
| C84 | Peripheral and cutaneous T-cell lymphoma |
| C85 | Other non-Hodgkin's lymphoma |
| C88 | Malignant immunoproliferative diseases |
| C90 | Multiple myeloma |
| C91 | Lymphoid leukemia (ALL, CLL) |
| C92 | Myeloid leukemias (AML M1–M4, CML) |
| C93 | Monocytic leukemias (AML M5) |
| C94 | Other leukemias (AML M6, AML M7) |
| C95 | Leukemias of unspecified cell type (AML M0) |
| D45 | Polycythemia vera |
| D46 | Myelodysplastic syndromes |
| D47 | Osteomyelofibrosis |
| D75.2 | Essential thrombocytosis |

**Ref:**   1.   WHO. International Classification of Diseases, 10th edn (ICD-10). WHO, Genf, 1996
            2.   WHO. ICD-0 International Classification of Diseases for Oncology, 3rd edn. WHO, Genf, 2000

**Web:**   1.   http://www.who.int/whosis/icd10/          World Health Organization (WHO)
            2.   http://www.cdc.gov/nchs                      National Center for Health Statistics (NCHS)
                                                             Center for Disease Control (CDC)

## 1.6    Tumor Classification and TNM System

**D.P. Berger, H. Henß**

**Def:** Tumor classification allows for the categorization of malignancies commensurate with different stages of a disease. The objective is to form defined, distinguishable groups of diagnostic, therapeutic, and prognostic relevance.

### Pathological Classification: TNM System

The TNM code is internationally established as the pathological classification of solid tumors. Hematological neoplasias are classified differently (see respective disease entities). For solid tumors, too, other clinically relevant staging systems are sometimes being used in addition to the TNM classification. They are essentially aligned with the TNM code:
- Testicular tumors: Lugano / Royal Marsden / Indiana stages
- Colorectal carcinoma: Dukes stages
- Ovarian carcinoma: FIGO stages
- Small cell lung cancer: limited / extensive disease

### Clinical Classifications: AJCC / UICC

Clinical classification (corresponding to stages 0, I, II, III, IV) aids further simplification and unites therapeutically and prognostically similar TNM stages. In general, in situ carcinomas are classified as stage 0 and tumors with evident distant metastasis as stage IV.

Depending on each disease entity, clinical categorization is carried out in accordance with recommendations by UICC (Union Internationale Contre le Cancer), AJCC (American Joint Committee on Cancer), or national organizations.

**Meth:**    **TNM System**

Internationally standardized system for the categorization and course documentation of solid tumors. The TNM system is based on a graduated description of tumor size (T), lymph node spread (N), and distant metastasis (M).

**General principles of the TNM classification (1992, modified 2002)**

| Parameter | Categories | General definition[a] |
|---|---|---|
| Tumor size | TX | Primary tumor cannot be assessed |
| | T0 | No evidence of primary tumor |
| | Tis | Carcinoma in situ (microscopic evidence) |
| | T1–4 | Increasing size / local extension of primary tumor |
| Lymph node metastasis | NX | Regional lymph nodes cannot be assessed |
| | N0 | No regional lymph node metastasis |
| | N1–3 | Increasing involvement of regional lymph nodes |
| | Detection | s: sentinel lymph node, i: isolated tumor cells, mol: molecular genetic testing |
| Distant metastasis | MX | Distant metastasis cannot be assessed |
| | M0 | No distant metastasis |
| | M1 | Distant metastasis |
| | Organs involved | ADR: adrenals, BRA: brain, HEP: hepatic, LYM: lymph nodes, MAR: bone marrow, OSS: osseous, PER: peritoneum, PLE: pleura, PUL: pulmonary, SKI: skin, OTH: others |

| Parameter | Categories | General definition[a] |
|---|---|---|
| Histopathological grading | GX | Grade of differentiation cannot be assessed |
| | G1 | Well differentiated |
| | G2 | Moderately differentiated |
| | G3 | Poorly differentiated |
| | G4 | Undifferentiated / anaplastic |
| Prefixes/suffixes | aTNM | Autoptic classification |
| | cTNM | Clinical classification |
| | pTNM | Pathological classification |
| | rTNM | Recurrent tumors |
| | yTNM | Classification during/after initial therapy |
| | T(m)NM | Multiple primary tumors |
| Resection status | RX | Presence of residual tumor cannot be assessed |
| | R0 | No residual tumor |
| | R1 | Microscopic residual tumor |
| | R2 | Macroscopic residual tumor |
| Venous invasion | VX | Venous invasion cannot be assessed |
| | V0 | No venous invasion |
| | V1 | Microscopic venous invasion |
| | V2 | Macroscopic venous invasion |
| Diagnostic certainty | C1 | Clinical examination |
| | C2 | Special diagnostic means |
| | C3 | Surgical exploration |
| | C4 | Exhaustive pathological examination |
| | C5 | Autopsy |

[a] For disease-specific stage definitions ▶ Chaps. 8.1–8.13

**Ref:**
1. Greene FL, Page DL, Fleming ID et al. (eds) AJCC Cancer Staging Handbook. TNM Classification of Malignant Tumors, 6th edn. Springer, New York, 2002
2. Gospodarowicz MK, Miller D, Groome PA et al. The process for continuous improvement of the TNM classification. Cancer 2004;100:1–5
3. Sobin LH, Wittekind C (eds). TNM Classification of Malignant Tumors, 6th edn. Wiley, New York, 2002
4. WHO. International Classification of Diseases, 10th edn (ICD-10). WHO, Genf, 1996

**Web:**
1. http://www.cancerstaging.org    American Joint Committee on Cancer (AJCC)
2. http://www.cancer.gov    National Cancer Institute (NCI), with Cancernet
3. http://www.uicc.org    Union Internationale Contre le Cancer (UICC)

**1.7** **Indications for Tumor Therapy**

D.P. Berger, H. Henß , R. Engelhardt

**Def:** Factors determining the indication for tumor therapy are:
- Diagnosis
- General health of the patient
- Tumor stage
- Available methods of treatment
- Goals of treatment
- Patient's wish to be treated

**Meth:** *Diagnosis*
Correct diagnosis is a fundamental prerequisite for antineoplastic treatment:
- Histological or cytological diagnosis is necessary
  Exception: acute emergency situations with clinically certain malignancy
- Pathological diagnosis and clinical diagnosis must be compatible

*General Health*
Scoring of general performance status by Karnofsky or WHO (▶ Chap. 1.8)

*Tumor Stages*
Staging systems (▶ Chap. 1.6)

*Methods of Treatment*
- Surgical treatment
- Drug treatment including chemotherapy
- Radiotherapy
- Interdisciplinary treatment: multimodal antineoplastic therapy including surgery, drug treatment, and radiation. Treatment is planned and performed by specialists cooperating in the involved fields (surgery, medical hematology and oncology, radiotherapy, gynecology, urology, etc.)
- Experimental methods of treatment (e.g., immunotherapy, gene therapy, hyperthermia): use within the framework of clinical trials when conventional treatment is not appropriate

*Terms of Interdisciplinary Tumor Therapy*
- *Adjuvant Treatment:* postoperative application of additional methods of treatment, aimed at the elimination of residual tumor, or micrometastases, usually via radiotherapy (locally effective treatment) or drug-based tumor therapy (systemically effective treatment)
- *Neoadjuvant Treatment:* preoperative application of additional methods of treatment, aiming at primary reduction of tumor size (to achieve operability) and systemic elimination of disseminated tumor foci

**Therapeutic goals and results of treatment**

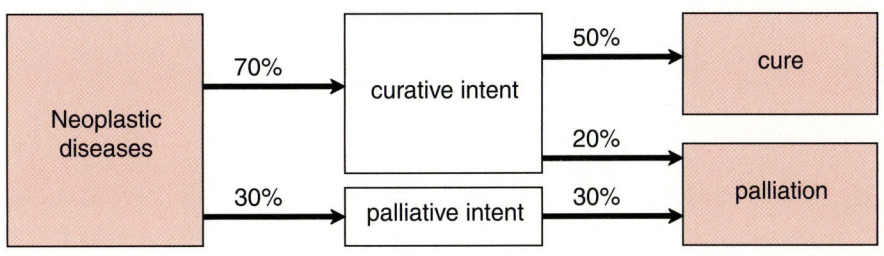

- *Curative treatment:* the objective of therapy is to cure the patient. Primary curative intention justifies intensive methods of treatment (e.g. extensive surgical resection, high-dose chemotherapy, interdisciplinary therapy) despite increased strain on the patient. Treatment must be carried out in accordance with international standards and guidelines
- *Palliative treatment:* aimed at improving the patient's quality of life, controlling symptoms and pain, as well as prolonging the life span. A palliative intention does not normally justify intensive or strenuous methods of treatment. Treatment is particularly adapted to the individual situation of the patient
- *Supportive treatment:* supportive care methods to improve the patient's quality of life and make treatment more tolerable rather than focusing on antineoplastic effectiveness in the narrow sense

The therapeutic objectives in patients with neoplasms may change throughout the course of the disease. If treatment with a primary curative intention fails, the therapeutic focus usually changes to palliative treatment in order to limit further invasive measures.

**Ref:**        1.    Julia H, Rowland JH, Hewitt M, Ganz PA. Cancer survivorship: a new challenge in delivering quality cancer care. J Clin Onc 2006;24:5101–4

**Web:**        1.    http://www.cancer.org                          ACS, Clinical Practice Guidelines
                2.    http://www.guideline.gov                       National Guideline Clearinghouse (NGC)
                3.    http://cancer.gov/cancerinformation           National Cancer Institute (NCI), with Cancernet
                4.    http://www.cebm.net                           Center for Evidence-Based Medicine

# 1.8    Performance Status of Tumor Patients ("Performance Status Scales")

D.P. Berger, H. Bertz

**Def:**

| WHO, SAKK, ECOG, Zubrod Definition | Grade | Karnofsky Definition | Index |
|---|---|---|---|
| No symptoms; fully active | 0 | Normal activity; no complaints; no symptoms of disease | 100% |
| Symptoms; moderate reduction in physical activity and capacity to work; not bed-ridden | 1 | Slight reduction in normal activity; minor symptoms of disease | 90% |
| | | Normal activity only with effort; some symptoms of disease | 80% |
| Unable to work; cares for self; increasing need for assistance, needs to be in bed < 50% of waking hours | 2 | Cares for self; unable to carry on normal activity or to do active work | 70% |
| | | Requires occasional assistance; mainly cares for self | 60% |
| Cannot care for self; requires permanent care or hospitalization; needs to be in bed > 50% of waking hours | 3 | Requires considerable assistance and frequent medical care | 50% |
| | | Disabled; requires special care and assistance | 40% |
| Rapid progression of disease; confined to bed | 4 | Severely disabled; hospitalization is indicated although death not imminent | 30% |
| | | Very sick; hospitalization necessary; active supportive treatment necessary | 20% |
| | | Moribund; fatal processes progressing rapidly | 10% |
| Dead | 5 | Dead | 0% |

*WHO* World Health Organization, *SAKK* Schweizerische Arbeitsgemeinschaft für Klinische Krebsforschung (Swiss Group for Clinical Cancer Research), *ECOG* Eastern Cooperative Oncology Group

**Ref:**

1. Buccheri G, Ferrigno D, Tamburini M. Karnofsky and ECOG performance status scoring in lung cancer: a prospective, longitudinal study of 536 patients from a single institution. Eur J Cancer 1996;32A:1135–41
2. Garman KS, Cohen HJ. Functional status and the elderly patient. Crit Rev Oncol Hematol 2002;43:191–298
3. Mor V, Laliberte L, Morris JN et al. The Karnofsky Performance Status Scale. An examination of its reliability and validity in a research setting. Cancer 1984;53:2002–7
4. Oken MM, Creech RH, Tormey DC et al. Toxicity and response criteria of the Eastern Cooperative Oncology Group. Am J Clin Oncol 1982;5:649–55

**Web:**

1. http://www.who.int     World Health Organization (WHO)
2. http://ecog.dfci.harvard.edu     Eastern Cooperative Oncology Group (ECOG)
3. http://www.fda.gov/cder/cancer     Food and Drug Administration (FDA) Oncology Tools

## 1.9      Response Evaluation in Solid Tumors

**D.P. Berger**

**Def:**      Clinical response evaluation in individual patients takes into consideration objective parameters as well as subjective criteria:
- Tumor regression in comparison to initial size (degree of remission, "response")
- Remission duration: progression / relapse-free interval
- Survival time: tumor-free survival time and overall survival time
- Toxicity
- Symptom control: regression of tumor-related symptoms (pain, etc.)
- Quality of life: changes in general health

In an overall evaluation of a treatment method within a patient population, the therapeutic response is assessed using similar parameters:
- Response rate: percentage of subjects with tumor remission within a given patient population
- Median remission duration
- Median survival time
- Survival rates (one-year survival rate, five-year survival rate)
- Cost-effectiveness in comparison to other methods of treatment

**Meth:**      *Response Evaluation in Solid Tumor Therapy*
- Monitoring of tumor size and comparison to pre-treatment baseline
- Definition of tumor progression parameters prior to start of therapy
- Implementation of follow-ups using pre-defined evaluation methods
- Imaging as a prerequisite for objective assessment (x-ray, CT, NMR, photography, etc.)

**Class:**      *Solid Tumor Response Parameters*
- *WHO Criteria (Miller 1981):* tumor response is evaluated on the basis of measurable tumor manifestations. Tumor size is measured bidimensionally (product of longest diameter × greatest perpendicular diameter, a × b). With multiple tumors, individual products are added up. For the overall response, non-measurable tumor manifestations are also being considered.
- *RECIST Criteria ("Response Evaluation Criteria In Solid Tumors", Therasse 2000):* response evaluation ("best response") only includes measurable tumors ("target lesions"). The evaluation of the tumor size is based on diameter (longest diameter). In case of multiple tumors, individual diameters are added up. Overall response includes the evaluation of target lesions, other non-measurable tumor manifestations ("non-target lesions"), and the occurrence of new tumor manifestations.
- *Measurable Tumor:* any tumor manifestation that can be measured in at least two dimensions.
- *Non-measurable Tumor:* any tumor manifestation which is detectable but can not be measured in two dimensions (e.g., metastasis < 1 cm diameter, lymphangitis carcinomatosa, peritoneal carcinosis, malignant pleural effusion, diffuse metastasis). A "non-measurable" tumor can still be evaluable, e.g., in case of unidimensional expansion (liver enlargement due to metastasis, etc), by the use of clinical parameters (dyspnea, pain, immobility, etc.) or "surrogate" markers (tumor markers, immunoglobulins, etc.).
- *Skeletal Metastasis:* bone metastases are regarded as tumor parameters. However, remission is defined differently (see Table).

**Definition of solid tumor remission**

| Remission status | Abbreviation | Measurable tumor (WHO criteria) | Measurable tumor (RECIST criteria) | Non-measurable tumor or skeletal metastasis |
|---|---|---|---|---|
| Complete remission | CR | Disappearance of all known disease, confirmed at ≥ 4 weeks[1] | Disappearance of all target lesions, confirmed at ≥ 4 weeks[1] | Disappearance of all target lesions and normalization of tumor markers, confirmed at ≥ 4 weeks[1] |
| Partial remission | PR | ≥ 50% decrease from baseline, confirmed at ≥ 4 weeks[1] | ≥ 30% decrease from baseline, confirmed at ≥ 4 weeks[1] | ≥ 30–50% decrease from baseline confirmed at ≥ 4 weeks[1] |
| | | No new metastasis | No new lesions | No new metastasis |
| | | No progression of other tumor parameters | No progression of non-target lesions | No increase in other tumor parameters |
| No change[2] = Stable disease | NC SD | Neither PR or PD criteria met, confirmed at ≥ 4 weeks[1] | Neither PR or PD criteria met, confirmed at ≥ 4 weeks[1] | Target lesion and tumor parameters unchanged compared to baseline, confirmed at ≥ 4 weeks[1] |
| | | No new metastasis | No new lesions | No new metastasis |
| | | No progression of other tumor parameters | No progression of non-target lesions | No increase in other tumor parameters |
| Progression = Progressive disease | P PD | ≥ 25% increase of one or more lesions and/or appearance of new lesions and/or progression of other tumor parameters | ≥ 30% increase over smallest sum observed and/or appearance of new lesions and/or progression of other tumor parameters | ≥ 25% increase in existent lesions compared to baseline and/or appearance of new lesions and/or appearance of other tumor parameters |

[1]Confirmed by 2 tests ≥ 4 weeks apart
[2]"Minor response (MR)": tumor size 50–75% compared to baseline, frequently used in clinical trials

### Definition of Therapeutic Response
- Therapeutic response of measurable and non-measurable tumors should be defined separately
- In the presence of several measurable tumor parameters, the single worst parameter is defining the response category. Example: three measurable tumors with partial remission (PR), but occurrence of new lesion ▶ overall response: "progression."

### Remission Duration
- The duration of complete remission (CR) is the time between the first day of documented CR and the first day of detectable progression
- The duration of partial remission is the time between the first day of treatment and the first day of documented progression ("overall response period")

### Therapeutic Response in Hematological Neoplasias

There are separate evaluation systems for different types of hematological neoplasias (leukemia, lymphomas). These are, however, based on similar principles:

- Response classification using complete remission, partial remission, stable disease, progression
- In the presence of genetic markers (e.g., Philadelphia chromosome with chronic myeloid leukemia): differentiation between clinical response and "cytogenetic response" (detectability of a cytogenetic or molecular genetic marker)

### Survival Time

- "Absolute survival": time between diagnosis / initiation of therapy and death
- "Event-free survival" (EFS): time between diagnosis / initiation of therapy / tumor response and occurrence of new tumor manifestation

**Ref:**

1. Green S, Weiss GR. Southwest Oncology Group standard response criteria, endpoint definitions and toxicity criteria. Invest New Drugs 1992;10:239–53
2. Jaffe CC. Measures of response: RECIST, WHO, and new alternatives. J Clin Oncol 2006;24:3245–51
3. Therasse P, Arbuck SG, Eisenhauer EA et al. New guidelines to evaluate the response to treatment in solid tumors. J Natl Cancer Inst 2000;92:205–16
4. WHO. WHO handbook for reporting results of cancer treatment. WHO, 1979

**Web:**

1. http://www.who.int                          World Health Organization (WHO)
2. http://www3.cancer.gov/dip/RECIST.htm       NCI, RECIST Criteria
3. http://www.swog.org                         Southwest Oncology Group (SWOG)

## 1.10 Common Toxicity Criteria (NCI)

**D.P. Berger**

Common Toxicity Criteria (NCI)

| Criteria | Grade 0 | Grade 1 | Grade 2 | Grade 3 | Grade 4 |
|---|---|---|---|---|---|
| Performance status | Fully active | Ambulatory, capable of light work activities | Capable of self-care but not of working, in bed ≤ 50% of time | Capable of only limited self-care, in bed > 50% of time | Completely bedridden |
| Weight loss | < 5% | 5–9.9% | 10–19.9% | > 20% | – |
| Weight gain | < 5% | 5–9.9% | 10–19.9% | > 20% | – |
| Leucocytes | ≥ 4,000/μl | 3,000–3,999/μl | 2,000–2,999/μl | 1,000–1,999/μl | < 1,000/μl |
| Neutrophils | ≥ 2,000/μl | 1,500–1,999/μl | 1,000–1,499/μl | 500–999/μl | < 500/μl |
| Lymphocytes | ≥ 2,000/μl | 1,500–1,999/μl | 1,000–1,499/μl | 500–999/μl | < 500/μl |
| Hemoglobin | ≥ 11.0 g/dl | 10.0–10.9 g/dl | 8.0–9.9 g/dl | 6.5–7.9 g/dl | < 6.5 g/dl |
| Platelets | ≥ 100,000/μl | 75,000–99,999/μl | 50,000–74,999/μl | 25,000–49,999/μl | < 25,000/μl |
| Bleeding | None | Mild No transfusion | Moderate 1–2 transfusions | Significant 3–4 transfusions | Severe > 4 transfusions |
| Prothrombin time | Normal | > 1.0–1.25 × N | > 1.25–1.5 × N | > 1.5–2.0 × N | > 2.0 × N |
| PTT | Normal | > 1.0–1.66 × N | > 1.66–2.33 × N | > 2.33–3.0 × N | > 3.0 × N |
| Fibrinogen | Normal | 0.75–0.99 × N | 0.5–0.74 × N | 0.25–0.49 × N | < 0.25 × N |
| Urea | Normal | < 30.0 mg/dl | 30.1–50.0 mg/dl | > 50.0 mg/dl | – |
| Creatinine | Normal | 1.1–1.5 × N | 1.6–3.0 × N | 3.1–6.0 × N | > 6.0 × N |
| Hypercalcemia | < 2.65 mmol/l | 2.65–2.87 mmol/l | 2.88–3.12 mmol/l | 3.13–3.37 mmol/l | > 3.37 mmol/l |
| Hypocalcaemia | > 2.10 mmol/l | 1.95–2.10 mmol/l | 1.75–1.94 mmol/l | 1.51–1.74 mmol/l | ≤ 1.50 mmol/l |
| Hypokalemia | > 3.50 mmol/l | 3.01–3.50 mmol/l | 2.51–3.00 mmol/l | 2.01–2.50 mmol/l | ≤ 2.00 mmol/l |
| Hyponatremia | > 135 mmol/l | 131–135 mmol/l | 126–130 mmol/l | 121–125 mmol/l | ≤ 120 mmol/l |
| Hypomagnesemia | > 1.40 mmol/l | 1.11–1.40 mmol/l | 0.81–1.10 mmol/l | 0.51–0.80 mmol/l | < 0.50 mmol/l |
| Proteinuria | None | < 3.0 g/l | 3.0–10.0 g/l | > 10.0 g/l | Nephrotic syndrome |
| Hematuria | None | Microhematuria | Macrohematuria | Macrohematuria with clots | Transfusion-dependent hematuria |
| Bilirubin | Normal | < 1.5 × N | 1.6–3.0 × N | 3.1–10.0 × N | > 10.0 × N |

*LVEF* left ventricular ejection fraction, *N* normal value, *PTT* partial thromboplastin time, *RR* blood pressure, *SGOT* serum glutamic–oxaloacetic transaminase, *SGPT* serum glutamic-pyruvic transaminase

**Common Toxicity Criteria (NCI) (continued)**

| Criteria | Grade 0 | Grade 1 | Grade 2 | Grade 3 | Grade 4 |
|---|---|---|---|---|---|
| SGOT / SGPT | Normal | $< 2.5 \times N$ | $2.6–5.0 \times N$ | $5.1–20.0 \times N$ | $> 20.0 \times N$ |
| Alkaline phosphatase | Normal | $< 2.5 \times N$ | $2.6–5.0 \times N$ | $5.1–20.0 \times N$ | $> 20.0 \times N$ |
| Hyperglycemia | $\leq 115$ mg/dl | 116–160 mg/dl | 161–250 mg/dl | 251–500 mg/dl | > 500 mg/dl, ketoacidosis |
| Hypoglycemia | $\geq 65$ mg/dl | 55–64 mg/dl | 40–54 mg/dl | 30–39 mg/dl | < 30 mg/dl, shock |
| Amylase | Normal | $\leq 1.5 \times N$ | $1.6–2.0 \times N$ | $2.1–5.0 \times N$ | $> 5.0 \times N$ |
| Nausea | None | Mild Normal food intake | Moderate Reduced food intake | Severe No oral food intake | Life-threatening |
| Vomiting | None | Mild, 1 /day | 2–5 /day | 6–10 /day | > 10 /day, life-threatening |
| Mucositis | None | Erythema, mild symptoms Normal food intake | Erythema Painful ulcers Solid food intake | Painful ulcers Liquid intake | Life-threatening Parenteral nutrition No oral intake |
| Diarrhea | None | 2–3 /day | 4–6 /day Moderate cramps | $\geq 7$ /day Incontinence, severe cramps | Life-threatening Hospital admission required |
| Obstipation | None | Mild | Moderate Laxative use | Pronounced, subileus | Ileus, obstruction Life-threatening |
| Arrhythmia | None | Asymptomatic No treatment | Symptomatic No treatment | Symptomatic Treatment necessary | Life-threatening, ventricular tachycardia, fibrillation |
| Cardiac ischemia | None | Non-specific T wave flattening, asymptomatic | Asymptomatic ST-T segment changes | Angina pectoris without signs of infarction | Myocardial infarction |
| Cardiac function | Normal | Asymptomatic LVEF 50–59% | Asymptomatic LVEF 40–49% | Symptomatic LVEF 20–39% | Severe or refractory insufficiency LVEF < 20% |
| Pericardium | Normal | Asymptomatic effusion | Pericarditis | Symptomatic effusion, tap necessary | Pericardial tamponade, emergency tap necessary |

*LVEF* left ventricular ejection fraction, *N* normal value, *PTT* partial thromboplastin time, *RR* blood pressure, *SGOT* serum glutamic-oxaloacetic transaminase, *SGPT* serum glutamic-pyruvic transaminase

**Common Toxicity Criteria (NCI) (*continued*)**

| Criteria | Grade 0 | Grade 1 | Grade 2 | Grade 3 | Grade 4 |
|---|---|---|---|---|---|
| Hypertension | None | Transient, RR diastole ↑ by > 20 mmHg RR > 150/100 mmHg | Recurrent / persisting, RR diastole ↑ by > 20 mmHg RR > 150/100 mmHg | Requiring treatment | Hypertensive crisis |
| Hypotension | None | Mild orthostatic dysregulation No treatment | Fluid-substitution necessary (< 24 h) | Inpatient treatment necessary (≥ 24 h) | Shock, life-threatening Organ failure |
| Pulmonary function | > 90% of baseline value, normal | 76–90% of baseline value, mild symptoms | 51–75% of baseline value, exertional dyspnea | 26–50% of baseline value, resting dyspnea | < 25% of baseline value, complete bed rest required |
| $pO_2$ | > 85 mmHg | 71–85 mmHg | 61–70 mmHg | 51–60 mmHg | ≤ 50 mmHg |
| $pCO_2$ | ≤ 40 mmHg | 41–50 mmHg | 51–60 mmHg | 61–70 mmHg | > 70 mmHg |
| Thrombosis / phlebitis | None | – | Superficial thrombophlebitis | Deep vein thrombosis | Pulmonary embolism, venous occlusion |
| Injection site reaction | Normal | Mild pain, pruritus, erythema | Moderate pain, swelling, phlebitis, inflammation | Ulcer, necrosis, surgical treatment necessary | – |
| Skin reaction, erythema, systemic | Normal | Asymptomatic erythema or scattered maculopapular efflorescences | Dense efflorescences, pruritus, erythema, desquamation | Generalized maculopapular alterations, strong desquamation | Exfoliative or ulcerative dermatitis |
| Hand-foot syndrome | None | Minimal alterations, no pain | Painful alterations, function maintained | Painful alterations, defective function | – |
| Alopecia | None | Moderate patchy alopecia, visible | Complete alopecia | – | – |
| Allergy | None | Intermittent chills, temperature < 38°C | Urticaria, chills, temperature > 38°C, mild bronchospasm | Bronchospasm, serum sickness, parenteral treatment | Anaphylactic reaction |
| Tiredness (fatigue) | None | Mild | Moderate, daily activities restricted | Severe, pronounced reduction of activities | No activities possible |

*LVEF* left ventricular ejection fraction, *N* normal value, *PTT* partial thromboplastin time, *RR* blood pressure, *SGOT* serum glutamic-oxaloacetic transaminase, *SGPT* serum glutamic-pyruvic transaminase

**Common Toxicity Criteria (NCI)** *(continued)*

| Criteria | Grade 0 | Grade 1 | Grade 2 | Grade 3 | Grade 4 |
|---|---|---|---|---|---|
| Fever | None | < 38°C | 38.1–40°C | > 40°C for < 24 h | > 40°C for > 24 h, hypotension |
| Febrile neutropenia | None | – | – | Existent | Life-threatening, sepsis |
| Infection | None | Mild infection<br>Not requiring treatment | Moderate infection<br>Oral antibiotics | Major infection<br>Intravenous antibiotics | Life-threatening, sepsis |
| Somnolence | Normal | Mild somnolence | Moderate somnolence | Pronounced somnolence, stupor | Coma |
| Confusion | Normal | Transient confusion, disorientation, attention deficit | Confusion, loss of orientation, attention deficit | Confusion, delirium | Life-threatening, hospital admission necessary |
| Sensory function | Normal | Mild paresthesia<br>Deep tendon reflexes ↓ | Moderate paresthesia, objective impairment | Severe paresthesia<br>Loss of function | Complete loss of function |
| Motor function | Normal | Mild subjective weakness without function impairment | Mild verified weakness without significantly impaired function | Verified weakness with function impairment | Life-threatening paralysis |
| Cerebellar / ataxia | Normal | Mild dyscoordination or dysdiadochokinesia | Intention tremor, dysmetria, nystagmus, blurred speech | Ataxia | Cerebellar necrosis, loss of function |
| Mood | Normal | Mild anxiety or depression | Moderate anxiety or depression | Severe anxiety or depression | Suicidal |
| Pain | None | Mild<br>No treatment necessary | Pronounced<br>Treatment necessary | Severe, morphine application necessary | Intractable |
| Degustation | Normal | Change of taste, normal nutrition | Loss of taste, restricted nutrition | – | – |
| Vision | Normal | Mildly decreased | Moderately decreased | Symptomatic, subtotal loss of vision | Blindness |
| Hearing | Normal | Asymptomatic, only audiometric verifiable impairment | Tinnitus, mild subjective hypacusis | Symptomatic hypacusis, corrigible with hearing aid | Deafness, irreversible |

*LVEF* left ventricular ejection fraction, *N* normal value, *PTT* partial thromboplastin time, *RR* blood pressure, *SGOT* serum glutamic–oxaloacetic transaminase, *SGPT* serum glutamic-pyruvic transaminase

**Ref:**

1. Brown EG, Wood L, Wood S. The medical dictionary for regulatory activities (MedDRA). Drug Saf 1999;20:109–17
2. Edwards IR, Aronson JK. Adverse drug reactions: definitions, diagnosis, management. Lancet 2000;356:1255–9
3. Hesslewood SR. European system for reporting adverse reactions to and defects in radiopharmaceuticals: annual report 1999. Eur J Nucl Med 2001;28:2–8
4. Pirmohamed M, Breckenridge AM, Kitteringham NR et al. Adverse drug reactions. BMJ 1998;316:1295–8
5. Trotti A, Colevas AD, Setser A et al. CTCAE v3.0: development of a comprehensive grading system for the adverse effects of cancer treatment. Semin Radiat Oncol 2003;13:176–81
6. Vincent C. Understanding and responding to adverse events. N Engl J Med 2003;348:1051–6

**Web:**

1. http://ctep.cancer.gov/reporting/ctc.html — NCI Common Toxicity Criteria
2. http://ecog.dfci.harvard.edu/~ecogdba/general/common_tox.html — ECOG Common Toxicity Criteria
3. http://www.accessdata.fda.gov/scripts/cder/onctools/toxicity.cfm — FDA, Common Toxicity Criteria

## 1.11        Assessing the Quality of Life of Tumor Patients

**S. Fetscher, H. Bertz**

**Def:**        There is no standardized definition of "quality of life". The definition suggested by the WHO describing "health" as "complete physical, psychological and social well-being" largely corresponds to the popular-medical understanding of the term "quality of life."
The following components of quality of life can be distinguished:
- Physical condition
- Psychological condition
- Social interaction
- Functioning in the everyday life, behavioral components

**Meth:**        Quality of life evaluation is based on patient self-assessment (usually questionnaire), structured interview procedures and outside assessment by relatives or medical personnel.

### Methods of Assessing the General Quality of Life
- Short-form 36 (SF-36), standard method for non-oncological questions
- Affect-balance scale
- Munich Quality of Life-Dimensions List
- Nottingham Health Profile (NHP)
- Lancaster Quality of Life Profile
- Sickness Impact Profile (SIP)
- Oregon Quality of Life Questionnaire
- International Quality of Life Assessment-Group Profile

### Special Methods of Quality of Life Assessment in Hematology / Oncology
- EORTC Questionnaire (EORTC QLQ-C30), standard method for oncological assessment in Europe
- Functional Assessment of Cancer Treatment (FACT), standard method for oncological assessment in the USA
- Rotterdam Symptom Checklist (RSCL)
- Quality of Life in Cancer Scale
- Lung Cancer Symptom Scale

**IMPORTANT:** It is a common misunderstanding that the Karnofsky Index or ECOG Score can be used for quality of life assessment (Chap. 1.8). Both methods are used for the evaluation of a patient's general physical health which is only one component of quality of life. In an individual case, a low Karnofsky index (poor general health) can go hand in hand with a good quality of life and good general health can coincide with poor quality of life.

**Ind:**        Quality of life assessment is particularly indicated in treatment studies or in the framework of modern quality management. In clinical research, implementation of quality of life measures is being increasingly demanded by ethics commissions and institutional review boards.
Quality of life assessment is mandatory with:
- Comparative trials on supportive therapy
- Multicentric phase III trials aimed at establishing new therapeutic standards
- Trials in geriatric oncology
- Trials of palliative therapy

Quality of life assessment with established methods (e.g., EORTC Questionnaire)—especially when used for the evaluation of new methods of therapy—has the following objectives:
- With only small differences in remission and survival data, improved quality of life may determine the choice of treatment
- Clear basis for assessing effects and side effects of a particular treatment
- Improvement of operational aspects and quality of tumor treatment and individual patient care.

- Clearly defined criteria for palliative treatment in patients with advanced malignancies, where toxic experimental therapies are not justified. Once life expectancy is limited, aspects of quality of life need to lead medical and therapeutic decision-making.

**Ref:**
1. de Haes J, Curran D, Young T et al. Quality of life evaluation in oncological clinical trials – the EORTC model. Eur J Cancer 2000;36:821–5
2. Giesler RB, Williams SD. Opportunities and challenges: assessing quality of life in clinical trials. J Natl Cancer Inst 1998;90:1498–9
3. Holzner B, Bode RK, Hahn EA et al. Equating EORTC QLQ–C30 and FACT–G scores and its use in oncological research. Eur J Cancer 2006;42:3169–77

**Web:**
1. http://www.fda.gov — Food and Drug Administration (FDA)
2. http://www.nci.nih.gov — National Cancer Institute (NCI)
3. http://www.eortc.be/home/qol/ — European Organization for Research and Treatment of Cancer (EORTC), "Quality of Life Web Site"
4. http://www.isoqol.org/ — International Society for Quality of Life Research

## 1.12          Evidence-based Medicine (EBM), Guidelines and Quality Management

**H. Henß**

**Def:**      "Evidence-based medicine" (EBM) describes the implementation of diagnostic and therapeutic methods which are based on assured knowledge (evidence), putting purpose and benefit of the respective method second. This is particularly important when several different methods are under consideration.

**Class:**    The evidence of clinical information is classified corresponding to the reliability of the underlying trials. Depending on the way data were obtained, different levels of evidence can be distinguished. Prospective randomized trials including control groups imply the highest reliability.

**Levels of evidence according to standard of knowledge**

| Level of evidence | Definition |
|---|---|
| 1 | Evidence obtained from at least one properly designed randomized controlled trial |
| 2 | Evidence obtained from well-designed controlled trials without randomization |
| 3 | Evidence obtained from well-designed cohort or case-control analytic studies, preferably from more than one center or research group |
| 4 | Evidence obtained from case series with or without intervention |
| 5 | Opinions of respected authorities, based on clinical experience, descriptive studies, or reports of expert committees |

EBM does not imply that only methods based on controlled randomized studies are legitimate. However, decision making should be based on the highest available level of evidence in each case.

### Standards and Guidelines in Oncology

**Def:**      Standards and guidelines, especially on the basis of assured evidence, are designed to support medical decision making in order to guarantee high quality healthcare. Guidelines are:
- Systematically developed tools which help decide on medically adequate approaches to diagnosis and therapy of certain diseases
- Consensus of several experts from various disciplines ("interdisciplinary guidelines") which was developed using defined, transparent procedures
- Scientifically established and practical recommendations for action
- Orientation guides, from which deviation is acceptable in justified circumstances

#### *Objectives of Guidelines and Standards:*
- Securing and improving the health care of the population
- Motivation to apply medical procedures that are scientifically established and economically appropriate
- Information about necessary and established medical procedures with regard to special health risks and disorders
- Reduction of undesirable fluctuation of quality in medical care

**Class:**

*Characteristics of Standards*

Standards are classified according to their reliability:

- Recommendations: describe options of acting and omission. Of minor normative nature and little scientific evidence.
- Guidelines: systematically developed tools which help decide on medically adequate approaches to specific problems. Science-based practical orientation guides ("action pathways") from which deviation is acceptable in justified cases
- Directives: code of conduct which is approved by a legally authorized institution, set out in writing, and published; legally binding for the legal and judicial area of a specific institution; non-compliance is punished by specific sanctions

*IMPORTANT:* Directives have to, guidelines should, and recommendations may be observed.

## Quality Management

**Def:**

"Quality" describes all characteristics of a product / service with regards to its ability to satisfy defined and required needs. It comprises:

- Structural quality (financial, technical, and personnel equipment)
- Process quality (here: quality of diagnostic and therapeutic measures, organization, and supervision of treatment procedures)
- Quality of outcome (quality of achieved results by diagnosis and therapy)

"Quality management" describes a dynamic process of continuous evaluation and optimization of all diagnostic and therapeutic measures. "Quality assurance" in the narrow sense merely ascertains compliance with once-defined standards. However, medicine in general and hematology / oncology in particular are subject to constant progress. Therefore, quality management is the preferred option.

**Meth:**

Quality management results from continuous processes:

- Quality analysis (measuring and registration of deficits)
- Quality improvement (adjustment to expected norms)

Quality is measured by indicators (e.g., treatment associated toxicity; remission rates, survival times, quality of life). Prerequisites are clearly defined indicators that are measured by consistent methods.

### Benchmarking

Continuous improvement of quality ("total quality management", TQM) describes the regular comparison of different hospitals or departments by the means of pre-defined indicators. It can initiate development and introduction of new procedures and / or lead to abandonment of obsolete practices. The two most important "parameters" are the patient and the respective disease course.

### Gap Analysis

Defective processes hinder smooth diagnosis and therapy. Usually, only a small number of flaws gives rise to a multitude of disruptions ("Single point of failure"). Errors should therefore be listed according to the frequency of their occurrence ("Pareto Diagram") before initiating a "reform." That way, the most significant defects can be detected and adequate measures necessary for their elimination can be decided upon swiftly.

### Good Clinical Practice (GCP)

GCP describes the execution of clinical procedures on the basis of tested and approved standard methods ("standard operating procedures"; SOP). GCP is of major importance with complex high-risk procedures (e.g., chemotherapy) and was initially developed for the conduct of clinical trials (▶ Chap. 3.7).

**Ref:**

1. Ayanian JZ, Crischilles EA, Wallace RB et al. Understanding cancer treatment and outcomes: the Cancer Care Outcomes Research and Surveillance Consortium. J Clin Oncol 2004;22:2992–6
2. Ray-Coquard I, Philip T, de Laroche G et al. A controlled before-after study: impact of a clinical guidelines program and regional cancer network organization on medical practice. Br J Cancer 2002;86:313–21
3. Schneider EC, Epstein AM, Malin JL et al. Developing a system to assess the quality of cancer care: ASCO's National Initiative on Cancer Care Quality. J Clin Oncol 2004;22:2985–91
4. Vardy J, Tannock IF. Quality of cancer care. Ann Oncol 2004;15:1001–6

**Web:**

| | | |
|---|---|---|
| 1. | http://www.cebm.net | Evidence-Based Medicine, Oxford |
| 2. | http://www.guideline.gov | National Guideline Clearinghouse (NGC) |
| 3. | http://cochrane.org/docs/ebm.htm | Cochrane Library, Reviews for EBM |

## 1.13     Electronic Media

**D.P. Berger**

**Def:**    Electronic media, especially the internet, provide an opportunity to rapidly distribute and access current data. This advantage has led to an increased amount of information on up-to-date studies, treatment concepts, and scientific results being online available to doctors and patients.

According to recent studies, there are 12.5 million online searches daily worldwide on health relevant topics. About 40% of tumor patients use the internet to gather information about their disease and approximately 2.3 million patients suffering from a malignant disease have access to the internet, especially in Europe, Asia, and North America.

**Meth:**    The table below lists websites relevant to the hemato-oncological field. We would like to point out that we cannot assume any responsibility for the contents of the listed pages and explicitly distance ourselves from content which is of a non-medical nature or not in accordance with the current state of the art or ethical standards. This list is not exhaustive. It emphasizes websites which have been continuously updated over recent years. Examples are:

### *"Cancer Topics" (www.cancer.gov/cancertopics)*

Up-to-date information by the National Cancer Institute (NCI), Washington, USA:

- Epidemiology, diagnosis, and treatment of hematological and oncological diseases
- Monthly review and updating of the disease-related databases
- Database of worldwide therapy studies
- Information on new treatment approaches and cytostatics
- Information on supportive care
- Separate information resources for doctors and patients

### *PubMed (www.ncbi.nlm.nih.gov/pubmed)*

Comprehensive literature database of the National Center for Biotechnology Information (NCBI) of the National Library of Medicine (NLM). Access to over 10 million manuscripts with abstracts. Includes Medline and several other databases. Search function with excellent access to relevant information.

**Hematology / oncology online**

| Provider / contents | Website |
|---|---|
| *International organizations:* | |
| AACR, American Assoc. for Cancer Research | http://www.aacr.org |
| ACS, American Cancer Society | http://www.cancer.org |
| AJCC, American Joint Committee on Cancer | http://www.cancerstaging.org |
| ASCO, American Society of Clinical Oncology | http://www.asco.org |
| ASH, American Society of Hematology | http://www.hematology.org |
| BMDW, Bone Marrow Donors Worldwide | http://bmdw.org |
| DFCI, Dana Farber Cancer Institute, Harvard | http://www.dfci.harvard.edu |
| Duke Comprehensive Cancer Center | http://cancer.duke.edu |
| EACR, European Assoc. for Cancer Research | http://eacr.org |
| ECOG, Eastern Cooperative Oncology Group | http://www.ecog.dfci.harvard.edu |
| EORTC, European Organisation for Research and Treatment of Cancer | http://www.eortc.be |
| ESMO, European Society of Medical Oncology | http://www.esmo.org |

**Hematology / oncology online** *(continued)*

| Provider / contents | Website |
| --- | --- |
| ESO, European School of Oncology | http://www.cancerworld.org |
| FDA, Food and Drug Administration | http://www.fda.gov |
| FECS, Federation of European Cancer Societies | http://www.fecs.be |
| FHCRC, Fred Hutchinson Cancer Research Center | http://www.fhcrc.org |
| IACR, International Association Cancer Registries | http://www.iacr.com.fr |
| IARC, International Agency for Research on Cancer | http://www.iarc.fr |
| MASCC, Mult. Assoc. Supportive Care in Cancer | http://www.mascc.org |
| MD Anderson Cancer Center | http://www.mdanderson.org |
| MSKCC, Memorial Sloan-Kettering Cancer Center | http://www.mskcc.org |
| NCCN, Natl Comprehensive Cancer Network | http://www.nccn.org |
| NCI, National Cancer Institute, USA | http://www.cancer.gov |
| "Oncolink", Univ. Pennsylvania Cancer Center | http://oncolink.upenn.edu |
| SEER, Surveillance Epidemiology End Results | http://seer.cancer.gov |
| SWOG, Southwest Oncology Group | http://www.swog.org |
| Telescan, Netherlands Cancer Institute | http://telescan.nki.nl |
| UICC, Union Internationale Contre le Cancer | http://www.uicc.org |
| WHO, World Health Organization | http://www.who.int |
| *General information:* | |
| NCI "Cancer Topics" | http://www.cancer.gov/cancertopics |
| Cancer Information Network | http://www.cancernetwork.com |
| FDA Oncology Tools | http://www.fda.gov/cder/cancer |
| Medline Plus | http://www.nlm.nih.gov/medlineplus |
| NCCN Clinical Practice Guidelines Oncology | http://www.nccn.org |
| Medscape Hematology Oncology | http://medscape.com/hematology-on-cologyhome |
| Blood Line | http://www.bloodline.net/ |
| Hematology Atlas, Sao Paulo | http://www.hematologyatlas.com |
| Hematology Atlas, Nagoya | http://pathy.med.nagoya-u.ac.jp/atlas/doc/atlas.html |
| *Disease-specific information:* | |
| Leukemia and Lymphoma Society | http://www.leukemia.org/ |
| Lymphoma Information Network | http://www.lymphomainfo.net |
| International Myeloma Foundation | http://myeloma.org |
| Brain Tumor Society | http://tbts.org |
| Brain Tumor Association | http://www.abta.org/ |
| National Breast Cancer Foundation | http://nationalbreastcancer.org |

**Hematology / oncology online** *(continued)*

| Provider / contents | Website |
|---|---|
| National Breast Cancer Coalition | http://natlbcc.org |
| Lung Cancer Online | http://lungcanceronline.org |
| Lung Cancer | http://lungcancer.gov |
| Colorectal Cancer Network | http://www.colorectal-cancer.net |
| Kidney Cancer Association | http://www.nkca.org/ |
| Prostate Cancer | http://www.prostate.com |
| American Prostate Society | http://www.ameripros.org/ |
| National Prostate Cancer Coalition | http://www.4npcc.org |
| Prostate Cancer Foundation | http://www.prostatecancerfoundation.org |
| Prostate Health Directory | http://www.prostatehealthdirectory.org |
| The Virtual Prostate | http://www.virtualprostate.com |
| TCRC, Testicular Cancer Resource Center | http://www.comed.com/Prostate |
| Management of Cancer Pain Guidelines | http://tcrc.acor.org |
| Carcinogens | http://ehp.niehs.nih.gov.roc |
| *Information on pharmaceuticals:* | |
| Drug Information Network | http://www.druginfonet.com/ |
| Medline Plus Drug Information | http://www.nlm.nih.gov/medlineplus |
| Cytokine Database | http://www.copewithcytokines.de/ |
| Chemfinder Database | http://chemfinder.cambridgesoft.com/ |
| Dose Calculation of Cytostatics | http://www.meds.com/DChome.html |
| *Literature / journals / information:* | |
| PubMed, National Library of Medicine | http://www.ncbi.nlm.nih.gov/pubmed |
| History of Biomedicine | http://wwwihm.nlm.nih.gov/ |
| Blood | http://www.bloodjournal.org |
| CA – A Cancer Journal for Clinicians | http://caonline.amcancersoc.org |
| Cell | http://www.cell.com |
| Journal of Clinical Oncology | http://www.jco.org |
| Journal of the National Cancer Institute | http://jncicancerspectrum/oupjournals.org |
| The Lancet | http://www.thelancet.com/ |
| Nature | http://www.nature.com |
| Nature Medicine | http://www.nature.com/nm |
| Nature Reviews Cancer | http://www.nature.com/nrc |
| The New England Journal of Medicine | http://www.nejm.org/ |
| Science | http://www.sciencemag.org |
| Seminars in Hematology | http://www.seminhematol.org |
| Seminars in Oncology | http://www.seminoncol.org |

**Hematology / oncology online** *(continued)*

| Provider / contents | Website |
|---|---|
| *Search engines / other medical servers:* | |
| Google | http://www.google.com |
| Yahoo | http://www.yahoo.com |
| Hotbot | http://www.hotbot.com |
| Dogpile | http://www.dogpile.com |
| CNN Health News | http://www.cnn.com/health |
| Cancer News | http://www.cancernews.com |
| Medscape | http://www.medscape.com |
| Healthgate | http://www.healthgate.com |
| Medical Matrix | http://www.medmatrix.org |
| Reuters Health | http://www.reutershealth.com |
| WebMD | http://www.webmd.com |
| DocCheck | http://www.doccheck.com |

**Ref:**

1.  Casali P, Licitra L, Tondini C et al. START: a European state-of-the-art on-line instrument for clinical oncologists. Ann Oncol 1999;10:769–73
2.  Eysenbach G. The impact of the internet on treatment outcomes. CA Cancer J Clin 2003;53:355–71

## 2.1 Cytogenetics and Fluorescence In Situ Hybridization (FISH)

**R. Kunzmann, M. Luebbert**

**Def:** Cytogenetics and fluorescence in situ hybridization (FISH) are methods of detecting clonal chromosomal aberrations in malignant cells → important for primary diagnosis, assessment of progression, therapy, and prognosis of hematological diseases.
The following abnormalities can be distinguished:
- Primary disease-specific abnormalities e.g., t(9;22), ("Philadelphia chromosome," sole chromosomal abnormality in the chronic phase of CML), pathogenetically of causal significance
- Secondary chromosomal abnormalities in connection with genomic instability and clonal evolution (e.g., multiple, unspecific structural aberrations), pathogenetically of no causal significance

**Dg:** **Chromosomal abnormalities in hematologic diseases**

| Disease[1] | Aberration | Prognosis |
|---|---|---|
| *Acute myeloid leukemia (AML):* | | |
| Acute myeloblastic leukemia (M2) | t(8;21) | Good |
| Acute promyelocytic leukemia (M3) | t(15;17) | Good |
| Acute myelomonocytic leukemia with abnormal eosinophils (M4Eo) | inv(16), t(16;16) | Good |
| AML type M4 or M5 | t(11q23;n) | Poor |
| Different subtypes, abnormal thrombopoiesis | inv(3), t(3;3) | Poor |
| Different subtypes, often secondary AML | -5, -7, del(5q), del(7q), del(17p), ≥ 3 anomalies | Poor |
| *Myelodysplastic syndromes (MDS):* | | |
| "Refractory anemia" | del(5q) | Good |
| Different subtypes | -Y, del(20q) | Good |
| Different subtypes | -7, del(7q), t(1;7), ≥ 3 anomalies | Poor |
| *Acute lymphocytic leukemia (ALL):* | | |
| Different subtypes | Hyperdiploid | Good |
| Pre-B-ALL | t(1;19) | Medium risk |
| B-ALL, Burkitt's lymphoma | t(8;14),t(2;8),t(8;22) | Poor |
| Pre-pre-B-ALL | t(4;11) | Poor |
| Mostly c-ALL | t(9;22) | Poor |
| *Immunoproliferative diseases:* | | |
| Multiple myeloma (MM) | del(13)(q14)(17p) | Poor |

[1] See also respective chapters: ALL ▶ 7.1.1, AML ▶ 7.1.2, MDS ▶ 7.2, CLL ▶ 7.5.2, MM ▶ 7.5.10

In principle, the presence of multiple chromosomal abnormalities (≥ 3 aberrations, "complex" anomalies) at the time of primary diagnosis or during the course of a disease constitutes a poor prognosis.

**Meth:**      ## Cytogenetics ("Karyotyping")

### Objective
Detection of numerical and structural chromosome aberrations in malignant cell clones.

### Indications
- *Primary diagnosis* of acute leukemias (AML, ALL), myelodysplastic syndromes (MDS), chronic myeloid leukemia (CML) and other myeloproliferative syndromes (MPS), multiple myeloma (MM), chronic lymphatic leukemia (CLL)
- *Post-therapeutic follow-up* – only if a cytogenetic marker has been identified and other diagnostic methods (morphology, immunocytology, molecular diagnosis with PCR) do not yield clear results
- *Evaluation of prognosis* for AML, MDS, ALL, MM, CLL, CML (see above)
- *Progression* or *transformation* of hematological diseases (e.g., MDS, CML)

### Methods
- Preparation of metaphase cells after establishing primary culture (unstimulated)
- Staining of condensed metaphase chromosomes using Giemsa staining or other methods
- Light microscopic evaluation of chromosomal shape, number and staining (20–30 metaphases per sample)

### Clonality Criteria
- Evidence of an identical structural chromosome abnormality or an additional chromosome in ≥ 2 cells
- Evidence of an identical numeric chromosome abnormality in ≥ 3 cells

### Nomenclature

| Symbol | Definition |
|--------|------------|
| p | Short arm of a chromosome |
| q | Long arm of a chromosome |
| + | Additional chromosome, e.g., "+8" = chromosome 8 trisomy |
| - | Loss of chromosome, e.g., "-7" = chromosome 7 monosomy |
| t | Translocation (interchromosomal exchange of fragments) |
| del | Deletion (loss of chromosome segment) |
| inv | Inversion (intrachromosomal rotation of fragments) |
| der | Structural rearrangement (e.g., unbalanced translocation) |
| i | Isochromosome (duplication of one chromosome arm) |
| dup | Duplication of a chromosome segment |
| mar | Marker chromosome |

### Limitations
- Tests dependent on availability of sufficient cell material (ideally first marrow aspirate) and conditions of sampling and dispatch (sterility) → risk of false-negative results due to insufficient material or < 10 analyzable metaphases
- Even if sufficient material, sensitivity is 1:20 to 1:30 due to limited number of analyzable cells, therefore detection of minimal residual disease (MRD) not possible when < 5% of cells show the cytogenetic marker
- Tests dependent on cell division → a normal karyotype does not rule out abnormal, non-dividing clones
- Submicroscopic structural aberrations non-detectable

- Labor-intensive method (cell isolation and culture, chromosome preparation and staining, interpretation of samples)

## Fluorescence In Situ Hybridization ("FISH")

### Objective
Detection (quantitative) of known numerical or structural abnormalities, especially in follow-up examinations

### Indications
See "Cytogenetics," especially in case of lack of significance of classic cytogenetic methods

### Methods
- Hybridization of fixed nuclei (interphase technique) using one or several chromosome- or gene-specific fluorescence-labeled DNA probes
- Fluorescence microscopic examination of > 100–400 cells

### Advantages Over Classic Cytogenetics
- Detection limit: 100–1,000 cells can be analyzed → higher sensitivity
- Compared with "classic" metaphase cytogenetics, interphase-FISH analysis does not depend on cell division and cell culture variations, hence allowing quantitative conclusions
- Suitable for follow-up tests with established cytogenetic markers
- Lower demands on quality regarding sampling and dispatch
- Conclusions about aberrations in diseases with otherwise unsuccessful karyotyping (e.g., MDS with marrow fibrosis, hypocellular AML)

### Limitations
- Specificity: only known or presumed numerical or structural aberrations which complement the used DNA probe can be detected (not a global test for the detection of all chromosomal aberrations), hence supplementary to chromosome analysis
- Quality of the used DNA probe

**Ref:**
1. Bordeleau L, Berinstein NL. Molecular diagnostics in follicular non-Hodgkin's lymphoma. Semin Oncol 2000;27(6 Suppl 12):42–52
2. Burmeister T, Thiel E. Molecular genetics in acute and chronic leukemias. J Cancer Res Clin Oncol 2001;127:80–90
3. Grimwade D, Walker H, Oliver F et al. The importance of diagnostic cytogenetics on outcome in AML: analysis of 1,612 patients entered into the MRC AML 10 trial. Blood 1998;92:2322–33
4. Harrison CJ. The management of patients with leukaemia: the role of cytogenetics in this molecular era. Br J Hematol 2000;108:19–30
5. Huret JL, Dessen P, LeMinor S et al. The "Atlas of Genetics and Cytogenetics in Oncology and Haematology" on the internet and a review on infant leukemias. Cancer Genet Cytogenet 2000;120:155–9
6. Kristensen TD, Wesenberg F et al. High-resolution comparative genomic hybridisation yields a high detection rate of chromosomal aberrations in childhood acute lymphoblastic leukaemia. Eur J Haematol 2003;70:363–72
7. Mrozek K, Heinonen K, Bloomfield CD. Prognostic value of cytogenetic findings in adults with acute myeloid leukemia. Int J Hematol 2000;72:261–71

**Web:**
1. http://www.ncbi.nlm.nih.gov/Genbank/GenbankOverview.html — NIH gene database
2. http://www.gdb.org/ — Human Genome Database
3. http://atlasgeneticsoncology.org/ — Atlas of Genetics and Cytogenetics
4. http://www.slh.wisc.edu/cytogenetics/index.php — Cancer Cytogenetics
5. http://www.biologia.uniba.it/rmc/ — Molecular Cytogenetics Resources
6. http://www.genenames.org/ — Human Gene Nomenclature

## 2.2    Molecular Diagnosis

### H. Veelken, M. Lübbert

**Def:** Detection and characterization of genetic and epigenetic alterations associated with malignancies. Specific nucleic acid modifications serve as molecular markers for malignant cell clones.

**Ind:**
- Confirmation of diagnosis via detection of tumor-associated molecular markers
- Identification of prognostically relevant subgroups / genotypes within a tumor entity for therapy planning
- Detection of minimal residual disease in the framework of follow-up tests to allow early therapeutic intervention

**Pphys:** **Examples for molecular markers of hematological neoplasias**

| Genetic marker | Disease | Indication | Prognosis |
| --- | --- | --- | --- |
| BCR-ABL, p210 | CML | Diagnosis, follow-up | Very poor |
| | Ph¹-AML | Risk stratification, follow-up | |
| BCR-ABL, p190 | Ph¹-ALL | Risk stratification, follow-up | Very poor |
| PML/RARα | AML M3 | Diagnosis, follow-up | Very good |
| AML1/ETO | AML M2 | Risk stratification, follow-up | Good |
| flt-3mutation | AML | Risk stratification, follow-up | Poor |
| CBFβ/MYH11 | AML M4Eo | Risk stratification, follow-up | Good |
| TEL/AML1 | prae-B-ALL | Risk stratification, follow-up | Good |
| AF4/MLL | pre-pre-B-ALL | Risk stratification, follow-up | Poor |
| E2A/PBX1 | pre-B-ALL | Risk stratification, follow-up | Medium risk |
| Ig/BCL2 | NHL | Diagnosis, follow-up | |
| Antigen receptor gene rearrangements | NHL, ALL | Differentiation of reactive lymphoproliferation, follow-up | |

- For a multitude of tumors, characteristic molecular aberrations have been described. Here, we are only listing marker genes which are clinically relevant and form part of standard diagnostic procedures
- With suspected germline mutations and possibly hereditary malignancies, genetic counseling should always precede decisions about the use of molecular diagnosis
- In routine diagnosis of hematological neoplasias, rearrangements of antigen receptor genes as well as fusion genes which are a result of gene rearrangement following chromosomal translocation are used as valuable molecular markers
- Cytogenetics, FISH, and molecular diagnostics can at present be regarded as complementary procedures, which cannot replace each other
- Gene expression profiles using oligonucleotides or cDNA microarrays allow conclusions about mRNA expression patterns with may be associated with specific malignancies (▶ Chap. 2.3)

**Meth:** Samples: blood (EDTA), bone marrow aspirate (EDTA), fresh or ethanol-fixed biopsy sample.
- Isolation of DNA or RNA (depending on indication and marker)
- RNA-based assays: reverse transcription of RNA into cDNA
- Amplification of DNA or cDNA via polymerase chain reaction (PCR) using specific oligonucleotides (primer)

- Quantitative analysis via "real-time" PCR of the amplification products; semiquantitative analysis via gel electrophoresis (agarose, polyacrylamide)
- In specific cases: analysis of genomic DNA (Southern blot), RNA analysis (Northern blot), ligase chain reaction, and other methods

**Ind:**

### Confirmation of Diagnosis
- CML, myeloproliferative syndromes: BCR/ABL fusion gene
- Malignant lymphoma: clonality of antigen receptor gene rearrangements
- Follicular lymphoma: Ig/BCL2 rearrangement, t(14;18), t(2;18), t(18;22)
- Microgranular variant of acute promyelocytic leukemia (AML M3v): PML/RARα

### AML (Primary Diagnosis): Identification of Prognostically Relevant Subgroups
- AML1/ETO fusion gene, t(8;21)(q22;q22)
- CBFβ/MYH11 fusion gene, inv(16) and t(16;16)(p13;q22)
- PML/RARα fusion gene, t(15;17)(q21;q22) with AML FAB M3
- flt-3 mutations (internal tandem duplication, TK domain) mostly with normal karyo type
- NPM1 mutation (mostly with normal karyo type)

### ALL (Primary Diagnosis): Identification of Prognostically Relevant Subgroups
- BCR/ABL fusion gene, t(9;22)(q34;q11)
- Translocations of the MLL gene, e.g., AF-4/MLL, t(4;11)(q21;q23)
- E2A/PBX fusion gene, t(1;19)(q23;p13)

### Soft Tissue Sarcomas (Primary Diagnosis): Identification of Prognostically Relevant Subgroups
- Ewing's sarcoma/PNET: EWS/FLI1 fusion gene, t(11;22)(q24;q12)
- Clear cell sarcoma: EWS/ATF fusion gene, t(12;22)(q13;12)
- Synovial sarcoma: SYT/SSX fusion gene, t(x;18)(p11;q11)
- Liposarcoma: TLS/CHOP10 fusion gene, t(12;16(q13;p11)
- Alveolar rhabdomyosarcoma: PAX3/FKHR fusion gene, t(2;13(q35;q14)

### Minimal Residual Disease (MRD) (sensitivity up to 1 malignant cell in $10^6$ normal cells)
- CML: BCR/ABL fusion gene (especially in cytogenetic complete response: imatinib or IFNα treatment following allogeneic or autologous hematopoietic transplantation, administration of donor lymphocytes)
- AML: depending on genotype at initial diagnosis (e.g., AML1/ETO, CBFβ/MYH11, PML/RARα)
- ALL: depending on genotype at initial diagnosis (especially with Ph$^1$-ALL, but also after translocations of the MLL gene, E2A/PBX), detection of the clonotypical antigen receptor gene rearrangement
- NHL: depending on genotype at initial diagnosis (e.g., Ig/BCL2), detection of the clonotypical antigen receptor gene rearrangement

### Advantages
- Only small amounts of material required for analysis; no specific fixation necessary
- High sensitivity of PCR-based methods; particularly suitable for the detection of minimal residual disease
- Compared with cytogenetics, no need for proliferating cells

### Disadvantages
- Formalin-fixed samples less suitable due to degradation of nucleic acids
- Analysis of only one molecular marker per assay
- Rigorous quality controls and intricate isolation are necessary measures due to the high sensitivity of PCR-based assays → contamination with foreign material would yield false-positive results

**Ref:**

1. Cassinat B, Zassadowski F, Balitrand N et al. Quantitation of minimal residual disease in acute promyelocytic leukemia patients with t(15;17) translocation using real-time RT–PCR. Leukemia 2000;14:324–8
2. Krauter J, Pascheberg U, Heinze B et al. Detection of karyotypic aberrations in acute myeloblastic leukemia (AML): a prospective comparison between PCR/FISH and standard cytogenetics in 140 patients with de novo AML. Br J Haematol 1998;103:72–8
3. Perez EA, Pusztai L, Van de Vijver M. Improving patient care through molecular diagnostics. Semin Oncol 2004;31(5 Suppl 10):14–20
4. Schoch C, Kohlmann A et al. Acute myeloid leukemias with reciprocal rearrangements can be distinguished by specific gene expressions profiles. Proc Natl Acad Sci U S A 2002;99:10008–13
5. Staudt LM. Molecular diagnosis of the hematologic cancers. N Engl J Med 2003;348:1777–85
6. Varella-Garcia M. Molecular cytogenetics in solid tumors: laboratorial tool for diagnosis, prognosis, and therapy. Oncologist 2003;8:45–58

**Web:**

1. http://jmd.amjpathol.org                    Journal of Molecular Diagnostics
2. http://www.acmg.net/                        American College of Medical Genetics
3. http://www.abgc.net/                        American Board of Genetic Counseling
4. http://www.eshg.org                         European Society of Human Genetics
5. http://www.eurogene.org/index.php           European Genetics Foundation
6. http://genetics.faseb.org/genetics/acmg/stds/g.htm    ACMG Standards and Guidelines

## 2.3  Gene Expression Analysis using Microarrays

J. Scheele, U. Martens

**Def:**  Simultaneous surveying of the expression of numerous defined genes of the human genome using microarray technology (biochips). The human genome consists of approximately 40,000 chromosomal genes.

**Meth:**  *Microarrays*

Hybridization of fluorescence-marked tumor RNA with defined genetic probes on a glass chip.

- The number of probes varies from several hundreds (low-density chips) to several thousands (high-density chips), depending on the chip. Probes consist of PCR-amplified cDNA fragments (100–3,000 base pairs) or oligonucleotides (25–80 base pairs)
- Hybridization of the sample RNA with the cDNA probe is indicated by a fluorescence signal
- Hybridization results (indicating gene expression patterns) are obtained by automated scanning of the microarray chip

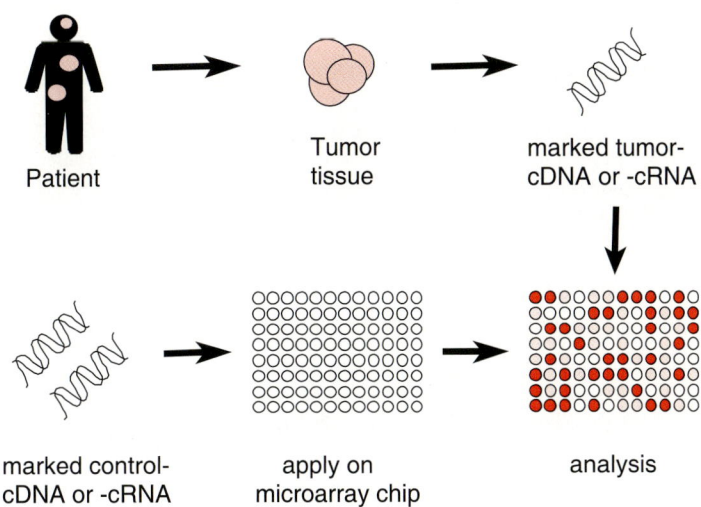

Patient → Tumor tissue → marked tumor-cDNA or -cRNA

marked control-cDNA or -cRNA → apply on microarray chip → analysis

*Data Analysis*

The large amount of data collected (with expression patterns of up to several thousand genes) requires automated evaluation procedures. Analysis of numeric gene expression is carried out using complex mathematical algorithms, e.g. cluster analysis. Cluster analysis results are presented as:

- "Dendrograms (Cluster Trees)": tree-like presentation of gene groups with similar expression patterns (cluster)
- "Heat Maps": colored matrices categorized into clusters that indicate gene expression levels of differentially expressed genes by different shades of color

**Ind:**  Microarray analysis is used mainly within the framework of clinical studies; potential applications in clinical practice are under investigation. Indications:

*Identification of Molecular Mechanisms of Tumor Development (▶ Chap. 1.2)*

Elucidation of genetic contexts in tumor development and progression in experimental model systems. Identification of tumor-specific targets forms the basis for the development of targeted therapies.

### Diagnosis and Prognosis of Malignancies

In addition to conventional diagnostic techniques (e.g., immunohistology and molecular genetic markers), global gene expression analysis allows for advanced classification and prognosis evaluation of human neoplasias. In the future, these findings might have an influence on therapeutic decisions. Clinical studies have proven the importance of genetic profiles ("molecular signature") for:

- Acute leukemias: subtyping and risk classification
- Diffuse large cell B-NHL: subtyping and risk classification
- Breast cancer: risk classification

### Pharmacogenomics

Gene expression analysis permits predictions about the effectiveness and resistance of pharmaceuticals (▶ Chap. 3.8), which could form the basis for future individualized hematological and oncological therapy

- The analysis of 95 genes possibly allows for the prediction of chemosensitivity or chemoresistance of imatinib therapy in Ph+ CML and ALL.

### Advantages of Gene Expression Analysis:

- Large amount of information due to parallel analysis: mapping of the entire transcriptome of a cell population

### Disadvantages:

- High costs of high-density chips
- Large amounts of data necessitating complex bioinformatic analyses
- For the majoity of tumor types, target genes, expression profiles and prognostic significance have not been established

**Ref:**

1. Baak JPA, Path FRC, Hermsen MAJA et al. Genomics and proteomics in cancer. Eur J Cancer 2003;39:1199–215
2. Bullinger L, Döhner K, Bair E et al. Use of gene expression profiling to identify prognostic subclasses in adult acute myeloid leukemia. N Engl J Med 2004;350:1605–16
3. Ebert BL, Golub TR. Genomic approaches to hematologic malignancies. Blood 2004;104:923–32
4. Hubank M. Gene expression profiling and its application in studies of haematological malignancy. Br J Haematol 2004;124:577–94
5. Quackenbush J. Microarray analysis and tumor classification. N Engl J Med 2006; 354:2463–72
6. Ramaswamy S, Ross KN, Lander ES et al. A molecular signature of metastasis in primary solid tumors. Nat Genet 2003;33:49–54
7. Rosenwald AR, Wright G, Chan WC et al. The use of molecular profiling to predict survival after chemotherapy for diffuse large-B-cell lymphoma. N Engl J Med 2002;346:1937–47
8. Van de Vijver MJ, He YD, van't Veer LJ et al. A gene-expression signature as a predictor of survival in breast cancer. N Engl J Med 2002;347:1999–2009

**Web:**

1. http://dc.nci.nih.gov/dc/                                     NCI, Molecular Classification of Cancer
2. http://genome-www5.stanford.edu/                    Stanford Microarray Database
3. http://www.ebi.ac.uk/arrayexpress/                     EBI Transciptional Database
4. http://www.genome.ad.jp/kegg/kegg2.html        KEGG, Biochemical Pathways
5. http://genmapp.org                                              GenMapp, Biochemical Pathways
6. http://affymetrix.com                                           Affymetrix Microarrays

## 2.4 Tumor Markers

**R. Engelhardt, S. Fetscher, F. Otto**

**Def:** Tumor markers are cellular products of malignant tumor tissue, which can be detected in peripheral blood and other body fluids. "Tumor markers" in a narrower sense are soluble antigens, hormones, or enzymes which are produced by solid tumors and can be detected in circulating blood.

**Phys:** *Tumor Products*
- Tumor-associated antigens: AFP, CEA, CA 19-9, CA 15-3, CA 125
- Hormones: gastrin, calcitonin, insulin, βHCG, catecholamines, VIP
- Enzymes: NSE, PSA, LDH
- Serum proteins: immunoglobulins, Bence Jones protein, thyroglobulin

*Tumor-induced Markers*
- Acute phase proteins: ferritin, haptoglobin, $\beta_2$-microglobulin, $\alpha_2$-globulin
- Enzymes: AP, γGT, LDH, GOT, GPT, CK

**Pphys:** Tumor marker serum levels are affected by:
- Tumor parameters: tumor weight, metabolic activity, marker release due to active secretion / necrosis / apoptosis, tumor perfusion / vascularization
- Therapy: effective treatment may cause transient marker release due to oncolysis (DD: tumor progression under therapy), followed by marker level decrease / normalization
- Metabolic parameters: raised levels in connection with renal insufficiency, liver insufficiency, and cholestasis
- Test methods: tumor marker test results can vary depending on the method applied → inconsistent reference values with different tests (esp. with CEA and CA 19-9), limited reproducibility with different methods

**Ind:** Due to low sensitivity and specificity, tumor marker analyses tend to be of limited clinical consequence. Specific indications for their use are therefore required. Usually, tumor markers are:
- *Unsuitable* for screening of asymptomatic patients (except PSA in connection with rectal digital examination and sonography in men over 50 years of age)
- *Unsuitable* for primary tumor diagnosis
- *Unsuitable* for proving malignancy in organ abnormalities (except βHCG detection or high AFP levels in men)
- *Potentially suitable* for assessment of risk groups or symptomatic patients
- *Suitable in individual cases* for prognostic evaluation (CEA in colorectal carcinoma, AFP and βHCG in germ cell tumors, $\beta_2$-microglobulin in multiple myeloma)

Tumor marker analysis is mainly used for *treatment evaluation and follow-up of treated patients* for better or earlier determination of tumor response (relapse, metastasis).
- Increase in tumor markers may be detectable several months before occurrence of clinical symptoms
- Clinically relevant conclusions may be derived from tumor marker kinetics, *not* individual values

*Whether tumor marker analysis is indicated depends on the clinical relevance. For example:*
- AFP and βHCG in germ cell tumors are meaningful due to therapeutic relevance.
- CA 19-9 in metastatic pancreatic carcinoma is of limited value → in palliative situations, the approach is determined primarily by clinical symptoms. Here, tumor marker analysis is not required.

## Tumors and "associated markers"

| Tumor | First-choice markers | Other markers (only indicated in individual cases) |
|---|---|---|
| Bronchial carcinoma | CEA, NSE | CA 15-3, SCC, CYFRA 21-1 |
| Biliary tract carcinoma | CA 19-9 | CEA, CA 125 |
| ENT tumors | CEA | SCC |
| Insulinoma | Insulin | – |
| Carcinoid | HIAA | – |
| Germ cell tumors | AFP, βHCG | NSE |
| Colorectal cancer | CEA | CA 19-9 |
| Hepatic carcinoma | AFP | CEA, CA 19-9, CA 125 |
| Gastric carcinoma | CA 19-9 | CEA, CA 72-4 |
| Breast cancer | CA 15-3 | CEA, CA 125 |
| Esophageal cancer | CEA | SCC |
| Ovarian cancer | CA 125 | CEA, CA 15-3, CA 19-9 |
| Pancreatic carcinoma | CA 19-9 | CEA, CA 125 |
| Pheochromocytoma | Catecholamines | Vanillylmandelic acid |
| Plasmocytoma | Immunoglobulins | β2-MG |
| Prostate cancer | PSA | PAP |
| Thyroid carcinoma | TG, calcitonin | CEA, NSE |

### *Recommended Time Points for Tumor Marker Analysis*
- Preoperatively
- Postoperatively: 2–10 days after surgery, then every 3 months, from third year on: every 6 months
- Before changing treatment
- In case of clinically suspected relapse or metastasis, or before continuing treatment of tumors that cannot be measured with imaging techniques
- Restaging
- 14–30 days after first detection of increased tumor marker levels

**Ref:**

1. Brawer MK. Prostate-specific antigen: current status. CA Cancer J Clin 1999;49:264–81
2. Gion M, Mione R, Barioli P et al. Dynamic use of tumor markers: rationale, clinical applications and pitfalls. Anticancer Res 1996;16:2279–84
3. Locker GY, Hamilton S, Harris J et al. ASCO 2006 Update of recommendations for the use of tumor markers in gastrointestinal cancer. J Clin Oncol 2006;24:5313–27
4. Rapkiewicz AV, Espina V, Petricoin EF et al. Biomarkers of ovarian tumours. Eur J Cancer 2004;40:2604–12
5. Scher HI, Eisenberger M, D'Amico AV et al. Eligibility and outcomes reporting guidelines for clinical trials for patients in the state of a rising prostate-specific antigen. Recommendations from the PSA Working Group. J Clin Oncol 2004;22:537–56
6. Sölétormos G, Nielsen D, Schioler V et al. Monitoring different stages of breast cancer using tumour markers CA 15-3, CEA and TPA. Eur J Cancer 2004;40:481–6

**Web:**

1. http://www.asco.org              ASCO Tumor Marker Guidelines
2. http://oncolink.upenn.edu/        Oncolink, Tumor Marker Fact Sheet
3. http://cancernet.nci.nih.org/     Tumor Marker Fact Sheets

**Tumor markers**

| Markers | Characterization Physiological occurrence | Normal value[a] | Serum-t½ | Increase in tumor type (sensitivity) | False-positive results with disease (specificity) |
|---|---|---|---|---|---|
| AFP | α₁-fetoprotein, Endodermal sinus, fetal liver | < 15 ng/ml | 3–6 days | Hepatocellular carcinoma (90%), germ cell tumors (50–80%), endodermal sinus tumors (100%) | Liver necrosis (80%), hepatitis (60%), cirrhosis (20%), pregnancy, spina bifida |
| βHCG | Human chorionic gonadotropin β Trophoblastic structures | ♂ < 5 U/l | 18–24 h | Nonseminomatous germ cell tumors (50–85%), choriocarcinoma (100%), hydatidiform mole (97%) | Pregnancy (100%) |
| β₂-MG | β₂-microglobulin Lymphocytes, macrophages | 1.2–2.5 mg/l | – | Multiple myeloma (70%), non-Hodgkin's lymphoma | Renal diseases with defective glomerular filtration |
| Calcitonin | Calcitonin Thyroid C cells | < 300 ng/l | 12 min | Medullary thyroid carcinoma | C-cell hyperplasia |
| CA125 | Cancer antigen 125 Ovarian and bronchial epithelia | < 65 U/ml | 4–5 days | Serous ovarian carcinoma (90%), lung cancer, colon carcinoma, breast cancer | Pregnancy, menstruation, benign diseases of the ovary, liver and pancreas, peritonitis |
| CA 15-3 | Cancer antigen 15-3 Epithelia | < 28 U/ml | 10–14 days | Breast cancer (30–60%) | Mastopathy, hepatic cirrhosis |
| CA 19-9 | Cancer antigen 19-9 Fetal gastrointestinal epithelium | < 37 U/ml | – | Pancreatic (75–85%), gastric (40–60%), colorectal (25–50%), hepatocellular carcinoma (40%) | Cholecystitis (50%), cholestasis, pancreatitis (30%), hepatitis (25%), cirrhosis (20%), colitis |
| CA 72-4 | Cancer antigen 72-4 Epithelia | < 4 U/ml | – | Gastric cancer (50%), ovarian carcinoma (60–70%) | Benign gastrointestinal diseases |
| CEA | Carcinoembryonic antigen Embryonic intestinal mucosa, pancreas and liver | < 5 ng/ml | 14–21 days | Colorectal cancer (50–80%), pancreatic arcinoma (55–60%), gastric cancer (45%), breast cancer (35–55%), lung cancer (30–50%) | Hepatic cirrhosis (30%), diseases of the intestine, liver, pancreas and lungs, hemodialysis (30%), smokers (3%) |
| CYFRA 21-1 | Pulmonary squamous epithelium | < 4 U/ml | – | Squamous cell lung cancer (60–80%) | Specificity 90% |

[a] Dependent on method used

**Tumor markers** *(continued)*

| Markers | Characterization Physiological occurrence | Normal value[a] | Serum-t½ | Increase in tumor type (sensitivity) | False-positive results with disease (specificity) |
|---|---|---|---|---|---|
| HIAA | 5-OH indole acetic acid | < 9 mg in 24-h urine collection | – | Carcinoid tumor | – |
| Ig | Immunoglobulins B-cells | – | – | Multiple myeloma, lymphomas, CLL | Chronic inflammatory reactions |
| Insulin | Insulin Pancreas | < 150 mU/l | – | Insulinoma | – |
| NSE | Neuron-specific enolase Neuroendocrine / neuronal cells, erythrocytes, thrombocytes | < 25 ng/ml | 12–14 days | Small cell lung cancer (80%), neuroblastoma (85%), APUDomas (35%), metastatic seminoma (70%) | Benign pulmonary diseases, pneumonia (35%), hemolysis |
| PSA | Prostate-specific antigen Prostatic ducts | < 3.7 ng/ml | 2–3 days | Prostatic cancer (90%) | Prostatic hypertrophy (65%), prostatitis, prostatic massage |
| PTH | Parathormone Parathyroid gland | < 55 ng/l | – | Parathyroid tumors | Secondary hyperparathyroidism |
| SCC | Squamous cell carcinoma antigen Squamous epithelia | < 2.5 ng/ml | – | Cervical carcinoma (85%), head and neck tumors (60%) | Hepatobiliary abnormalities, terminal renal insufficiency |
| TG | Thyroglobulin Thyroid gland | < 50 mg/l | > 14 days | Differentiated thyroid carcinoma | Benign thyroid diseases |
| TPA | Tissue polypeptide antigen Epithelia | < 120 U/l | 2–3 days | Bladder carcinoma (80–100%), epithelial tumors | Benign diseases of the liver, lungs, and urogenital tract |
| VMS | Catecholamines / vanillylmandelic acid | – | – | Pheochromocytoma, sympathetic neuroblastoma | – |

[a] Dependent on method used

## 2.5    CD Antigens and Immunocytological Diagnosis

### D. Behringer, E. Jüttner, J. Burger, M. Burger

**Def:**    *CD Antigens*

Surface antigens which have been designated "clusters of differentiation" (CD). International workshops periodically update the systematization of antigens on hematological cells and antibodies suitable for their detection. The objective is to group antibodies which recognize the same antigen into clusters, thereby providing an essential classification for diagnostic and therapeutic purposes. So far, a total of 350 cell surface antigens are classified in the CD nomenclature. The function of some of the identified antigens is not known. CD classification forms the basis of immunocytological diagnosis.

*Immunocytology*

Identification of membrane and intracytoplasmic molecules (antigens) on and in different cell types using specific antibodies.

**Ind:**    Besides cytology and cytochemistry, immunocytology is an established complementary method in the diagnosis of leukemias and lymphomas. Immunocytology information is incorporated in the REAL and WHO classifications of lymphomas (► Chap. 7.5) and in the French-American-British Group (FAB) classification of leukemias (► Chap. 7.1). Interpretation of immunocytological findings is based on the knowledge of the antigen expression patterns of normal cells.

*Indications*
- Acute leukemias: essential for primary diagnosis; follow-up only with "informative phenotype" (i.e., if the immunocytological findings contribute to the diagnosis)
- Lymphomas: non-Hodgkin's lymphomas, hairy cell leukemia, plasmacytoma
- Myeloproliferative syndromes (MPS)/myelodysplastic syndromes (MDS): characterization of blasts in the development of acute leukemia
- Organ infiltration by epithelial tumor cells: detection of cytokeratin-positive cells. The prognostic value of "minimal tumor infiltration" (TNM stage M(i)) of the bone marrow is under debate
- Cellular immune defect constellations
- Quantification of hematopoietic progenitor cells (CD34$^+$)
- Paroxysmal nocturnal hemoglobinuria (PNH)

**Meth:**    *Suitable Samples*
- Peripheral blood (e.g., in EDTA)
- Lymph node aspirate or biopsy (in 0.9% saline, room temperature)
- Bone marrow aspirate (e.g., in 0.25% EDTA, 0.9% saline)
- Body fluids (at least 50 ml, in EDTA tubes)
- Liquor (at least 5 ml, in plain sterile tube)
- Other aspirates, e.g., from skin (in 0.9% saline, with EDTA)

*Immunocytological Analysis*
- Quality / informative value of the analysis greatly depends on the promptness of sample processing → transportation of samples immediately after collection. Generally, samples have to be processed within 24 h.
- Immunocytological analysis is usually carried out with fluorochrome-labeled antibodies and a flow cytometer. Availability of a limited number of cells (e.g., liquor, lymph nodes, organ aspirates, detection of epithelial cells in tissues) requires immunocytological staining of single cells on a slide.
- Immunocytological methods (use of unfixed cells) can make use of a larger antibody panel than immunohistochemistry (use of formalin-fixed cells, paraffin embedding).

**Dg:**    For an appropriate interpretation of immunocytology additional diagnostic test results and the clinical picture generally have to be taken into account.

### Acute Leukemias

#### Objectives of Immunophenotyping of Acute Leukemias

Acute leukemias are classified according to the recommendations of the European Group for the Immunophenotyping of Leukemias (EGIL).

- Classification: myeloid versus lymphatic, subgroups of AML and ALL (▶ Chap. 7.1)
- Definition of prognostically relevant subtypes, especially in B-lymphatic leukemia, less established in AML
- Follow-up for the detection of residual leukemia cells (minimal residual disease, no routine test as yet)

#### Classification of acute lymphatic leukemias

| Type | | Criteria |
|---|---|---|
| B-lymphocytic[a] | | ≥ 2 positive markers: CD19+, CD79a+, CD22+ |
| Pro-B-ALL | B-I | No other positive B-cell markers |
| Common ALL (c-ALL) | B-II | In addition: CD10+ |
| Pre-B-ALL | B-III | In addition: cytoplasmic IgM+ |
| Mature B-ALL | B-IV | Cytoplasmic / membranous, kappa+ or lambda+ |
| T-lymphocytic[b] | | Cytoplasmic or membranous CD3+ |
| Pro-T-ALL | T-I | CD7+ |
| Pre-T-ALL | T-II | CD2+ / CD5+ / CD8+ |
| Cortical T-ALL | T-III | CD1a+ |
| Mature T-ALL | T-IV | Membranous CD3+ and CD1a- |
| α/β T-ALL | T-IVa | TCRα/β |
| γ/δ T-ALL | T-IVb | TCRγ/δ |
| ALL with myeloid markers | My+ ALL | Coexpression of 1–2 myeloid markers; however, no sufficient criteria for biphenotypic acute leukemia |

[a] Usually TdT+ (except B-IV)
[b] Usually TdT+, HLA-DR-, and CD34-

#### Classification of acute myeloid leukemias

| Type | FAB | | Criteria |
|---|---|---|---|
| Myelomonocytic | – | – | ≥ 2 positive markers: myeloperoxidase, CD13, CD33, CD65, CD117 |
| Erythocytic, immature | – | M6 | Immunophenotypically non-classifiable |
| Erythrocytic, mature | – | M6 | Glycophorin A positive |
| Megakaryocytic | – | M7 | CD41+ and/or mCD61+ / cyCD61+ |
| Poorly differentiated AML | M0-AML | M0 | Peroxidase / esterase / CD3 / CD79a / CD22 negative |
| TdT-positive AML | Tdt+ AML | – | TdT+ |
| AML with lymphatic markers | AML | – | Coexpression of 1–2 lymphatic markers; no criteria for biphenotypic acute leukemia |

**Biphenotypic acute leukemias (BAL)**

| Points | B-cells | T-cells | Myeloid cells |
|---|---|---|---|
| 2 | CD79a, cyIgM, cyCD22 | mCD3, cyCD3, TCRα/β, TCRγ/δ | Myeloperoxidase, (lyso-zyme) |
| 1 | CD10, CD19, CD20 | CD2, CD5, CD8, CD10 | CD13, CD33, CD65 |
| 0.5 | TdT, CD24 | TdT, CD7, CD1a | CD14, CD15, CD64, CD117 |

BAL is defined as > 2 points for myeloid cells and > 1 point for lymphatic cells. Each positive marker results in corresponding points

### Undifferentiated Acute Leukemias

Rare subgroup of acute leukemias which cannot be further classified using the above mentioned criteria. Usually CD34+, HLA-DR+, CD38+, and CD7+.

## Leukemic Lymphomas

Neoplastic lymphocytes and secondary (reactive) lymphatic proliferation are distinguished by:
- Detection of monoclonality (kappa or lambda light chain restriction)
- Overexpression or absence of markers (mature T-cell leukemias)

Diagnosis of a specific disease / lymphoma is only possible in conjunction with the morphology and the clinical constellation. However, preliminary data with an immunophenotypic grading system have shown that particularly for distinguishing CLL from other leukemic B-cell lymphomas, immunophenotypic classification is highly consistent with the clinical diagnosis.

**Classification of leukemic B-cell lymphomas**

| Antigen | Diagnosis | | | | | | | |
|---|---|---|---|---|---|---|---|---|
| | CLL | PLL | HCL | FL | MCL | LPIC | SLVL | PCL |
| CD5 | +++ | + w | − | − | +++ | − | + | − |
| CD10 | − | − | − | ++ | − | − | + | − |
| CD11c | ++ w | + | +++ s | − | − | + | + | − |
| CD19 | +++ | +++ | +++ | +++ | +++ | +++ | +++ | − |
| CD20 | +++ | +++ | +++ | +++ | +++ | +++ | − | − |
| CD23 | +++ | + | − | + | − | + | + | − |
| CD38 | − | − | + w | + w | − | ++ | + | +++ s |
| CD103 | − | − | +++ s | − | − | − | + | − |
| FMC7 | + w | +++ | +++ | +++ | +++ | + | +++ | − |

*CLL* chronic lymphatic leukemia, *PLL* prolymphocytic leukemia, *HCL* hairy cell leukemia, *FL* follicular lymphoma, *MCL* mantle cell lymphoma, *LPIC* lymphoplasmacytoid immunocytoma, *SLVL* splenic lymphoma with villous lymphocytes, *PCL* plasma cell leukemia, − no antigen expression, + antigen expression in < 50% of cases, ++ antigen expression in > 50% of cases, +++ full antigen expression, *w* weak antigen expression, *s* strong antigen expression

**Classification of leukemic T-cell lymphomas**

| Antigen | Diagnosis | | | |
|---------|-----------|---|---|---|
|         | T-PLL | SS / MF | LGLL | Adult TCL |
| TdT    | –   | –   | –   | –   |
| CD1a   | –   | –   | –   | –   |
| CD2    | +++ | +++ | +++ | +++ |
| CD3    | +++ | +++ | +++ | +++ |
| CD4    | +   | +++ | +   | +++ |
| CD5    | +++ | +++ | +++ | +++ |
| CD7    | +++ | –   | +   | +   |
| CD8    | +   | –   | ++  | –   |
| CD25   | –   | –   | –   | +++ |
| CD56   | –   | –   | ++  | –   |
| CD57   | –   | –   | ++  | –   |
| HLA-DR | –   | –   | –   | +   |

*T-PLL* T-prolymphocytic leukemia, *SS / MF* Sézary's syndrome / mycosis fungoides, *LGLL* large granular lymphocyte leukemia, *TCL* T-cell leukemia, – no antigen expression, + antigen expression in < 50% of cases, ++ antigen expression in > 50% of cases, +++ full antigen expression, *w* weak antigen expression, *s* strong antigen expression

**CD antigens and non-classified antigens**

|         | Antigen | Normal cellular reactivity | Comments |
|---------|---------|---------------------------|----------|
| CD1  | Gp49 | Thymocytes, DC, B (sub) | Immature T-cell marker |
| CD2  | Gp50, LFA-3 ligand | T, NK (sub) | T-cell marker |
| CD3  | T-cell receptor associated | T | T-cell marker |
| CD4  | MHC class II receptor, HIV receptor | T (sub), mono, myeloid precursor | Helper T-lymphocytes |
| CD5  | | T, B (sub) | T-cell marker, typical for B-CLL |
| CD7  | 40 kDa protein | T, NK, myeloid precursor (sub) | |
| CD8  | MHC class I receptor (gp32) | T (sub), NK (sub) | Cytotoxic or suppressor T-cells |
| CD9  | P24 | Mono, thrombocytes, pre-B | |
| CD10 | Gp100, common acute leukemia antigen (CALLA) | B- and T-precursors, neutrophils | Typical c-ALL marker |
| CD11b | Gp155/95, C3bi receptor | Mono, macrophages, neutrophils, NK | |

*B* B-lymphocytes, *DC* dendritic cells, *Mono* monocytes, *NK* natural killer cells, *Sub* subpopulation, *T* T-lymphocytes

**CD antigens and non-classified antigens** *(continued)*

| | Antigen | Normal cellular reactivity | Comments |
|---|---|---|---|
| CD11c | Gp150/95, adhesion molecule | Mono, neutrophils, NK, B (sub) | Strongly expressed in hairy cell leukemia |
| CD13 | Aminopeptidase N | Mono, neutrophils | Myeloid marker |
| CD14 | Gp55 | Mono, (neutrophils) | LPS receptor, monocyte marker |
| CD15 | X hapten | Neutrophils, (mono) | Myeloid marker |
| CD16 | FcγRIII, gp50-65 | NK, neutrophils, mono (sub) | |
| CD19 | Gp95 | B | B-cell marker |
| CD20 | p37/32 | Mature B | Mature B-cell marker |
| CD21 | C3d/EBV receptor | B (sub) | |
| CD22 | Gp135 | B | B-cell marker |
| CD23 | FcγRII, low-affinity IgE receptor | B (sub) | B-CLL marker |
| CD24 | Gp41/38 | B, T (activated), neutrophils | |
| CD25 | IL-2 receptor (α chain) | T (activated), B (activated) | |
| CD30 | Ki-1 | T | Hodgkin's cells and Ki-1 NHL |
| CD33 | 67 kDa glycoprotein | Mono, progenitor cells, neutrophils | Myeloid marker |
| CD34 | 105–120 kDa glycoprotein | Myeloid / lymphatic progenitors | stem cell marker |
| CD38 | 45 kDa protein | T / B (activated), B (sub), plasma cells | |
| CD40 | Gp50 | B | |
| CD41 | GPIIb/IIIa, GPIIb | Thrombocytes | |
| CD43 | Leukosialin, gp95 | T, neutrophils | |
| CD44 | Pgp-1, gp 80-95 | T, neutrophils, erythrocytes | |
| CD45 | Leukocyte common antigen | Leukocytes | Leukocyte marker |
| CD54 | Intercellular adhesion molecule | Activated cells | |
| CD55 | Decay accelerating factor | Various cell types | May be absent in PNH |
| CD56 | Gp220/135, isoform of NCAM | NK, activated lymphocytes | |
| CD57 | HNK1 | NK, T, B (sub) | |
| CD59 | Prolectin | Various cell types | |
| CD61 | Integrin β3, Thr GPIIIa | Thrombocytes | |

*B* B-lymphocytes, *DC* dendritic cells, *Mono* monocytes, *NK* natural killer cells, *Sub* subpopulation, *T* T-lymphocytes

**CD antigens and non-classified antigens** (*continued*)

| | Antigen | Normal cellular reactivity | Comments |
|---|---|---|---|
| CD64 | FcγRI, gp75 | Mono | |
| CD65 | Ceramide dodecasaccharide | Neutrophils, (mono) | Line-specific myeloid marker |
| CD68 | Gp110 | Macrophages | |
| CD69 | Gp32/28 | Activated B, activated T | |
| CD71 | Gp110 | Proliferating cells, macrophages | |
| CD79a | Ig-α/Mb-1, part of B-cell receptor | B (immature, cytoplasmic) | B-cell marker |
| CD79b | Part of B-cell receptor | B (mature) | B-cell marker |
| CD103 | Receptor for E-cadherin (HML-1) | Lymphocytes, B (sub), activated T | Characteristic of hairy cell leukemia |
| CD117 | c-kit, stem cell factor receptor | Myeloid precursor | |
| CD138 | Syndecan-1 | Plasma cells, epithelial cells | Plasma cell marker |
| FMC-7 | 105 kDa glycoprotein | B (mature) | |
| HLA-DR | Part of MHC-II complex | B, activated T, mono, precursor | |
| Glycophorin A | Sialinic acid-rich polypeptide | Erythrocytes, proerythroblasts | Erythroid marker |
| Lactoferrin | Lactoferrin | Granulocytes, mature myeloid cells | Marker for mature myeloid cells |
| Myeloperoxidase | Myeloperoxidase | Neutrophils, (mono), cytoplasmic | Myeloid marker |
| Lysozyme | Lysozyme | Mono, cytoplasmic only | Monocytic marker |
| TdT | Terminal deoxynucleotidyl transferase | Lymphoid T- and B-precursor | |
| TCRα/β | α/β chains of the T-cell receptor | 95% of all T | |
| TCRγ/δ | γ/δ chains of the T-cell receptor | 5% of all T | |
| Kappa | Ig light chain type kappa | B (sub, membranous) | |
| Lambda | Ig light chain type lambda | B (sub, membranous) | |
| Ig μ chain | IgM heavy chain | B | |
| Cytokeratin | | Epithelial cells | Cytoplasmic epithelial cell marker |
| HEA | Human epithelial antigen | Epithelial cells | Membrane-bound epithelial marker |

*B* B-lymphocytes, *DC* dendritic cells, *Mono* monocytes, *NK* natural killer cells, *Sub* subpopulation, *T* T-lymphocytes

**Classification of B-cell lymphomas: immunocytology by REAL / WHO**

| Real / WHO, Kiel | B-cell antigens: CD | | | | T-cell antigens: CD | | | | | | sIg | cIg | Other, cytogenetics |
|---|---|---|---|---|---|---|---|---|---|---|---|---|---|
| | 19 | 20 | 79a | 22 | 5 | 10 | 11c | 23 | 43 | 103 | | | |
| Mature B-cells | +++ | +++ | +++ | +++ | | | | | | | +++ | | CD45+++, HLA-DR+++, FMC7+++ |
| Plasma cells | | | | | | | | | | | | +++ | CD38++, CD138+++, CD45+ |
| B-LBL, B-lympho-blastic | +++ | + | +++ | +++ | | +++ | | | | | - | | TdT+++, HLA-DR+++, cMu+, CD34++, IgH / IgL / TCR rearrangement |
| B-CLL, B-SLL, lymphoplasmacytoid immunocytoma B-PLL | +++ | +++ | +++ | +++ | +++ (-) | - | + | +++ | +++ | | M+++ D++ | + | FMC7, +12 (30%), 13q- (25%), IgH / IgL rearrangement, t(11;14) |
| Lymphoplasma-cytoid lymphoma, immunocytoma, Lymphoplasmacy-toid immunocytoma | +++ | +++ | +++ | +++ | - | - | | + | ++ | | M+++ D- | M+++ D- | IgH / IgL rearrangement |
| Mantle cell lym-phoma, centrocytic | +++ | +++ | +++ | +++ | +++ | + | - | - | +++ | | M+++ D+++ | | Ig lambda>kappa, FDZ t(11;14) |
| Follicle center lym-phoma (I,II,III) Follicular lym-phoma, cb cc | +++ | +++ | +++ | +++ | | ++ | - | + | - | | M++ D>G | | FDZ, B-cell associated antigen t(14;18) (70–95%) |
| Marginal zone B-cell lymphoma, extranodal (MALT), nodal, monocytoid, immunocytoma | +++ | +++ | +++ | +++ | - | - | ++ | - | + | | M>G, D- | ++ | Trisomy 3, t(11;18) |

*B-LBL* precursor B-lymphoblastic leukemia / lymphoma, *B-CLL* B-cell chronic lymphocytic leukemia, *B-SLL* small lymphocytic lymphoma, *B-PLL* prolymphocytic leukemia, *cc* centro-blastic centrocytic, *cb* centroblastic, *VL* villous lymphocytes, *B-ib* B-immunoblastic, *cb* centroblastic, *FDZ* follicular dendritic cells, +++ positive in > 90% of cases, ++ positive in > 50% of cases, + positive in < 50% of cases, - positive in < 10% of cases, ( ) = rare cases, *Ig* immunoglobulins (A, M, D, G immunoglobulin classes), red characteristics important for definition or differential diagnosis

**Classification of B-cell lymphomas: immunocytology by REAL / WHO (continued)**

| Real / WHO, Kiel | B-cell antigens: CD | | | | T-cell antigens: CD | | | | | | sIg | cIg | Other, cytogenetics |
|---|---|---|---|---|---|---|---|---|---|---|---|---|---|
| | 19 | 20 | 79a | 22 | 5 | 10 | 11c | 23 | 43 | 103 | | | |
| Splenic marginal zone lymphoma ± VL | ++ | +++ | +++ | +++ | - | - | + | - | + | | M>G, D- | ++ | No trisomy 3 |
| Hairy cell leukemia | ++ | +++ | +++ | +++ | - | - | +++ | - | | +++ | +++ | | CD25+++, FMC7+++ IgH / IgL rearrangement |
| Plasmacytoma, plasma cell myeloma | - | - | ++ | - | | | | | ++ | | - | +++ | CD45+, HLA-DR+, CD38+++, EMA+, CD56++, IgH / IgL rearrangement |
| Diffuse large B-cell lymphoma cb; B-ib; large-cell, anaplastic | +++ | +++ | +++ | +++ | + | + | | | | | ++ | + | CD45+ bcl-2 rearrangement (20–30%) |
| Large BL subtype: primary mediastinal | +++ | +++ | +++ | +++ | | | | | | | - | - | CD45+, CD30+, CD15- IgH, IgL rearrangement |
| Burkitt's lymphoma | +++ | +++ | +++ | +++ | - | +++ | | | | | M+++ | | CD77+++, t(8;14), t(2;8), t(8;22) bcl-2 rearrangement (30%) |
| High-grade BL, Burkitt-like lymphoma | +++ | +++ | +++ | +++ | - | - | | | | | + | | |

*B-LBL* precursor B-lymphoblastic leukemia / lymphoma, *B-CLL* B-cell chronic lymphocytic leukemia, *B-SLL* small lymphocytic lymphoma, *B-PLL* prolymphocytic leukemia, *cb cc* centroblastic centrocytic, *VL* villous lymphocytes, *cb* centroblastic, *B-ib* B-immunoblastic, *FDZ* follicular dendritic cells, ( ) = rare cases, - positive in < 10% of cases, + positive in < 50% of cases, ++ positive in > 50% of cases, +++ positive in > 90% of cases, *Ig* immunoglobulins (A, M, D, G immunoglobulin classes), red characteristics important for definition or differential diagnosis

**Classification of T-cell lymphomas: immunocytology by REAL / WHO**

| Real / WHO, Kiel | T-cell antigens: CD | | | | | | | | | | TdT | B-cell | Other, cytogenetics |
|---|---|---|---|---|---|---|---|---|---|---|---|---|---|
| | 1a | 2 | 3 | 4 / 8 | 5 | 7 | 16 | 25 | 56 | 57 | | | |
| Mature T-cells | - | +++ | +++ | +++ | +++ | +++ | | | | | - | | |
| T-LBL, T-lymphoblastic | ++ | var | +++ | +++ / - | var | +++ | +++ | | | +++ | ++ | - | Ig-, TCR rearrangement var., (IgH rearrangement) |
| T-CLL / T-PLL | - | +++ | +++ | +++ | +++ | +++ | | (-) | | | | | inv14(q11;q32) (75%), trisomy 8q |
| LGL leukemia, T-cell type, T-CLL NK cell type | | +++ / +++ | +++ / - | 4- / 8++ | - | - | +++ / +++ | - | - / ++ | ++ / ++ | | | TCRαβ+++, TCR- rearrangement / TCRβ-, germ cell lineage |
| Mycosis fungoides / Sézary syndrome | +++ | +++ | +++ | 4+++ (8+) | +++ | + | | | | | | | S-100+++, Langerhans cells, TCR rearrangement |
| Peripheral T-cell lymphomas, unspecified T-zone lymphoma, lymphoepitheloid, pleomorphic small-, medium-, large-cell, T-ib | | ++ | ++ | 4>8, (-) | ++ | + | | | | | | - | Common TCR rearrangement |
| Angioimmunoblastic lymphoma | | | | 4+++ | | | | | | | | | FDZ, TCR associated antigens +, TCR (75%) / IgH (10%) rearrangement, EBV +, rare trisomy 3 / 5 |
| Angiocentric lymphoma | | +++ | - | +++ | ++ | ++ | | | +++ | | | | EBV+ Ig rearrangement in pulmonary cases |

*T LBL* precursor T-lymphoblastic leukemia / lymphoma, *T-CLL* T-cell chronic lymphocytic leukemia, *T-PLL* T-cell prolymphocytic leukemia, *LGL* large granular lymphocyte, *T-ib* T-immunoblastic, *TCR* T-cell receptor, *FDZ* follicular dendritic cells, *var* variable, +++ positive in > 90% of cases, ++ positive in > 50% of cases, + positive in > 50% of cases, - positive in < 50% of cases, - positive in < 10% of cases, ( ) = rare cases, red characteristics important for definition or differential diagnosis

**Classification of T-cell lymphomas: immunocytology by REAL / WHO (continued)**

| Real / WHO, Kiel | T-cell antigens: CD | | | | | | | | | | TdT | B-cell | Other, cytogenetics |
|---|---|---|---|---|---|---|---|---|---|---|---|---|---|
| | 1a | 2 | 3 | 4 / 8 | 5 | 7 | 16 | 25 | 56 | 57 | | | |
| Intestinal T-cell lymphoma (± enteropathy) | | | +++ | 4- 8++ | | +++ | | | | | | | CD103+++, TCRβ rearrangement |
| Adult T-cell lymphoma/ leukemia Pleomorphic small-, medium-, large-cell, HTLV+ | | +++ | +++ | 4+++ 8+ | +++ | - | | +++ | | | | | TCR rearrangement, Integrated HTLV1 |
| Anaplastic large cell lymphoma (T-/null cell types) Large cell anaplastic (Ki-1) T-cell lymphoma | | var | + | | var | var | | ++ | | | | | CD30+++, EMA++, CD15+, CD43+, CD45++, CD68-, t(2;5), TCR rearrangement (~50%) |

*T LBL* precursor T-lymphoblastic leukemia / lymphoma, *T-CLL* T-cell chronic lymphocytic leukemia, *T-PLL* T-cell prolymphocytic leukemia, *LGL* large granular lymphocyte, *T-ib* T-immunoblastic, *TCR* T-cell receptor, *FDZ* follicular dendritic cells, *var* variable, +++ positive in > 90% of cases, ++ positive in > 50% of cases, + positive in < 50% of cases, - positive in < 10% of cases, ( ) = rare cases, red characteristics important for definition or differential diagnosis

**Ref:**

1. Bene M, Castoldi G, Knapp W et al. Proposals for the immunological classification of acute leukemias. Leukemia 1995;9:1783–6
2. Bennett J, Catovskz D, Daniel M et al. Proposed revised criteria for the classification of acute myeloid leukemias. Ann Intern Med 1985;103:626–9
3. Cheson B, Cassileth P, Head D et al. Report of the National Cancer Institute-sponsored workshop on definitions of diagnosis and response in acute myeloid leukemia. J Clin Oncol 1990;8:813–9
4. Gratama JW, Sutherland DR, Keeney M. Flow cytometric enumeration and immunophenotyping of hematopoietic stem and progenitor cells. Semin Hematol 2001;38:139–47
5. Harris NL, Jaffe E, Stein H et al. A Revised European-American Classification of lymphoid neoplasms: a proposal from the International Lymphoma Study Group. Blood 1994;84:1361–92
6. Harris NL, Jaffe ES, Diebold J et al. World Health Organization classification of neoplastic diseases of the hematopoietic and lymphoid tissues: report of the Advisory Committee meeting, Airlie House, Virginia, November 1997. J Clin Oncol 1999;17:3835–49
7. Mason D et al (eds). Leucocyte Typing VII. Oxford University Press, 2001
8. Stetler-Stevenson M, Braylan RC. Flow cytometric analysis of lymphomas and lymphoproliferative disorders. Semin Hematol 2001;38:111–23
9. Vardiman J, Harris NL, Brunning RD; the World Health Organization (WHO) classification of the myeloid neoplasms. Blood 2002;100:2292–2302
10. Zola H, Swart B, Nicholson I et al. CD molecules 2005: Human cell differentiation molecules. Blood 2005;106:3123–3126

**Web:**

1. http://image.bloodline.net/               Picture Atlas, Bloodline
2. http://www.hlda8.org                       HLDA Workshop
3. http://mpr.nci.nih.quv/prow               Flow Cytometry Database

## 2.6        HLA System and MHC

### C. Grüllich, L. Houet, J. Finke

**Def:**        MHC = Major Histocompatibility Complex
HLA System = Human Leukocyte Antigen System, human MHC

**Class:**        The MHC is an array of highly polymorphic genes whose products (polymorphic membrane glycoproteins) are expressed on a multitude of cells. These are important for the immunological distinction of self (endogenous) and non-self (exogenous). The HLA system, the human MHC, is
located on the short arm of chromosome 6 (region 6p21.31) and comprises approximately 200
genes divided into three classes. More than 40 genes of class I and class II encode for the classic
histocompatibility antigens.

**Structure of MHC antigens**

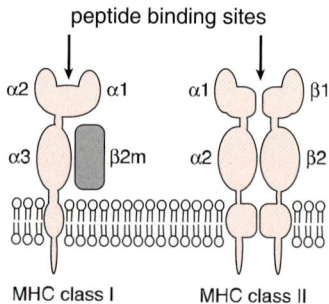

### HLA Class I Antigens (MHC Class I)
- *Classic types:* HLA-A, -B, -C (serologically defined)
- *Others:* HLA-E (T-lymphocytes), HLA-F, HLA-G (extravillous trophoblasts), HLA-H, HLA-J
  (unknown function)
- *Expression:* nucleated cells, especially cell types holding immunological function. Low expression on endocrine and mesenchymal cells (fibroblasts, neurons, myocytes). No expression on
  sperm cells and placental trophoblasts
- *Structure:* heavy α-chain (44 kDa), non-covalently attached to β2-microglobulin. Three extracellular domains, a transmembranous region, and an intracellular component. The two outer
  domains of the α-chain are binding sites for specific antigens (peptides of 8–10 amino acids)

### HLA Class II Antigens (MHC Class II)
- *Classic types:* HLA-DR, -DQ, -DP
- *Others:* HLA-DM, -DO, molecular chaperones mediating the binding of peptides to MHC
  molecules in the context of antigen presentation
- *Expression:* constitutively expressed on B-cells, activated T-cells, macrophages, dendritic cells,
  and thymic epithelial cells. Cytokine (TNF, IFNγ)-induced expression on mononuclear phago-
  cytes, endothelial and epithelial cells
- *Structure:* heterodimers, heavy α-chain (33 kDa) and light β-chain (29 kDa). Both chains exhibit two extracellular domains (α1, α2 and β1, β2), a transmembranous region, and an intracytoplasmic region. The binding site is open on both sides, consequently allowing attachment
  of peptides of variable length (15–25 amino acids)

### HLA Class III
- Historic term. Genes of class III do not code for histocompatibility antigens but mostly for
  soluble molecules (complement system, tumor necrosis factor α and β, cytochrome P450,
  HSP 70) which have a function in antigen processing

**Meth:**

### Population Genetics of HLA Antigens:
- Location of HLA genes on chromosome 6, recombinations are very rare.
- Each individual carries two alleles of every HLA locus, the expression is codominant. If the two alleles differ, the individual is "heterozygous" in relation to this locus. If they are identical, the individual is "homozygous"
- Children inherit one paternal and one maternal haplotype of HLA genes each; hence, regarding HLA characteristics, siblings can be fully identical (theoretical probability 25%), haploidentical (50%), or not identical (25%)

### Nomenclature of HLA Antigens
- The notation of the HLA phenotype usually considers the HLA groups A, B, C, and DR, e.g., HLA-A1,2;B45,44;Cw4,6;DR1,7
- The notation of the HLA genotype is based on patterns according to the parental antigens, e.g., HLA-A1,B33,Cw6,DR1 / A2,B35,Cw4,DR7
- The antigen names are a combination of the gene locus (e.g., DQ-B1) and the allele number (e.g., 03-03). The allele number comprises four digits indicating major group and subgroup. A sometimes present fifth digit indicates a silent mutation which does not cause changes in the amino acid sequence (e.g., DQB1*03031)

**Phys:**

The remarkable allele polymorphism of the HLA genes concentrates on the region of the antigen binding site and hence has decisive influence on antigen presentation. It is of central importance in regulating the immune system by contributing to the differentiation between "self" and "nonself" and molding the development of a mature T-cell repertoire

In contrast to B-lymphocytes, T-lymphocytes do not recognize antigens in their free, soluble form, but only as peptides attached to a certain MHC molecule on the cell surface ("MHC Restriction"). The MHC-antigen complex specifically interacts with the T-cell receptor (TCR)

### Antigen Presentation
In principle, antigenic material can derive from exogenous (e.g., bacterial antigens) and endogenous (e.g., intracellularly synthesized viral proteins, tumor antigens, self-peptides) sources. Processing and presentation of both types of antigen differ:
- *Exogenous antigens:* phagocytically incorporated by antigen presenting cells. After fusion of phagosomes with lysosomes, the native protein is degraded with the aid of cellular proteases. In the endoplasmic reticulum (ER), attachment of the peptide to MHC class II molecules takes place. The peptide-MHC II complex is expressed on the cell surface and recognized by CD4+ T-cells
- *Endogenous antigens:* processing of endogenous antigens (after prior "ubiquitination," i.e., binding to ubiquitin) in the proteasome. Transport of the processed peptides into the ER (with the help of the TAP1/TAP2 heterodimer), where they are linked with de novo-synthesized HLA class I and $\beta_2$-microglobulin molecules. The peptide-MHC I complex is transported to the cell surface via the Golgi apparatus, where it is specifically recognized by CD8+ T-cells

**Dg:**

### HLA Typing
Analysis of the expression of HLA antigens by:
- *Conventional serology:* usage of monoclonal antibodies or HLA-specific alloantisera (complement-dependent lymphocytotoxicity test). Primarily used for typing the major groups HLA-A and -B, low resolution. Serological methods depend on expression of MHC molecules on the cell surface and fail in case of non-vital cells or low MHC expression
- *Molecular typing methods based on PCR* utilize sequence-specific primers ("PCR-SSP") and oligonucleotides ("PCR-SSO"), respectively, for low / medium / high resolution
- *DNA sequencing* of HLA loci for detection of individual alleles. Molecular biological methods of typing are better reproducible and should generally be used for typing HLA class II and HLA-C
- *Mixed lymphocyte culture (MLC)* for analysis of donor-recipient differences of class II genes
- An overview of HLA alleles currently detectable via serological and molecular biological techniques can be accessed via the following address: www.worldmarrow.org

**Ind:**     *Indications for HLA Typing*

HLA antigens/MHC molecules play an important role in:

- Typing and choosing recipient and donor in case of allogeneic bone marrow or blood stem cell transplantation (▶ Chap. 5.3). Especially relevant for transplantation are the four HLA groups A, B, DR, and DQ
- Typing and choosing recipient and donor in case of organ transplantation (heart, kidney, etc.)
- Transfusion: HLA-matched substitution of thrombocytes in case of sensitization against foreign HLA class I molecules
- Characterization of antigen-specific cellular response of the immune system (T-cell response).
- Cellular immunotherapy: active specific immunotherapy in tumor patients (malignant melanoma, bladder carcinoma, etc.) with defined HLA / tumor antigens in the framework of clinical studies
- Forensics: e.g., paternity testing
- Disease association: association of specific HLA genotypes and/or phenotypes with certain diseases (e.g., ankylosing spondylitis HLA-B27, Reiter's disease HLA-B27, idiopathic hemochromatosis HLA-A 3, chronic hepatitis HLA-B B35, narcolepsy HLA-DR15-DQ6, diabetes mellitus type I HLA-DR4, rheumatoid arthritis HLA-DR4, psoriasis vulgaris HLA-Cw6)

**Ref:**

1. Fisch P, Moris A, Rammensee HG et al. Inhibitory MHC class I receptors on gammadelta T cells in tumour immunity and autoimmunity. Immunol Today 2000;21:187–191
2. Godsell DS. The molecular perspective: MHC. Oncologist 2005;10:80–1
3. Klein J, Sato A. The HLA System. N Engl J Med 2000;243:702–9, 782–6
4. Marsh SG, Bodmer JG, Albert ED et al. Nomenclature for factors of the HLA system, 2000. Tissue Antigens 2001;57:236–83

**Web:**

1. http://www.ashi-hla.org/              American Society for Histocompatibility and Immunogenetics
2. http://www.ihwg.org/                   International Histocompatibility Working Group
3. http://www.worldmarrow.org            WMDA, World Marrow Donor Association

# 3.1 Basic Principles of Chemotherapy

D.P. Berger, R. Engelhardt, H. Henß

**Pharm:** Pharmacokinetics and pharmacodynamics. Fundamental terms and influencing variables in application, distribution, metabolism, and elimination of cytostatic drugs

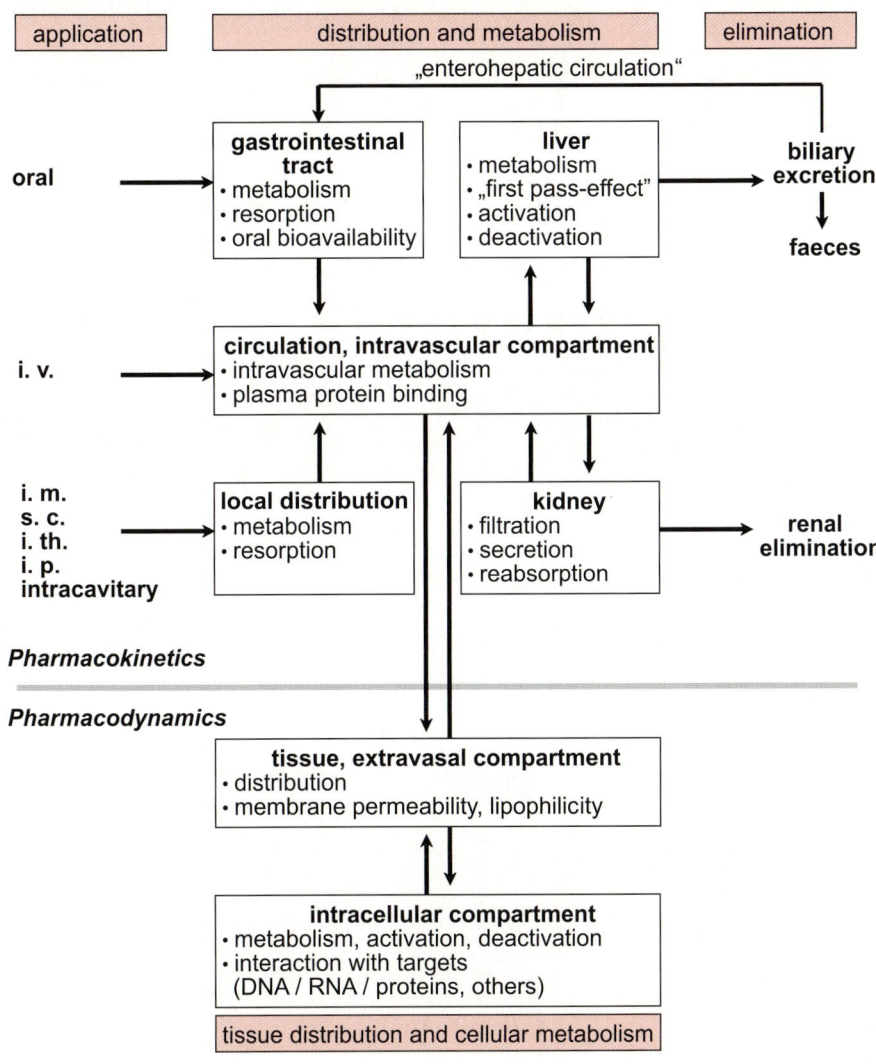

**Ma:**     **Targets of clinically used cytostatic drugs**

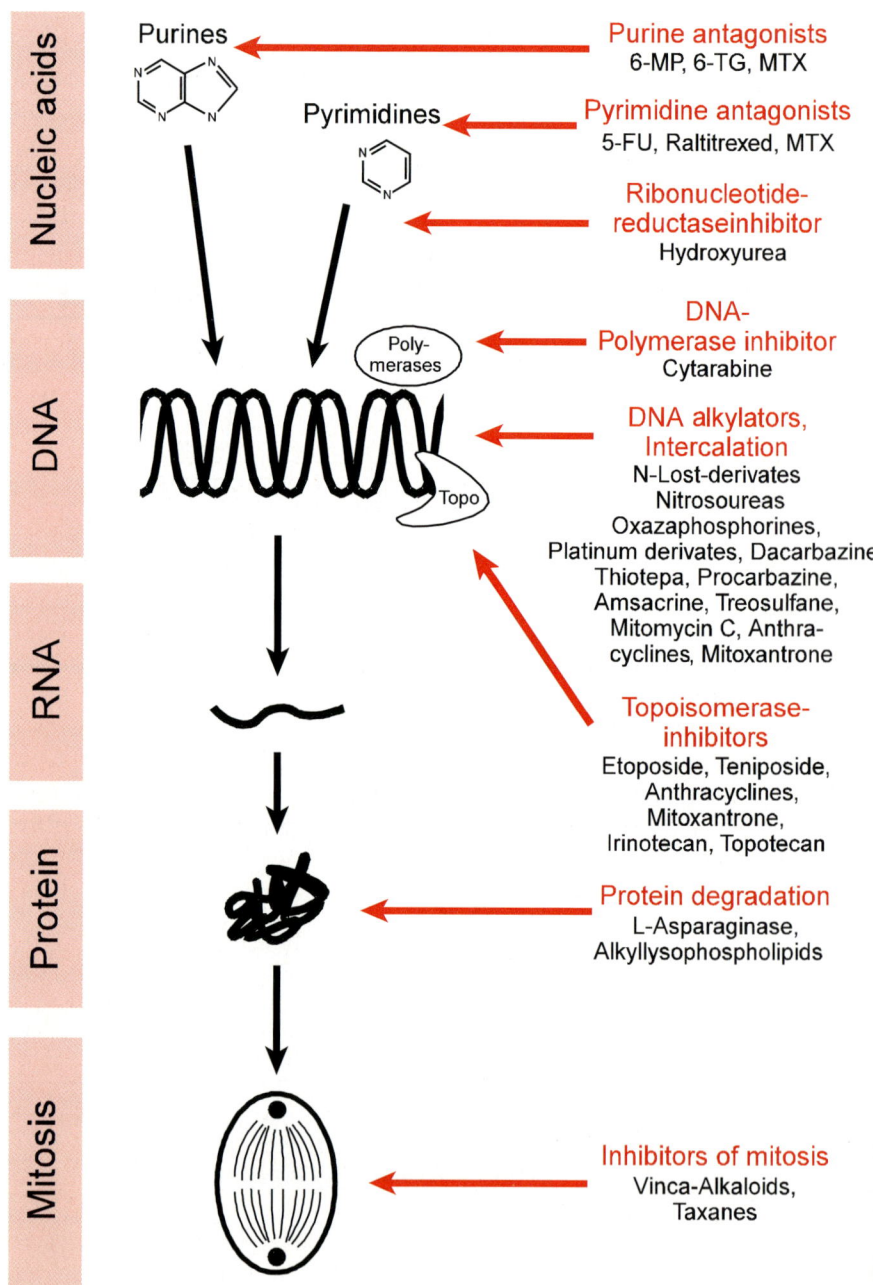

*Topo* topoisomerases, *MP* mercaptopurine, *TG* thioguanine, *MTX* methotrexate, *FU* fluorouracil

**Cell cycle and phase specifity of cytostatic drugs**

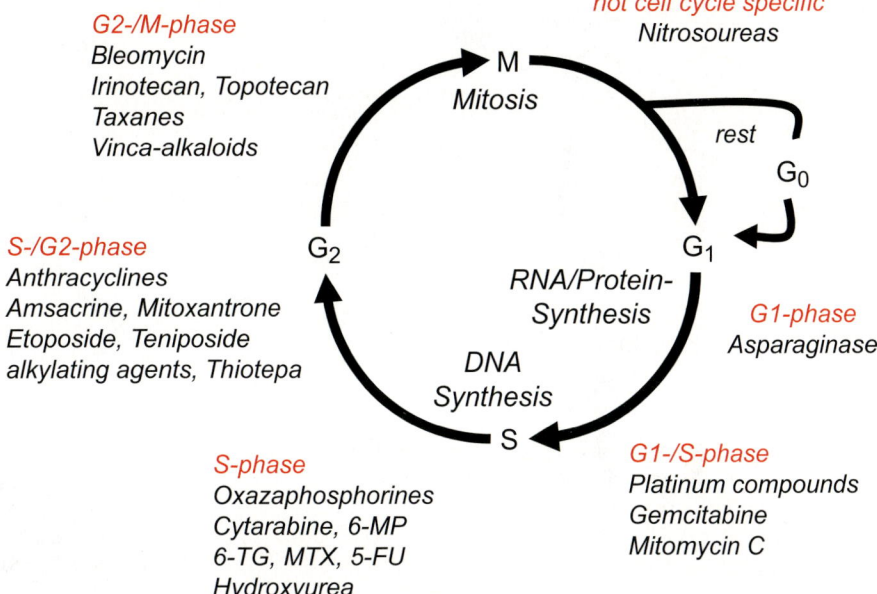

*MP* mercaptopurine, *TG* thioguanine, *MTX* methotrexate

## Mechanisms of Resistance

Resistance to cytostatic drugs limits the effect of chemotherapy. Types of resistance:

- Primary resistance ("a priori resistance"): pre-existing resistance against certain compounds
- Secondary resistance: acquired resistance following chemotherapy

## Specific Mechanisms of Resistance

- *"Multidrug resistance (MDR)"* via P-glycoprotein (P170, membrane protein, 170 kDa): ATP-dependent transport of naturally occurring toxins out of the cell → inhibition of effect of anthracyclines, vinca alkaloids, taxanes, epipodophyllotoxins. Physiological expression of P170 in gastrointestinal tract, biliary ducts, kidney. Induction of expression in malignant cells by cytostatics.
- *Topoisomerase II resistance* due to changes of the target molecule DNA-topoisomerase II → reduced effect of epipodophyllotoxins and anthracyclines.
- *Antimetabolite resistance:* altered expression of target enzymes (e.g., thymidylate synthase TS, dihydrofolate reductase DHFR) → reduced effect of 5-FU, methotrexate, etc.
- *Glutathione (GSH) and glutathione-S transferase (GST):* reduced glutathione and GST contribute to intracellular detoxification of alkylating agents and platinum compounds → reduced effect caused by increased intracellular GSH levels or increased expression of GST.
- *$O^6$-Alkyltransferase (AT):* DNA-repairing enzyme, corrects alkylation of $O^6$ position of guanine induced by nitrosoureas → reduces effect of carmustine, lomustine, nimustine.

**Mechanisms of cytoplasmic effect and resistance**

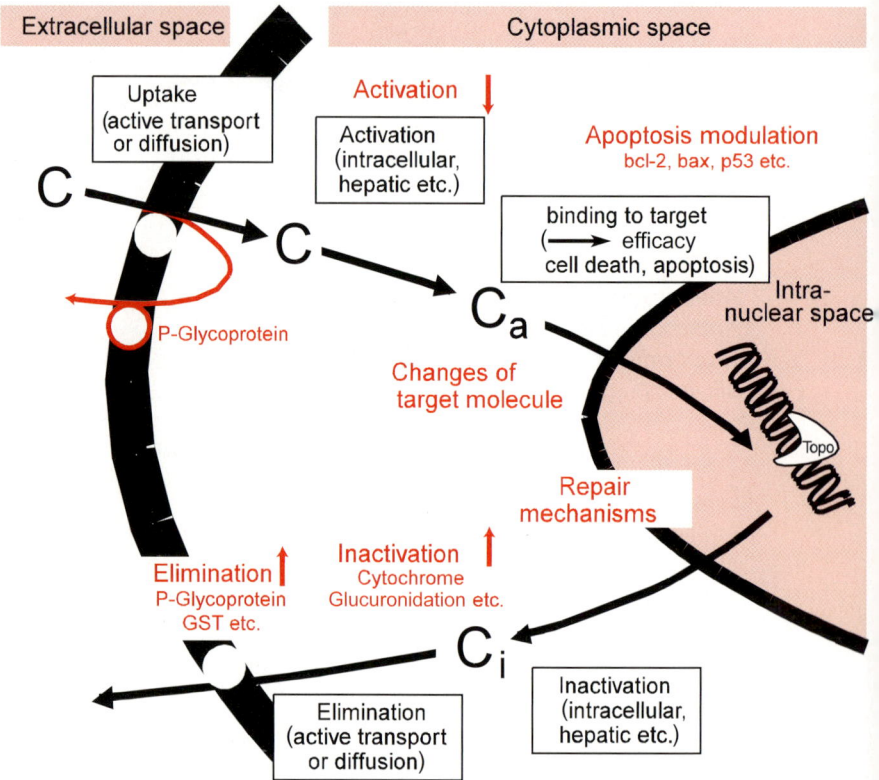

*C* cytostatic, *Ca* active metabolite, *Ci* inactive metabolite, *black* cellular pharmacokinetic effects, *red* resistance mechanisms

**Ref:**

1. Anderson CM. Drug profiles. In: Perry MC, Anderson CM, Doll DC et al. (eds) Companion Handbook to the Chemotherapy Sourcebook, 2nd edn. Lippincott Williams & Wilkins, Philadelphia, 2004, pp 419–72
2. Chauncey TR. Drug resistance mechanisms in acute leukemia. Curr Opin Oncol 2001;13:21–6
3. Egorin MJ. Overview of recent topics in clinical pharmacology of anticancer agents. Cancer Chemother Pharmacol 1998;42(Suppl):22–30
4. Fischer DS, Knobf MT, Durivage HJ et al. The Cancer Chemotherapy Handbook. Mosby, Philadelphia, 2003, pp 48–241
5. Rowinsky EK. The pursuit of optimal outcomes in cancer therapy in a new age of rationally designed target-based anticancer agents. Drugs 2000;60(Suppl 1):1–14
6. Skeel RT. Antineoplastic drugs and biological response modifiers. Classification, use and toxicity of clinically useful agents. In: Skeel RT (ed) Handbook of Cancer Chemotherapy, 6th edn. Lippincott Williams & Wilkins, Philadelphia, 2003, pp 53–156

**Web:**

1. http://www.druginfonet.com/          Drug Information, Information on Antineoplastic Agents
2. http://www.meds.com/DChome.html    Information on cytostatics
3. http://chemfinder.cambridgesoft.com  Chemical Data Base

# 3.2 Cytostatic Drugs

**D.P. Berger, R. Engelhardt, H. Henß**

| Substance class | Group | Compound | Abbreviation / synonym |
|---|---|---|---|
| Alkylating agents | Nitrogen mustard derivatives | Busulfan | BUS, BU |
| | | Chlorambucil | CBL |
| | | Melphalan | L-PAM, MPL |
| | | Bendamustine | BM |
| | Nitrosourea derivatives | Nimustine | ACNU |
| | | Carmustine | BCNU |
| | | Lomustine | CCNU |
| | Oxazaphosphorines | Cyclophosphamide | CY, CTX |
| | | Ifosfamide | IFO |
| | | Trofosfamide | |
| | Platinum derivatives | Cisplatin | CDDP, DDP |
| | | Carboplatin | CBCDA |
| | | Oxaliplatin | |
| | Triazine | Altretamine | HMM |
| | Tetrazines | Dacarbazine | DTIC |
| | | Temozolomide | |
| | Aziridines | Thiotepa | |
| | Other | Amsacrine | AMSA, m-AMSA |
| | | Estramustine phosphate | |
| | | Procarbazine | PBZ |
| | | Treosulfan | TREO |
| Antibiotics | Anthracyclines | Daunorubicin | DNR |
| | | Doxorubicin | Adriamycin, ADR, DXR |
| | | Epirubicin | EPI |
| | | Idarubicin | IDA |
| | Anthracenediones | Mitoxantrone | MITOX |
| | Other | Actinomycin D | Dactinomycin, DACT, ActD |
| | | Bleomycin | BLEO |
| | | Mitomycin C | MMC |
| Antimetabolites | Antifolates | Methotrexate | MTX |
| | | Raltitrexed | |
| | | Pemetrexed | |
| | Purine antagonists | 6-Mercaptopurine | 6-MP |
| | | 6-Thioguanine | 6-TG |

[a] RNR ribonucleoside reductase

| Substance class | Group | Compound | Abbreviation / synonym |
|---|---|---|---|
| | | 2'-Deoxycoformycin | Pentostatin, DCF |
| | | Fludarabine phosphate | F-Ara-ATP |
| | | 2-Chlorodeoxyadenosine | 2-CDA, cladribine |
| | Pyrimidine antagonists | 5-Fluorouracil | 5-FU |
| | | Capecitabine | |
| | | Cytosine arabinoside | Cytarabine, AraC |
| | | Difluorodeoxycytidine | Gemcitabine, DFDC |
| | | UFT | Tegafur-uracil |
| | RNR[a] inhibitors | Hydroxyurea | Hydroxycarbamide, HU |
| Alkaloids | Podophyllotoxin derivatives | Etoposide | VP-16 |
| | | Teniposide | VM26 |
| | Vinca alkaloids | Vinblastine | VBL |
| | | Vincristine | VCR |
| | | Vindesine | VDS |
| | | Vinorelbine | VRLB |
| | Taxanes | Docetaxel | Taxotere |
| | | Paclitaxel | Taxol |
| | Camptothecin derivatives | Irinotecan | CPT-11 |
| | | Topotecan | |
| Enzymes | | L-asparaginase | ASP |
| Other | Arsenic derivative | Arsenic trioxide | $As_2O_3$ |
| | Alkylphosphocholine | Miltefosine | HDPC |

[a] RNR ribonucleoside reductase

**Web:**

1. http://www.druginfonet.com/        Drug Information Network
2. http://chemfinder.cambridgesoft.com/        Chemfinder Database
3. http://www.meds.com/DChome.html        Dose Calculation of Cytostatics

## 3.2.1 Characteristics of Clinically Used Cytostatic Drugs

H. Henß, J. Scheele, R. Engelhardt, D.P. Berger

### Altretamine (Hexamethylmelamine, HMM)

**Chem:** N,N,N',N',N,N-hexamethyl-1,3,5-triazine-2,4,6-triamine, hexamethylmelamine

**MOA:** DNA alkylation and intercalation, inhibition of DNA and RNA synthesis

**Pkin:**
- *Kinetics:* good oral absorption (75–90%), half-life: t½ 4–13 h
- *Metabolism:* extensive first-pass hepatic metabolism to active metabolites, hepatic degradation (cytochrome P450-dependent), renal excretion of demethylated metabolites

**Se:**
- *Bone marrow:* myelosuppression (20–40%), with neutropenia, thrombocytopenia, anemia
- *Gastrointestinal:* nausea, vomiting, abdominal cramps, diarrhea, loss of appetite
- *Liver:* transaminase elevation (rare), impaired liver function
- *Skin:* alopecia (rare), erythema, pruritus, urticaria, allergic reactions
- *Nervous system:* dose-limiting peripheral and central neurotoxicity with irreversible neuropathies, paresthesia, sensory disturbances, hallucinations, confusion, ataxia, lethargy, somnolence
- *Local toxicity:* damaged capsules extremely irritating to mucous membranes
- *Other:* cystitis (rare), severe hypotension with concurrent administration of altretamine and monoamine oxidase inhibitors

**Ci:** Impaired liver function

**Th:** *Approved indications:* ovarian cancer
*Other areas of use:* lymphomas, solid tumors (endometrial cancer, cervical cancer, small cell lung cancer)

#### Dosage and Administration
- Oral administration after food, 260–320 mg/m²/day (8–12 mg/kg/day) p.o., in 3–4 daily divided doses, for 14–21 days, repeat every 4–6 weeks; in combination therapy 150–200 mg/m²/day (4 mg/kg/day)
- Dose modification ▶ Chap. 3.2.4
- ATTN: cimetidine and barbiturates alter effect (t½) due to cytochrome P450 induction or inhibition
- BEFORE TREATMENT: full blood count, liver and renal function tests, neurological evaluation

**Amsacrine (AMSA, m-AMSA)**

**Chem:**     4'-(9-Acridinylamino)-3'-methoxymethanesulfonanilide, alkylating agent, topoisomerase II inhibitor

**MOA:**
- DNA alkylation and intercalation, inhibition of topoisomerase II
- Cell-cycle-specific: S/G2 phases

**Pkin:**
- *Kinetics:* Half-life: t½ 2 h, prolonged with impaired liver function
- *Elimination:* biliary and renal excretion of unchanged drug and metabolites

**Se:**
- *Bone marrow:* myelosuppression dose-limiting, especially leukopenia, moderate thrombocytopenia, anemia
- *Cardiovascular:* arrhythmias, heart failure, cardiac arrest (especially in presence of hypokalemia)
- *Gastrointestinal:* nausea, vomiting (30%), mucositis (10%), diarrhea (10%)
- *Liver:* transient elevation of transaminases
- *Skin:* alopecia, jaundice, erythema (rare), urticaria, allergic reactions
- *Nervous system:* rare, peripheral and central neurotoxicity with headache, confusion, seizures
- *Local toxicity* (extravasation ▶ Chap. 9.9): phlebitis, necrosis
- *Other:* orange urine

**Ci:**
- Hypokalemia, electrolyte disturbances
- Impaired liver and renal function

**Th:**     *Approved indications:* AML

**Dosage and Administration**
- Standard dose: 75–150 mg/m²/day i.v. on days 1–5, repeat every 1–3 weeks
- Dose modification ▶ Chap. 3.2.4, incompatibility ▶ Chap. 3.2.6, stability ▶ Chap. 3.2.7
- BEFORE TREATMENT: full blood count, urea and electrolytes, liver and renal function tests, cardiac evaluation

### Arsenic Trioxide

**Chem:**   Arsenic trioxide, $As_2O_3$

**MOA:**   Induction of differentiation, apoptosis and DNA fragmentation of PML-RARα-positive cells in acute promyelocytic leukemia, antiangiogenetic effect

**Pkin:**
- *Kinetics:* intravenous administration, intravascular binding to hemoglobin (96%), half-life: t½ 12 h
- *Metabolism:* hepatic degradation (90%), renal excretion (10%)

**Se:**
- *Bone marrow:* myelosuppression (15%), with anemia, neutropenia, thrombocytopenia
- *Cardiovascular:* tachycardia (50%), QT prolongation, AV block, ventricular arrhythmia (torsades de pointes)
- *Gastrointestinal:* nausea, vomiting, mucositis, sore throat, diarrhea, abdominal pain (50%), gastrointestinal bleeding (rare), weight loss
- *Liver:* elevated transaminases, impaired liver function, hyperglycemia
- *Kidney:* hypokalemia, hypocalcemia, hypomagnesemia, impaired renal function (rare)
- *Skin:* dermatitis, erythema, urticaria, pruritus, cutaneous bleeding (ecchymosis, petechiae (rare)), epistaxis (25%)
- *Nervous system:* headache (60%), insomnia, anxiety disorders, arthralgia, paresthesias
- *Local toxicity:* phlebitis, local edema, erythema
- *Other:* "differentiation syndrome": fever, leukocytosis, cough, dyspnea, hypoxia, thoracic pain, pleural / pericardial effusions, hypotension, edema. Treatment with corticosteroids (e.g., dexamethasone 10 mg twice a day). Coagulation disorders (rare), DIC (disseminated intravascular coagulation)

**Ci:**
- Severely impaired liver or renal function
- Electrolyte disturbances, QT prolongation (especially > 500 ms), AV conduction disorders

**Th:**   *Approved indications:* acute promyelocytic leukemia (APL, AML FAB M3) with translocation t(15;17) or PML-RARα expression

#### Dosage and Administration
- Induction 0.15 mg/kg/day until remission, 8 weeks maximum, then no therapy for 3–6 weeks, consolidation 0.15 mg/kg/day for 4–5 weeks
- BEFORE TREATMENT: full blood count, urea and electrolytes, liver and renal function tests, ECG (exclude QT prolongation)

## L-Asparaginase (L-ASP), PEG-Asparaginase (Pegaspargase)

**Chem:**    Enzyme derived from *Escherichia coli* or *Erwinia carotovora*. Covalently linked with polyethylene glycol (PEG) to form PEG-asparaginase

**MOA:**
- Catalyses hydrolysis of L-asparagine to L-asparaginic acid and ammonia, intravascular depletion of asparagine and inhibition of protein synthesis of malignant lymphatic cells (normal cells are capable of asparagine synthesis by induction of asparagine synthetase)
- Cell-cycle-specific: G1 phase

**Pkin:**
- *Kinetics:* terminal half-life: t½ 8–30 h (depending on dose and compound), t½ prolonged to 3–6 days with PEG-asparaginase
- *Elimination:* metabolic degradation (proteolysis)

**Se:**
- *Gastrointestinal:* moderate nausea / vomiting (60%), mucositis, loss of appetite, diarrhea (rare)
- *Liver / pancreas:* impaired liver function, elevated transaminases (50% of patients), hepatitis, pancreatitis, hyperglycemia, impairment of clotting factor synthesis (especially fibrinogen and antithrombin III), thromboembolic events, hemorrhage
- *Kidney:* transient increase of serum creatinine and uric acid, acute renal failure (rare) or severely impaired renal function (rare)
- *Nervous system:* acute: reversible encephalopathy in 25–50% of patients: lethargy, somnolence, confusion; chronic: psychotic organic brain syndrome
- *Other:* dose-limiting allergic reactions: fever, chills, urticaria, skin reactions, bronchospasm, laryngospasm, asthma, anaphylactic shock. Reduced immunogenicity with PEG-asparaginase

**Ci:**
- Known intolerance
- Pancreatitis
- Impaired liver function, pre-existing coagulation disorders

**Th:**    *Approved indications:* ALL
*Other areas of use:* AML, NHL, CML in lymphatic blast crisis, CLL

### Dosage and Administration
- L-Asparaginase 5,000–20,000 IU/m²/day i.v. for 10–20 days, i.m. application possible
- PEG-asparaginase: 2,500 IU/m²/day i.v. every 14 days, i.m. application possible
- Dose modification ▶ Chap. 3.2.4, incompatibility ▶ Chap. 3.2.6, stability ▶ Chap. 3.2.7
- ATTN: coagulation disorders: if fibrinogen < 0.8 g/l or ATIII < 70%, give fresh frozen plasma (FFP) or ATIII. If fibrinogen < 0.5 g/l or Quick's test < 30%, end treatment. Allergic Reactions: close observation of the patient, monitor blood pressure. Allergic reactions must be treated acutely with antihistamines and corticosteroids. Change preparation if necessary (allergic reactions commonly due to bacterial impurities)
- BEFORE TREATMENT: full blood count, liver and renal function tests, blood glucose, clotting studies. Pretherapy intradermal skin test (dose: 2 IU) to exclude possible hypersensitivity is recommended

### Azacytidine (5-aza-cytidine)

**Chem:** 4-Amino-1-β-D-ribofuranosyl-s-triazin-2(1H)-one, pyrimidine nucleoside analog

**MOA:**
- Causes demethylation and hypomethylation of DNA, potentially with functional changes of genes regulating differentiation and proliferation of hematopoietic cells → direct cytotoxicity on abnormal hematopoietic cells in the bone marrow

**Pkin:**
- *Kinetics:* terminal half-life t½ after subcutaneous administration 2.5–4.2 h
- *Elimination:* hepatic metabolism, renal elimination 85%, fecal excretion < 1%

**Se:**
- *Bone marrow:* anemia, leucopenia, neutropenia, thrombocytopenia
- *Respiratory:* cough, dyspnea, respiratory tract infections, pharyngitis
- *Cardiovascular:* tachycardia, hypotension, atrial fibrillation (rare), cardiac failure (rare)
- *Gastrointestinal:* nausea / vomiting, diarrhea, constipation, anorexia, abdominal pain
- *Liver / pancreas:* impaired liver function, hepatic coma (rare)
- *Kidney:* serum creatinine ↑, impaired renal function, renal tubular acidosis (rare), hypokalemia
- *Skin:* erythema, rash, injection site reactions, ecchymosis, pruritus
- *Nervous system:* headache, confusion, dizziness, anxiety, depression, lethargy, insomnia, syncope
- *Other:* fever, infections, fatigue, weakness, rigors, arthralgia, myalgia, back pain, edema

**Ci:**
- Known intolerance to azacytidine or mannitol
- Severe hepatic impairment, advanced malignant hepatic tumors
- Severe renal impairment

**Th:** *Approved indications:* MDS
*Other areas of use:* AML, CML, sickle cell disease, β-thalassemia, malignant mesothelioma

#### Dosage and Administration
- 75 mg/m²/day s.c. days 1–7 every 4 weeks, or 105 mg/m²/day s.c. days 1–5 every 4 weeks. Intravenous application possible
- ATTN: azacytidine may be embryotoxic, teratogenic, and mutagenic in humans. Appropriate precautions should be taken to avoid pregnancy and fathering. Monitoring of blood counts, liver enzymes, and renal function required
- BEFORE TREATMENT: full blood count, liver and renal function tests, electrolytes

## Bendamustine

**Chem:** Gamma-(1-methyl-5-bis(beta-chloroethyl)aminobenzimidazole-(2)-butyric acid, alkylating agent, nitrogen mustard derivative

**MOA:** Cross-linking of DNA single and double strands by alkylation, DNA-protein and protein-protein linking

**Pkin:**
- *Kinetics:* initial half-life: t½ 6–10 min, terminal t½ 28–36 min
- *Metabolism:* hepatic hydrolysis to cytotoxically active β-hydroxy-bendamustine (β-OH-BM), predominantly renal elimination

**Se:**
- *Bone marrow:* myelosuppression
- *Cardiovascular:* arrhythmias, myocardial infarction (isolated cases)
- *Gastrointestinal:* nausea, vomiting, loss of appetite, constipation, diarrhea
- *Skin:* erythema, skin changes, alopecia, mucous membrane irritation
- *Nervous system:* weakness, fatigue, tiredness, peripheral neuropathy
- *Local toxicity* (extravasation ▶ Chap. 9.9): phlebitis, necrosis with perivascular administration

**Ci:**
- Impaired renal function
- Severely impaired liver function

**Th:** *Approved indications:* NHL, CLL, plasmacytoma, breast cancer

### Dosage and Administration
- Standard dose: 25 mg/m²/day i.v. for 3 weeks or longer
- Dose modification ▶ Chap. 3.2.4, stability ▶ Chap. 3.2.7
- BEFORE TREATMENT: full blood count, liver and renal function tests

**Bleomycin**

**Chem:** Antibiotic, mix of different bleomycins

**MOA:**
- DNA strand breaks, inhibition of DNA ligase, DNA intercalation
- Cell-cycle-specific: G2/M phase

**Pkin:**
- *Kinetics:* initial half-life: t½ 30 min, terminal t½ 2–5 h
- *Metabolism:* cytochrome P450-dependent hepatic activation, intracellular degradation (50%) by aminohydrolase (low levels in lung and skin → organotoxic), renal excretion of unchanged drug (50%) and metabolites

**Se:**
- *Bone marrow:* mild myelosuppression
- *Pulmonary:* dose-limiting interstitial pneumonitis and pulmonary fibrosis in up to 10% of cases with cough, dyspnea, hypoxia. Cumulative toxicity especially with total doses > 300 mg, increased in patients aged < 15 years and > 65 years
- *Gastrointestinal:* nausea / vomiting, loss of appetite, mucositis, diarrhea
- *Skin:* dose-dependent in 50% of patients: alopecia, erythema, urticaria, exanthema, striae, hyperpigmentation, edema, hyperkeratoses, nail changes, pruritus
- *Local toxicity:* phlebitis, pain at injection site
- *Other:* flu-like symptoms (fever, chills, myalgia). In 1% of patients allergic reactions up to anaphylaxis. Raynaud's syndrome

**Ci:**
- Pre-existing lung disease (especially chronic obstructive pulmonary disease), previous lung radiation, assisted ventilation with increased $O_2$ concentration
- Severely impaired liver or renal function

**Th:** *Approved indications:* testicular cancer, Hodgkin's disease, NHL, squamous cell carcinoma (head and neck region, esophagus, penis, cervix, vulva)
*Other areas of use:* solid tumors, instillation (malignant effusions)

### Dosage and Administration
- Standard dose: 15–30 mg absolute, 1–2×/week, administration i.v. / i.a. / s.c. or i.m. possible
- With intracavitary administration (pleural effusion, pericardial effusion, urinary bladder) 30–180 mg absolute
- Dose modification ▶ Chap. 3.2.4, incompatibility ▶ Chap. 3.2.6, stability ▶ Chap. 3.2.7
- ATTN: not to be given in combination with nephrotoxic or pneumotoxic drugs (busulfan, cyclophosphamide, melphalan, mitomycin)
- BEFORE TREATMENT: full blood count, liver and renal function tests (creatinine clearance), pulmonary function tests. Pretherapy test dose (1–2 mg) to exclude possible hypersensitivity is recommended

## Busulfan

**Chem:** Tetramethylene dimethane sulfonate, bifunctional alkylating agent

$$H_3C - \overset{\displaystyle O}{\underset{\displaystyle O}{\overset{\|}{\underset{\|}{S}}}} - O - CH_2 - CH_2 - CH_2 - CH_2 - O - \overset{\displaystyle O}{\underset{\displaystyle O}{\overset{\|}{\underset{\|}{S}}}} - CH_3$$

**MOA:**
- DNA and RNA alkylation (N7 position of guanine), DNA strand breaks and cross-linking
- Cell-cycle-specific: S/G2 phase

**Pkin:**
- *Kinetics:* oral or intravenous administration, terminal half time t½ 2.5 h, entering cerebrospinal fluid
- *Metabolism:* hepatic degradation to inactive metabolites (tetrahydrofuran, methane sulfonic acid), renal excretion of unchanged drug and metabolites

**Se:**
- *Bone marrow:* myelosuppression dose-limiting, long neutropenic phase (following treatment, nadir between days 11 and 30), thrombocytopenia, anemia
- *Cardiovascular:* hypertension, hypotension, tachycardia, thromboembolic events
- *Pulmonary:* pulmonary fibrosis ("busulfan lung," rare), especially with cumulative dose > 3,000 mg (threshold dose 500 mg). Increased risk with lung radiation and assisted ventilation with increased $O_2$ concentration
- *Gastrointestinal:* moderate nausea / vomiting, mucositis, loss of appetite
- *Liver:* transient disturbances of liver function, hepatic veno-occlusive disease (VOD) after high-dose therapy
- *Skin:* erythema, hyperpigmentation, alopecia
- *Nervous system:* central nervous system toxicity (rare), with visual disturbances, confusion, seizures, especially with high-dose therapy
- *Other:* infertility, cataracts, gynecomastia (rare), other fibroses (rare): pulmonary, retroperitoneal, endocardial. Hemorrhagic cystitis (rare)

**Ci:** Pre-existing lung disease (especially chronic obstructive pulmonary disease)

**Th:** *Approved indications:* CML (palliative), polycythemia vera
*Other areas of use:* other myeloproliferative diseases, conditioning prior to autologous / allogeneic transplantation in patients with leukemia or lymphoma

### Dosage and Administration
- Standard dose: 0.5–8 (–12) mg/day p.o. or 0.05–0.06 mg/kg body weight/day p.o.
- High-dose therapy: 4 mg/kg body weight/day for 4 days (*ATTN:* only in transplant centers)
- Stability ▶ Chap. 3.2.7
- ATTN: cumulative dose of > 500 mg: increased risk of pulmonary fibrosis
- BEFORE TREATMENT: full blood count, liver and renal function tests (creatinine clearance), pulmonary function tests

## Capecitabine

**Chem:** Pyrimidine analog, antimetabolite

**MOA:**
- Inhibition of thymidylate synthetase by FdUMP and thymidine synthesis
- Incorporated into RNA, inhibition of RNA synthesis by FUTP
- Cell-cycle-specific: S phase

**Pkin:**
- *Kinetics:* half-life: t½ 0.7–1.2 h
- *Metabolism:* oral administration, rapid and complete absorption. Intracellular conversion of the prodrug by hepatic carboxylesterase to 5'-deoxy-5-fluorocytidine (5'DFCR), subsequent intracellular metabolism by thymidine phosphorylase to 5-fluorouracil (5-FU), intracellular activation and phosphorylation (formation of FdUMP, FUTP). Degradation in liver and intestinal mucosa by dihydropyrimidine dehydrogenase (DPD)
- *Excretion:* renal elimination of unchanged drug and metabolites

**Se:**
- *Bone marrow:* myelosuppression with neutropenia, thrombocytopenia, anemia
- *Cardiovascular:* lower limb edema, cardiac ischemia (rare, may occur with pre-existing coronary heart disease), ECG changes
- *Gastrointestinal:* diarrhea (40%), mild nausea / vomiting (40%), mucositis, abdominal pain, stomatitis, loss of appetite
- *Liver:* elevated transaminases (reversible), hyperbilirubinemia
- *Skin:* hand-foot syndrome (palmar-plantar erythrodysesthesia, 50%), dermatitis (25%), alopecia
- *Nervous system:* headache, paresthesias, dysgeusia, vertigo, insomnia, confusion (rare), ataxia
- *Other:* fatigue, loss of appetite, fever, weakness, lethargy, mucositis, dehydration

**Ci:** Known hypersensitivity to fluorouracil (DPD deficiency)

**Th:** *Approved indications:* colorectal cancer, breast cancer
*Other areas of use:* head and neck tumors, pancreatic cancer

### Dosage and Administration
- Standard dose: 2,000–2,500 mg/m²/day p.o. on days 1–14, every 3 weeks. To be taken with water in 2 daily divided doses, 30 min after food
- Dose modification ▶ Chap. 3.2.4
- BEFORE TREATMENT: full blood count, liver and renal function tests (creatinine clearance)

## Carboplatin (CBCDA)

**Chem:**  cis-Diamine(1,1-cyclobutanedicarboxylato)platinum (II), platinum derivative

**MOA:**
- Covalent binding of DNA and protein, DNA intercalation, strand breaks
- Cell-cycle-specific: G1/S phases

**Pkin:**
- *Kinetics:* enters cerebrospinal fluid, initial half-life t½ 60–90 min, terminal t½ 3–6 h
- *Metabolism:* intracellular formation of reactive platinum complexes, renal excretion of unchanged drug (60%) and metabolites (40%)

**Se:**
- *Bone marrow:* myelosuppression, especially prolonged thrombocytopenia (dose-limiting), leukopenia and cumulative disturbances of erythropoiesis
- *Gastrointestinal:* nausea / vomiting, loss of appetite, mucositis
- *Liver:* transient elevation of transaminases
- *Kidney:* nephrotoxicity (rare), electrolyte disturbances ($Na^+\downarrow$, $K^+\downarrow$, $Mg^{2+}\downarrow$)
- *Skin:* alopecia (rare), erythema, pruritus
- *Nervous system:* peripheral neurotoxicity (rare, mainly in patients > 65 years), hearing disorders (rare) or optic neuritis (rare)
- *Local toxicity:* pain at injection site
- *Other:* infertility, fever, chills, allergic reactions (rare)

**Ci:**
- Impaired renal function, dehydration
- Pre-existing hearing disorders, acute infections

**Th:**   *Approved indications:* epithelial ovarian cancer, cervical cancer, lung cancer, head and neck tumors
*Other areas of use:* other solid tumors, refractory leukemia, lymphoma

### Dosage and Administration
- Standard dose: 300–400 mg/m²/day i.v. on day 1, every 4 weeks
- Pharmacological dose calculation: calculation of total dose in mg according to the target AUC ("area under the curve," area under the concentration-time curve in mg/ml × min) and the renal function (GFR, glomerular filtration rate in ml/min):

$$\text{Dose} = \text{AUC} \times (\text{GFR} + 25)$$

- The target AUC for carboplatin is 5–7 mg/ml/min in monotherapy protocols and 4–6 mg/ml/min in polychemotherapy protocols
- High-dose therapy: 500 mg/m²/day i.v. on days 1–3 (*ATTN:* only in transplant centers)
- Dose modification ▶ Chap. 3.2.4, incompatibility ▶ Chap. 3.2.6, stability ▶ Chap. 3.2.7
- ATTN: not to be given in combination with nephrotoxic or ototoxic drugs (aminoglycosides, NSAIDs, loop diuretics, etc.). Fluid replacement
- BEFORE TREATMENT: full blood count, liver and renal function tests (creatinine clearance)

### Carmustine (BCNU)

**Chem:** 1,3-Bis(2-chloroethyl)-1-nitrosourea, bifunctional alkylating agent

$$Cl-H_2C-H_2C-HN-CO-N\underset{N=O}{\overset{CH_2-CH_2-Cl}{\big<}}$$

**MOA:**
- DNA and RNA alkylation ($O^6$ position of guanine), DNA strand breaks, cross-linking
- Cell cycle non-specific (including G0 phase)

**Pkin:**
- *Kinetics:* lipophilic compound, enters cerebrospinal fluid, initial half-life: t½ 4–7 min, terminal t½ 20–70 min
- *Metabolism:* spontaneous hepatic degradation into inactive metabolites (isocyanate, diazohydroxide), renal excretion of unchanged drug and metabolites

**Se:**
- *Bone marrow:* prolonged and cumulative myelosuppression (dose-limiting), leukocyte and thrombocyte nadir 3–5 weeks after administration
- *Pulmonary:* with repeated administration, interstitial pneumonitis, pulmonary infiltrates and pulmonary fibrosis (cumulative toxicity)
- *Gastrointestinal:* nausea / vomiting for 8–24 h, mucositis, diarrhea; rarely: esophagitis, ulcers, gastrointestinal bleeding
- *Liver:* transient elevation of transaminases, hepatic veno-occlusive disease (VOD) with high-dose therapy
- *Kidney:* impaired renal function
- *Skin:* alopecia, dermatitis, erythema, hyperpigmentation
- *Nervous system:* peripheral and central neurotoxicity with confusion, psychotic organic brain syndrome, neuroretinitis, optic neuritis, ataxia
- *Local toxicity* (extravasation ► Chap. 9.9): venous irritation, necrosis
- *Other:* infertility

**Ci:**
- Pre-existing disorders of bone marrow function, acute infections
- Severe liver or renal disorders

**Th:** *Approved indications:* CNS tumors, cerebral metastases, multiple myeloma, lymphomas, gastrointestinal tumors
*Other areas of use:* breast cancer, melanoma

#### Dosage and Administration
- Standard dose: 100 mg/m²/day i.v. with protection from light, on days 1–2, every 6–8 weeks
- High-dose therapy: 300–600 mg/m²/day i.v. on day 1 (*ATTN:* only in transplant centers)
- Dose modification ► Chap. 3.2.4, incompatibility ► Chap. 3.2.6, stability ► Chap. 3.2.7
- ATTN: cumulative, delayed, and prolonged myelotoxicity. Increased risk of pulmonary toxicity with total cumulative dose > 1,000 mg/m². Increased toxicity with concurrent administration of metronidazole, cimetidine, or verapamil.
- BEFORE TREATMENT: full blood count, liver and renal function tests (creatinine clearance), pulmonary function tests

### Chlorambucil

**Chem:**  4-(4-[Bis(2-chloroethyl)amino]phenyl)butanoic acid, alkylating agent

$$HOOC-H_2C-H_2C-H_2C-\bigcirc-N\begin{array}{c} CH_2-CH_2-Cl \\ CH_2-CH_2-Cl \end{array}$$

**MOA:**
- DNA and RNA alkylation, DNA strand breaks, cross-linking
- Cell cycle non-specific (including G0 phase)

**Pkin:**
- *Kinetics:* oral bioavailability 60–100%, terminal half-life: t½ 1.5–2.5 h
- *Metabolism:* hepatic degradation into active (aminophenylacetic acid) and inactive metabolites, renal excretion of unchanged drug (1%) and metabolites

**Se:**
- *Bone marrow:* myelosuppression dose-limiting, neutropenia, thrombocytopenia with standard dose (see below) usually only moderate
- *Pulmonary:* pulmonary fibrosis (rare), especially with cumulative dose > 2,000 mg
- *Gastrointestinal:* mild nausea / vomiting, loss of appetite
- *Liver:* transient elevation of transaminases, severe hepatotoxicity (very rare)
- *Skin:* erythema, urticaria, alopecia
- *Nervous system:* rarely, peripheral / central neurotoxicity
- *Other:* infertility (especially with cumulative dose > 400 mg), fever, cystitis (rare)

**Ci:**  Pre-existing myelosuppression, acute infections

**Th:**  *Approved indications:* CLL, NHL, Hodgkin's disease
*Other areas of use:* multiple myeloma, Waldenström's macroglobulinemia, ovarian cancer, breast cancer, testicular tumors, trophoblastic tumors

#### Dosage and Administration
- Standard dose: oral administration, once a day with food, various protocols, e.g.:
  - 0.05–0.2 mg/kg body weight/day p.o. for 3–6 weeks, thereafter daily maintenance dose of 2 mg absolute p.o.
  - 0.4 mg/kg body weight/day p.o. on day 1, every 2–4 weeks
  - 18–30 mg/m²/day p.o. on day 1, every 2 weeks
  - 16 mg/m²/day p.o. on days 1–5, every 4 weeks
- ATTN: cumulative dose > 2,000 mg: increased risk of pulmonary fibrosis. Increased side effects with concurrent administration of phenylbutazone derivatives or phenobarbital
- BEFORE TREATMENT: full blood count, liver and renal function tests

## Cisplatin (CDDP)

**Chem:** cis-Diamminedichloroplatinum(II), platinum derivative

$$Cl\diagdown\diagup NH_3$$
$$Pt$$
$$Cl\diagup\diagdown NH_3$$

**MOA:**
- Covalent binding of platinum complexes to DNA, RNA, and proteins, cross-linking
- Cell-cycle-specific: G1/S phases

**Pkin:**
- *Kinetics:* half-life: initial t½ 25–50 min, terminal t½ 60–90 h
- *Metabolism:* formation of reactive platinum complexes, renal excretion (90%) of unchanged drug and metabolites, biliary excretion (10%)

**Se:**
- *Bone marrow:* myelosuppression, leukopenia, thrombocytopenia, anemia
- *Cardiovascular:* arrhythmias (rare), heart failure
- *Gastrointestinal:* severe nausea / vomiting (prolonged, duration > 24 h), loss of appetite, mucositis, diarrhea, enteritis
- *Liver:* transient elevation of transaminases
- *Kidney:* electrolyte changes ($Ca^{2+}$ ↓, $Mg^{2+}$ ↓, $K^+$ ↓, $Na^+$ ↓), cumulative nephrotoxicity with renal tubular damage (dose-limiting), probably from inadequate hydration
- *Skin:* alopecia, dermatitis
- *Nervous system:* ototoxicity and peripheral neurotoxicity (dose-limiting, cumulative, with total doses > 100–200 mg/m²), dysgeusia, focal encephalopathy (rare), visual disturbances, optic neuritis, vertigo
- *Local toxicity* (extravasation ▶ Chap. 9.9): phlebitis, necrosis
- *Other:* infertility, allergic reactions (rare)

**Ci:** Impaired renal function, dehydration, hearing disorders, acute infections

**Th:** *Approved indications:* testicular tumors, ovarian cancer, bladder cancer
*Other areas of use:* solid tumors (head and neck region, lungs, esophagus, cervix, endometrium, prostate, osteosarcoma, melanoma), NHL

### Dosage and Administration
- Standard dose: various protocols:
  - Low dose: 15–20 mg/m²/day i.v. on days 1–5, every 3–4 weeks
  - Medium dose: 50–75 mg/m²/day i.v. on days 1 + 8, every 3–4 weeks
  - High dose: 80–120 mg/m²/day i.v. on day 1, every 3–4 weeks
- Dose modification ▶ Chap. 3.2.4, incompatibility ▶ Chap. 3.2.6, stability ▶ Chap. 3.2.7
- ATTN: not to be given in combination with nephrotoxic drugs (aminoglycosides, NSAIDs, loop diuretics, etc.). Fluid replacement, aim: urine volume > 200 ml/h, with electrolyte replacement ($K^+$, $Mg^{2+}$) if necessary. Cumulative neurotoxicity and ototoxicity (with total dose > 100–200 mg/m²).
- BEFORE TREATMENT: full blood count, electrolytes, liver and renal function tests (creatinine clearance), audiometry and neurological evaluation, if necessary. Fluid administration 1,000–2,000 ml (with KCl and $MgSO_4$), osmotic diuresis

### Cladribine (2-CDA)

**Chem:** 2-Chloro-deoxyadenosine, purine analog, antimetabolite

**MOA:**
- Inhibition of DNA polymerase β and ribonuclease reductase
- Induction of DNA strand breaks, depletion of NAD and ATP
- Cell cycle non-specific (including G0 phase)

**Pkin:**
- *Kinetics:* enters cerebrospinal fluid, half-life: initial t½ 35 min, terminal t½ 7 h
- *Metabolism:* intracellular formation of the active triphosphate derivative, 2-chlorodeoxy-ATP, by deoxycytidine kinase
- *Elimination:* renal excretion

**Se:**
- *Bone marrow:* myelosuppression dose-limiting, with neutropenia (30%) and thrombocytopenia, lymphopenia (100%)
- *Gastrointestinal:* moderate nausea / vomiting (15% of patients), diarrhea
- *Liver:* transient elevation of transaminases
- *Kidney:* impaired renal function, especially with inadequate fluid replacement
- *Skin:* erythema (rare), up to toxic epidermolysis
- *Nervous system:* peripheral or central neurotoxicity in 15% of patients
- *Other:* immunosuppression with T-cell deficiency (CD4+ ↓↓, CD8+ ↓), infections, fever (60%), tiredness (50%), headaches

**Ci:** Severely impaired renal function

**Th:** *Approved indications:* hairy cell leukemia
*Other areas of use:* NHL, CLL, CML, acute leukemia, mycosis fungoides

#### Dosage and Administration
- Standard dose: usually given for one cycle only, no repeat. Various protocols:
    - 0.1 mg/kg body weight/day c.i.v., on days 1–7 (continuous infusion)
    - 0.14 mg/kg body weight/day i.v. on days 1–5 (2-h infusion)
- Dose modification ▶ Chap. 3.2.4, incompatibility ▶ Chap. 3.2.6, stability ▶ Chap. 3.2.7
- BEFORE TREATMENT: full blood count, liver and renal function tests (creatinine clearance)

## Cyclophosphamide

**Chem:** 2-[Bis(2-chloroethylamino)]-tetrahydro-2H-1,3,2-oxazaphosphine-2-oxide
Oxazaphosphorine, alkylating agent

**MOA:**
- DNA and RNA alkylation, DNA strand breaks, cross-linking, DNA synthesis ↓
- Cell-cycle-specific: S phase

**Pkin:**
- *Kinetics:* oral bioavailability 90–100%, half-life: terminal t½ 4–8 h
- *Metabolism:* initial hepatic hydroxylation by the microsomal cytochrome P450 monooxygenase system, release of active metabolite (phosphoramide mustard) in plasma and tissue, hepatic degradation into inactive metabolites. Renal excretion of active and inactive metabolites, dialyzable

**Se:**
- *Bone marrow:* myelosuppression dose-limiting, leukopenia (nadir 8–14 days after administration) and thrombocytopenia, anemia
- *Cardiovascular:* in 5–10% of cases with high-dose therapy, acute myocarditis / pericarditis, heart failure, hemorrhagic myocardial necrosis
- *Pulmonary:* with high-dose therapy, pulmonary fibrosis (rare), pneumonitis
- *Gastrointestinal:* nausea, vomiting (especially with doses > 600 mg/m²/day), mucositis, stomatitis, loss of appetite
- *Liver:* transient elevation of transaminases, cholestasis (rare)
- *Kidney / genitourinary tract:* hemorrhagic cystitis (dose-limiting), especially with high-dose therapy, bladder fibrosis, impaired renal function
- *Skin:* alopecia, erythema, hyperpigmentation, nail changes, dermatitis
- *Nervous system:* with high-dose therapy: acute encephalopathy
- *Other:* infertility, immunosuppression, fever, allergic reactions

**Ci:** Severely impaired liver or renal function, acute infections, cystitis, urinary tract obstruction

**Th:** *Approved indications:* lymphomas, multiple myeloma, ovarian cancer, breast cancer
*Other areas of use:* leukemias, solid tumors, immunosuppression, severe autoimmune diseases

### Dosage and administration
- Standard dose: oral or intravenous administration, various protocols:
  - 50–200 mg/m²/day p.o. on days 1–14 in the morning, every 28 days
  - 500–1,000 mg/m²/day i.v. on day 1 in the morning, every 21 days
- High-dose therapy: up to 16,000 mg/m²/day i.v. (*ATTN:* only in hematology / oncology centers)
- Dose modification ▶ Chap. 3.2.4, incompatibility ▶ Chap. 3.2.6, stability ▶ Chap. 3.2.7
- ATTN: prophylaxis of hemorrhagic cystitis starting with a dose of > 400 mg/m²/day: fluid replacement (urine volume > 200 ml/h), mesna. Effects enhanced by barbiturates (cytochrome P450 activation) and cimetidine
- BEFORE TREATMENT: full blood count, liver and renal function tests (creatinine clearance)

## Cytarabine (Cytosine Arabinoside, Arabinosylcytosine, AraC)

**Chem:**   4-Amino-1-β-D-ribofuranosyl-2(1H)-pyrimidinone, deoxycytidine analog, antimetabolite

**MOA:**
- Incorporated into DNA, inhibition of DNA polymerases, DNA synthesis ↓
- Cell-cycle-specific: S phase

**Pkin:**
- *Kinetics:* Half-life: initial t½ 12 min, terminal t½ 2 h, enters cerebrospinal fluid
- *Metabolism:* intracellular phosphorylation to active ara-CMP and ara-CTP, hepatic degradation into inactive metabolites (ara-U, ara-UMP) by deamination, renal excretion of metabolites

**Se:**
- *Bone marrow:* myelosuppression dose-limiting, leukopenia, thrombocytopenia, anemia
- *Pulmonary:* with high-dose therapy acute pulmonary toxicity, pulmonary edema, ARDS ("acute respiratory distress syndrome") → intensive care unit necessary
- *Gastrointestinal:* nausea / vomiting, mucositis, diarrhea, loss of appetite. Rarely with high-dose therapy, pancreatitis, ulcers, bowel necrosis, esophagitis
- *Liver:* transient elevation of transaminases, cholestasis
- *Skin:* alopecia, dermatitis, erythema, exanthema, keratitis
- *Nervous system:* peripheral and central neurotoxicity. Cerebral and cerebellar disorders, especially in older patients (> 60 years) and with high-dose therapy. With intrathecal administration: acute arachnoiditis, leukoencephalopathy
- *Other:* fever, myalgia, arthralgia, bone and muscle pain, flu-like symptoms, conjunctivitis

**Ci:**   Severely impaired liver or renal function, pre-existing CNS disease

**Th:**   *Approved indications:* AML, ALL, CML in blast crisis, NHL

### Dosage and Administration
- Standard dose: various protocols:
    - Low-dose AraC: 10–20 mg/m²/day s.c. daily, for 21 days
    - Medium-dose AraC: 100 mg/m² twice a day i.v. on days 1–7 or 200 mg/m²/day c.i.v. on days 1–7
    - High-dose AraC: 1,000–3,000 mg/m² twice a day i.v. on days 1–6 (*ATTN:* only in hematology centers), with prophylactic administration of dexamethasone i.v. and as eye drops
    - Intrathecal (40–50 mg absolute) or intramuscular administration possible
- Dose modification ▶ Chap. 3.2.4, incompatibility ▶ Chap. 3.2.6, stability ▶ Chap. 3.2.7
- BEFORE TREATMENT: full blood count, liver and renal function tests (creatinine clearance), neurological evaluation if necessary

## Dacarbazine (DTIC)

**Chem:** 5-(3,3-Dimethyl-1-triazeno)imidazole-4-carboxamide, tetrazine derivative, alkylating agent

$$CH_3$$

H_2N—CO

**MOA:**
- DNA methylation and direct DNA toxicity, alkylating agent
- Cell cycle non-specific (including G0 phase)
- Inhibition of purine, RNA and protein synthesis

**Pkin:**
- *Kinetics:* half-life: initial t½ 20–80 min, terminal t½ 3–5 h
- *Metabolism:* hepatic activation (by microsomal oxidases) into MTIC (monomethyl triazeno imidazole carboxamide), renal excretion of unchanged drug (40%) and metabolites (50%), minor hepatobiliary and pulmonary excretion

**Se:**
- *Bone marrow:* myelosuppression dose-limiting, leukopenia, thrombocytopenia
- *Pulmonary:* pneumonitis (rare)
- *Gastrointestinal:* severe nausea / vomiting, loss of appetite, mucositis (rare), diarrhea
- *Liver:* transient elevation of transaminases, hepatic veno-occlusive disease (VOD, rare), hepatic necrosis
- *Kidney:* impaired renal function (rare)
- *Skin:* erythema, exanthema, photosensitivity, alopecia (rare)
- *Nervous system:* rarely central nervous system disorders (headache, visual disturbances, confusion, lethargy, seizures), paresthesias
- *Local toxicity* (extravasation ▶ Chap. 9.9): local thrombophlebitis, necrosis
- *Other:* rarely, flu-like symptoms (fever, chills, myalgia), allergic reactions, hypotension

**Ci:** Severely impaired liver or renal function

**Th:** *Approved indications:* malignant melanoma, Hodgkin's disease
*Other areas of use:* soft tissue sarcoma, osteosarcoma, renal cell carcinoma

### Dosage and Administration
- Standard dose: intravenous administration, with protection from light, various protocols:
  - 150–250 mg/m²/day i.v. on days 1–5, every 3–4 weeks
  - 375 mg/m²/day i.v. on days 1 + 15, every 3–4 weeks
  - 750–850 mg/m²/day i.v. on day 1, every 4 weeks
- Dose modification ▶ Chap. 3.2.4, incompatibility ▶ Chap. 3.2.6, stability ▶ Chap. 3.2.7
- ATTN: patients should avoid sunlight (photosensitivity). Antiemetic prophylaxis mandatory
- BEFORE TREATMENT: full blood count, liver and renal function tests (creatinine clearance)

## Dactinomycin (Actinomycin D)

**Chem:**    Peptide antibiotic

**MOA:**
- DNA intercalation, inhibition of RNA and protein synthesis
- Inhibition of topoisomerase II

**Pkin:**
- *Kinetics:* strong tissue binding, half-life: terminal t½ 30–40 h
- *Metabolism:* hepatic degradation, renal and biliary excretion of unchanged drug (70%) and metabolites

**Se:**
- *Bone marrow:* prolonged myelosuppression (dose-limiting), neutropenia, thrombocytopenia, anemia
- *Gastrointestinal:* severe nausea / vomiting, mucositis, gastrointestinal ulcers, diarrhea, loss of appetite, dysphagia
- *Liver:* hepatitis (rare), impaired liver function, hepatomegaly, ascites
- *Kidney:* impaired renal function (rare)
- *Skin:* alopecia, acne, erythema, exanthema, desquamation, hyperpigmentation, delayed tissue reaction in a previously irradiated site ("radiation recall reaction"), rarely allergic reactions up to anaphylaxis
- *Local toxicity* (extravasation ► Chap. 9.9): phlebitis, necrosis
- *Other:* rarely, flu-like symptoms (fever, myalgia)

**Ci:**
- Severely impaired liver or renal function
- Acute infections (especially varicella, *Herpes zoster*)

**Th:**    *Approved indications:* Wilms' tumor, soft tissue sarcomas, testicular cancer, choriocarcinoma, uterine cancer
*Other areas of use:* trophoblastic tumors, AML, osteosarcomas, melanomas, endometrial cancer, ovarian cancer

### Dosage and Administration
- Standard dose: various protocols:
    - 0.25–0.6 mg/m²/day i.v. on days 1–5, every 3–5 weeks
    - 1.0–2.0 mg/m²/day i.v. on day 1, every 3–5 weeks
    - 35–50 µg/kg as an isolated limb perfusion
- Dose modification ► Chap. 3.2.4, incompatibility ► Chap. 3.2.6, stability ► Chap. 3.2.7
- BEFORE TREATMENT: full blood count, liver and renal function tests (creatinine clearance)

## Daunorubicin (DNR, Rubidomycin), Liposome-encapsulated Daunorubicin

**Chem:**  Anthracycline, antineoplastic glycoside antibiotic

**MOA:**
- DNA intercalation, induction of DNA strand breaks, generation of free oxygen radicals, inhibition of topoisomerase II
- Cell-cycle-specific: S/G2 phases

**Pkin:**
- *Kinetics:* half-life: terminal t½ 15–48 h
- *Metabolism:* hepatic degradation to active (daunorubicinol) and inactive metabolites, aglycon formation, biliary (50%) and renal (< 20%) excretion

**Se:**
- *Bone marrow:* myelosuppression (dose-limiting), leukopenia and thrombocytopenia
- *Cardiovascular:* acute and chronic cardiotoxicity (dose-limiting)
  - *Acute:* ECG changes, arrhythmias, ischemia, infarction
  - *Chronic:* congestive cardiomyopathy with decreased left ventricular ejection fraction (LVEF)
  - *Risk factors:* pre-existing cardiac disorders, age < 15 or > 60 years, fast bolus injection, mediastinal radiation, total dose of > 500–600 mg/m². Liposome-encapsulated daunorubicin shows reduced cardiotoxicity
- *Gastrointestinal:* nausea, vomiting, mucositis, stomatitis, diarrhea (rare)
- *Liver:* transient elevation of transaminases
- *Skin:* exanthema, urticaria, alopecia, delayed tissue reaction in a previously irradiated site ("radiation recall reaction"), nail changes, hyperpigmentation (rare)
- *Local toxicity* (extravasation ▶ Chap. 9.9): causes severe necrosis
- *Other:* infertility, peripheral neuropathy (rare), red urine

**Ci:**
- Cardiac disease (arrhythmias, myocardial infarction, coronary heart disease, heart failure)
- Severely impaired liver function, acute infections

**Th:**
*Approved indications:* ALL, AML (daunorubicin), AIDS-associated Kaposi's sarcoma (liposome-encapsulated daunorubicin)
*Other areas of use:* NHL, CML, neuroblastoma

### Dosage and Administration
- *Daunorubicin:* 45–60 mg/m²/day i.v. on days 1–3, every 4 weeks
- *Liposome-encapsulated daunorubicin:* 40 mg/m²/day i.v. every 2 weeks
- Dose modification ▶ Chap. 3.2.4, incompatibility ▶ Chap. 3.2.6, stability ▶ Chap. 3.2.7
- ATTN: cumulative threshold dose 500–600 mg/m² with daunorubicin
- BEFORE TREATMENT: full blood count, liver and renal function tests (creatinine clearance), cardiac evaluation, echocardiogram / radionuclide ventriculography

### Decitabine (5-aza-2′-deoxycytidine)

**Chem:**   4-Amino-1-(2-deoxy-β-D-erythro-pentofuranosyl)-1,3,5-triazin-2(1H)-one, pyrimidine nucleo-side analog

**MOA:**
- Inhibition of DNA methyltransferase after incorporation into DNA
- Causes demethylation and hypomethylation of DNA, potentially with functional changes of genes regulating differentiation, proliferation, and apoptosis

**Pkin:**
- *Kinetics:* terminal half-life t½ 0.5 ± 0.3 h
- *Elimination:* deamination by cytidine deaminase (liver, granulocytes, intestinal epithelia)

**Se:**
- *Bone marrow:* anemia, leucopenia, neutropenia, thrombocytopenia
- *Respiratory:* cough, dyspnea, respiratory tract infections, pneumonia, pharyngitis
- *Cardiovascular:* tachycardia, atrial fibrillation (rare), cardiac failure (rare), myocardial infarction (rare)
- *Gastrointestinal:* nausea / vomiting, diarrhea, constipation, anorexia, abdominal pain
- *Liver / pancreas:* transient elevation of liver enzymes, bilirubin ↑
- *Kidney:* dysuria (rare), impaired renal function, hypokalemia, hypomagnesemia
- *Skin:* erythema, rash, ecchymosis, pruritus, alopecia
- *Nervous system:* headache, dizziness, confusion, anxiety, depression, lethargy, insomnia
- *Other:* fever, infections, fatigue, weakness, rigors, arthralgia, back pain, edema, hyperglycemia

**Ci:**
- Known hypersensitivity to decitabine
- Uncontrolled active infection

**Th:**   *Approved indications:* MDS (intermediate-1, intermediate-2, high-risk IPSS groups)
*Other areas of use:* AML, CML, sickle cell anemia

#### Dosage and Administration
- 15 mg/m²/day i.v. over 3 h every 8 h for 3 days, repeat every 6 weeks for a minimum of 4 cycles
- ATTN: decitabine may be embryotoxic, teratogenic, and mutagenic in humans. Appropriate precautions should be taken to avoid pregnancy and fathering. Monitoring of blood counts, liver enzymes, and renal function recommended
- BEFORE TREATMENT: full blood count, liver and renal function tests, electrolytes

### Docetaxel

**Chem:** Taxane derivative, plant alkaloid, mitotic inhibitor

**MOA:**
- Stabilization of tubulin polymers, inhibition of spindle formation, mitotic arrest
- Cell-cycle-specific: M phase

**Pkin:**
- *Kinetics:* highly protein bound, half-life: terminal $t\frac{1}{2}$ 10–19 h
- *Metabolism:* hepatic degradation, cytochrome P450-dependent hydroxylation, biliary excretion (> 80–90%), renal excretion (< 10–20%)

**Se:**
- *Bone marrow:* myelosuppression dose-limiting, neutropenia, thrombocytopenia, anemia
- *Cardiovascular:* arrhythmias (rare), symptoms of ischemia
- *Gastrointestinal:* nausea / vomiting, mucositis, diarrhea, constipation
- *Liver:* transient elevation of transaminases, liver impairment (rare)
- *Skin:* alopecia, dermatotoxicity (50–75%): erythema, exanthema, pruritus, dysesthesia, nail changes, epidermolysis (rare)
- *Nervous system:* peripheral neurotoxicity (40–70%) with paresthesias and motor disturbances, paralytic ileus (rare), rarely central nervous system disorders (weakness, visual disturbances, seizures)
- *Local toxicity* (extravasation ▶ Chap. 9.9): phlebitis, necrosis
- *Other:* hypersensitivity reactions (flushing, urticaria, transient myalgia, hypotension (rare), bronchospasm, angioedema). Fatigue, reduced performance status, loss of appetite, fluid retention (increased capillary permeability) with weight gain, edema, hypotension, pleural effusion, ascites (especially with cumulative dose > 400 mg/m²)

**Ci:** Severely impaired liver function, pre-existing cardiac disease

**Th:** *Approved indications:* lung cancer, breast cancer
*Other areas of use:* ovarian cancer, gastrointestinal tumors, bladder cancer, prostate cancer, head and neck tumors, sarcomas

#### Dosage and Administration
- Standard dose: 60–100 mg/m²/day i.v. on day 1, every 3 weeks or 35 mg/m²/day, weekly for 6 weeks
- Dose modification ▶ Chap. 3.2.4, incompatibility ▶ Chap. 3.2.6, stability ▶ Chap. 3.2.7
- ATTN: fluid retention with cumulative dose > 400 mg/m²
- BEFORE TREATMENT: full blood count, electrolytes, liver and renal function tests, cardiac evaluation. Premedication with dexamethasone; H1 blockers, H2 blockers, and diuretics may be given if required

## Doxorubicin (DXR, Adriamycin, ADR), Liposome-encapsulated Doxorubicin

**Chem:**     Anthracycline, hydroxydaunorubicin, antineoplastic glycoside antibiotic

**MOA:**
- DNA intercalation, induction of DNA strand breaks, generation of free oxygen radicals, inhibition of topoisomerase II
- Cell-cycle-specific: S/G2 phases

**Pkin:**
- *Kinetics:* 70% plasma protein-bound, half-life: triphasic pattern, terminal t½ 21–90 h
- *Metabolism:* hepatic degradation to active (doxorubicinol) and inactive metabolites, aglycon formation. Biliary (50%) and renal (< 10%) excretion

**Se:**
- *Bone marrow:* myelosuppression (dose-limiting), leukopenia, thrombocytopenia
- *Cardiovascular:* cardiotoxicity (dose-limiting)
    - *Acute cardiotoxicity:* ECG changes, arrhythmias, ischemia, infarction
    - *Chronic cardiotoxicity:* congestive cardiomyopathy with decreased LVEF
    - *Risk factors:* pre-existing cardiac disorders, age < 15 or > 60 years, rapid bolus injection, mediastinal radiation, total dose of 400–550 mg/m²
- *Gastrointestinal:* nausea / vomiting, mucositis, stomatitis, diarrhea (rare)
- *Skin:* exanthema, urticaria, alopecia, delayed tissue reaction in a previously irradiated site ("radiation recall reaction"), nail changes, hyperpigmentation (rare); reversible erythrodysesthesia with liposome-encapsulated doxorubicin
- *Local toxicity* (extravasation ▶ Chap. 9.9): causes severe necrosis
- *Other:* fever, allergic reactions, red urine

**Ci:**
- Cardiac disease (arrhythmias, myocardial infarction, coronary heart disease, heart failure)
- Severely impaired liver function, acute infections

**Th:**     *Approved indications:* solid tumors (e.g., small cell lung cancer, breast cancer, ovarian cancer, endometrial cancer, bladder cancer, thyroid cancer, sarcomas, Wilms' tumor), malignant lymphomas (e.g., Hodgkin's disease, multiple myeloma, NHL), AML, ALL

### Dosage and Administration
- Doxorubicin: 45–75 mg/m²/day every 21–28 days, 10–20 mg/m²/day i.v. weekly
  High-dose therapy: 90–150 mg/m²/day (*ATTN:* only in transplant centers)
- Liposome-encapsulated doxorubicin: 20–50 mg/m²/day i.v. every 3–4 weeks
- Dose modification ▶ Chap. 3.2.4, incompatibility ▶ Chap. 3.2.6, stability ▶ Chap. 3.2.7
- ATTN: cumulative threshold dose 400–550 mg/m² with doxorubicin
- BEFORE TREATMENT: full blood count, liver and renal function tests (creatinine clearance). Cardiac evaluation with echocardiography or radionuclide ventriculography

### Epirubicin (EPI)

**Chem:**    Anthracycline, antineoplastic glycoside antibiotic

**MOA:**
- DNA intercalation, induction of DNA strand breaks, generation of free oxygen radicals, inhibition of topoisomerase II
- Cell-cycle-specific: S/G2 phases

**Pkin:**
- *Kinetics:* half-life: triphasic pattern, terminal t½ 18–45 h
- *Metabolism:* hepatic degradation, glucuronidation, biliary (50%) and renal (< 10%) excretion

**Se:**
- *Bone marrow:* myelosuppression (dose-limiting), leukopenia and thrombocytopenia
- *Cardiovascular:* less cardiotoxic than daunorubicin or doxorubicin:
  - *Acute cardiotoxicity:* ECG changes, arrhythmias, ischemia, infarction
    *Chronic cardiotoxicity:* congestive cardiomyopathy with decreased LVEF
  - *Risk factors:* pre-existing cardiac disorders, age < 15 or > 60 years, rapid bolus injection, mediastinal radiation, cumulative dose > 900–1,000 mg/m²
- *Gastrointestinal:* nausea / vomiting, mucositis, stomatitis, diarrhea (rare)
- *Skin:* exanthema, urticaria, delayed tissue reaction in a previously irradiated site ("radiation recall reaction"), nail changes, hyperpigmentation (rare). Moderate alopecia
- *Local toxicity* (extravasation ▶ Chap. 9.9): causes severe necrosis
- *Other:* infertility, allergic reactions, red urine

**Ci:**
- Cardiac disease (arrhythmias, myocardial infarction, coronary heart disease, heart failure)
- Severely impaired liver function

**Th:**    *Approved indications:* solid tumors: (lung cancer, breast cancer, ovarian cancer, gastrointestinal tumors, prostate cancer, soft tissue sarcoma), lymphomas

#### Dosage and Administration
- Standard dose: 40–100 mg/m²/day i.v. every 3–4 weeks or 15–30 mg/m²/day i.v. weekly
- High-dose therapy: 120–180 mg/m²/day (*ATTN:* only in transplant centers)
- Topical administration: intravesical instillation in bladder cancer
- Dose modification ▶ Chap. 3.2.4, incompatibility ▶ Chap. 3.2.6, stability ▶ Chap. 3.2.7
- ATTN: cumulative threshold dose 900–1,000 mg/m²
- BEFORE TREATMENT: full blood count, liver and renal function tests (creatinine clearance). Cardiac evaluation with echocardiogram or radionuclide ventriculography

### Estramustine Phosphate

**Chem:** Estra-1,3,5(10)-triene-3,17-diol(17beta)-, 3-[bis(2-chloroethyl)carbamate]
Combination molecule with estradiol and alkylating moieties

**MOA:**
- Estrogen-like effect, antigonadotropic effect
- Alkylating agent: DNA and RNA alkylation, DNA strand breaks, cross-linking
- Interaction with tubulin, interference with formation of microtubules, mitotic arrest

**Pkin:**
- *Kinetics:* oral bioavailability 75%, absorption inhibited by calcium-rich beverages / foods (milk, etc.). Half-life: initial t½ 90 min, terminal t½ 20–24 h
- *Metabolism:* dephosphorylation, cleavage of carbamide bond with release of estrogen moiety and bifunctional alkylating agent, biliary and renal excretion of metabolites

**Se:**
- *Bone marrow:* moderate myelosuppression (rare)
- *Cardiovascular:* cardiovascular disorders in 10–25% of patients: phlebitis, thromboembolism, angina pectoris symptoms, ischemia, heart failure, edema
- *Gastrointestinal:* nausea / vomiting, loss of appetite, diarrhea (rare)
- *Liver:* transient elevation of transaminases, cholestasis (rare)
- *Skin:* erythema, skin irritation, pruritus, alopecia
- *Local toxicity* (extravasation ► Chap. 9.9): local phlebitis
- *Other:* gynecomastia (50% of patients, prophylactic breast irradiation possible before therapy). Loss of libido, impotency (20–50%), paresthesia in perineum or prostatic area. Allergic reactions

**Ci:**
- Thrombophilia, thromboembolism, cardiovascular disease
- Impaired liver function, gastrointestinal ulcers, *Herpes zoster*

**Th:** *Approved indications:* prostate cancer

#### Dosage and Administration
- *Intravenous administration:* 350–450 mg/day i.v. daily, for 5–10 days
- *Oral administration:* 3 × 280 mg/day for 28 days. With response, continue treatment with 2 × 280 mg/day
- Dose modification ► Chap. 3.2.4, incompatibility ► Chap. 3.2.6, stability ► Chap. 3.2.7
- ATTN: reduced absorption with oral intake of calcium-containing foods or beverages (milk, calcium-containing water, etc.)
- BEFORE TREATMENT: full blood count, liver and renal function tests, cardiac evaluation

### Etoposide (VP-16), Etoposide Phosphate

**Chem:** 4'-Demethylepipodophyllotoxin 9-(4,6-0-ethylidene-beta-D-glucopyranoside)
Epipodophyllotoxin derivative, plant alkaloid, topoisomerase II inhibitor. Etoposide phosphate is a water-soluble phosphate ester of the plant alkaloid etoposide.

**MOA:**
- Inhibition of topoisomerase II → mitotic arrest → DNA strand breaks
- Cell-cycle-specific: G2/S/M phases

**Pkin:**
- *Kinetics:* oral bioavailability 30–70%, half-life: terminal t½ 4–14 h. Etoposide phosphate is phosphorylated to etoposide with t½ 7 min
- *Metabolism:* hepatic degradation, renal and biliary excretion of unchanged drug and metabolites

**Se:**
- *Bone marrow:* myelosuppression (dose-limiting), neutropenia, thrombocytopenia
- *Cardiovascular:* arrhythmias (rare), hypotension with intravenous administration, ischemia
- *Gastrointestinal:* nausea / vomiting (mainly with oral administration), mucositis, dysphagia, diarrhea, constipation, loss of appetite
- *Liver:* transient elevation of transaminases
- *Skin:* moderate alopecia, erythema (rare), hyperpigmentation, pruritus
- *Nervous system:* rarely peripheral neuropathy or central nervous systems disorders
- *Other:* infertility, allergic reactions (fever, chills, bronchospasm, skin reactions), anaphylaxis

**Ci:**
- Severely impaired liver or renal function, neurological disorders
- Pre-existing cardiac disease (especially angina pectoris / coronary heart disease)

**Th:** *Approved indications:* lung cancer, testicular cancer, ovarian cancer, choriocarcinoma, Hodgkin's disease, NHL, AML
*Other areas of use:* gastrointestinal tumors, sarcomas, breast cancer

#### Dosage and Administration
- *Etoposide:* 50 mg/m²/day p.o. on days 1–21, or 50–120 mg/m²/day i.v. on days 1–5, every 3–4 weeks
  - High-dose therapy: 500 mg/m²/day i.v. on days 1–3 (*ATTN:* only in transplant centers)
- *Etoposide phosphate:* 100 mg etoposide is equivalent to 113.6 mg etoposide phosphate
- Dose modification ▶ Chap. 3.2.4, incompatibility ▶ Chap. 3.2.6, stability ▶ Chap. 3.2.7
- ATTN: calcium antagonists may enhance etoposide cytotoxicity
- BEFORE TREATMENT: full blood count, liver and renal function tests (creatinine clearance)

## Fludarabine (2-Fluoro-ara-AMP, Fludarabine Phosphate)

**Chem:**     9-β-D-Arabinosyl-2-fluoroadenine, purine analog, antimetabolite

**MOA:**     Incorporated into DNA and RNA, inhibition of DNA polymerase α, ribonucleotide reductase, DNA primase and ligase

**Pkin:**
- *Kinetics:* half-life: initial $t\frac{1}{2}$ 0.6–2 h, terminal $t\frac{1}{2}$ 7–20 h
- *Metabolism:* dephosphorylation in plasma, intracellular rephosphorylation by deoxycytidine kinase, formation of active triphosphate derivative F-Ara-ATP, renal excretion

**Se:**
- *Bone marrow:* myelosuppression dose-limiting, leukopenia, thrombocytopenia, anemia
- *Cardiovascular:* acute cardiotoxicity with arrhythmias (rare), hypotension
- *Pulmonary:* acute pulmonary toxicity (rare), dyspnea, interstitial infiltrates
- *Gastrointestinal:* nausea / vomiting (rare), mucositis, loss of appetite, diarrhea
- *Liver:* transient elevation of transaminases, cholestasis (rare)
- *Skin:* moderate alopecia (rare), erythema (rare), dermatitis
- *Nervous system:* peripheral neuropathy with paresthesias (15% of patients), central nervous system disorder with somnolence, weakness, confusion, delayed CNS toxicity with higher doses, demyelination, visual disturbances, seizures, coma
- *Other:* immunosuppression with T-cell deficiency (CD4+ ↓↓, CD8+ ↓) and increased incidence of opportunistic infections. Fever, myalgia. Isolated cases of tumor lysis syndrome (▶ Chap. 9.6)

**Ci:**     Severely impaired renal function

**Th:**     *Approved indications:* B-CLL
*Other areas of use:* other low malignant NHL, cutaneous T-cell lymphomas, Hodgkin's disease High-dose therapy before stem cell transplantation

### Dosage and Administration
- Standard dose: 20–30 mg/m²/day i.v. on days 1–5, repeat every 3–4 weeks
- Dose modification ▶ Chap. 3.2.4, incompatibility ▶ Chap. 3.2.6, stability ▶ Chap. 3.2.7
- BEFORE TREATMENT: full blood count, liver and renal function tests (creatinine clearance), exclude pre-existing neuropathy

### Fluorouracil (5-FU)

**Chem:** 5-Fluoro-2,4(1H, 3H)-pyrimidinedione, pyrimidine analog, antimetabolite

**MOA:**
- Inhibition of thymidylate synthetase by FdUMP → thymidine synthesis ↓, incorporated into RNA, inhibition of RNA synthesis by FUTP
- Cell-cycle-specific: S phase

**Pkin:**
- *Kinetics:* enters cerebrospinal fluid, half-life: initial $t\frac{1}{2}$ 8–14 min, terminal $t\frac{1}{2}$ 5 h
- *Metabolism:* intracellular activation and phosphorylation (formation of FdUMP, FUTP etc.). Degradation in liver and intestinal mucosa by dihydropyrimidine dehydrogenase (DPD). Metabolic elimination (90%), renal excretion (10%)

**Se:**
- *Bone marrow:* myelosuppression dose-limiting, mainly with bolus administration, leukopenia, thrombocytopenia, anemia
- *Cardiovascular:* acute cardiotoxicity with arrhythmias (rare), angina pectoris, ischemia up to myocardial infarction in isolated cases
- *Gastrointestinal:* nausea / vomiting, loss of appetite, in some cases severe mucositis / diarrhea (delayed toxicity), dose-limiting, especially following continuous infusion
- *Skin:* conjunctivitis, lacrimation ↑, dermatitis, erythema, palmar-plantar erythrodysesthesia, hyperpigmentation, moderate alopecia
- *Nervous system:* rarely central nervous system disorder (somnolence, confusion), reversible cerebellar disorder (ataxia, vertigo, tiredness, speech disorders)
- Other: allergic reactions, thrombophlebitis, fever

**Ci:**
- Severely impaired liver function, pre-existing stomatitis / diarrhea
- DPD deficiency

**Th:**
*Approved indications:* gastrointestinal tumors, breast cancer
*Other areas of use:* ovarian cancer, cervical cancer, prostate cancer, bladder cancer, head and neck tumors. Topical application: solar keratoses, Bowen's disease, basal cell carcinoma

#### Dosage and Administration
- Standard dose: various protocols:
  - 400–1,000 mg/m²/day i.v. on days 1–5, every 2–4 weeks
  - 600–1,000 mg/m²/day i.v. on day 1, every 7–14 days
  - Continuous infusion 2,600 mg/m²/week c.i.v.
  - Intra-arterial administration as regional chemotherapy (e.g., liver perfusion)
- Dose modification ► Chap. 3.2.4, incompatibility ► Chap. 3.2.6, stability ► Chap. 3.2.7
- BEFORE TREATMENT: full blood count, liver and renal function tests (creatinine clearance)

#### Folinic Acid (Calcium Folinate):
- Folinic acid increases cytotoxic effect of 5-FU
- Combination therapy 5-FU + folinic acid: always administer folinic acid before 5-FU

### Gemcitabine (DFDC)

**Chem:**     2′,2′-Difluorodeoxycytidine, pyrimidine analog, antimetabolite

**MOA:**
- Inhibition of ribonucleotide reductase, inhibition of deoxycytidine deaminase, incorporated into DNA by DNA polymerases, induction of DNA strand breaks
- Cell-cycle-specific: G1/S phases

**Pkin:**
- *Kinetics:* negligible plasma protein binding, half-life: initial $t\frac{1}{2}$ 8 min, terminal $t\frac{1}{2}$ 14 h
- *Metabolism:* intracellular activation by phosphorylation. Deamination in plasma. Metabolized into cytostatically inactive metabolite 2′-deoxydifluorouridine in liver, kidney, and other tissues. Renal (10%) and metabolic (90%) excretion

**Se:**
- *Bone marrow:* pronounced myelotoxicity (dose-limiting) with neutropenia in 25% of patients, thrombocytopenia (rare) in 25% of patients, anemia
- *Pulmonary:* pulmonary edema (rare)
- *Gastrointestinal:* nausea, vomiting (15%), diarrhea (rare), mucositis (rare)
- *Liver:* transient elevation of transaminases
- *Kidney:* moderate proteinuria / hematuria, hemolytic uremic syndrome (rare)
- *Skin:* erythema, pruritus, alopecia (rare), edema
- *Other:* peripheral edema, flu-like symptoms (may be treated with paracetamol); in rare cases infusion reactions (flushing, dyspnea, facial edema, headache, hypotension)

**Ci:**     Severely impaired liver and renal function

**Th:**     *Approved indications:* non-small cell lung cancer, breast cancer, pancreatic cancer, bladder cancer, ovarian cancer, lymphoma
*Other areas of use:* testicular tumors

#### Dosage and Administration
- Standard dose: 1,000 mg/m²/day i.v. on days 1, 8, 15, repeat on day 29
- Dose modification ▶ Chap. 3.2.4, incompatibility ▶ Chap. 3.2.6, stability ▶ Chap. 3.2.7
- BEFORE TREATMENT: full blood count, liver and renal function tests

### Hydroxyurea (Hydroxycarbamide)

**Chem:** Hydroxycarbamide, antimetabolite

$$H_2N - CO - NH - OH$$

**MOA:**
- Inhibition of ribonucleotide reductase, inhibition of DNA synthesis
- Cell-cycle-specific: S phase

**Pkin:**
- *Kinetics:* oral bioavailability 80–90%, enters cerebrospinal fluid, half-life: t½ 2–5 h
- *Metabolism:* rapid hepatic inactivation, predominantly renal excretion of unchanged drug (50%) and inactive metabolites (50%)

**Se:**
- *Bone marrow:* myelosuppression dose-limiting with leukopenia, thrombocytopenia, anemia, megaloblastosis in bone marrow
- *Pulmonary:* acute pulmonary toxicity with diffuse pulmonary infiltration (rare), pulmonary edema
- *Gastrointestinal:* moderate nausea, vomiting, loss of appetite. In rare cases mucositis, diarrhea, constipation
- *Liver:* transient elevation of transaminases, cholestasis (rare)
- *Kidney:* renal function disorders (rare) with proteinuria, hyperuricemia
- *Skin:* exanthema, erythema (especially face and neck), hyperpigmentation (rare), nail changes, alopecia, delayed tissue reaction in a previously irradiated site ("radiation recall reaction")
- *Nervous system:* peripheral / central neurotoxicity (rare)
- *Other:* flu-like symptoms (rare), fever

**Ci:** Severely impaired liver or renal function

**Th:** *Approved indications:* CML
*Other areas of use:* myeloproliferative syndromes, cervical cancer, prostate cancer

#### Dosage and Administration
- Standard dose: 500–1,000 mg/m²/day (or 15–30 mg/kg body weight/day) daily p.o.; with long-term therapy, dose is adjusted according to leukocyte count
- With solid tumors: 2,000–3,000 mg/m²/day (or 60–80 mg/kg body weight/day) every third day
- Dose modification ► Chap. 3.2.4
- BEFORE TREATMENT: full blood count, liver and renal function tests (creatinine clearance)

### Idarubicin (IDA)

| | |
|---|---|
| **Chem:** | 4-Demethoxydaunorubicin, anthracycline, antineoplastic glycoside antibiotic |

**MOA:**
- DNA intercalation, induction of DNA strand breaks, generation of free oxygen radicals, inhibition of topoisomerase II
- Cell-cycle-specific: S/G2 phases

**Pkin:**
- *Kinetics:* oral bioavailability 30–35%, enters cerebrospinal fluid, half-life: triphasic pattern, terminal $t\frac{1}{2}$ 6–25 h
- *Metabolism:* hepatic degradation, active (idarubicinol) and inactive metabolites, aglycon formation, biliary (50%) and renal (10%) excretion

**Se:**
- *Bone marrow:* myelosuppression (dose-limiting), leukopenia and thrombocytopenia
- *Cardiovascular:* less cardiotoxic than other anthracyclines:
  - *Acute cardiotoxicity:* ECG changes, arrhythmias, ischemia, infarction
  - *Chronic cardiotoxicity:* congestive cardiomyopathy (rare)
  - *Risk factors:* pre-existing cardiac disorders, age < 15 or > 60 years, rapid bolus injection, mediastinal radiation, cumulative dose > 150–290 mg/m²
- *Gastrointestinal:* nausea, vomiting (80%), mucositis, stomatitis, diarrhea (rare)
- *Liver:* transient elevation of transaminases
- *Skin:* dermatitis, exanthema, urticaria, alopecia, delayed tissue reaction in a previously irradiated site ("radiation recall reaction"), palmar-plantar erythrodysesthesia (rare)
- *Local toxicity* (extravasation ▶ Chap. 9.9): causes severe necrosis
- *Other:* infertility, fever, allergic reactions, red urine

**Ci:**
- Severe cardiac disorders (arrhythmias, myocardial infarction, coronary heart disease, heart failure, etc.)
- Severely impaired liver and renal function, acute infections

**Th:**
*Approved indications:* AML, ALL
*Other areas of use:* breast cancer, CML in blast crisis

#### Dosage and Administration
- Standard dose: 10–12 mg/m² i.v. or 35–50 mg/m² p.o. on days 1–3, every 3–4 weeks
- Dose modification ▶ Chap. 3.2.4, incompatibility ▶ Chap. 3.2.6, stability ▶ Chap. 3.2.7
- ATTN: cumulative threshold dose of 150–290 mg/m²
- BEFORE TREATMENT: full blood count, liver and renal function tests. Cardiac evaluation, echocardiogram or radionuclide ventriculography if risk factors present

## Ifosfamide

**Chem:** N,3-Bis(2-chloroethyl)tetrahydro-2H-1,3,2-oxazaphosphorin-2-amine 2-oxide
Oxazaphosphorine, bifunctional alkylating agent

$$\text{O} \overset{\underset{\displaystyle \|}{\text{O}}}{\underset{\underset{\displaystyle \text{N}-\text{CH}_2-\text{CH}_2-\text{Cl}}{|}}{\text{P}}}-\text{N}-\text{CH}_2-\text{CH}_2-\text{Cl}$$

**MOA:**
- DNA and RNA alkylation, DNA strand breaks, DNA intercalation, DNA synthesis $\downarrow$
- Cell-cycle-specific: S phase

**Pkin:**
- *Kinetics:* half-life: terminal t½ 5–6 h
- *Metabolism:* slow hepatic hydroxylation by microsomal cytochrome P450 oxidase, release of active metabolite (isophosphoramide mustard) in plasma and tissue, hepatic degradation into inactive metabolites, renal excretion of unchanged drug (15–55%) and metabolites

**Se:**
- *Bone marrow:* myelosuppression dose-limiting, leukopenia and thrombocytopenia
- *Gastrointestinal:* acute and delayed nausea (50%), vomiting, mucositis, diarrhea, loss of appetite
- *Liver:* transient elevation of transaminases, cholestasis (rare)
- *Genitourinary:* hemorrhagic cystitis, impaired renal function
- *Skin:* alopecia (80%), erythema (rare), urticaria (rare), nail changes, hyperpigmentation, dermatitis
- *Nervous system:* acute encephalopathy and cerebellar neurotoxicity, especially in the presence of impaired renal function or acidosis: confusion, psychosis, ataxia, seizures, somnolence, coma (prophylaxis: sodium carbonate, treatment: methylene blue)
- *Other:* infertility, fever

**Ci:**
- Severely impaired liver or renal function, acute infections
- Cystitis, urinary tract obstruction

**Th:** *Approved indications:* testicular tumor, lung cancer, ovarian cancer, cervical cancer, pancreatic cancer, soft tissue sarcomas, lymphomas
*Other areas of use:* breast cancer, osteosarcoma

### Dosage and Administration
- Standard dose: various protocols:
  - 1,200–2,400 mg/m²/day i.v. mornings, for 3–5 days
  - 4,000–8,000 mg/m²/day c.i.v. for 24 h
- Dose modification ▶ Chap. 3.2.4, incompatibility ▶ Chap. 3.2.6, stability ▶ Chap. 3.2.7
- ATTN: prophylaxis of hemorrhagic cystitis: fluid replacement (aim: urine volume > 200 ml/h), administration of mesna. Effects enhanced by barbiturates (cytochrome P450 activation) and cimetidine
- BEFORE TREATMENT: full blood count, liver and renal function tests (creatinine clearance); alkalinization

## Irinotecan (CPT-11)

**Chem:**  Camptothecin analog, topoisomerase I inhibitor

**MOA:**
- Inhibition of topoisomerase I, DNA religation ↓↓ → DNA strand breaks and DNA intercalation
- Cell-cycle-specific: G2/M phases

**Pkin:**
- *Kinetics:* ubiquitous distribution, enters cerebrospinal fluid, third space fluid accumulation (pleural effusions, ascites), half-life: t½ 14–18 h
- *Metabolism:* intracellular activation by carboxylesterase to active metabolite SN-38 (7-ethyl-10-hydroxy-camptothecin), hepatic degradation to inactive metabolites, biliary and renal excretion of active and inactive metabolites

**Se:**
- *Bone marrow:* myelosuppression dose-limiting, neutropenia, eosinophilia, thrombocytopenia, anemia
- *Cardiovascular:* thromboembolic events (rare)
- *Gastrointestinal:* nausea, vomiting, loss of appetite, delayed and in some cases severe diarrhea with mucositis (5–10 days after administration) in 10–20% of patients
- *Liver:* transient elevation of transaminases
- *Kidney:* reversible decrease of renal function, microscopic hematuria
- *Hematology:* alopecia, erythema
- *Other:* acute cholinergic syndrome (acute diarrhea, salivation, lacrimation, etc. within 24 h of administration) especially with doses > 300 mg/m²; treat with atropine 0.25–1 mg. Fever, weakness, reduced performance status.

**Ci:**  Pre-existing diarrhea, acute infections

**Th:**  *Approved indications:* metastatic colorectal cancer
*Other areas of use:* gastrointestinal tumors, lung cancer, ovarian cancer, cervical cancer

### Dosage and Administration
- Standard dose: various protocols:
  - 250–350 mg/m²/day i.v. on day 1, every 3 weeks
  - 100–125 mg/m²/day i.v. on days 1, 8, 15, 22, every 6 weeks
- Dose modification ▶ Chap. 3.2.4, incompatibility ▶ Chap. 3.2.6, stability ▶ Chap. 3.2.7
- ATTN: for severe delayed diarrhea, loperamide may be given. With diarrhea in the neutropenic phase, increased risk of gram-negative sepsis
- BEFORE TREATMENT: full blood count, liver and renal function tests (creatinine clearance)

### Lenalidomide

**Chem:** 3-(4-Amino-1-oxo 1,3-dihydro-2H-isoindol-2-yl)piperidine-2,6-dione, thalidomide analog

**MOA:** Mechanism of action not fully characterized. Proposed mechanisms include:
- Immunomodulation: immunosuppressive properties, proinflammatory cytokines ↓, anti-inflammatory cytokines ↑, tumor necrosis factor ↓, cyclooxygenase-2 (COX-2) ↓
- Anti-angiogenic properties
- Direct antineoplastic / cytotoxic activity in cells of lymphatic origin

**Pkin:**
- *Kinetics:* rapid oral absorption, peak plasma concentration after 0.6–1.5 h, protein binding 30%, half-life t½ 3 h
- *Metabolism:* renal excretion (> 65% as unchanged drug)

**Se:**
- *Bone marrow:* severe myelosuppression (80%), with leukopenia, neutropenia (59%), thrombocytopenia (62%), anemia
- *Pulmonary:* cough, dyspnea, upper respiratory tract infections, pneumonia
- *Cardiovascular:* edema, chest pain, atrial fibrillation, cardiac failure, myocardial infarction, hypertension, thromboembolic events, pulmonary embolism
- *Gastrointestinal:* nausea / vomiting, diarrhea, anorexia, constipation, abdominal pain
- *Hepatic:* transient increase of liver enzymes, hyperbilirubinemia
- *Kidney:* dysuria, serum creatinine ↑, hypokalemia, hypomagnesemia
- *Skin:* erythema, pruritus, rash, dry skin, ecchymosis, petechiae, sweating
- *Nervous system:* headache, dizziness, confusion, depression, insomnia, peripheral neuropathy
- *Other:* fever, fatigue, infections, arthralgia, myalgia, back pain, asthenia, hypothyroidism

**Ci:**
- Pregnant women or women capable of becoming pregnant. Female patients must use two different methods of contraception. Male patients must use condoms.
- Hypersensitivity to lenalidomide

**Th:** *Approved indications:* MDS with deletion 5q- and transfusion-dependent anemia, multiple myeloma
*Other areas of use:* MDS (non-5q-)

#### Dosage and Administration
- Standard dose: 10 mg p.o. daily
- ATTN: potential for life-threatening human birth defects. Appropriate precautions should be taken to avoid pregnancy and fathering. In order to avoid fetal exposure to lenalidomide, in the US the drug is only available under a special restricted distribution program. Hematological toxicity (neutropenia, thrombocytopenia) requires weekly monitoring. Significantly increased risk of deep venous thrombosis and pulmonary embolism
- BEFORE TREATMENT: full blood count, liver and renal function tests, electrolytes, thyroid function tests, pregnancy test (in women of childbearing potential)

## Lomustine (CCNU)

**Chem:**  1-(2-Chloroethyl)-3-cyclohexyl-1-nitrosourea, alkylating agent

$$\bigcirc\!-\text{HN}-\text{CO}-\text{N}\begin{array}{l}\nwarrow \text{CH}_2-\text{CH}_2-\text{Cl}\\ \searrow \text{N}=\text{O}\end{array}$$

**MOA:**
- DNA and RNA alkylation ($O^6$ position of guanine), DNA strand breaks, cross-linking, inhibition of DNA polymerase and RNA synthesis
- Cell cycle non-specific (including G0 phase)

**Pkin:**
- *Kinetics:* high oral availability, lipophilic compound, enters cerebrospinal fluid, half-life: t½ 2 h, t½ of the metabolites 5–72 h
- *Metabolism:* hepatic hydroxylation (cytochrome P450) to active metabolites, spontaneous degradation to inactive metabolites, renal excretion of unchanged drug and metabolites

**Se:**
- *Bone marrow:* prolonged and cumulative myelosuppression (dose-limiting), leukopenia and thrombocytopenia after 4–6 weeks, anemia
- *Pulmonary:* pulmonary infiltrates and pulmonary fibrosis (cumulative)
- *Gastrointestinal:* nausea / vomiting (within 6–24 h), mucositis, diarrhea, loss of appetite
- *Liver:* transient elevation of transaminases
- *Kidney:* impaired renal function (cumulative nephrotoxicity)
- *Skin:* erythema, pruritus, moderate alopecia, dermatitis, hyperpigmentation
- *Nervous system:* peripheral and central neurotoxicity, psychotic organic brain syndrome, optic neuritis, confusion, ataxia
- *Other:* infertility, amenorrhea, fatigue

**Ci:**
- Pre-existing bone marrow dysfunction, acute infections
- Severely impaired liver or renal function

**Th:**  *Approved indications:* Hodgkin's disease, CNS tumors, melanomas, lung cancer
*Other areas of use:* brain metastases, NHL, multiple myeloma, breast cancer, ovarian cancer, colorectal cancer

### Dosage and Administration
- Standard dose: 80–130 mg/m²/day p.o. on day 1, every 6–8 weeks
- Dose modification ▶ Chap. 3.2.4
- ATTN: cumulative, delayed and prolonged myelotoxicity. Cumulative nephrotoxicity and pulmonary toxicity (with doses > 1,200–1,500 mg/m²)
- BEFORE TREATMENT: full blood count, liver and renal function tests (creatinine clearance), pulmonary function tests

### Melphalan (MPL)

| | |
|---|---|
| **Chem:** | 4-[Bis(2-chloroethyl)amino]-L-phenylalanine<br>L-phenylalanine mustard (L-PAM), alkylating agent |

$$H_2C-H_2C-\bigcirc-N\begin{cases}CH_2-CH_2-Cl\\CH_2-CH_2-Cl\end{cases}$$

with $H_2N$ and $HOOC$ on the side chain.

**MOA:**
- DNA and RNA alkylation, DNA strand breaks, cross-linking
- Cell-cycle-specific: S/G2 phases

**Pkin:**
- *Kinetics:* oral bioavailability, interindividual variation (20–90%), half-life: initial $t\frac{1}{2}$ 6–8 min, terminal $t\frac{1}{2}$ 1–4 h
- *Metabolism:* spontaneous degradation by hydrolysis to inactive dechlorinated metabolites, renal excretion of unchanged drug (10–15%) and metabolites

**Se:**
- *Bone marrow:* delayed myelosuppression (dose-limiting), leukopenia, thrombocytopenia, lasting up to 4–6 weeks, hemolytic anemia (rare)
- *Pulmonary:* pulmonary fibrosis (rare), pneumonitis, especially with high-dose therapy
- *Gastrointestinal:* nausea, vomiting, mucositis, loss of appetite, diarrhea, especially after high-dose therapy
- *Liver:* hepatic veno-occlusive disease (VOD) after high-dose therapy
- *Skin:* alopecia (rare), exanthema, erythema, urticaria, pruritus, edema
- *Other:* infertility (amenorrhea, oligospermia). Allergic reactions/anaphylaxis (rare). Inadequate ADH secretion syndrome (rare), hyponatremia

**Ci:** Severely impaired renal function

**Th:** *Approved indications:* multiple myeloma, ovarian cancer
*Other areas of use:* breast cancer, thyroid cancer, testicular tumors, limb perfusion (melanoma), high-dose therapy before stem cell transplantation

### Dosage and Administration
- Standard dose: various protocols:
  - 0.1–0.2 mg/kg body weight/day (8–10 mg/m$^2$/day) p.o., for 4–5 days
  - 0.25 mg/kg body weight/day (10–15 mg/m$^2$/day) p.o. for 4–7 days, every 4–6 weeks
- High-dose therapy: 140–200 mg/m$^2$/day i.v. on day 1 (*ATTN:* only in transplant centers)
- Dose modification ▶ Chap. 3.2.4, incompatibility ▶ Chap. 3.2.6, stability ▶ Chap. 3.2.7
- BEFORE TREATMENT: full blood count, liver and renal function tests (creatinine clearance)

## Mercaptopurine (6-MP, Purinethol)

**Chem:**   1,7-dihydro-6H-purine-6-thione, purine analog (hypoxanthine analog), antimetabolite

**MOA:**
- Inhibition of de novo purine synthesis and purine conversion, chromosome breaks
- Cell-cycle-specific: S phase

**Pkin:**
- *Kinetics:* oral bioavailability 5–35% (interindividual variation), first-pass hepatic metabolism, half-life: terminal t½ 0.5–3 h
- *Metabolism:* intracellular activation with formation of various active metabolites (ribonucleotide derivatives). Hepatic degradation by xanthine oxidase ($\rightarrow$ half-life prolonged if xanthine oxidase inhibitors given, e.g., allopurinol), biliary (80–85%) and renal (5–20%) excretion

**Se:**
- *Bone marrow:* myelotoxic (dose-limiting), leukopenia, thrombocytopenia, anemia
- *Gastrointestinal:* moderate nausea, vomiting, loss of appetite in 25% of patients, mucositis, diarrhea, abdominal pain
- *Liver:* transient elevation of transaminases, cholestasis in 30% of patients, severe liver impairment in isolated cases, hepatic veno-occlusive disease (VOD)
- *Kidney:* reversible decrease of renal function, hyperuricemia
- *Skin:* dermatitis (rare), exanthema, hyperpigmentation, moderate alopecia
- *Other:* fever, immunosuppression

**Ci:**   Severely impaired liver function

**Th:**   *Approved indications:* ALL
*Other areas of use:* AML, CML, NHL, polycythemia vera, chronic inflammatory diseases

### Dosage and Administration
- Standard dose: 70–100 mg/m²/day p.o. daily (1.5–2.5 mg/kg body weight/day)
- Dose modification ▶ Chap. 3.2.4
- ATTN: reduce dose to 25% with concurrent administration of allopurinol
- BEFORE TREATMENT: full blood count, liver and renal function tests (creatinine clearance)

## Methotrexate (MTX, Amethopterin)

**Chem:** 4-Amino-10-methylfolic acid derivative, antimetabolite

**MOA:**
- Dihydrofolate reductase $\downarrow$ → tetrahydrofolic acid formation $\downarrow$ → DNA synthesis $\downarrow$
- Cell-cycle-specific: S phase

**Pkin:**
- *Kinetics:* 50–70% plasma protein-bound, half-life: terminal t½ 8–10 h
- *Metabolism:* hepatic inactivation by 7-hydroxylation (20–45%), renal and biliary excretion of unchanged drug (80%) and metabolites (20%)

**Se:**
- *Bone marrow:* myelosuppression (dose-limiting), leukopenia, thrombocytopenia
- *Pulmonary:* pneumonitis (rare), pulmonary fibrosis
- *Gastrointestinal:* pronounced mucositis (dose-limiting), moderate nausea / vomiting, diarrhea, gastrointestinal bleeding (rare)
- *Liver:* impaired liver function, elevated transaminases
- *Kidney:* renal tubular damage (dose-limiting), especially with acidic urine (pH < 7.0)
- *Skin:* dermatitis, erythema, exanthema, pruritus, conjunctivitis, alopecia (rare), palmar-plantar erythrodysesthesia
- *Nervous system:* reversible acute encephalopathy, leukoencephalopathy, confusion, motor and sensory disturbances, seizures, coma
- *Other:* allergic reactions, anaphylaxis, vasculitis

**Ci:**
- "Third space" fluid deposits: pleural effusions, ascites, etc.
- Impaired renal and liver function, gastrointestinal ulcers

**Th:** *Approved indications:* leukemias, malignant lymphomas, meningeal leukemia, solid tumors, psoriasis vulgaris, rheumatoid arthritis
*Other areas of use:* immunosuppression with allogeneic stem cell transplantation

### Dosage and Administration
- Low-dose: 20–60 mg/m²/day i.v. weekly or 4–6 mg/m²/day p.o. on days 1–3
- Medium-high dose: 500 mg/m²/day i.v. every 2–3 weeks with leucovorin rescue
- High-dose: up to 12,000 mg/m² i.v. with leucovorin rescue. ATTN: only at hematology/oncology centers. High risk of severe side effects
- May be administered intrathecally (maximum 15 mg absolute), orally or intramuscularly
- Dose modification ► Chap. 3.2.4, incompatibility ► Chap. 3.2.6, stability ► Chap. 3.2.7
- ATTN: not to be given in combination with nephrotoxic drugs. Not to be given in combination with acetylsalicylic acid, penicillin, sulfonamides, phenytoin (renal excretion $\downarrow$). Accumulates in fluid-filled spaces (pleural effusions, ascites) → t½ $\uparrow\uparrow$ → toxicity $\uparrow\uparrow$
- BEFORE TREATMENT: full blood count, liver and renal function tests (creatinine clearance). Fluid replacement (urine volume > 200 ml/h), alkalinization (urine pH > 7.4)

### Folinic Acid (Calcium Folinate, Leucovorin):
- Folinic acid is an antidote for medium-high dose and high-dose methotrexate therapy
- Folinic acid is usually started 24 h after methotrexate and given for at least 36 h (with close monitoring of the serum methotrexate level)

### Miltefosine

**Chem:**  2-(Hexadecoxy-oxido-phosphoryl)oxyethyl-trimethyl-ammonium
Alkylphosphocholine

$$CH_3 - (CH_2)_{15} - O - PO_3^- - (CH_2)_2 - N^+(CH_3)_3$$

**MOA:**
- Inhibition of the membrane-based enzyme systems

**Pkin:**
- Topical application → no evidence of effective systemic levels

**Se:**
- *Skin:* with local application: pruritus, erythema, tense feeling in skin, skin dryness, desquamation, burning

**Ci:**
- Concurrent radiotherapy
- Large nodular / deep-seated metastases with simultaneous skin involvement

**Th:**  *Approved indications:* cutaneous metastases of breast cancer

### Dosage and Administration
- Standard dose: 1 × /day in the first week to the involved skin area, thereafter twice a day, 1–2 drops per 10 cm², not more than 5 ml/day in total
- Hormone therapy or chemotherapy may be given concurrently

### Mitomycin C (MMC)

**Chem:** Antineoplastic antibiotic, aziridine derivative, bifunctional alkylating agent

**MOA:**
- DNA alkylation, cross-linking, DNA depolymerization, generation of free radicals → strand breaks
- Cell-cycle-specific: G1/S phases

**Pkin:**
- *Kinetics:* half-life: initial t½ 8 min, terminal t½ 50 min
- *Metabolism:* intracellular activation by opening of the aziridine ring, hepatic degradation to inactive metabolites, renal excretion of unchanged drug (25%) and metabolites

**Se:**
- *Bone marrow:* cumulative myelosuppression (dose-limiting), often severe and prolonged leukopenia and thrombocytopenia (lasting up to 6–8 weeks). In rare cases microangiopathic hemolytic anemia (MAHA)
- *Cardiovascular:* heart failure (rare), ischemia
- *Pulmonary:* pulmonary toxicity (pneumonitis, fibrosis) in up to 10% of patients
- *Gastrointestinal:* moderate nausea / vomiting, loss of appetite, mucositis
- *Liver:* impaired liver function (rare), transient elevation of transaminases
- *Kidney:* impaired renal function (rare), hemolytic uremic syndrome
- *Skin:* alopecia, erythema, photosensitivity
- *Nervous system:* headache (rare), visual disturbances, paresthesia
- *Local toxicity* (extravasation ▶ Chap. 9.9): local phlebitis, necrosis
- *Other:* fever (rare), allergic reactions, fatigue

**Ci:**
- Severely impaired liver or renal function
- Pre-existing cardiac or pulmonary disease (coronary heart disease, COPD, etc.)

**Th:** *Approved indications:* gastric cancer, pancreatic cancer
*Other areas of use:* head and neck tumors, gastrointestinal tumors, lung cancer, bladder cancer, breast cancer, prostate cancer, cervical cancer

### Dosage and Administration
- Standard dose: various protocols:
  Monotherapy: 10–20 mg/m²/day i.v. on day 1, every 6–8 weeks
  Polychemotherapy: 5–10 mg/m²/day i.v. on day 1, every 6 weeks
- Topical use: bladder instillation: 20–40 mg absolute
- Dose modification ▶ Chap. 3.2.4, incompatibility ▶ Chap. 3.2.6, stability ▶ Chap. 3.2.7
- BEFORE TREATMENT: full blood count, liver and renal function tests (creatinine clearance), cardiopulmonary evaluation

### Mitoxantrone

**Chem:**  1,4-Dihydroxy-5,8-bis[[2-[(2-hydroxyethyl)amino]ethyl]amino]anthraquinone dihydrochloride
Dihydroxyanthracenedione, synthetic anthracycline analog

**MOA:**
- DNA intercalation, induction of DNA strand breaks, inhibition of topoisomerase II
- Cell-cycle-specific: S/G2 phases

**Pkin:**
- *Kinetics:* enters cerebrospinal fluid, tissue accumulation, half-life: terminal t½ 40–190 h
- *Metabolism:* hepatic degradation, side chain oxidation, renal and biliary excretion of unchanged drug and metabolites

**Se:**
- *Bone marrow:* myelosuppression dose-limiting, especially leukopenia
- *Cardiovascular:* chronic cardiotoxicity: cardiomyopathy, heart failure (less pronounced in comparison to doxorubicin) from total cumulative dose > 160 mg/m²
- *Gastrointestinal:* moderate nausea / vomiting, mucositis, gastrointestinal bleeding (rare), abdominal pain, diarrhea
- *Liver:* transient elevation of transaminases, cholestasis (rare)
- *Kidney:* transient disturbances of renal function
- *Skin:* moderate alopecia, allergic reactions, dermatitis, pruritus, blue discoloration of sclera / finger nails / injection site and urine (reversible after 48 h)
- *Other:* infertility, headache, allergic reactions (rare)

**Ci:**
- Severely impaired liver and renal function, acute infections
- Pre-existing cardiac disease, myocardial impairment, previous anthracycline administration at the maximum tolerated cumulative dose

**Th:**
*Approved indications:* prostate cancer, AML
*Other areas of use:* CML, NHL, cerebral tumors, lung cancer, breast cancer, hepatocellular cancer, high-dose therapy before stem cell transplantation

#### Dosage and Administration
- Standard dose: various protocols:
  - Solid tumors: 12–14 mg/m²/day i.v. on day 1, every 3 weeks
  - Acute leukemia (in combination with cytarabine): 10–12 mg/m²/day i.v. on days 1–5
- Dose modification ▶ Chap. 3.2.4, incompatibility ▶ Chap. 3.2.6, stability ▶ Chap. 3.2.7
- ATTN: cumulative threshold dose 160 mg/m² (increased risk of cardiotoxicity)
- BEFORE TREATMENT: full blood count, liver and renal function tests (creatinine clearance). Cardiac evaluation, echocardiogram / radionuclide ventriculography if risk factors present

### Nimustine (ACNU)

**Chem:** 1-(4-Amino-2-methyl-5-pyrimidinyl)methyl-3-(2-chloroethyl)-3-nitrosourea
Alkylating agent

**MOA:**
- DNA and RNA alkylation ($O^6$ position of guanine), DNA strand breaks, cross-linking, inhibition of DNA polymerase and RNA synthesis
- Cell cycle non-specific (including G0 phase)

**Pkin:**
- *Kinetics:* lipophilic compound, enters cerebrospinal fluid, half-life: t½ 30–60 min
- *Metabolism:* spontaneous degradation into inactive metabolites, renal excretion of unchanged drug and metabolites

**Se:**
- *Bone marrow:* prolonged and cumulative myelosuppression (dose-limiting), leukopenia and thrombocytopenia, with slow recovery
- *Gastrointestinal:* nausea / vomiting, mucositis, diarrhea
- *Liver:* transient elevation of transaminases
- *Kidney:* impaired renal function (rare)
- *Skin:* alopecia, dermatitis, hyperpigmentation
- *Nervous system:* peripheral and central neurotoxicity
- *Other:* infertility

**Ci:**
- Pre-existing bone marrow dysfunction, acute infections
- Severely impaired liver or renal function

**Th:** *Approved indications:* malignant gliomas, cerebral metastases, lung cancer, breast cancer, gastric cancer, colorectal cancer, CML, Hodgkin's disease, NHL

#### Dosage and Administration
- Standard dose: 90–100 mg/m²/day (or 2–3 mg/kg body weight/day) i.v. on day 1, every 4–8 weeks
- Dose modification ▶ Chap. 3.2.4, incompatibility ▶ Chap. 3.2.6, stability ▶ Chap. 3.2.7
- ATTN: cumulative, delayed and prolonged myelotoxicity
- BEFORE TREATMENT: full blood count, liver and renal function tests (creatinine clearance)

### Oxaliplatin

**Chem:**      Trans-1-diaminocyclohexane oxalato-platinum, platinum derivative

**MOA:**
- Platinum-DNA adduct with inhibition of DNA synthesis, DNA intercalation, cross-links, inhibition of RNA synthesis, inhibition of DNA repair mechanisms
- Cell cycle non-specific (including G0 phase)

**Pkin:**
- *Kinetics:* highly protein bound (70–95%), half-life: terminal $t\frac{1}{2}$ 9 days
- *Metabolism:* spontaneous formation of active metabolites, predominantly renal excretion of platinum and oxaliplatin metabolites

**Se:**
- *Bone marrow:* moderate myelosuppression, neutropenia
- *Gastrointestinal:* nausea, vomiting, diarrhea
- *Liver:* transient elevation of transaminases
- *Kidney:* reversible decrease of renal function (rare)
- *Skin:* moderate alopecia (rare)
- *Nervous system:* acute (< 1%): peripheral paresthesias and acute laryngeal / pharyngeal dysesthesia with a feeling of suffocation, induced / exacerbated by exposure to cold. Chronic (45%): cumulative peripheral sensory neuropathy (dose-limiting) with dysesthesia, paresthesia of the limbs, after total dose > 900–1,000 mg/m², exacerbated by exposure to cold, reversible after a few months in some cases
- *Local toxicity* (extravasation ▶ Chap. 9.9): causes necrosis
- *Other:* allergic reactions, fatigue, arthralgia

**Ci:**
- Severely impaired renal function
- Pre-existing bone marrow dysfunction
- Pre-existing peripheral sensory neuropathy
- Known intolerance to platinum

**Th:**      *Approved indications:* colorectal carcinoma
*Other areas of use:* lung cancer, esophageal cancer, ovarian cancer, head and neck tumors

#### Dosage and Administration
- Standard dose: various protocols:
    - 100–130 mg/m²/day i.v. on day 1, every 3 weeks
    - 85–100 mg/m²/day i.v. on day 1, every 2 weeks
- Dose modification ▶ Chap. 3.2.4, incompatibility ▶ Chap. 3.2.6, stability ▶ Chap. 3.2.7
- ATTN: cumulative, dose-limiting peripheral neurotoxicity with total cumulative dose > 1,000 mg/m²
- BEFORE TREATMENT: full blood count, liver and renal function tests (creatinine clearance), neurological evaluation

## Paclitaxel

**Chem:** Taxane derivative, plant alkaloid, mitotic inhibitor

**MOA:**
- Stabilization of tubulin polymers, inhibition of the spindle function, mitotic arrest
- Cell-cycle-specific: M phase

**Pkin:**
- *Kinetics:* highly protein-bound, half-life: initial t½ 20 min, terminal t½ 6 h (paclitaxel) to 27 h (protein-bound paclitaxel)
- *Metabolism:* hepatic degradation, cytochrome P450-dependent hydroxylation, biliary excretion (25%), renal excretion (< 10%)

**Se:**
- *Bone marrow:* myelosuppression dose-limiting, especially neutropenia, moderate thrombocytopenia, anemia
- *Cardiovascular:* cardiac conduction disorders (rare), arrhythmias, ischemia
- *Gastrointestinal:* nausea / vomiting, mucositis / diarrhea (rare)
- *Liver:* transient elevation of transaminases, hepatic impairment (rare)
- *Skin:* alopecia, erythema, nail changes
- *Nervous system:* peripheral neurotoxicity with paresthesias (especially with single doses > 175 mg/m²/day or total cumulative dose > 1,000 mg/m²), paralytic ileus (rare), in rare cases central nervous system disorders (headache, weakness, visual disturbances, seizures)
- *Local toxicity* (extravasation ▶ Chap. 9.9): phlebitis, necrosis
- *Other:* hypersensitivity reactions in 1–3% of patients (flushing, urticaria, transient myalgia / arthralgia, hypotension (rare), bronchospasm, angioedema, anaphylaxis), fatigue, reduced performance status, loss of appetite

**Ci:** Severely impaired liver function, pre-existing cardiac disease, neuropathy

**Th:** *Approved indications (paclitaxel):* breast cancer, ovarian cancer, lung cancer, Kaposis's sarcoma
*Approved indications (protein-bound paclitaxel):* metastatic breast cancer
*Other areas of use:* esophageal cancer, gastric cancer, bladder cancer, cervical cancer, prostate cancer, head and neck tumors, melanomas

### Dosage and Administration
- Monotherapy: 175–200 mg/m²/day i.v. on day 1 every 21 days or 80–100 mg/m²/day i.v. on day 1 weekly
- Polychemotherapy: 135–185 mg/m²/day i.v. on day 1 every 21 days or 60–100 mg/m²/day i.v. on day 1 weekly
- Protein-bound paclitaxel: 260 mg/m²/day i.v. on day 1 every 3 weeks
- Dose modification ▶ Chap. 3.2.4, incompatibility ▶ Chap. 3.2.6, stability ▶ Chap. 3.2.7
- ATTN: administration sequence important: always administer paclitaxel prior to cisplatin / carboplatin, but after anthracyclines (doxorubicin / epirubicin)
- BEFORE TREATMENT: full blood count, urea and electrolytes, liver and renal function tests (creatinine clearance), cardiac evaluation. Premedication with steroids (dexamethasone), H1/ H2 inhibitors (clemastine, famotidine), diuretics if necessary

### Pemetrexed

**Chem:** L-Glutamic acid, N-[4-[2-(2-amino-4,7-dihydro-4-oxo-1H-pyrrolo[2,3-d]pyrimidin-5-yl)ethyl]-benzoyl], folic acid antagonist, antimetabolite

**MOA:**
- Inhibition of thymidylate synthetase, dihydrofolate reductase and glycinamide ribonucleotide formyltransferase → inhibition of RNA synthesis
- Cell-cycle-specific: S phase

**Pkin:**
- *Kinetics:* half-life: terminal t½ 20 h
- *Metabolism:* negligible hepatic degradation, renal excretion of unchanged drug (70–90%) and metabolites

**Se:**
- *Bone marrow:* myelosuppression with neutropenia, thrombocytopenia, anemia
- *Cardiovascular:* pericarditis (rare)
- *Gastrointestinal:* nausea / vomiting (35%), mucositis, diarrhea, loss of appetite
- *Liver:* transient elevation of transaminases, hepatic impairment/hepatitis (rare)
- *Skin:* alopecia, erythema, palmar-plantar erythrodysesthesia (hand-foot syndrome)
- *Nervous system:* sensory peripheral neuropathy and acute neurotoxicity from functional folate deficiency → folic acid / vitamin $B_{12}$ prophylaxis
- *Other:* fatigue, reduced performance status

**Ci:** Pre-existing neurological disorders

**Th:** *Approved indications:* pleural mesothelioma, lung cancer (NSCLC)
*Other areas of use:* breast cancer, colon cancer, pancreatic cancer, head and neck tumors

#### Dosage and Administration
- Standard dose: 500 mg/m²/day i.v. on day 1, every 3 weeks
- Dose modification ▶ Chap. 3.2.4
- BEFORE TREATMENT: full blood count, liver and renal function tests. Prophylactic administration of folic acid 350–1,000 µg (starting 5 days before therapy and until 21 days after therapy) and vitamin B12 1,000 µg i.m. (1 week before therapy, as well as after every 3rd therapy cycle)

**Pentostatin (DCF)**

**Chem:**     2'-Deoxycoformycin, purine analog, antimetabolite

**MOA:**
- Inhibition of adenosine deaminase, inhibition of ribonucleotide reductase → inhibition of DNA synthesis
- Inhibition of homocysteine hydrolase, lymphocytotoxic effects

**Pkin:**
- *Kinetics:* half-life: initial t½ 9 min, terminal t½ 5–14 h
- *Metabolism:* intracellular degradation to nucleotides, renal excretion (> 90%)

**Se:**
- *Bone marrow:* myelosuppression dose-limiting, pronounced leukopenia, lymphopenia, thrombocytopenia, anemia
- *Cardiovascular:* arrhythmias (rare), ECG changes, heart failure
- *Pulmonary:* cough, dyspnea, pulmonary infiltrates (rare)
- *Gastrointestinal:* moderate nausea / vomiting (50%), diarrhea (rare) / mucositis, dysgeusia
- *Liver:* transient elevation of transaminases, hepatitis (rare)
- *Kidney:* decreased renal function (increased incidence with inadequate hydration), renal tubular damage (rare), renal failure
- *Skin:* erythema / exanthema (25%), with increased photosensitivity in some cases, pruritus, exfoliative dermatitis, keratoconjunctivitis, periorbital edema
- *Nervous system:* central nervous system disorders (headache, tiredness, etc.), progressive encephalopathy (rare), seizures, coma
- *Other:* immunosuppression with T-cell deficiency, peripheral edema, fever, myalgia, headache, allergic reactions

**Ci:**
- Impaired renal function (creatinine clearance < 60 ml/min)
- Skin changes, central nervous system disorders

**Th:**     *Approved indications:* hairy cell leukemia
*Other areas of use:* cutaneous T-cell lymphomas, NHL

### Dosage and Administration
- Standard dose: 4 mg/m²/day i.v. every 14 days
- Dose modification ► Chap. 3.2.4, incompatibility ► Chap. 3.2.6, stability ► Chap. 3.2.7
- ATTN: due to the risk of decreased renal function, adequate fluid replacement necessary (1,000–2,000 ml). Not to be given in combination with fludarabine or cytarabine (pneumotoxic)
- BEFORE TREATMENT: full blood count, liver and renal function tests (creatinine clearance)

### Procarbazine

**Chem:**     N-Isopropyl-alpha-(2-methylhydrazino)-p-toluamide

$$H_3C-NH-NH-CH_2-\bigcirc-CO-NH-\underset{\underset{CH_3}{|}}{\overset{\overset{CH_3}{|}}{CH}}$$

**MOA:**
- DNA alkylation and depolymerization, methylation, inhibition of DNA, RNA and protein synthesis
- Cell-cycle-specific: S phase

**Pkin:**
- *Kinetics:* oral bioavailability 95–100%, enters cerebrospinal fluid, half-life: t½ 7 min, initial t½ 30–90 min, terminal t½ 60 min
- *Metabolism:* hepatic cytochrome P450-dependent activation, degradation to inactive metabolites, renal excretion

**Se:**
- *Bone marrow:* delayed myelosuppression (dose-limiting), nadir after 3–5 weeks
- *Cardiovascular:* tachycardia, hypotension
- *Gastrointestinal:* nausea / vomiting, mucositis (rare), dysphagia, diarrhea, loss of appetite
- *Liver:* transient elevation of transaminases
- *Skin:* alopecia (rare), erythema, exanthema, photosensitivity, hyperpigmentation, allergic reactions
- *Nervous system:* central nervous system disorders (headache, somnolence, agitation, depression, visual disturbances, hallucinations, ataxia, nystagmus, seizures) or mild reversible peripheral neurotoxicity
- *Other:* flu-like symptoms (fever, chills, myalgia, arthralgia), gynecomastia, infertility (amenorrhea, azoospermia)

**Ci:**
- Severely impaired liver or renal function
- Glucose-6-phosphate dehydrogenase (G6PD) deficiency

**Th:**     *Approved indications:* Hodgkin's disease, NHL
*Other areas of use:* plasmacytoma, CNS tumors, lung cancer, melanoma, polycythemia vera

#### Dosage and Administration
- Standard dose: 100 mg/m²/day p.o. on days 1–14, every 21–28 days
- Dose modification ► Chap. 3.2.4
- ATTN: Procarbazine is a monoamine oxidase inhibitor; interactions:
  - Alcohol: intolerance, flushing, tachycardia, neurological disorders
  - Antihistamines, barbiturates, phenothiazines, narcotics: synergistic effects, overdosage
  - Tricyclic antidepressants, L-dopa, sympathomimetics, tyramine-containing foods (milk products, red wine, etc.): hypertension, hypertensive crisis, coma
- BEFORE TREATMENT: full blood count, liver and renal function tests

### Raltitrexed

**Chem:** Folate analogue, quinazoline derivative

**MOA:**
- Inhibition of thymidylate synthetase $\rightarrow$ de novo thymidine synthesis $\downarrow$ $\rightarrow$ DNA synthesis $\downarrow$ DNA fragmentation
- Cell cycle specific: S phase

**Pkin:**
- *Kinetics*: 93% plasma protein-bound, half-life: terminal $t\frac{1}{2}$ 168 h
- *Metabolism*: intracellular conversion to polyglutamate forms, long-term intracellular retention
- *Elimination*: predominantly renal (>50%)

**Nw:**
- *Bone marrow*: myelosuppression dose-limiting, especially neutropenia, mostly mild to moderate
- *Gastrointestinal*: nausea, vomiting, anorexia, less frequently mucositis, diarrhea
- *Liver*: reversible increase in transaminases
- *Skin*: alopecia, dermatitis, erythema
- *Other*: asthenia, fever

**Ci:** Severe hepatic and renal impairment

**Th:** *Approved indications*: colorectal cancer

### *Dosage and Administration*
- Standard dose: 3 mg/m²/day i.v. on day 1, every 3 weeks
- Dose modification ▶ Chap. 2.2.4, incompatibility ▶ Chap. 2.2.7, stability ▶ Chap. 2.2.8
- ATTN: folic acid, folinic acid or vitamin preparations must not be given immediately prior to or during drug administration
- BEFORE TREATMENT: full blood count, liver and renal function tests

## Temozolomide

**Chem:**   3,4-Dihydro-3-methyl-4-oxoimidazo(5,1-d)-as-tetrazine-8-carboxamide
Methazolastone, alkylating agent

**MOA:**    Alkylating drug, DNA methylation at $O^6$ and $N^7$ positions of guanine, DNA strand breaks

**Pkin:**
- *Kinetics:* enteric absorption after protonation in the stomach, 100% bioavailability, enters cerebrospinal fluid, half-life: t½ 90–130 min
- *Metabolism:* activation to monomethyl triazeno imidazole carboxamide (MTIC), hepatic degradation, renal excretion of unchanged drug and metabolites, minor hepatobiliary and pulmonary excretion

**Se:**
- *Bone marrow:* myelosuppression dose-limiting, with leukopenia, lymphopenia, thrombocytopenia, anemia
- *Gastrointestinal:* nausea, vomiting, loss of appetite, constipation, mucositis (rare), diarrhea
- *Liver:* transient elevation of transaminases
- *Skin:* erythema, exanthema, photosensitivity, alopecia (rare)
- *Nervous system:* rarely, central nervous system disorders: headache, fatigue, vertigo, dysgeusia, paresthesias, seizures
- *Other:* fever, edema (rare)

**Ci:**     Severe myelosuppression

**Th:**     *Approved indications:* malignant gliomas: glioblastoma multiforme, anaplastic astrocytoma
*Other areas of use:* cerebral tumors, melanomas

### Dosage and Administration
- Standard dose: 200 mg/m²/day p.o. on days 1–5, repeat after 4 weeks
- For patients who have previously received chemotherapy, initial dose is 150 mg/m²/day on days 1–5 with repeat after 4 weeks, increasing dose to 200 mg/m²/day
- Dose modification ▶ Chap. 3.2.4
- ATTN: avoid sunlight
- BEFORE TREATMENT: full blood count, liver and renal function tests

### Teniposide (VM-26)

**Chem:** 4'-Demethylepipodophyllotoxin 9-(4,6-O-2-thenylidene-beta-D-glucopyranoside)
Epipodophyllotoxin derivative, plant alkaloid, topoisomerase II inhibitor

**MOA:**
- Inhibition of topoisomerase II → DNA strand breaks → mitotic arrest
- Cell-cycle-specific: G2 / S / M phases

**Pkin:**
- *Kinetics:* > 95% protein-bound, half-life: terminal t½ 5–14 h
- *Metabolism:* cytochrome P450 hepatic degradation (90%), renal excretion (10%)

**Se:**
- *Bone marrow:* myelosuppression dose-limiting, especially neutropenia, anemia (rare) and thrombocytopenia (rare)
- *Cardiovascular:* hypotension with rapid intravenous administration
- *Gastrointestinal:* nausea / vomiting (25%), mucositis (rare), diarrhea, gastrointestinal / perforation (rare)
- *Liver:* transient elevation of transaminases, hepatic veno-occlusive disease (VOD, rare)
- *Skin:* moderate alopecia, erythema (rare), hyperpigmentation
- *Nervous system:* rarely, peripheral neuropathy (paresthesias) or central nervous system disorders (headache, confusion, weakness, fatigue, seizures)
- *Other:* infertility, allergic reactions (fever, chills, bronchospasm, skin reactions), anaphylaxis

**Ci:** Severely impaired liver or renal function, pre-existing neurological disorders

**Th:** *Approved indications:* ALL, lymphomas, CNS tumors
*Other areas of use:* small cell lung cancer

### *Dosage and Administration*
- Standard dose: various protocols:
  - 20–60 mg/m²/day i.v. on days 1–5, every 2–3 weeks
  - 100–250 mg/m²/day i.v. on day 1, weekly for 4–8 weeks
  - 165 mg/m²/day i.v. on days 1 + 4, weekly for 4 weeks
- Dose modification ▶ Chap. 3.2.4, incompatibility ▶ Chap. 3.2.6
- BEFORE TREATMENT: full blood count, liver and renal function tests

## Thalidomide

**Chem:**  Alpha-(N-phthalimido)glutarimide

**MOA:**  Mechanism of action not fully characterized. Proposed mechanisms include:
- Immunomodulation: immunosuppressive properties, proinflammatory cytokines ↓, anti-inflammatory cytokines ↑, tumor necrosis factor α ↓, leukocyte migration ↓
- Anti-angiogenic properties, endothelial cell proliferation ↓

**Pkin:**
- *Kinetics:* oral bioavailability 90%, peak plasma concentration reached after 2.9–5.7 h, protein binding 55–66%, half-life t½ 5.5–7.3 h
- *Metabolism:* non-enzymatic hydrolysis in plasma

**Se:**
- *Bone marrow:* leukopenia, neutropenia
- *Pulmonary:* cough, dyspnea, upper respiratory tract infections, pneumonia
- *Cardiovascular:* edema, chest pain, atrial fibrillation, cardiac failure, myocardial infarction, tachycardia, bradycardia, orthostatic hypotension, thromboembolic events, pulmonary embolism
- *Gastrointestinal:* nausea, anorexia, constipation, abdominal pain
- *Hepatic:* transient increase of liver enzymes, hyperbilirubinemia
- *Kidney:* dysuria, hypocalcemia
- *Skin:* erythema, pruritus, rash, alopecia, Stevens-Johnson syndrome / toxic epidermal necrolysis (rare)
- *Nervous system:* headache, dizziness, drowsiness, somnolence, anxiety, tremor, confusion, peripheral neuropathy, seizures (rare)
- *Other:* fever, fatigue, infections, arthralgia, myalgia, back pain, asthenia, hypothyroidism

**Ci:**
- Pregnant women or women capable of becoming pregnant. Female patients must use two different methods of contraception. Male patients must use condoms.
- Hypersensitivity to thalidomide

**Th:**  *Approved indications:* multiple myeloma (newly diagnosed, first line with dexamethasone), erythema nodosum leprosum (ENL)
*Other areas of use:* MDS, Crohn's disease, graft-versus-host disease (GvHD)

### Dosage and Administration
- Standard dose: 100–800 mg p.o. daily
- ATTN: potential for life-threatening human birth defects. Appropriate precautions should be taken to avoid pregnancy and fathering. In order to avoid fetal exposure to thalidomide, in the US the drug is only available under a special restricted distribution program. Significantly increased risk of deep venous thrombosis and pulmonary embolism. Avoid concomitant use of alcohol, CNS depressants, and medications associated with peripheral neuropathy
- BEFORE TREATMENT: full blood count, liver and renal function tests, electrolytes, thyroid function, neurological status, pregnancy test (in women of childbearing potential)

### 6-Thioguanine (6-TG)

**Chem:**  2-Aminopurine-6(1H)-thione, purine analog (guanine analog), antimetabolite

**MOA:**
- Inhibition of de novo purine synthesis and purine conversion, chromosome breaks
- Cell-cycle-specific: S phase

**Pkin:**
- *Kinetics:* oral bioavailability variable (10–60%), interindividual variation in absorption over 8–12 h, half-life: terminal t½ 1.5–11 h
- *Metabolism:* intracellular activation and formation of various effective metabolites (ribonucleotide and deoxyribonucleotide derivatives), hepatic degradation, biliary excretion of metabolites

**Se:**
- *Bone marrow:* myelotoxicity dose-limiting, leukopenia, thrombocytopenia, anemia (rare)
- *Gastrointestinal:* mild nausea, vomiting, loss of appetite, mucositis, diarrhea, intestinal perforation in isolated cases
- *Liver:* transient elevation of transaminases, cholestasis (rare), hepatic veno-occlusive disease (VOD) in isolated cases
- *Kidney:* impaired renal function (rare), renal failure (rare)
- *Skin:* erythema (rare), dermatitis
- *Nervous system:* loss of vibration sensitivity, gait disorders

**Ci:**  Severely impaired liver function

**Th:**  *Approved indications:* ALL, AML, CML

### Dosage and Administration
- Standard dose: 80–200 mg/m²/day (2–3 mg/kg body weight/day) p.o. daily, for 5–20 days, to be taken on an empty stomach with fluids
- Dose modification ▶ Chap. 3.2.4
- BEFORE TREATMENT: full blood count, liver function tests

### Thiotepa

**Chem:**        Tris(1-aziridinyl)phosphine sulfide, aziridine, alkylating agent

**MOA:**
- DNA, RNA and protein alkylation, DNA strand breaks, cross-linking, inhibition of nucleic acid synthesis and protein synthesis
- Cell-cycle-specific: S / G2 phases

**Pkin:**
- *Kinetics:* readily enters cerebrospinal fluid, half-life: initial t½ 8 min, terminal t½ 2–3 h
- *Metabolism:* rapid decay in plasma, formation of bifunctional alkylating metabolites (main metabolite is TEPA, i.e., triethylenephosphoramide), renal excretion of unchanged drug (< 10%) and metabolites

**Se:**
- *Bone marrow:* myelosuppression dose-limiting, cumulative, leukopenia, thrombocytopenia and anemia (rare)
- *Gastrointestinal:* nausea, vomiting, mucositis, loss of appetite, diarrhea, enteritis, especially after high-dose therapy
- *Liver:* transient elevation of transaminases
- *Genitourinary:* impaired renal function (especially with high-dose therapy); with intravesical instillation: abdominal pain, hematuria, dysuria, ureteric obstruction
- *Skin:* erythema, dermatitis, alopecia (rare) after high-dose therapy, hyperpigmentation
- *Nervous system:* central neurotoxicity (headache, confusion, paresthesias, muscle weakness, somnolence, coma), especially with cumulative doses > 1,100 mg/m²
- *Other:* infertility, hyperuricemia, fever (rare), allergic reactions

**Ci:**        Severely impaired liver or renal function

**Th:**        *Approved indications:*
- *Systemic:* breast cancer, ovarian cancer, chronic leukemias, lymphomas
- *Local:* bladder tumors, condylomata, malignant effusions

### Dosage and Administration
- Due to good local tolerance, intravenous, intra-arterial, subcutaneous, intravesical, intrathecal, and intracavitary (intrapleural, intraperitoneal) administration possible
- Standard dose:
  - Systemic: 12–16 mg/m²/day i.v. on day 1 weekly or every 2–4 weeks
  - Local application: instillation of 15–60 mg absolute weekly, for 4 weeks
- High-dose therapy regimens: 125–150 mg/m²/day i.v. for 4 days on days 1–4 (*ATTN:* only in transplant centers)
- Incompatibility ▶ Chap. 3.2.6, stability ▶ Chap. 3.2.7
- BEFORE TREATMENT: full blood count, liver and renal function tests (creatinine clearance)

### Topotecan

**Chem:** Camptothecin analog, topoisomerase I inhibitor

**MOA:**
- Inhibition of topoisomerase I, DNA religation ↓↓ → DNA strand breaks and intercalation
- Cell-cycle-specific: G2 / M phases

**Pkin:**
- *Kinetics:* ubiquitous distribution, enters cerebrospinal fluid, accumulates in "third space" fluid deposits (pleural effusions, ascites), half-life: terminal t½ 2–6 h
- *Metabolism:* plasma degradation, renal excretion of unchanged drug (40–50%) and metabolites

**Se:**
- *Bone marrow:* myelosuppression dose-limiting, leukopenia (80%) and thrombocytopenia, anemia
- *Gastrointestinal:* diarrhea (30%), nausea, vomiting (10%), loss of appetite, mucositis
- *Liver:* transient elevation of transaminases, hyperbilirubinemia
- *Kidney:* impaired renal function, microscopic hematuria
- *Skin:* alopecia, erythema, urticaria (rare), pruritus
- *Nervous system:* headache, peripheral neurotoxicity (rare)
- *Other:* fever, fatigue, reduced performance status, dyspnea (rare), arthralgia (rare), myalgia

**Ci:**
- Acute infection
- "Third space" fluid deposits (ascites, pleural effusions)

**Th:**
*Approved indications:* ovarian cancer, small cell lung cancer, cervical carcinoma
*Other areas of use:* AML, NHL, cerebral metastases

#### Dosage and Administration
- Standard dose: 1.5 mg/m²/day i.v. on days 1–5, every 3 weeks
- Dose modification ► Chap. 3.2.4, incompatibility ► Chap. 3.2.6, stability ► Chap. 3.2.7
- ATTN: with combination therapy regimens, topotecan must be administered prior to cisplatin. Dose must be increased with concurrent administration of anticonvulsive therapy
- BEFORE TREATMENT: full blood count, liver and renal function tests (creatinine clearance)

### Treosulfan

**Chem:**  L-Threitol-1,4-bis (methanesulfonate), bifunctional alkylating agent

$$H_3C-\overset{\overset{\displaystyle O}{\|}}{\underset{\underset{\displaystyle O}{\|}}{S}}-O-CH_2-\overset{\overset{\displaystyle OH}{|}}{CH}-\overset{\overset{}{}}{\underset{\underset{\displaystyle OH}{|}}{CH}}-CH_2-O-\overset{\overset{\displaystyle O}{\|}}{\underset{\underset{\displaystyle O}{\|}}{S}}-CH_3$$

**MOA:**
- DNA and RNA alkylation ($N^7$ position of guanine), DNA strand breaks, cross-linking
- Cell-cycle-specific: S / G2 phases

**Pkin:**
- *Kinetics:* oral bioavailability 90%, half-life: terminal t½ 1.5–2 h
- *Metabolism:* spontaneous activation in plasma, degradation to inactive metabolites, renal excretion of unchanged drug (15%) and metabolites

**Se:**
- *Bone marrow:* myelosuppression dose-limiting, long neutropenic phase, thrombocytopenia
- *Pulmonary:* pulmonary fibrosis (rare), allergic alveolitis, pneumonia
- *Gastrointestinal:* moderate nausea / vomiting, mucositis, diarrhea
- *Liver:* transient disturbances of liver function, cholestasis
- *Skin:* erythema, urticaria, pruritus, hyperpigmentation, alopecia
- *Nervous system:* paresthesias
- *Local toxicity* (extravasation ▶ Chap. 9.9): phlebitis, necrosis
- *Other:* hemorrhagic cystitis (rare), allergic reactions, flu-like symptoms

**Ci:**  Pulmonary function disorders, pre-existing bone marrow dysfunction

**Th:**  *Approved indications:* ovarian tumors
*Other areas of use:* lung cancer (NSCLC), esophageal cancer, head and neck tumors

### Dosage and Administration
- Standard dose: various protocols:
    - *Intravenously:* 5,000–8,000 mg/m²/day i.v. on day 1, every 21–28 days
    - *Orally:* 750–1,250 mg/day p.o. on days 1–28, every 56 days to be taken with food
- Incompatibility ▶ Chap. 3.2.6, stability ▶ Chap. 3.2.7
- BEFORE TREATMENT: full blood count, liver and renal function tests, pulmonary function evaluation

## Trofosfamide

**Chem:** N,N,3-Tris(2-chloroethyl)tetrahydro-2H-1,3,2-oxazaphosphorin-2-amine 2-oxide
Oxazaphosphorine, alkylating agent

$$\text{O} \quad CH_2 - CH_2 - Cl$$
$$O \quad \parallel \qquad | $$
$$\diagdown P - N - CH_2 - CH_2 - Cl$$
$$\diagdown \quad | $$
$$N - CH_2 - CH_2 - Cl$$

**MOA:**
- DNA and RNA alkylation, DNA strand breaks, cross-linking, inhibition of DNA synthesis
- Cell-cycle-specific: S phase

**Pkin:**
- *Kinetics:* oral bioavailability > 95%, half-life: terminal t½ 4–8 h
- *Metabolism:* hepatic hydroxylation by microsomal cytochrome P450 monooxygenase to 4-hydroxytrofosfamide, active metabolites released in plasma and tissues, hepatic degradation, renal excretion of unchanged drug (5–15%) and metabolites

**Se:**
- *Bone marrow:* Myelosuppression dose-limiting, leukopenia and thrombocytopenia
- *Gastrointestinal:* moderate nausea / vomiting, loss of appetite
- *Liver:* transient elevation of transaminases
- *Genitourinary:* hemorrhagic cystitis with high-dose therapy or prolonged treatment (dose-limiting)
- *Skin:* alopecia
- *Other:* moderate immunosuppression

**Ci:**
- Severely impaired liver or renal function, acute infections
- Cystitis, urinary tract obstruction

**Th:** *Approved indications:* maintenance therapy for hematological neoplasms (e.g., CLL, Hodgkin's disease, NHL, plasmacytoma, Waldenström's macroglobulinemia) and solid tumors (e.g., ovarian cancer, breast cancer, small cell lung cancer, seminoma)

### Dosage and Administration
- Oral administration with plenty of fluids, standard dose:
    - Initial therapy: 150–200 mg/m²/day p.o.
    - Maintenance dose: 25–100 mg/m²/day p.o.
- Dose modification ▶ Chap. 3.2.4
- ATTN: enhances the effects of sulfonylureas. Effects enhanced by barbiturates (cytochrome P450 activation) and cimetidine
- BEFORE TREATMENT: full blood count, liver and renal function tests

### UFT (Tegafur-Uracil)

**Chem:**    Tegafur: 5-fluoro-1-tetrahydro-2-furanyl-2,4(1H,3H)-pyrimidinedione
Uracil: 2,4(1H,3H)-pyrimidinedione

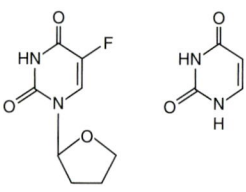

Tegafur          Uracil

**MOA:**
- Tegafur (Ftorafur) is metabolized in vivo to 5-FU. Uracil inhibits further degradation of 5-FU → t½ prolonged
- Inhibition of thymidylate synthetase by FdUMP → thymidine synthesis ↓
- Incorporated into RNA, inhibition of RNA synthesis by FUTP
- Cell-cycle-specific: S phase

**Pkin:**
- *Metabolism:* Conversion to 5-FU, intracellular activation and phosphorylation (formation of FdUMP, FUTP, etc.). Degradation in liver and intestinal mucosa by dihydropyrimidine dehydrogenase is reduced by uracil, metabolic (90%), renal (10%) excretion

**Se:**
- *Bone marrow:* mild myelosuppression
- *Cardiovascular:* rarely acute cardiotoxicity with arrhythmias, ischemia, myocardial infarction in isolated cases
- *Gastrointestinal:* nausea, vomiting, diarrhea, abdominal pain
- *Liver:* elevated transaminases, bilirubin ↑ (rare)
- *Kidney:* proteinuria (rare) and hematuria
- *Skin:* erythema, pruritus, dermatitis, pigmentation disorders, alopecia (especially with long-term use), palmar-plantar erythrodysesthesia
- *Nervous system:* in rare cases central nervous system changes (headache, vertigo, somnolence, confusion), dysgeusia
- *Other:* fever, fatigue, reduced performance status, arthralgia

**Ci:**
- Severely impaired liver function
- Pre-existing stomatitis / diarrhea / myelosuppression
- CyP2A6 deficiency

**Th:**    *Approved indications:* colorectal cancer
*Other areas of use:* gastrointestinal tumors, breast cancer, other solid tumors

#### Dosage and Administration
- Standard dose: 300 mg/m²/day p.o. for 28 days, then no therapy for 7 days
- Dose modification ▶ Chap. 3.2.4, stability 2 years at room temperature
- BEFORE TREATMENT: full blood count, liver and renal function tests

### Vinblastine

**Chem:** Vincaleukoblastine, alkaloid extracted from *Vinca rosea*, mitotic inhibitor

**MOA:**
- Binds to tubulin $\rightarrow$ formation of mitotic spindle microtubules $\downarrow$ $\rightarrow$ mitotic arrest
- Inhibition of DNA-dependent RNA polymerases $\rightarrow$ RNA synthesis $\downarrow$
- Cell-cycle-specific: G2 / M phases

**Pkin:**
- *Kinetics:* half-life: initial t½ < 5 min, terminal t½ 20–64 h
- *Metabolism:* hepatic activation (deacetylation), hepatic metabolism (cytochrome P450-dependent), biliary (30%) and renal (25%) excretion

**Se:**
- *Bone marrow:* myelosuppression dose-limiting, neutropenia, thrombocytopenia (rare) / anemia
- *Cardiovascular:* cardiovascular disorders, hypertension, hypotension
- *Pulmonary:* pulmonary toxicity with acute interstitial pneumonitis / bronchospasm when given in combination with mitomycin
- *Gastrointestinal:* mild nausea / vomiting, diarrhea, mucositis, constipation (in severe cases paralytic ileus), intestinal spasm (rare), gastrointestinal bleeding (rare)
- *Skin:* moderate alopecia, erythema, exanthema, photosensitivity
- *Nervous system:* moderate peripheral neurotoxicity (cumulative) with paresthesias, motor disturbances (rare), less pronounced than with vincristine or vindesine
- *Local toxicity* (extravasation ▶ Chap. 9.9): phlebitis, necrosis
- *Other:* muscle spasms in mandible/ neck / back / limbs

**Ci:** Impaired liver function, hepatic radiation, neuropathies, acute infections

**Th:** *Approved indications:* malignant lymphomas, testicular cancer, breast cancer, choriocarcinoma, Kaposi's sarcoma
*Other areas of use:* other solid tumors, CML

#### Dosage and Administration
- Standard dose: various protocols:
  - *Polychemotherapy:* 6 mg/m²/day i.v. on day 1 every 7–14 days
  - Monotherapy: 4 mg/m²/day i.v. on day 1 every 7 days, gradually increase by 2 mg/m²/day each week up to a maximum of 18 mg/m²/day
- Dose modification ▶ Chap. 3.2.4, incompatibility ▶ Chap. 3.2.6, stability ▶ Chap. 3.2.7
- ATTN: Cumulative neurotoxicity, enhanced by cisplatin, etoposide, paclitaxel. Regular neurological examination. Increased risk of paralytic ileus with administration of opiates
- BEFORE TREATMENT: full blood count, liver and renal function tests (creatinine clearance), neurological evaluation. Constipation prophylaxis

## Vincristine

**Chem:**    22-Oxovincaleukoblastine, alkaloid extracted from *Vinca rosea*, mitotic inhibitor

**MOA:**
- Binds to tubulin → formation of mitotic spindle microtubules ↓ → mitotic arrest
- Inhibition of DNA-dependent RNA polymerases → RNA synthesis ↓
- Cell-cycle-specific: G2 / M phases

**Pkin:**
- *Kinetics:* half-life: initial t½ < 5 min, terminal t½ 23–85 h
- *Metabolism:* hepatic metabolism, biliary excretion (> 70–80%), minor renal excretion

**Se:**
- *Bone marrow:* mild myelosuppression, especially neutropenia
- *Cardiovascular:* cardiovascular disorders, hypertension, hypotension
- *Pulmonary:* interstitial pneumonitis / bronchospasm (esp. when given in combination with mitomycin C)
- *Gastrointestinal:* constipation / ileus, nausea / vomiting, mucositis
- *Kidney:* polyuria (ADH secretion ↓), dysuria, urinary retention (bladder atony)
- *Skin:* moderate alopecia, erythema
- *Nervous system:* peripheral neurotoxicity (cumulative, dose-limiting), autonomic neurotoxicity, in some cases cranial nerve deficits and central nervous system disorders: hypesthesia, paresthesias, motor disorders, areflexia, in rare cases paralysis, ataxia, ileus, optic atrophy, blindness, seizures
- *Local toxicity* (extravasation ► Chap. 9.9): phlebitis, necrosis
- *Other:* muscle spasms / pain in mandible / neck / back / limbs, fever (rare), pancreatitis (rare)

**Ci:**    Impaired liver function, hepatic radiation, manifest neuropathies, constipation

**Th:**    *Approved indications:* lymphomas, leukemias, solid tumors (e.g., breast cancer, lung cancer, sarcomas, Wilms' tumor, neuroblastoma)
*Other areas of use:* other solid tumors

### Dosage and Administration
- Standard dose: 1.0–1.4 mg/m²/day i.v. on day 1, maximum single dose 2 mg (1 mg in patients over 65 years)
- Dose modification ► Chap. 3.2.4, incompatibility ► Chap. 3.2.6, stability ► Chap. 3.2.7
- ATTN: regular neurological examination. Cumulative neurotoxicity (especially with total doses > 20 mg). Neurotoxicity enhanced by cisplatin, etoposide, paclitaxel. Increased risk of ileus with administration of opiates
- BEFORE TREATMENT: full blood count, liver and renal function tests (creatinine clearance) neurological evaluation. Constipation prophylaxis

### Vindesine

**Chem:** 3-Carbamoyl-4-deacetyl-3-de(methoxy-carbonyl) vincaleukoblastine sulfate
Mitotic inhibitor

**MOA:**
- Binds to tubulin → formation of mitotic spindle microtubules ↓ → mitotic arrest
- Inhibition of DNA-dependent RNA polymerases → RNA synthesis ↓
- Cell-cycle-specific: G2 / M phases

**Pkin:**
- *Kinetics:* half-life: initial t½ < 5 min, terminal t½ 20–24 h
- *Metabolism:* hepatic metabolism (cytochrome P450-dependent), biliary excretion (> 80–90%) and renal excretion (10–15%)

**Se:**
- *Bone marrow:* myelosuppression (dose-limiting), especially neutropenia
- *Cardiovascular:* cardiovascular disorders, hypertension, hypotension
- *Pulmonary:* interstitial pneumonitis / bronchospasm (esp. when given in combination with mitomycin C)
- *Gastrointestinal:* constipation, nausea / vomiting (rare), mucositis
- *Skin:* alopecia (more pronounced than with vincristine), erythema
- *Nervous system:* peripheral, autonomic and central neurotoxicity similar to vincristine, but less pronounced: hypesthesia, paresthesias, motor disorders, areflexia
- *Local toxicity* (extravasation ▶ Chap. 9.9): phlebitis, necrosis
- *Other:* muscle spasms / pain in mandible / neck / back / limbs, fever (rare), pancreatitis (rare)

**Ci:** Impaired liver function, hepatic radiation, neuropathies, constipation

**Th:** *Approved indications:* leukemias, lymphomas, melanoma, lung cancer, breast cancer, esophageal cancer, testicular tumors, head and neck tumors
*Other areas of use:* other solid tumors, plasmacytoma

#### Dosage and Administration
- Standard dose: various protocols:
  - 3–4 mg/m²/day i.v. on day 1, every 7–14 days, maximum single dose: 5 mg absolute
  - 1.0–1.3 mg/m²/day i.v. for 5–7 days, every 3 weeks
- Dose modification ▶ Chap. 3.2.4, incompatibility ▶ Chap. 3.2.6, stability ▶ Chap. 3.2.7
- ATTN: regular neurological examination. Cumulative neurotoxicity enhanced by cisplatin, etoposide, paclitaxel. Risk of ileus with administration of opiates
- BEFORE TREATMENT: full blood count, liver and renal function tests, neurological evaluation. Constipation prophylaxis

### Vinorelbine

**Chem:**    3',4'-Didehydro-4'-deoxy-8'-norvincaleukoblastine, mitotic inhibitor

**MOA:**
- Binds to tubulin → formation of mitotic spindle microtubules ↓ → mitotic arrest
- Inhibition of DNA-dependent RNA polymerases → RNA synthesis ↓
- Cell-cycle-specific: G2 / M phases

**Pkin:**
- *Kinetics:* oral bioavailability 20–40%, half-life: initial t½ < 5 min, terminal t½ 18–49 h
- *Metabolism:* hepatic metabolism to active and inactive metabolites, biliary excretion (35–80%), minor renal excretion (15–30%)

**Se:**
- *Bone marrow:* myelosuppression dose-limiting, neutropenia, thrombocytopenia / anemia (rare)
- *Gastrointestinal:* nausea / vomiting / diarrhea / mucositis / constipation (rare)
- *Skin:* moderate alopecia
- *Nervous system:* peripheral neurotoxicity (cumulative) with paresthesias, motor disorders (rare), less pronounced than with vincristine or vindesine
- *Local toxicity* (extravasation ▶ Chap. 9.9): phlebitis, necrosis
- *Other:* muscle spasms / pain in mandible / neck / back / limbs (rare)

**Ci:**    Impaired liver function, radiotherapy, neuropathies

**Th:**    *Approved indications:* non-small cell lung cancer, breast cancer
*Other areas of use:* other solid tumors

#### Dosage and Administration
- Standard dose: 30 mg/m²/day i.v. on day 1, weekly
- Dose modification ▶ Chap. 3.2.4, incompatibility ▶ Chap. 3.2.6, stability ▶ Chap. 3.2.7
- ATTN: regular neurological examination. Cumulative neurotoxicity, enhanced by cisplatin, etoposide, paclitaxel. Risk of paralytic ileus with administration of opiates
- BEFORE TREATMENT: full blood count, liver and renal function tests, neurological evaluation. Constipation prophylaxis

**3.2.2**     **Check List Cytostatic Treatment**

**D.P. Berger**

**Def:**    Every cytostatic treatment carries the risk of adverse and potentially life-threatening effects. Therefore, it is imperative to observe general treatment guidelines as well as specific precautions for certain cytostatics.

**Meth:**    The procedures listed below are mandatory in all patients before and during cytostatic treatment. However, this list is not exhaustive. Additional measures may be indicated, depending on the patient's general condition, pre-existing disorders, and the disease situation.

**Recommended procedures / check-ups in cytostatic therapy**

| Compounds | Procedures / tests |
|---|---|
| All cytostatics | Case history, clinical examination; exhaustive patient counseling and obtaining of informed consent before treatment; information on sperm / oocyte preservation (▶ Chaps. 4.10.1, 4.10.2), and potentially necessary supportive measures (transfusion therapy, antiemesis, etc.) Blood count, liver / renal function tests, inflammation parameters |
| • Anthracyclines, amsacrine, mitoxantrone | Serum bilirubin, ECG, with suspected cardiopathies / cardiac insufficiency: echocardiography or radionuclide ventriculography |
| • Asparaginase | Blood glucose, lipase, coagulation status, neurostatus |
| • Bleomycin, busulfan | Pulmonary function, chest x-rays |
| • Carmustine, lomustine | Pulmonary function, chest x-rays, neurostatus |
| • Cisplatin | Creatinine clearance, serum magnesium, neurostatus, possibly audiometry, fluid therapy, osmotic diuresis |
| • Cladribine, fludarabine, pentostatin | Lymphocyte subpopulations (especially CD4- / CD8-positive T-cells), neurostatus |
| • Cyclophosphamide, ifosfamide | Fluid therapy, mesna, alkalization |
| • Methotrexate | Creatinine clearance, rule out ascites and pleural effusion, fluid therapy, alkalization, possibly leucovorin rescue, methotrexate serum levels |
| • 6-Mercaptopurine | Dose reduction in case of simultaneous administration of allopurinol |
| • Pemetrexed | Prophylactic administration of folic acid and vitamin $B_{12}$ |
| • Taxanes | Cardiac check-up, neurostatus, premedication with steroids and H1/H2 blocker |
| • Vinca alkaloids | Serum bilirubin, neurostatus, constipation prophylaxis |

**Ref:**    1.   Ginsberg JP, Womer WB. Preventing organ-specific chemotherapy toxicity. Eur J Cancer 2005;41:2690–700
        2.   Lee WM. Drug-induced hepatotoxicity. N Engl J Med 2003;349:474–85

**Web:**    1.   http://www.druginfonet.com/       Drug information
        2.   http://www.meds.com/DChome.html     Information on Cytostatics

### 3.2.3    Drug Dosage Calculation Based on Body Surface Area (BSA)

**C.I. Müller, D.P. Berger, M. Engelhardt**

**Def:**    Many important pharmacokinetic parameters (e.g., renal function, liver function) correlate particularly with the body surface area (BSA). Therefore, dosage recommendations for cytostatics are generally based on the patient's body surface area (in $m^2$). Height and weight are used to calculate BSA.

**Meth:**    *Normal-weight Patients*
Body surface area (BSA) calculation is based on empirical formulas:

*Body Surface Area Calculation by Mosteller*

$$\text{Body Surface Area } (m^2) = (\text{ Height (cm)} \times \text{Weight (kg)} / 3{,}600 )^{0.5}$$

*Body Surface Area Calculation by Gehan and George*

$$\text{Body Surface Area } (m^2) = 0.0235 \times \text{Height (cm)}^{0.42245} \times \text{Weight (kg)}^{0.51456}$$

Simplified formulas are not sufficiently accurate for clinical use and should not be used for calculating the dosage of cytostatics. Sufficiently accurate alternatives used in everyday clinical practice are slide charts, BSA tables, or so called nomograms. Alternatively, many internet pages provide online body surface area calculations or offer BSA calculators for download.

*Obese Patients*
In obese patients, various cytostatic dosages have to be adapted to the body weight.
Rule of thumb:
- With palliative indication: limiting of body surface area-based cytostatic dosage to a maximum of 2 $m^2$
- With curative indication: dosage calculation based on "ideal body weight" (IBW) or "adapted IBW" (▶ Chap. 3.2.4)

**Ref:**
1. Bailey BJ, Briars GL. Estimating the surface area of the human body. Stat Med 1996;15:1325–32
2. Baker SD, Verweij J, Rowinsky EK et al. Role of body surface area in dosing of investigational anticancer agents in adults, 1991-2001. J Natl Cancer Inst 2002;94:883–8
3. Gehan EA, George SL. Estimation of human body surface area from height and weight. Cancer Chemother Rep 1970;54:225–35
4. Mosteller RD. Simplified calculation of body-surface area. N Engl J Med 1987;317:1098
5. Reilly JJ, Workman P. Normalization of anti-cancer drug dosage using body weight and surface area: is it worthwhile? Cancer Chemother Pharmacol 1993;32:411–8

**Web:**
1. http://www.halls.md/body-surface-area/refs.htm        BSA, Formulas and Comments
2. http://www.halls.md/body-surface-area/bsa.htm        BSA Calculation
3. http://www.ultradrive.com/bsac.htm        BSA Calculation

**Nomogram for determination of the body surface area of an adult**

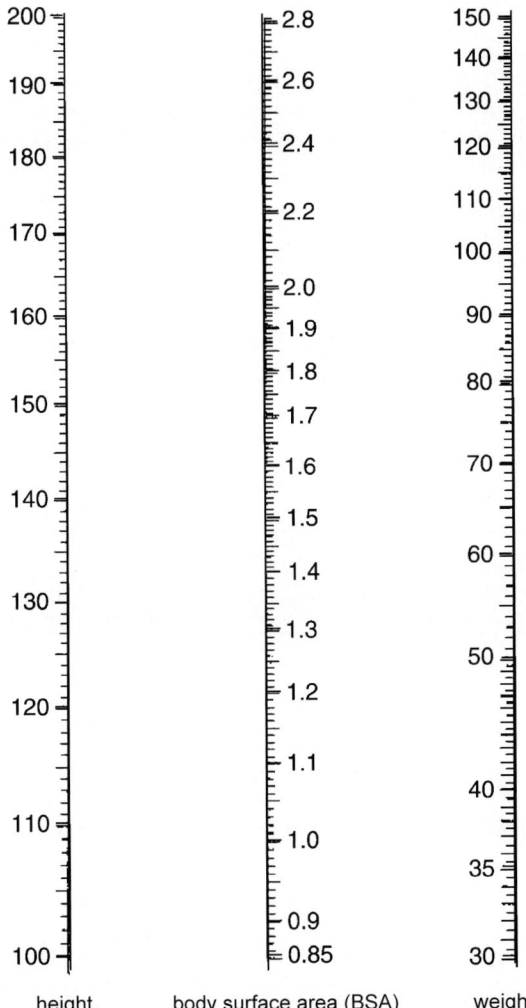

| height | body surface area (BSA) | weight |

## 3.2.4     Dose Adjustment of Cytostatic Drugs

**W. Digel**

The individual doses of cytostatic drugs should be adapted to the current status of the patient. Primarily, the following parameters should be taken into consideration: hematological situation, liver function, renal function, performance status, expected toxicity (e.g., cardiotoxicity, oto-, neurotoxicity, mucosal toxicity) and comorbidities.

**Phys:**

### Renal Parameters: Creatinine Clearance

#### Calculation

$$\text{Creatinine Clearance (ml/min)} = \frac{\text{Creatinine}_{Urine}\ (\text{mg/dl}) \times \text{Urine Volume (ml)}}{\text{Creatinine}_{Serum}\ (\text{mg/dl}) \times \text{Time (min)}}$$

#### Estimation

$$\male \quad \text{Creatinine Clearance (ml/min)} = \frac{\text{Body Weight (kg)} \times (140 - \text{Age})}{\text{Creatinine}_{Serum}\ (\text{mg/dl}) \times 72}$$

$$\female \quad \text{Creatinine Clearance (ml/min)} = \frac{\text{Body Weight(kg)} \times (120 - \text{Age})}{\text{Creatinine}_{Serum}\ (\text{mg/dl}) \times 72}$$

### Liver Parameters

The following parameters are used to evaluate liver function:
- Bilirubin, alkaline phosphatase
- Transaminases (AST, ALT), $\gamma$GT
- Synthetic capacity (coagulation parameters, Quick's test score)

### Bone Marrow Function

Generally, bone marrow toxicity is the dose-limiting side effect of cytostatic treatment (exceptions: bleomycin, vincristine, L-asparaginase).

*ATTENTION:*
- Whether dose adjustment is necessary or whether it is preferable to extend the treatment interval, has to be decided in each individual case.
- In cases of prolonged neutropenia after chemotherapy, the administration of hematopoietic growth factors (e.g., G-CSF) should be considered.
- If bone marrow damage / suppression of normal hematopoiesis can be attributed to the primary disease (leukemia, lymphoma with bone marrow involvement, etc.), dose reduction based on blood count parameters is not indicated.

**Recommended dose adjustment according to bone marrow function**

| Leukocyte count (/µl) | Thrombocyte count (/µl) | Dose (%) |
|---|---|---|
| > 3,500 | > 100,000 | 100 |
| 3,000–3,500 | 75,000–100,000 | 75 |
| 2,500–3,000 | 50,000–75,000 | 50 |
| < 2,500 | < 50,000 | 0 |

### Body Weight and Chemotherapy

In obese patients, dose adjustment of cytostatics to body weight is required. This is of particular importance for cyclophosphamide and etoposide / VP-16 in the frame of high-dose chemotherapy.

- In these cases, dose should be based on the "ideal body weight" (IBW).
- If the IBW is more than 15 kg below the real body weight (which is usually the case with highly obese patients), dose adjustment should be based on the "adapted ideal body weight" (AIBW).

### Ideal Body Weight (IBW)

$$\text{♂} \quad IBW = 50 \text{ kg} + 2.3 \times \left( \frac{\text{Height in cm}}{2.53} - 60 \right)$$

$$\text{♀} \quad IBW = 45.5 \text{ kg} + 2.3 \times \left( \frac{\text{Height in cm}}{2.53} - 60 \right)$$

### Adjusted Ideal Body Weight (AIBW)

$$AIBW = IBW + 0.4 \times (\text{Actual Body Weight} - IBW)$$

### Dose Modification Table

General rules of cytostatic drug dose adjustment based on hepatic and renal functions are given in the table below. Manufacturers' recommendations and relevant literature have been incorporated. Since data can vary considerably, the cytostatic dosage should be determined discerningly, taking into consideration the patient's general status.

All data are percentages of the standard dosages specified in the respective therapy protocols.

**Ref:**

1. Canal P, Chatelut E, Guichard S. Practical treatment guide for dose individualisation in cancer chemotherapy. Drugs 1998;56:1019–38
2. Donelli MG, Zucchetti M, Munzone E et al. Pharmacokinetics of anticancer agents in patients with impaired liver function. Eur J Cancer 1998;34:33–46
3. Ibrahim S, Honig P, Huang SM et al. Clinical pharmacology studies in patients with renal impairment: past experience and regulatory perspectives. J Clin Pharmacol 2000;40:31–8
4. Lichtman SM, Villani G. Chemotherapy in the elderly: pharmacologic considerations. Cancer Control 2000;7:548–56
5. Marx GM, Blake GM, Galani E et al. Evaluation of the Cockroft-Gault, Jelliffe and Wright formulae in estimating renal function in elderly cancer patients. Ann Oncol 2004;15:291–5
6. Stevens LA, Coresh J, Greene Tet al. Assessing kidney function – measured and estimated glomerular filtration rate. N Engl J Med 2006; 354:2473–83

**Web:**

1. http://www.druginfonet.com/ — Drug Information (with specialist information)
2. http://chemfinder.camsoft.com/ — Data Base of Chemical Compounds
3. http://www.meds.com/DChome.html — Information on Cytostatics
4. http://www.manuelsweb.com/IBW.htm — IBW calculator
5. http://medcal3000.com/CreatinineCl.htm — Creatinine Clearance Calculator
6. http://nephron.com/ — GFR calculator

**Dose modification table: recommended dose adjustment of cytostatics in case of reduced organ function**

| Compound | Dose modification with renal dysfunction | | | Dose modification with liver dysfunction | | |
|---|---|---|---|---|---|---|
| | Parameter | Limit | Dose | Bilirubin (mg/dl) | AST (IU/l) | Dose |
| Altretamine (HMM) | Use cautiously in patients with renal insufficiency | | | Use cautiously in patients with liver dysfunction | | |
| Amsacrine | Crea$_{Serum}$ (mg/dl) | > 1.5 | 75% | < 1.5<br>1.5–3.0<br>> 3.0 | < 60<br>60–180<br>>180 | 100%<br>50%<br>Relative CI |
| Asparaginase | None | | | Use cautiously in patients with liver dysfunction | | |
| Bendamustine | Use cautiously in patients with renal insufficiency | | | Use cautiously in patients with liver dysfunction | | |
| Bleomycin | GFR (ml/min)<br><br>No reduction when given twice weekly | > 60<br>10–60<br>< 10 | 100%<br>75–50%<br>50–25% | Use cautiously in patients with liver dysfunction | | |
| Capecitabine | GFR (ml/min) | > 50<br>30–50<br>< 30 | 100%<br>75%<br>Not specified | Use cautiously in patients with liver dysfunction | | |
| Carboplatin | GFR (ml/min) | ≥ 60<br>41–59<br>16–40<br>≤ 15 | 100%<br>60%<br>40%<br>Relative CI | Use cautiously in patients with liver dysfunction | | |
| Carmustine | GFR (ml/min) | > 10<br>< 10 | 100%<br>Relative CI | < 1.5<br>1.5–3.0<br>3.1–5.0<br>> 5.0 | < 60<br>60–180<br>> 180 | 100%<br>75%<br>50%<br>Relative CI |
| Cisplatin | GFR (ml/min) | > 60<br>< 60 | 100%<br>Absolute CI | Use cautiously in patients with liver dysfunction | | |
| Cladribine (2-CDA) | Use cautiously in patients with renal insufficiency | | | Use cautiously in patients with liver dysfunction | | |

[a] With alkaline phosphatase > 2.5 × upper normal value
[b] With alkaline phosphatase > 6 × upper normal value
AST aspartate transaminase, CI contraindication, Crea creatinine, GFR glomerular filtration rate

**Dose modification table: recommended dose adjustment of cytostatics in case of reduced organ function (continued)**

| Compound | Dose modification with renal dysfunction | | | Dose modification with liver dysfunction | | |
|---|---|---|---|---|---|---|
| | Parameter | Limit | Dose | Bilirubin (mg/dl) | AST (IU/l) | Dose |
| Cyclophosphamide | GFR (ml/min) | >60<br>10–60<br><10 | 100%<br>75%<br>50% | <3.0<br>3.1–5.0<br>>5.0 | <180<br>>180<br>>180 | 100%<br>75%<br>Relative CI |
| Cytarabine | GFR (ml/min) | <10 | 50–75% | Possible dose reduction (incomplete data) | | |
| Dacarbazine | GFR (ml/min) | >60<br>10–60<br><10 | 100%<br>75%<br>50% | <1.5<br>1.5–3.0<br>3.1–5.0<br>>5.0 | <60<br>60–180<br>>180 | 100%<br>75%<br>50%<br>Relative CI |
| Dactinomycin | GFR (ml/min) | <10 | 75% | Use cautiously in patients with liver dysfunction | | |
| Daunorubicin | Crea$_{serum}$ (mg/dl) | >3.0 | 50% | <1.5<br>1.5–3.0<br>3.1–5.0<br>>5.0 | <60<br>60–180<br>>180 | 100%<br>75%<br>50%<br>Relative CI |
| | *NOTE:* dose reduction recommended in geriatric patients | | | | | |
| Docetaxel | No dose adjustment (insignificant renal elimination) | | | –<br>–<br>>1.5 | <30<br>30–60[a]<br>>60[b] | 100%<br>75%<br>Relative CI |
| Doxorubicin | GFR (ml/min) | <10 | 75% | <1.5<br>1.5–3.0<br>3.1–5.0<br>>5.0 | <60<br>60–180<br>>180 | 100%<br>50%<br>25%<br>Relative CI |
| Epirubicin | Dose reduction in patients with major renal dysfunction | | | <1.5<br>1.5–3.0<br>3.1–5.0<br>>5.0 | <60<br>60–180<br>>180 | 100%<br>50%<br>25%<br>Relative CI |
| Estramustine | Use cautiously in patients with renal insufficiency | | | Use cautiously in patients with liver dysfunction | | |

[a] With alkaline phosphatase > 2.5 × upper normal value
[b] With alkaline phosphatase > 6 × upper normal value
*AST* aspartate transaminase, *CI* contraindication, *Crea* creatinine, *GFR* glomerular filtration rate

**Dose modification table: recommended dose adjustment of cytostatics in case of reduced organ function (continued)**

| Compound | Dose modification with renal dysfunction | | | Dose modification with liver dysfunction | | |
|---|---|---|---|---|---|---|
| | Parameter | Limit | Dose | Bilirubin (mg/dl) | AST (IU/l) | Dose |
| Etoposide | GFR (ml/min) | > 60<br>10–60<br>< 10 | 100%<br>75%<br>50% | < 1.5<br>1.5–3.0<br>3.1–5.0<br>> 5.0 | < 60<br>60–180<br>> 180<br>– | 100%<br>75%<br>50%<br>Relative CI |
| Fludarabine | GFR (ml/min) | < 50<br>< 10 | 75%<br>Relative CI | Not specified | | |
| Fluorouracil | GFR (ml/min) | > 10<br>< 10 | 100%<br>50–75% | < 5.0<br>> 5.0 | –<br>– | 100%<br>Relative CI |
| Gemcitabine | Use cautiously in patients with renal insufficiency | | | Use cautiously in patients with liver dysfunction | | |
| Hydroxyurea | GFR (ml/min) | > 50<br>10–50<br>< 10 | 100%<br>50%<br>25% | > 5.0 | – | Relative CI |
| Idarubicin | Use cautiously in patients with renal insufficiency | | | > 2.5<br>2.5–5.0<br>>5.0 | –<br>–<br>– | 100%<br>50%<br>Relative CI |
| Ifosfamide | Use cautiously in patients with renal insufficiency | | | Use cautiously in patients with liver dysfunction | | |
| Irinotecan | Use cautiously in patients with renal insufficiency | | | > 1.5 | – | Absolute CI |
| Lomustine | GFR (ml/min) | > 50<br>10–50<br>< 10 | 100%<br>75%<br>50% | Use cautiously in patients with liver dysfunction | | |
| Melphalan | GFR (ml/min) | > 60<br>10–60<br>< 10 | 100%<br>50%<br>25% | Use cautiously in patients with liver dysfunction | | |
| Mercaptopurine | GFR (ml/min) | > 60<br>10–60<br>< 10 | 100%<br>10–50%<br>Relative CI | < 1.5<br>1.5–3.0<br>3.1–5.0<br>> 5.0 | 60–180<br>> 180<br>– | 100%<br>50%<br>25%<br>Relative CI |

[a] With alkaline phosphatase > 2.5 × upper normal value
[b] With alkaline phosphatase > 6 × upper normal value
AST aspartate transaminase, CI contraindication, Crea creatinine, GFR glomerular filtration rate

**Dose modification table: recommended dose adjustment of cytostatics in case of reduced organ function (continued)**

| Compound | Dose modification with renal dysfunction | | | Dose modification with liver dysfunction | | |
|---|---|---|---|---|---|---|
| | Parameter | Limit | Dose | Bilirubin (mg/dl) | AST (IU/l) | Dose |
| Methotrexate (low dose) | GFR (ml/min) | > 60<br>10–60<br>< 10 | 100%<br>10–50%<br>Relative CI | Use cautiously in patients with liver dysfunction | | |
| Methotrexate (high dose) | GFR (ml/min) | < 60 | Absolute CI | 1.0–3.0<br>3.1–5.0<br>> 5.0 | 60–180<br>> 180<br>– | 100%<br>75%<br>Relative CI |
| Mitomycin C | Crea$_{Serum}$ (mg/dl) | > 1.5<br>> 1.7 | Follow-up<br>Relative CI | Contraindicated in patients with severe liver dysfunction | | |
| Mitoxantrone | With mild to medium renal dysfunction, no dose reduction necessary | | | < 1.5<br>1.5–3.0<br>3.1–5.0<br>> 5.0 | < 60<br>60–180<br>> 180<br>– | 100%<br>50%<br>25%<br>Relative CI |
| Nimustine | Use cautiously in patients with renal insufficiency | | | Use cautiously in patients with liver dysfunction | | |
| Oxaliplatin | GFR (ml/min) | < 30 | Relative CI | Use cautiously in patients with liver dysfunction | | |
| Paclitaxel | With mild to medium renal dysfunction, no dose reduction necessary (renal elimination < 10%) | | | < 3.0<br>> 3.0 | –<br>– | 100%<br>50% |
| Pemetrexed | GFR (ml/min) | ≥ 45<br>< 45 | 100%<br>Relative CI | Use cautiously in patients with liver dysfunction | | |
| Pentostatin | GFR (ml/min)<br>Positive correlation between pentostatin clearance and creatinine clearance | < 60 | Relative CI | Use cautiously in patients with liver dysfunction | | |
| Procarbazine | Use cautiously in patients with renal insufficiency | | | Use cautiously in patients with liver dysfunction | | |
| Temozolomide | Use cautiously in patients with renal insufficiency | | | Use cautiously in patients with liver dysfunction | | |

[a] With alkaline phosphatase > 2.5 × upper normal value
[b] With alkaline phosphatase > 6 × upper normal value
AST aspartate transaminase, CI contraindication, Crea creatinine, GFR glomerular filtration rate

**Dose modification table: recommended dose adjustment of cytostatics in case of reduced organ function (continued)**

| Compound | Dose modification with renal dysfunction | | | Dose modification with liver dysfunction | | |
|---|---|---|---|---|---|---|
| | Parameter | Limit | Dose | Bilirubin (mg/dl) | AST (IU/l) | Dose |
| Teniposide | Use cautiously in patients with renal insufficiency | | | < 1.5<br>1.5–3.0<br>3.1–5.0<br>> 5.0 | < 60<br>60–180<br>> 180<br>– | 100%<br>75%<br>50%<br>Relative CI |
| 6-Thioguanine | Use cautiously in patients with renal insufficiency | | | Contraindicated in patients with severe liver dysfunction | | |
| Topotecan | GFR (ml/min) | > 40<br>20–40<br>< 20 | 100%<br>50%<br>Absolute CI | < 10 | | No dose adjustment |
| Trofosfamide | Contraindicated in patients with severe renal dysfunction | | | Use cautiously in patients with liver dysfunction | | |
| UFT (tegafur-uracil) | Use cautiously in patients with renal insufficiency | | | Contraindicated in patients with severe liver dysfunction | | |
| Vinblastine | GFR (ml/min) | > 10<br>< 10 | 100%<br>75% | < 1.5<br>1.5–3.0<br>3.1–5.0<br>> 5.0 | < 60<br>60–180<br>> 180<br>– | 100%<br>50%<br>25%<br>Relative CI |
| Vincristine | GFR (ml/min) | > 10<br>< 10 | 100%<br>75% | < 1.5<br>1.5–3.0<br>3.1–5.0<br>> 5.0 | < 60<br>60–180<br>> 180<br>– | 100%<br>50%<br>25%<br>Relative CI |
| Vindesine | No dose reduction necessary | | | < 1.5<br>1.5–3.0<br>3.1–5.0<br>> 5.0 | < 60<br>60–180<br>> 180<br>– | 100%<br>50%<br>25%<br>Relative CI |
| Vinorelbine | No dose reduction necessary | | | < 2.0<br>2.1–3.0<br>> 3.0 | –<br>–<br>– | 100%<br>50%<br>25% |

[a] With alkaline phosphatase > 2.5 × upper normal value
[b] With alkaline phosphatase > 6 × upper normal value
AST aspartate transaminase, CI contraindication, Crea creatinine, GFR glomerular filtration rate

**3.2.5**  **Chemotherapy During Pregnancy and Lactation**

H. Henß

**Def:** Antineoplastic treatment during pregnancy or lactation.

**Ep:** Chemotherapy in pregnant or breastfeeding women is indicated in rare cases. The most common tumor types are:
- Breast cancer
- Cervical carcinoma
- Lymphoma
- Malignant melanoma

**Prg:** Risks of malignancies in pregnant women:
- Threat to the mother's life
- Threat to the child's life
- Spread of disease to the child
- Side effects of treatment on mother and child

Beside medical aspects, ethical and psychosocial considerations are to be taken into account when determining whether antineoplastic chemotherapy in pregnant / breastfeeding women is indicated. Of paramount importance is the interdisciplinary cooperation of the chemotherapist with the obstetrician, pediatrician, and, if necessary, with the medical ethicist.

**Th:** ### Principles of Therapy

Decisions on chemotherapy during pregnancy have to be taken on an individual patient basis. The patient and her relatives are to be included in the decision-making process. Of practical importance are, in particular:
- Stage of pregnancy
- Stage / prognosis of malignancy
- Patient's general health / secondary disorders
- Therapeutic options
- Postchemotherapy fertility / urgency of wanting a child

### First to 20th Week of Gestation (WOG)

Cytostatic chemotherapy up to the 20th WOG bears a high risk of fetal malformation (15–20%). Termination of pregnancy should therefore be seriously considered. In deciding between abortion and deferment of chemotherapy, the therapeutic situation of both mother and child needs to be taken into consideration. Treatment is absolutely indicated when, due to expected rapid progression (acute leukemia, highly malignant lymphoma), it is unlikely that the mother will survive until the earliest possible delivery date.

#### Curative Therapeutic Intention
- As far as possible, deferment of curative chemotherapy should be avoided.
- Immediate initiation of treatment after termination of pregnancy.
- If the parents object to an abortion, chemotherapy should nonetheless be started immediately (*ATTN:* with highly elevated risk of malformation). Through frequent sonographic monitoring, malformations can be detected before the 24th WOG and the pregnancy can subsequently be terminated. It is important to inform the patient of the risk of non-detection of malformations by ultrasound examination.

### Palliative Therapeutic Intention

- Immediate initiation of treatment after termination of pregnancy.
- If in light of the palliative situation immediate treatment is not desired, deferment until completion of organogenesis may be considered. The possible risks for both mother (tumor progression) and child (transplacental tumor metastasis into fetus) must be pointed out.

## Twentieth to 32nd Week of Gestation (WOG)

Chemotherapy between the 20th and 32nd WOG rarely leads to fetal malformation. The main therapeutic risks are organ toxicity, intrauterine growth retardation (IUGR) and preterm delivery. Precautions:

- Monitoring of pregnancy at a perinatal center
- Planning of early delivery
- Consideration of possible myelosuppression in both mother and child
- Consideration of prenatal surfactant therapy to enhance pulmonary maturation

### Curative Therapeutic Intention

Immediate initiation of chemotherapy.

### Palliative Therapeutic Intention

Possible deferment of antineoplastic therapy until infant is viable. Postpartum initiation of treatment. Patient information on risks and possible consequences of therapy delay for both mother (tumor progression) and child (risk of metastasis).

## From 32nd Week of Gestation (WOG)

Usually, the fetus is viable from the 32nd WOG on → delivery before initiation of chemotherapy.

## Lactation

Infants should be weaned before chemotherapy is initiated. For the majority of cytostatic drugs, the transfer into breast milk is not specified. However, potential damage to the child can not be ruled out completely.

**Ref:**

1. Germann N, Goffinet F, Goldwasser F. Anthracyclines during pregnancy: embryo-fetal outcome in 160 patients. Ann Oncol 2004;15:146–50
2. Giacalone PL, Laffargue F, Benos P. Chemotherapy for breast carcinoma during pregnancy. A French national survey. Cancer 1999;86:2266–72
3. Loibl S, von Minckwitz G, Gwyn K et al. Breast carcinoma during pregnancy. Cancer 2006; 106:237–46
4. Partridge AH, Garber JE. Long-term outcomes of children exposed to antineoplastic agents in utero. Semin Oncol 2000;27:712–26
5. Salooja N, Szydio RM, Socie G et al. Pregnancy outcomes after peripheral blood or marrow transplantation: a retrospective survey. Lancet 2001;358:271–6
6. Williams SF, Schilsky RL. Antineoplastic drugs administered during pregnancy. Semin Oncol 2000;27:618–22

**Web:**

1. http://www.cancer.gov/cancertopics/pdq/treatment/breast-cancer-and-pregnancy/    NCI Cancernet
2. http://www.sogc.org/guidelines/public/111E-CPG-February2002.pdf    SOGC Guideline

**3.2.6    Selected Cytostatic Drug Incompatibilities**

A. Göbel, B. Lubrich

**Def:**    Physicochemical incompatibility of antineoplastic compounds may lead to, e.g., precipitation, discoloration, decomposition. These processes can be triggered by even brief contact with other compounds, e.g., when using the same infusion pump, injection via a Y-piece, or parallel infusion via a manifold set.

*Prevention of Drug Incompatibility*

In principle, mixing different cytostatic drug solutions as well as mixing cytostatics with parenteral nutrition solutions should be avoided. When using complex therapeutic regimens, manufacturers' recommendations and drug incompatibility databases should be consulted.

*Incompatibility Table*
- Cytostatic drugs and substances listed below are physicochemically incompatible.
- Consecutive administration of incompatible compounds without changing the infusion pump or injection via a Y-piece has to be avoided.
- Incompatibilities are negligible if the infusion set is replaced before each drug administration or flushed with 0.9% saline or 5% glucose solution.
- Drugs not listed in this table cannot generally be seen as compatible. In case of incompatibility questions, the responsible pharmacy should be contacted.

Physicians and nurses administrating chemotherapy have the obligation to regularly and carefully check infusions for incompatibilities.

| Cytostatic | Incompatible with: |
| --- | --- |
| Amsacrine | Saline and other chlorine solutions, acyclovir, amphotericin B, aztreonam, ceftazidime, ceftriaxone, cimetidine, furosemide, ganciclovir, heparin, methylprednisolone-21-hydrogen succinate, metoclopramide, ondansetron, sargramostim |
| Asparaginase | Not specified |
| Bleomycin | Aminophylline, amino acids, ascorbic acid, carbenicillin, cefalotin, cefazolin, dexamethasone, diazepam, furosemide, 5% glucose, hydrocortisone-21-hydrogen succinate, methotrexate, mitomycin, nafcillin, penicillin G, riboflavin, sulfhydryl-containing drugs (e.g., glutathione), terbutaline, divalent and trivalent cations |
| Carboplatin | Aluminum (e.g., in infusion cannulas), 5-FU, mesna, sodium bicarbonate |
| Carmustine | Alkaline solutions, allopurinol, sodium bicarbonate, PVC (infusion container and application set) |
| Cisplatin | Amino acids, water for injection, alkaline solutions, aluminum (e.g., in infusion cannulas), amifostine, cefepime, chelating agents (e.g., penicillamine), 5-FU, gallium nitrate, 5% glucose, mesna, metoclopramide, sodium bicarbonate, sodium bisulfite-, -hydrogen sulfite- and -thiosulfate-containing drugs, piperacillin / tazobactam, thiotepa |
| Cladribine | 5% glucose |
| Cyclophosphamide | Aluminum (e.g., in infusion cannulas), amphotericin B, benzyl alcohol |

| Cytostatic | Incompatible with: |
|---|---|
| Cytarabine | Allopurinol, carbenicillin, cefalotin, 5-FU, gallium nitrate, ganciclovir, gentamicin, heparin, hydrocortisone-21-hydrogen succinate, insulin, methotrexate, nafcillin, penicillin G, methylprednisolone-21-hydrogen succinate, oxacillin |
| Dacarbazine | Alkaline solutions, allopurinol, cefepime, heparin, hydrocortisone-21-hydrogen succinate, L-cysteine, mercaptoethanol, methoxypsoralen, sodium bicarbonate, piperacillin sodium / tazobactam |
| Dactinomycin | Benzyl alcohol, cellulose ester (in filter), filgrastim, paraben, riboflavin |
| Daunorubicin | Allopurinol, aluminum, aztreonam, cefepime, dexamethasone, fludarabine, 5-FU, furosemide, heparin, methotrexate, piperacillin sodium / tazobactam, pH < 4.0 or pH > 7.0 |
| Daunorubicin liposomal | Benzyl alcohol or other bacteriostatics, dexamethasone, heparin, solvents other than 5% glucose, detergents and similar substances, electrolyte-containing solvents and drugs |
| Docetaxel | Amphotericin B, liposomal doxorubicin, methylprednisolone sodium succinate, nalbuphine |
| Doxorubicin | Alkaline solutions, allopurinol, aluminum (e.g., in infusion cannulas), aminophylline, amino acids, cefalotin, cefepime, dexamethasone, diazepam, 5-FU, furosemide, gallium nitrate, ganciclovir, heparin, hydrocortisone-21-hydrogen succinate, pH < 4.0 or pH > 7.0, methotrexate, sodium bicarbonate, piperacillin sodium / tazobactam, vincristine |
| Doxorubicin liposomal | Amphotericin B, benzyl alcohol / other bacteriostatics, docetaxel, mannitol, metoclopramide, mitoxantrone, morphine, sodium bicarbonate, detergents, electrolyte-containing solvents and drugs |
| Epirubicin | Alkaline solutions, 5-FU, heparin, ifosfamide, methotrexate, mesna |
| Estramustine | 0.9% saline and other infusion solutions (other than 5% glucose), calcium-containing preparations |
| Etoposide | ABS synthetics, solutions with pH > 6, cefepime, filgrastim, gallium nitrate, idarubicin, sodium bicarbonate, PVC (infusion container and application set) |
| Etoposide phosphate | pH > 7, amphotericin B, cefepime, chlorpromazine, imipenem-cilastatin, methylprednisolone sodium succinate, mitomycin |
| Fludarabine | Acyclovir, amphotericin B, chlorpromazine, daunorubicin, ganciclovir, hydroxyzine, miconazole, prochlorperazine edisylate, pH < 4.5 or pH > 8 |
| Fluorouracil | Calcium folinate, carboplatin, chlormethine, chlorpromazine, cisplatin, cytarabine, daunorubicin, diazepam, droperidol, doxorubicin, epirubicin, etoposide, fentanyl, filgrastim, folinic acid, gallium nitrate, leucovorin calcium, methotrexate, metoclopramide, morphine sulfate, ondansetron, spirogermanium, sulfobenzoic penicillin, vincristine, vinorelbine |
| Gemcitabine | Acyclovir, amphotericin B, furosemide, ganciclovir, irinotecan, methotrexate, methylprednisolone sodium succinate, mitomycin |
| Idarubicin | Acyclovir, alkaline solutions, allopurinol, ampicillin/sulbactam, cefazolin, cefepime, ceftazidime, clindamycin, dexamethasone-21-hydrogen phosphate, etoposide, furosemide, gentamicin, heparin, hydrocortisone-21-hydrogen succinate, imipenem, cilastin, lorazepam, methotrexate, mezlocillin, sodium bicarbonate, pethidine, piperacillin sodium / tazobactam, sargramostim, teniposide, vancomycin, vincristine |
| Ifosfamide | Benzyl alcohol, cefepime, methotrexate, mesna |
| Irinotecan | Alkaline solutions, gemcitabine, sodium folinate |

ABS: Acrylnitril Butadien Styrol Polymer

| Cytostatic | Incompatible with: |
|---|---|
| Melphalan | Amphotericin B, chlorpromazine, 5% glucose |
| Methotrexate | Aluminum, bleomycin, chlormethine, chlorpromazine, cytarabine, daunorubicin, dexamethasone, doxorubicin, droperidol, 5-FU, gemcitabine, heparin, hydrocortisone-21-hydrogen succinate, idarubicin, ifosfamide, metoclopramide, methotrexate, midazolam, nalbuphine, prednisolone-21-dihydrogen phosphate, promethazine, propofol, ranitidine, vancomycin |
| Mitomycin | Aztreonam, bleomycin, cefepime, etoposide phosphate, filgrastim, gemcitabine, 5% glucose, piperacillin sodium / tazobactam, sargramostim, vinorelbine |
| Mitoxantrone | Alkaline solutions, amino acid-containing solutions, aztreonam, cefepime, heparin, hydrocortisone-21-dihydrogen phosphate, paclitaxel, piperacillin sodium / tazobactam, propofol, thiotepa |
| Nimustine | Not specified |
| Oxaliplatin | 0.9% saline |
| Paclitaxel | Amphotericin B, chlorpromazine, liposomal doxorubicin, hydroxyzine, methylprednisolone-21-hydrogen succinate, mitoxantrone, PVC (infusion container and application set) |
| Pentostatin | Acidic solutions |
| Teniposide | ABS synthetics, heparin, idarubicin, PVC (infusion container and giving set), solvents other than 0.9% saline and 5% glucose |
| Thiotepa | Cisplatin, filgrastim, minocycline, mitoxantrone, acidic solutions, vinorelbine |
| Topotecan | Not specified |
| Treosulfan | Alkaline solutions |
| Vinblastine | Cefepime, furosemide, heparin, pH < 3.5 or pH > 5 |
| Vincristine | Cefepime, doxorubicin, furosemide, idarubicin, sodium bicarbonate, pH < 3.5 or pH > 5 |
| Vindesine | 5-FU, sodium bicarbonate, pH < 3.5 or pH > 5 |
| Vinorelbine | Acyclovir, alkaline solutions, allopurinol, aminophylline, amphotericin B, ampicillin, cefazolin, cefoperazone, ceforanide, cefotaxime, cefotetan, ceftriaxone, cefuroxime, 5-FU, furosemide, ganciclovir, methylprednisolone-21-hydrogen succinate, mitomycin, sodium bicarbonate, piperacillin, thiotepa, trimethoprim / sulfamethoxazole |

ABS: Acrylnitril Butadien Styrol Polymer

**Ref:**

1. Trissel LA. Handbook on Injectable Drugs, 14th edn. American Society of Health-System Pharmacists, Bethesda, 2007.

**Web:**

1. http://www.druginfonet.com/ — Drug Information (with specialist information)
2. http://chemfinder.camsoft.com/ — Database of Chemical Compounds
3. http://rxlist.com — Internet Drug Index
4. http://www.meds.com/DChome.html — Information on Cytostatics

## 3.2.7    Preparation and Stability of Cytostatics

**B. Lubrich, A. Göbel**

**Def:**    Precautions for the safe handling of cytostatics involve preparation, use, and disposal. Of particular importance is systemic exposure of staff to cytostatics via inhalation, ingestion, and cutaneous absorption. Potential threats include:
- Local and systemic toxicity
- Acute and chronic toxicity
- Genotoxicity / teratogenicity / mutagenicity

**Meth:**    *Proper and Safe Handling of Cytostatics: Minimum Requirements*
- Staff safety, occupational health and safety
- Patient safety
- Product safety
- Environmental protection

### Occupational Safety
Cytostatics must be prepared and used by trained staff only.

### Preparation and Use of Cytostatics
Cytostatic drug solutions are prepared in the pharmacy in accordance with the pharmaceutical law, pharmacy rules, and approved principles of pharmaceutical science.

Preparations for the use of cytostatics are the responsibility of the physician and are carried out by him-/herself or by members of staff based on approved principles of medical science.

### Facilities
Cytostatic drug solutions should be prepared at a central location, e.g., in the hospital pharmacy:
- In rooms separated from other sectors, with limited access for authorized staff only.
- There must be no eating, drinking, or smoking in the designated rooms.
- There must be no other activities taking place in the room during preparation of cytostatics.
- Doors and windows must be kept closed during preparation: draft-free work environment.

### Safety Cabinets
Preparation must be carried out in category 2 safety cabinets.
- Safety cabinets are to be regularly inspected in accordance with current policies. Inspections are to be documented in a log book.
- A user manual must be provided for work at the cabinets.
- The user manual must contain directives for cleaning and disinfection of all work surfaces.
- Supply and exhaust air in the preparation room must correspond with the cabinet. The exhaust air ventilation system must be ducted outside.
- Air flow modification during work (e.g., covering of ventilation slots, addition of voluminous or large numbers of items to the cabinet, vigorous movements) is to be avoided as it could negatively influence the retention capacity / product safety / entrainment prevention.

### Protective Clothing
- Protective clothing is mandatory to avoid direct contact between skin or mucous membranes and cytostatics.
- Liquid-proof, long-sleeved, high-necked, non-fuzzing gowns with fitting cuffs. Suitable clothing includes liquid-proof disposable gowns or textile disposable gowns with liquid-proof gauntlets.
- Gowns must only be worn within the designated rooms.
- Gowns must be changed at least on a daily basis.

### Gloves
- Liquid-proof disposable gloves, e.g., latex and/or nitrile gloves of at least 0.2 mm thickness and of documented quality (double gloving recommended).

- Gloves must be long enough to remain tight above the cuff during work.
- In the event of visible contamination or leakage and after working with amsacrine, carmustine, irinotecan, mitoxantrone, and thiotepa, gloves must be changed immediately.

### Protective Glasses with Side Shields
When handling cytostatics outside the safety cabinet, e.g., to remove a major spillage of cytostatics, protective glasses with side shields must be worn.

### Inhalation Protection
When handling cytostatics outside the safety workbench, e.g., to remove a major spillage of cytostatics, a particle filtration half-mask must be worn.

### Textile Aids
For easy removal of contamination, cytostatics should be prepared on a liquid-proof absorbent mat. In addition:
- Use compresses when opening ampoules.
- When retracting cannulas from pierceable rubber stoppers or removing residual air from syringes, use compresses or gauze swabs in order to avoid contamination from spraying or aerosol formation.

### Technical Aids
- As far as possible, choose cytostatics in "cytosafe packaging."
- Strict use of disposable syringes and needles with Luer-Lok connections.
- Use pressure release devices with filters (spikes) for venting injection bottles.
- Cytostatics should be dissolved in a closed system. Cytostatics and solvents or vehicles are transferred between containers using transfer caps or needles, providing internal pressure equalization. That way, containers can be disconnected without pressure differences, preventing splashing or release of cytostatic aerosols.

### Transport
Drug solutions must be transported in shatter-proof, water-proof, and sealable containers.

### Storage and Stability of Cytostatics
The following factors impact cytostatic drug storage and stability:
- Expiry date of primary product (dry substance or solution)
- Physicochemical stability of cytostatic stock solution
- Physicochemical stability of the ready-prepared cytostatic compound
- Hygienic aspects, i.e., microbiological fitness
- Cool storage or storage at room temperature
- Light protection
- Shelf-life of prepared solution

*Storage limits and conditions for compounds prepared in the pharmacy are to be specified by the responsible pharmacy and stated on the drug label. Cytostatic drug solutions must be stored according to these specifications. After expiry, compounds must be discarded.*

*Details on physicochemical stability of common cytostatic solutions are given in the table below.*

### Preparation and Administration of Cytostatic Infusions and Injections
- When connecting, changing, venting, or removing an infusion system, contamination of staff members must be avoided (e.g., by wearing protective gloves), as well as contamination of the room and aerosol formation.
- For this purpose, technical aids (pressure release systems with aerosol filters) should be used.
- Vent the infusion system only with carrier solution.

### Dispensing of Cytostatics for Oral Application
When dispensing drugs into containers designated for patients (e.g., dispenser), certain precautions have to be observed, e.g.:

- Wearing of protective gloves
- Use of tweezers or spoons
- Splitting of tablets, pulverization, etc. should be carried out using suitable aids (closed systems) and with particular care (preparation usually in the pharmacy).
- When cleaning and handling containers and items used for dispensing drugs, contamination of staff members must be avoided. Full details should be given in a user manual.

### Administration of Liquid and Semisolid Cytostatic Formulations
Use suitable protective gloves or applicators.

### Spillage
Spilled cytostatics must be removed immediately and carefully and in compliance with the preventive measures specified for the preparation of cytostatics:
- When lifting contaminated broken glass use an extra pair of gloves to prevent physical risks. Preferably, lift shards with tongs.
- Use dry disposable cloths to soak up spilled solutions.
- Use wet disposable cloths for spilled powder.
- Afterwards, clean with soapy water.
- Dispose of all contaminated materials using a leak-proof single-use container.
- Sets of the necessary equipment (protective gown, safety goggles, gloves and masks, cellulose, waste container, scoop) – including instructions – should be held ready.

### Skin Contamination
Areas of skin contaminated with cytostatics must be irrigated immediately with copious quantities of cold water.

### Eye Contamination
In case of eye contamination, irrigate with copious quantities of water or isotonic saline solution for 10 min. Then, consult an ophthalmologist.

### Disposal of Cytostatics
Cytostatics are collected and disposed of according to local regulations.
- Collection and disposal of cytostatic residue requires particular supervision and is to be carried out in accordance with waste regulations and the Hazardous Substances Ordinance using labeled, robust, and leak-proof containers.
- Collection should be separate and in a central location. Disposal should be carried out in hazardous waste incinerators.
- Materials contaminated with cytostatics (textile aids, disposable gowns, applicators, etc.) can be treated as household waste.
- Contaminated reusable clothes or reusable textile materials must be changed, collected without further manipulation, and laundered.
- Cytostatics-containing excrements are not regarded hazardous but should be disposed of on the ward in compliance with hygiene guidelines and health and safety regulations.

**Ref:**

1.    ASCO. Criteria for facilities and personnel for the administration of parenteral systemic antineoplastic therapy. J Clin Oncol 2004;22:4613–5
2.    Connor TH, McDiarmid MA. Preventing occupational exposures to antineoplastic drugs in health care settings. CA Cancer J Clin 2006;56:354–65
3.    Trissel LA. Handbook on Injectable Drugs, 14th edn. American Society of Health-System Pharmacists, Betherda, 2007

**Web:**

1.    http://www.druginfonet.com/          Drug Information
2.    http://www.meds.com/DChome.html    Information on Cytostatics

**Physicochemical stability of ready-prepared cytostatic and antibody preparations**

| Cytostatics | Stock solution | | | Solution for application | | | Storage / details |
|---|---|---|---|---|---|---|---|
| | Solvent | Concentration | Stability / temperature | Carrier | Stability at RT | Stability at 2–8°C | |
| Alemtuzumab | | 10 mg/ml | 28 d / cool | Saline or G5 | 24 h | 24 h | Cool, protect from light |
| Amsacrine | Lactic acid 0.035m | 5 mg/ml | 48 h / RT | G5 (!) | 72 h | Unspecified | RT |
| L-Asparaginase | Water for injection | 2,500 U/ml | 5 d / cool | Saline | 8 h | 24 h | Cool, avoid vigorous shaking (!) |
| Bendamustine | Water for injection | 3 mg/ml | Dilute in 0.9% saline immediately after reconstitution | Saline (!) | 9 h | 5 d | Cool |
| Bevacizumab | – | 25 mg/ml | 5 d / cool | Saline | – | 48 h | Cool, protect from light |
| Bleomycin | Saline (!) | 3 mg/ml | 28 d / cool | Saline (!) | 14 d | 28 d | Cool, protect from light |
| Bortezomib | Saline | 1 mg/ml | 8 h / cool | Dilution not recommended; application of stock solution | | | |
| Busulfan | – | 6 mg/ml | 28 d / cool | Saline | 8 h | 15 h | Cool, stability details are for concentrations 0.5 mg/ml, use plastic material free of polycarbonate |
| Carboplatin | – | 10 mg/ml | 28 d / cool | G5 (!) | 14 d | 28 d | Cool |
| Carmustine | 1. Absolute ethanol 2. Water for injection | 3.33 mg/ml | 24 h / cool | G5 (!) | 6 h | 48 h | Cool, protect from light adsorption on synthetics (except PE) |
| Cetuximab | – | 2 mg/ml | 24h / cool | – | 24 h | 28 d | Cool, protect from light, use special inline-filters |
| Cisplatin | – | 0.5 mg/ml | 28 d / cool | Saline (!) | 21 d | 21 d | Cool, protect from light |
| Cisplatin | – | 1 mg/ml | 28d / cool | Saline | 21 d | 21 d | Cool protect from light; dilute not more than 1:2 with saline |

RT room temperature, d day, h hour, G5 5% glucose, Saline 0.9% saline, (!) compulsory. Solvents in brackets refer to the relevant dry substance. These specifications are applicable for parenteral application and conditions of microbiologically validated central preparation of cytostatics

**Physicochemical stability of ready-prepared cytostatic and antibody preparations** *(continued)*

| Cytostatics | Stock solution | | | Solution for application | | | |
|---|---|---|---|---|---|---|---|
| | Solvent | Concentration | Stability / temperature | Carrier | Stability at RT | Stability at 2–8°C | Storage / details |
| Cladribine | – | 1 mg/ml | 7 d / cool | Saline (!) | 28 d | 28 d | Cool, protect from light |
| Cyclophosphamide | Saline | 20 mg/ml | 28 d / cool | Saline or G5 | 4–7 d | 28 d | Cool |
| Cytarabine | Saline | 50 or 100 mg/ml | 14 d / cool | Saline or G5 | 7 d | 28 d | Cool |
| Dacarbazine | (Water for injection) | 10 mg/ml | 72 h / cool | Saline or G5 | 8 h | 24 h | Cool, protect from light |
| Dactinomycin | Water for injection | 0.5 mg/ml | 28 d / cool | Saline or G5 | 72 h | 72 h | Cool, protect from light |
| Daunorubicin | Saline or G5 | 2 mg/ml | 28 d / cool | Saline or G5 | 28 d | 28 d | Cool, protect from light |
| Daunorubicin, liposomal | – | 50 mg/ml | – | G5 | – | 6 h < 0.5 mg/ml  24 h 0.5–1 mg/ml | Cool, protect from light |
| Docetaxel | Special solvent | 10 mg/ml | 28 d / RT or cool | Saline or G5 | 28 d | 28 d | RT, protect from light |
| Doxorubicin | (G5) | 2 mg/ml | 28 d / cool | Saline or G5 | 28 d | 28 d | Cool, protect from light, pH 5 |
| Doxorubicin, liposomal (PEGylated) | – | 2 mg/ml | 28 d / cool | G5 (!) | 48 h | 7 d | Cool, protect from light |
| Doxorubicin, liposomal (non-PEGylated) | – | 2 mg/ml | 5 d / cool | G5 (!) | 24 h | 24 h | Cool, protect from light |
| Epirubicin | (G5) | 2 mg/ml | 28 d/cool | G5 | 28 d | 28 d | Cool, protect from light, pH 5 |
| Erwinia-asparaginase | Saline | 5,000 IU/ml | 20 d / cool | Saline or G5 | 7 d | 28 d | Cool |
| Estramustine | Water for injection | 37.5 mg/ml | 10 d / cool | G5 (!) | 24 h | 48 h | Cool, avoid vigorous shaking (!) |

*RT* room temperature, *d* day, *h* hour, *G5* 5% glucose, *Saline* 0.9% saline, *(!)* compulsory. Solvents in *brackets* refer to the relevant dry substance. These specifications are applicable for parenteral application and conditions of microbiologically validated central preparation of cytostatics

**Physicochemical stability of ready-prepared cytostatic and antibody preparations *(continued)***

| Cytostatics | Stock solution | | | Solution for application | | | |
|---|---|---|---|---|---|---|---|
| | Solvent | Concentration | Stability / temperature | Carrier | Stability at RT | Stability at 2–8°C | Storage / details |
| Etoposide | – | 20 mg/ml | 28 d / cool | Saline or G5 | 96 h (0.2 mg/ml) 48 h (0.4 mg/ml) 24 h (0.5 mg/ml) | – | RT |
| Etoposide phosphate | Water for injection | 10 mg/ml | 28 d / cool | Saline or G5 | 28 d | 28 d | Cool, protect from light |
| Fludarabine phosphate | Water for injection | 25 mg/ml | 16 d / cool | Saline or G5 | 16 d | 16 d | Cool |
| 5-Fluorouracil | – | 50 mg/ml | 28 d / RT | Saline or G5 | 28 d | 28 d | Cool if diluted solutions, RT if concentration > 40 mg/ml |
| Gemcitabine | Saline | 28 mg/ml | 28 d / RT (!) | Saline | 28 d | 28 d | Cool, protect from light |
| Idarubicin | Saline | 1 mg/ml | 28 d / cool | Saline or G5 | 28 d | 28 d | Cool, protect from light |
| Ifosfamide | Water for injection | 40 mg/ml | 28 d / cool | Saline or G5 | 28 d | 28 d | Cool |
| Irinotecan | – | 20 mg/ml | 28 d / cool | Saline or G5 | 28 d | 28 d | Cool, protect from light |
| Melphalan | Added solvent | 5 mg/ml | 19 h / RT | Saline (!) | 3 h | 24 h | Cool (!) |
| Methotrexate | – | 25 or 100 mg/ml | 28 d / cool | Saline or G5 | 7 d | 28 d | Cool, protect from light, risk of crystallization in G5 |
| Mitomycin | Water for injection | 0.5 mg/ml | 7 d / cool | Saline | 48 h | 5 d | Cool, pH 7 (!) |
| Mitoxantrone | – | 2 mg/ml | 28 d / cool | Saline or G5 | 28 d | 28 d | Cool, risk of crystallization |
| Nimustine | Water for injection | 5 mg/ml | 72 h / cool | Saline or G5 | 7 h | 6 d | Cool, protect from light |

*RT* room temperature, *d* day, *h* hour, *G5* 5% glucose, *Saline* 0.9% saline, (*!*) compulsory. Solvents in *brackets* refer to the relevant dry substance. These specifications are applicable for parenteral application and conditions of microbiologically validated central preparation of cytostatics

**Physicochemical stability of ready-prepared cytostatic and antibody preparations (continued)**

| Cytostatics | Stock solution | | | Solution for application | | | |
|---|---|---|---|---|---|---|---|
| | Solvent | Concentration | Stability / temperature | Carrier | Stability at RT | Stability at 2–8°C | Storage / details |
| Oxaliplatin | Water for injection | 2 mg/ml | 28 d / cool | G5 (!) | 28 d | 28 d | Cool, protect from light |
| Paclitaxel | – | 6 mg/ml | 28 d / cool | Saline or G5 | 72 h | 72 h | RT, prepare in polypropylene or glass containers only, avoid PVC |
| PEG-asparaginase | – | 750 IU/ml | 10 d / cool | Saline or G5 | 4 h | 96 h | Cool |
| Pemetrexed | Saline | 50 mg/ml | 72 h /cool | Saline | 24 h | 72 h | Cool, protect from light |
| Pentostatin | Saline | 2 mg/ml | 96 h / cool | Saline (!) | 48 h | 96 h | Cool |
| Rituximab | – | 10 mg/ml | 28 d / cool | Saline or G5 | 24 h | 24 h | Cool, concentration 1–4 mg/ml |
| Thiotepa | Water for injection | 10 mg/ml | 28 d / cool | G5 | 3 d (> 5 mg/ml) 8 h (< 0.5 mg/ml) | 15 d 8 h | Cool |
| Topotecan | Water for injection | 1 mg/ml | 28 d / cool | Saline or G5 | 28 d | 28 d | Cool, protect from light |
| Trastuzumab | Water for injection | 21 mg/ml | 28 d / cool | Saline (!) | 24 h | 24 h | Cool |
| Treosulfan | Water for injection | 50 mg/ml | 5 d / RT | Dilution not recommended, infusion of stock solution | | | |
| Vinblastine | Saline | 1 mg/ml | 28 d / cool | Saline or G5 | 28 d | 28 d | Cool, protect from light |
| Vincristine | Saline | 1 mg/ml | 28 d / cool | Saline or G5 | 28 d | 28 d | Cool, protect from light |
| Vindesine | Saline | 1 mg/ml | 28 d / cool | Saline or G5 | 21 d | 21 d | Cool, protect from light |
| Vinorelbine | – | 10 mg/ml | 28 d / cool | Saline or G5 | 28 d | 28 d | Cool, protect from light |

*RT* room temperature, *d* day, *h* hour, *G5* 5% glucose, *Saline* 0.9% saline, (*!*) compulsory. Solvents in *brackets* refer to the relevant dry substance. These specifications are applicable for parenteral application and conditions of microbiologically validated central preparation of cytostatics

## 3.3 Hormone Therapy

### H. Henß, R. Engelhardt

**Def:** Use of hormones and hormonally active compounds (stimulating or inhibiting) in tumor therapy. Areas of application:
- Antineoplastic therapy
- Supportive or substitution therapy

**Pharm:** **Hormone therapy**

| Type | Mode of action |
|---|---|
| *GnRH Analogs* | |
| Buserelin, goserelin, leuprolide | Inhibition of gonadotropin secretion by continuous stimulation of the pituitary gland → release of gonadotropins (LH, FSH) ↓ → estrogen ↓, testosterone ↓ |
| *Antiestrogens, SERM* | |
| Tamoxifen, raloxifene | Estrogen receptor competitive binding → inhibition of estradiol-specific effects, estradiol ↓, TGFβ ↑, TGFα ↓, EGF receptor expression ↓, IL-2 secretion ↑ |
| *Aromatase Inhibitors* | |
| *Unspecific:* aminoglutethimide *Specific:* fadrozole, exemestane, vorozole, anastrozole, letrozole | Inhibition of aromatization of androstenedione to estrone → cellular estrogen biosynthesis ↓ |
| *Gestagens* | |
| Megestrol acetate, medroxyprogesterone acetate | Estrogen level ↓, estrogen receptor synthesis ↓, pituitary secretion of LH / FSH / ACTH ↓ → cortisol / androstenedione / testosterone / estrone / estradiol and estrone sulfate levels ↓, dihydrotestosterone synthesis ↓ |
| *Antiandrogens* | |
| *Unspecific:* cyproterone acetate *Specific:* flutamide, nilutamide, bicalutamide | Blockade of androgen receptors → inhibition of androgenic proliferative stimulation of prostatic epithelia |

*ACTH* adrenocorticotropic hormone, *EGF* epidermal growth factor, *FSH* follicle-stimulating hormone, *GnRH* gonadotropin-releasing hormone, *IL* interleukin, *LH* luteinizing hormone, *SERM* selective estrogen receptor modulators, *TGF* tumor growth factor

### Antineoplastic Therapy

**MOA:** *Hormone Therapy*
Specific hormonal effects following interaction with cell-surface receptors, e.g., estrogen / progesterone / steroid receptors.

*Antihormonal Therapy*
Inhibition of specific hormonal effects via:
- Administration of hormonally active compounds → suppression of endocrine regulatory systems
- Application of specific inhibitors (e.g., competitive inhibition of hormone receptors)

**Ind:**     ***Areas of Application***
Hormone-sensitive neoplasias (verified receptor expression):
- Breast cancer (antiestrogens, gestagens, LHRH analogs)
- Prostate cancer (estrogens, antiandrogens, LHRH analogs)
- Carcinoma of the uterine corpus (antiestrogens)
- Thyroid carcinoma (thyroxine for TSH suppression, also: substitution therapy)
- Lymphomas, multiple myeloma (corticosteroids)
- Carcinoid tumors (octreotide)

**Th:**     For therapy details, see respective chapters.


## Substitution Therapy

**Ma:**     Use of hormones to replace hormone production which has completely or partially ceased as a result of antineoplastic therapy.

**Ind:**
- Estrogen / gestagen preparations in cases of premature menopause following chemotherapy
- Testosterone after bilateral orchiectomy
- Thyroxine after thyroidectomy
- Cortisone after bilateral adrenalectomy (e.g., due to bilateral adrenal tumors)


## Estrogen Substitution in Premature Menopause

**Pphys:**     In women, chemotherapy and high-dose chemotherapy in particular, can lead to gonadal damage with subsequent estrogen deficiency and premature menopause. Risks include:
- Menopausal symptoms
- Osteoporosis
- Cardiovascular complications

**Ind:**     Estrogen substitution may be indicated in women with early menopausal symptoms and evidence of reduced hormone levels (estrogen).

**Ci:**     ATTENTION: Continuous estrogen and combined (estrogen + gestagen) therapy constitutes an increased risk of breast cancer and cardiovascular events in healthy menopausal women (WHI study). Treatment should only be initiated after careful evaluation of risks and benefits as well as detailed patient information.

**Se:**     Side effects of long-term estrogen substitution:
- Thrombosis, thromboembolism, cardiovascular events
- Increased breast tissue density → reduced sensitivity for mammography
- Increased risk for relapse of breast cancer and endometrial carcinoma

**Th:**     Alternatives to estrogen substitution:
- Osteoporosis: bisphosphonates, tamoxifen, selective estrogen receptor modulators (e.g., raloxifene)
- Cardiovascular prevention: increased physical activity, dietary measures, tobacco abstinence, lipid-lowering compounds (statins) where indicated
- Menopausal symptoms: oral or transdermal clonidine, gabapentin against hot flushes, topical estrogen application (creams) against vaginal dryness (attention: systemic resorption if used long-term)
- In severe cases: gabapentin

### Testosterone Replacement After Bilateral Orchiectomy

**Pphys:** Testicular carcinoma initially requires unilateral orchiectomy. Loss of the contralateral testicle due to unrelated causes or a second metachronous testicular carcinoma results in anorchia with subsequent testosterone deficiency.

**Ind:** Testosterone therapy has no influence on prognosis and progression of testicular carcinoma → long-term testosterone replacement after bilateral orchiectomy definitely indicated.

**Ci:** Prostate cancer

### Thyroxine Replacement After Thyroidectomy in Thyroid Carcinoma

**Pphys:** Thyroid carcinoma commonly requires total thyroidectomy with life-long thyroid hormone replacement (L-thyroxine).

**Ind:** Administration of high dose of L-thyroxine (175–250 µg/d). Treatment goals:
- Substitution of thyroid hormones
- Suppression of TSH (thyroid-stimulating hormone): TSH can stimulate growth of thyroid carcinomas → L-thyroxine inhibits TSH secretion of pituitary gland

**Ref:**
1. Boekhout AH, Beijnen JH, Schellens JHM. Symptoms and treatment in cancer therapy-induced early menopause. Oncologist 2006;11:641–54
2. Miller WR. Aromatase inhibitors: mechanism of action and role in the treatment of breast cancer. Semin Oncol 2003;30(suppl 14):3–11
3. Smith RE. A review of Selective Estrogen Receptor Modulators and National Surgical Adjuvant Breast and Bowel Projects clinical trials. Semin Oncol 2003;30(suppl 16):4–13
4. Writing Group for the Women's Health Initiative (WHI) Investigators. Risks and benefits of estrogen plus progestin in healthy postmenopausal women. JAMA 2002;288:321–33
5. Zlotta AR, Schulman CC. Neoadjuvant and adjuvant hormone therapy for prostate cancer. World J Urol 2000;18:179–82

**Web:**
1. http://www.prostateinfo.com/ — Hormone Therapy in Prostate Cancer
2. http://www.acor.org/TCRC/tclinks6.html — Hormone Therapy in Testicular Tumors
3. http://www.aace.com/ — American Association of Clinical Endocrinologists
4. http://www.duj.com/Article/Hellstrom2/Hellstrom2.html — Testosterone Replacement Therapy

## 3.3.1    Characterization of Hormone Treatments in Oncology

H. Henß

### Anastrozole

**Chem:**    a,a,α,α-Tetramethyl-5-[(1,2,4-triazol-1-yl)methyl]benzol-1,3-diacetonitrile, non-steroidal aromatase inhibitor

$$(CH_3)_2NCC \qquad CCN(CH_3)_2$$

**MOA:**
- Competitive aromatase inhibition → conversion of androgens into estrogens ↓ → estradiol serum level ↓
- No gestagenic, androgenic, or estrogenic effect

**Pkin:**
- *Kinetics:* good oral resorption (85%), independent of food intake, half-life: t½ 50 h
- *Metabolism:* hepatic degradation, dealkylation, glucuronidation, predominantly renal elimination of original compound (10%) and metabolites (90%)

**Se:**
- *Cardiovascular:* vasodilatation (25%), peripheral edema, infrequent hypertension, thromboembolic events (rare)
- *Lung:* dyspnea (rare)
- *Gastrointestinal:* moderate nausea, vomiting, diarrhea, loss of appetite
- *Liver:* increase of transaminases, hypercholesterolemia
- *Skin:* erythema, pruritus, mild alopecia
- *Nervous system:* headaches (10%), paresthesia, sleep disturbances
- *Other:* fatigue (15%), reduced performance, flush (20%), back pain, bone pain. In rare cases flu-like symptoms

**Ci:**
- Premenopause
- Pregnancy and breast feeding
- Liver dysfunction, renal failure

**Th:**    *Approved indications:* advanced breast cancer in postmenopausal women. Adjuvant treatment of estrogen receptor positive breast cancer.

### Dosage and Administration
Oral administration: 1 mg (1 tablet) daily

## Bicalutamide

**Chem:** (RS)-N-[4-Cyan-3-(trifluormethyl)phenyl]-3-(4-fluorphenylsulfonyl)-2-hydroxy-2-methylpro-panamide, non-steroidal antiandrogen

**MOA:**
- Competitive binding to androgen receptor → inhibition of testosterone effect on prostate cancer cells
- Binding to central androgen receptors (pituitary gland)

**Pkin:**
- *Kinetics:* slow oral resorption (independent of food intake), peak plasma level about 30 h following oral application, half-life: t½ 50 h
- *Metabolism:* hepatic degradation, biliary and renal excretion of original compound and metabolites

**Se:**
- *Bone marrow:* anemia (rare)
- *Cardiovascular:* hypertension (infrequent), edema
- *Lung:* dyspnea (rare)
- *Gastrointestinal:* nausea (10%), vomiting, diarrhea, constipation
- *Liver:* increase of transaminases, cholestasis
- *Skin:* occasional erythema, exanthema, perspiration, alopecia (rare)
- *Nervous system:* diminished libido, occasional vertigo, tiredness, somnolence
- *Other:* hot flushes (45%), gynecomastia (35%) impotence, pain syndromes (25–30%, thoracic region, back, pelvis), fatigue, reduced performance

**Ci:** Not to be taken by women or children

**Th:** *Approved indications:* advanced prostate cancer, in combination with LHRH analogues ("total androgen blockade")

### Dosage and Administration
- Oral administration, 50 mg daily
- Dose modification: use cautiously in patients with severe liver dysfunction
- ATTN: increase of effect of coumarin derivatives

### Buserelin

**Chem:**    5-Oxo-$l$-prolyl- $l$-histidyl- $l$-tryptophyl- $l$-seryl- $l$-tyrosyl- $l$-$O$-tert-butyl-d-seryl- $l$-leucyl- $l$-argi-nyl- $N$-ethyl- $l$-prolinamide, GnRH-analog

$$\text{L-Glp}-\text{L-His}-\text{L-Trp}-\text{L-Ser}-\text{L-Tyr}-\text{D-Ser}-\text{L-Leu}-\text{L-Arg}-\text{L-Pro}-\text{NH}-\text{C}_2\text{H}_5$$
$$\underset{\text{C(CH}_3)_3}{|}$$

**MOA:**    GnRH / LHRH analog with continuous stimulation of pituitary receptors → desensitization of pituitary gland → LH / FSH secretion ↓ → estrogen / testosterone synthesis ↓ ("drug-induced castration")

**Pkin:**
- *Kinetics:* subcutaneous injection, slow-release drug with effective serum levels for 10–14 weeks
- *Metabolism:* hepatic degradation
- *Elimination:* degradation by peptidases, biliary and renal excretion

**Se:**
- *Gastrointestinal:* constipation, nausea, vomiting, loss of appetite
- *Liver:* transient increase of transaminases, hypercholesterolemia
- *Kidney:* hypercalcemia (rare)
- *Skin:* erythema, exanthema, perspiration, acne, seborrhea
- *Nervous system:* diminished libido, occasional vertigo, tiredness, somnolence
- *Other:* hot flushes (45%), gynecomastia (35%) impotence, pain syndromes (25–30%, thoracic region, back, pelvis), fatigue, reduced performance

**Ci:**    Hypersensitivity to buserelin

**Th:**    *Approved indications:* advanced hormone responsive prostate cancer (not after bilateral orchiectomy)
*Other areas of use:* metastatic breast cancer

### Dosage and Administration
- Subcutaneous injection every 3 months, one applicator with 9.45 mg (corresponding to 3 implant rods)
- ATTN: short initial stimulation of estrogen or testosterone excretion, prior to hormone blockage → simultaneous antiestrogen / antiandrogen treatment for initial 3–4 weeks recommended

## Exemestane

**hem:** 6-Methylenandrosta-1,4-diene-3,17-dione, steroidal aromatase inhibitor

**MOA:**
- Irreversible aromatase inhibition → conversion of androgens into estrogens ↓ → estradiol serum level ↓
- No effect on corticosteroid or aldosterone synthesis

**kin:**
- *Kinetics:* good oral resorption (> 80%), esp. with simultaneous food intake, half-life: t½ 24 h
- *Metabolism:* hepatic degradation (cytochrome P450 3A4), biliary and renal elimination of metabolites

**e:**
- *Bone marrow:* lymphopenia (rare)
- *Cardiovascular:* hypertension (infrequent)
- *Lung:* dyspnea, cough
- *Gastrointestinal:* nausea (18%), occasional vomiting, diarrhea, loss of appetite, abdominal pain
- *Liver:* transient increase of transaminases
- *Skin:* erythema, perspiration, alopecia (infrequent)
- *Nervous system:* headaches, vertigo, sleep disturbances, depression
- *Other:* fatigue (20%), reduced performance, flushes (10%), back pain, bone pain. In rare cases flu-like symptoms

**i:**
- Premenopause
- Pregnancy and breast feeding

**h:** *Approved indications:* breast cancer in postmenopausal women.
*Other areas of use:* prevention of prostate cancer

### Dosage and Administration
- Oral administration, 25 mg (1 tablet) daily, following meal
- Dose reduction in severe liver or renal failure
- ATTN: induction of cytochrome P450 system (e.g., by phenytoin, rifampicin, barbiturates) reduces effect. Inhibition of cytochrome P450 system (e.g., itraconazole, cimetidine, macrolides) increases effect and toxicity

**Flutamide**

**Chem:**    4'-Nitro-3'-(trifluormethyl)isobutyranilide, non-steroidal antiandrogen

**MOA:**
- Competitive binding to androgen receptor → inhibition of testosterone effect on prostate cancer cells
- Binding to central androgen receptors (pituitary gland)

**Pkin:**
- *Kinetics:* good oral resorption (independent of food intake), peak plasma level 0.5–2 h following oral application, active metabolite 2-OH-flutamide, half-life: t½ 8–10 h
- *Metabolism:* hepatic degradation, hydroxylation, biliary and renal elimination of initial compound (50%) and metabolites

**Se:**
- *Bone marrow:* anemia (rare)
- *Cardiovascular:* hypertension, edema
- *Gastrointestinal:* nausea (10%), vomiting, diarrhea
- *Liver:* transient increase of transaminases, liver function disorders, cholestasis, hepatitis
- *Skin:* erythema
- *Nervous system:* vertigo, headaches
- *Other:* hot flushes (60%), diminished libido (35%), gynecomastia (prophylactic radiation of nipples with 10 Gy feasible), galactorrhea, impotence (10–35%) fatigue, reduced performance cramps

**Ci:**
- Not to be taken by women or children
- Liver function disorders

**Th:**    *Approved indications:* advanced prostate cancer, in combination with LHRH analogues ("total androgen blockade")

### Dosage and Administration
- Oral administration, 750 mg/day (3 × 1 tablet/day)
- ATTN: increased effect of coumarin derivatives

## Fulvestrant

**hem:** 7-Alpha-[9-(4,4,5,5,5-pentafluoropentylsulfinyl) nonyl]estra-1,3,5-(10)-triene-3,17-beta-diol, estradiol analog, steroidal antiestrogen

**IOA:**
- Competitive binding to estrogen receptors without estrogen like activity → complete blocking of all estrogen effects, with simultaneous downregulation of estrogen receptors
- No cross-resistance to classic antiestrogens

**kin:**
- *Kinetics:* slow distribution following intramuscular injection, peak plasma level after 7–9 days, half-life: t½ 40 h
- *Metabolism:* hepatic degradation (in part by cytochrome P450 3A4 system), predominantly biliary elimination

**e:**
- *Bone marrow:* anemia (10%)
- *Cardiovascular:* venous thrombosis (rare)
- *Lung:* dyspnea, pharyngitis, cough
- *Gastrointestinal:* nausea, vomiting, diarrhea, loss of appetite, up to 50% of patients
- *Liver:* transient increase of transaminases
- *Skin:* erythema, exanthema, angioneurotic edema, urticaria
- *Nervous system:* headaches (15%), vertigo, sleep disturbances, depression
- *Local toxicity:* injection site (reactions)
- *Other:* fatigue (65%), reduced performance, hot flushes (25%), back pain, arthralgia. In rare cases flu-like symptoms

**i:**
- Pregnancy and breast feeding
- Severe liver dysfunction

**h:** *Approved indications:* estrogen receptor positive breast cancer in postmenopausal women

### Dosage and Administration
Intramuscular injection of 250 mg (5 ml) monthly

## Goserelin

**Chem:**  1-(5-Oxo-l-prolyl- l-histidyl- l-tryptophyl- l-seryl- l-tyrosyl- l-O-tert-butyl-d-seryl- l-leucyl- l-arginyl- l prolyl)semicarbazide, GnRH analog

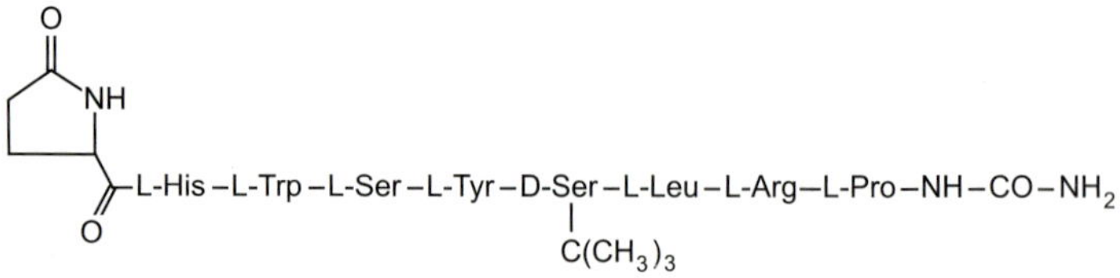

$$\text{L-His}-\text{L-Trp}-\text{L-Ser}-\text{L-Tyr}-\text{D-Ser}-\text{L-Leu}-\text{L-Arg}-\text{L-Pro}-\text{NH}-\text{CO}-\text{NH}_2$$
$$\underset{C(CH_3)_3}{|}$$

**MOA:**  GnRH / LHRH analog with continuous stimulation of pituitary receptors $\rightarrow$ desensitization of pituitary gland $\rightarrow$ LH / FSH secretion $\downarrow$ $\rightarrow$ estrogen / testosterone synthesis $\downarrow$ ("drug-induced castration")

**Pkin:**
- *Kinetics:* subcutaneous injection, slow-release drug with slow resorption for 27 days, half-life $t\frac{1}{2}$ 4–5 h
- *Metabolism:* renal elimination of original compound

**Se:**
- *Cardiovascular:* hypertension
- *Gastrointestinal:* constipation, nausea, vomiting, loss of appetite
- *Liver:* transient increase of transaminases, hypercholesterolemia
- *Kidney:* hypercalcemia
- *Skin:* erythema, exanthema, perspiration, acne, seborrhea, allergic reactions (rare)
- *Nervous system:* headaches (75%), vertigo, sleep disturbances, somnolence, depression
- *Bones:* osteoporosis, bone pain (rare)
- *Other:* fatigue, reduced performance. In men: hot flushes (60%), gynecomastia, impotence, loss of libido. In women: amenorrhea, uterine bleeding

**Ci:**
- Pregnancy and lactation
- Not for use in children

**Th:**  *Approved indications:* advanced prostate cancer, endometriosis, metastatic breast cancer

### Dosage and Administration
Subcutaneous injection monthly 3.6 mg, or every 3 months 10.8 mg
**ATTN:** short initial stimulation of estrogen or testosterone excretion, prior to hormone blockage $\rightarrow$ simultaneous antiestrogen / antiandrogen treatment for initial 3–4 weeks recommended

**Letrozole**

**hem:** 4,4'-(1H-1,2,4-Triazol-1-ylmethylene)dibenzonitrile, non-steroidal aromatase inhibitor

**MOA:**
- Competitive aromatase inhibition → conversion of androgens into estrogens ↓ → estradiol serum level ↓
- No gestagenic, androgenic, or estrogenic effect. No influence on corticosteroid or aldosterone synthesis

**kin:** *Kinetics:* good oral resorption (85%), independent of food intake, half-life: t½ 2 days
*Metabolism:* hepatic degradation, glucuronidation, predominantly renal excretion of original compound (5%) and metabolites (> 80%)

**e:**
- *Cardiovascular:* vasodilatation (25%), tachycardia, thromboembolic events (rare)
- *Lung:* dyspnea, cough
- *Gastrointestinal:* nausea (15%), vomiting, diarrhea, loss of appetite
- *Liver:* transient increase of transaminases, hypercholesterolemia
- *Skin:* erythema, exanthema, pruritus, perspiration
- *Nervous system:* headaches (10%), depression, anxiety disorders
- *Other:* fatigue (10%), reduced performance, flush, pain syndromes (thoracic region, back, joints, myalgia)

**Ci:**
- Premenopausal women
- Pregnancy and breast feeding
- Liver dysfunction, renal failure

**h:** *Approved indications:* advanced breast cancer in postmenopausal women. Adjuvant treatment of estrogen receptor positive breast cancer

### Dosage and Administration
- Oral administration, 2.5 mg (1 tablet) daily
- Dose reduction in severe liver or renal function impairment

## Leuprorelin

**Chem:**    5-Oxo-l-prolyl- l-histidyl- l-tryptophyl- l-seryl- l-tyrosyl- d- leucyl - l-leucyl- l-arginyl- *N*-ethy. l-prolinamide, GnRH analog

**MOA:**    GnRH / LHRH analog with continuous stimulation of pituitary receptors → desensitization pituitary gland → LH / FSH secretion ↓ → estrogen / testosterone synthesis ↓ ("drug-induce castration")

**Pkin:**
- *Kinetics:* subcutaneous injection, slow-release drug, half-life t½ 2–4 h
- *Metabolism:* hepatic degradation, biliary and renal elimination

**Se:**
- *Bone marrow:* anemia, leucopenia (rare)
- *Cardiovascular:* ECG changes (20%), hypertension, peripheral edema, thromboemboli events
- *Gastrointestinal:* constipation, nausea, vomiting, loss of appetite
- *Liver:* transient increase of transaminases, hypercholesterolemia
- *Kidney:* hypercalcemia (rare)
- *Skin:* erythema, exanthema, perspiration, acne, seborrhea, allergic reactions (rare)
- *Nervous system:* headaches, vertigo, sleep disturbances, somnolence, depression
- *Bone:* osteoporosis, bone pain (rare)
- *Other:* fatigue, reduced performance. In men: hot flushes (50%), gynecomastia (35%) impc tence, loss of libido. In women: amenorrhea, uterine bleeding

**Ci:**
- Pregnancy and lactation
- Not for use in children (except girls with precocious puberty vera)

**Th:**    *Approved indications:* breast cancer, endometriosis, uterus myomatosis
*Other areas of use:* prostate cancer

### Dosage and Administration
- 3.75 mg monthly, or 11.25 mg every 3 months i.m. (dual-chamber injection)
- ATTN: short initial stimulation of estrogen or testosterone excretion, prior to hormon blockage → simultaneous antiestrogen / antiandrogen treatment for initial 3–4 weeks recom mended

## Medroxyprogesterone acetate, MPA

**hem:** 17-Hydroxy-6α-methyl-4-pregnene-3,20-dione, gestagen

**MOA:**
- Gestagen and androgenic activity
- Reduction of pituitary FSH / LH secretion
- Stimulation of estrogen and androgen degradation

**kin:**
- *Kinetics:* oral or intramuscular administration, oral bioavailability 10%, following intramuscular administration stable plasma levels for 7 days, terminal t½ 14–60 h
- *Metabolism:* hepatic degradation, biliary and renal elimination of original compound and metabolites

**e:**
- *Cardiovascular:* edema, arterial hypertension, thromboembolic events
- *Gastrointestinal:* nausea, vomiting, diarrhea, constipation
- *Liver:* transient increase of transaminases, cholestasis
- *Skin:* alopecia, dermatitis, acne, hirsutism (rare)
- *Nervous system:* headaches, sleep disturbances, tremor, depression, mania
- *Other:* fatigue, reduced performance, cramps, development of diabetes mellitus, allergic reactions, anaphylaxis. In men: gynecomastia, breast pain, galactorrhea, hot flushes. In women: menstrual disorders, amenorrhea

**i:**
- Pregnancy and lactation
- Previous thromboembolic events or stroke
- Severe liver or renal impairment, hypercalcemia
- Severe hypertension, diabetes mellitus

**h:** *Approved indications:* metastatic breast cancer, advanced endometrial cancer
*Other areas of use:* advanced renal cancer

### Dosage and Administration
- *Breast cancer:* 300–1,500 mg/day p.o, or 500–1,000 mg/week i.m. for 28 days, followed by maintenance dose (according to plasma level, goal > 100 ng/ml)
- *Endometrial cancer:* 300–600 mg/day p.o. or 500–1,000 mg/week i.m.

### Megestrol acetate

**Chem:**    6-Methyl-3,20-dioxo-4,6-pregnadiene-17α-yl-acetate, gestagen

**MOA:**
- Gestagen and androgenic activity
- Reduction of pituitary FSH / LH secretion
- Stimulation of estrogen and androgen degradation

**Pkin:**
- *Kinetics:* oral administration, good oral bioavailability, terminal t½ 15–20 h
- *Metabolism:* hepatic degradation, renal elimination of original compound and metabolites

**Se:**
- *Cardiovascular:* edema, arterial hypertension, thromboembolic events
- *Gastrointestinal:* nausea, vomiting, diarrhea, constipation
- *Liver:* transient increase of transaminases
- *Skin:* alopecia, erythema
- *Nervous system:* headaches, carpal tunnel syndrome
- *Other:* fatigue, reduced performance. Development of diabetes mellitus, hypercalcemia. In men: gynecomastia, breast pain, galactorrhea, hot flushes. In women: menstrual disorders, amenorrhea

**Ci:**
- Pregnancy and lactation
- Previous thromboembolic events or stroke
- Severe liver or renal impairment, hypercalcemia
- Severe hypertension, diabetes mellitus

**Th:**    *Approved indications:* metastatic breast cancer, advanced endometrial cancer
*Other areas of use:* cancer-induced cachexia

### Dosage and Administration
- Oral administration, 160 (–320) mg/day p.o. in breast and endometrial cancer
- In cancer-induced cachexia, doses up to 400–800 mg/day have been applied

### Raloxifene

**Chem:** 6-Hydroxy-2-(4-hydroxyphenyl)benzol[b]thiene-3-yl-4-(2-piperidinoethoxy)phenylketone, non-steroidal antiestrogen

**MOA:**
- Competitive binding to cytoplasmic estrogen receptors, selective agonistic and antagonistic effects (selective estrogen receptor modulation, SERM): estradiol ↓ TGFβ ↑, TGFα ↓, EGF receptor expression ↓, IL-2 secretion ↑
- Agonist of bone and cholesterol metabolism
- No effect on pituitary gland, breast, or uterus tissue

**Pkin:** *Metabolism:* hepatic degradation, renal elimination

**AE:**
- *Cardiovascular:* vasodilatation, hypertension, venous thromboembolism (deep venous thrombosis, pulmonary embolism)
- *Gastrointestinal:* nausea, vomiting, dyspepsia
- *Skin:* erythema, exanthema
- *Nervous system:* headaches
- *Musculoskeletal:* calf cramps
- *Other:* hot flushes, breast pain, vaginitis

**Ci:**
- Use in premenopausal women
- Previous thromboembolic events
- Liver function impairment, cholestasis, renal impairment
- Endometrial cancer, uterine bleeding of unknown origin

**Th:** *Approved indications:* osteoporosis in postmenopausal women
*Other areas of use:* hormone-dependent breast cancer in postmenopausal women

**Dosage and Administration**
60 mg/day p.o.

### Tamoxifen

**Chem:**      (Z)-2-[4-(1,2-Diphenyl-1-butenyl)phenoxyl]-N,N-dimethylethylamine, non-steroidal antiestrogen

**MOA:**
- Competitive inhibition of estrogen binding to cytoplasmic estrogen receptors, selective agonistic and antagonistic effects (selective estrogen receptor modulation, SERM), in estrogen-dependent tissues inhibition of proliferation. Estradiol ↓ TGFβ ↑, TGFα ↓, EGF receptor expression ↓, IL-2 secretion ↑
- Agonist of bone and cholesterol metabolism

**Pkin:**
- *Kinetics:* high bioavailability following oral administration, enterohepatic circulation, terminal t½ 7 days
- *Metabolism:* hepatic degradation, biliary elimination

**Se:**
- *Bone marrow:* mild thrombocytopenia, leucopenia (5%)
- *Cardiovascular:* edema, thromboembolic events (rare)
- *Gastrointestinal:* loss of appetite, nausea (5–20%), vomiting
- *Liver:* transient increase of transaminases, cholestasis, hypertriglyceridemia
- *Skin:* rash, mild alopecia, erythema multiforme
- *Nervous system:* visual disturbances (cataract, corneal changes, retinopathy), headaches
- *Musculoskeletal:* calf cramps
- *Other:* in patients with bone metastases hypercalcemia possible, hot flushes (25–30%), in premenopausal women menstrual cycle disturbances, endometrial proliferation (polyps, malignancies)

**Ci:**
- Known hypersensitivity, children
- Severe thrombocytopenia or leucopenia
- Hypercalcemia
- History of thromboembolic events
- Endometrial cancer, uterine bleeding of unknown origin

**Th:**      *Approved indications:* osteoporosis in postmenopausal women
*Other areas of use:* breast cancer (adjuvant, advanced) hormone dependent

### Dosage and Administration
20–40 mg/day p.o.

### Toremifene

**Chem:**  2-{4-[(Z)-4 Chlor-1,2-diphenyl-1-butenyl]phenoxyl}-N,N-dimethyl-ethylamine, non-steroidal antiestrogen

**MOA:**
- Competitive inhibition of estrogen binding to cytoplasmic estrogen receptors, selective agonistic and antagonistic effects (selective estrogen receptor modulation, SERM), in estrogen-dependent tissues inhibition of proliferation. Estradiol ↓ TGFβ ↑, TGFα ↓, EGF receptor expression ↓, IL-2 secretion ↑
- Agonist of bone and cholesterol metabolism
- Cytostatic effect

**Pkin:**
- *Kinetics:* high bioavailability following oral administration, enterohepatic circulation, albumin binding (92%), terminal t½ 5–6 days
- *Metabolism:* hepatic degradation, biliary elimination

**Se:**
- *Bone marrow:* mild thrombocytopenia, leucopenia
- *Cardiovascular:* edema, thromboembolic events (rare)
- *Gastrointestinal:* nausea, vomiting, loss of appetite
- *Liver:* transient increase of transaminases, cholestasis
- *Skin:* pruritus, erythema
- *Nervous system:* vertigo, sleep disturbances, tiredness, headaches
- *Other:* Hot flushes (10–30%), perspiration, vaginal bleeding / fluor, bone pain, hypercalcemia, endometrial proliferation (rare)

**Ci:**
- Endometrial cancer, uterine bleeding of unknown origin
- History of thromboembolic events
- Severe liver impairment

**Th:**  *Approved indications:* metastatic breast cancer, hormone dependent

### *Dosage and Administration*
60 mg/d p.o.

# 3.4     Cytokines

**A.K. Kaskel, H. Veelken**

**Def:**     Intercellular mediators synthesized by immune cells and mesenchymal cells (fibroblasts, endothelial cells, stroma cells) which modulate immune responses, cellular proliferation, and differentiation. Characteristics:
- Soluble proteins or glycoproteins, 15–40 kDa molecular weight
- Pleiotropic, overlapping, and/or synergistic effects

**Class:**     Cytokines

| Factor | Characterization |
|--------|------------------|
| *Interleukins (IL):* | |
| IL-1 | Inflammation mediator |
| IL-2 | T-cell expansion and activation, IL-2 receptor expression ↑ |
| IL-3 | Proliferation of pluripotent stem cells |
| IL-4 | B-/T-cell proliferation / differentiation, TH2 cells ↑, dendritic cells ↑ |
| IL-5 | Activation and differentiation of eosinophils |
| IL-6 | Acute-phase reaction, thrombopoiesis stimulation |
| IL-7 | Lymphopoiesis induction, T-cell proliferation / differentiation |
| IL-8 | Activation / chemotaxis of neutrophils |
| IL-9 | B-cell activation, antibody production |
| IL-10 | Suppression of macrophage function, TH2 induction |
| IL-11 | Inflammation mediator, thrombopoiesis stimulation |
| IL-12 | T-cell activation / differentiation, TH1 induction |
| IL-13 | B-cell activation / differentiation, dendritic cells ↑ |
| IL-14 | B-cell proliferation / differentiation |
| IL-15 | T-/NK cell activation/differentiation |
| IL-16 | CD4 ligand, inflammation mediator |
| IL-17 | Cytokine secretion by mesenchymal cells ↑ |
| IL-18 | "IFNγ-inducing factor," inflammation mediator |
| IL-19 | Secretion of IL-6 and TNFα in monocytes ↑, proapoptotic |
| IL-20 | Proliferation of keratinocytes ↑, mediator of inflammation |
| IL-21 | B-cell apoptosis, production of IFNγ ↑ in T- and NK cells |
| IL-22 | "T-cell-derived inducible factor," inflammation mediator |
| IL-23 | Associated with TH1 response, IL-12 secretion ↑ |
| IL-24 | Growth-inhibiting, proapoptotic in tumor cell lines |
| IL-25 | Associated with TH2 response, IL-4, IL-5, IL-13 ↑, eosinophils |
| IL-26 | T- and NK cells |
| IL-27 | Proliferation of naive CD4 cells, TH1 differentiation |
| IL-28 | Antiviral activity |
| IL-29 | Antiviral activity |

Hematopoietic growth factors ▶ Chap. 4.3

**Class:**   **Cytokines** *(continued)*

| Factor | Characterization |
|--------|------------------|
| *Interferons (IFN) and other:* | |
| IFNα | Antiproliferative, antiviral |
| IFNβ | Antiproliferative, antiviral |
| IFNγ | Antiproliferative, antiviral, monocyte stimulation |
| TNFα | Tumor necrosis factor α (cachectin), inflammation mediator |
| TNFβ | Tumor necrosis factor β (= lymphotoxin α, LTα), inflammation mediator |

Hematopoietic growth factors ► Chap. 4.3

## Interferon α (IFNα)

**Chem:** Type 1 interferon, "leukocyte interferon"; glycoprotein, > 20 variants, 156–172 amino acids, 19–26 kDa. Peginterferon is a polyethylene-glycol conjugated form with an increased half-life.

**Phys:**
- *Gene locus:* chromosome 9p22, variable expression of IFNα variants
- *Expression:* leukocytes, monocytes / macrophages, B-lymphocytes, fibroblasts

**MOA:** All IFNα types display antiviral, antiparasitic, and antiproliferative activity:
- *T-cells:* T-suppressor activity, activation of cytotoxic T-cells, TH1 induction
- Modulation of B- and NK cell function, monocyte activation / macrophages
- Antigen expression ↑, oncogene expression ↓, inhibition of angiogenesis

**Pkin:**
- *Kinetics:* half-life: terminal t½ IFNα$_{2a}$: 4–8 h, IFNα$_{2b}$: 2–3 h, peg-IFN: 40–80 h
- *Metabolism:* proteolysis, renal elimination

**Se:**
- *Bone marrow:* moderate anemia, granulocytopenia, thrombocytopenia
- *Thyroid gland:* hyper/hypothyroidism (partly irreversible), thyroiditis
- *Cardiovascular:* arrhythmia, myocardial infarction, cardiomyopathy, cardiac failure, hypotension, hypertension, hemorrhages, cerebrovascular disorders
- *Pulmonary:* cough, dyspnea, pulmonary edema, pneumonia
- *Gastrointestinal tract:* moderate nausea, diarrhea, loss of appetite
- *Liver / pancreas:* reversible increase of transaminases, hyperglycemia
- *Kidney:* fluid retention, edema, hypocalcemia
- *Skin:* erythema, pruritus, dry skin, scaling, alopecia
- *Nervous system:* central nervous disorders, depression (increased risk of suicide), dizziness, insomnia, somnolence, peripheral neuropathy, paresthesia, optic neuritis
- *Other:* flu-like symptoms (fever, sweating, chills, fatigue), myalgia, arthralgia, headaches, arthritis

**Ci:**
- Human protein allergy, autoimmune diseases, immunosuppression
- Severe cardiopulmonary or vascular disease
- Severe hepatic or renal dysfunction
- Diseases of the central nervous system
- Untreated hyper/hypothyroidism (TSH / T3 / T4 evaluation before treatment)
- Severe bone marrow damage
- Lactation, pregnancy (effective contraception during treatment)

**Th:** *Indications:* chronic active hepatitis B/C, CML, NHL, multiple myeloma, melanoma, Kaposi's sarcoma, renal cell carcinoma
*Clinical trial use:* solid tumors, myeloproliferative syndromes

*Dosage:* application s.c., i.v., or i.m., e.g.:
- IFNα 2–9 × 10$^6$ IU/day, 3–7 × per week, slowly increasing dose
- High-dose IFNα up to 20 × 10$^6$ IU/m²/day
- PEGylated IFNα 40–150 μg once a week with hepatitis C

ATTN: Patients on high-dose IFNα treatment need to be closely monitored. Chest x-ray if cough or dyspnea develop. Laboratory tests including full blood count, liver and renal function, blood glucose. Development of antibodies possible.

### Interferon β (IFNβ)

**Chem:** Type 1 interferon, "fibroblast interferon"; glycoprotein, 166 amino acids, 20 kDa

**Phys:**
- *Gene locus:* chromosome 9p22, close to interferon α gene group
- *Expression:* fibroblasts

**MOA:** Antiviral, antiparasitic, antiproliferative, and immune-modulating properties like interferon α, T-suppressor-cell activation

**Pkin:**
- *Kinetics:* terminal half-life $IFN\beta_{1a}$ 8–10 h, $IFN\beta_{1b}$ 1–4 h
- *Metabolism:* proteolysis, renal excretion

**Se:**
- *Bone marrow:* granulocytopenia, lymphopenia, thrombocytopenia (rare), anemia
- *Cardiovascular:* arrhythmia, tachycardia, hypotension, hypertension
- *Gastrointestinal:* nausea, vomiting, loss of appetite, stomatitis
- *Liver:* transient increase of transaminases
- *Kidney:* urea ↑, creatinine ↑
- *Skin:* exanthema, pruritus, alopecia, dry skin, injection site reactions, re-activation of herpes virus infections
- *Nervous system:* central nervous disorders, paresthesia, neuropsychiatric changes (depression, somnolence, confusion, risk of suicide) possible
- *Other:* flu-like symptoms: fever, sweating, chills, fatigue, myalgia, arthralgia, headaches (may be treated with paracetamol)

ATTN: Close monitoring of patients when using high dose. Possible antibody formation against recombinant IFNβ. Single cases of rapidly progressing glomerulonephritis after combined treatment with IFNβ and interleukin 2.

**Ci:**
- Human protein allergy
- Pre-existing cardiac disease
- Severe hepatic dysfunction, renal insufficiency

**Th:** *Indications:* multiple sclerosis, severe viral disease (e.g., encephalitis, generalized *Herpes zoster*)
*Clinical trial use:* nasopharyngeal carcinoma, other solid tumors, cutaneous T-cell lymphomas

*Dosage:* s.c. or i.v. application, e.g.:
- $0.5–5 \times 10^6$ IU/day i.v., 3–6 × per week, maximum $25 \times 10^6$ IU/day
- With multiple sclerosis: 44 μg $IFN\beta_{1a}$ i.m. 3 × per week

## Interferon γ (IFNγ)

**Chem:**    Type 2 interferon, "T-lymphocyte interferon"; protein dimer, subunits of 146 amino acids, 6 variants, 20–25 kDa

**Phys:**
- *Gene locus:* chromosome 12q24.1
- *Expression:* T-cells, NK cells

**MOA:**    Antiviral, antiparasitic, and proliferation-modulating properties:
- *T-cells:* stimulation of proliferation, modulation of T-cell differentiation, activation of cytotoxic T-cells, and induction of IL-2 receptors
- *B-cells:* induction of immunoglobulin synthesis
- *Monocytes / macrophages, NK cells:* activation
- Stimulation of MHC class I *and* class II antigen expression, modulation (increase) of tumor antigen expression
- Modulation of hematopoiesis and lipid metabolism

**Pkin:**
- *Kinetics:* half-life: s.c. application: 6 h, i.m.: 3 h, i.v.: 38 min
- *Metabolism:* proteolysis, renal excretion

**Se:**
- *Bone marrow:* moderate leukopenia, anemia (rare)
- *Cardiovascular:* arrhythmias, tachycardia, hypotension, hypertension, thromboembolic events (rare), myocardial infarction
- *Gastrointestinal:* nausea, vomiting, diarrhea, loss of appetite
- *Liver:* transient increase of transaminases
- *Kidney:* urea ↑, creatinine ↑
- *Skin:* exanthema, pruritus, injection site reactions
- *Nervous system:* central nervous system disorders, hallucinations, depression, confusion, tremor, impaired vision, paresthesias
- *Other:* flu-like symptoms: fever, sweating, chills, fatigue, myalgia, arthralgia, headaches (may be treated with paracetamol)

**Ci:**
- Human protein allergy
- Severe cardiovascular disease
- CNS disorders, epilepsy
- Severe hepatic dysfunction, renal insufficiency

**Th:**    *Indications:* progressive septic granulomatosis (chronic granulomatous disease, CGD)
*Clinical trial use:* invasive aspergillosis, infection with mycobacteria, solid tumors (renal cell carcinoma, pleural mesothelioma)

*Dosage:* application s.c., i.m., or i.v., usually
- Progressive septic granulomatosis (CGD): 50 µg/m²/day s.c. 3 × per week
- Renal cell carcinoma: 50–100 µg s.c. once a week

## Interleukin 2 (IL-2), Aldesleukin

**Chem:** Glycoprotein, 133 amino acids, 15 kDa

**Phys:**
- *Gene locus:* chromosome 4q26-28
- *Expression:* T-cells (CD4+)

**MOA:**
- *T-cells:* proliferation, clonal expansion, chemotaxis, activation, induction of non-MHC restricted cytotoxic T-cells, binding to IL-2 receptor
- *B- and NK cells:* proliferation, differentiation, activation
- Induction / release of several other cytokines (interferon γ)
- Stimulation of cytotoxic tumor infiltrating monocytes / macrophages

**Pkin:**
- *Kinetics:* rapid distribution after parenteral administration, terminal half-life t½ 30–90 min
- *Metabolism:* proteolysis, renal elimination

**Se:**
- *With high-dose treatment:* capillary leak syndrome (dose-limiting), neurological / renal / gastrointestinal / cardiovascular symptoms
- *Bone marrow:* anemia, thrombocytopenia, leukopenia, eosinophilia
- *Cardiovascular:* hypotension, edema, endocarditis, cardiac arrhythmias, angina pectoris, cardiac arrest, thromboembolic events
- *Pulmonary:* dyspnea, pulmonary edema, cough, hemoptysis, ARDS, bronchospasm
- *Gastrointestinal:* nausea, vomiting, diarrhea, mucositis, gastritis, gastrointestinal hemorrhage, constipation, meteorism, loss of appetite
- *Kidney:* oligo- / anuria, interstitial nephritis, acute renal failure, hypocalcemia
- *Liver / pancreas:* transient increase of transaminases, hyperglycemia
- *Skin:* pruritus, dermatitis, alopecia, conjunctivitis
- *Nervous system (central and peripheral neuropathy):* depression, confusion, agitation, hallucination, neuralgia, paresthesia, sensory and motor dysfunction, seizures, somnolence, coma
- *Cerebrovascular disorders:* TIA, cerebral hemorrhage, cerebral infarction
- *Other:* flu-like symptoms: fever, sweating, chills, fatigue, myalgia, arthralgia, headaches

ATTN: Nephrotoxic, cardiotoxic, and myelotoxic drugs and hypertensives can enhance the side effects. Glucocorticoids decrease the effects of IL-2.
High-dose IL-2 treatment only under strict monitoring: cardiovascular system, neurostatus, renal function, liver function, full blood count, thyroid function.

**Ci:**
- Performance status ECOG > 2, cerebral metastasis
- Human protein allergy, severe infections
- Severe cardiovascular or pulmonary disorders (pO$_2$ < 60 mmHg)
- Lactation, pregnancy (strict contraception is mandatory)

**Th:**
*Indications:* metastatic renal cell carcinoma
*Clinical trial use:* malignant melanoma, NHL, solid tumors, donor lymphocyte infusion after allogeneic transplantation, AIDS-associated malignancies

*Dosage and administration:* i.v. or s.c., e.g.:
- Continuous infusion: 3–24 × 10$^6$ IU/m$^2$/day (18 × 10$^6$IU = 1 mg) c.i.v. for 2–5 days
- S.c.: 1–5 × 10$^6$ IU/m$^2$/day s.c. once or several times a week

### Interleukin 11 (IL-11)

**Chem:** Protein, 178 amino acids, 19 kDa

**Phys:**
- *Gene locus:* chromosome 19q13.3-q13.4
- *Expression:* bone marrow fibroblasts, various mesenchymal and epithelial cell types (e.g., bronchial / alveolar and gastrointestinal epithelial cells, osteoblasts, CNS)

**MOA:**
- *Inflammation mediator* (mainly in lung)
- *Hematopoiesis:* synergistically with other cytokines, stimulation of megakaryopoiesis, erythropoiesis, myelopoiesis, lymphopoiesis, and (in vitro) bone marrow stroma cells, increase of thrombocytes usually 5–9 days after application
- *Gastrointestinal:* in vitro inhibition of the proliferation of intact crypt stem cells, in vivo stimulation of proliferation / apoptosis inhibition in damaged crypt cells
- *Other:* adipogenesis inhibitor, modulator of the metabolism of extracellular matrix (fibrosis-enhancing)

**Pkin:**
- *Kinetics:* rapid distribution after s.c. application, terminal half-life: $t\frac{1}{2}$ 7 h
- *Metabolism:* proteolysis, renal excretion

**Se:** Usually, only mild and transient side effects:
- *Cardiovascular:* supraventricular arrhythmias, tachycardia
- *Pulmonary:* dyspnea, pulmonary edema, cough, pleural effusion
- *Gastrointestinal:* nausea / vomiting, diarrhea
- *Kidney:* fluid retention → dilution anemia, electrolyte imbalance, effusions, edema, papillary edema (visual disturbances)
- *Skin:* erythema
- *Nervous system:* amentia, insomnia, headache
- *Other:* flu-like symptoms, increase of acute phase proteins, anaphylaxis

**Ci:**
- Cardiac insufficiency, absolute arrhythmia
- Electrolyte / fluid imbalance

**Th:** *Indications:* prevention of severe thrombocytopenia and reduction of the need for platelet transfusions following myelosuppressive chemotherapy (USA)

*Dosage:* 50 µg/kg body weight/day s.c., application 6–24 h after chemotherapy, daily application until thrombocytes > 50,000/µl, maximum 21 days

## Tumor Necrosis Factor α (TNFα)

**Chem:** 157 amino acids, 17.3 kDa

**Phys:**
- *Gene locus:* chromosome 6 (within MHC complex)
- *Expression:* activated monocytes, macrophages

**MOA:**
- *Inflammation mediator:* induction of cytokines and low molecular weight mediators (prostaglandin, PaF) ↑, leukocyte migration ↑
- *B- and T-cells:* proliferation and activation, phagocytosis / cytotoxicity ↑
- *Vascular effect:* endothelial cell proliferation ↓, vessel wall damage, modulation of adhesion molecule and cytokine expression → local procoagulant effects → microthrombosis

**Pkin:**
- *Kinetics:* half-life dose-dependent, i.v. application of 150 µg/m²: 15–30 min

**Se:**
- *Bone marrow:* leukopenia, anemia, thrombocytopenia
- *Cardiovascular:* hypotension and tachycardia, arrhythmia, shock
- *Kidney:* acute renal failure
- *Nervous system:* central nervous system disorders, peripheral neuropathy
- *Other:* flu-like symptoms (fever, chills, sweating, fatigue, nausea), thromboembolic events, DIC (disseminated intravascular coagulation) in isolated cases

**Ci:**
- Severe cardiovascular or pulmonary diseases, simultaneous treatment with cardiotoxic drugs
- Peptic ulcer, severe ascites, limited bone marrow function
- Renal or hepatic dysfunction, hypercalcemia

**Th:** *Indications:* isolated limb perfusion in combination with melphalan and hyperthermia in non-resectable soft tissue sarcoma

ATTN: Isolated limb perfusion must be carried out in specialized centers under intensive surveillance and permanent monitoring of systemic drug concentrations (objective: leakage of drugs into the systemic circulation < 10%).

*Dosage:* i.v. application for isolated limb perfusion in combination with chemotherapy (e.g., melphalan), 3–4 mg TNFα per liter of perfused volume (maximum 150 mg)

**Ref:**
1. Atkins MB, Regan M, McDermott D. Update on the role of interleukin 2 and other cytokines in the treatment of patients with stage IV renal carcinoma. Clin Cancer Res 2004;10(18 Pt 2):6342S–6S
2. Anderson GM, Nakada MT, DeWitte M. Tumor necrosis factor-alpha in the pathogenesis and treatment of cancer. Curr Opin Pharmacol 2004;4:314–20
3. Dranoff G. Cytokines in cancer pathogenesis and cancer therapy. Nat Rev Cancer 2004;4:11–22
4. Morcellin S, Rossi CR, Pilati P et al. Tumor necrosis factor, cancer and anticancer therapy. Cytokine Growth factor Rev 2005;16:35–53
5. Pestka S, Krause CD, Walter MR. Interferons, interferon-like cytokines, and their receptors. Immunol Rev 2004;202:8–32

**Web:**
1. http://www.weizmann.ac.il/cytokine — International Cytokine Society
2. http://www.sciencedirect.com/science/journal/10434666 — Cytokines Journal
3. http://www.elsevier.com/wps/product/cws_home/868 — Cytokine Growth Factor Reviews
4. http://cytokine.medic.kumamoto-u.ac.jp — Cytokine Family Database

## 3.5     Monoclonal Antibodies

**K. Potthoff, H. Veelken**

**Def:**     Monoclonal immunoglobulin preparations with specific effects directed against defined target structures (antigens). Monoclonal antibody production is usually based on "recombinant" DNA technology.

### Antibody Nomenclature

Notations for monoclonal antibodies consist of several components and follow internationally valid systematics. In general, they are formed by one prefix and three suffixes (according to the following pattern: "prefix – suffix 1 – suffix 2 – suffix 3"):

- Suffix 1: indicating the target structure: colon ("col"), mammary ("ma"), testis ("got"), prostate ("pr" / "pro"), cardiovascular ("cir"), viral ("vir"), immune system ("lim" / "li"), infect associated ("les"), mixed / diverse tumors ("tum" / "tu")
- Suffix 2: indicating the species of origin: human ("u"), mouse ("o"), rat ("a"), hamster ("e"), primate ("i"), chimeric ("xi"), humanized ("zu")
- Suffix 3: "mab" indicating a monoclonal antibody or antibody fragment

Example: *Alem-tu-zu-mab:* humanized antibody against an antigen that is expressed by different malignant tumors.

**Th:**     ### Potential Mechanism of Action of Monoclonal Antibodies

- Competitive receptor blockade → blockage of receptor-mediated effects (e.g., inhibition of cytokines or growth factors)
- Receptor activation → induction of receptor-mediated effects (e.g., apoptosis induction)
- Complement activation and complement-mediated cytotoxicity (CDC)
- Antibody-mediated cellular cytotoxicity (ADCC)
- Conjugation of antibodies and radioactive ("radioimmunoconjugates") or cytotoxic components ("immunotoxins")

### Use of Monoclonal Antibodies

Since 1998, several different monoclonal antibodies have been licensed for treatment of solid tumors and hematological neoplasias. Application as monotherapy or in combination, e.g., with chemotherapy.

### Species Specificity

Antibodies are usually specific for each species. Application of murine antibodies in humans might lead to loss of effect due to generation of antibodies as well as to incompatibility reactions. Several different types of antibodies with human parts are clinically used:

- "Chimeric" antibodies: constant region of human origin, variable region (including antigen-binding site) of primary species of origin
- "Humanized" antibodies: antigen-binding region of primary species of origin, remainder of human origin (95%)
- "human" antibodies: 100% human sequence

**New monoclonal antibodies in clinical trials (selection)**

| Compound | Target structure (cell type) | Indication |
| --- | --- | --- |
| Apolizumab (Hu1D10) | HLA-DR-β-chain (B-cells, macrophages, dendritic cells) | B-NHL, CLL |
| Basiliximab | Interleukin-2 receptor (activated T-cells) | GVHD prophylaxis |
| Daclizumab | Interleukin-2 receptor α (T-cells) | T-NHL, T-cell leukemia |

**New monoclonal antibodies in clinical trials (selection)** *(continued)*

| Compound | Target structure (cell type) | Indication |
|---|---|---|
| Epratuzumab | CD22 (B-cells) | B-NHL, autoimmune diseases |
| HuM291 | CD3 (mature T-cells) | T-NHL |
| Infliximab | TNFα (monocytes, macrophages, lymphocytes) | GVHD treatment |
| $^{131}$I-Lym-1 | HLA-DR10 | B-NHL |
| Pertuzumab (rhuMAb-2C4) | HER dimerization (HER1/ EGFR, HER1/HER4) | Solid tumors |

**Ref:**

1. Baselga J. Monoclonal antibodies directed at growth factor receptors. Ann Oncol 2000;11(suppl 3):187–90
2. Giaccone G. Epidermal growth factor receptor inhibitors in the treatment of non-small cell lung cancer. J Clin Oncol 2005;23:3235–42
3. Hicklin DJ, Ellis LM. Role of the vascular endothelial growth factor pathway in tumor growth and angiogenesis. J Clin Oncol 2005;23:1011–27
4. Hynes NE, Lane HA. ERBB receptors and cancer: the complexity of targeted inhibitors. Nat Rev Cancer 2005;5:341–54
5. López-Guillermo A, Mercadal S. The clinical use of antibodies in haematological malignancies. Ann Oncol 2007;18 ( Suppl. 9): ix51–7
6. Plosker G, Figgitt, D. Rituximab: a review of its use in non-Hodgkin's lymphoma and chronic lymphocytic leukaemia. Drugs 2003, 63:803–43
7. Reichert JM, Valge-Archer VE. Development trends for monoclonal antibody cancer therapeuties. Nat Rev Drug Discov 2007;6:349–355
8. Villamor N, Montserrat E, Colomer D. Mechanism of action and resistance to monoclonal antibody therapy. Semin Oncol 2003;30:424–33

**Web:**

1. http://www.oncolink.upenn.edu — Oncolink Information
2. http://www.cancer.org/ — American Cancer Society
3. http://www.nci.nih.gov/ — National Cancer Institute, Bethesda, USA
4. http://www.fda.gov/cber/ — FDA, Center for Biologics Evaluation and Research
5. http://www.gallartinternet.com/mai — Monoclonal Antibody Index
6. http://www.cancerbackup.org.uk/treatments/ biologicaltherapies/monoclonalantibodies — Cancer Backup UK
7. http://en.wikipedia.org/wiki/ monoclonal_antibodies — Wikipedia, Monoclonal Antibodies

### Alemtuzumab

**Chem:** Humanized, recombinant, monoclonal IgG1-κ antibody (rat / human), specifically binding to the CD52 antigen

**MOA:**
- Binding to CD52 (on B- / T- / NK cells, monocytes, macrophages)
  - → complement-mediated cytotoxicity (CDC), antibody-mediated cytotoxicity (ADCC), apoptosis induction, depletion particularly of CD52-positive lymphocytes
  - → peripheral T-cell depletion for 3–6 months. Recovery of CD4+ T-cells to 75% of baseline within 6–12 months after treatment
- Strong CD52 expression on T-cells → effective in T-CLL

**Pkin:** *Kinetics:* half-life: median t½ 12 days

**Se:**
- *Bone marrow:* prolonged myelosuppression (neutropenia, lymphocytopenia, thrombocytopenia, 50–70%) → infections (in 10–15% of cases, dose-limiting), esp. HSV, CMV, Candida, aspergillosis, *Pneumocystis carinii* pneumonia (PcP), mycobacterioses
- *Cardiovascular:* hypotension, hypertension, tachycardia, arrhythmia, vascular spasms
- *Pulmonary:* pneumonia, bronchitis, pulmonary edema, bronchospasms, dyspnea
- *Gastrointestinal:* nausea (50%), vomiting, diarrhea, constipation, abdominal pain, gastrointestinal hemorrhage, loss of appetite
- *Liver:* transient increase of transaminases, hyperglycemia
- *Nervous system:* headache, dysgeusia, tremor, rigor, paresthesia, dizziness, confusion, anxiety, depression, insomnia
- *Infusion-induced reactions:* fever (85%), chills, hot flushes, sweating, erythema, urticaria, pruritus, rhinitis, conjunctivitis, sore throat, angioedema
- *Other:* night sweat, fatigue, reduced performance status, peripheral edemas, arthralgia, myalgia, bone pain, LDH ↑, coagulation disorders

**Ci:**
- Hypersensitivity to murine proteins
- Severely impaired cardiac, renal, or hepatic function
- Florid systemic infections, immune deficiency, HIV infection
- Pregnancy, lactation

**Th:** *Indications:* CLL, second line treatment
*Clinical trial use:* first-line and consolidation therapy for CLL, T-cell NHL, T-cell depletion in GVHD prophylaxis, ITP, immunocytopenia

*Dosage:* i.v. application (infusion over 2 h), with dose escalation:
- Week 1: 3 mg i.v. day 1, 10 mg i.v. day 2, 30 mg i.v. day 3; weeks 2–12: 30 mg i.v. 3 × per week, over 4–12 weeks
- ATTN: risk of severe infusion-induced reactions including fever, chills, thrombocytopenia, decrease of blood pressure, tumor lysis syndrome. Premedication with paracetamol and antihistamines (e.g., clemastine). No dose escalation in case of severe infusion-associated side effects. Close monitoring of vital parameters
- Infection prophylaxis with cotrimoxazole and virustatics from day 8 until CD4 cell count is ≥ 200/µl

### Bevacizumab

**Chem:** Chimeric, recombinant, monoclonal IgG1 antibody (mouse / human), specifically binding to VEGF (vascular endothelial growth factor)

**MOA:**
- VEGF binds to VEGF receptors (VEGF-R1, -R2, -R3) on endothelial cells → endothelial cell proliferation → development of blood vessels (angiogenesis)
- Bevacizumab binds to VEGF → inhibiting VEGF-VEGF receptor binding (esp. VEGF-R1 = Flt-1 and VEGF2 = KDR) → inhibiting tumor neoangiogenesis → inhibiting tumor growth and metastasis

**Pkin:** *Kinetics:* median half-life t½ 20 days (11–50 days)

**Se:**
- *Bone marrow:* leukopenia and anemia (rare)
- *Cardiovascular:* hypotension, hypertension, cardiac insufficiency (esp. in combination with anthracyclines), myocardial infarction, thromboembolic events
- *Pulmonary:* cough, bronchitis, pneumonia, hemoptysis (esp. in patients with squamous cell carcinoma), dyspnea
- *Gastrointestinal tract:* nausea, vomiting, diarrhea, constipation, mucositis, gastrointestinal perforation (2–4%), abdominal pain, loss of appetite
- *Liver:* transient increase of transaminases, cholestasis
- *Kidney:* proteinuria (15–30%), nephrotic syndrome, hypocalcemia, hyponatremia
- *Nervous system:* headache, tumor pain, dizziness, syncopes
- *Infusion-induced reactions ("cytokine release syndrome"):* fever, chills, hot flushes, rigor, urticaria, pruritus, rhinitis, sore throat, dyspnea, bronchospasm, stridor
- *Other:* hemorrhages (epistaxis, hemoptysis, gastrointestinal bleeding), fatigue, reduced performance status, infections, myalgia, arthralgia, peripheral edema

**Ci:**
- Hypersensitivity to mouse proteins, severe cardiac disease
- Increased risk for bleeding or previous hemorrhages
- Uncontrolled hypertension
- Pregnancy, lactation

**Th:** *Indications:* metastatic colorectal carcinoma, non-small cell lung cancer
*Clinical trial use:* breast cancer, ovarian cancer, glioblastoma, pancreatic carcinoma, renal cell carcinoma

*Dosage:* i.v. application over 90 min
- 5 mg/kg i.v. every 2 weeks, initial intravenous infusion over 90 min, consecutive infusions over 30–60 min
- ATTN: application at the earliest 28 days following surgery (impaired wound healing)

## Cetuximab

**Chem:** Recombinant, monoclonal, chimeric IgG1 antibody (mouse / human), high affinity binding to the extracellular domain of human epidermal growth factor receptor 1 (EGF-R1, HER1)

**MOA:** Binding to EGF-R1 (on solid tumor cells):
- Inhibition of endogenous ligands (EGF, TGFα), competitive inhibition of EGF-R1-tyrosine kinase, signal transduction ↓
- Receptor internalization and downregulation
- Antibody-mediated cytotoxicity, apoptosis induction, tumor neoangiogenesis ↓
- Inhibition of tumor growth and metastasis

**Pkin:** *Kinetics:* median half life t½: 60–100 h with standard dose

**Se:**
- *Bone marrow:* moderate myelosuppression
- *Cardiovascular:* hypertension, hypotension, tachycardia
- *Pulmonary:* dyspnea, bronchospasm, stridor
- *Gastrointestinal:* nausea / vomiting, diarrhea (esp. in combination with irinotecan), constipation, abdominal pain, loss of appetite
- *Liver:* transient increase of transaminases
- *Nervous system:* headache, insomnia
- *Skin:* acne-like eczema, nail changes (up to 80%, reversible), skin dryness, pruritus, alopecia (rare)
- *Infusion-induced reactions:* severe hypersensitivity reactions (5%) during or 1 h after first infusion, with pulmonary obstruction (bronchospasm, stridor, hoarseness), hypotension, fever, chills, urticaria, exanthema
- *Other:* fatigue, reduced performance status, infections, headache, peripheral edema

**Ci:**
- Hypersensitivity to cetuximab
- Pregnancy, lactation

**Th:** *Indications:* metastasized colorectal carcinoma, head and neck cancer
*Clinical trial use:* breast cancer, non-small cell lung cancer

*Dosage:* i.v. application:
- Initially 400 mg/m² i.v. over 2 h
- Consecutive infusions: 250 mg/m² i.v. over 1 h
- EGFR expression analysis in tumor tissue recommended prior to treatment (e.g., immunohistochemistry)
- ATTN: risk of infusion-induced reaction with fever, chills, thrombocytopenia, hypotension, tumor lysis syndrome. Premedication with paracetamol 500–1,000 mg p.o. and antihistamines (e.g., clemastine 2 mg i.v.) recommended

### Eculizumab

**Chem:** Recombinant humanized monoclonal IgG$_{2/4}$κ antibody specifically binding to the complement protein C5, molecular weight 148 kDa.

**MOA:**
- Binding to complement protein C5
  - → Inhibition of cleavage of C5 to C5a and C5b
  - → Prevention of formation of terminal complement complex C5b-9
- Inhibition of terminal complement mediated intravascular hemolysis in patients with paroxysmal nocturnal hemoglobinuria (PNH) (▶ Chap. 6.4.3)

**Pkin:**
- *Kinetics:* elimination half-life t½ 272 ± 82 h
- *Metabolism:* proteolysis

**Se:**
- *Bone marrow:* anemia (2%)
- *Pulmonary:* cough, nasopharyngitis, respiratory tract infection, sinusitis
- *Gastrointestinal:* nausea (16%), vomiting, constipation
- *Nervous system:* headache (44%)
- *Infusion-induced reactions ("cytokine-release syndrome"):* fever, chills, rigor, rhinitis, conjunctivitis, sore throat, bronchospasm, angioedema
- *Other:* serious hemolysis after discontinuation (LDH ↑), systemic infections, serious meningococcal infections, viral infections (including herpes simplex), backache, arthralgia, myalgia, limb pain, fatigue, influenza-like symptoms

**Ci:**
- Patients who are not vaccinated against *Neisseria meningitidis*
- Unresolved *Neisseria meningitidis* infection

**Th:** *Approved indications:* paroxysmal nocturnal hemoglobinuria (PNH)

*Dosage and application:*
- 600 mg i.v. infusion weekly for 4 weeks, then 900 mg every 14 days
- ATTN: increased risk of meningococcal infections → patients must receive a meningococcal vaccine at least 2 weeks prior to initiation of eculizumab therapy
- Monitor for signs and symptoms of infusion reactions
- Monitor for signs of hemolysis, serum LDH levels

### Gemtuzumab Ozogamicin

**Chem:** Immunotoxin conjugate, humanized, recombinant, monoclonal IgG4-κ antibody specifically binding to the antigen CD33, conjugated with the cytostatic antibiotic calicheamicin

**MOA:**
- Binding to CD33 on leukemic myeloblasts and myeloid cells (myelomonocytic progenitors, neutrophils, erythrocytes, thrombocytes, monocytes / macrophages). In AML, over 80% of cells are CD33 positive. CD34-positive hematopoietic stem cells are CD33 negative.
- Internalization of CD33 with gemtuzumab ozogamicin → release of calicheamicin derivatives in lysosomes → DNA strand breaks → cytotoxic effect.
- Simultaneously, antibody-mediated cytotoxicity (ADCC), apoptosis induction.

**Pkin:**
- *Kinetics:* median serum half-life t½ of gemtuzumab ozogamicin 45–60 h, t½ of unconjugated calicheamicin 100 h
- *Metabolism:* internalization and hydrolysis, hepatic and renal elimination

**Se:**
- *Bone marrow:* severe myelosuppression (neutropenia, thrombocytopenia, anemia), bone marrow recovery after approximately 40 days. Infections due to neutropenia (50%), hemorrhages (15% of cases, cerebral, gastrointestinal, epistaxis, hematuria, in rare cases disseminated intravascular coagulation)
- *Cardiovascular:* hypotension, hypertension, tachycardia
- *Pulmonary:* cough, dyspnea, pharyngitis, bronchitis, pneumonia, pulmonary edema, ARDS
- *Gastrointestinal:* nausea / vomiting (70%), diarrhea (40%), constipation, abdominal pain, loss of appetite
- *Liver:* transient increase of transaminases, cholestasis (25%), hyperglycemia
- *Skin:* local reactions, erythema, pruritus, petechiae
- *Infusion-induced reactions ("cytokine release syndrome"):* fever (85%), chills (75%), hot flushes, sweat, erythema, urticaria, hypo- or hypertension, dyspnea
- *Other:* tumor lysis syndrome (rare, risk of acute renal failure), arthralgia, myalgia, hypercalcemia

**Ci:**
- Hypersensitivity to gemtuzumab ozogamicin
- Pregnancy, lactation
- Severely impaired liver function (bilirubin > 2 g/dl)

**Th:** *Indication (USA):* relapse of CD33-positive AML in patients ≥ 60 years
*Clinical trial use:* AML patients < 60 years

*Dosage:* i.v. application (infusion over 2 h)
- 9 mg/m²/day i.v. on days 1, 15
- ATTN: risk of infusion-induced reactions including fever, chills, thrombocytopenia, hypotension, tumor lysis syndrome. Premedication with paracetamol 500–1000 mg p.o. and antihistamines (e.g., clemastine 2 mg i.v.)

### Rituximab

**Chem:** Recombinant, monoclonal, chimeric IgG1-antibody (mouse / human) specifically binding to the transmembrane antigen CD20

**MOA:**
- Binding to CD20 (on normal pre-B- / B-cells and 95% of malignant B-NHL) → complement-mediated cytotoxicity (CDC) and antibody-mediated cellular cytotoxicity (ADCC), apoptosis induction, depletion of CD20-positive lymphocytes → B-cell depletion, serum immunoglobulins ↓, commencing regeneration after 2 weeks, complete reconstitution after 9–12 months
- Direct antiproliferative effect against malignant B-cell lines shown in vitro
- Sensitization against cytotoxic compounds (combination therapy)

**Pkin:**
- *Kinetics:* median half-life t½ after first infusion: 68–76 h, after fourth infusion t½ 190–200 h. Pronounced intra- and interindividual variability of serum concentration, detection of rituximab in serum 3–6 months after treatment possible
- *Metabolism:* proteolysis

**Se:**
- *Bone marrow:* lymphopenia (50%), marginal myelosuppression
- *Cardiovascular:* hypotension, hypertension, arrhythmia, rare cuses of angina pectoris, cardiac insufficiency, myocardial infarction, mainly with pre-existing heart disease
- *Pulmonary:* cough, dyspnea, sinusitis, bronchitis, bronchiolitis obliterans, pulmonary infiltrates, ARDS ("acute respiratory distress syndrome")
- *Gastrointestinal:* nausea / vomiting, diarrhea, abdominal pain
- *Liver:* transient increase of transaminases, hyperglycemia
- *Nervous system:* central neuropathy, headache, paresthesia, dizziness, anxiety, insomnia, somnolence, nervousness
- *Skin:* erythema, pruritus, urticaria
- *Infusion-induced reactions ("cytokine-release syndrome"):* fever (50%), chills, rigor, rhinitis, conjunctivitis, sore throat, bronchospasm, angioedema
- *Other:* infections, night sweat, fatigue, reduced performance status, edema, arthralgia, myalgia, skeletal pain, hypercalcemia, LDH ↑, lymphadenopathy, coagulation disorders, dysgeusia, tumor lysis syndrome

**Ci:**
- Hypersensitivity to murine proteins, severe pre-existing cardiac disease

**Th:**
*Approved indications for use:* refractory / relapsed B-cell lymphoma
*Clinical trial use:* multiple myoma, ITP, rheumatoid arthritis, autoimmune disease

*Dosage and application:*
- 375 mg/m²/day i.v. weekly with monotherapy, in combination with CHOP on day 1 of each cycle
- ATTN: infusion-induced reaction prophylaxis: premedication with paracetamol 500–1,000 mg p.o. and clemastine 2 mg i.v., slow increase of infusion rate (initially 50 mg/h, gradually increasing up to maximum 400 mg/h). Close monitoring. Discontinue antihypertensive medication 12 h before treatment
- ATTN: in case of high tumor load (lymphomas > 10 cm, lymphocytosis > 50,000/µl, leukocytosis > 50,000/µl): acute tumor lysis syndrome possible (→ Chap. 9.6)

**Panitumumab**

**Chem:**  Recombinant, monoclonal, fully human IgG2 antibody, with selective high affinity binding to the human epidermal growth factor receptor  (EGF-R, HER1), inhibiting ligand binding.

**MOA:**  Binding to EGF-R (on solid tumor cells):
- Inhibiting the effect of endogenous EGF-R ligands (EGF, TGFα), competitive inhibition of EGF-R tyrosine kinase, signal transduction ↓
- Receptor internalization and downregulation
- Antibody-mediated cytotoxicity, apoptosis induction, tumor neoangiogenesis ↓
- Inhibiting tumor growth and metastasis

Efficacy of panitumumab monotherapy in metastatic colorectal carcinoma is increased with expression of the wild-type KRAS gene. Tumors with expression of mutated KRAS show reduced response rates. KRAS status should be considered in selecting patients with metastatic colorectal carcinoma as candidates for panitumumab therapy.

**Pkin:**  *Kinetics:* elimination half life (t½): 7.5 days (3.6 – 10.9 d)

**Se:**
- *Pulmonary:* dyspnea, cough, pulmonary fibrosis (rare)
- *Gastrointestinal:* nausea / vomiting, diarrhea (esp. in combination with irinotecan), constipation, abdominal pain, mucositis
- *Skin:* acneiform skin rash, pruritus, erythema, exfoliation, nail disorders, dry skin
- *Other:* fatigue, reduced performance status, infections, peripheral edema, hypomagnesemia, infusion reactions (rare), allergic reactions (rare)

**Ci:**  Pregnancy, lactation

**Th:**  *Indications for use:* metastasized colorectal carcinoma
*Clinical trial use:* breast cancer, non-small cell lung cancer

*Dosage:*
- 6 mg/kg i.v. every 14 days, 1 h-infusion
- Examination of EGFR and KRAS status in tumor tissue recommended prior to treatment (e.g. immunohistochemistry)
- ATTN: reduced risk of infusion-reduced reactions as compared to other EGFR inhibitors, due to fully human nature of the antibody.

## Trastuzumab

**Chem:** Humanized, recombinant, monoclonal IgG1-κ antibody (mouse / human), selectively binding with high affinity to the extracellular domain of the human epidermal growth factor receptor 2 (EGF-R2, HER2)

**MOA:**
- HER2 protooncogene encodes the transmembrane receptor protein p185 (185 kD, HER2/neu) with intrinsic tyrosine kinase activity. HER2 overexpression in 25–30% of primary breast cancer and in other epithelial neoplasias, e.g., non-small cell lung cancer, bladder / gastric / ovarian / prostate cancer
- Specific binding of trastuzumab to extracellular domain of p185 → complement-mediated cytotoxicity (CDC) and antibody-mediated cytotoxicity (ADCC), apoptosis induction, inhibition of signal transduction, receptor downregulation, cell cycle arrest

**Pkin:** *Kinetics:* median half-life t½: 28 days (1–32 days), elimination period up to 24 weeks

**Se:**
- *Bone marrow:* mild myelosuppression
- *Cardiovascular:* acute cardiotoxicity (dose-limiting): hypotension, syncope, tachycardia, cough, dyspnea, edema, 3rd heart sound, reduced cardiac ejection fraction, decompensated cardiac insufficiency (monotherapy: 5%, combination treatment with anthracyclines: 19%); ischemia, pericardial effusion, arrhythmia, cardiomyopathy, cardiac arrest. Vascular thrombosis
- *Pulmonary:* cough, dyspnea, rhinitis, sinusitis, pharyngitis, pleural effusion, pulmonary infiltrates, ARDS
- *Gastrointestinal:* nausea (30%), vomiting, abdominal pain, diarrhea, loss of appetite
- *Nervous system:* headache, dizziness, insomnia, paresthesias, neuropathy, tremor, anxiety, depression
- *Infusion-induced reactions ("cytokine release syndrome," 40%):* fever, chills, cough, erythema, urticaria, pruritus, angioedema, anaphylaxis
- *Other:* infections (mainly rhinitis, bronchopulmonary infections, catheter infections, mastitis), flu-like symptoms, arthralgia, myalgia, pruritus, back pains, transient tumor pain, fatigue, reduced performance status, antibody formation

**Ci:**
- Hypersensitivity to mouse proteins
- Pre-existing cardiac disease, dyspnea at rest
- Combination treatment trastuzumab + anthracyclines is not recommended due to increased cardiotoxicity

**Th:** *Indications:* breast cancer

*Dosage and application:*
- Initially 4 mg/kg over 90 min i.v., then 2 mg/kg once a week over 30 min i.v., no premedication necessary
- ATTN: cardiotoxicity, esp. in combination with anthracyclines and with pre-existing cardiac disease (e.g., cardiac diseases, thoracic radiotherapy)
- BEFORE TREATMENT: ECG, echocardiography (LVEF determination), diagnosis of HER2 overexpression (immunohistochemistry and/or fluorescence in situ hybridization (FISH) in tumor tissue)

## 3.6    Specific Protein Kinase Inhibitors ("Targeted Therapies")

### K. Potthoff, R. Waesch, J. Scheele, U. Martens

In addition to therapeutically used antibodies (▶ Chap. 3.5), low molecular weight antineoplastic compounds specifically binding to biologically relevant target structures are also classified a "targeted therapies."

The identification of classic cytostatic drugs was based on a multitude of empirical studies ("screening") in tumor model systems (e.g., murine tumors). In contrast, the development of "targeted therapies" is based on the knowledge of pathogenesis and pathophysiology of malignant disease ("rational drug design").

Main approaches:

- *Modification of gene function:* gene therapy, antisense oligonucleotides, ribozymes
- *Modification of protein function:* monoclonal antibodies, receptor antagonists, binding proteins, angiogenesis inhibitors
- *Specific toxic effect:* combination of specific "cognition" molecules (e.g., receptor ligands, monoclonal antibodies) and toxins (synthetic or natural toxins), so-called "drug targeting" e.g., with immunotoxins

*Signal transduction inhibitors* inhibit specific protein kinases, other enzymes or effector molecules of intracellular signal transduction.

Ma:

### *Mode of Action and Target Structures*

The effects of specific inhibitors depend on the cellular target structures. Molecules targeting different structures are used in preclinical and clinical trials.

| Point of attack | Target structure (selection) |
| --- | --- |
| Regulation of angiogenesis | VEGF, angiopoietin, tie, HIF |
| Regulation of apoptosis | TRAIL-R1, bcl-2, p53, NFκ-B, PI3-kinase, ubiquitin |
| Oncogenes | ras, raf, jun, fos, kinases |
| Regulation of proliferation | Growth factors, e.g., EGF, IGF |
| Signal transduction | Tyrosine kinases (EGF-R, VEGF-R, PDGF-R), serine-threonine kinases (TOR) |
| Cell cycle regulation | Cyclins, cyclin-dependant kinases (CDK), mitotic kinases |

*VEGF* vascular endothelial growth factor, *HIF* hypoxia-inducible factor, *TRAIL* tumor necrosis factor-related apoptosis-inducing ligand, *NFκ-B* nuclear factor kappa B, *PI3* phosphatidylinositol-3, *EGF* epidermal growth factor, *IGF* insulin-like growth factor, *PDGF* platelet-derived growth factor, *TOR* target of rapamycin

### *Tyrosine Kinases*

Kinases are enzymes which phosphorylate specific substrates (e.g., tyrosine residues). Tyrosine kinases play an important role in signal transduction. Differentiation between:

- Receptor tyrosine kinases
- Intracellular tyrosine kinases

Tyrosine kinase inhibitors are the most important clinically used "targeted therapies."

Ref:

1. Bells HS, Ryan KM. Intracellular signalling and cancer: complex pathways lead to multiple targets. Eur J Cancer 2005;41:206–15
2. Benson C, Kaye S, Workman P et al. Clinical anticancer drug development: targeting the cyclin-dependent kinases. Br J Cancer 2005;92:7–12
3. Deininger M, Buchdunger E, Druker BJ. The development of imatinib as a therapeutic agent for chronic myeloid leukemia. Blood 2005;105:2640–53

4. Ghobrial IM, Witzig TE, Adjej AA. Targeting apoptosis pathways in cancer therapy. CA Cancer J Clin 2005;55:178–94

5. Giaccone G. Epidermal growth factor receptor inhibitors in the treatment of non-small cell lung cancer. J Clin Oncol 2005;23:3235–42

6. Lancet JE, Karp JE. Farnesyltransferase inhibitors in hematologic malignancies: new horizons in therapy. Blood 2003;102:2880–9

7. Nencioni A, Grünebach F, Patrone F et al. Proteasome inhibitors: antitumor effects and beyond. Leukemia 2007;21:20–6

8. Pollak MN, Schernhammer ES, Hankinson SE. Insulin-like growth factors and neoplasia. Nat Rev Cancer 2004;4:505–18

9. Sabatini DM. mTOR and cancer. Nat Rev Cancer 2006;6:729–34

**Web:**

| | | |
|---|---|---|
| 1. | http://cis.nci.nih.gov/fact/7_49.htm | National Cancer Institute |
| 2. | http://www.nature.com/nrc/focus/targetedtherapies | Nature Reviews Cancer |
| 3. | http://www.oncolink.com/treatment/treatment.cfm?c=12 | Oncolink "Targeted Therapies" |
| 4. | http://www.fda.gov/cder/drug/infopage/gleevec | FDA, Glivec Information |

### Bexarotene

**Chem:**   Retinoid receptor X activator, 4-[1-(5,6,7,8-tetrahydro-3,5,5,8,8,-pentamethyl-2-naphthalenyl) ethenyl]benzoic acid

**MOA**
- Selective activation of retinoid X receptors (RXR) α, β, and γ
  - → Activated receptors function as transcription factors
  - → Impact on apoptosis, cellular proliferation and differentiation
- Growth inhibition of specific malignant cells lines in vitro and vivo

**Pkin:**
- *Kinetics:* moderate oral absorption, peak plasma levels reached after 2 h, plasma protein binding > 99%, terminal half-life t½ 7 h
- *Metabolism:* hepatic degradation via cytochrome P450 system (CYP3A4) and glucuronidation, hepatobiliary elimination

**Se:**
- *Bone marrow:* leukopenia, neutropenia, anemia
- *Cardiovascular:* peripheral edema
- *Pulmonary:* dyspnea, cough, pneumonia
- *Gastrointestinal:* nausea, vomiting, diarrhea, abdominal pain
- *Liver / pancreas:* transient elevation of transaminases, cholestasis, lipid abnormalities (triglycerides ↑, cholesterol ↑, LDL ↑, HDL ↓), acute pancreatitis
- *Nervous system:* headaches, confusion
- *Skin:* rash, dry skin, pruritus, exfoliative dermatitis
- *Other:* fatigue, asthenia, infections, muscle cramps, hypothyroidism (TSH ↓, thyroxin ↓), posterior subcapsular cataracts

**DDI:**
- Cytochrome P450 (CYP3A4) inhibiting substances (ketoconazole, itraconazole, voriconazole, erythromycin, clarithromycin) are expected to increase bexarotene plasma concentrations
- CYP3A4-inducing substances (dexamethasone, phenytoin, carbamazepine, rifampicin, phenobarbital, St. John's wort) are expected to decrease bexarotene plasma concentrations
- Effects of insulin may be enhanced → risk of hypoglycemia

**Ci:**
- Hypersensitivity to retinoids, pregnancy, lactation
- Relative CI: patients with risk factors for pancreatitis

**Th:**   *Approved indications:* cutaneous manifestations of cutaneous T-cell lymphoma (CTCL)
*Clinical trial use:* head and neck cancer, NSCLC, renal cell carcinoma, Kaposi's sarcoma

*Dosage:* oral application (300 mg/m²/day p.o.) or topical application
- *ATTN:* bexarotene may cause fetal harm when administered to pregnant women. Appropriate precautions should be taken to avoid pregnancy and fathering
- *BEFORE TREATMENT:* full blood count, hepatic and renal function tests, thyroid function, blood lipids

## Bortezomib (PS-341)

**Chem:** Proteasome inhibitor, [(1R)-3-methyl-1-[[(2S)-1-oxo-3-phenyl-2-[(pyrazinylcarbonyl)amino]-propyl]amino]butyl]boric acid

**MOA:**
- Reversible inhibitor of 26S-proteasome → inhibiting degradation of ubiquitinated proteins → apoptosis induction in cells with bcl-2 overexpression, angiogenesis inhibition, IL-6 mediated effects ↓, adhesion molecules ↓
- Proteasome inhibition reversible after 72 h

**Pkin:**
- *Kinetics:* median half-life t½ 9–15 h
- *Metabolism:* hepatic degradation via several cytochrome P450 enzymes

**Se:**
- *Bone marrow:* neutropenia, anemia, thrombocytopenia (15–40%)
- *Cardiovascular:* orthostatic hypotension, syncope, hypertension, arrhythmia, cardiac failure, myocardial infarction
- *Gastrointestinal tract:* diarrhea (dose-limiting, 51%), nausea (65%), vomiting, abdominal cramps, loss of appetite
- *Kidney:* renal function disorders, electrolyte disorders (rare)
- *Nervous system:* peripheral neuropathy (dose-limiting), headaches, drowsiness
- *Other:* fever, fatigue, reduced performance status (65%), arthralgia, myalgia, conjunctivitis, hyperbilirubinemia, tumor lysis syndrome, allergic reactions (rare)

**DI:**
- Cytochrome P450 (CYP3A4) inhibiting substances (ketoconazole, itraconazole, voriconazole, erythromycin, clarithromycin) → bortezomib concentration ↑
- CYP3A4 induction (dexamethasone, phenytoin, carbamazepine, rifampicin, phenobarbital, St. John's wort) → effect of bortezomib ↓
- *ATTN:* no simultaneous administration of phenprocoumon (metabolization via CYP2C9) → patients with anticoagulation therapy should switch to low molecular weight heparin

**Ci:**
- Hypersensitivity to bortezomib, boric compounds, or mannitol
- Pregnancy, lactation
- Cardiac or neuropathic disorders

**Th:**
*Indication:* multiple myeloma, cutaneous T-cell lymphoma
*Clinical trial use:* solid tumors

*Dosage:* 1.3 mg/m²/day i.v. on days 1, 4, 8, 11, repetition on day 22

## Dasatinib

**Chem:**  Tyrosine kinase inhibitor, N-(2-chloro-6-methylphenyl)-2-[6-[4-(2-hydroxyethyl)-1-piperazinyl]amino]-5-thiazolcarboxamide

**MOA:**
- Inhibiting tyrosine kinases BCR-ABL, c-kit, EPHA2, PDGFRβ as well as kinases that belong to SRC family (SRC, LCK, YES, FYN)
- Inhibiting proliferation / apoptosis induction in Philadelphia-positive CML and ALL by inhibiting BCR-ABL fusion protein and in gastrointestinal stromal tumors (GIST) by inhibiting c-kit-protein (CD117, stem cell factor receptor)

**Pkin:**
- *Kinetics:* oral bioavailability, plasma protein binding 93–96%, median half-life t½ 3–5 h
- *Metabolism:* hepatic inactivation (cytochrome P450 3A4) and elimination (glucuronidation)

**Se:**
- *Bone marrow:* neutropenia, thrombocytopenia (48–83%), impaired thrombocyte function, anemia
- *Cardiovascular:* QT elongation
- *Gastrointestinal:* nausea, vomiting, abdominal pain, diarrhea, loss of appetite, gastrointestinal bleeding (7–14%)
- *Liver:* transient increase of transaminases, cholestasis
- *Nervous system:* headaches, somnolence, insomnia
- *Skin:* dermatitis, exanthema, pruritus, alopecia
- *Other:* fluid retention (50%, with effusions, peripheral edema, pulmonary edema), dyspnea, fever, fatigue, reduced performance status, weight loss, hemorrhages

**DDi:**
- Cytochrome P450 (CYP3A4) inhibiting substances (ketoconazole, itraconazole, voriconazole, erythromycin, clarithromycin) → dasatinib concentration ↑
- CYP3A4 induction (dexamethasone, phenytoin, carbamazepine, rifampicin, phenobarbital, St. John's wort) → effect of dasatinib ↓
- Antacids reduce the oral bioavailability of dasatinib

**Ci:**  Use cautiously in patients with QT elongation, hypokalemia, hypomagnesemia, therapy with antiarrhythmics

**Th:**  *Indications:* CML, Ph+ ALL, if refractory to primary treatment

*Dosage:*
- 140 mg/day p.o. (70 mg tablets in the morning and evening)
- Dose increase up to 200 mg/day possible

## Erlotinib

**Chem:**   Tyrosine kinase inhibitor, N-(3-ethynylphenyl-)-6,7-bis(2-methoxyethoxy)-4-quinazolinamine

**MOA:**
- EGFR (epidermal growth factor receptor) expression on solid tumors, especially with non-small cell lung cancer, esophageal carcinoma, head and neck tumors, renal cell carcinoma, gastrointestinal carcinoma, breast cancer
- Inhibiting epidermal growth factor receptor type 1 (HER1/EGFR1) tyrosine kinase → inhibiting EGFR activation / signal transduction → inhibiting proliferation and angiogenesis, apoptosis induction

**Pkin:**
- *Kinetics:* oral bioavailability 60–80%, median half-life t½ 36 h
- *Metabolism:* hepatic degradation (cytochrome P450 3A1/1A2) and renal excretion

**Se:**
- *Pulmonary:* dyspnea, cough, interstitial pneumonia, pneumonitis, bronchiolitis obliterans, pulmonary fibrosis
- *Gastrointestinal:* nausea, vomiting, abdominal pain, diarrhea, loss of appetite, gastrointestinal hemorrhages
- *Liver:* transient increase of transaminases, cholestasis, impaired coagulation
- *Nervous system:* headaches
- *Eyes:* conjunctivitis, keratitis, visual disturbances, lacrimation ↑
- *Skin:* erythema (70%), dermatitis, exanthema, pruritus
- *Other:* fatigue, reduced performance status

**IDi:**
- Cytochrome P450 (CYP3A4) inhibiting substances (ketoconazole, itraconazole, voriconazole, erythromycin, clarithromycin) → erlotinib concentration ↑
- CYP3A4 induction (dexamethasone, phenytoin, carbamazepine, rifampicin, phenobarbital, St. John's wort) → effect of erlotinib ↓
- *ATTN: do not use phenprocoumon with erlotinib due to metabolization by CYP2C9. Anticoagulated patients should receive low molecular weight heparin.*

**Ci:**   Hypersensitivity, pregnancy, lactation, impaired liver function

**Th:**   *Approved indications (USA):* non-small cell lung cancer, pancreatic cancer
*Clinical trial use:* solid tumors

*Dosage:* oral application, 1 h before or 2 h after meals
150 mg/day p.o.

### Imatinib Mesylate

**Chem:**   Tyrosine kinase inhibitor, 4-[(4-methyl-1-piperazinyl)methyl]-N-[4-methyl-3-[[4-(3-pyridinyl) 2-pyrimidinyl]amino]-phenyl]benzamide methanesulfonate

**MOA:**
- Inhibition of the Bcr-Abl fusion protein (tyrosine kinase) in Philadelphia chromosome positive CML and ALL cells → proliferation inhibition and apoptosis induction
- Inhibition of the c-kit protein (CD117, stem cell factor receptor SCF-R, tyrosine kinase) in gastrointestinal stromal tumors (GIST)
- Inhibition of the activated PDGF receptor (platelet-derived growth factor receptor)

**Pkin:**
- *Kinetics:* oral bioavailability 98%, plasma protein binding 95%, median half-life t½ 18 h (imatinib) to 40 h (active metabolite N-demethyl-imatinib)
- *Metabolism:* renal and hepatic elimination via cytochrome P450 (CYP3A4)

**Se:**
- *Bone marrow:* neutropenia, thrombocytopenia, anemia
- *Gastrointestinal tract:* nausea, vomiting, abdominal pain
- *Liver:* reversible increase of transaminases, cholestasis
- *Nervous system:* headaches, drowsiness, dysgeusia, fatigue, paresthesia, dizziness, insomnia, conjunctivitis, visual disturbances, lacrimation ↑
- *Skin:* dermatitis, exanthema, pruritus, alopecia, allergic reactions
- *Other:* fluid retention (60%, effusions, peripheral edema, pulmonary edema), dyspnea, fatigue, reduced performance status, muscle cramps, arthralgia, myalgia, gastrointestinal and intratumoral hemorrhages (GIST)

**DDi:**
- Cytochrome P450 (CYP3A4) inhibiting substances (ketoconazole, itraconazole, voriconazole, erythromycin, clarithromycin) → imatinib plasma concentration ↑
- CYP3A4-inducing substances (dexamethasone, phenytoin, carbamazepine, rifampicin, phenobarbital, St. John's wort) → effect of imatinib ↓
- *ATTN:* do not use phenprocoumon with imatinib mesylate due to metabolization by CYP2C9. Anticoagulated patients should receive low molecular weight heparin.

**Ci:**   Hypersensitivity, pregnancy, lactation, impaired liver function

**Th:**   *Indications:* Philadelphia chromosome positive (Ph+) CML, Ph+ ALL, c-kit-positive gastrointestinal stromal tumors (GIST)
*Clinical trial use:* mastocytosis, hypereosinophilic syndrome, solid tumors

*Dosage:* oral application with meals
- GIST: 400–800 mg/day p.o.
- CML: 400 mg/day p.o. (chronic phase), 600 mg/day p.o. (accelerated phase / blast crisis), 800 mg/day (in case of progression after at least 3 months of treatment)

### Sorafenib Tosylate

**Chem:** Multikinase inhibitor, 4-(4-[3-[4-chloro-3-(trifluoromethyl)phenyl]ureido]phenoxy-N-methyl-pyridine-2-carboxamide

**MOA:**
- Inhibiting multiple intracellular kinases (CRAF, BRAF) and receptor tyrosine kinases (c-kit, FLT-3, VEGFR-2, VEGFR-3, PDGFR-β)
- Inhibiting signal transduction of VEGF (vascular endothelial growth factor) → angiogenesis inhibition → inhibiting growth of angiogenesis-dependent solid tumors

**kin:**
- *Kinetics:* oral bioavailability 38–49%, plasma protein binding > 99%, median half-life t½ 25–48 h
- *Metabolism:* hepatic degradation (cytochrome P450 3A4, glucuronidation via UGT1A9), fecal and renal elimination

**Se:**
- *Bone marrow:* neutropenia, lymphopenia, thrombocytopenia
- *Cardiovascular:* hypertension, myocardial ischemia (rare)
- *Gastrointestinal:* nausea, vomiting, diarrhea, loss of appetite, amylase ↑, lipase ↑, mucositis, dysphagia, gastrointestinal hemorrhage (rare)
- *Liver:* transient increase of transaminases, cholestasis
- *Nervous system:* headaches, sensory neuropathy
- *Skin:* erythema, dermatitis, skin edema, dysesthesia, paresthesia, hand-foot syndrome, in rare cases with desquamation and ulceration
- *Other:* fatigue, reduced performance status, fever, weight loss, arthralgia, myalgia, hemorrhages, hypophosphatemia

**Di:**
- CYP3A4-inducing substances (dexamethasone, phenytoin, carbamazepine, rifampicin, phenobarbital, St. John's wort) → effect of sorafenib ↓

**Ci:**
- Hypersensitivity, pregnancy, lactation

**Th:** *Approved indications:* advanced renal cell carcinoma
*Clinical trial use:* solid tumors

*Dosage:* oral application, 1 h before or 2 h after meals
800 mg/day p.o. (400 mg in the morning and evening)

### Sunitinib Malate

**Chem:**  Multikinase inhibitor, N-[2-(diethylamino) ethyl]-5-[(z)-(5-fluoro-1,2-dihydro-2-oxo-3H-indol 3-ylidin)methyl]-2,4-dimethyl-1H-pyrrol-3-carboxamide

**MOA:**
- Inhibition of > 80 tyrosine kinases, including PDGF receptors α and β, VEGF receptor 1-3 SCF receptor (kit), FLT-3, CSF-1 receptor, and GCDNF receptor (RET)
- Inhibiting signal transduction of VEGF (vascular endothelial growth factor) → angiogenesi inhibition → inhibiting growth of angiogenesis-dependent solid tumors

**Pkin:**
- *Kinetics:* plasma protein binding 90–95%, terminal half-life t½ 40–60 h, t½ of active metabo lite 80–110 h
- *Metabolism:* hepatic activation and degradation via cytochrome P450 system (CYP3A4), feca (61%) and renal (16%) elimination

**Se:**
- *Bone marrow:* neutropenia, lymphopenia, anemia, thrombocytopenia
- *Cardiovascular:* hypertension, LVEF ↓, peripheral edema, myocardial ischemia, thromboem bolic events (rare)
- *Pulmonary:* dyspnea, cough
- *Gastrointestinal:* nausea, vomiting, diarrhea, constipation, loss of appetite, amylase ↑, lipase ↑ mucositis, dysphagia, abdominal pain
- *Liver:* transient increase of transaminases, cholestasis
- *Kidney:* creatinine ↑, hyperuricemia, hypokalemia, hypernatremia
- *Nervous system:* headaches, dysgeusia, amentia
- *Skin:* dermatitis, erythema, skin edema, hand-foot syndrome, pigmentation, change of hai color, alopecia
- *Other:* fatigue, reduced performance status, fever, weight loss, arthralgia, myalgia, hemor rhage, hypophosphatemia

**DDi:**
- Cytochrome P450 (CYP3A4) inhibiting substances (ketoconazole, itraconazole, voriconazole erythromycin, clarithromycin) → sunitinib plasma concentration ↑, consider dose reduction to 37.5 mg/day
- CYP3A4-inducing substances (dexamethasone, phenytoin, carbamazepine, rifampicin, phe nobarbital, St. John's wort) → effect of sunitinib ↓, consider dose increase to 87.5 mg

**Ci:**
- Hypersensitivity, pregnancy, lactation
- Relative CI: pre-existing cardiac disorders, left ventricular insufficiency

**Th:**  *Approved indications:* gastrointestinal stromal tumors (GIST), advanced renal cell carcinoma *Clinical trial use:* solid tumors

*Dosage:* oral application, 50 mg/day p.o.

**Temsirolimus**

**Chem:**  mTOR ("mammalian target of rapamycin") inhibitor

**MOA:**
- Intracellular binding to protein FKBP-12
  - → Protein–drug complex inhibits activity of mTOR
  - → Blocking of PI3/AKT pathway through decreased phosphorylation of p70S6k and S6 ribosomal proteins
  - → Inhibition of cell division, cell cycle phase G1 growth arrest

**Pkin:**
- *Kinetics:* hepatic formation of metabolites via cytochrome P450 system (CYP3A4), active metabolite sirolimus, terminal half-life $t\frac{1}{2}$ 17 h ($t\frac{1}{2}$ of sirolimus 55 h)
- *Metabolism:* hepatobiliary elimination

**Se:**
- *Bone marrow:* leukopenia, neutropenia, lymphopenia, anemia, thrombocytopenia
- *Cardiovascular:* peripheral edema
- *Pulmonary:* dyspnea, cough, pneumonia, interstitial lung disease (ILD)
- *Gastrointestinal:* nausea, vomiting, mucositis, anorexia, abdominal pain, bowel perforation
- *Liver / pancreas:* transient increase of transaminases, lipid abnormalities, hyperglycemia
- *Kidney:* creatinine ↑, hyperphosphatemia, renal failure
- *Skin:* rash, dry skin, pruritus
- *Other:* hypersensitivity reactions, fatigue, asthenia, infections, delayed wound healing, arthralgia, myalgia

**IDi:**
- Cytochrome P450 (CYP3A4) inhibitors (ketoconazole, itraconazole, voriconazole, erythromycin, clarithromycin) → sirolimus plasma concentration ↑, consider dose reduction of temsirolimus to 12.5 mg/day
- CYP3A4 inducers (dexamethasone, phenytoin, carbamazepine, rifampicin, phenobarbital, St. John's wort) → effect of temsirolimus ↓, consider dose increase to 37.5–50 mg

**Ci:**  Hypersensitivity, pregnancy, lactation

**Th:**  *Approved indication:* advanced renal cell carcinoma

*Dosage:* 25 mg/day i.v. once weekly
- *ATTN:* temsirolimus may cause fetal harm when administered to pregnant women. Appropriate precautions should be taken to avoid pregnancy and fathering. Antihistamine pretreatment is recommended
- *BEFORE TREATMENT:* full blood count, hepatic and renal function tests, blood lipids. Monitor blood lipids and blood glucose

## 3.7    Drug Development and Clinical Studies

### C. Schmoor, S. Stoelben, H. Maier-Lenz, D. Berger, H. Henß

**Def:**   Clinical development of a drug takes place after completion of preclinical development and involves a series of clinical trials and defined test phases. It should be conducted in accordanc with:

- Ethical principles (Declaration of Helsinki, local ethics commission)
- Legal regulations (e.g., pharmaceutical law, administrative regulations)
- "Good clinical practice," GCP (international GCP guidelines of the "International Conferenc on Harmonization," ICH-GCP)
- "Good manufacturing practice," GMP
- "Good laboratory practice," GLP

Adequate statistical methods and scientifically accurate analysis of results are essential for th design and evaluation of clinical studies of all phases.

**Meth:**   **Phases of drug testing**

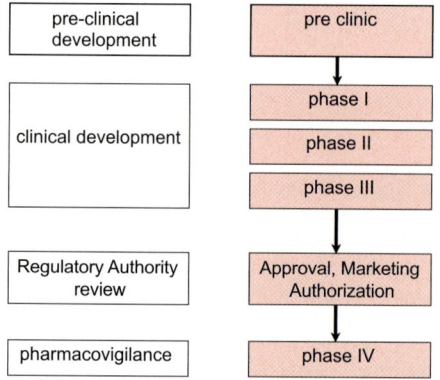

### Preclinical Phase
- Chemical / biochemical / biotechnological development
- Pharmacological evaluation, stability
- Toxicology: acute toxicity, long-term toxicity, carcinogenic / mutagenic / teratogenic effects in animal models
- Preclinical in vitro and in vivo efficacy testing

### Phase I
- "First in human" testing after successful preclinical development.
- In the majority of clinical settings, phase I trials are conducted with healthy volunteers at specific clinical research organizations (CROs). However, due to the potential for side effects (e.g. cytostatic toxicity), classic oncological phase I trials are frequently conducted in hospital units providing experimental treatment to inpatients. Test group: usually 15–20 patients per trial.
- Primary questions: acute tolerance, dosage ("maximum tolerable dose," MTD), initial dose for phase II trials.
- Other questions: acute toxicity, pharmacokinetics, pharmacodynamics, development of formulations.

### Phase II
- After successful phase I trial
- Evaluation of experimental drugs in patients with specific target indications, e.g., selected tumor types
- Test group: usually < 100 patients; trial design open or blinded, randomized, placebo-controlled
- Primary questions: efficacy, dose-response-relationship, safety

### Phase III
- After successful phase II trial
- Comparison of treatment group (experimental treatment) versus control group (standard treatment), generally conducted as prospective randomized, double-blind trials; test group: usually > 100 patients
- Primary objective: efficacy in specific target indications compared with standard treatment, long-term safety
- Other objectives: drug safety, side effects, drug interactions

### Regulatory Authority Approval
- After successful preclinical and clinical (phase I to III) testing, the drug development data can be submitted to Regulatory Authorities for review and approval.
- European approval:
  - Centralized procedure: submission of data to the European Medicines Agency (EMEA) in London.
  - Decentralized procedure: submission of data to a national licensing authority.
- US approval: FDA, Food and Drug Administration
- After successful evaluation by the regulatory authorities, a product license (Marketing Authorization) is issued.

### Phase IV
- Clinical studies *after* drug has been licensed
- Primary objective: efficacy in particular situations, rare side effects and interactions, rare contraindications
- Pharmacovigilance: continuous monitoring of drug-related adverse reactions at national and international Regulatory Authority level as well as by the manufacturer

## Good Clinical Practice (GCP)

"Good clinical practice" (GCP) refers to international ethical and scientific standards that must be complied with when planning, executing, and documenting clinical studies with human beings. Objectives are:
- Protection of the study participants' rights
- Protection of safety and wellbeing of the study participants
- Correct documentation and presentation of the study results

GCP guidelines were originally developed for clinical trials with registrational intent. However, there is agreement among the scientific community that GCP principles are relevant for all clinical research, including investigator-initiated studies and cooperative group trials.

### ICH-GCP
The current GCP guidelines were developed by the ICH (International Conference on Harmonization of Technical Requirements for Registration of Pharmaceuticals for Human Use, 1st May 1996) and are referred to as ICH-GCP. The following recommendations were incorporated:
- Ethical principles for medical research involving human subjects (Declaration of Helsinki)
- GCP guidelines by the WHO (World Health Organization), the European Union, USA, Japan, Australia, Canada, and Scandinavia

## Principles of Good Clinical Practice (ICH-GCP) (excerpts)

### Clinical trial requirements

- Clinical trials should be conducted in accordance with the ethical principles that have their origin in the Declaration of Helsinki, and that are consistent with GCP and the applicable regulatory requirement(s)
- Before a trial is initiated, foreseeable risks and inconveniences should be weighed against the anticipated benefit for the individual trial subject and society. A trial should be initiated and continued only if the anticipated benefits justify the risks
- The rights, safety, and wellbeing of the trial subjects are the most important considerations and should prevail over interests of science and society
- The available nonclinical and clinical information on an investigational product should be adequate to support the proposed clinical trial
- Clinical trials should be scientifically sound, and described in a clear, detailed protocol
- A trial should be conducted in compliance with the protocol that has received prior institutional review board (IRB) / independent ethics committee (IEC) approval / favorable opinion
- Freely given informed consent should be obtained from every subject prior to clinical trial participation
- All clinical trial information should be recorded, handled, and stored in a way that allows its accurate reporting, interpretation, and verification
- The confidentiality of records that could identify subjects should be protected, respecting the privacy and confidentiality rules in accordance with the applicable regulatory requirement(s)
- Investigational products should be manufactured, handled, and stored in accordance with applicable good manufacturing practice (GMP). They should be used in accordance with the approved protocol
- Systems with procedures that assure the quality of every aspect of the trial should be implemented

### Requirements for Investigators

- The medical care given to, and medical decisions made on behalf of subjects should always be the responsibility of a qualified physician or, when appropriate, of a qualified dentist
- Each individual involved in conducting a trial should be qualified by education, training, and experience to perform his or her respective task(s)

**Ref:**

1. Dixon JR. The International Conference on Harmonization Good Clinical Practice Guideline. Qual Assur 1998;6:65–74
2. EEC note for guidance: good clinical practice for trials on medicinal products in the European Community. CPMP Party on Efficacy of Medicinal Products. Pharmacol Toxicol 1990;67:361–72
3. Gajic A, Herrmann R, Salzberg M. The international quality requirements for the conduct of clinical studies and the challenges for study centers to implement them. Ann Oncol 2004;15:1305–9
4. Idanpaan-Heikkila JE. WHO guidelines for good clinical practice (GCP) for trials on pharmaceutical products: responsibilities of the investigator. Ann Med 1994;26:89–94
5. World Medical Association. Helsinki Declaration, 1975. In: Beauchamp TL, Walters LW (eds) Contemporary Issues in Bioethics, 2nd edn. Wadsworth, Belmont, CA, 1982

**Web:**

1. http://eudract.emea.europa.eu/       European Clinical Trials Database
2. http://www.clinicaltrials.gov        US Clinical Trials Database
3. http://www.controlled-trials.com/    Study Register
4. http://www.centerwatch.com           Clinical Trials Listing Service
5. http://www.emea.europa.eu/           EMEA, European Agency for Evaluation of Medicinal Products
6. http://www.fda.gov/                  FDA, Food and Drug Administration, USA
7. http://www.ich.org                   ICH, International Conf. Harmonization

## 3.8 Pharmacogenetics and Pharmacogenomics

**J.S. Scheele , A. Müller , U. Martens**

**Def:** *Pharmacogenetics:* study of genetic factors determing efficacy and safety of drugs
*Pharmacogenomics:* study of the entire spectrum of genes which can influence pharmacodynamics and pharmacokinetics of specific drugs

**Meth:** *Pharmacogenetic Methods*
- Genotyping of "single nucleotide polymorphisms" (SNPs): selective genetic polymorphisms impact the activity of key proteins essential for drug response and drug metabolism. With some cytostatics, SNPs allow rational predictions about response and toxicity.
- Gene expression analysis (► Chap. 2.3): global gene expression analysis using DNA arrays → genetic determinants of efficacy and toxicity of chemotherapeutics can be empirically identified. The term pharmacogenomics encompasses not only the influence of gene expression on a drug, but also the effect drugs have on the gene expression pattern.
- Drug development: identification of potential targets for new drugs.

**Phys:** Identification of genetic determinants of efficacy and toxicity of chemotherapeutics is useful if the following conditions are met:
- Wide interindividual differences in pharmacokinetic parameters (e.g., oral bioavailability, half-life, etc.)
- Bimodal AUC distribution ("area under the curve") for the concentration-time curve of active metabolites
- Occurrence of severe toxicities, with lack of dose-response relationship

**Examples of Pharmacogenetic determinants of chemotherapy-induced toxicity**

| Substance | Enzyme | Mutation | Mode of action |
|---|---|---|---|
| 6-Mercaptopurine (6-MP) | Thiopurine methyl-transferase (TPMT) | SNPs: TPMT*2 TPMT*3A TPMT*3C | 6-MP catabolism ↓ |
| 5-fluorouracil (5-FU) | Dihydropyrimidine dehydrogenase (DPD) | SNPs: DPYD*2A DPYD*9A | 5-FU catabolism ↓ |
| Irinotecan (CPT11) | UDP- glucurono-syltransferase 1A1 (UGT1A1; Gilbert's syndrome) | Insertion in promoter and SNPs | Catabolism of the active metabolite SN-38 ↓ |
| Methotrexate + 5-fluorouracil (e.g., CMF protocol) | Methylenetetrahy-drofolate reductase (MTHFR) | C677T | MTHFR ↓ → $CH_2$-THF ↑ |

**Examples of Pharmacogenetic determinants of chemotherapy response**

| Substance | Enzyme | Mutation | Mode of action |
|---|---|---|---|
| Cytosine arabinoside | Human equilibrative nucleoside transporter 1 (hENT1) | MLL-gene rearrangement | hENT1 expression ↑ → response ↑ |
| Doxorubicin | Glutathione-S-transferase (GST) | GSTP1 gene | GSTP1 expression ↑ → response ↓ |
| 5-Fluorouracil | Thymidylate synthase (TS) | Promoter polymorphism | TS induction, amplification → response ↓ |
| Prednisone | Glutathione-S-transferase | GSTP1 gene | SNPs with amino acid changes → response ↑ |

**Pharmacogenetics of 5-fluorouracil (5-FU)**

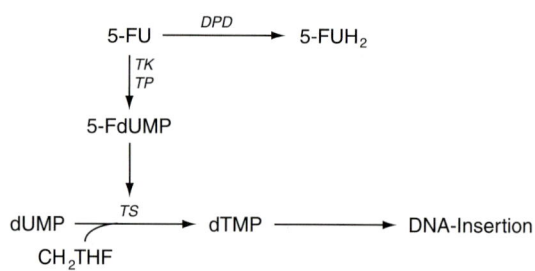

- Formation of inactive 5-fluoro-5,6-dihydrouracil ($5\text{-FUH}_2$) by dihydropyrimidine dehydrogenase (DPD) is the rate-limiting step in the catabolism of 5-FU.
- The antineoplastic effect of 5-FU in the tumor cell is mediated by the active metabolite 5-fluorodeoxyuridine monophosphate (5-FdUMP). FdUMP is formed in two steps, involving thymidine phosphorylase (TP) and thymidine kinase (TK). Inhibition of thymidylate synthase (TS) by 5FdUMP represents the critical step of 5-FU cytotoxicity. TS catalyses the transformation of dUMP into deoxythymidine 5' monophosphate (dTMP), which is the rate-limiting step of DNA synthesis. TS inhibition depends on the cofactor 5,10-methylenetetrahydrofolate ($CH_2THF$) which forms a ternary complex with 5-FdUMP and TS.
- A defect in the catabolic enzyme DPD, which occurs in its complete form in 0.1% of patients and in its partial form in 3–5% of patients, triggers a life-threatening toxic syndrome encompassing severe myelotoxicity, neurotoxicity, and gastrointestinal toxicity.
- The DPD genotype has an autosomal recessive pattern of inheritance. An allelic inactivation leading to 50% reduction of normal DPD activity is sufficient for the development of 5-FU toxicity. At least 20 mutations have been found in the DPD coding region and promoter. Two mutations with proven clinical relevance are DPYD*2A and DPYD*9A. DPYD*2A is a splice site mutation resulting in the production of shortened mRNA. DPYD*9A is a common missense T85C mutation in exon 2, leading to a C29R amino acid exchange. Correlation between the two mutations and the clinical phenotype together with other SNPs in enzymes of the 5-FU metabolism should yield improved prediction of 5-FU-associated toxicity.

## Pharmacogenetics of 6-mercaptopurine (6-MP)

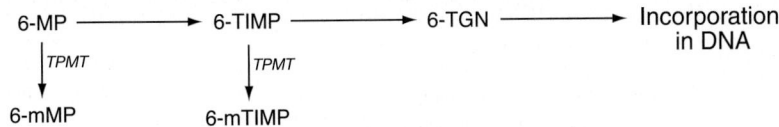

- At the cellular level, 6-mercaptopurine (6-MP) is converted into 6-thioinosine monophosphate (6-TIMP) and 6-thioguanine triphosphate nucleotide (TGN). The incorporation of 6-TGN into DNA mediates the antileukemic activity of 6-MP.
- At the same time, steps of deactivation take place. How much 6-MP can be activated in the bone marrow depends on the extent of deactivating methylation by thiopurine methyltransferase (TPMT).
- Patients with genetic deficiency in TPMT accumulate 6-TGN to toxic concentrations, leading to severe and prolonged myelosuppression. Due to the long latency period of this toxicity, pharmacogenetic prediction of TPMT activity is clinically relevant.
- Ten TPMT variants with diminished enzyme activity have been described. TPMT*2, TPMT*3A, and TPMT*3C are responsible for 80–95% of the phenotype in TPMT deficiencies. Patients with the wildtype genotype show high TPMT activity. Patients who are heterozygous or homozygous for variant alleles display medium or low enzyme activity.
- The TPMT*3A allele contains two SNPs in exon 7 (G460A) and exon 10 (A719G). With a frequency of 3–6%, it is the most prevalent variant amongst the Caucasian population. TPMT*3A was found in 55% of patients with a phenotype for this enzyme deficiency. Patients with this deficiency should only receive 5–10% of the planned 6-MP dose.

**Ref:**

1. Dervieux T, Meshkin B, Neri B. Pharmacogenetic testing: proofs of principle and pharmacoeconomic implications. Mutat Res 2005;31:90–105
2. Desai AA, Innocenti F, Ratain MJ. Pharmacogenomics: roads to anticancer therapeutics nirvana? Oncogene 2003;22:6621–8
3. Lee W, Lockhart AC, Kim RM et al. Cancer pharmacogenomics: powerful tools in cancer chemotherapy and drug development. Oncologist 2005;10:104–11
4. Loni L, De Braud F, Zinzani PL et al. Pharmacogenetics and proteomics of anticancer drugs in non-Hodgkin's lymphoma. Leuk Lymphoma 2003;44(suppl 3):S115–22
5. Marsh S. Pharmacogenomics. Ann Oncol 2007;18(suppl 9):ix24–8
6. Stam RW, den Boer ML, Meijerink JP et al. Differential mRNA expression of Ara-C-metabolizing enzymes explains Ara-C sensitivity in MLL gene-rearranged infant acute lymphoblastic leukemia. Blood 2003;101:1270–6
7. Tan BR, McLeod HL. Pharmacogenetic influences on treatment response and toxicity in colorectal cancer. Semin Oncol 2005;32:113–9
8. Weinshilboum R, Wand L. Pharmacogenomics: from bench to bedside. Nat Rev Drug Discovery 2004;3:739–48

**Web:**

1. http:// www.nature.com/tpj/index.html — Pharmacogenomics Journal
2. http://www.ncbi.nlm.nih.gov/About/primer/pharm.html — Pharmacogenomics Primer
3. http://www.pharmgkb.org — Pharmacogenetics Database
4. http://www.nigms.nih.gov/Initiatives/PGRN — Pharmacogenetics Research Network
5. http://snp.cshl.org — SNP Consortium

## 4.1    Antiemetic Prophylaxis and Therapy

### M. Daskalakis, H. Bertz

**Def:**    Symptom triad, "ANE syndrome": Anorexia (loss of appetite), Nausea, and Emesis (vomiting). Most common adverse effects patients encounter after cytostatic treatment.

### Types of Cytostatic Drug-induced ANE Syndrome

- Acute: during chemotherapy and up to 24 h afterwards
- Delayed: more than 24 h after chemotherapy
- Anticipatory: prior to chemotherapy, triggered by classic conditioning after occurrence of nausea and vomiting during previous chemotherapy cycles; mainly due to cortical stimulation

**Pphys:**    ### Pathophysiological Concept of Acute Nausea and Vomiting

The vomiting center, located in the lateral reticular formation of the medulla oblongata, initiates and coordinates the mechanisms of emesis. It receives impulses from vestibular nuclei, visceral and cortical afferents, and the adjacent chemoreceptor trigger zone (CTZ, area postrema of the fourth ventricle). The CTZ is the primary mediator of the chemotherapy-associated ANE syndrome. Cytostatic drugs and radiotherapy can stimulate the CTZ either

- Directly/centrally by directly activating the CTZ receptor systems (e.g., via substance P + Neurokinin-1-receptor), or
- Indirectly/peripherally by damaging enterochromaffine cells of the gastrointestinal tract
  - → Release of serotonin which binds to local $5-HT_3$ receptors
  - → Activation of visceral afferents connected with the CTZ / vomiting center
  - → Release of substance P

### Mode of Action of Antiemetic Drugs

$5-HT_3$ antagonists mediate their effects centrally and peripherally through inhibition of serotonin effects. Other receptor systems (dopamine / opiate / neurokinin / acetylcholine / histamine receptors) also act as mediators of the ANE syndrome and provide targets for antiemetic drugs. Some antiemetics targeting specific receptors show a polytropic mode of action. High doses of metoclopramide, for example, also have antiserotoninergic effects while neuroleptic drugs show different degrees of antidopaminergic and anticholinergic activity. Neurokinin-1 (NK1) receptor blockers antagonize the emetogenic effect of substance P in the CNS. In current clinical studies, they have been shown to enhance the antiemetic effects of $5-HT_3$ antagonists and steroids.

**Pg:**    ### Risk Factors for the ANE Syndrome

- Negative experiences during previous chemotherapy cycles
- Age < 35 years
- Female gender
- History of kinetosis, history of hyperemesis gravidarum
- Anxiousness as a primary personality trait

Patients who abuse alcohol are less likely to develop an ANE syndrome.

**Acute emetogenic potential of cytostatic drugs (Hesketh 1997)**

| Stage[a] | Emesis[b] | Substance |
|---|---|---|
| 5 | > 90% | AraC > 1 g/m², carboplatin > 1 g/m², carmustine > 250 mg/m², cisplatin ≥ 50 mg/m², cyclophosphamide > 1,500 mg/m², dacarbazine > 500 mg/m², ifosfamide > 3 g/m², melphalan 100–200 mg/m², thiotepa 5 mg/kg/day, streptozotocin |

[a] Stages: 1–2 (weakly emetogenic), 3–4 (moderately emetogenic), 5 (highly emetogenic)
[b] Percentage of patients who experience vomiting if not given antiemetic prophylaxis

**Acute emetogenic potential of cytostatic drugs (Hesketh 1997)** *(continued)*

| Stage[a] | Emesis[b] | Substance |
|---|---|---|
| 4 | 60–90% | Actinomycin D, AraC 250–1,000 mg/m$^2$, carboplatin 300–1,000 mg/m$^2$, carmustine $\leq$ 250 mg/m$^2$, cisplatin < 50 mg/m$^2$, cyclophosphamide 750–1,500 mg/m$^2$, dacarbazine < 500 mg/m$^2$, daunorubicin, doxorubicin > 60 mg/m$^2$, epirubicin > 90 mg/m$^2$, ifosfamide 1–3 g/m$^2$, lomustine, methotrexate > 1 g/m$^2$, nimustine, pentostatin, procarbazine |
| 3 | 30–60% | AraC 20–250 mg/m$^2$, carboplatin < 300 mg/m$^2$, cyclophosphamide $\leq$ 750 mg/m$^2$, doxorubicin 20–60 mg/m$^2$, epirubicin $\leq$ 90 mg/m$^2$, 5-fluorouracil > 1 g/m$^2$, idarubicin, ifosfamide < 1 g/m$^2$, melphalan, methotrexate 250–1,000 mg/m$^2$, mitoxantrone > 15 mg/m$^2$, topotecan, oral cyclophosphamide |
| 2 | 10–30% | Asparaginase, AraC < 20 mg/m$^2$, bleomycin, docetaxel, doxorubicin < 20 mg/m$^2$, etoposide, 5-fluorouracil < 1 g/m$^2$, gemcitabine, irinotecan, melphalan (p.o.), mercaptopurine, methotrexate 50–250 mg/m$^2$, mitomycin C, mitoxantrone < 15 mg/m$^2$, oxaliplatin, paclitaxel, thiotepa, teniposide |
| 1 | < 10% | Busulfan, chlorambucil, cladribine, fludarabine, goserelin, hydroxyurea, methotrexate < 50 mg/m$^2$, thioguanine, vinblastine, vincristine, vinorelbine, capecitabine, rituximab, trastuzumab |

[a] Stages: 1–2 (weakly emetogenic), 3–4 (moderately emetogenic), 5 (highly emetogenic)
[b] Percentage of patients who experience vomiting if not given antiemetic prophylaxis

### *Estimation of the Emetogenic Potential of Combination Chemotherapy*
Based on the drug with the strongest emetogenic effect in monotherapy, the emetogenic potential of combination chemotherapy is estimated as follows:
- No change with addition of stage 1 cytostatics
- Increase by one degree in total with addition of any number of stage 2 substances
- Increase by one degree per added stage 3 or 4 substance

*ATTENTION:* The addition of radiotherapy may increase emetogenicity

**Time to Onset and duration of emesis**

| Cytostatic drug | Time to Onset (h) | Duration (h) |
|---|---|---|
| Bleomycin | 3–6 | – |
| Carboplatin | 6–14 | 24–48 |
| Cisplatin | 1–6 | 24–120 |
| Cyclophosphamide | 6–12 | 24–48 |
| Cytosine arabinoside | 1–3 | 3–8 |
| Daunorubicin | 2–6 | 22–48 |
| Doxorubicin | 4–6 | 24–36 |
| DTIC / dacarbazine | 1–3 | 12–24 |
| Epirubicin | 4–6 | 12–24 |
| Etoposide / VP-16 (i.v.) | 3–8 | – |
| 5-Fluorouracil | 3–6 | 48–72 |

**Time to Onset and duration of emesis** *(continued)*

| Cytostatic drug | Time to Onset (h) | Duration (h) |
|---|---|---|
| Gemcitabine | 3–6 | – |
| Irinotecan | 1–8 | – |
| Bleomycin | 3–6 | – |
| Carboplatin | 6–14 | 24–48 |
| Cisplatin | 1–6 | 24–120 |
| Cyclophosphamide | 6–12 | 24–48 |
| Cytosine arabinoside | 1–3 | 3– 8 |
| Daunorubicin | 2–6 | 22–48 |
| Doxorubicin | 4–6 | 24–36 |
| DTIC / dacarbazine | 1–3 | 12–24 |
| Epirubicin | 4–6 | 12–24 |
| Etoposide / VP-16 (i.v.) | 3–8 | – |
| 5-Fluorouracil | 3–6 | 48–72 |
| Gemcitabine | 3–6 | – |
| Irinotecan | 1–8 | – |
| Methotrexate | 4–12 | 3–12 |
| Mitomycin C | 1–4 | 48–72 |
| Mitoxantrone | 2–6 | < 24 |
| Procarbazine | 24–27 | Variable |
| Vinblastine | 4–8 | < 24 |
| Vincristine | 4–8 | – |

**Sy:**      *Severity of Nausea and Emesis according to WHO Common Toxicity Criteria*

Nausea:
- Grade I      mild, normal food intake
- Grade II      moderate, reduced food intake
- Grade III      severe, food intake impossible
- Grade IV      life-threatening

Vomiting:
- Grade I      mild, once daily
- Grade II      moderate, 2–5 times daily
- Grade III      severe, 6–10 times daily
- Grade IV      life-threatening, > 10 times daily

**DDx:**      *Differential Diagnosis: Nausea*
- *Gastrointestinal:* gastroenteritis, stenosis, ileus, cholestasis
- *Central / peripheral nervous system:* increased intracranial pressure (e.g., due to brain tumors, toxic or inflammatory cerebral edema); central and peripheral vertigo, migraine
- *Metabolic:* electrolyte imbalance (especially hypercalcemia), acid-base imbalance, hepatic and adrenocortical insufficiency, uremia, hyperemesis gravidarum
- *Functional:* sensory stimuli, psychological factors (exhaustion, depression)
- *Drugs:* cytostatics, antibiotics, opiates, cardiac glycosides

**Th:**    **Antiemetic Prophylaxis and Therapy**

### Basic Principles
- Antiemetic prophylaxis is more efficient than therapy: start effective antiemesis from the first chemotherapy cycle (prevention of "conditioned emesis"). Oral antiemetics are preferable.
- Treatment according to emesis risk (individual factors, emetogenicity of the treatment), 15 min (i.v.) or 30 min (p.o.) prior to administration of cytostatics.
- History of emesis in the previous therapy cycle: anxiolytic medication on the evening before chemotherapy (lorazepam), intensification of antiemetic prophylaxis.
- If required (e.g., with "salvage therapy," prophylaxis of delayed emesis), continue treatment after the chemotherapy has finished.
- *ATTENTION:* Do not use corticosteroids in combination with stimulatory immunotherapy (e.g., interleukin-2 or interferon) or in patients with decompensated diabetes.
- In 70% of cases, effective prophylaxis of acute vomiting prevents the development of a delayed ANE syndrome.

**Antiemetic prophylaxis according to emetogenic risk (ASCO MASCC 2006)**

| Emetogenic risk (%) | Prophylaxis of acute emesis | Prophylaxis of delayed emesis |
|---|---|---|
| High risk (> 90%) | 5-HT$_3$ antagonist + dexamethasone 20 mg/day + aprepitant 125 mg/day p.o. | Dexamethasone 8 mg 2 × per day for 3–4 days + aprepitant 80 mg/day p.o. for 2 days |
| Moderate risk (30–60%) | 5-HT$_3$ antagonist + dexamethasone 8 mg/day (with AC in breast cancer; aprepitant) | Dexamethasone 4–8 mg 1–2 × per day according to patient's need |
| Low risk (10–30%) | Dexamethasone 4–8 mg/day or 5-HT$_3$ antagonist | Dexamethasone 4–8 mg 1–2 × per day according to patient's need |
| Minimal risk (< 10%) | Dexamethasone 4–8 mg/day according to patient's need | |

## Antiemetic Drugs

### 5-HT$_3$ Antagonists
- Dolasetron, granisetron, ondansetron, tropisetron, palonosetron
- Within the recommended dosage, all compounds are equipotent
- If absorption is normal, oral and intravenous administration are equipotent
- Despite variations in half-life (serum t½: ondansetron 3 h, tropisetron 7 h, dolasetron 8 h, granisetron 9 h, palonosetron 40 hrs) and duration of efficacy (receptor affinity), a once-daily dose is usually sufficient; only ondansetron 8 mg may need to be boosted
- Increased effect if combined with dexamethasone (synchronous administration)

### Benzamide Derivative
- Metoclopramide, 0.5 mg/kg BW p.o.
- *ATTN:* occurrence of dose-independent dyskinesias, particularly with younger patients
- Therapy: biperiden (Akineton) 2.5–5 mg bolus i.v.
- Prophylaxis of adverse effects if required: combination with an antihistamine (e.g., dimenhydrinate)
- If adverse effects occur: change antiemetic treatment to 5-HT$_3$ antagonists in subsequent cycles

### *Neurokinin-1 Receptor Antagonists*
- The neurokinin-1 receptor antagonist, aprepitant, complements the effects of 5-HT$_3$ antagonists and corticosteroids in highly emetogenic chemotherapy. Aprepitant is effective in the treatment of both acute and delayed emesis (e.g., cisplatin-induced).
- Dosage: day 1: 125 mg aprepitant p.o. (1 h prior to chemotherapy), day 2–3: 80 mg p.o. (mornings).
- *ATTN:* Neurokinin-1 receptor antagonists interact with the cytochrome P450 system (esp. CYP3A4) and can potentially increase the plasma concentration of various cytostatics (e.g., taxanes, etoposide, irinotecan, vinca alkaloids) and targeted therapies.
- Consider reducing the steroid dose (interference with steroid pharmacokinetics).

## "Salvage Therapy" for the Treatment of Acute Emesis

Antiemetic treatment after insufficient prophylaxis is based on the use of more potent antiemetics or combinations of antiemetics and additives with different modes of action. Dose escalation of individual antiemetics is ineffective. Patients treated on an outpatient basis are to be provided with medication and instructions necessary for "salvage therapy." In cases of prolonged acute emesis, maximum treatment must be continued.

| Primary antiemetic | Synergistic secondary antiemetic drug | Additive |
|---|---|---|
| 5-HT$_3$ antagonist | Corticosteroid, phenothiazine, butyrophenone, benzodiazepine | – |
| Benzamide derivative | Corticosteroid | Antihistamine, benzodiazepine |
| Phenothiazine | Corticosteroid | Antihistamine |
| Butyrophenone | Corticosteroid | Antihistamine |
| Corticosteroid | Benzodiazepine | – |

In patients with a history of kinetosis, the primary combination should include an antihistamine

## Prophylaxis of Delayed-onset ANE Syndrome

### *Indications*
- Highly emetogenic chemotherapy (stage 5, risk > 90%)
- History of emesis during previous cycles

### *Treatment*
- Administration of oral antiemetics preferable, starting the morning after the last chemotherapy treatment
- Chemotherapy involving cisplatin: dexamethasone 8 mg/day p.o. for 2 days + 5-HT$_3$ antagonist for 3–5 days
- Chemotherapy without cisplatin: 5-HT$_3$ antagonist + dexamethasone or metoclopramide + dexamethasone

## Prophylaxis of Anticipatory Vomiting

- Lorazepam 1–2 mg on the evening before chemotherapy as well as 1–2 × daily during chemotherapy
- Behavioral therapy where appropriate

## Antiemesis with High-dose Chemotherapy

### High-risk Constellation
- Highly to moderately emetogenic chemotherapy, possibly for several days and in combination with radiotherapy (TBI)
- Several previous chemotherapy courses, with nausea and vomiting
- Reduced performance status, extensive concomitant medication

### Treatment
Combination of $5\text{-}HT_3$ antagonist + dexamethasone; possibly more effective if combined with phenothiazines

## Antiemesis with Radiotherapy

- High-risk situation (TBI, total nodal irradiation, abdominal bath technique): $5\text{-}HT_3$ antagonist + dexamethasone before and 24 h after the treatment fractions
- Intermediate risk (cranial radiosurgery, radiotherapy to the lower thoracic region, the upper abdominal region and the pelvis): $5\text{-}HT_3$ antagonist or benzamide derivative ± dexamethasone before each treatment fraction
- Low risk (irradiation of the head / neck, extremities, upper thoracic region): no prophylaxis, treatment only if required

**Ref:**

1. ESMO Guidelines Working Group. Chemotherapy-induced nausea and vomiting: ESMO Clinical Recommendations for prophylaxis. Ann Oncol 2007;18(suppl 2):ii83–5
2. Grunberg SM, Deuson RR, Mavros P et al. Incidence of chemotherapy-induced nausea and emesis after modern anti-emetics. Cancer 2004;100:2261–8
3. Hesketh PJ, Kris MG, Grünberg SM et al. Proposal for classifying the acute emetogenicity of cancer chemotherapy. J Clin Oncol 1997;15:103–9
4. Jordan K, Kasper C, Schmoll HJ. Chemotherapy-induced nausea and vomiting: current and new standards in the antiemetic prophylaxis and treatment. Eur J Cancer 2005;41:199–205
5. Kris MG, Heskett PJ, Somerfield MR et al. ASCO Guideline for antiemetics in oncology. J Clin Oncol 2006;24:2932–47
6. Oettle H, Riess H. Treatment of chemotherapy-induced nausea and vomiting. J Cancer Res Clin Oncol 2001;127:340–5
7. Schnell FM. Chemotherapy-induced nausea and vomiting: the importance of acute antiemetic control. Oncologist 2003;8:187–98

**Web:**

1. http://www.mascc.org    Supportive Care in Cancer, MASCC
2. http://www.guideline.gov    National Guideline Clearinghouse
3. http://www.nccn.org/professionals/physician_gls/PDF/antiemesis.pdf    NCCN Guidelines Antiemesis
4. http://www.nlm.nih.gov/medlineplus/ency/article/003117.htm    Medline Plus, Nausea / Vomiting

**Antiemetic drugs**

| Antiemetic group | Drug | Administration | Dosage / day | Side effects |
|---|---|---|---|---|
| **High antiemetic potency** | | | | |
| 5-HT$_3$ antagonists | Ondansetron | p.o. | 2–3 times 8 mg | Fatigue, headache, constipation *ATTENTION*: gastrointestinal tumors, older patients, opiate medication, postoperative |
| | | i.v. | 1–3 times 8 mg | |
| | Tropisetron | p.o., i.v. | Once 5 mg | |
| | Granisetron | p.o. | Once 2 mg | |
| | | i.v. | Once 1–3 mg | |
| | Dolasetron | p.o. | Once 200 mg 60 min before Cx | |
| | | i.v. | Once 100 mg 30 min before Cx | |
| Neurokinin-1 receptor antagonists | Aprepitant | p.o. | Day 1: once 125 mg 60 min before Cx Day 2–3: once 80 mg, mornings | Fatigue, constipation, diarrhea, interaction with cytochrome P450 system |
| Benzamide derivatives, dopamine-D2 receptor antagonists | Metoclopramide HCl | p.o., i.v., rectal | 0.5–2 mg/kgBW, max. 5–6 times | Sedation, hypertension, extrapyramidal symptoms (antidote: biperiden i.v.) |
| | Alizapride | p.o., i.v. | 6 times 50–100 mg | |
| **Moderate antiemetic potency** | | | | |
| Glucocorticoids | Dexamethasone | i.v., i.m. | Once 20 mg or 3 times 8 mg | Sedation, perianal irritation, headache, flush, increased blood pressure and blood glucose |
| | | p.o. | 1–3 times 4–8 mg | |
| | Methylprednisolone | p.o., i.v. | 40–250 mg | |
| Phenothiazine, neuroleptics | Levomepromazine | p.o., i.v., i.m. | 4 times 10–25 mg | Extrapyramidal symptoms, sedation, headache |
| | Triflupromazine | p.o., i.v., i.m., rectal | 3–4 times 5–10 mg | |
| | Promethazine | p.o. | 4 times 25 mg | |
| Butyrophenone, neuroleptics | Domperidone | p.o. | 3 times 10–20 mg | See phenothiazines |
| | Haloperidol | p.o. | 3 times 1–2 mg | |
| **Mild antiemetic potency** | | | | |
| Antihistamines | Dimenhydrinate | p.o. | 1–2 tablets/8 h | Sedation, anticholinergic symptoms |
| | | Rectal | 3–4 times 1 suppository | |
| | | i.v., i.m. | 1–2 ampoules/dose | |
| Benzodiazepine | Diazepam | p.o., i.v., rectal | 3 times 2.5–5 mg | Sedation |
| | Lorazepam | p.o., i.v. | Twice 1–2 mg | |

## 4.2 Antibiotic Treatment and Neutropenic Fever

H. Bertz

**Def:** *Neutropenia:* leukocytes $< 1 \times 10^9/l$ or granulocytes $< 0.5 \times 10^9/l$
*Fever:* temperature (oral or axillary) once $> 38.5°C$ or twice $> 38.0°C$ in 24 h

**ATTENTION:** Avoid taking temperature rectally as it poses additional risks of infection. Sepsis (► Chap. 9.1) may cause hypothermia.

Despite the ever-increasing effectiveness of antibiotics and antimycotics, infections remain a common cause of increased mortality in neutropenic patients. The duration and extent of neutropenia determine to which degree the patient is at risk:
- Low risk: granulocytes $0.5–1 \times 10^9/l$, granulocytopenia for 2–7 days → in the case of sepsis: lethality 14%
- High risk: granulocytes $< 0.1 \times 10^9/l$, granulocytopenia for $\geq 7–10$ days → in the case of sepsis: lethality 47%

**Ep:** Incidence of the different causes of fever during granulocytopenia (de Pauw 1996)
- Microbiologically documented bacteremia      27%
- Clinically documented infection      42%
- Fever of unknown origin (FUO)      31%

Most common sources of infection (EORTC):
- Oral cavity and pharynx      25%
- Lung, lower respiratory tract      25%
- Intravenous catheters, skin, soft tissues      15%
- Gastrointestinal tract      15%
- Perianal region      10%
- Urogenital tract      5–10%
- Nose and paranasal sinuses      5%

**Pg:** *Pathogenesis*
Relevant components in the development of infections in patients with malignancies:
- Mucositis and subsequent damage to the natural mucosal barrier of the digestive tract, lung, and urinary bladder
- Catheters and intravascular access devices (central venous catheters, venous ports, Quinton catheters, intra-arterial catheters, urinary catheters, etc.)
- Neurological abnormalities (bladder / colon function, swallowing reflex, etc.) → pyelonephritis, cystitis, aspiration pneumonia
- Impaired cellular immunity (lymphoma) → increased risk of infection especially with *Pneumocystis carinii*, *Nocardia*, CMV
- Splenic dysfunction, e.g., splenomegaly, lymphoma infiltration, after splenectomy, functional asplenia (Howell-Jolly bodies) → increased risk of infection with streptococci, *Haemophilus influenzae*
- Granulocytopenia after radiotherapy / chemotherapy or due to bone marrow infiltration by the primary disease
- Use of purine analogs (fludarabine) and monoclonal antibodies against T-lymphocytes (alemtuzumab) or B-lymphocytes (rituximab) → lymphocytic dysfunction

Approximately 80% of infections in neutropenic patients are of endogenous origin (i.e., caused by the body's own bacterial flora).

**General spectrum of pathogens**

| | |
|---|---|
| Gram-negative bacteria | Enteric bacteria (*Escherichia coli, Salmonella, Klebsiella, Enterobacter cloacae, Serratia, Proteus*, etc.), *Pseudomonas, Haemophilus, Bacteroides* |
| Gram-positive bacteria | Coagulase-negative staphylococci, *Staphylococcus aureus*, streptococci (pneumococcus spec.), *Listeria*, anaerobic bacteria (peptostreptococci, propionibacteria, clostridia) |
| Other bacteria | Mycobacteria, *Pneumocystis carinii*, toxoplasmosis |
| Viruses | *Herpes simplex, Herpes zoster*, cytomegalovirus, hepatitis |
| Fungi | *Candida* species, *Aspergillus* species |

More than 50% of all initial gram-negative infections are caused by *Escherichia coli, Klebsiella pneumoniae*, and *Pseudomonas aeruginosa*. The most common gram-positive pathogens (increasing frequency) are: coagulase-negative staphylococci, *Staphylococcus aureus*, streptococci, and *Bacillus* species. Anaerobes usually only occur in mixed infections.

### Specific Spectrum of Pathogens
The properties of "hospital-specific" pathogens isolated in a medical institution must be considered. Besides the specific pathogen spectrum, the "specific resistance" of hospital pathogens is of importance. For example:
- Occurrence of oxacillin-resistant staphylococci
- Resistance to vancomycin or imipenem

**Sy:**
### Fever
Due to the insufficient immune response, fever is often the only symptom of infection during neutropenia. The course of the fever may be indicative of the pathogenesis of the infection:
- Temperature increase within a few hours, patient impaired → gram-negative bacteria
- Gradual increase → gram-positive bacteria or fungi
- *ATTN*: patients treated with corticosteroids or analgesics (metamizole, paracetamol) may not develop fever

### Specific Signs of Infection
- Local inflammation around catheters / access devices → coagulase-negative staphylococci
- Skin infections → gram-positive cocci
- Ulcers of the mucous membranes, mucositis → *Candida*, streptococci, herpes virus
- Acral necrosis (fingers, toes) due to thromboembolism → aspergillosis
- Focal inflammation (on fingers, toes) → endocarditis, e.g., streptococci
- Localized pain in case of hepatic involvement (mycosis, *Candida* spp. and *Aspergillus* spp.) or gastrointestinal infection (usually gram-negative)
- Necrotizing gingivitis, acute abdominal pain, diarrhea → anaerobes
- Severe diarrhea during antibiotic treatment → *Clostridium difficile*, rotavirus
- Sinusitis, pulmonary (coin-shaped) infiltrates → *Aspergillus*, mucormycosis
- Sepsis: drop in blood pressure, tachycardia, hypothermia (▶ Chap. 9.1)

**Dg:**
### Medical History, Clinical Examination
- Case history including fever, diarrhea, dysuria, etc.
- Physical examination: intravenous access sites, catheter ports, skin, oral mucous membranes, perianal region, pulmonary auscultation and percussion, abdominal pressure pain, pain on palpitation / pressure pain of the paranasal sinuses, lymphadenopathy, monitoring of blood pressure and pulse, meningism

### Laboratory Tests
Routine laboratory tests, parameters of inflammation

*Microbiology*
- Peripheral blood cultures and cultures using intravenous access devices (► Chap. 10.8)
- From peripheral puncture sites (preferably two puncture sites): 4 aerobic and 1 anaerobic blood culture bottle
- With suspected catheter sepsis: draw an isolator tube from each access as well as from a peripheral vein and collect two aerobic blood cultures; remove catheter, microbiological analysis of the catheter tip
- With prevailing clinical signs: culture of urine, culture of sputum, swabs from suspicious lesions, lumbar / pleural / ascites puncture and culture
- With pulmonary infiltrates: bronchoalveolar lavage (BAL); in rare cases lung biopsy
- With diarrhea: stool culture, detection of enterotoxins from *Clostridium difficile*, Gruber-Widal reaction

*Imaging*
- Chest x-ray, if required x-ray of paranasal sinuses
- If required abdominal ultrasound
- If required high-resolution CT scan

*ATTENTION:* invasive diagnostic techniques always carry the risk of (new) infections → sterile sampling techniques, thorough disinfecting of hands and puncture sites.

DDx:
- Malignancy-associated fever (lymphoma, leukemia, renal cell carcinoma, etc.)
- Drug-associated fever ("drug fever," e.g., from intolerance to antibiotics)
- Allergic reaction to blood products or amphotericin B

Th: *Course of Treatment*

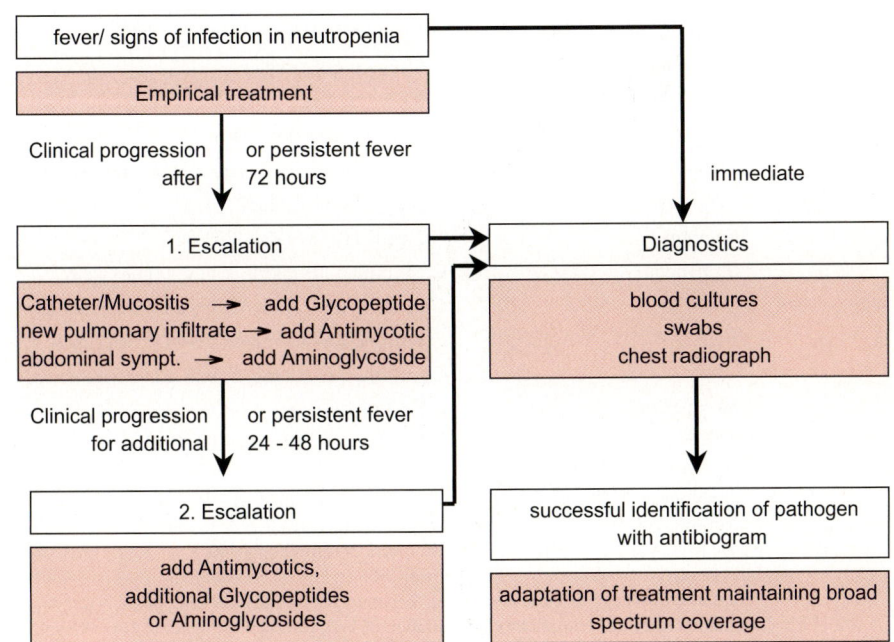

## Treatment Initiation

With fever during neutropenia, rapid initiation of treatment is essential:

- Immediate initiation of empirical antibiotic treatment upon occurrence of fever or any clinically detectable signs of infection (even without fever)
- Differential diagnostic considerations are secondary; blood cultures and possibly swabs should be taken immediately before administration of antibiotics; further diagnostic investigations (imaging, ultrasound, bronchoalveolar lavage (BAL), abscess puncture, etc.) may be carried out afterwards

The initial treatment strategy must be individually decided upon the basis of the available information (antibiotic prophylaxis, high- / low-risk situation, danger of nephro- / ototoxicity, anti-*Pseudomonas aeruginosa* activity).

- *Standard:* combination of broad-spectrum penicillin (piperacillin or cefepime) or gyrase inhibitors (ciprofloxacin or levofloxacin) and aminoglycosides (gentamicin or netilmicin).
- *Equivalent alternative:* monotherapy with ceftazidime or piperacillin / tazobactam.
- Also suitable for monotherapy: carbapenems.
- In relation to survival, the use of vancomycin in the initial empirical treatment is of no advantage. Its use carries the risk of establishing vancomycin-resistant strains.

**Dosages for empirical antibiotic treatment of patients with fever during neutropenia**

| *Patient without renal insufficiency* | | |
|---|---|---|
| Piperacillin | 4 g i.v. 3 times a day | 250–300 mg/kg/day |
| Piperacillin and tazobactam | 4.5 g i.v. 3 times a day | |
| Ceftriaxone | 2 g i.v. once a day | |
| Ceftazidime[a] | 2 g i.v. 3 times a day | |
| Gentamicin[b] | 360 mg i.v. once a day | 3–5 mg/kg/day |
| Netilmicin | 400 mg i.v. once a day | 6–7.5 mg/kg/day |
| Cefepime | 2 g i.v. 3 times a day | |
| Vancomycin[c] | 1 g i.v. twice a day | 20–30 mg/kg/day |
| Amphotericin B[d] | 0.75–1 mg/kg/day i.v. | |
| Ciprofloxacin | 500–750 mg twice a day | |
| Levofloxacin | 500 mg once or twice daily | |
| *Patients with renal insufficiency or simultaneous use of nephrotoxic compounds* | | |
| Ceftazidime[a] | 2 g i.v. 3 times a day | |
| Cefepime | 2 g i.v. 3 times a day | |
| Imipenem | Creatinine < 1.5 mg/dl: 1 g i.v. 3 times a day | |
| | Creatinine 1.5–2.5 mg/dl: 0.5 g i.v. 3 times a day | |
| | Creatinine 2.6–3.5 mg/dl: 0.5 g i.v. twice daily | |
| | Creatinine 3.6–6.0 mg/dl: 0.25 g i.v. twice daily | |
| Meropenem | 1 g 3 times a day | |
| Teicoplanin[e] | 800 mg day i.v. ("loading dose"), then 400 mg/day | |

[a] May be given to patients with non-anaphylactoid penicillin allergy. However, potential cross allergies

[b] Caution: nephrotoxicity. Determine level before administration of 3rd dose; target: trough level < 2 mg/l

[c] Strictly i.v. over 1 h (if paravenous injection: risk of thrombophlebitis); determine level, trough level < 5–10 mg/l

[d] Initiate treatment with close monitoring (hepatotoxicity, potassium loss), possibly test dose and dose escalation, toxicity can be reduced by administration of 1–2 l NaCl 0.9%, pethidine, paracetamol, clemastine

[e] If *S. aureus* is found in blood culture: treat over 14–21 days

### Catheter Removal

Of paramount importance if *Staphylococcus aureus*, mycobacteria, *Candida*, *Corynebacterium jejuni* and *Acinetobacter baumannii*, *Stenotrophomonas maltophilia*, *Pseudomonas aeruginosa*, or *Bacillus* species are detected in the catheter culture.

### Escalation in the Case of Fever of Unknown Origin (FUO)

In the case of clinical progression, escalation with glycopeptides (vancomycin or teicoplanin) and aminoglycosides.

With persistent fever and clinically stable course, start empirical treatment after 48–72 h:

- Catheter and/or mucositis → glycopeptides
- New lung infiltrates → antimycotics (e.g., lipid-formulation amphotericin B, azoles)
- Primary glycopeptide therapy and persistent temperature: discontinue glycopeptides, escalation with aminoglycosides; if fever still persists after 48 h: antimycotics

### Pathogen-specific Adaptation of Treatment

Once the results of the diagnostic measures have been obtained (blood cultures with antibiotic resistance testing, swabs, etc.), treatment may be specifically adapted, particularly if it has been insufficient so far:

- Positive bacterial cultures → treatment according to antibiogram
- Infections caused by gram-positive bacteria (e.g., infected catheter, port) → immediate administration of vancomycin or teicoplanin
- Infections caused by anaerobes → metronidazole, imipenem or meropenem
- Herpes infections → acyclovir
- CMV infections → ganciclovir or foscarnet
- Fungal infections → lipid-formulation amphotericin B, azoles, echinocandins (change of catheter)
- Infections caused by atypical agents → erythromycin or clarithromycin

**ATTENTION:** in patients with fever during neutropenia, restricting the antibiotic spectrum when adapting the treatment must be strictly avoided, i.e., no monotherapy with vancomycin / teicoplanin or an antimycotic only.

**Dosages for pathogen-specific treatment**

| | |
|---|---|
| ***Cytomegalovirus (CMV)*** | |
| Ganciclovir | 5 mg/kg i.v. twice daily for 14 days, then maintenance therapy once daily |
| Foscarnet | 60 mg/kg i.v. twice daily for 14 days, possibly maintenance therapy |
| ***Herpes simplex virus (HSV)*** | |
| Acyclovir | 5–10 mg/kg i.v. 3 times daily for 5–10 days<br>Alternatively, 800 mg p.o. 4 times a day |
| Brivudine | 125 mg/day |
| ***Varicella zoster virus (VZV)*** | |
| Acyclovir | 10 mg/kg i.v. 3 times a day for 5–10 days |
| Brivudine | 125 mg/day |
| Foscarnet | 60 mg/kg i.v. twice daily for 14 days |
| ***Candida*** | |
| Fluconazole | 400 mg/day (up to 800 mg/day) i.v. or p.o |
| Caspofungin | 70 mg/day i.v. on day 1, then 50 mg/day i.v. |
| ***Pneumocystis jiroveci*** | |
| Trimethoprim-sulfamethoxazole | 30 mg/kg i.v. 3–4 times a day for 14–21 days |

**Dosages for pathogen-specific treatment** *(continued)*

| *Aspergillus, Candida species* | |
|---|---|
| Amphotericin B | 0.75–1 mg/kg/day |
| Liposomal Ampho B[a] | 3–5 mg/kg/day |
| Voriconazole | 2 × 6 mg/kg/day i.v. on day 1, then 4 mg/kg twice daily i.v. / p.o. |
| Posaconazole | 2 × 400 mg/d |
| Caspofungin | 70 mg/day i.v. on day 1, then 50 mg/day i.v. |
| *Atypical pathogens (Mycoplasma, Legionella)* | |
| Erythromycin | 500–1,000 mg 4 times a day |
| Clarithromycin | 500 mg twice daily p.o. / i.v. |

[a] *ATTENTION*: high costs, use only if treatment with amphotericin B is unsuccessful or toxic

### Treatment Duration

Basic principle: "As short as possible, as long as necessary". If the therapy is too short, the infection might relapse (associated with a poor prognosis). If the duration of treatment is too long, resistance and fungal infections may develop. Recommendations:

- Leukocytes > $1 \times 10^9$/l: stop antibiotic treatment 3 days after cessation of fever; however, minimum course: 5 days.
- Leukocytes < $1 \times 10^9$/l: continue treatment until leukocytes > $1 \times 10^9$/l (independent of the patient's temperature status); if patient has been afebrile for 5 days, slowly deescalate the antibiotic treatment; if fever persists: continue treatment to up to 3 days after cessation of fever, possibly change to oral medication (gyrase inhibitors plus penicillin).

**Prg:**    Ninety percent of all patients respond well to antimicrobial treatment. The prognosis is dependent on:

- Patient's performance status
- Underlying disease (in general, infections in patients with solid tumors carry a better prognosis)
- Type of pathogen (poor prognosis with gram-negative infections; multiresistant hospital-acquired infections or *Pseudomonas aeruginosa*)
- Degree and duration of granulocytopenia
- Location of the source of infection (worst prognosis: lower respiratory tract)
- Toxicity of chemotherapy / radiotherapy
- In low-risk situations, oral combination therapy alone (gyrase inhibitors + penicillin) may be sufficient
- In low-risk situations, rapid change from i.v. to oral medication possible (see above)

**Px:**    ### Basic Hospital Hygiene

- Regular and thorough washing / disinfecting of hands
- Rooms with low bacterial / fungal levels: no potted plants / flowers, no humidifiers, no cold steam nebulizers, protection against dust from building sites (*Aspergillus*)
- Invasive procedures are to be carried out under sterile conditions
- Patient hygiene, especially skin care, dental care, mucositis prophylaxis; avoid foods with high bacterial / fungal counts
- Adaptation of therapeutic procedures: no suppositories, avoid taking rectal temperature
- Isolation if required
- If neutropenia persists for more than 7 days: regular monitoring, even if patient is afebrile – cultures of blood, stool, sputum, and throat swabs once weekly

### Hematopoietic Growth Factors

- Hematopoietic growth factors (e.g., G-CSF) should be administered according to current guidelines (ASCO, ESMO, ► Chap. 4.3).

- Granulocyte transfusions may be given as supportive treatment under controlled conditions within studies (▶ Chap. 5.4).

### Prophylactic Treatment

- The benefits of *prophylactic intestinal decontamination* are uncertain → not recommended.
- *Prophylactic use of antibiotics with levofloxacin is now recommended for patients expecting a neutropenic phase > 7 days.* Other antibiotics (e.g., ciprofloxacin or trimethoprim-sulfa-methoxazole) prior to an expected neutropenia period are not indicated. Despite reducing the incidence of fever during neutropenia and delaying the occurrence of infection, they do not reduce infection-associated mortality. Antibiotic-associated side effects, selection of therapy-resistant strains and occurrence of mycoses and infections caused by *Clostridium difficile* are common.
- *Prophylactic antimycotic treatment* has only been proven to be beneficial in connection with allogeneic transplantation → fluconazole 200 mg p.o. twice daily. Posaconazol shows favorable results in reducing the incidence of invasive fungal infections in leukemia pts. and pts. with therapy of acute GvHD > grade 2
- Patients who have had tuberculosis should receive antituberculosis prophylaxis prior to immunosuppressive treatment → isoniazid (INH) 300 mg/day p.o., if necessary also rifampicin 600 mg/day p.o.

**Ref:**

1. Crawford J, Dale DC, Lyman GH. Chemotherapy-induced neutropenia: risks, consequences, and new directions for its management. Cancer 2004;100:228–37
2. De Pauw BE. Strategies in the treatment of infections in neutropenic patients. Med Microbiol Lett 1996;5:305–9
3. Hughes WT, Armstrong D, Bodey GP et al. 2002 Guidelines for the use of antimicrobial agents in neutropenic patients with cancer. Clin Infect Dis 2002;34:730–51
4. Kern WV, Cometta A, De Bock R et al. Oral versus intravenous empirical antimicrobial therapy for fever in patients with granulocytopenia who are receiving cancer chemotherapy. N Engl J Med 1999;341:312–8
5. Neuburger S, Maschmeyer G. Update on managment of infections in cancer and stem cell transplant patients. Ann Hematol 2006;85:345–56
6. Pizo PA. Fever in immunocompromised patients. N Engl J Med 1999;341:893–900
7. Smith TJ, Khatcheressian J, Lyman GH et al. 2006 Update of recommendations for the use of white blood cell growth factors. An evidence-based clinical practice guideline. J Clin Oncol 2006;24:3187–205

**Web:**

1. http://www.guideline.gov — National Guideline Clearinghouse
2. http://www.mascc.org — Supportive Care in Cancer, MASCC
3. http://www.neutropenia.ca/ — Neutropenia Support Association
4. http://www.nccn.org/professionals/physician_gls/ PDF/myeloid_growth.pdf — NCCN Guideline

## 4.3     Growth Factors

### V. Thierry, C.I. Müller, M. Engelhardt

**Def:**     Cytokines (polypeptides or glycopeptides) which can increase proliferation, differentiation, and function of certain types of hematopoietic cells (▶ Chap. 1.3) or other cell types.

### Types
- Granulopoietic growth factors: G-CSF (filgrastim, lenograstim), GM-CSF (molgramostim)
- Erythropoietic growth factors: erythropoietin, darbepoetin α
- Thrombopoietic growth factors: IL-11, thrombopoietin
- Growth factors of early hematopoiesis: SCF, Flt-3, IL-1, IL-3, IL-6
- Keratinocyte growth factor: palifermin

**Ind:**     Evidence-based guidelines give clear indications for use of hematopoietic growth factors in hematology and oncology. Growth factors may be a prerequisite for specific types of therapy (e.g. hematopoietic stem cell transplantation, dose dense therapy) or may be used in supportive care indications (e.g., chemotherapy-induced anemia). The benefits and potential risks of growth factors need to be weighed for every individual patient.

### Use of Granulopoietic Growth Factors

#### Guidelines
- Guidelines of the European Society of Medical Oncology (ESMO) and the European Organization for Research and Treatment of Cancer (EORTC)
- Guidelines of the American Society of Clinical Oncology (ASCO), American Society of Hematology (ASH), " National Comprehensive Cancer Network" (NCCN)

#### Indications for Granulopoietic Growth Factors

*Definite indications:*
- Mobilization of hematopoietic progenitors / stem cells from bone marrow into peripheral blood (allogeneic and autologous)
- Severe chronic neutropenia: idiopathic, with metabolic defects, with combined immunodeficiencies, congenital or cyclic neutropenia (G-CSF)

*Other appropriate indications:*
- Primary prophylaxis following myelotoxic chemotherapy, especially if neutropenia ≤ 500/μl is expected
- After myeloablative therapy and autologous and allogeneic transplantation of bone marrow or peripheral blood stem cells, graft failure
- Aplastic anemia
- Neutropenia related to Felty's syndrome, T-γ-lymphoproliferative syndrome, hairy cell leukemia
- HIV infection: primary neutropenia or drug-induced neutropenia
- Dose-dense protocols, especially in breast cancer, lymphomas, and in older patients
- Secondary prophylaxis after chemotherapy, if neutropenic complication occurred after first cycle
- Prolonged neutropenia after radiotherapy
- Autoimmune neutropenia
- Neutropenia related to low-risk myelodysplastic syndromes

*Risk factors supporting prophylactic use:*

Expected neutropenia ≤ 500/µl and febrile neutropenia risk ≥ 20%

- Acute leukemia, high-grade lymphoma, CLL with antibody deficiency
- Age > 65 years, significant comorbidity / impaired general health, hypotension
- High-dose therapy, polychemotherapy, limited bone marrow reserve after intense prior treatment
- Duration of chemotherapy cycles < 4 weeks
- Treatment of relapse
- Severely myelotoxic or mucosa-toxic chemotherapy
- Existing infections: pneumonia, fungal infections

**IMPORTANT:** discontinue granulopoietic growth factors at least 2 days before new chemotherapy cycle starts.

## Use of Erythropoietic Growth Factors

### Guidelines

The following recommendations are based on guidelines from:
- European Organization for Research and Treatment of Cancer (EORTC), European Society for Medical Oncology (ESMO)
- American Society of Hematology (ASH), American Society of Clinical Oncology (ASCO), "National Comprehensive Cancer Network" (NCCN), "US Veterans' Administration"

### Indications for Erythropoietic Growth Factors

*Indications:*

- Chronic renal failure (renal anemia): → hemoglobin increase, reduced cardiovascular morbidity and mortality, improved quality of life
- Symptomatic chemotherapy-induced anemia (Hb ≤ 10 g/dl): decreased need for transfusions, improved quality of life

*Other areas of use:*

- Bone marrow failure (aplastic anemia, HIV infection): decreased need for transfusions
- Sepsis and intensive care
- Anemia in low-risk myelodysplastic syndromes (MDS)

### ASH / ASCO Guidelines for the Use of Epoetins (darbepoetin, erythropoietin)

- Recommended as alternative to packed red cell transfusion in patients with chemotherapy-induced anemia (Hb ≤ 10 g/dl)
- In patients with declining Hb (Hb 10–12 g/dl) up to clinical judgment
- With insufficient response (Hb increment < 1–2 g/dl) epoetins should not be administered for more than 6–8 weeks (exclude tumor progression, iron deficiency)
- Target hemoglobin: 10–12 g/dl
- Check parameters of iron metabolism (iron, ferritin, transferrin, TIBC). Iron supplementation may reduce the need for epoetins, improve clinical course, and help diagnose causes for poor response
- Recommended in patients with anemia associated with low-risk myelodysplasia (with or without simultaneous chemotherapy).

**Co:**        Recently, an increase in the rate of thromboembolic events and a decrease in survival has been observed in individual clinical trials in epoetin-treated patients with anemia of cancer, who did not receive chemotherapy. In this patient population, erythropoetins should only be used in the framework of clinical trials.

Antibody formation against erythropoietin α with pure red cell aplasia has been observed in patients with renal anemia (rare).

**Ref:**
1.   Aapro MS. Cameron DA, Pettengell R et al. EORTC guidelines for the use of granulocyte-colony stimulating factor to reduce the incidence of chemotherapy-induced febrile neutropenia in adult patients with lymphomas and solid tumours. Eur J Cancer 2006;42:2433–53
2.   Bokemeyer M, Aapro MS, Courdia A et al. EORTC guidelines for the use of erythropoietic proteins in anaemic patients with cancer: 2006 update. Eur J Cancer 2007;43:258–70
3.   Clark OAC, Lyman GH, Castro AA et al. Colony-stimulating factors for chemotherapy-induced febrile neutropenia: a meta-analysis of randomised controlled trials. J Clin Oncol 2005;23: 4198–214
4.   Crawford J et al. Myeloid growth factors in cancer treatment. NCCN, Clinical Practice Guidelines in Oncology - v.2.2005
5.   ESMO Guidelines Working Group. Hematopoietic growth factors: ESMO recommendations for the application. Ann Oncol 2007;18(suppl 2):ii89–91
6.   ESMO Guidelines Working Group. Erythropoietins in cancer patients: ESMO recommendations for use. Ann Oncol 2007;18(suppl 2):ii86–8
7.   Rizzo JD, Somerfield MR, Hagerty KL et al. Use of epoetin and darbepoetin in patients with cancer: 2007 ASCO/ASH Clinical Practice Guideline Update. J Clin Oncol 2008;26:132–49
8.   Smith TJ, Khatcheressian J, Lyman GH et al. 2006 Update of Recommendations for the Use of White Blood Cell Growth Factors: an evidence-based clinical practice guideline. J Clin Oncol 2005;24:3187–205
9.   Spielberger R, Stiff P, Bensinger W et al. Palifermin for oral mucositis after intensive therapy for hematologic cancer. N Engl J Med 2004;351:2590–8

**Web:**
1.   http://www.asco.org                      ASCO, Am Soc Clin Oncol
2.   http://www.mascc.org                     Supportive Care in Cancer
3.   http://www.hematology.org                ASH, Am Soc Clin Oncol
4.   http://www.esmo.org                      ESMO, Eur Soc Med Oncol
5.   http://www.guideline.gov                 National Guideline Clearinghouse
6.   http://wwwahrq.gov/clinic/epcix.htm      Agency for Healthcare Research and Quality

### Erythropoietin (EPO), Darbepoetin α

**Chem:**  *Erythropoietin α/β:* hematopoietic growth factors of red blood cell lineage, 166 amino acids, 34–37 kDa
*Darbepoetin α:* erythropoietic growth factor. Glycoprotein, hypersialated, 38.5 kDa, carbohydrated fraction 52%

**Pg:**
- *Gene locus of erythropoietin:* chromosome 7q21-q22
- *Synthesis:* 85–90% by tubular and juxtatubular capillary endothelial renal cells and interstitial renal cells. 10–15% are synthesized extrarenally (liver)

**MOA:**
- Binding to erythropoietin receptor
- Proliferation, differentiation, and inhibition of apoptosis of erythropoietic cells of red blood cell lineage → erythropoiesis ↑

**Pkin:**
- Erythropoietin α/β: terminal t½ 4–13 h. Darbepoetin α: terminal t½ 25–49 h

**Se:**
- *Bone marrow:* thrombocytosis (rare)
- *Cardiovascular:* tachycardia, hypertension, thromboembolic events
- *Gastrointestinal:* nausea, vomiting, diarrhea
- *Blood Chemistry:* potassium ↑, phosphate ↑, iron deficiency, ferritin ↓
- *Skin:* pruritus, erythema
- *Nervous system:* paraesthesia, dysesthesia, dysgeusia
- *Other:* fever, headache, peripheral edema, myalgia, arthralgia

**CAUTION:** In case of overdose or rapid hemoglobin increase cardiovascular complications possible (hypertension, thromboembolic events). Risk of shunt thrombosis in dialysis patients.

Recently, an increase in the rate of thromboembolic events and a decrease in survival has been observed in individual clinical trials with erythtropoetins in patients with anemia of cancer, who did not receive chemotherapy. In this patient population, erythropoetins should only be used in the framework of clinical trials.

**Ci:**
- Hypersensitivity, uncontrolled hypertension, pregnancy
- Vascular disease / ischemia (peripheral, cerebral or coronary)

**Th:**
### Approved Indications
- Anemia (renal anemia, chemotherapy-induced anemia in malignancies or AIDS)
- For autologous blood transfusion or prevention of anemia in elective operative procedures

### Dosing and Application
- Target hemoglobin: 10–12 g/dl, dose ↑ with insufficient response to treatment. 50% dose reduction if Hb increases > 2 g/dl per month.
- *Erythropoietin α/β:* subcutaneous application. Chemotherapy-induced anemia: 10,000 IU 3× per week or 40,000 IU 1× per week s.c. Renal anemia: 20–25 IU/kg body weight s.c. 3× per week for 1 month, then dose adaptation.
- *Darbepoetin α:* s.c. or i.v. application. Chemotherapy-induced anemia: 500 µg once every 3 weeks s.c. / i.v. Alternatively 300 µg every 2 weeks or 150 µg/week. Renal anemia: initially 1.35 µg/kg s.c. / i.v. every 3 weeks, then dose adaptation.
- *CAUTION:* iron deficiency and infections are the most common causes for an insufficient therapeutic effect of epoetins. Assess causes of anemia prior to initiation of therapy, if required supplement iron, vitamin $B_{12}$, folic acid, exclusion of bleeding.

## G-CSF (Granulocyte Colony-stimulating Factor)

**Chem:**    Hematopoietic growth factor. Glycoprotein, 207 amino acids, 20 kDa
Glycosylated (lenograstim), non-glycosylated (filgrastim) and polyethylene glycol-linked (pegfilgrastim) derivatives are used clinically.

**Pg:**
- *Gene locus:* chromosome 17q21-q22
- *Synthesis:* stromal cells of bone marrow, endothelial cells, monocytes

**MOA:**
- Stimulation of proliferation and differentiation of neutrophils and hematopoietic progenitor cells
- Increased release of neutrophils from bone marrow
- Activation of mature granulocytes, chemotaxis, phagocytosis, antibody-dependent cytotoxicity (ADCC) ↑

**Pkin:**
- *Filgrastim, lenograstim:* terminal t½ 3–4 h. Hepatic and renal elimination
- *Pegfilgrastim:* maximum serum concentration after 16–120 h, receptor-mediated clearance by neutrophils, terminal t½ 15– > 80 h. Serum concentration correlates with duration of neutropenia

**Se:**
- *Bone marrow:* transient thrombocytosis, leucocytosis
- *Cardiovascular:* tachycardia (rare) and hypertension
- *Liver:* LDH ↑, alkaline phosphatase ↑, γGT ↑
- *Other:* bone pain, myalgia, in individual cases fever, fatigue, sweats
- *With long-term therapy* (e.g., chronic congenital neutropenia): nausea, vomiting, diarrhea, mild alopecia, fluid retention, fatigue, hepatomegaly, splenomegaly, allergic reactions, cutaneous vasculitis

*CAUTION:* stimulation of proliferation and differentiation of leukemic cells has been demonstrated in rare cases.

**Ci:**
- Hypersensitivity against human protein
- Liver and renal function impairment

**Th:**
### Approved Indications
- Reduction of duration of neutropenia with chemotherapy / high-dose chemotherapy
- Mobilization of peripheral blood stem cells (► Chap. 5.1)
- Long-term therapy of congenital or acquired neutropenia
- In clinical studies: mobilization of granulocytes (► Chap. 5.4)

### Dosing and Application
- *Filgrastim, lenograstim:* daily application after chemotherapy, 5–10 µg/kg body weight/day s.c. Continuation until ANC nadir has resolved (e.g., total leukocyte count > 2,000/µl)
- *Pegfilgrastim:* 6 mg s.c. once (prefilled syringe) 24 h after chemotherapy

## GM-CSF (Granulocyte Macrophage Colony-stimulating Factor)

**hem:** Hematopoietic growth factor. Protein monomer, 127 amino acids, molecular weight 14–35 kDa, depending on glycosylation

**g:**
- *Gene locus:* chromosome 5q22-31
- *Synthesis:* stromal cells of bone marrow, fibroblasts, endothelial cells, T-cells

**MOA:**
- Stimulation of proliferation and differentiation of monocytes / granulocytes
- Stimulation of erythroid and megakaryocytic progenitor cells
- Activation and chemotaxis of mature monocytes and granulocytes
- Amplification of antibody-dependent cytotoxicity (ADCC) of neutrophils
- Stimulation of dendritic cells
- Stimulation of cytokine release (M-CSF, TNFα) by monocytes

**kin:**
- *Kinetics:* terminal t½: 1–2 h after i.v. application, 2–3 h after s.c. application
- *Metabolism:* hepatic and renal elimination

**e:**
- *Bone marrow:* eosinophilia, transient thrombocytopenia
- *Cardiovascular:* arrhythmia, tachycardia, hypertension, hypotension. Rare: cardiac insufficiency, vascular disorders, capillary leak syndrome, fluid retention, edema
- *Gastrointestinal:* nausea, vomiting, anorexia
- *Liver:* transaminases ↑, alkaline phosphatase ↑, γGT ↑, LDH ↑
- *Kidney:* creatinine ↑, urea ↑, uric acid ↑
- *Skin:* erythema, exanthema, pruritus, alopecia
- *Nervous system:* central nervous disorders, seizures, paraesthesia, headache, neuropathy, sleep disorders
- *Other:* bone pain, arthralgia, myalgia, flu-like symptoms with fever, fatigue, sweats, depressive mood, headache (more frequent than with G-CSF)
- *Rare:* allergic reactions, anaphylaxis, splenomegalia

**CAUTION:** stimulation of proliferation and differentiation of leukemic cells has been demonstrated in rare cases. Compared to G-CSF, GM-CSF shows reduced proliferative / hematopoietic potential, and increased immunomodulating / inflammatory properties.

**i:**
- Hypersensitivity to human protein
- Serious cardiovascular disease, liver and renal function impairment

**h:**
### Approved Indications
- Reduction of duration of neutropenia with chemotherapy / high-dose chemotherapy
- Mobilization of peripheral blood stem cells (▶ Chap. 5.1)
- In experimental studies: stimulation of immune system, induction of dendritic cells

### Dosing and Application
5–10 µg/kg body weight/day s.c. after completion of chemotherapy. Continuation until ANC nadir has resolved

**Palifermin, KGF**

**Chem:**     Recombinant epithelial growth factor, keratinocyte growth factor (KGF), fibroblast growth factor 7 (FGF-7). Protein, 140 amino acids, 16.3 kDa

**MOA:**
- Binding to KGF receptor on epithelial cells
- Proliferation, differentiation, and migration of epithelial cells → proliferation of mucosal cell
- Prevention of mucous tissue damage during high-dose chemotherapy or total body irradiation (TBI)

**Pkin:**     *Kinetics:* terminal t½: 4.5 h

**Se:**
- *Skin:* erythema, local swelling, pruritus
- *Oral changes:* dysesthesia, taste disorders
- *Blood chemistry:* amylases ↑, lipases ↑
- *Other:* headache, arthralgia

**Ci:**
- Hypersensitivity
- Pregnancy, lactation

**Th:**     *Indications*
Approved indication: prevention of mucositis in hematopoietic stem cell transplantation

*Dosing and Application*
60 µg/kg body weight/day s.c. for 3 days before induction chemotherapy (± TBI) and after transplantation

## 4.4 Nutrition in Cancer Patients

## 4.4.1 Malnutrition in Cancer Patients

### A. Müller, G. Zürcher

**Def:** Unintentional significant weight loss with signs of disease activity as a consequence of insufficient food intake and inflammatory reactions with metabolic alterations. The weight loss constitutes a loss of skeletal muscle and body fat with preservation of visceral organs and a compensatory increase in extracellular fluid.

**Epo:** In cancer patients, weight loss is a common finding with an incidence of 30–90%, depending on tumor entity, location, stage of disease, tumor size, and treatment. More than 80% of all patients suffer during the course of the disease from anorexia, nausea, and emesis. Autopsies have shown that malnutrition is one of the most common causes of death, accounting for 10–20%.

**phys:**
### Causes of Weight Loss
- Insufficient energy and nutrients intake (due to anorexia, taste changes, pain, nausea; adverse effects of cancer therapy, psychological problems etc.)
- Pathologic alterations in nutrient metabolism (e.g., protein turnover ↑, muscle protein synthesis ↓, lipolysis ↑, fatty acid oxidation ↑, hepatic glucose production ↑, hepatic protein synthesis ↑, acute phase proteins ↑)

In contrast to hunger conditions, tumor patients cannot adapt their energy and nutritional requirements to the food supply. Anorexia and metabolic alterations are induced by cytokines (TNFα, IL-1, IL-6, IL-8, interferon γ, ciliary neurotrophic factor (CNTF)), and tumor-specific factors (proteolysis-inducing factor (PIF), lipid-mobilizing factor (LMF)).

### Consequences of Malnutrition
- Impaired immunological function (lymphocyte count and function ↓, macrophage / B- ,T-, and NK cell function ↓, chemotaxis / migration of neutrophils ↓)
- Chemotherapy-/Radiotherapy-induced toxity ↑
- Mortality ↑
- Quality of life ↓
- Costs ↑, duration of hospital stay ↑

**y:**

| Initial symptoms (at time of tumor diagnosis) | Percent (%) of patients |
| --- | --- |
| Weight loss | 50 |
| Anorexia | 40 |
| Epigastric fullness | 60 |
| Early satiety | 40–60 |
| Impaired taste | 46 |
| Dry mouth (xerostomia) | 41 |
| Nausea | 39 |
| Vomiting | 27 |

When antineoplastic treatment is initiated, 16% of patients show signs of severe malnutrition. Forty-five percent of patients lose more than 10% of their initial weight during their hospital stay.

**Dg:**     *Medical History, Clinical Examination*
There are no internationally accepted standard methods for assessing the nutritional status of on
cological patients.

**Grading of unintentional weight loss, Morrison and Hark (1999)**

| Time frame | Significant weight loss (%) | Severe weight loss (%) |
|---|---|---|
| 1 week | 1–2 | > 2 |
| 1 month | 5 | > 5 |
| 3 months | 7.5 | > 7.5 |
| 6 months | 10 | > 10 |
| 12 months | 20 | > 20 |

*Subjective Global Assessment (SGA) (Detsky, 1987)*

## Case History
1. Weight Changes:     Weight loss in last 6 months: _____ (kg) ( _____ %)
   Changes in last 2 weeks:     □ gain     □ loss     □ unchanged

2. Changes in Food Intake (compared to normal)
   □ unchanged     □ change: duration _____ weeks
   Diet change:     □ suboptimal solids  □ full liquid diet
                    □ hypocaloric fluid  □ NPO (starvation)

3. Gastrointestinal Symptoms (persisting daily for > 2 weeks)
   □ none     □ vomiting     □ loss of appetite     □ nausea     □ diarrhea

4. Functional Impairment
   □ none     □ impairment: duration _____ weeks
   Type:     □ limited fitness to work     □ ambulatory (walking or wheelchair)
             □ bedridden

5. Effect of Disease on Nutritional Requirement
   Main diagnosis:_____
   Metabolic requirements:     □ no stress          □ mild stress
                               □ moderate stress    □ severe stress

## Physical Examination     (0 well; 1+ mild; 2+ moderate; 3+ severe)
_____ Subcutaneous fat loss (triceps, thorax)
_____ Muscle wasting (quadriceps, deltoid)
_____ Ankle edema
_____ Presacral edema (anasarca)
_____ Ascites

## Subjective Assessment of the Nutritional Status
   □ A = Well nourished
   □ B = Mildly / moderately undernourished or suspected malnutrition
   □ C = Severely undernourished (evident physical signs of malnutrition, e.g., loss of sub-
   cutaneous adipose tissue, edema with weight loss > 10%, amyotrophia)

Clinically relevant malnutrition can be assumed in case of:
- Body weight loss > 10%
- Subjective global assessment, group C

Assessment of oral nutrition should at least include a quantitative survey but also a qualitative evaluation of energy and food intake (preferably carried out by a dietician / nutritionist), ideally using dietary history or nutrition protocols.
- Starvation = daily oral energy intake < 500 kcal
- Insufficient energy intake = daily oral energy intake < 60% of required intake

## Objectives of Nutrition Therapy

- Maintenance / improvement of nutritional status
- Maintenance / improvement of subjective quality of life
- Increase in treatment efficacy and reduction of side effects
- Improvement of prognosis, prevention of treatment breaks or delays

## Indications for Oral / Enteral Nutrition Therapy

There is no correlation between the degree of malnutrition and tumor size, tumor differentiation, or duration of disease. Hence, it is impossible to predict when cancer cachexia is going to occur in the individual case. Nutritional intervention to optimize oral / enteral nutrition is indicated from the first signs of malnutrition and moderate weight loss, e.g., in the following situations:
- Weight Loss > 5%
- Food intake < 500 kcal/day, expected duration > 5 days
- Food intake < 60% of the calculated nutritional needs, expected duration > 10 days

## Oral Nutrition Therapy in Cancer Patients

### Individual Planning of Nutrition Therapy
- Assessment of nutritional needs based on the current weight or normal / ideal weight according to body mass index (BMI) (▶ Chap. 4.4.2)
- Oral / enteral nutrition is to be preferred over parenteral nutrition → oral nutrition should be optimized first
- Special nutritional guidelines exist in the case of hepatic / renal dysfunction, after gastrointestinal surgery, and with specific metabolic defects
- If energy and nutrient intake is insufficient complement with formula diets / nutritional supplements
- After long periods without food: gradual increase of food intake
- After allogeneic bone marrow or peripheral blood stem cell transplantation: no fresh fruit / vegetables / raw foods / raw milk products / mold cheese

### Oral Nutrition in Cancer Patients

- Wholefood / light wholefood in form of a varied mixed diet or special preparation (e.g., strained, liquid)
- "Controlled" favored diet, i.e., allowing for aversions and preferences
- If necessary, special diet, e.g., lactose-free or MCT diet
- Complementary food (formula diets, supplements)

### Fluid Intake
Requirements: 20–40 ml/kg/d (equivalent to 1.5 l/m² body surface area)
- Fluid intake through solid foods                                800 ml/day

- Loss of fluids through skin and lungs      1,000 ml/day
- Loss of fluids through feces      150 ml/day
- Fluid gain with nutrient oxidation      300 ml/day
- Recommended oral fluid intake (normal requirements)      1,500–2,000 ml/day
- Increased requirements with fever, vomiting, diarrhea, heat, high protein intake, high salt intake, high energy metabolism

### Energy Intake

Required energy intake = weight × energy factor

In patients with normal or subnormal weight, energy requirements are calculated using the actual weight. In overweight patients, calculation is based on the normal / ideal body weight (▶ Chap. 4.4.2).

Energy factors: basic metabolic rate: 25 kcal/kg/d, bed rest 26–(29) kcal/kg/d, light activity 30 kcal/kg/d, moderate activity 35 kcal/kg/d, heavy activity 40 kcal/kg/d

- Oncological patients have reduced, normal or increased energy requirements (⅓ of patients are hypometabolic, ¼ of patients are hypermetabolic)
- Recommended energy intake for active patients: 30–35 kcal/kg/d, steady weight usually at 30 kcal/kg/d

### Intake of Nutrients

Based on the recommendations of the German Nutrition Society (Deutsche Gesellschaft für Ernährung, DGE) for healthy individuals:

- Protein: in tumor patients, increase recommended intake to 1.2–1.5 g/kg/d
- Fat: 1.0 g/kg; in tumor patients, high fat intake desirable (> 35% fat in total energy intake)
- Carbohydrates: approximately 50% of total energy intake
- Higher or lower requirements must be determined individually, e.g., with hepatic or renal insufficiency

### Oral Intake of Vitamins / Minerals / Trace Elements

**DACH recommendations (German and Austrian Nutrition Society, Swiss Society for Nutrition Research, Swiss Nutrition Foundation), 2000, for healthy adolescents and adults from 15 years of age**

| Nutrient | Recommended intake/day |
|---|---|
| *Fat-soluble vitamins* | |
| A (retinol) | 0.8–1.1 mg retinol equivalent (= 3,300 IU) |
| D (calciferol) | < 65 years 5 µg (= 200 IU), > 65 years 10 µg (= 400 IU) |
| E (tocopherol) | ♂ 15–12 mg, ♀ 11–12 mg |
| K (phylloquinone) | ♂ 70–80 µg, ♀ 60–65 µg |
| *Water-soluble vitamins* | |
| B₁ (thiamin) | ♂ 1.0–1.3 mg, ♀ 1.0 mg |
| B₂ (riboflavin) | ♂ 1.2–1.5 mg, ♀ 1.2 mg |
| Niacinamide | ♂ 13–17 mg, ♀ 13 mg |
| B₅ (pantothenate) | 6 mg |
| B₆ (pyridoxine) | ♂ 1.4–1.6 mg, ♀ 1.2 mg |
| B₁₂ (cyanocobalamin) | 3.0 µg |
| Folic acid | 400 µg folic acid equivalent |
| C (ascorbic acid) | 100 mg |
| Biotin | 30–60 µg |

**DACH recommendations (German and Austrian Nutrition Society, Swiss Society for Nutrition Research, Swiss Nutrition Foundation), 2000, for healthy adolescents and adults from 15 years of age** *(continued)*

| Nutrient | Recommended intake/day |
|---|---|
| *Minerals* | |
| Sodium | 2 g (80 mmol)[a] |
| Potassium | 2 g (50 mmol)[a] |
| Calcium | < 19 years 1,200 mg (30 mmol), from 19 years 1,000 mg (22.75 mmol) |
| Phosphorus | < 19 years 1,250 mg (41 mmol), from 19 years 700 mg |
| Magnesium | ♂ 350–400 mg (14–16 mmol), ♀ 300–350 mg (12–14 mmol) |
| *Trace elements* | |
| Iron | ♂ 10–12 mg, ♀ 10–15 mg |
| Zinc | ♂ 10 mg, ♀ 7 mg |
| Fluoride | ♂ 3.2–3.8 mg, ♀ 2.9–3.1 mg |
| Iodine | ♂ 180–200 µg, ♀ 150 µg |
| Copper | 1.0–1 mg[b] |
| Manganese | 2.0–5.0 mg[b] |
| Selenium | 30–70 µg[b] |
| Chromium | 30–100 µg[b] |
| Molybdenum | 50–100 µg[b] |

[a] Estimated minimal intake
[b] Estimated appropriate intake

## Special Nutritional Requirements in Cancer Patients

### Lack of Appetite (Anorexia), Impaired Taste (Dysgeusia), Loss of Taste (Hypogeusia, Ageusia)
- Small portions, food intake every 2–3 h (also at night if patient is hungry)
- Test taste acceptability and allow for individual taste
- Use spices sparingly, allow individual seasoning
- Avoid strong food odors (well-ventilated rooms)
- Aperitifs, wine or beer 1 h before eating stimulate the appetite

### Nausea / Vomiting
- Frequent small portions of light food
- Avoid hasty eating or drinking
- No sweet / fatty / bloating / strong-odor foods
- No starchy soups or sauces
- Do not offer favorite foods (avoid "acquired aversion")
- Dry foods (crackers, toast) have an antiemetic effect
- Cold drinks

### Dysphagia / Mucositis / Xerostomia
- Viscous or pureed foods, possibly industrially prepared baby food (low in acid and sodium, strained)
- Avoid spicy and salty, acidic foods (fruit with high acid content, fruit juices, tomatoes), fizzy drinks
- Avoid fresh milk (stimulates mucus production); use sour milk, sour milk products, kefir, and soybean drinks

- Stimulate salivation by frequent drinking (still water, tea), chewing gum, sugar-free lemo
  sweets
- For caries prophylaxis, observe good dental hygiene when using acidic foods

### Flatulence / Fullness / Diarrhea
- In case of severe diarrhea, light foods with low lactose / fat and fiber content
- Fennel tea, black tea, oatmeal and rice, white flour products, grated apple, bananas are recom
  mended
- Avoid juice, coffee, fizzy drinks, raw vegetables, fresh fruit, wholemeal products, nuts, fres
  milk and sour milk products, fatty and fried foods, hot spices

## Parenteral Nutrition

Parenteral nutrition becomes necessary when optimal oral nutrition fails to provide suf
ficient amounts of energy and nutrients. Enteral nutrition is preferable to parenteral nutritio
(▶ Chap. 4.4.2) as enteral nutrition is:
- Easier to implement, more cost effective
- Maintains intestinal function, stimulates intestinal hormones, improves activity of the gastro
  intestinal mucosa, preventing intestinal villus atrophy and bacterial translocation
- Has a lower infection and complication rate

When not absolutely contraindicated, a "minimal enteral nutrition" should be maintained (for
mula diet, possible via gastric / jejunal tube).

## Enteral Nutrition

### Absolute Contraindications
- Intestinal ischemia
- Intestinal perforation
- Acute abdomen / mechanical ileus / gastrointestinal hemorrhage

### Relative Contraindications
- Paralytic ileus (minimal enteral nutrition possible)
- High reflux rate (minimal enteral nutrition possible)
- Severe diarrhea, high output enterocutaneous fistulas

### Method
- Via feeding tube: nasal or percutaneous access. In case of frequent tube dislocation or duratio
  of enteral nutrition > 2–3 weeks, a gastrostoma (PEG) or jejunostoma (PEJ) should be consid
  ered. Use feeding tubes made of polyurethane (soft, use for up to 90 days) or silicon rubbe
  (for long-term use).
- Enteral diets: industrially produced formula diets. The different types of formulas vary in en
  ergy concentration (1.0–2.0 kcal/ml), type of protein, fats, carbohydrates, fiber, osmolarity
  viscosity, immune-modulating substrates ("nutraceutics").
- For oral use, formulas are usually supplied in various flavors. For enteral feeding, use neutra
  formulas as taste enhancers lead to increased osmolarity.
- Substrate supply: for calculation of nutritional requirements see oral nutrition.
- When assessing fluid intake, consider fluid content of enteral formulas (approximately 75%).
- Use still mineral water, boiled water, and chamomile or fennel tea.
- Continuous food supply or bolus; continuous application is mandatory with duodenal an
  jejunal tubes. The duration of enteral feeding depends on the energy requirements.

**Ref:**

1. Arends J, Bodoky G, Bozzetti F et. al. ESPEN guidelines on enteral nutrition: non-surgical oncology. Clin Nutr 2006;25:245–59
2. Davis MP, Dreicer R, Walsh D et al. Appetite and cancer associated anorexia. J Clin Oncol 2004;22:1510–7
3. Detsky A, Mc Laughlin J. Baker J et al. What is Subjective Global Assessment of Nutritional Status? JPEN 1987;11:8–13
4. Doyle C, Kushi LH, Byers T et al. Nutrition and physical activity during and after cancer treatment. CA Cancer J Clin 2006;56:323–53
5. Morrison G, Hark L. Medical Nutrition and Disease. Blackwell Science, 1999
6. Nitenberg G, Raynard B. Nutritional support of the cancer patient: issues and dilemmas. Crit Rev Hematol Oncol 2000;34:137–68
7. Skipworth R, Fearon KCK. The scientific rationale for otimizing nutritional support in cancer. Eur J Gastroenterol Hepatol 2007;19:371–7

**Web:**

1. http://www.mascc.org                                    Multinational Association of Supportive Care in Cancer
2. http://www.nutritioncare.org                          Am Soc Parental and Enteral Nutrition
3. http://www.nutrition.org                                American Society for Clinical Nutrition
4. http://www.cancer.org/docroot/MBC/MBC_6.asp  Am Cancer Society, Nutrition
5. http://www.espen.org                                    Eur Soc Clin Nutrition Metabolism

## 4.4.2　　Parenteral Nutrition

**A. Müller, G. Zürcher**

**Def:**　Balanced intravenous administration of nutrients, bypassing the gastrointestinal tract

**Ind:**　*Indications for Parenteral Nutrition in Hematology / Oncology*
Individual need depending on:

- Nutritional status
- Comorbidities (concomitant diseases)
- Type of antineoplastic treatment
- Patient's performance status

Parenteral nutrition is indicated when:

- Oral / enteral nutrition < 500 Kcal/d expected for at least 5 days
- Oral / enteral nutrition < 60% of the calculated nutritional needs expected for at least 10 days

**Phys:**　*Substrate Supply*
The *substrate supply* has to be determined individually for each patient. Energy and nutrient requirements depend on the individual nutritional status, type of disease, treatment, clinical status and, in particular, substrate utilization. Since under the current clinical conditions substrate utilization cannot be measured, determination of adequate supply is based on the patient's individual degree of substrate elimination. Substrate elimination (carbohydrates, fat, amino acids) can easily be clinically monitored in the form of plasma levels of blood glucose, triglycerides, urea, or blood urea nitrogen (= BUN = urea × 0.46).

The *actual weight (AW)* and in obese patients (body mass index, BMI > 30 kg/m²) the normal / ideal weight are suitable reference parameters for a preliminary substrate dosage guideline. In extremely cachectic patients (BMI < 16 kg/m²) and patients having undergone longer fasting, nutrition has to be built up very slowly (initial intake based on 50% of AW, frequent laboratory monitoring).

**Calculation of body weight parameters**

| Parameter | Calculation |
|---|---|
| Body mass index (BMI) (kg/m²) | Body weight (kg) / body height (m)² |
| BMI normal / ideal weight (kg) | ♂: (Body height (m))² × 23[a] |
| | ♀: (Body height (m))² × 21,5[a] |

[a] Adolescents and adults from 19 years of age

**Calculation of required parenteral nutrition (per kg of normal weight (NW) / ideal weight and day)**

- **Fluids:**　　20–40 ml (1.5 l/m² body surface area, equivalent to fluid loss through urine and perspiration)
- **Energy:**　　25–35 kcal
- **Protein:**　　1.0–1.5, 2.0 g max. (0.1 g/kg/h amino acids max.)
- **Fat:**　　0.5–1.5, 1.8 g max. (0.15 g/kg/h max.)
　　> 35% of total calorie intake
- **Carbohydrates:**　　Maximum 5 g glucose (0.3 g/kg/h)
　　Maximum 3 g xylitol (0.125 g/kg/h)

**Calculation of required parenteral nutrition (per kg of normal weight (NW) / ideal weight and day *(continued)***

- Vitamin K: 100–150 µg daily
- Trace elements: (▶ Chap. 4.4.1)

**Estimated daily energy / protein requirements based on height and normal weight (NW) in men**

| Patient | | Energy requirement (kcal) at: | | | Protein requirement (g) at: | |
|---|---|---|---|---|---|---|
| Height (cm) | NW (kg) | 25 kcal | 30 kcal | 35 kcal | 1.2 g | 1.5 g |
| 160 | 61 | 1525 | 1830 | 2135 | 73 | 91 |
| 165 | 65 | 1625 | 1950 | 2275 | 78 | 97 |
| 170 | 69 | 1725 | 2070 | 2415 | 83 | 103 |
| 175 | 73 | 1825 | 2190 | 2555 | 88 | 109 |
| 180 | 78 | 1950 | 2340 | 2730 | 94 | 117 |
| 185 | 82 | 2050 | 2460 | 2870 | 98 | 123 |
| 190 | 87 | 2175 | 2610 | 3045 | 104 | 130 |
| 195 | 91 | 2275 | 2730 | 3185 | 109 | 136 |

**Estimated daily energy / protein requirements based on height and NW in women**

| Patient | | Energy requirement (kcal) at: | | | Protein requirement (g) at: | |
|---|---|---|---|---|---|---|
| Height (cm) | NW (kg) | 25 kcal | 30 kcal | 35 kcal | 1.2 g | 1.5 g |
| 150 | 49 | 1225 | 1470 | 1715 | 59 | 73 |
| 155 | 53 | 1325 | 1590 | 1855 | 64 | 79 |
| 160 | 56 | 1400 | 1680 | 1960 | 67 | 84 |
| 165 | 60 | 1500 | 1800 | 2100 | 72 | 90 |
| 170 | 64 | 1600 | 1920 | 2240 | 77 | 96 |
| 175 | 67 | 1675 | 2010 | 2345 | 80 | 100 |
| 180 | 71 | 1775 | 2130 | 2485 | 85 | 106 |
| 185 | 75 | 1875 | 2250 | 2625 | 90 | 1112 |

**Meth:**

## Ways of Administering Parenteral Nutrition

### *Peripheral Venous*
Hypocaloric, protein-sparing nutrition to guarantee protein supply. Required osmolarity of infusion solution: < 800 mOsm/l. Use of complete solutions.
Indications:
- First step toward total parenteral nutrition
- Limited period of fasting (maximum 1 week; fasting is defined as < 500 kcal oral calorie intake)
- Mild to moderate catabolism (daily nitrogen loss 10–15 g)
- Supplementation of oral / enteral nutrition

### Central Venous

Total parenteral normocaloric nutrition (TPN, total parenteral nutrition) continuously administered via a central venous line. Use of complete solutions or individually balanced nutrition with
single components (obligatory with diminished organ function).

Indications:

- Poor general health and nutrition status
- Moderate to severe catabolism
- Infusion and nutrition therapy with diminished organ function

**Dg:**

## Laboratory Monitoring of Parenteral Nutrition

### Protein Supply

- Monitoring via measurement of urea / blood urea nitrogen (BUN). Target: daily BUN increase
  < 30 mg/dl.
- Elevated BUN levels: reduction of amino acid supply
- With hepatic insufficiency: determination of ammonia levels

### Carbohydrates

- Monitoring via blood glucose determination
- Desired level: 145 mg/dl, (8.04 mmol/l)
- *ATTENTION:* a higher insulin dose does not increase glucose oxidation. Therefore, with raised
  blood glucose, reduce glucose supply

### Fat

- Monitoring via serum triglyceride determination
- Threshold value: during infusion: < 350–400 mg/dl (4.2–4.8 mmol/l)

**Ref:**

1.  ASPEN: Board of directors. Specific guidelines for disease adults: Cancer JPEN 2002;26:82SA–83SA
2.  ASPEN: Board of directors. Specific guidelines for disease adults: Cancer - hematopoietic cell transplanta-
    tion. JPEN 2002;26:83SA–85SA
3.  Bozetti F, Cavazzi C, Mariani L et al. Artificial nutrition in cancer patients: which route, what composition
    World J Surg 1999;23:577–83
4.  Wilson RL. Optimizing nutrition for patients with cancer. Clin J Oncol Nurs 2000;4:23–8

**Web:**

1.  http://www.mascc.org/                Multinational Association of Supportive Care in Cancer
2.  http://cancernet.nci.nih.gov/        CancerNet, with Information on Parenteral Nutrition
3.  http://www.nutritioncare.org/        Am Soc Parenteral Enteral Nutrition
4.  http://www.nutrition.org/            American Society for Clinical Nutrition

## 4.5 Pain Control

**U. Brunnmüller, K. Potthoff, J. Heinz**

**Def:** Pain is a demanding and limiting complication of malignancy, which is subjective in nature and requires an individual approach to diagnosis and treatment.

**Ep:** Depending on type, stage, and location of the malignancy, 50–80% of cancer patients experience chronic pain.

**Pain in tumor patients**

**Pg:**

| Cause of pain | Frequency (%)[a] |
|---|---|
| Tumor related / associated | > 80 |
| Treatment related | 15–20 |
| Non-tumor / non-treatment related | 10 |

[a] More than one option possible

**Dg:** *Medical History, Clinical Examination*
The following parameters should be recorded for each episode of pain:
- Location — to be indicated by patient; segmental, spreading, etc.
- Quality — e.g., burning, sharp, dull, colicky
- Intensity — e.g., use of visual analog scales (VAS) 0–10
- Course — duration, frequency, rhythm
- Affected systems — e.g., bones, soft tissue
- Etiology — e.g., depending on movement, stress, temperature, etc.

**Class:** *Types of Pain*
- Acuity — acute, chronic
- Etiology — tumor related, treatment related, independent
- Pathogenesis — nociceptive pain: bone, periosteum, soft tissue, inflammation, ischemia, neuropathic pain: burning pain
- Time course — short duration, continuous

**Th:** **Basic Principles of Pain Management**

Consistent pain control should be provided at an early stage:
- Adequate and full assessment of the cause of pain
- Initial dose and dose tritration based on patient symptoms, preferably oral medication
- Adequate dose and analgesic used (patients should be pain-free)
- Medication according to the principle of anticipation, i.e., medicate before pain occurs
- Regular medication at specific intervals
- Prophylaxis and therapy of side effects (e.g., nausea)
- Regular re-evaluation of extent and character of pain, assessment of treatment efficacy (e.g., via pain diary kept by the patient)

Not using analgesics until pain occurs is a sign of insufficient pain treatment. Tumor-specific measures (considering benefit versus risk) and psychological support (psychosocial component of pain) are recommended.

**WHO analgesic ladder**

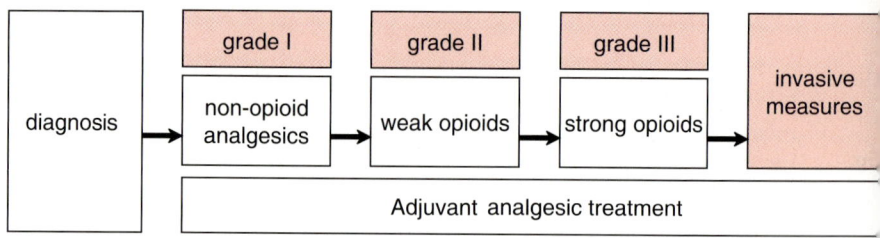

### WHO Step I: Non-opioid Analgesics

**Chem:** Non-acidic antipyretic anti-inflammatory drugs: paracetamol, metamizole
Non-steroidal anti-inflammatory drugs: diclofenac, ibuprofen
Analgesics without antipyretic / anti-inflammatory action: flupirtin

**MOA:** Inhibition of prostaglandin synthesis, spinal and peripheral analgesia, anti-inflammatory and spasmolytic effects (metamizole)

**Pkin:** Hepatic and renal elimination

**Se:** Ulcerogenic, inhibition of thrombocyte aggregation, temperature decrease (*ATTENTION*: masking of fever), hepatotoxicity (paracetamol), renal toxicity (especially diclofenac, ibuprofen)

*ATTN:* simultaneous corticosteroid therapy requires gastric mucosa protection.

| Compound | Single dose (mg p.o.) | Duration of action (h) | Maximum daily dose |
|---|---|---|---|
| Diclofenac | 50–100 | 8 | 200 mg |
| Flupirtin | 100–200 | 8 | 600 mg |
| Ibuprofen | 400–800 | 8–12 | 2,400 mg |
| Metamizole | 500–1,000 | 4–6 | 4–6 g |
| Paracetamol | 500–1,000 | 4–6 | 4–6 g |

### WHO Step II: Weak Opioids

**Chem:** Morphine derivatives

**MOA:** Morphine receptor μ-agonists; efficacy: morphine = 1, dihydrocodeine = 0.3, tilidine / naloxone = 0.2, tramadol = 0.1

**Pkin:** Hepatic metabolization

**Se:** Dose dependent: constipation (except tilidine / naloxone), nausea / vomiting, urticaria, miosis, hypotension, bradycardia, urinary retention, sedation, tremor, hallucination, respiratory depression

| Compound | Single dose (mg p.o.) | Duration of action (h) | Maximum daily dose (mg) |
|---|---|---|---|
| Dihydrocodeine | 60–180 | 8 | 540 |
| Tilidine / naloxone | 50–300 | 8–12 | 600 |
| Tramadol | 50–100 | 8 | 400 |

## WHO Step III: Strong Opioids

**Chem:**   Morphine and morphine derivatives

**MOA:**   Morphine receptor μ-agonists; efficacy: morphine = 1, fentanyl = 100, oxycodone = 2, hydromorphone = 7.5

**Pkin:**   Hepatic metabolization

**Se:**   Dose dependent: constipation, nausea / vomiting, urticaria, miosis, hypotension, bradycardia, urinary retention, sedation, tremor, hallucination, respiratory depression
Antidote: in the event of overdosage / respiratory depression: 0.4 mg naloxone i.v. titrated to response, repeat every 3–5 min, repeat at longer intervals once respiration is stabilized

| Compound | Single dose | Duration of action | Maximum daily dose |
|---|---|---|---|
| *Oral administration* | | | |
| Morphine sulfate | ≥ 10 mg p.o. | 8–12 h | None[a] |
| Oxycodone | ≥ 10 mg p.o. | 12 h | None[a] |
| Hydromorphone | ≥ 4 mg p.o. | 12 h | None[a] |
| Buprenorphine | 0.216–0.432 mg s.l. | 8–12 h | None[a] |
| *Continuous intravenous administration* | | | |
| Morphine sulfate | 2 mg/h | Syringe driver | None[a] |
| Pethidine | 25 mg/h | Syringe driver | None[a] |
| Piritramide | 15–150 mg/day (0.01–0.03 mg/kg/h) | Syringe driver | None[a] |
| *Transdermal application* | | | |
| Fentanyl-TTS | 25–100 μg/h | Skin patch | None[a] |
| Buprenorphine | 35–70 μg/h | Skin patch | None[a] |

[a] Until freedom from cancer pain is achieved, *p.o.* (per os), *s.l.* (sublingual)

**Th:**   ***Principles of Opioid Therapy***
- Overdosage is rare. The most common mistake in opioid therapy is underdosing.
- Due to the nature of opioid side effects, treatment should always be combined with laxatives (e.g., lactulose, macrogol). Antiemetics may be necessary initially (e.g., metoclopramide).
- It is advisable to conduct opioid treatment with a pure opioid agonist (all WHO step III opioids are pure agonists, except buprenorphine). As the combination of an opioid agonist with buprenorphine has a partial antagonistic effect, this combination is not recommended.
- Once pain intensity decreases with effective antineoplastic therapy, signs of overdosing may appear (sedation, respiratory depression). In that case, the opioid dose must be reduced.

- For acute pain attacks under continuous or slow-release opioid therapy: additive administration of an immediate-release opioid (e.g., oral immediate-release morphine sulfate), 10 mg or 1/6 of daily oral dose is recommended.
- With severe side effects or insufficient analgesic treatment: change opioid.

### Initiation of Intravenous Opioid Therapy

- In case of severe cancer pain, rapid initiation of therapy via intravenous titration: 2 mg morphine every 5 min until pain resolves. For calculation of required daily dose, multiply dose necessary for pain reduction by a factor of 6.
- Continued treatment with syringe driver: convert to hourly dosing.
- Continued oral treatment: multiply daily i.v. dose by 3, administer as two doses of modified-release morphine sulfate per os.

### Initiation of Oral Opioid Therapy

- In case of moderate pain, initial dose of 10 mg of retarded morphine; with severe pain initial dose of 30 mg retarded morphine.
- Repeat every 12 h with successive dose adaptation: increase previous dose by 30–50% until sufficient pain reduction is achieved.
- If pain occurs before completion of 12-h interval: add immediate-release oral morphine sulfate
- Slow-release tilidine / naloxone at a maximum daily dose of 600 mg equals 120 mg of modified-release morphine. Advantage: less constipation.

### Transdermal Fentanyl

Indications: dysphagia, malabsorption, steady level of pain
Advantages: continuous pain reduction, only mild constipation
Disadvantage: long dose adjustment period; limited options for dose titration, possible need for additional medication

Side effects (dose dependent): nausea, vomiting, miosis, respiratory depression, sedation

**Analgesic adjuvants (adjusted to type of pain)**

| Compound | Dose | Indication |
| --- | --- | --- |
| Amitriptyline[a] | 25–75 mg/day, p.o. | Neuropathic pain |
| Butylscopolamine | 20 mg/day p.o. | Colic pain, acute |
| Carbamazepine[a] | 600–1,200 mg/day, p.o | Neuropathic pain |
| Dexamethasone | 3–6 × 4–8 mg/day, p.o, for 2–3 weeks | Neurocompression, cerebral pressure, capsular pain, bone metastases |
| Gabapentin[a] | 900–3,600 mg/day, p.o. | Neuropathic pain |
| Pregabalin | 150–600 mg/day p.o. | Neuropathic pain |
| Pamidronate | 30–90 mg i.v, every 28 days | Bone metastasis |
| Zoledronate | 30–60 mg i.v., every 28 days | Bone metastasis |

[a] Gradually increase doses of amitriptyline, gabapentin, carbamazepine because of initial side effects

**Prophylaxis of constipation during opioid therapy**

| Compound | Dose | Intensity |
| --- | --- | --- |
| Sodium picosulfate | 10–20 gtt, 1–2× per day | Grade I |
| Lactulose | 15–30 ml, 3× per day | Grade I |
| Macrogol | 1 pack, 1–2× per day | Grade I |

**Prophylaxis of constipation during opioid therapy** *(continued)*

| Compound | Dose | Intensity |
|----------|------|-----------|
| Paraffin | 0.5–1 tablespoon, 2× per day | Grade II |
| Sennoside | 1 tablespoon, 2× per day | Grade II |
| Sorbitol | Enema | Grade III |

**Antiemesis during opioid therapy**

| Compound | Dose | Intensity |
|----------|------|-----------|
| Metoclopramide | 3 × 10 mg | Grade I |
| Haloperidol | 3 × 0.5 mg | Grade I |
| Dimenhydrinate | 3 × 100–200 mg | Grade II |
| Scopolamine | 1 mg / 72 h | Grade II |
| Granisetron | 1–2 mg p.o., 2 mg i.v. | Grade III |
| Tropisetron | 5 mg p.o / i.v. | Grade III |
| Ondansetron | 4–8 mg p.o. / i.v. | Grade III |
| Dexamethasone | 4–8 mg p.o. / i.v. | Grade III |
| Midazolam | 5 mg p.o. | Grade IV |

### Anesthesiological Methods

- Sympathetic nerve block, cryoneurolysis, celiac plexus neurolysis, indications: neuropathic pain and visceral pain, ischemia-related pain
- Continuous epidural analgesia, continuous plexus analgesia, neurolysis of somatic nerves and sacral roots, indication: insufficient pain control despite all conservative measures

## Specific Types of Pain

### Soft Tissue / Bone Pain (Nociceptive Pain)

**Pphys:**
- Pressure stimulation of nociceptors → nociceptive pain
- Inflammation, prostaglandin E, bradykinin, substance P, potassium, pH

**Sy:**
- Easily traceable pain, stabbing, nagging
- Often associated with localized inflammation, pressure pain, erythema, swelling
- Exacerbation through exercise / motion, relieve through decompression / rest

**Dg:**
- Laboratory studies: analysis of inflammatory markers, alkaline phosphatase, calcium
- Histology of tissue from inflammation site
- Imaging: plain x-ray, sonography, CT / NMR, skeletal scintigraphy

**Th:**
- Systemic treatment according to WHO analgesic ladder, non-steroidal anti-inflammatory drugs are highly effective. Adjuvant treatment: dexamethasone, bisphosphonates
- Adjuvant physical therapy, use of muscle relaxants
- Local treatment: radiotherapy

### Visceral Pain (Nociceptive Pain)

**Pphys:**
- Stimulation of mechano- and chemosensitive nociceptors
- Common afferent with sympathetic nerves
- Spinal convergence with somatic afferents

**Sy:**
- Dull, hard-to-localize pain, improving on exercise
- Hollow organ involvement: cramp-like or colicky pain
- Concomitant vegetative symptoms
- Hyperalgesia of skin according to Head's zones

**Dg:**
- Pressure pain, dysfunctional peristalsis, bowel obstruction
- Laboratory studies: routine analysis of inflammatory parameters
- Imaging: detectable tumor invasion (abdominal sonography, CT / NMR)

**Th:**
- Systemic treatment according to WHO analgesic ladder
- Adjuvant treatment: amitriptyline; for colicky pain: metamizole (spasmolytic effect) or adjuvant treatment with 10 mg butylscopolamine 10 mg every 6–8 h
- Invasive measures (e.g., celiac plexus neurolysis in pancreatic carcinoma)

### Neuropathic Pain

**Pphys:**
- Spinal reduction of pain threshold, pain coding in spinal dorsal horn wide dynamic range (WDR) neurons

**Sy:**
- Spontaneous pain, burning, shooting, stabbing, with hyperalgesia and allodynia
- Independent of movement
- Neurological deficits possible

**Dg:**
- Laboratory studies: usually without pathological findings, normal inflammation markers
- Neurophysiology: usually without pathological findings
- Imaging: invasion of nerves / plexus by tumor (detectable via CT / NMR)

**Th:**
- Systemic treatment according to WHO analgesic ladder; adjuvant treatment: gabapentin, carbamazepine, amitriptyline, and dexamethasone
- Invasive methods (ganglionic local opioid analgesia, GLOA) should be considered at an early stage
- Local treatment: radiotherapy

**Ref:**
1.  Goldberg GR, Morrison RS. Pain management in hospitalized cancer patients. J Clin Oncol 2007;25: 1792–801
2.  Jost LM. Management of cancer pain. ESMO Clinical Recommendations. Ann Oncol 2007;18(suppl 2): ii92–4
3.  Levy MH, Samuel TA. Management of cancer pain. Semin Oncol 2005;32:179–93
4.  McNicol E, Strassels S, Goudas L et al. Nonsteroidal anti-inflammatory drugs, alone or in combination with opioids, for cancer pain: a systematic review. J Clin Oncol 2004;22:1975–92
5.  McQuay H. Opioids in pain management. Lancet 1999;353:2229–32
6.  Mercadante S. The use of anti-inflammatory drugs in cancer pain. Cancer Treat Rev 2001;27:51–61
7.  Van den Beuken-Van Everdingen MHJ, De Rijke JM, Kessels AG et al. Prevalence of pain in patients with cancer. Ann Oncol 2007;18:1437–49

**Web:**
1.  http:// www.dgss.org                                    DGSS, German Assoc. for the Study of Pain
2.  http://www.painresearch.utah.edu/cancerpain             Cancer Pain Resource
3.  http://www.ampainsoc.org                                APS, American Pain Society
4.  http://www.painmed.org/                                 AAPM, American Academy of Pain Medicine
5.  http://www.cancer-pain.org/                             Cancer Pain Organisation
6.  http://www.who.org                                      WHO Pain Ladder
7.  http://www.nccn.org                                     Cancer Pain Guidelines

## 4.6 Fatigue

**E. Reinert, H. Henß**

**Def:** Tumor-related form of weakness and tiredness (exhaustion), inadequate in its extent and characteristics. Fatigue interferes with normal daily activities and severely diminishes quality of life.

**ICD-10:** G 93.3: chronic fatigue

**Ep:** Of all cancer patients, 30–60% suffer from chronic fatigue. An incidence up to 60–90% can be found during therapy cycles (chemotherapy, radiotherapy) or with progressive disease.

**Pg:** The exact pathomechanisms are largely unknown. In cancer patients, fatique has been attributed to a variety of factors.

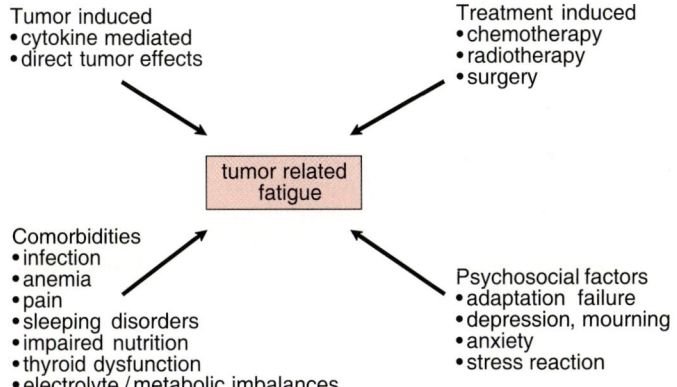

**Sy:** Most patients perceive fatigue equally as burdensome as treatment-associated nausea, vomiting, or pain (different perception of physicians and patients).
- Physical: physical exhaustibility, weakness, asthenia, increased need for sleep (but sleep is not restorative), sleep disturbances
- Affective: reduced motivation, lack of energy, depressive mood, sadness, anxiety
- Cognitive: decreased vigilance and attention, memory problems

**Dg:** *Medical History, Clinical Examination*
- Complete medical history including all symptoms, e.g., by fully standardized self-assessment questionnaire: Fatigue Assessment Questionnaire (FAQ) by Glaus or Functional Assessment of Cancer Therapy – Fatigue Subscale (FACT-F)
- Ask for premorbid psychological disorders, e.g., depression

*Laboratory Tests*
- Exclude anemia (Hb, Hct, bleeding, ferritin / transferrin status)
- Thyroid parameters
- Electrolytes, renal function
- Parameters of inflammation

**Dd:**
- Anemia
- Hypothyroidism (e.g., induced by radiotherapy)
- Chronic infections

- Depression: differentiation from depression is often difficult. Mild to moderate depression is accompanied by fatigue symptoms. Differential criteria include additional symptoms of depression (mood swings, fluctuation during the day, feelings of guilt, pessimistic views of the future, ideas or acts of self-harm or suicide), which are quantitatively less developed in fatigue

**Th:**

### Supportive Therapy
- Maximum antiemesis (▶ Chap. 4.1)
- Effective pain treatment (▶ Chap. 4.5)
- Anemia treatment (▶ Chap. 4.3), possibly transfusion, iron supplementation
- Myasthenia: physical exercise, e.g., gradual endurance training by aerobic exercise (▶ Chap. 4.12)
- Anorexia /cachexia: many small low fat meals, vitamin supplements if required, treatment with megestrol acetate or medroxyprogesterone acetate (▶ Chap. 4.4.1)
- Treatment of comorbidities. infections, cardiac dysfunction, renal function impairment
- Antidepressants: especially with associated sleep disturbances: nortriptyline / amitriptyline, other: bupropion, selective serotonin reuptake inhibitors (e.g., paroxetine or sertraline)

### Psycho-oncological Care
- Individual counseling
- Relaxation techniques, group counseling
- Psychoeducation: economization of time and energy, e.g., performing household chores in small steps, making time for small walks, saving energy for social activities
- Patient brochures or information materials, as available
- Psychostimulation, e.g., methylphenidate

*ATTENTION:* In the terminal phase of cancer or in palliative situations, it is important to adopt an adequate approach, i.e., acceptance of fatigue

**Ref:**

1. Carrol KK, Kohli S, Mustian KM et al. Pharmacologic treatment of cancer- related fatigue. Oncologist 2007;12(suppl 1):43–52
2. Escalante CP. Treatment of cancer-related fatigue: an update. Support Care Cancer 2003;11:79–83
3. Glaus A. Fatigue in Patients with Cancer. Analysis and Assessment. Springer, Berlin Heidelberg New York, 1998
4. Iop A, Manfredi AM, Bonura S. Fatigue in cancer patients receiving chemotherapy. Ann Oncol 2004;15:712–20
5. Morrow GR, Shelke AR, Roscoe JA et al. Management of cancer-related fatigue. Cancer Invest 2005;22:229–39
6. Stasi R, Abriani L, Beccaglia P et al. Cancer-related fatigue. Cancer 2003;98:1786–801
7. Wagner LI, Cella D. Fatigue and cancer: causes, prevalence and treatment approaches. Br J Cancer 2004;91:822–8

**Web:**

1. http://www.nci.nih.gov/cancerinfo/pdq/supportivecare/          NCI PDQ, Fatigue
2. http://www.nccn.org/professionals/physican_gls/PDF/fatigue.pdf   NCCN Fatigue Guidelines
3. http://www.cancer.org/docroot/MIT/MIT_2_2x_Fatigue.asp          ACS, Fatigue

## 4.7 Bisphosphonates

**C.I. Müller, D.P. Berger, M. Engelhardt**

**Def:** Pyrophosphate analogs with a high affinity for structures of the bone, especially in regions of increased bone turnover; osteoclast inhibitors. Clinically used in destructive processes of the bone (e.g., osteolytic bone metastasis) and hypercalcemia.

**Chem:** Pyrophosphate analogs consisting of two phosphate groups connected by a central carbon atom.

**Bisphosphonate structure**

$$\begin{array}{ccc} HO & R1 & OH \\ | & | & | \\ O=P-C-P=O \\ | & | & | \\ HO & R2 & OH \end{array}$$

Various types can be distinguished by their R1 and R2 groups:
- Bisphosphonates without nitrogen substitution (etidronate, clodronate)
- Aminobisphosphonates (pamidronate, alendronate)
- Amino-substituted bisphosphonate (ibandronate)
- Heterocyclic bisphosphonates (zoledronate, risedronate)

For clodronate, ibandronate, pamidronate, and zoledronate, clinical studies support usage in treatment of bone metastases and/or tumor-induced hypercalcemia.

Potency of drug effect: clodronate < pamidronate < ibandronate < zoledronate

**Pg:** In bone metastasis and tumor-related hypercalcemia (▶ Chap. 8.12.5)
- → Release of osteoclast activating cytokines (IL-1, IL-6, TNFα, TGFα)
- → Osteoclast-induced bone destruction with osteolysis (solid tumors, multiple myeloma) / decrease of bone density
- → "Skeletal-related events": pathological fractures, microfractures / sintering (vertebrae), hypercalcemia

**MOA:** *Inhibition of Bone Resorption*
Bisphosphonates bind to the bone matrix, especially in regions of increased bone turnover.
- Release from bone matrix and uptake by osteoclasts during bone resorption
- Osteoclast activity ↓, osteoclast differentiation ↓, apoptosis ↑
- Bone pain ↓, incidence of skeletal-related events ↓
- Quality of life ↑, performance status ↑

*Antineoplastic Effects*
Beside the inhibition of osteoclast activity, recent preclinical studies indicate an antineoplastic effect, in particular with aminobisphosphonates (pamidronate, ibandronate, zoledronate). The clinical relevance of this observation has not been established.
- Inhibition of tumor cell proliferation, invasion and adhesion, apoptosis ↑
- Inhibition of tumor angiogenesis
- Activation of γδ-T-cells ↑

**Th:**      *Areas of Use*

- Prevention and therapy of tumor-induced hypercalcemia (e.g., patients with metastases of lung cancer, renal cell carcinoma, prostate cancer, breast cancer, multiple myeloma)
- Decrease of skeletal-related morbidity (bone pain, fractures, etc.), including osteolytic bone metastasis (e.g., breast cancer, prostate cancer, multiple myeloma) and bone destruction (multiple myeloma and other hematological neoplasia)
- Prevention of steroid-induced osteoporosis with long-term corticoid therapy (e.g., immunosuppression after allogeneic stem cell transplantation)

The occurrence of osteonecrosis of the jaw (ONJ) has been described in up to 5–10% of multiple myeloma patients receiving long-term bisphosphonate treatment. New treatment schedules with limited duration of bisphosphonate use (1–2 years) have been proposed. The impact of reduced bisphosphonate treatment duration or less frequent use on ONJ incidence has not been established.

**Ref:**
1.  Berenson JR, Hillner BE, Kyle RA et al. American Society of Clinical Oncology clinical practice guidelines: the role of bisphosphonates in multiple myeloma. J Clin Oncol 2002;20:3719–36
2.  Clézardin P, Ebetino FH, Fournier PGJ. Bisphosphonates and cancer-induced bone disease: beyond their antiresorptive activity. Cancer Res 2005;65:4971–4
3.  Coleman RE. Bisphosphonates in breast cancer. Ann Oncol 2005;16:687–95
4.  Hillner BE, Ingle JN, Chlebowski RT et al. American Society of Clinical Oncology 2003 update on the role of bisphosphonates and bone health issues in women with breast cancer. J Clin Oncol 2003;21:4042–57
5.  Lüftner D, Henschke P, Possinger K. Clinical value of bisphosphonates in cancer therapy. Anticancer Res 2007;27:1759–68
6.  Santini D, Vespasiani Gentilucci U, Vincenzi B et al. The antineoplastic role of bisphosphonates: from basic research to clinical evidence. Ann Oncol 2003;14:1468–76
7.  Wu S, Dahut WL, Gulley, JL. The use of bisphosphonates in cancer patients. Acta Oncol 2007;46:581–91

**Web:**
1.  http://www.asco.org/                                          ASCO Guidelines
2.  http://www.multiplemyeloma.org/                              Multiple Myeloma Research
3.  http://www.ama-assn.org/                                      American Medical Association
4.  http://courses.washington.edu/bonephys/opbis.html            Bisphosphonates
5.  http://www.cancerbackup.org.uk/
    Treatments/Supportivetherapies/Bisphosphonates               Cancer Backup
6.  http://www.cochrane.org/reviews/en/index_list_b.html         Cochrane Library

## Clodronate

**Chem:** Dichlormethylene (bi)phosphonate

$$
\begin{array}{ccc}
\text{HO} & \text{Cl} & \text{OH} \\
| & | & | \\
\text{O} = \text{P} - \text{C} - \text{P} = \text{O} \\
| & | & | \\
\text{HO} & \text{Cl} & \text{OH}
\end{array}
$$

**MOA:** Binding to calcium salts of the bone matrix $\rightarrow$ osteoclast activity $\downarrow$ $\rightarrow$ bone resorption $\downarrow$

**Pkin:**
- *Distribution:* terminal t½ 1–16 h, 2–5% bioavailability after oral administration. High interindividual variability. Half-life in skeleton > 1 year
- *Metabolism and excretion:* 70% renal elimination of unmetabolized drug, 30% binds to bone matrix

**Se:**
- *Bone marrow:* lymphocytopenia
- *Gastrointestinal:* nausea, vomiting, diarrhea
- *Liver:* transient increase of transaminases, LDH ↑
- *Kidney:* hypocalcemia, hypophosphatemia, with rapid infusion: renal impairment, proteinuria
- *Skin:* allergic reaction
- *Other:* hypersensitivity reaction

**Ci:**
- Severe renal impairment
- Acute infection of the gastrointestinal tract
- Children, pregnancy, lactation

**Th:**
### Approved Indications
- Osteolysis resulting from bone metastases or hematological neoplasia
- Hypercalcemia of malignancies (bone metastases, bone destruction)

### Dosing and Application (i.v. or p.o.)
- Bone metastasis: initial therapy 300 mg/day i.v., day 1–5, followed by oral maintenance dose (800–1,600 mg/day p.o.) or i.v. maintenance therapy (1,500 mg every 3 weeks)
- Hypercalcemia: 1,500 mg i.v. over 4 h
- *CAUTION:* additive effect in combination with aminoglycosides (severe hypocalcemia)

**Ibandronate**

**Chem:** [1-Hydroxy-3-(methylpentylamino)propylidene]diphosphonate

$$O=P-C-P=O$$

**MOA:** Binding to calcium salts of the bone matrix → osteoclast activity ↓ → bone resorption ↓

**Pkin:**
- *Distribution:* terminal t½ 10–60 h, 1% bioavailability after oral administration. High interindividual variability. Half-life in skeleton > 1 year
- *Metabolism and excretion:* 60% renal elimination of unmetabolized drug, 40% binds to bone matrix

**Se:**
- *Bone marrow:* anemia
- *Gastrointestinal:* nausea, vomiting, diarrhea, xerostomia, dysphagia, esophagitis, dyspepsia, abdominal pain
- *Kidney:* hypocalcemia, hypophosphatemia
- *Skin:* pruritus
- *Nervous system:* paresthesia, dysesthesia, dysgeusia
- *Other:* hypersensitivity reactions, thoracic pain, flu-like symptoms, fever, myalgia, arthralgia

**Ci:**
- Hypersensitivity
- Children, pregnancy, lactation

**Th:** *Approved Indications*
- Tumor-induced hypercalcemia, with or without bone metastasis
- Prevention of skeletal-related events (fractures) in breast cancer

*Dosing and Application (i.v. or p.o.)*
- Bone metastasis: 50 mg/day p.o. in the morning, or 4 mg i.v. once per month. *ATTENTION* Creatinine clearance < 30 ml/min: → dose reduction to 50 mg p.o. once a week
- Hypercalcemia: 4–6 mg i.v. over 30 min

### Pamidronate

**Chem:**    3-Amino-1-hydroxypropylidendiphosphonate

$$
\begin{array}{ccc}
 & NH_2 & \\
 & | & \\
HO & (CH_2)_2 & OH \\
| & | & | \\
O=P & -C- & P=O \\
| & | & | \\
HO & OH & OH
\end{array}
$$

**MOA:**    Binding to calcium salts of the bone matrix $\rightarrow$ osteoclast activity $\downarrow$ $\rightarrow$ bone resorption $\downarrow$

**Pkin:**
- *Distribution:* terminal t½ 27 h. Half-life in skeleton > 1 year
- *Metabolism and excretion:* 50% renal elimination of unmetabolized drug, 50% binds to bone matrix

**Se:**
- *Bone marrow:* lymphocytopenia, thrombocytopenia, anemia
- *Cardiac / vascular:* cardiovascular disorders, decreased blood pressure, hypertension, tachycardia, syncope, atrial fibrillation, cardiac insufficiency
- *Gastrointestinal:* nausea, vomiting, diarrhea, loss of appetite, abdominal pain
- *Liver:* transient increase of transaminases, cholestasis, LDH ↑
- *Kidney:* hypocalcemia, hypokalemia, hypophosphatemia, hypomagnesemia, with rapid infusion: renal impairment, proteinuria
- *Skin:* allergic reaction, exanthema, pruritus
- *Nervous System:* central nervous impairment, insomnia, impaired vision (rare), seizures (rare), vertigo, agitation, headache
- *Other:* hypersensitivity reactions up to anaphylactic shock, thoracic pain, flu-like symptoms in 20–40%, fever, myalgia, arthralgia, conjunctivitis, uveitis, scleritis, episcleritis, osteonecrosis of the jaw

**Ci:**
- Renal impairment
- Acute infection of the gastrointestinal tract
- Children, pregnancy, lactation

**Th:**
#### Indications: Diseases with Increased Osteolytic Activity
- Tumor-induced hypercalcemia
- Osteolysis resulting from bone metastases in breast cancer
- Osteolysis resulting from bone metastases in multiple myeloma
- Paget's disease of the bone

#### Dosing and Application (i.v)
- Bone lesions: 60 mg i.v. every 3 weeks or 90 mg i.v. every 4 weeks, infusion over 2–4 h
- Hypercalcemia: 90–120 mg i.v. 15 ml/h

### Zoledronate

**Chem:**        1-Hydroxy-2-(imidazol-1-ylethyliden]diphosphonate

$$O=P-C-P=O$$

**MOA:**        Binding to calcium salts of the bone matrix → osteoclast activity ↓ → bone resorption ↓

**Pkin:**
- *Distribution:* terminal t½ 146 h. Half-life in skeleton > 1 year
- *Metabolism and excretion:* 50% renal elimination of unmetabolized drug, 50% binds to bone matrix

**Se:**
- *Bone marrow:* lymphocytopenia, thrombocytopenia, anemia
- *Cardiac / vascular:* cardiovascular disorders, hypotension, hypertension, bradycardia
- *Gastrointestinal:* nausea, vomiting, diarrhea, xerostomia, loss of appetite, dyspepsia, abdominal pain
- *Kidney:* hypocalcemia, hypokalemia, hypophosphatemia, hypomagnesemia, with rapid infusion: renal impairment, proteinuria
- *Skin:* allergic reaction, exanthema, pruritus, erythema
- *Nervous System:* central nervous complications, fatigue, insomnia, confusion, vertigo, paresthesia, impaired taste, headache
- *Other:* hypersensitivity reaction up to anaphylactic shock, thoracic pain, flu-like symptoms, fever, myalgia, arthralgia, conjunctivitis, uveitis, scleritis, episcleritis, osteonecrosis of the jaw

**Ci:**
- Renal impairment
- Acute infection of the gastrointestinal tract
- Children, pregnancy, lactation

**Th:**        ***Indications: Diseases with Increased Osteolytic Activity***
- In patients with progressive disease affecting the skeleton: prevention of skeletal-related complications (pathological fractures, compression of vertebrae, etc.)
- Tumor-induced hypercalcemia

***Dosing and Application (i.v)***
- Bone lesions: 4 mg i.v. every 4 weeks, infusion over 15 min
- Hypercalcemia: 4–8 mg i.v. infusion over 15 min
- *CAUTION:* additive effect in combination with aminoglycosides (severe hypocalcemia)

**4.8** **Malignant Effusions**

A. Kiani, R. Engelhardt

**Def:** *Effusions:* accumulation of fluid in pleural, pericardial, or peritoneal cavities.
*Malignant effusion:* malignant pericardial effusion / pleural effusion / ascites due to tumor infiltration (detection of malignant cells in the effusion).
*Paramalignant effusion:* formation due to indirect consequences of a malignancy (e.g., hypoproteinemia, pulmonary embolism, obstructive pneumonia, or after radiotherapy).

**Phys:** Small amount of physiological fluid is normally found in the pleural, pericardial, and peritoneal cavity. Drainage via local lymph vessels.

**Pg:** Pathogenetic mechanisms:
- Increased fluid formation: capillary permeability ↑, direct secretion by tumor cells, intravascular pressure ↑
- Decreased fluid drainage: impairment of the lymphatic system (compression or infiltration of lymph vessels)

**Sy:** Characteristic symptoms: displacement or compression and diminished function of organs.
- Pleural effusion: impaired pulmonary function, dyspnea, thoracic pain
- Pericardial effusion: impaired cardiac function, cardiac tamponade
- Ascites: diaphragmatic eversion, dyspnea, abdominal complaints

**Dg:** Besides diagnosing the effusion, diagnosis of the underlying malignancy (histology) is of primary importance.
- Diagnosis of effusion: clinical examination, imaging (sonography, echocardiography)
- Histology: effusion cytology, immunocytology

### Differentiation Between Transudate and Exudate
- *Transudate:* serous fluid, mostly of non-inflammatory origin, protein content < 30 g/l, specific gravity < 1.016
- *Exudate:* fluid secretion of mostly inflammatory origin, protein content > 30 g/l, specific gravity > 1.016

Malignant pleural effusions are always exudates (as opposed to paramalignant effusions which can also be transudates). Transudates do not require further effusion analysis, but additional diagnostic procedures may be necessary.

**Th:** ### Therapeutic Principles
Malignant effusions generally indicate advanced cancer. Most cases therefore require palliation of burdensome symptoms via local and possibly systemic therapeutic approaches. Of paramount importance is the improvement of the patient's quality of life with a minimum of strain.

### Specific Treatment
▶ Chaps. 4.8.1–4.8.3

**Ref:**
1. Convey AM. Management of malignant pleural effusions and ascites. J Support Oncol 2005;3:169–76
2. Nelson KA, Walsh D, Abdullah O et al. Common complications of advanced cancer. Semin Oncol 2000;27:34–44

**Web:**
1. http://www.uic.edu/classes/pmpr/pmpr652/Final/bressler/maligeffu.html — University of Illinois Education
2. http://www.cancer.gov/cancertopics/pdq/supportivecare/cardiopulmonary/HealthProfessional/page3 — NCI

## 4.8.1    Malignant Pleural Effusion

A. Kiani, R. Engelhardt

**Def:**   Malignancy-induced accumulation of fluid in the pleural cavity (between the visceral and the parietal pleura).

**Phys:**   *Pleural Fluid*
- Small amount of physiological intrapleural fluid (5–15 ml per hemithorax)
- Low-protein (protein < 15 g/l) capillary filtrate of the parietal pleura
- Drainage via pleural lymph vessels
- Daily pleural fluid exchange: 15–30 ml per hemithorax (reserve capacity: up to 500 ml per hemithorax)

**Pphys:**   *Pleural Effusion*
Increase of the pleural fluid volume as a result of fluid imbalances due to:
- Increased capillary fluid filtration (e.g., pleural negative pressure ↑, hydrostatic capillary pressure ↑, pleural fluid oncotic pressure ↑, capillary oncotic pressure ↓)
- Impaired lymph drainage

*Malignant Pleural Effusion*
- Capillary permeability ↑ or lymph drainage ↓ due to tumor cell invasion of the parietal or visceral pleura
- Pleural lymph drainage ↓ due to mediastinal lymph node metastases
- Pleural negative pressure ↑ due to atelectasis / bronchial obstruction
- Chylothorax formation due to thoracic duct obstruction

*Paramalignant Pleural Effusion*
Formation due to indirect consequences of a malignancy (hypoproteinemia, pulmonary embolism, obstructive pneumonia, or after radiotherapy).

**Causes of malignant pleural effusions**

| Disease | Frequency (%) |
| --- | --- |
| Lung cancer | 35 |
| Breast cancer | 25 |
| Lymphomas | 10 |
| Ovarian carcinoma | 5 |
| Unknown primary tumor / other | 25 |

**Sy:**   Symptom triad: dyspnea + thoracic pain (often respiration dependent) + cough
Twenty percent of patients are not symptomatic.

**Dg:**   *Clinical Diagnosis*
- Case history (dyspnea)
- Physical examination: pleural effusions from 300 to 500 ml are detectable by clinical examination: percussion dullness, decreased breath sounds and vocal fremitus, egophony at the upper border of the fluid

*Imaging*
- Chest x-ray: obligatory, detection limit of approximately 150–200 ml pleural fluid
- Sonography: most sensitive method, detection of up to 10 ml pleural fluid
- Thoracic CT: optional, detection of intrathoracic abnormalities

### Invasive Measures: Tissue Sampling for Histology

Of particular importance with pleural effusions of unknown origin and for the evaluation of pleural abnormalities (spread, etc.).

- Diagnostic thoracentesis: obligatory with pleural effusions of unknown origin (▶ Chap. 10.1)
- Percutaneous pleural biopsy (blind or CT-guided)
- Thoracoscopic pleural biopsy (under intubation anesthesia, highest diagnostic reliability)

## Analysis of Pleural Fluid

### Differentiation Between Transudate and Exudate

- *Transudate:* serous fluid, mostly of non-inflammatory origin, protein content < 30 g/l, specific gravity < 1.016
- *Exudate:* fluid secretion of mostly inflammatory origin, protein content > 30 g/l, specific gravity > 1.016

Malignant pleural effusions are always exudates (as opposed to paramalignant effusions which can also be transudates). Transudates do not require further analysis, but additional diagnostic procedures may be necessary.

### Light's Criteria

Exudates have to fulfill at least one of the following criteria:

- Pleural fluid protein / serum protein ratio > 0.5
- Pleural fluid LDH / serum LDH ratio > 0.6
- Pleural fluid LDH greater than two-thirds the upper limit of normal for serum LDH

### Detection of Malignant Cells in the Pleural Fluid

- Cytological examination, 50% sensitivity
- Immunocytological examination, 80% sensitivity
- Amount and quality of the sample determine the test validity → minimum of 25–50 ml (heparinized sample)
- Approximately 20% of tumor-associated pleural effusions are paramalignant → no detectable tumor cells

### pH

Normal value of pleural fluid: pH 7.6. Differentiation between transudate / exudate:

- pH 7.4–7.55: transudate, non-malignant
- pH 7.3–7.45: mostly exudate, suspected malignancies or infection
- pH < 7.3: poor prognosis with malignant effusions

### Bacteriological Examination

Obligatory to rule out tuberculosis or infected effusion (pleural empyema)

### Optional Tests

- Cholesterol: helpful to distinguish exudate from transudate (> 1.55 mmol/l, 60 mg/dl, respectively)
- Glucose: low values (< 20–30 mg/dl) are typical for pleural effusions in rheumatoid arthritis; with malignant effusions, glucose values of < 60 mg/dl constitute a poor prognosis
- Amylase: DD pancreatitis (pancreatic amylase), ruptured esophagus (salivary amylase)
- Triglycerides: with chylothorax, triglyceride levels > 110 mg/dl
- Adenosine deaminase (ADA): helpful in diagnosis of tuberculosis-induced pleural effusions (ADA > 70m IU/l)
- CEA, other tumor markers: helpful in differentiating between adenocarcinoma and pleural mesothelioma

**Dd:**        **Differential diagnosis of pleural effusion (industrial nations)**

| Disease | Frequency (%) |
|---|---|
| Cardiac insufficiency | 40 |
| Pneumonia ("parapneumonic" effusion) | 30 |
| Malignancies ("malignant" or "paramalignant" effusion) | 15 |
| Pulmonary embolism | 10 |
| Hepatic cirrhosis | 4 |
| Autoimmune diseases | 0.5 |
| Tuberculosis (in developing countries up to 40%) | 0.2 |

**Th:**        ## Therapeutic Principles

Malignant pleural effusions usually indicate dissemination of the primary tumor → local treatment is always palliative, systemic treatment is possibly curative.
- Systemic treatment according to the histology of the primary disease
- In chemotherapy-sensitive malignancies: chemotherapy with curative intention
- With resistant disease: palliative treatment according to symptoms

### Treatment

#### Therapeutic Pleuracentesis
- *Indication:* rapid relief for the patient prior to further measures (e.g., chemotherapy in breast cancer)
- *Technique:* ▶ Chap. 10.1
- *Disadvantages:*
  - Only short-term effect
  - Danger of compartment formation with repeated centesis
  - Danger of decompression-induced pulmonary edema with aspiration of > 1,000 ml

#### Pleural Drainage and Pleurodesis
- *Indication:* Treatment of choice for symptomatic malignant pleural effusions which cannot be treated conservatively
- *Technique:* ▶ Chap. 10.2

#### Pleuroperitoneal Shunt
Subcutaneously inserted pump with two catheters through which pleural fluid is manually pumped into the peritoneal cavity.
- *Indication:* failure of the lung to reexpand after drainage; failed pleurodesis
- *Disadvantages:* intubation anesthesia usually required; occasional shunt blockage
- *Long-term pleural drainage:* via a tunneled catheter (e.g., Pleurx system; Denver shunt).

#### Pleurectomy
Effective but rarely indicated as a way of controlling malignant pleural effusions. It involves removing the parietal pleura.

**Prg:**        Malignant pleural effusion: median survival 3–4 months (depending on tumor entity).

**Ref:**

1. Alexandrakis MG, Passam FH, Kyriakou DS et al. Pleural effusions in hematologic malignancies. Chest 2004;125:1546–55
2. Antony VB, Loddenkemper R, Astoul P et al. Management of malignant pleural effusions. Eur Respir J 2001;18:402–19
3. Antunes G, Neville E, Duffy J et al. BTS guidelines for the management of malignant pleural effusions. Thorax 2003;58:29–38
4. Light RW. Pleural effusion. N Engl J Med 2002;346:1971–7
5. Pollak JS. Malignant pleural effusions: treatment with tunneled long-term drainage catheters. Curr Opin Pulm Med 2002;8:302–7
6. Rahman NM, Chapman SJ, Davies RJ. Pleural effusion: a structured approach to care. Br Med Bull 2005;72:31–47
7. Tarn AC, Lapworth R. Biochemical analysis of pleural analysis of pleural fluid: what should we measure? Ann Clin Biochem 2001;38:311–22
8. Tassi GF, Cardillo G, Marchetti GP et al. Diagnostic and therapeutical management of malignant pleural effusion. Ann Oncol 2006;17(suppl 2):ii11–2

**Web:**

1. http://www.merck.com/mmpe/sec05/ch060/ch060d.html    Merck Manual
2. http://www.meds.com/pdq/effusion_pro.html    Medicine Online
3. http://www.emedicine.com/EMERG/topic462.htm    Emedicine
4. http://www.emedicine.com/med/topic1843.htm    Pleural Effusion, Emedicine
5. http://www.nlm.nih.gov/medlineplus/ency/article/000086.htm    Medline Plus

## 4.8.2     Malignant Pericardial Effusion

### A. Kiani, R. Engelhardt

**Def:** Malignancy-induced accumulation of fluid in the pericardial cavity (between the visceral and the parietal pericardium).

**Ep:** Myocardial or pericardial involvement in up to 15% of patients with solid tumors.

**Phys:** *Intrapericardial Fluid*
- Small amount of physiological intrapericardial fluid (15–50 ml)
- Drainage via lymph vessels

**Pphys:** *Pericardial Effusion*
Intrapericardial accumulation of fluid, e.g. as a result of acute pericarditis.

*Malignant Pericardial Effusion*
Intrapericardial fluid accumulation due to direct tumor invasion or metastasis to the parietal visceral pericardium, with blockage of draining lymph vessels.

*Paramalignant Pericardial Effusion*
Not caused by malignant pericardial infiltration, but by indirect consequences of a malignancy (e.g., radiotherapy, drugs, infection, obstruction of the mediastinal lymph drainage); approximately 50% of symptomatic pericardial effusions in patients with known malignancies.

*Most Common Causes of Malignant Pericardial Effusions*
- Lung cancer
- Breast cancer
- Leukemias
- Malignant lymphomas

**Sy:** *Initial Unspecific Symptoms*
Dyspnea, cough, orthopnea, thoracic pain

*In Case of Cardiac Tamponade*
Tachycardia, hypotension, increased jugular venous pressure, possibly pulsus paradoxus (inspiratory decrease in blood pressure > 10 mmHg) and Kussmaul's sign (inspiratory increase in jugular venous pressure)

**Dg:** *Clinical Diagnosis*
- Patient history: malignancy, dyspnea, signs of cardiac insufficiency
- Physical examination: signs of venous congestion / cardiac insufficiency

*Imaging*
- Echocardiography: method of choice allowing localization and quantification of the effusion
- Chest x-ray: widened cardiac silhouette (differential diagnosis: myogenic dilatation)
- CT, MRI: optional, detection of compartment formation in the effusion

*Invasive Procedures / Histology*
Pericardiocentesis and aspiration of fluid for histology and possibly for therapeutic purposes — only by experienced staff, with echocardiographic and ECG monitoring.

*Fluid Diagnosis*
- Macroscopic aspect: malignant pericardial effusions are often hemorrhagic (non-specific finding)
- Cytological (possibly immunocytological) tumor cell detection

- Test validity determined by amount and quality of the sample (minimum 25–50 ml, heparinized)
- *ATTENTION:* no tumor cells in paramalignant pericardial effusions
- Bacteriological analysis to rule out infection

### Most Common Causes of Acute Pericarditis
- Infections (viral, bacterial, including tuberculosis)
- Myocardial infarction
- Uremia
- Rheumatic disease (e.g., SLE, rheumatic fever)

### Cardiac Tamponade (▶ Chap. 9.4)
Hemodynamically significant pericardial effusion with a large or rapidly increasing amount of fluid causing ventricular flow obstruction
→ Clinical signs of left-sided heart failure and venous congestion (see above)
→ Clinical diagnosis, echocardiography, possibly invasive diagnostic procedures

Cardiac tamponade is a life-threatening emergency requiring rapid pericardiocentesis (▶ Chap. 9.4). After hemodynamic stabilization, further therapeutic measures may be carried out (see below).

### Therapeutic Principles

- Patients with asymptomatic pericardial effusion: close monitoring
- Patients with symptomatic pericardial effusion (with or without signs of pericardial tamponade):
  - Pericardiocentesis, followed by further therapeutic measures
  - Chemotherapy or radiotherapy sensitive tumors: antineoplastic treatment
  - Refractory tumors: intrapericardial sclerotherapy and/or surgical intervention

### Treatment

#### Therapeutic Pericardiocentesis
- *Indication:* initial intervention in case of symptomatic pericardial effusion
- *Technique:*
  - Should be performed by a specialist or other experienced individuals, with echocardiographic and ECG monitoring
  - Under local anesthesia and sterile conditions, a pigtail catheter is percutaneously inserted through the subxiphoid approach into the pericardial cavity where it remains to provide permanent drainage
- *Disadvantage:* usually short-term effect

#### Intrapericardial Sclerotherapy
- *Indication:* patients with symptomatic, malignant pericardial effusion after percutaneous drainage
- *Technique:*
  - Intrapericardial installation of a sclerosing drug via a percutaneous catheter after pericardial drainage best results with doxycycline (up to 80% success), bleomycin, cisplatin, and carboplatin
  - Clamping of the catheter for several hours, then continuous drainage until drainage fluid volume < 25 ml per 24 h
  - In many cases, repeated sclerotherapy is necessary
- *Mode of action:* triggering of an inflammatory reaction with subsequent adhesion of visceral and parietal pericardia

### Surgical Techniques

- *Indication:* symptomatic pericardial effusion and failure of conservative therapeutic measures including intrapericardial sclerotherapy
- *Technique:*
  - Subxyphoid pericardiotomy ("pericardial window") under general anesthesia or local anesthesia with sedation → pericardial drainage into pleural cavity
  - Due to high morbidity, extensive surgical procedures (pericardiotomy via thoracoscopy or anterior thoracotomy) are rarely indicated

**Prg:**   Malignant pericardial effusion: median survival 2–3 months

**Ref:**
1. Chen EP, Miller JI. Modern approaches and use of surgical treatment for pericardial disease. Curr Cardiol Rep 2002;41:4–6
2. Keefe DL. Cardiovascular emergencies in the cancer patient. Semin Oncol 2000;27:244–55
3. Maher EA. Pericardial sclerosis as the primary management of malignant pericardial effusion and cardiac tamponade. J Thorac Cardiovasc Surg 1996;112:637–43
4. Maisch B, Sererovic PM, Ristic AD et al. Guidelines on the diagnosis and management of effusions. Eur Soc Cardiol, 2004
5. Martinoni A, Cipolla CM, Civelli M et al. Intrapericardial treatment of neoplastic pericardial effusions. Herz 2000;25:787–93
6. Retter AS. Pericardial disease in the oncology patient. Heart Dis 2002;4:387–91
7. Shepherd FA. Malignant pericardial effusion. Curr Opin Oncol 1997;9:170–4

**Web:**
1. http://www.emedicine.com/med/topic1786.htm          Pericardial Effusion, e-medicine
2. http://www.nlm.nih.gov/medlineplus/ency/article/000194.htm   Medline Plus
3. http://www.nci.nih.gov/cancertopics/pdq/supportivecare/
   cardiopulmonary/HealthProfessional                NCI PDQ

## 4.8.3 Malignant Ascites

**A. Kiani, R. Engelhardt**

**Def:** Malignancy-induced fluid accumulation in the peritoneal cavity. Occurrence in 20% of patients with intra-abdominal tumors.

**Phys:** *Intraperitoneal Fluid*
- Small amount of physiological intra-abdominal fluid (< 10 ml)
- Drainage via intra-peritoneal lymph vessels

**Pphys:** *Ascites*
Increased amount of abdominal fluid due to:
- Fluid imbalance (increased portal pressure, hypoalbuminemia, increased capillary permeability)
- Impaired lymph drainage (thoracic duct)

*Malignant Ascites*
- Capillary permeability ↑ (due to cytokine secretion, e.g., VEGF, TNFα) or lymphatic drainage ↓ (due to tumor cell invasion)
- Increased exudation of fluids and proteins into the abdomen (directly, by tumor cells or indirectly, due to secreted humoral factors)
- Portal hypertension / hypoalbuminemia in case of hepatic metastases or hepatocellular carcinoma

*Most Common Causes of Malignant Ascites*
- Gastrointestinal tumors (stomach, colon, pancreas, liver, bile ducts)
- Ovarian carcinoma

**Sy:** In early stages, only nonspecific signs. Typical symptoms at > 2 l of ascitic fluid:
- Body weight ↑, abdominal girth ↑, diaphragmatic eversion, dyspnea
- Anorexia, abdominal complaints / tension

**Dg:** *Clinical Diagnosis*
- Patient history (malignancy, dyspnea, weight gain, abdominal complaints)
- Physical examination: detection limit of approximately 1,000 ml; shifting dullness, periumbilical dullness in knee-elbow position, fluid wave (ballottement), diaphragmatic eversion, possibly umbilical hernia

*Imaging*
- Sonography: most sensitive method; in supine position, ascites detectable from 300 ml (perihepatic / perisplenic spaces), in knee-elbow position from 10 to 20 ml
- Abdominal x-ray: low sensitivity
- Abdominal CT scan: optional, detection of concomitant intra-abdominal disorders

*Invasive Procedures / Histology*
Diagnostic paracentesis: obligatory in ascites of unknown origin (▶ Chap. 10.3)

### Ascites Fluid Analysis

*Macroscopic Aspect*
Sanguineous (often malignant), serous (e.g., portal hypertension), turbid (infected), chylous (e.g., with malignant lymphomas).

### Determination of the Serum-Ascites Albumin Gradient (SAAG)

SAAG = albumin$_{serum}$ / albumin$_{ascites}$ ratio; differentiates between ascites with or without portal hy‐
pertension with > 90% accuracy and replaces the traditional classification of ascites into exuda‐
and transudate.

- SAAG > 1.1: *portal hypertension.* DD: hepatic cirrhosis, cardiac insufficiency, portal vein
  thrombosis, veno-occlusive disease (VOD), hepatic metastases, hepatic failure
- SAAG < 1.1: *no portal hypertension.* DD: peritoneal carcinomatosis, peritoneal tuberculosis,
  nephrotic syndrome, biliary ascites

### Cytology / Differentiation

- Total cell count: low specificity, but useful in the follow-up of antibiotic treatment of spontane‐
  ous bacterial peritonitis.
- Differentiation: predomination of neutrophils or total neutrophil count > 250/µl are signs of
  bacterial infection → indication for antibiotic treatment even without positive bacterial cul‐
  ture.
- Cytology and immunocytology: in case of suspected peritoneal carcinomatosis. Validity de‐
  pendent on amount and quality of the sample → minimum 25–50 ml ascitic fluid (heparinized
  sample).
- *ATTENTION:* cytology results turn out negative in all cases of malignant ascites without peri‐
  toneal carcinomatosis (hepatic metastases, hepatocellular carcinoma, chylous ascites, etc.).
  Cytological examination of malignant ascites has a sensitivity of approximately 65%.

### Total Protein in the Ascites Fluid

In case of suspected bacterial infection (neutrophilia ↑, see above):

- Total protein$_{ascites}$ < 1.0 g/dl: most likely spontaneous bacterial peritonitis (SBP)
- Total protein$_{ascites}$ > 1.0 g/dl: most likely secondary peritonitis, investigate cause

### Microbiology

Culture of ascites (e.g., in blood culture vials): in case of suspected peritoneal infection. Culturing
is significantly more sensitive than other methods (e.g., blood smear).

### Cholesterol, Fibronectin

Besides cytology, plasma cholesterol (> 45 mg/dl) and fibronectin (> 7.5 mg/dl) are the most sen‐
sitive parameters for differentiating between malignant and portal ascites.

    *ATTENTION:* false-positive results with inflammatory ascites, false-negative results with ma‐
lignant ascites *without* peritoneal carcinomatosis.

### Optional Tests

- Amylase → DD: pancreatitis (pancreatic amylase), intestinal perforation (salivary amylase)
- CEA, other tumor markers: indicative of adenocarcinoma
- Glucose, LDH, ascitic fluid pH: of little diagnostic significance

**Dd:**          **Differential diagnosis of ascites (industrial nations)**

| Disease | Frequency (%) |
|---|---|
| Hepatic cirrhosis (portal ascites) | 80 |
| Malignancy | 10 |
| Cardiac insufficiency | 3 |
| Tuberculosis | 2 |
| Other | 5 |

h:

## Therapeutic Paracentesis

### Indication
Short-term relief in patients with symptomatic ascites, prior to further investigations and treatment.

### Techniques
▶ Chap. 10.3

### Disadvantages
- Only short-term effect
- Loss of protein, hence more rapid reformation of ascites and risk of intravascular hypovolemia with prerenal failure → prophylactic intravenous substitution of human albumin, particularly with repeated paracentesis: e.g., 50 ml of 25% human albumin per 1,000 ml extracted ascitic fluid
- Loss of fluid and electrolytes

## Sodium Restriction, Diuretics

### Indication
Malignant ascites with portal hypertension (SAAG < 1.1 g/dl, e.g., due to hepatic metastases), but not in cases of pure peritoneal carcinomatosis.

### Methods
- Sodium restriction: maximum daily intake 3 g NaCl
- Fluid restriction: only in case of hyponatremia (serum $Na^+$ < 130 mmol/l)
- Diuretics: spironolactone 25 mg 4 × daily
- If no weight reduction after 3 days: addition of 20 mg xipamide (alternatively 40 mg furosemide) daily, gradual dose increase to maximum 400 mg spironolactone and 40 mg xipamide (alternatively 160 mg furosemide) possible

*ATTENTION:* with diuretic use, check electrolytes!

## Systemic Chemotherapy

### Indication
Ascites associated with chemotherapy-sensitive malignancies.

### Methods
Chemotherapy according to the underlying malignancy.

## Intraperitoneal Chemotherapy

### Indication
Symptomatic ascites.

### Methods
Intraperitoneal instillation of cytostatic drugs, via semipermanent or temporary lines, in connection with repeated paracentesis.
- Choice of cytostatic drug: compounds with low local toxicity and good local efficacy: e.g., mitoxantrone, cisplatin, carboplatin, paclitaxel, 5-FU, melphalan, and bleomycin
- Efficacy dependent on: tumor entity, size of the peritoneal tumor, distribution of the cytostatic drug in the abdomen (may be limited, e.g., due to adhesions)
- Advantage: permits high local drug concentrations (e.g., lack of hepatic first-pass effect), lower systemic (e.g., hematological) toxicity

### Complications
- Systemic: myelosuppression, nephrotoxicity, emesis, neurotoxicity
- Local: infections (mostly skin bacteria), chemical peritonitis (pain, fever), ileus (adhesion fibrosis due to local inflammation)

## Peritoneovenous Shunt

### Indication
Therapy-resistant symptomatic ascites.

### Technique
Drainage of ascitic fluid into the superior vena cava via a valve-operated surgically implanted line (LeVeen or Denver shunt).

### Complications
Shunt obstruction, infections, tumor dissemination (usually of little clinical importance), DIC (disseminated intravascular coagulation, rare occurrence in conjunction with malignant ascites)

## Experimental Methods

- Intraperitoneal chemohyperthermia, particularly with gastrointestinal tumors
- Intraperitoneal instillation of radioisotopes (e.g., $^{32}$P, $^{198}$Au)
- Intraperitoneal immunotherapy: administration of immunologically active substances, e.g., TNFα (50 μg per 500 ml infusion solution), interferon α/β/γ, interleukin 2, *Corynebacterium parvum*, VEGF, and matrix metalloproteinase inhibitors; most effective with minimal tumor burden; toxicity: fever, pain
- TIPS (transjugular intrahepatic portosystemic shunt): as an alternative to peritoneovenous shunt in diuretic refractory ascites with increased portal pressure
- Permanent drainage catheter: potential therapeutic option for patients who are unable to tolerate repeated paracentesis (e.g., due to electrolyte shifts) and in whom a peritoneovenous shunt is contraindicated; complications (common): infections, peritonitis

**Prg:** In case of malignant ascites: median survival approximately 2–4 months, depending on tumor entity.

**Ref:**
1.  Becker G, Galandi D, Blum HE. Malignant ascites: Systematic review and guideline for treatment. Eur J Cancer 2006;42:589–97
2.  Jeffery J, Murphy MJ. Ascitic fluid analysis: the role of biochemistry and haematology. Hosp Med 2001;62:282–6
3.  Markmann M. Intraperitoneal chemotherapy. Semin Oncol 1991;18:248–54
4.  McHutchinson JG. Differential diagnosis of ascites. Semin Liver Dis 1997;17:191–202
5.  Parsons SL, Watson SA, Steele RJ. Malignant ascites. Br J Surg 1996;83:6–14
6.  Runyon BA. Care of patients with ascites. N Engl J Med 1994;330:337–42
7.  Smith EM, Jayson GC. The current and future management of malignant ascites. Clin Oncol 2003;15:59–72

**Web:**
1.  http://www.cancerweb.ncl.ac.uk/cancernet/103862.html      Malignant Ascites, Cancernet
2.  http://www.surgicaloncology.com/psmreslt.htm          Surgical Oncology
3.  http://www.emedicine.com/med/topic173.htm            Emedicine

**.9** **Transfusion Therapy**

**.9.1** **Cellular Blood Products**

A. Leo, E. Leo, H. Bertz

**ef:**

*Specific replacement of individual blood components according to the patient's requirements ("targeted hemotherapy"):*
- Cellular blood products: packed red blood cells (RBC), platelet concentrate
- Acellular blood products: fresh frozen plasma (FFP), coagulation factors, immunoglobulins, human albumin
- Granulocyte transfusion: experimental treatment procedure (▶ Chap. 5.4)

All human blood products are:
- Classified as treatments for human application, and their preparation, distribution, and use are safe-guarded by pharmaceutical and transfusion laws
- Only available on prescription
- Liable for batch documentation (including albumin and recombinant coagulation factors)

**Packed Red Cells**

**ef:**

Leukocyte-depleted erythrocyte suspension in additive solution.

**leth:**

### Preparation and Storage
- *Packed red cells:* standard preparation from a single unit of whole blood (plasma residue < 15 ml, hematocrit approximately 60%, leukocyte count per unit < $1 \times 10^6$) in additive solution (e.g., SAG-mannitol, PAGGS-mannitol); shelf-life: 35–49 days depending on manufacturer
- *Washed packed red cells (plasma content < 1 ml):* shelf-life dependent on preparation. Indications: congenital IgA deficiency (with anti-IgA antibodies), patients with severe allergic reactions after administration of foreign protein, paroxysmal nocturnal hemoglobinuria
- *Irradiated packed red cells:* radiation with 30 Gy, for prevention of transfusion-associated graft-versus-host disease (see below)

**hys:**

### Serological Compatibility of Packed Red Cells

Serological compatibility testing:
- Major crossmatch: obligatory compatibility testing between patient serum and donor red cells
- Minor crossmatch: optional compatibility testing between patient red cells and donor serum (now replaced by antibody screening of donor samples)
- Antibody screening of the recipient (obligatory with each compatibility test)

### Blood Group Antigens and Antibodies

#### ABO System
- Antigens: A, B, O
- Antibodies (isoagglutinins): anti-A, anti-B, formed early in life, mainly IgM- but also IgG-type antibodies
- Most important antigen system in blood transfusions due to preformed ("regular") antibodies against blood groups different from that of the individual (Landsteiner's rule, e.g., anti-A and anti-B in blood group O); in major ABO-mismatched transfusions, these antibodies (e.g., donor A, recipient O) may cause severe acute hemolytic transfusion reactions (▶ Chap. 9.8)

**AB0 compatibility (major compatibility)**

| Patient (recipient) | Compatible Donor (packed red cells) |
|---|---|
| A | A, O[a] |
| B | B, O[a] |
| AB | A, B[a], AB[a], O[a] |
| O | O |

[a] Minor incompatibility practically irrelevant due to negligible donor plasma residue in packed red cells

### Rhesus (Rh) System
- Antigens: D antigen (most potent blood group immunogen), C/c, E/e
- Rhesus antibodies (IgG type, rarely IgM type) are generally formed after immunization ("ir regular antibodies")

**Rhesus compatibility (D antigen)**

| Patient (recipient) | Compatible Donor (packed red cells) |
|---|---|
| Rh(D) negative | Rh(D) negative[a,b] |
| Rh(D) positive | Rh(D) positive or negative[a] |

[a] According to current guidelines, patients requiring regular transfusions and women <45 years of age should receive Rh (D, C, and E) compatible serum

[b] In case of shortage of Rh(D)-negative units, transfusion with Rh(D)-positive blood is possible (except in preimmunized patients and in pre-menopausal women).

### Other Systems
Irregular antibodies against antigens of low immunogenicity (e.g., Kidd system, Duffy system) rarely cause severe transfusion reactions.

### Autoimmune Hemolytic Anemia
In patients with hematological or oncological diseases, interference with cross-matching due to cold- or warm-type autoimmune hemolytic anemia with free irregular autoantibodies and positive direct antiglobulin (Coombs') test may occur.

**Ind:**        ## Acute / Chronic Anemia

### Indications for Transfusion: Guidelines
- In patients with hematological or oncological diseases, transfusion should be considered at hemoglobin concentrations below 8.0 g/dl
- In chronic anemia, lower hemoglobin concentrations (6–8 g/dl) are often tolerated without any further symptoms → packed red cells not indicated
- In patients with coronary heart disease or at risk of reduced cerebral perfusion: transfusion indicated at hemoglobin levels below 10 g/dl
- Patients requiring modified transfusion regimes due to exceptional circumstances (surgery, thalassemia major, etc.) may require a different approach

*CAUTION:* Indications for transfusion have to be adapted to clinical symptoms. Asymptomatic blood loss does not constitute a general indication for transfusion. Prior to allogeneic stem cell transplantation, transfusions should be avoided in order to prevent alloimmunization.

**Co:**        ▶ Chap. 9.8

h:

## Packed Red Cell Transfusion: Procedure

1. *Prerequisites for transfusion*
- Clear indication
- Specification of the ordering criteria: blood required on site or on standby at the blood bank, urgency, patient / donor CMV status, irradiated units
- Correct labeling of blood samples for serological compatibility testing, avoidance of mix-ups at collection (most common cause of ABO maltransfusion)

2. *Patient information* / informed consent (signature)

3. *Inspection of the blood product and accompanying documentation*
- Strict adherence to maintaining the cold chain
- Compare patient data with data on blood product
- Validity period of serological compatibility testing / irregular antibodies (check accompanying documentation)
- Expiry date, external damage, visible hemolysis
- Anti-CMV status
- Warming-up of the blood product prior to transfusion is necessary for transfusion rates of > 50 ml/min, recipients with increased cold agglutinins, and massive transfusions. A blood warming device may be required.

**ATTENTION:** washed / irradiated blood products must be clearly labeled by the manufacturer.

4. *ABO identity testing (bedside test):* Mandatory testing of the recipient's ABO identity directly at the hospital bedside / on the ward under the immediate supervision or carried out by the physician in charge of blood transfusion. The results must be documented in writing. Bedside testing of the blood product is not compulsory (may be carried out for comparison purposes).

5. *Use of transfusion equipment with filter* (pore size 170–230 μm):
- In rare cases (e.g., impaired pulmonary perfusion in association with massive transfusions), microaggregate filters (pore size 40 μm) are required
- Administration via separate access, no further additives
- Once opened, the blood product must be used within maximum 6 h; after transfusion, the blood bag must be kept in a cool place for 24 h for forensic purposes
- *Initiation of transfusion must be supervised by a physician:* adequate monitoring of the patient before, during, and after transfusion (blood pressure, allergic reactions, etc.)
- *Transfusion rate* normally 250–500 ml/h, exception: patients with cardiovascular or pulmonary disease → risk of volume overload → monitor even more closely, slower infusion

6. *Evaluation of transfusion effect – rule of thumb:* hemoglobin increase by 1.0–2.0 g/dl or hematocrit increase by 3–5% per red cell concentrate.

7. *Batch documentation*

8. *Post-transfusion monitoring:* be aware of possible transfusion-associated complications (hemoglobin decrease of unknown cause, post-transfusion purpura, jaundice, etc.)

## Platelet Concentrates (PC)

ef:

Leukocyte-depleted platelet suspension in human plasma and/or additive solution.

Meth:

### Preparation
- Platelet concentrates from single donor platelet apheresis or from pooled buffy coats of 4–6 donors
- Platelet content of both types of preparation: $2–4 \times 10^{11}$ per unit in up to 300 ml plasma, leukocyte content $< 1 \times 10^6$ per unit

### Storage

- At 22 ± 2°C under continuous agitation for up to 5 days (*ATTENTION:* do not chill)
- However, quality impairment caused by several hours without agitation (e.g., during transport) is negligible

**Phys:**     ### ABO Compatibility

Platelets should normally be given as ABO-compatible transfusions. However, ABO-incompatible transfusions cannot always be avoided:

- Minor-mismatched platelet transfusions are equally successful and show no or little adverse effects. They can, however, trigger hemolysis which in rare cases may be severe. Adults can generally tolerate up to 500 ml minor-incompatible plasma.
- Major-incompatible transfusions are on average 40% less successful (platelets express ABO antigens). However, degradation is usually without clinical symptoms.

### Rh Compatibility

Due to the low erythrocyte content of adequately prepared platelet concentrates, Rh immunization after incompatible blood transfusions (Rh(D)-positive blood and Rh(D)-negative recipient) is unlikely. However, as precaution, Rh(D)-negative female patients < 45 years of age should prophylactically be given intravenous anti-D (dose: 100 μg).

**Ind:**     ### Therapeutic Use

Overt signs of hemorrhage (e.g., petechial bleeding, mucosal bleeding, nose bleed) or hemorrhage in cases of proven thrombocytopenia or thrombocyte dysfunction

### Prophylactic Use

The value of prophylactic platelet administration and the threshold for use are under discussion. Criteria:

- Rule of thumb: platelet count < 10,000 to 20,000/μl constitutes an increased risk of hemorrhage and an indication for transfusion.
- Concomitant disorders, especially fever, sepsis, splenomegaly, etc., increase the risk of hemorrhage even at a higher platelet count.
- Platelet dysfunction or leukemic infiltration of vascular walls in patients with acute leukemias constitute an increased risk of hemorrhage even with a significantly higher platelet count (> 30,000/μl).
- In some institutions, a lower threshold (5,000–10,000 platelets/μl) is accepted for prophylactic platelet administration in patients with prolonged thrombocytopenia without concomitant symptoms (fever, splenomegaly, etc.). The indication for platelet transfusion has to be decided upon in each individual case, taking into account all clinical aspects and the potentially increased risk of hemorrhage.
- For invasive procedures (installation of venous line, puncture, etc.), a higher platelet count is desirable (40,000–60,000/μl).

**Ci:**     Relative contraindications for platelet transfusion (use in individual cases may be considered):

- Allergy to human plasma proteins
- Post-transfusion purpura (PTP)
- Idiopathic thrombocytopenic purpura (ITP; ► Chap. 6.3.1)
- Heparin-induced thrombocytopenia type II (HIT; ► Chap. 6.3.2)
- Thrombotic thrombocytopenic purpura (Moschcowitz disease, TTP; ► Chap. 6.3.3)

Prior to allogeneic hematopoietic stem cell transplantation, transfusions should be avoided in order to prevent alloimmunization.

**Co:**     ► Chap. 9.8

**Th:**     ## Platelet Concentrate Transfusion: Procedure

1. *Patient information* / informed consent (signature)

*2. Inspection of the blood product and accompanying documentation*
- Compare data on blood product with documentation (no serological compatibility testing required), expiry date
- External damage, platelet "swirling" phenomenon
- Bedside testing of recipient not mandatory
- Anti-CMV status

*3. Use of transfusion equipment with filter* (pore size 170–230 μm)
- Initiation of transfusion under medical supervision
- After transfusion, blood bags must be kept in a cool place for 24 h for forensic purposes

*4. Batch documentation*

*5. Transfusion outcome*
- Monitor post-transfusion platelet count (1-h count, 24-h count)
- Rule of thumb: platelet count increase by 25,000/μl per administered platelet concentrate

### Platelet-refractory Patients

#### Definition
No increase in platelet count after at least 2 adequate platelet transfusions.

#### Possible Causes
- *Non-immunological:* hemorrhage, fever, sepsis, DIC, splenomegaly, antibiotics.
- *HLA antibodies:* present in multitransfused patients and women with previous pregnancies. Primary immunization depends on the degree of leukocyte contamination of blood products → adequate leukocyte depletion ($< 1 \times 10^6$) prevents primary HLA immunization. However, in the case of prior immunization, the presence of incompatible platelets is sufficient to cause a booster response.
- *Platelet-specific antibodies:* antibodies against platelet-specific antigens (glycoproteins) rarely occur alone but coexist with HLA antibodies.
- *Others:* ABO isoagglutinin, drug-induced antibodies.

#### Approach to Refractory Patients
- Exclusion of non-immunological causes
- HLA antibody screening → if positive: use HLA compatible platelets
- Possibly platelet cross-matching (restricted to special laboratories)
- Possibly platelet antibody screening

**Meth:**

### Methods

### Leucocyte Depletion of Cellular Blood Products

In-line filtration during preparation (leukocyte reduction to $< 1 \times 10^6$ per unit of blood).

#### Advantages of Leukocyte Depletion
- Prevention of sensitization to histocompatibility antigens (alloimmunization)
- In-line-filtrated products are equivalent to CMV-negative products → suitable for recipients of allogeneic hematopoietic stem cell transplantation (in anti-CMV-negative recipients of anti-CMV-negative stem cell transplants, use of anti-CMV-negative blood products is recommended)
- Low rate of febrile non-hemolytic transfusion reactions (FNHTR; most common transfusion reaction, ▶ Chap. 9.8)

## Irradiation of Blood Products for the Prevention of GVHD

### Technique
Gamma irradiation, recommended dose: 30 Gy.

### Indications
Prevention of transfusion-associated graft-versus-host disease (TA-GVHD; ▶ Chap. 9.8) in connection with:
- Allogeneic hematopoietic stem cell transplantation
- High-dose chemotherapy with or without total body irradiation in leukemias, malignant lymphomas, and solid tumors
- Chemotherapy in Hodgkin's disease, non-Hodgkin's lymphomas, and acute leukemias
- Severe immunodeficiency (hereditary or acquired)
- Transfusion before autologous peripheral blood stem cell harvesting
- Intrauterine transfusion, premature infants
- Transfusions between first-grade relatives
- Aplastic anemia

### Disadvantages
In rare cases, radiation damage to cellular components of packed red cells: potassium leakage, formation of free radicals → reduction of shelf life of RBCs (according to manufacturers' specifications). So far, there is no concrete evidence of cellular damage occurring during thrombocyte irradiation. The value of fresh frozen plasma (FFP) irradiation in the prevention of graft-versus-host reaction is disputable (sporadic reports on detection of actively proliferating cells).

## Prevention of CMV Transmission by Cellular Blood Products

### Indications (risk groups)
- Recipients of hematopoietic stem cell transplants
- Recipients of organ transplants
- Immunodeficient patients, anti-CMV-negative HIV-infected patients
- Premature infants, fetuses (intrauterine transfusion)
- Anti-CMV-negative pregnant women

### Recommendation
Generally, leukocyte-depleted cellular blood products and anti-CMV-negative blood products are equally suitable to prevent CMV infection (according to guidelines). However, for 'anti-CMV-negative recipients of anti-CMV-negative stem cell transplants' and 'intrauterine transfusion recipients' strict use of anti-CMV-negative blood products is strongly recommended.

*ATTENTION:* for batch documentation and quality management regarding the use of blood products, follow national transfusion laws.

**Ref:**
1. American Association of Blood Banks, Association Bulletins #97/2 and #02-4
2. BCSH (British Committee for Standards in Hematology). Guidelines for the use of platelet transfusions. B J Haematol 2003;122:10–23
3. Goodnough LT, Brecher ME, Kantner MH et al. Transfusion medicine. N Engl J Med 1999;340:438–47, 525–33
4. Klein HG, Spahn DR, Carson JL. Red blood cell transfusion in clinical practice. Lancet 2007;370:415–26
5. Stroncek DF, Rebulla P. Platelet transfusions. Lancet 2007;370:427–38
6. Triulzi DJ. Blood Transfusion Therapy: A Physician's Handbook, 7th edn. AABB Bookstore, 2002
7. Wandt H, Ehninger G, Gallmeier WM. New strategies for prophylactic platelet transfusion in patients with hematologic diseases. The Oncologist 2001;6:446–50

**Web:**
1. http://www.aabb.org/                                          American Association of Blood Banks
2. http://www.bbts.org.uk/                                       British Blood Transfusion Society
3. http://www.ohsu.edu/pathology/transman/index.html            Transfusion Manual
4. http://www.who.int/bloodsafety/en/                           WHO Site on Blood Safety

## 4.9.2 Non-cellular Blood Products

**A. Leo, E. Leo, H. Bertz**

**Def:** *Specific replacement of individual blood components according to the patient's requirements ("targeted hemotherapy"):*
- Cellular blood products: packed red cells, platelet concentrate
- Non-cellular blood products: fresh frozen plasma (FFP), coagulation factors, immunoglobulins, human albumin
- Granulocyte transfusion: experimental therapeutic procedure (▶ Chap. 5.4)

All human blood products are:
- Classified as treatments for human application and their preparation, distribution, and use are safe-guarded by the pharmaceutical and transfusion laws
- Only available on prescription
- Liable for batch documentation (including albumin and recombinant coagulation factors)

### Fresh Frozen Plasma (FFP)

**Def:** Quarantine-stored or virus-inactivated fresh frozen plasma prepared from whole blood or collected by apheresis and stabilized with citrate.

**Meth:** ***Preparation and Storage***
After collection, fresh plasma from single-donor whole blood is frozen solid at a minimum of $-30°C$. Shelf-life 1–2 years. Release after at least 4 months quarantine and retesting of the donor for anti-HIV1/2, anti-HCV, HCV genome, and HBs antigen. Coagulation factor and inhibitor activity 0.6–1.4 E/ml.
Special type: virus-inactivated pooled plasma (e.g., solvent-detergent method).

**Ind:** ***Indication***
Thrombotic thrombocytopenic purpura (TTP; ▶ Chap. 6.3.3) with plasmapheresis

***Empiric Indications (not supported by clinical studies)***
- Complex hemostatic disorders (e.g., hemorrhage due to hepatic parenchymal damage)
- Consumption or dilution coagulopathy with extensive blood loss
- Factor V and factor XI deficiency (single factor concentrates not available)
- Exchange transfusions

***ATTENTION:*** Fresh frozen plasma should not be used for volume or protein replacement or parenteral nutrition.

**Ci:** ***Absolute Contraindication***
Patients with plasma incompatibilities, especially with IgA deficiency syndrome

***Relative Contraindications***
- Consumption coagulopathy with untreated underlying disease
- Hypervolemia

**Co:** ▶ Chap. 9.8

**Th:**    **Transfusion of Fresh Frozen Plasma: Procedure**

1. *Prerequisite for transfusion:* clear indication

2. *Patient information* / informed consent (signature)

3. *Defrosting and check*
   – Rapid defrosting at maximum 37°C
   – Inspect blood product for external damage
   – Plasma should be clear and free of precipitates

4. *Transfusion* immediately after thawing
   – Initiation under medical supervision
   – Use transfusion device with filter, rapid administration
   – Following transfusion, store bag in a cool place for 24 h for forensic purposes

5. *Dosage / transfusion response*
   – Rule of thumb: coagulation factor increase by approximately 1–2% per 1 ml FFP/kg → averag
     dosage: 12–15 ml FFP/kg body weight
   – In adults, initial administration of 3–4 units FFP is required to achieve clinical effect (equiva
     lent to 15–20 ml FFP/kg)
   – Factor V or XI substitution: target 15–20% of normal plasma level; note the biological half-lif
     of the coagulation factors
   – TTP: immediate treatment with FFP, daily replacement of 50 ml/kg FFP (preferably poole
     plasma or cryosupernatant) via therapeutic plasma exchange

6. *Batch documentation*

## Prothrombin Complex Concentrates (PPSB)

**Def:**    Coagulation factors of the prothrombin complex (factors II, VII, IX, and X), proteins C and S
plus heparin and ATIII

**Meth:**    *Preparation*
Obtained from cryoprecipitate-reduced plasma via ion-exchange chromatography; PPSB concen
trate is standardized for factor IX.

**Ind:**    Deficiency of coagulation factors listed above (hepatic failure, reversal of coumarin effect, etc.).

*ATTENTION:* Only use PPSB if other therapeutic measures fail (e.g., administration of vitamin
or FFP).

**Ci:**    *Absolute Contraindications*
   • Disseminated intravascular coagulation (DIC; ▶ Chap. 6.5.5), except in cases of deficiency o
     coagulation factors contained in PPSB (factors II, VII, IX, X, proteins C and S)
   • Heparin-induced thrombocytopenia type II (HIT; ▶ Chap. 6.3.2)

**Th:**    *Dosage*
Rule of thumb for initial dose: initial dose (units) = body weight (kg) × desired factor increase (%
maintenance dose is lower (e.g., half the initial dose), depending on the half-life of the coagulatio
factors and desired minimum activity levels

**Co:**    ▶ Chap. 9.8

*ATTENTION:* PPSB may contain small residual quantities of activated coagulation factors whic
can be potentially thrombogenic. Therefore, PPSB should only be administered by physician
experienced in hemostaseology.

### Immunoglobulins

ef: Immunoglobulin-enriched preparations for intramuscular or intravenous injection. *ATTENTION:* specified route of administration must be strictly adhered to → different specification due to different methods of preparation.

Meth:
#### Preparation
- Intramuscular immunoglobulin preparations contain a minimum of 90% immunoglobulins with a protein concentration of 100–180 g/l
- Intravenous immunoglobulin preparations contain 85% IgG, 10% IgA, and 5% IgM
- Obtained from plasma pools of at least 1,000 individual donors → balanced antibody content

#### Preparations
- Immunoglobulin preparations with complete antibody spectrum
- Pepsin-treated preparations → loss of Fc-mediated functions (e.g., Fc receptor interaction and opsonization)
- Preparations for intramuscular or intravenous applications
- Specific hyperimmunoglobulins from selected donors → concentration of specific immunoglobulins approximately 10-fold higher than in normal preparations, due to higher initial titer (e.g., anti-D prophylaxis)

nd:
#### Indications for Immunoglobulin Administration
- Primary immune deficiencies (Bruton's agammaglobulinemia, severe combined immunodeficiency syndrome SCID, Wiskott-Aldrich syndrome, etc.)
- Clinically relevant antibody deficiency in malignant lymphomas, CLL, and multiple myeloma
- Neonates and infants with HIV
- Selected autoimmune diseases (ITP, Guillain-Barré syndrome, Kawasaki syndrome, myasthenia gravis, post-transfusional purpura)

There are also a number of controversial indications for immunoglobulins, e.g., sepsis in children and adults, multiple sclerosis, premature infants born before 32 weeks, lupus erythematosus, autoimmune hemolytic anemia, etc.

i:
#### Absolute Contraindication
IgA deficiency with known anti-IgA antibodies

#### Relative Contraindications
- Transient childhood hypogammaglobulinemia
- Simultaneous administration of immunoglobulins and live-attenuated vaccines (risk of decreased formation of active antibodies)

h:
#### Dosing
Dosage varies with indication; underdosing must be avoided

o: ► Chap. 9.8


### Human Albumin (HA)

Def: Human serum albumin

Meth:
#### Preparation
- Obtained from human pooled plasma via alcohol precipitation (Cohn)
- Available preparations: 5% and 20% solutions

**Phys:**        *Effects*
- Volume expansion: effective for several hours
- Colloid osmotic effect
- Transport function

**Ind:**        Massive blood loss, severe hypoalbuminemia, therapeutic plasma exchange. Use of HA for volume replacement, if non-protein preparations (e.g., crystalloids) are insufficient.

**Ci:**        Hypervolemia

**Co:**        ▶ Chap. 9.8

**Ref:**        1.    Farrugia A, Poulis P. Intravenous immunoglobulin: regulatory perspectives on use and supply. Transfus Med 2001;11:63–74

2.    Hellstern P, Halbmayer WM, Köhler M et al. Prothrombin complex concentrates: indications, contraindications and risks. Thromb Res 1999;95:S3–6

3.    Key NS. Coagulation factor concentrates. Lancet 2007;370:439–48

4.    Staudinger T, Frass M, Rintelen C et al. Influence of prothrombin complex concentrates on plasma coagulation in critically ill patients. Intensive Care Med 1999;25:1105–10

**Web:**        1.    http://www.med.unc.edu/isth                    International Society on Thrombosis and Haemostasis

# .10 Human Sperm Cryopreservation

## C. Keck, H.P. Zahradnik

**ef:** Prophylactic banking of human sperm in liquid nitrogen where male infertility is expected. Successful cryopreservation allows sperm to be used for attempts at assisted insemination at a later date, with the aim of inducing pregnancy.

**d:** Sperm banking is indicated in cases of:
- Fertility impairment due to chemotherapy or radiotherapy
- Sperm reserve prior to planned vasectomy
- Preservation of donor sperm for heterologous insemination

**ath:**
### Fertility Status of Oncology Patients
Approximately 40–70% of patients with malignancy show reduced ejaculate parameters (e.g., volume, viability) even before chemo- or radiotherapy. So far, the reasons for this fertility impairment are unknown. The extent of further reduction of testicular function by chemo- or radiotherapy depends on various factors:
- Disease stage, pretherapeutic fertility status
- Dosage and combination of chemotherapeutic drugs
- Type of radiotherapy (radiation field / fractionation / single and total dose)
- Individual vulnerability of the testicular parenchyma

**eth:**
### Sperm Preservation Guidelines
Prior to treatment, it is impossible to predict the exact extent of fertility impairment to be expected in the individual patient.

Therefore, *all male patients of reproductive age* should be informed about the possibility of sperm cryopreservation before starting antineoplastic treatment. This aspect is regularly neglected, especially with younger patients. The patient must be informed in detail about the procedure and expense of cryopreservation as well as options regarding the future use of the cryopreserved sperm and the medical, ethical, and legal aspects of the procedure.

### Procedure
- After a waiting period of 2–7 days, sperm is collected via masturbation
- Ejaculate analysis for quality assessment according to WHO guidelines (WHO 1992)
- Addition of cryoprotective medium
- Freezing, storage in liquid nitrogen at −196°C
- Optimum storage conditions allow the sperm to be stored indefinitely, without impairment of quality

### Processing of Cryopreserved Samples
- Samples are thawed to a temperature of 37°C and purified (if necessary)
- A pregnancy from cryopreserved sperm can only be achieved with the help of assisted reproductive techniques
- Treatment should be carried out at specialized centers experienced in the use of cryopreserved sperm

**Selection of commonly used assisted reproductive techniques**

*Sperm extraction*
- Microepididymal sperm extraction (MESE)
- Testicular sperm extraction (TESE)
- Percutaneous epididymal / testicular sperm extraction (PESE)

**Selection of commonly used assisted reproductive techniques** *(continued)*

*Fertilization and insemination*
- Intrauterine insemination (IUI)
- Gamete intrafallopian transfer (GIFT)
- Zygote intrafallopian transfer (ZIFT[a])
- Artificial insemination with donor sperm (AID)
- Subzonal injection of sperm (SUZI[a])
- Intracytoplasmic sperm injection (ICSI)
- In vitro fertilization (IVF)

[a] Rarely used technique, relevance declining

Before ascertaining the optimal technique for achieving a pregnancy for a particular couple, it is necessary to precisely evaluate the reproductive function of the female partner.
Techniques commonly used for insertion of cryopreserved sperm are IUI, IVF, and ICSI.

## Intrauterine Insemination (IUI)

### Technique
- Ovarian stimulation and ovulation induction
- Transcervical insertion of a fraction of selected sperm into the uterus at the time of ovulation

### Advantages
- Minimally invasive technique

### Disadvantages
- Compared with other techniques, low pregnancy rate (approximately 5–10% per treatment cycle)

## In Vitro Fertilization (IVF)

### Technique
- Ovarian stimulation and ovulation induction
- Ultrasound-guided transvaginal follicle aspiration, oocyte retrieval
- In vitro incubation of oocytes and sperm
- Transcervical intrauterine transfer of up to three 2- to 8-cell-stage embryos

### Advantages
- Pregnancy rate with cryopreserved sperm: 10–15%

### Disadvantages
- High level of stress for the female patient
- High costs (5–8 times more expensive than IUI)

## Intracytoplasmic Sperm Injection (ICSI)

### Technique
- Ovarian stimulation and ovulation induction
- Ultrasound-guided transvaginal follicle aspiration, oocyte retrieval
- Microscopic injection of a single sperm into oocyte cytoplasm
- Transcervical intrauterine transfer of up to three 2- to 8-cell-stage embryos

## Advantages
- Pregnancy rate with cryopreserved sperm: 20–30%

## Disadvantages
- High level of stress for the female patient
- High costs (10–15 times more expensive than IUI)

**Minimum andrological requirements and approximate pregnancy rates in common assisted reproductive techniques**

|  | IUI | IVF | ICSI |
|---|---|---|---|
| *Requirements* | | | |
| Sperm concentration | $> 5 \times 10^6$/ml | $1–5 \times 10^6$/ml | $1 \times 10^6$/ml |
| Sperm motility | > 40% | > 25% | 0–5% |
| Sperm morphology | > 20% | > 15% | 0–5% |
| *Pregnancy rate (per cycle)* | | | |
| Fresh sperm sample | 10–15% | 20–25% | 20–30% |
| Cryopreserved sperm sample | 5–10% | 10–15% | 20–30% |

*IUI* intrauterine insemination, *IVF* in vitro fertilization, *ICSI* intracytoplasmic sperm injection

### Risk of Malformation Due to Cryopreservation?
- So far, there is no evidence of an increased malformation rate in children of patients with malignancy compared with other groups.
- Insemination or in vitro fertilization techniques using both fresh or cryopreserved sperm have no significant bearing on the malformation rate in children. Current data on intracytoplasmic sperm injection do not suggest an increased risk of malformation either. However, due to the limited data available, final conclusions cannot yet be drawn.

### Perspectives
- *Infertility prophylaxis via medication:* stimulation or inhibition of gonad function prior to chemo- / radiotherapy; protective effect not yet established in clinical studies → use outside of clinical studies is obsolete
- *Autotransplantation:* possible extraction of gonad tissue prior to gonadotoxic therapeutic measures, autotransplantation of the cryopreserved tissue after completiton of treatment; so far, data from preclinical studies only

**ef:**

1. Anger JT, Gilbert BR, Goldstein M. Cryopreservation of sperm: indications, methods and results. J Urol 2003;170:1079–84
2. Crockin SL. Legal issues related to parenthood after cancer. J Natl Cancer Inst Monogr 2005;34:111–13
3. Lee SJ, Schover LR, Partridge AH et al. ASCO recommendations on fertility preservation in cancer patients. J Clin Oncol 2006;24:2917–31
4. Orwig KE, Schlatt S. Cryopreservation and transplantation of spermatogonia and testicular tissue for the preservation of male fertility. J Natl Cancer Inst Monogr 2005;34:51–6
5. Postovsky S, Lightman A, Aminpour D et al. Sperm cryopreservation in adolescents with newly diagnosed cancer. Med Pediatr Oncol 2003;40:355–9
6. Puschek E, Philip PA, Jeyendran RS. Male fertility preservation and cancer treatment. Cancer Treat Rev 2004;30:173–80
7. Wallace WH, Anderson RA, Irvine DS. Fertility preservation for young patients with cancer: who is at risk and what can be offered ? Lancet Oncol 2005;6:209–18

**Veb:**

1. http://www.givf.com/ — Genetics and IVF Institute
2. http://www.nci.nih.gov/cancertopics/pdq/supportivecare/ sexuality/HealthProfessional/page6 — NCI PDQ

## 4.11    Cryopreservation of Human Pronuclear Oocytes

### C. Keck, H.P. Zahradnik

**Def:**    Preservation of extracorporeally fertilized pronuclear oocytes (2-PN stage), i.e., before final fusion of the genetic information of oocyte and sperm. Successful cryopreservation allows completion of fertilization and transfer of the embryo into the uterus at a later stage.

**Ind:**
- Infertility prophylaxis in female cancer patients of reproductive age who have not yet completed family planning, before initiation of chemotherapy or radiotherapy
- Preservation of excess oocytes collected after ovarian stimulation for in vitro fertilization (IVF) in infertile couples

*ATTENTION:* legal aspects of oocyte preservation and in vitro fertilization, see national laws.

**Pphys:**    *Principles of Oocyte Cryopreservation in Female Cancer Patients*
Chemo- and radiotherapy in women of reproductive age affected by malignancies (e.g., breast cancer, Hodgkin's disease or non-Hodgkin's lymphomas) may cause premature reduction of ovarian function with early menopause and loss of reproductive ability.
The exact extent of individual fertility impairment as a result of chemo- or radiotherapy cannot be predicted but depends on various factors:
- Disease stage
- Dosage, type, and combination of chemotherapeutic drugs
- Type and dosage of radiotherapy
- Individual vulnerability of the ovarian tissue

**Meth:**    **Pronuclear Oocyte Preservation Technique**

*Ovarian Stimulation*
Prior to in vitro fertilization it is necessary to perform ovarian stimulation in order to achieve sufficient yield of mature oocytes → gonadotropin administration (FSH, LH) for 10–20 days and simultaneous pituitary suppression with GnRH analogs or GnRH antagonists.
- Increased serum estradiol concentrations → possible stimulation of receptor-positive breast cancer
- Ovarian hyperstimulation syndrome (in approximately 0.3% of patients): cystic enlargement of the ovaries, ascites, leukocytosis, transaminase increase, electrolyte imbalance

*Sampling and Cryopreservation of Pronuclear Oocytes*
- Ovulation induction via HCG administration (human chorionic gonadotropin) or GnRH
- Ultrasound-guided transvaginal follicle puncture and oocyte aspiration
- In vitro fertilization of the oocytes with sperm from the patient's partner
- In case of poor sperm quality, consider intracytoplasmic sperm injection (ICSI)
- Confirmation of successful fertilization of the oocyte via microscopic detection of 2 or more pronuclei approximately 18 h after in vitro insemination
- Addition of cryoprotective medium in special containers (plastic or glass ampoules)
- Freeze at −196°C, store in liquid nitrogen

*Processing of Cryopreserved Samples*
- Monitor female cycle to determine optimum time of transfer, possibly low-dose stimulation therapy to induce ovulation
- Gradual thawing of oocytes and washing out of cryoprotective medium
- Incubation of oocytes under controlled conditions until time of transfer
- Transcervical intrauterine transfer of maximum 3 embryos
- Possible luteal support with HCG or progesterone

## Recommended Approach to Female Cancer Patients of Reproductive Age

1. Inform patient about the possibility of oocyte cryopreservation.

2. Highlight the disadvantages of cryopreservation (delay in antineoplastic treatment by a minimum of 2–4 weeks).

3. Refer the patient and her partner to a center for reproductive medicine for further advice.

## Outcome of Cryopreservation

### Success Rate of Cryopreservation of Excess Oocytes after IVF or ICSI
- After freezing and thawing, 70–80% of oocytes are morphologically intact.
- Pregnancy rate between 10–20% per treatment cycle.
- The collection method for sperm used to fertilize the oocyte (ejaculate, epididymis, or testis) has no influence on the pregnancy rate.

### Factors Influencing the Pregnancy Rate after Transfer of Cryopreserved Oocytes
- Age of the patient
- Number and quality of transferred oocytes
- Endometrial receptivity

### Pregnancies after Transfer of Cryopreserved Pronuclear Oocytes
- Pregnancies resulting from IVF or ICSI with cryopreserved or freshly transferred embryos show no significant difference in perinatal mortality.
- The rate of malformation in children from pregnancies with cryopreserved embryos is not significantly higher than that of "normal" pregnancies (1% versus 3%, respectively).

### Perspectives
- *Evaluation of infertility prophylaxis* with new generations of GnRH analogs or GnRH antagonists.
- *Improvement of the outcome of cryopreservation of human unfertilized oocytes:* oocytes cryopreserved independent of the fertilization process and patient's current partner.
- *Ovarian tissue cryopreservation (autotransplantation):* in animal experiments, cryopreserved ovarian tissue was successfully autotransplanted after gonadotoxic radiotherapy.
- *Cultivation of fertilized oocytes up to the blastocyst stage* (i.e., day 5/6) → improved assessibility of preservation-induced cellular damage and selection of embryos prior to transfer resulting in improved pregnancy rates.

1. Falcone T, Bedaiwy MA. Fertility preservation and pregnancy outcome after malignancy. Curr Opin Obstet Gynecol 2005;17:21–6
2. Lee SJ, Schover LR, Partridge AH et al. ASCO recommendations on fertility preservation in cancer patients. J Clin Oncol 2006;24:2917–31
3. Patrizio P, Butts S, Caplan A. Ovarian tissue preservation and future fertility: emerging technologies and ethical considerations. J Natl Cancer Inst Monogr 2005;34:107–10
4. Practice Committee of the American Society for Reproductive Medicine. Ovarian tissue and oocyte cryopreservation. Fertil Steril 2004;82:933–8
5. Roberts JE, Oktay K. Fertility preservation: a comprehensive approach to the young woman with cancer. J Natl Cancer Inst Monogr 2005;34:57–9

1. http://www.givf.com/     Genetics and IVF Institute
2. http://www.nci.nih.gov/cancertopics/pdq/supportivecare/ sexuality/HealthProfessional/page6     NCI PDQ

## 4.12    Sexual Dysfunction

**U. Wetterauer, H. Henß**

**Def:**    Disturbances in female or male sexuality in connection with malignancy and/or antineoplastic treatment, including loss of libido and excitability (in men, erectile dysfunction), orgasmic inadequacy, and sexual dissatisfaction.

**Ep:**    Sexual dysfunction is a common occurrence in cancer patients. The incidence is dependent on gender, type of malignancy, and treatment. In the following groups, more than 50% of patients are affected:
- Breast cancer (especially after mastectomy)
- Tumors of the female reproductive organs (vagina / vulva / cervix / uterus / ovaries)
- Tumors of the male reproductive organs (prostate cancer, testicular tumors; especially after orchiectomy, prostatectomy)
- After surgery (e.g., retroperitoneum), chemo- or radiotherapy leading to diminished sexual function

Studies in oncology departments have shown > 50% of male and female patients wish to be told about possible effects of their disease and treatment on their sexuality.

**Pg:**    *Physical Causes*
- Reduced performance status due to underlying disease, fatigue
- Anatomical / postoperative damage to the sexual organs (mastectomy, vulvectomy, penile surgery, rectal surgery, prostatectomy)
- Postoperative pain, tumor-associated pain
- Painful cohabitation (tumor-associated / postoperative / treatment-associated)
- Tumor- or treatment-associated functional changes (e.g., dryness after radiotherapy)
- Side effects of drugs (analgesics, opioids, antidepressants, serotonin inhibitors, monoamine oxidase inhibitors, antiestrogens, antiandrogens)
- Tumor- or treatment-associated infertility (after radiotherapy, hysterectomy)

*Psychosocial Causes*
- Tumor diagnosis
- Feeling of unattractiveness (e.g., after mastectomy, patients with stoma)
- Tumor- or treatment-associated depressive disorders
- Fear of sexual failure
- Disease-associated conflicts within the partnership

**Class:**    Sexual dysfunction is generally categorized according to the specific phases of sexual interaction (Masters, Johnson, 1996).

| Disturbance | Sexual interaction phase |
| --- | --- |
| Sexual aversion | Approach |
| Inadequate arousal | Stimulation |
| Erectile dysfunction, vaginismus, painful intercourse (dyspareunia) | Coitus |
| Orgasmic inadequacy, anejaculation, retrograde ejaculation (into bladder) | Orgasm |
| Postorgasmic depression | Postorgasmic reaction |

**Dg:**    With sexual dysfunction, a combined psychosomatic and medical diagnostic approach is essential.

Of particular importance is an open approach to the subject of sexuality during consultation, e.g., by asking "Have you experienced any changes in your sexuality due to your illness?". This allows the patient to block ("No, not at all.") or gradually approach the subject ("Yes, but it is hard for me to talk about it.").

*GUIDELINE:* Appropriate counseling should always be offered, even though not all patients may request it or make use of it.

### Case History, Physical Examination
- Clinical symptoms, including sexuality before development of cancer
- Physical examination including genitalia

### Laboratory Tests
- Estrogen / androgen / gonadotropin levels

**d:**

Twenty-five to 30% of patients exhibit signs and symptoms of sexual dysfunction prior to cancer diagnosis, e.g., in connection with:
- Diabetes mellitus
- Hypertension
- Vascular abnormalities, arteriosclerosis
- Alcohol / nicotine abuse
- Neurological disorders, multiple sclerosis

**h:**

### Therapeutic Principles
The necessary therapeutic measures have to be decided upon on an individual basis. The patient and possibly his/her sexual partner should be involved in the decision-making process.

### Therapeutic Measures
- Psychological / psychotherapeutic care
- Local estrogen treatment in cases of dyspareunia and female genital atrophy
- Systemic estrogen or androgen replacement after ovariectomy or orchiectomy (▶ Chap. 3.3)
  *ATTENTION:* No hormonal replacement in breast cancer or prostate cancer
- Drug treatment of erectile dysfunction with phosphodiesterase-5 inhibitors, e.g., sildenafil, tadalafil, vardenafil
- Injection of alprostadil into the cavernous body of the penis (after radical prostatectomy)
- Plastic surgery after mastectomy / orchiectomy

**x:**

Prophylaxis of sexual dysfunction is of particular importance and includes:
- Prior to treatment, inform the patient in detail about possible sexual dysfunction
- Where infertility is expected: sperm / oocyte preservation (▶ Chaps. 4.10, 4.11)

**ef:**

1. Basson R, Schultz WW. Sexual sequelae of general medical disorders. Lancet 2007;369:409–24
2. Derogatis LR, Kourlesis SM. An approach to evaluation of sexual problems in the cancer patient. CA Cancer J Clin 1981;31:46–50
3. Hollenbeck BK, Dunn RL, Wei JT et al. Sexual health recovery after prostatectomy, external radiation, or brachytherapy for early stage breast cancer. Curr Urol Rep 2994;5:212–19
4. Kornblith AB, Ligibel J. Psychosocial and sexual functioning of survivors of breast cancer. Semin Oncol 2003;30:799–913
5. Lue TF. Erectile dysfunction. N Engl J Med 2000;342:1802–13
6. Wilmoth MC, Botchway P. Psychosexual implications of breast and gynecologic cancer. Cancer Invest 1999;17:631–6

**Veb:**

1. http://www.meb.uni-bonn.de/cancer.gov/CDR0000062859.html    Cancernet
2. http://cancernet.nci.nih.gov/cancertopics/pdq/supportivecare    Cancernet
3. http://www.cancerbackup.org.uk/info/sexuality.htm    CancerBACKUP

## 4.13     Physiotherapy and Sports Medicine

R. Schindler, S. Stobrawa, A. Schmid, U. Blattmann

**Def:**     Supportive treatment of cancer patients based on physical therapy and sports.

**Pg:**     Fatigue and reduced performance are common problems in patients with solid tumors or hematologic neoplasia. Mechanisms leading to reduced performance are:
- Effects of the underlying disease
- Treatment-associated effects (chemotherapy, radiotherapy, surgery, analgesics, hypnotic drugs etc.)
- Deliberate "protection" of the patient, lack of mobility
- Concomitant diseases (reduced pulmonary function, chronic cardiomyopathy, neurologic disorders)

**Vicious circle**

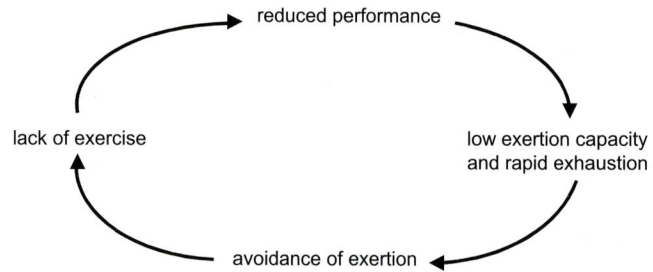

**Ind:**     Individual physiotherapy, sports medicine support, and endurance training may lead to improved performance and quality of life.
- *During hospital stay:* physical therapy including breathing / relaxation / exercise techniques individual or group sessions.
- *After completion of treatment:* e.g., after myeloablative chemotherapy and subsequent bone marrow or stem cell transplantation. Several clinical studies demonstrated a 30% performance increase in transplant patients after 6 weeks of medically supervised daily treadmill training.

### Physical Exercise in Cancer Long-Term Follow-Up
- The need for physical exercise has to be pointed out to the patient.
- Sports facilities may offer rehabilitation programs for cancer patients, e.g., after completion of chemotherapy and/or following resection of solid tumors (breast, larynx, intestine). Besides improving specific impaired functions (arm movement after radical mastectomy, respiratory gymnastics after pneumonectomy, etc.), the social and integrative aspects of sports activities are of particular importance.
- Provided there are no medical or orthopedic contraindications, patients can engage in all kinds of physical activity. The main emphasis should be on endurance training. The types of sports may be varied and training can be carried out several times a week.

**Ci:**     *In certain situations, physical exercise may be contraindicated or may need to be adjusted:*
- Nutritional deficiency, acute infections and/or fever, cardiac impairment
- Skeletal metastases
- Severe thrombocytopenia, anemia, or leukopenia

h:

## Therapeutic Concept

The right intensity of physical activity may lead to rapid improvement of both physical wellbeing and quality of life. An optimal training program must take into account changes in performance as well as the individual situation of each patient (reduced performance after chemotherapy, weakened muscles after bed rest, diminished mobility after surgery, etc.) as well as being creative and motivating.

Focal points of an integrated physiotherapy and sports medicine concept are:
- Physiotherapy breathing and relaxation techniques coupled with exercise
- Specific performance improvement via medically supervised endurance training, e.g., outdoor walking, cycling or ergometric training

Individual therapeutic concepts for each patient require interdisciplinary cooperation. Knowledge of diagnosis, current disease status, general condition, and blood count is important when planning physical therapy.

## Key Components of Physiotherapy

### Breathing Techniques
- Pneumonia prophylaxis and therapy
- Increase of respiratory depth and secretion clearance: active and passive
- Respiratory training
- Respiratory exercises to promote body consciousness and relaxation (aimed at active pain control)

### Relaxation Techniques
Aimed at promoting a psychophysical state of relaxation and pain control.
- Passive measures like massage, heat, bathing, passive movement techniques, etc.
- Positive body perception by concentrating on the body and picturing it → opportunity to experience the body in a positive light; use of progressive relaxation techniques by e.g., Jacobsen, Feldenkrais, Schaarschuch-Haase

### Exercise
- Mobility training: promotion of mobility and flexibility of passive and active joint structures, thromboembolic event prophylaxis, prevention of pressure sores
- Cardiovascular and endurance training: cardiovascular stimulation depending on the patient's condition, from various starting positions with or without special equipment, e.g., pedal exerciser, exercise bike, step home trainer, cross-trainer, treadmill
- "Weight training": maintenance and increase of the patient's physical strength by active training, possibly with the help of special equipment

### Group Therapy
In addition to individual training, patients can avail themselves of group physiotherapy. Working in a group promotes social contacts within the hospital, strengthens the patient's feeling of identity, and increases motivation.

## Criteria for Planning Individual Endurance Training Programs

### Duration of Training
- Physical performance can only be improved by using the major muscle groups rhythmically and persistently (20–30 min).
- It is recommended that exercise should be in intervals: 1–3 min of medium- to high-intensity exercise, followed by rest until complete recuperation. This method is also suitable for weaker patients who are unable to exercise for longer time periods at the beginning of their training program.

### Training Intensity

- In order to increase performance, the intensity of physical stress has to exceed a certain lim The intensity of most active and passive rehabilitation exercise programs in cancer follow-u lies well below this limit. Spontaneous daily activity requires only 30–50% of the maximu oxygen intake, which is insufficient for increasing performance. Passive treatments such balneotherapy, lymph drainage, and massage have no performance-increasing effect.
- Exercise bike or treadmill ergometry in the form of an incremental test measuring heart rat lactate concentrations, and oxygen uptake can be used to assess physical performance ar determine the appropriate intensity of training. In practice, training at 60–70% of the max mum performance level or $3 \pm 0.5$ mmol/l lactate concentration has proven effective. Ideall training should be controlled by continuous heart rate monitoring following these guideline Patients should experience training as being stimulating but not strenuous.

### Progression of Training

In order to achieve a continuous increase in performance, the level of training must be raise gradually, i.e., longer training periods or longer training intervals with the same rest periods ar higher training intensity according to the increase in performance. Training should not excee 1 h in total.

### Frequency of Training

Performance increase will be more pronounced and achieved faster, the more often training is ca ried out. Good results can be obtained with training at least 3 to 4 times a week for approximate 30–40 min.

### Type of Training

- Patient preference should be considered.
- Good results have been achieved with endurance training using an ergometer (e.g., exerci bike, treadmill, cross-trainer) or outdoor walking or cycling.
- Active sports such as ball games, team sports, or traumatic sports should be avoided.

**Ref:**

1. Dimeo F, Stieglitz RD, Novelli-Fischer U et al. Effects of physical activity on the fatigue and psychologic status of cancer patients during chemotherapy. Cancer 1999;85:2273–7
2. Knols R, Aaronson NK, Uebelhart D et al. Physical exercise in cancer patients during and after medical treatment. J Clin Oncol 2005;23:3830–42
3. McTiernan A. Physical activity after cancer: physiologic outcomes. Cancer Invest 2004;22:68–81
4. Meyerhardt JA, Heseltine D, Niedzwiecki D et al. Impact of physical activity on cancer recurrence and survival in patients with stage III colon cancer. J Clin Oncol 2006;24:3535–41
5. Stevinson C, Lawlor DA, Fox KR. Exercise interventions for cancer patients. Cancer Causes Control 2004;15:1035–56

**Web:**

1. http://www.apta.org                              Am Physical Therapy Assoc

## .14 Principles of Oncology Nursing Care

S. Rüter, K. Heeskens, H. Henß

**ef:**

Cancer patients require a high degree of nursing care. Nursing staff must have experience in handling infusion and cytostatic therapy as well as supportive medical care. In addition, cancer patients require specific psychological care, e.g., correct estimation of the level of psychological coping at the time of diagnosis or in palliative situations with the provision of appropriate levels of support. Furthermore, a professional approach with respect to closeness and distance as well as the ability to work as part of a comprehensive medical team are important requirements.

Relevant aspects of oncology nursing care:
1. Pancytopenia
2. Mucosal defects, esp. mucositis
3. Nausea and vomiting
4. Constipation and diarrhea
5. Pain
6. Dyspnea
7. Palliative situations / terminal care

### 1. Patients with Pancytopenia

**ef:**

Chemo- or radiotherapy-induced neutropenia (leukocytes < 1,000/µl or granulocytes < 500/µl), thrombocytopenia (< 100,000/µl) and anemia (Hb < 10 g/dl).

### 1a. Neutropenia

**x:**

Objective: reduction of risk factors for infection
- Regular disinfection of hands (staff and visitors), medical equipment (such as stethoscopes, etc.), daily disinfection of surfaces
- Rooms with en-suite facilities
- Change bed linen every 3 days
- Prevention of exogenous infections (avoidance of sick visitors, awareness of *Aspergillus* contamination in connection with building work, etc.)
- Limitation of invasive procedures (e.g., injections)
- Thorough daily washing of the patient, daily fresh clothing
- Personal hygiene after every bowel movement
- With indwelling intravenous lines, regular changes of dressing
- Thorough oral hygiene (see Section 2)
- "Low-germ foods", i.e., boiled or packaged foods only, no salads or fresh fruit, no mold cheese or cream cheese, discard open drinks after 24 h

**g:**

Objective: early detection of infections
- Regular assessment of vital signs (at least twice a day, avoid taking rectal temperature)
- Regular checking of skin (skin folds) and mucous membranes for signs of infection

### 1b. Thrombocytopenia

**x:**

Objective: prevention and detection of internal / external hemorrhage
- Avoid wet shaving
- Careful when cutting nails
- Avoid suppositories
- Avoid undue physical strain
- Caution with cooling compresses around the calves or use of ice

- Use soft toothbrush
- Twice-daily nose care, gentle nose blowing only
- Watch out for hematuria and blood in feces
- Check skin at least twice a day for petechial bleeding (entire body)
- In case of impaired vision / dizziness: consider brain hemorrhage

**Th:**      *Nose Bleed / Epistaxis (Common)*
- Move patient into an upright position with legs down (reduces blood pressure in nasal vessels)
- Apply ice to back of neck (contraction of mucous membrane blood vessels)
- Compress vessels by firmly pinching the soft part of the nostril together with thumb and index finger
- Possibly apply adrenaline-containing cream (additional contraction stimulation)
- If bleeding persists: tamponade (ENT specialist)
- Possibly thrombocyte transfusion (monitoring, allergic reactions)

## 1c. Anemia

**Sy:**      Fatigue, decrease in performance, dyspnea, palpitations, tachycardia

**Th:**      Patients need to be carefully monitored and instructed. The level of activity should be adjusted according to the patient's general condition. Packed red cell transfusions must be closely monitored (allergic reaction). If indicated, erythropoietin / darbepoetin treatment (▶ Chap. 4.3).

## 2. Patients with Mucous Membrane Lesions

**Pg:**      1. Direct toxicity of chemo- and/or radiotherapy
2. GVHD after allogeneic bone marrow transplantation
3. Poor general condition in terminal phase

The most common mucous membrane lesion—mucositis / esophagitis—occurs in approximately 40% of chemotherapy patients after 5–7 days.

**Px:**      Good oral and dental hygiene, local disinfection with fresh sage tea at least 3 times daily, nicotine and alcohol abstinence.

**Class:**   **Stages of Oral Mucositis (WHO)**

| Stage | Definition |
| --- | --- |
| 0 | Rosy moist oral mucosa, no abnormalities, no pain |
| 1 | Redness (erythema), swelling, mild soreness |
| 2 | Erythema, painful ulcers of the mucous membrane, patient can swallow solid diet |
| 3 | Extensive erythema, ulcers, patient can only swallow liquids |
| 4 | No oral alimentation possible, patient cannot swallow |

**Th:**      Nursing patients with mucositis / esophagitis
- Precise documentation of disease progression and measures taken
- Care must be constantly adjusted to the stage of the disease
- *Stage 0–4:* disinfecting oral irrigation, see "Prophylaxis"
- *From stage 1:* remove films and crusts (ideal microbial environment), take smears to test for oral candidiasis and herpes

- *From stage 2:* ulceration treatment. Local treatment with povidone iodine applied with cotton buds; with advanced mucositis or with patients having difficulty opening their mouth: oral irrigation 1:10 (stage tea in distilled water) at least 4 times daily
- *Pain control:*
  - Application of local anesthetics, 15 min before eating or wound treatment; in addition, anesthetic lozenges and ice cubes (to suck)
  - From stage 2, systemic analgesics may be indicated (e.g., piritramide via syringe pump)
- *Oral intake:* maintain oral nutrition as long as possible, take into consideration patients' requests (possibly pureed food), avoid irritants (hot spices), bear parenteral nutrition in mind
- *Herpes infection:* inform physician immediately, apply acyclovir cream to lips, take smear; in case of neutropenia: acyclovir i.v.
- *Fungus prophylaxis:* 4 times daily, after completion of oral hygiene, 1 pipette of amphotericin B suspension is spread around the mouth for 1 min and then swallowed

### 3. Patients with Nausea and Vomiting

Nausea and vomiting are a common occurrence in cancer patients with negative effects on quality of life.

**Pg:**
- Cytostatic treatment and/or radiotherapy
- Tumor-related nausea and vomiting (e.g., CNS or gastrointestinal tumors)

The nursing staff must have good comprehension of the emetogenic potential of cytostatic drugs (▶ Chap. 4.1). Thorough information for each individual patient about chemotherapy, expected side effects, and planned antiemetic measures is of major importance.

**Th:**
Principles of care:
- Allow bedridden patients to sit upright (as much as possible)
- Ensure comfortable room temperature
- Avoid noisiness
- Remove dentures
- After vomiting, offer mouth washes, hand and face refreshing, ensure peace and quiet
- Pain control (retching and vomiting → pain threshold ↓)
- Ensure antiemetics are given at the correct time before meals
- Impart a feeling of calm and not being rushed, calm the patient, remain at the bedside, do not leave patient to deal with the situation alone

### 4. Patients with Constipation and Diarrhea

**Def:**
Constipation: < 3 bowel movements per week
Diarrhea: > 3 bowel movements per day
Both are symptoms of abnormal bowel function and are a common occurrence in cancer patients.

#### Constipation

**Pg:**
- Mechanical interference (tumor compression)
- Caused by cytostatic therapy (vinca alkaloids, high-dose AraC)
- Drug-induced: e.g., opioids or antidepressants
- Psychological influences: depression, missing privacy
- Pains around anal area, e.g., fissures or hemorrhoids
- Immobility
- Dehydration

**Th:**
- Documentation of patient's bowel movements
- Explore underlying causes (in collaboration with physician)
- Increase fluid supply

- Administration of laxatives according to instructions
- Support mobility (physiotherapy)
- With vinca alkaloid treatment, simultaneous administration of mild laxatives, e.g., lactulose 1–3 times daily (ileus prophylaxis)

### Diarrhea

**Pg:**
- Chemotherapy-induced diarrhea
- Bacterial infections (esp. with neutropenia, *Clostridium difficile* colitis)
- Drug-induced: antibiotics, laxatives, analgesics (NSAIDs)
- GVHD-induced (Graft-versus-Host-Disease)
- Malabsorption, nervousness (stress)

**Th:**
- Close monitoring of frequency, volume, consistency, color, and added substances
- Laboratory fecal analyses (germs, blood, etc.)
- Possibly balancing of input and output
- Ensure meticulous anal hygiene and monitor skin (fissures, abscesses, eczema)
- Sufficient fluid supply (oral and i.v.)
- Nutrient and vitamin supplementation
- Enteral nutrition support
- Drug treatment
- Local pain control (anesthetic creams)

## 5. Patients with Pain

Fifty to 80% of cancer patients experience pain in the course of their disease. In addition, psychological factors can play an important role, so that caring for these patients remains a challenge. Most important tasks:
- Continuous pain monitoring and documentation (in cooperation with the patient, using pain scales /visual analog scales)
- Accurate administration of analgesics
- Nursing staff should reassure patients that their pain is being taken seriously; trust can positively influence the efficacy of pain control treatment
- Tranquility, relaxation, time for conversations, and distraction are valuable additional means of pain control

Nursing staff must have basic knowledge of pain management (▶ Chap. 4.5).

## 6. Patients with Dyspnea

**Def:**
Subjective dyspnea is often not in line with objectively readable measurements (e.g., blood gas analysis). Dyspnea may be difficult to assess for nursing staff and physicians.

**Sy:**
Varying from shortness of breath in conjunction with physical activity (stress dyspnea) to severe breathlessness during rest (orthopnea).

**Th:**
- Monitor respiration (respiratory frequency, depth, rhythm)
- Adopt a sensitive and calm approach to the patient and his/her family, anxiety can often contribute to dyspnea
- Help patient into a comfortable position
- Administration of oxygen
- Drug treatment (e.g., blood transfusion with anemia, tranquilizers)
- Involve physiotherapists for practice of respiratory techniques

## 7. Patients in Palliative Care / Terminal Disease Settings

One of the most important challenges of oncological care is nursing and supporting terminally ill patients.

Confrontation with finiteness, suffering and dying, despair and hopelessness must be endured and coped with (exchange amongst the care team is of vital importance).

Furthermore, despite increasing demands in the workplace, staff have to find the time and calmness to care for and individually support the patient and his/her entire family.

In the final stage, the wishes and needs of the dying take absolute priority.

**Ref:**
1. Keefe DM, Schubert MM, Elting LS et al. Updated clinical practice guidelines for prevention and treatment of mucositis. Cancer 2007;109:820–31
2. Stevenson J, Abernethy P A, Miller C, Currow DC. Managing comorbidities in patients at the end of life. BMJ 2004;329;909–12

**Web:**
1. http://www.ons.org      Oncology Nursing Society
2. http://www.harcourt-international.com/journals/ejon/      European Journal of Oncology Nursing

## 4.15    Psycho-oncological Care

**T. Gölz, B. Stein, A. Wünsch**

**Def:**   Cancer changes the lives of those affected by it in a physical, psychological, and social way. Patients experience distress related to both the malignancy and its treatment throughout the course of the disease. Considerable adjustment of the patient and his/her significant others is required in each stage of the disease, such as diagnosis, initiation of chemotherapy, cessation of therapeutic intervention, release, relapse, or the process of dying. Psycho-oncological care can support patients and their relatives to cope with different sources of distress. Psycho-oncological treatment is of particular importance for patients with pre-existing psychiatric disorders which affect the process of coping with cancer.

**Path:**   ### Psychological Stress

Depending on the stage of the disease, patients have to cope with the following factors of distress
- Latent and manifest threat to life
- Reduced physical, psychological, and social functioning and performance
- Loss of physical integrity
- Hospitalization, separation from significant others and familiar social contacts
- Professional and economic changes
- Pain
- Dependency on the medical system

### Psychological Reactions

The initial shock of being diagnosed with cancer is often followed by a phase of emotional instability, anxiety or depression, sometimes aggression or complete denial. These reactions are part of the process of coping with the disease. However, insufficient coping and its consequences can lead to temporary or permanent maladjustment and psychological disorders.
    In the coping process the following psychological reactions might occur:
- Existential problems accompanied by anxiety, depression, aggression, emotional instability, increased irritability, or suicidal tendency
- Problems regarding self-esteem and identity, such as reduced self-esteem or loss of self-confidence
- Decreased neuropsychological and cognitive functioning, e.g., lack of concentration
- Problems in partnership and family
- Sexual dysfunction (► Chap. 4.12)
- Poor compliance with medical treatment and recommendations
- Loss of ability to work with the consequence of financial problems, altered social status, and change of social roles
- Reduced social contacts and leisure activities

More than half of all oncological patients develop clinically relevant psychological symptoms during their course of treatment, mostly signs of anxiety or depression. Suicide risk is usually not increased, but should not be underestimated. Psychological treatment is indicated in approximately one third of patients.

### Need for Psycho-oncological Treatment

The need for support is increased in disease-related critical situations, such as disclosing diagnosis and prognosis, acute disease-related crises, relapse, therapy-induced dysfunction, or shift to palliative treatment. When planning and implementing psycho-oncological treatment, it is important to realize that psychological reactions can be an effort to cope with the situation, and do not have to be symptoms of a psychological disorder. Psycho-oncological treatment is necessary when patients ask for help or develop an acute stress reaction, depression, anxiety disorder, an adjustment disorder, or react with non-compliance and disturbed patient–physician interaction patterns.

Psychosocial risk factors for maladjustment or mental disorders in cancer patients are:
- Psychosomatic or psychiatric comorbidity
- Poor emotional status such as depressive or aggressive mood
- Suicidality, suicidal ideation or previous attempted suicide
- Chronic disease in family history
- Recent experiences of loss (e.g., death of partner, divorce)
- Substance abuse or addiction in the past
- Refusal of treatment or non-compliance
- Strong denial
- Poorly controlled pain
- Lack of social support (social isolation, unstable relationships, family crises, etc.)
- Socioeconomic crises e.g., unemployment, early retirement

**Th:**

## Psychological Interventions

Psycho-oncological care includes the support of patients as well as of their significant others. Psycho-oncological interventions focus on the reduction of symptoms of maladjustment and on improvement of quality of life despite physical problems.

### Individual Therapy

The most common form of psycho-oncological treatment is a flexible patient-oriented approach focusing on the current crisis situation. Important issues in that situation are usually emotional problems such as anxiety, depression, and aggression, often accompanied by thoughts about dying, self-esteem or identity crises, and compliance problems. The activation of resources is important to support the coping process.

In case of premorbid psychiatric disorders and biographical conflicts, the focus will be on coping with the current situation rather than treating the primary psychiatric disorder.

### Systemic Therapy / Approach: Considering Family and Significant Others

Cancer not only affects individuals; patients have partners, children, parents, and friends (significant others). Often, they are severely affected by the fact that their loved one is seriously ill, and need to cope with multiple factors of distress. Significant others might have strong sympathy with the patient and may experience intense feelings of hope, sadness, helplessness, anxiety, or desperation facing impending loss. They have to manage everyday life when the patient is in hospital, perhaps have to rearrange social roles and deal with socioeconomic changes. Therefore, about 30% of significant others need psychological support.

Often, patient and significant others try to protect each other against negative feelings; talking about them becomes a taboo and patients as well as significant others may feel isolated. Many adults do not know how to deal with the needs of children in this particular situation. Couple- and family-therapeutic interventions support the entire family system. Key aims are to stimulate emotional and meaningful communication between spouses, family members, or friends, and to activate resources for collective disease management. In case of severe adjustment problems individual therapy for significant others may be indicated. Additionally, systemic interventions may also be helpful for the therapeutic team, such as coaching or supervision.

### Focused Group Therapy

Psycho-oncological groups are aimed at promoting communication between patients in a similar situation to gain relief from emotional distress and to reduce social isolation or withdrawal. Within the group, similar experiences are shared and patients can benefit from each other's experiences and coping strategies. It can be helpful to introduce topics for discussion and reflection, e.g., coping with the initial diagnosis, relapses or treatment associated side effects, body consciousness, and partnership.

## Psychological Intervention Techniques

The choice of psychological intervention technique should depend on the problem and match the personality and specific requirements of the patient and his/her significant others. Techniques which focus on the patient's intrapsychological processes may be combined with more symptom-oriented behavioral techniques.

### Supportive Techniques

As for all psychological treatment a therapeutic alliance is required to support the patient, based on a therapist's attitude of acceptance and appreciation. Therefore, it is important to recognize prevailing coping strategies such as repression, regression, or rationalization as ways of adapting to the situation. The stabilizing effect of the therapeutic alliance is enhanced by techniques of empathizing with the patient's frame of reference and paraphrasing and verbalization of emotional experiences. The patient is encouraged to talk about negative thoughts and emotions to experience feelings of relief. Furthermore, intrapsychological and interpersonal resources are focused. Supportive techniques are commonly applied in crisis intervention, after the initial shock, and for the care of the dying.

### Symptom-oriented Techniques

Symptom-oriented techniques focus on behavior, thoughts, and emotions and are therefore more structured and directive. This approach is indicated in cases of anxiety, depression, sleeplessness, negative automatic thoughts, agitation, therapy-associated side effects, and pain. Commonly used techniques include a variety of cognitive-behavioral interventions, e.g., cognitive restructuring, as well as relaxation techniques, e.g., progressive muscle relaxation, autogenic training, or visualization exercises. Hypnotherapeutic interventions can be helpful to manage pain and nausea as well as to activate resources. It is recommended to apply psychoeducative techniques from an early treatment stage on, giving information about the illness, treatment procedures, and side effects. An informed patient can deal better with anxiety and is more compliant with the medical treatment.

**Ref:**

1. Faller H, Bülzebruck H. Coping and survival in lung cancer: a 10-year follow-up- Am J Psychiatry 2002;159:2105–7
2. Fawzy FI, Fawzy NW. A structured psychoeducational intervention for cancer patients. Gen Hosp Psychiatry 1994;16:149–92
3. Fritzsche K, Stein B, Herzog T et al. Psychosocial care of oncological in-patients. An empirical study of psychiatric and psychosomatic consultation services. Onkologie 1998;21:150–5
4. Greer S, Moorey S, Baruch JD, Watson M, Robertson BM, Mason A, Rowden L, Law MG, Bliss JM. Adjuvant psychological therapy for patients with cancer: a prospective randomised trial. Br Med J 1992;304:675–80
5. Jenkins V, Fallowfield L, Saul J. Information need of patients with cancer: results from a large study in UK cancer centres. Br J Cancer 2001;84:48–51
6. Kendall WS. Suicide and cancer: a gender-comparative study. Ann Oncol 2007;18:381–7

**Web:**

1. http://www.dapo-ev.de          German Association of Psychosocial-oncology
2. http://www.ipos-society.org/    International Psychooncology Society
3. www.psycho-oncology.net        International Directory of Psycho-oncology Programs

**4.16    Rehabilitation**

G. Adam, C. Zeller

**Def:**    Oncological rehabilitation entails not only the recovery from existing dysfunction but also prevention of future functional disorders. Key priority is the improvement of quality of life, rather than the successful restoration of gainful employment.

Basic requirements for provision of medical rehabilitation benefits:
- *Rehabilitation capacity:* rehabilitation capacity is given when a patient is mobilized and ready for an effective rehabilitation process.
- *Need for rehabilitation*
- *Willingness to rehabilitate:* requires the patient to be motivated as well as mentally and psychologically able to actively participate in the rehabilitation process.

The rehabilitation prognosis depends on the likelihood of the aspired goal being achieved.

### Access to Rehabilitation

As a prerequisite for using inpatient or outpatient rehabilitation services, funding must be secured, e.g., in the form of a comprehensive insurance.

**Dg:**    ## Diagnostic Guidelines in Oncological Rehabilitation

For adequate planning and conduct of oncological rehabilitation, complete tumor documentation (including previous treatments and course of disease) is necessary. Documentation requirements include:
- Primary diagnosis
- Tumor location and stage (e.g., TNM, FIGO, Ann Arbor, FAB)
- Previous treatment (surgery, chemotherapy, radiotherapy, supportive therapy, others)
- Treatment progress and current remission status

In accordance with the WHO concept of functional health, the International Classification of Functioning, Disability and Health (ICF) documents restrictions in:
- Physical function and structures, including mental funtioning
- Participation in all aspects of daily living. The object of full reconstitution of these daily activities defines the rehabilitation goal and the treatment concept

### Function-oriented Diagnosis

#### Somatic Dysfunction
- Reduced performance and degree of mobilization and mobility (ergometry, pulmonary function, neutral zero method etc.)
- Lymphedema (circumference measurement, etc.)
- Fatigue syndrome
- Pain (quality and quantity, e.g., visual analog scales)
- Dietary and digestive dysfunction

#### Psychological Disorders
- Acute stress
- Coping, information status, compliance
- Quality of life, e.g., EORTC questionnaire QLQ-C30
- Social contact

#### Indication-specific Diagnosis
- Disease-related impairment
- Diagnosis of relapse and emergency situations by qualified staff

- Additional diagnostic procedures depending on indication
- Awareness of possible diagnosis-related psychological effects

### Social Assessment

- Impact on professional life and reintegration
- Impact on everyday life and care requirements
- Social report after completion of rehabilitation, taking into account diagnosis, prognosis, rehabilitation progress, and rehabilitation outcome

**Th:**     ## Goals and Therapeutic Concepts of Oncological Rehabilitation

Besides the consequences of cancer and the long-term effects of therapeutic intervention, previous disabilities and illnesses must also be taken into account when establishing a therapeutic concept. The individual treatment approach with therapeutic measures and complementary information (e.g., talks, seminars) pursues three main goals:

- Somatic stabilization, e.g., physical and drug therapy
- Cognitive and emotional processing and coping with the illness as well as reorientation
- Mobilization of resources beneficial for active health promotion, including independence and personal responsibility, initiative, and participation in the process of health maintenance and healing

### Physicians

- Treatment planning, follow-up, and documentation
- Drug therapy: pain control, adjuvant and palliative chemotherapy, immunotherapy, cytokines, blood products
- Therapeutic continuity in agreement with primary and secondary healthcare institutions
- Advice, information, tertiary prevention

### Psychological Intervention (▶ Chap. 4.15)

- Support in coping with the disease
- Individual and group therapy offering advice on loss of physical integrity, sexual dysfunction, fear of relapse, partnership problems
- Relaxation techniques
- Promotion of a positive outlook, reorientation in everyday life
- Complementary art therapy, music therapy, ergotherapy

### Physiotherapy

- Mobilization, improvement of mobility, muscular exercises
- Promotion of physical strength and stamina
- Pain reduction (scars, polyneuropathy, musculoskeletal symptoms, etc.)
- Lymph drainage, lymphedema treatment
- Respiratory therapy
- Incontinence training

### Speech Therapy

- Treatment of disease- or therapy-induced motor or neurogenic aphasic disorders
- Voice rehabilitation in laryngectomy patients

### Oncological Nursing Care

- Information and training in relation to prostheses, incontinence aids
- Stoma therapy, ileo- / colo- / urostoma, tracheostoma
- Self-injection of drugs, introduction to pain management via infusion pumps
- Management of port catheters, enteral tubes

### Dietary Treatment

- With all forms of eating disorders, dietary treatment and advice according to guidelines of Nutritional Societies

- Adjustment to disease- or therapy-associated gastrointestinal dysfunction, e.g., postgastrectomy syndrome, small-bowel syndrome
- Energy supplementation
- With immunosuppressed patients, avoid foods that increase infection risk

### Professional Life
- Advice from career counselors or social services, support when returning to professional life
- Professional rehabilitation measures

### Social Support
- Advice and support for all social, legal and financial questions, questions on legal regulations for the severely disabled, practical questions in relation to daily life
- Practical aids
- Home care
- Contacting of local social services (self-help groups, integrative care)

### Information, Training, Health Promotion
Informative, motivating, and educational talks and seminars, indication-based and with a global approach to the illness, aimed at:
- Conveying the basics for understanding the disease process
- Fostering the patient's personal responsibility
- Actively involving the patient in the process of coping with cancer
- Promoting healthy features and remaining functional reserves in terms of "positive adaptation" instead of focusing exclusively on the disease process

### Hospital Spiritual Guidance
Individual counseling, non-denominational spiritual support groups

### Indication-specific Rehabilitation Concepts
Individual disease entities require specifically structured therapy concepts, e.g., for patients with gynecological, gastrointestinal, urological tumors, lung, and head / neck tumors or hematological malignancies, especially after transplantation procedures.

## Rehabilitation Services: Quality Requirements

### Structural Requirements
- *Personnel:* sufficient numbers of professionally qualified staff; specialist medical care according to indication; established consultation system for other specialist areas
- *Premises:* rooms for individual and group therapy equipped for all types of physical and psychological treatment, art therapy, ergotherapy, social counseling, indoor pool; additional rooms for therapy-free periods and leisure
- *Technical equipment:* intensive surveillance system with ECG monitoring, central oxygen supply; facilities for infection prophylaxis by reverse isolation of immunosuppressed patients; emergency diagnostic equipment, drug monitoring, microbiology
- *Networking:* cooperation with tumor centers, specialist oncology hospitals

### Process Quality
Therapeutic strategies and concepts are indication-based and follow specific national guidelines. These are aimed at validating the treatment process, thus contributing to attainment of the therapy target and quality assurance. A minimum number of annual rehabilitation processes per specific indication is required.

### Quality Assurance
The following are suitable methods for assessment and optimization of oncological rehabilitation concepts and maintenance of high quality standards:
- Cooperation with scientific institutes dealing with rehabilitation to promote efficacy assessment in oncological rehabilitation, including catamnestic studies on long-term effects

- Use of validated measuring instruments for assessment of somatic and psychological effects
- Programs for quality assurance of pension insurances, e.g., peer review analysis of process quality
- Certification of rehabilitation clinics, e.g., EFQM

**Ref:**        1.    Cheville AL. Cancer rehabilitation. Semin Oncol 2005;32:219–24
       2.    World Health Organization (WHO) 2001. International Classification of Functioning, Disability and Health (ICF). WHO Publication, Geneva

**Web:**        1.    http://www.emedicine.com/pmr/topic226.htm          emedicine
       2.    http://www.northeastrehab.com/Programs/oncology.htm    Northeast Rehab Health Network

## 5.1 Hematopoetic Stem Cell Technology (Harvesting, Culture, Purging)

**B. Deschler, C.I. Müller, C. F. Waller, M. Engelhardt**

**Def:** **Stem Cells**

Hematopoetic stem cells are a small and predominantly dormant population of undifferentiated cells. They are characterized by the ability to self renew by continuous cell division and to differentiate into lymphoid, myeloid, erythroid, or megakaryocytic cells (▶ Chap. 1.3). Hematopoietic stem cells transplanted after radiotherapy radiotherapy (total body irradiation) and/or high-dose chemotherapy from autologous or allogeneic sources are subjected to intense proliferation and differentiation inside the recipient. The contribution of individual cell types to short- and long-term bone marrow recovery after transplantation has not been fully elucidated, however, stem cells are responsible for maintaining continuous hematopoiesis.

**Meth:** *Stem Cell Mobilization ("Stem Cell Harvest")*
Hematopoietic stem cells can be harvested by various methods:
- Leukapheresis → peripheral blood stem cells
- Bone marrow aspiration → bone marrow stem cells
- Placenta / umbilical cord blood harvest → umbilical cord blood stem cells
- Embryonic / mesenchymal stem cells

### Stem Cell Purging

**Def:** Removal of clonogenic neoplastic cells from a stem cell transplant product.

**Phys:** Tumor cell contamination of autologous stem cell preparations may limit curative potential of high-dose chemotherapy. The presence of malignant cells in stem cell transplants was shown in various diseases, via cytological, histological, immunocytological, and molecular analyses. The contribution of transfused tumor cells to the occurrence of relapse was demonstrated in gene marking studies. However, relapse rates with "purged" stem cell products have not been significantly reduced as compared to "unpurged" stem cells. Endogenous relapse, due to, e.g., insufficient elimination of malignant cells within the patient, occurring despite high-dose chemotherapy, appears to be of greater significance. The use of "purged" stem cell products is not recommended outside of clinical studies.

**Meth:** *Stem Cell Selection*
Reduction of tumor cells in the graft can be achieved in vivo (i.e., treatment of the donor) or ex vivo / in vitro (i.e., treatment of the harvested cell sample).

*"Positive Selection"*
Attempt to purify hematopoietic progenitor cells using specific surface markers, e.g., CD34 or AC133.
*NOTE:* This method is of limited use if malignant cells and stem cells express similar surface markers (e.g., CD34 on leukemia cells).

*"Negative Selection"*
Attempt to specifically eliminate tumor cells from the graft:
- In vitro use of monoclonal antibodies utilizing complement, immunotoxin, magnetic particles, or cytostatics (e.g., mafosfamide). *NOTE:* potential damage to healthy hematopoietic cells as well as malignant cells
- Experimental approaches: use of antisense oligonucleotides or specific tyrosine kinase inhibitors, in vitro differentiation induction in leukemias

### *"Ex Vivo Expansion"*

Purification attempt involving in vitro expansion of hematopoietic cells and inhibition of malignant clones. In CML, but also in solid tumors and multiple myeloma, enhancement of the growth of non-malignant progenitor cells has been demonstrated under certain conditions, achieving a significant reduction in the number of malignant cells.

The most efficient methods as well as the clinical relevance of stem cell purging for specific disease entities can only be established by randomized trials.

### Stem Cell Expansion

**Def:** In preclinical and clinical studies attempts have been made to grow ("expand") cultured stem cells (ex vivo) in order to provide new treatment options. While it is possible to increase cell numbers, relevant stem cell expansion has not been achieved yet. In addition, clinical studies did not demonstrate a significant cost / benefit advantage despite the option of tumor cell depletion.

#### *Possible Targets of Stem Cell Cultures*

The following potential areas of use are being evaluated in clinical studies:
- Removal of contaminated tumor cells from autologous stem cell grafts
- Gene transfer into repopulating stem cells to correct hereditary enzyme deficiencies or for gene marking analyses
- Expansion of stem cells and partially differentiated progenitor cells from a single stem cell harvest for repeated clinical use in sequential therapy or tandem transplantation
- Expansion of lineage-determined progenitor cells (e.g., myeloid or megakaryopoietic postprogenitor cells) to accelerate hematopoietic regeneration or for differentiation into antigen-presenting dendritic cells
- Expansion of bone marrow repopulating stem and progenitor cells from umbilical cord blood samples for transplantation in adult patients
- Cell support in allogeneic transplantation
- De-/redifferentiation into other organ-type cells ("stem cell plasticity")

**Meth:** *Prerequisites*
- Preparation laboratory (equipped according to national and international guidelines) which allows production of cultivated and gene-transfected cells according to standards
- Central filing of all protocols of studies concerned with somatic cell and gene therapy

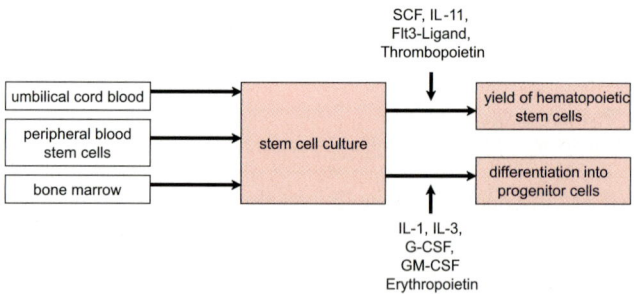

#### *Methods*
- Suspension culture using unseparated or CD34$^+$-separated stem cells (advantage of reduced culture volume).
- Addition of recombinant growth factors. Optimal cytokine combinations are currently being tested. Stem cell factor (SCF), FLT3 ligand, thrombopoietin, and IL-11 seem to preserve

and expand the undifferentiated stem cell population, while IL-3, IL-1, G-CSF, GM-CSF, and erythropoietin lead to expansion of differentiated cells.
- Suspension cultures (from peripheral or umbilical blood) require no serum.
- The duration of the cultivation period remains the limiting factor of suspension cultures: safe interval approximately 3–5 days, while stroma-containing cultures have led to successful hematopoietic reconstitution even after 12–14 days of culture.

### Quality Control
- Bacteriology, virology (EBV, CMV)
- Methyl cellulose culture assays for lineage-committed colony formation (CFU assay)
- Determination of progenitor cell/"stem cell" content, e.g., of CD34$^+$ cells or subsets (e.g., CD34$^+$/CD38$^-$ cells) via flow cytometric analysis

NOTE: Phenotypic determination of repopulating stem cells is not possible. After cultivation, there is no definite correlation between CD34 antigen expression or the frequency of in vitro colony-forming cells (CFC), long-term culture initiating cells (LTC-IC), and the number of repopulating stem cells.

### Storage
Cultivated cells are generally used immediately (without further storage). Successful cryopreservation (liquid N$_2$) has been described.

### Stem Cell Transfusion
After 3–5 days in suspension culture or 12–14 days in bone marrow culture, cells are administered in the form of filtered single cell suspensions, analog to fresh or cryopreserved stem cells. Cytokines are removed by centrifugation and washing of the cell suspension. Commonly, premedication with corticosteroids and antihistamines is administered.

1. Oakley EJ, Vant Zant G. Unraveling the complex regulation of stem cells: implications for aging and cancer. Leukemia 2007;21:612–21
2. Papayannapoulou T. Current mechanistic scenarios in hematopoietic stem/progenitor cell mobilization. Blood 2004;103:1580–5
3. Rocha V, Labopin M, Sanz G et al. Transplants of umbilical cord blood or bone marrow from unrelated donors in adults with acute leukemia. N Engl J Med 2004;351:2276–85
4. Sauvageau G, Iscove NN, Humphries RK. In vitro and in vivo expansion of hematopoietic stem cells. Oncogene 2004;23:7223–32
5. Siena S, Schiavo R, Pedrazzoli P et al. Therapeutic relevance of CD34$^+$ cell dose in blood cell transplantation for cancer therapy. J Clin Oncol 2000;18:1360–77
6. Sorrentino BP. Clinical strategies for expansion of haematopoietic stem cells. Nat Rev Immunol 2004;4:878–88
7. Weissman IL. Translating stem and progenitor cell biology to the clinic: barriers and opportunities. Science 2000;287:1442–6

1. http://stemcells.alphamedpress.org/     Stem Cells
2. http://www.marrow.org/     National Marrow Donor Program
3. http://www.bmtinfonet.org/     BMT InfoNet
4. http://stemcells.nih.gov/index.asp     NIH Stem Cell Info
5. http://stemcell.princeton.edu     Stem Cell Database

## 5.2    Autologous Hematopoetic Stem Cell Transplantation

**C.I. Müller, C.F. Waller, M. Lübbert, M. Engelhardt**

**Def:**    Hematological treatment aimed to accelerate bone marrow and blood reconstitution by use of autologous peripheral blood hematopoetic stem cells (PBSC) after intense (myeloablative) chemotherapy and / or radiotherapy (total body irradiation, TBI).

**Ep:**    In 2004, 22,216 autologous transplantations in Europe (EBMT)

**Phys:**    *Background*
The intensity of conventional chemotherapy is limited, in particular due to hematotoxcity (myelosupression) with neutropenia and thrombocytopenia. Dose-intensive myeloablative therapies require transplantation of hematopoietic stem cells from the patient (autologous transplantation) or a donor (allogeneic transplantation, ▶ Chap. 5.3).
- In early studies, hematopoietic stem cells (HSC) were obtained from the bone marrow by aspiration.
- Meanwhile, HSC are mainly harvested via blood cell separation (leukapheresis) after stimulation with colony-stimulating factors (CSF) and mobilization into the peripheral blood. Cells are cryopreserved and retransfused after high-dose therapy (peripheral blood stem cells transplantation, PBSCT).

In healthy donors (no stimulation with hematopoietic growth factors, i.e., steady-state conditions), HSCs are a rare population primarily located within the bone marrow. They do not circulate within the peripheral blood without mobilization.
- The number of circulating PBSC increases during the phase of hematopoietic reconstitution after conventional chemotherapy.
- The use of hematopoietic growth factors (e.g., granulocyte colony-stimulating factor, G-CSF) after conventional chemotherapy leads to a further increase and is used as a standard method for mobilizing and collecting PBSC.
- A sufficient PBSC yield is the prerequisite for high-dose chemotherapy with stem cell transplantation (PBSCT).

**Peripheral stem cell transplantation after high-dose chemotherapy**

*Hematopoietic Stem Cells or Progenitor Cells*
- Identification of hematopoietic progenitor cells by detection of CD34 antigen expression (1–4% of mononuclear cells in the bone marrow or mobilized blood are CD34-positive; however, recent data have shown the existence of CD34-negative hematopoietic stem cells, characterized by CD133, Thy-1, Oct-4, c-kit/CD117, SP phenotype).

- Over 90% of these cells are "committed progenitor cells" which have lost the ability to renew themselves. Only pluripotent stem cells hold this feature and have the potential for complete hematopoietic reconstitution (▶ Chap. 1.3).
- In mice, sufficient numbers of pluripotent stem cells for complete hematopoietic reconstitution can be attained with 100 highly purified cells. In humans after myeloablative chemotherapy (conditioning), $2-4 \times 10^6$ CD34-positive cells/kg body weight (BW) are regarded as sufficient. Optimal reconstitution of all cell lineages is achieved by transplantation of $\geq 4 \times 10^6$ CD34-positive cells/kg BW.

### Mobilization of Autologous PBSC

Patients who are candidates for high-dose chemotherapy with peripheral blood stem cell transplantation (PBSCT) should initially be treated with conventional chemotherapy in order to combine maximum clinical response with early PBSC mobilization and harvesting. Myelosuppression generated by PBSC mobilizing chemotherapy should ideally be brief (without affecting the stem cell compartment) and have a maximum effect on the underlying disease:

- So far, there is no optimal mobilization protocol which could be used for the entire range of cancer patients. Most commonly, cyclophosphamide is used to facilitate PBSC mobilization, e.g., in the VCP-E Protocol (Etoposide (VP16), Cyclophosphamide, Cisplatin, and Epirubicin ▶ Protocol 13.1.1) followed by administration of recombinant human G-CSF.
- Administration of rh G-CSF increases the number of circulating multipotent progenitor cells by factor 10. Maximum PBSC mobilization occurs concomitantly with an increase in neutrophil granulocytes after the leukocyte nadir has been passed.

**Meth:**

### Leukapheresis

PBSC are harvested as an outpatient procedure when the leukocyte count (WBC) is > 5,000–10,000/µl and CD34$^+$ cells are > 10–20/µl blood, using a standard cell separator ("leukapheresis"). The procedure is well tolerated. Possible electrolyte imbalances can be compensated.

- In patients without prior chemo- or radiotherapy, sufficient numbers of PBSC can usually be harvested with 1–2 leukaphereses.
- For reasons of quality control, volume, differential leukocyte count, percentage of CD34-positive cells, viability, and sterility of every stem cell apheresis sample must be determined.
- Leukapheresis PBSC may be further processed (e.g., CD34-positive or -negative selection ▶ Chap. 5.1) or directly preserved in liquid nitrogen (at −196°C). Cryopreserved cells can be stored for many years prior to transplantation.
- Both processing and storage of the cell samples are carried out under GMP conditions (Good Manufacturing Practice, EU GMP guidelines) in accordance with national laws.

**Ind:**

Randomized studies have shown high-dose chemotherapy to be advantageous in the treatment of high-grade (and indolent) non-Hodgkin's and Hodgkin's lymphoma compared with standard-dose chemotherapy. EBMT (European Group for Blood and Marrow Transplantation) has published guidelines for autologous stem cell transplantation as follows:

- In certain patient groups with high-grade non-Hodgkin's lymphomas (NHL), Hodgkin's disease, multiple myeloma, and chemosensitive relapses of germ cell tumors, high-dose chemotherapy with autologous transplantation is effective and regarded as standard of care.
- In solid tumors (e.g., sarcoma, breast cancer, or ovarian carcinoma), high-dose chemotherapy should only be carried out within clinical studies.
- High-dose chemotherapy with stem cell support has been proven to be a potentially effective treatment for various other malignancies. However, the clinical benefit as compared to standard treatment has to be established in randomized clinical trials for each individual disease entity.

**Recommendations on autologous hematopoietic stem cell transplantation in adults (EBMT, European Group for Blood and Marrow Transplantation)**

| Disease | | Disease Stage | Degree of recommendation |
|---|---|---|---|
| Leukemias | AML | 1st to 3rd CR, standard risk | Trials only |
| | | Relapse | Not recommended |
| | Secondary AML / MDS | – | Not recommended |
| | ALL | 1st or 2nd CR | Not recommended |
| | CML | Chronic phase | Not recommended |
| | | Acceleration, blast crisis | Not recommended |
| Lympho-proliferative diseases | NHL | Lymphoblastic (high risk) | Recommended |
| | | High grade: 2nd CR, PR, relapse | Recommended |
| | | Low grade: ≥ 1st CR, relapse | Trials only |
| | CLL | – | Trials only |
| | Multiple myeloma | Stage I | Trials only |
| | | Stage II–III | Recommended |
| | Hodgkin's disease | 1st CR | Trials only |
| | | ≥ 2nd CR, PR | Recommended |
| Solid tumors | Germ cell tumors | Chemosensitive relapse | Recommended |
| | | Refractory | Not recommended |
| | Sarcomas | Chemosensitive relapse / high risk | Trials only |
| | Breast cancer | Adjuvant, high risk | Trials only |
| | | Metastatic | Not recommended |
| | Ovarian carcinoma | Minimal residual disease | Trials only |
| | | Refractory | Not recommended |
| Autoimmune diseases | Progressive sclerosis | | Trials only |
| | Multiple sclerosis | | Trials only |
| | SLE | | Trials only |
| | Amyloidosis | | Trials only |

*AML* acute myeloid leukemia, *MDS* myelodysplastic syndrome, *ALL* acute lymphatic leukemia, *CML* chronic myeloid leukemia, *CLL* chronic lymphatic leukemia, *NHL* non-Hodgkin's lymphoma, *SLE* systemic lupus erythematosus, *CR* complete remission, *PR* partial remission

Co: Transplantation-associated mortality is 1–5%, depending on comorbidity factors and age of the patient. Normally, patients are discharged from hospital approximately 2–3 weeks after autologous PBSC transplantation.

### Acute Complications
- *Bone marrow aplasia:* high-dose chemotherapy causes bone marrow aplasia, which is overcome within approximately 10 (granulocytes) to 14 days (thrombocytes) after autologous PBSC transplantation. Infections and hemorrhage may occur within this period, and most

patients require antibiotics and blood products for 4–8 days. Fungal infections are rare. Viral infections may occur due to reactivation (HSV, VZV, rarely CMV).

- *Gastrointestinal toxicity:* oropharyngeal mucositis, gastroenteritis
- *Pulmonary toxicity:* with use of certain cytostatics (e.g., busulfan, cyclophosphamide, thiotepa, BCNU), inflammatory changes (fibrosis, alveolar hemorrhage, infection), pulmonary edema, pulmonary damage, and "acute respiratory distress syndrome" (ARDS)
- *Cardiotoxicity:* cardiac damage due to cytostatics, e.g., cyclophosphamide (cardiac insufficiency, transmural hemorrhagic myocardial necrosis), anthracyclines (acute and chronic cardiotoxicity); cardiac complications may be intensified in cases of preceding radiotherapy or anthracycline treatment
- *Renal dysfunction:* renal insufficiency or acute renal failure due to cytostatic drugs, antibiotic treatment with aminoglycosides, insufficient hydration during treatment, tumor lysis, and blood pressure fluctuations; renal insufficiency is usually reversible
- *Hepatic dysfunction:* besides fully reversible short-term increases in hepatic enzymes, rare occurrences of veno-occlusive disease (VOD)

### Long-term Side Effects and Recommendations for Follow-Up
- *Secondary malignancies:* particularly after high-dose chemotherapy with alkylating agents and after total body irradiation (TBI); the likelihood of secondary malignancies occurring after 15 years is up to 6% in conditioning protocols without TBI and up to 20% in protocols with TBI
- *Immunologic dysfunction:* monitoring of infections (CMV, VZV, *Pneumocystis carinii* pneumonia)
- *Vaccinations:* pneumococci, influenza, tetanus, diphtheria
- *Endocrine dysfunction:* monitoring of thyroid function, ovaries, testes, osteoporosis

Th:

### Therapy Protocols: Mobilization

| "VCP(E)" ▶ Protocol 13.1.1 | | | |
|---|---|---|---|
| Etoposide phosphate | 500 mg/m²/day | i.v. | Day 1, infusion 1 h |
| Cyclophosphamide | 1350 mg/m²/day | i.v. | Day 1, infusion 1 h |
| Cisplatin | 50 mg/m²/day | i.v. | Day 1, infusion 1 h |
| Epirubicin | 50 mg/m²/day | i.v. | Day 1, bolus injection |
| Before leukapheresis: G-CSF 5 µg/kg daily s.c., from day 5 | | | |

| "VIP(E)" ▶ Protocol 13.1.2 | | | |
|---|---|---|---|
| Etoposide phosphate | 500 mg/m²/day | i.v. | Day 1, infusion 1 h |
| Ifosfamide | 4000 mg/m²/day | i.v. | Day 1, infusion 18 h |
| Cisplatin | 50 mg/m²/day | i.v. | Day 1, infusion 1 h |
| Epirubicin | 50 mg/m²/day | i.v. | Day 1, bolus injection |
| Before leukapheresis: G-CSF 5 µg/kg daily s.c., from day 5 | | | |

| "IEV" ▶ Protocol 13.1.6 <60 years (>60 years) | | | |
|---|---|---|---|
| Etoposide phosphate | 150 (120) mg/m²/day | i.v. | Day 1–3, infusion 1 h |
| Ifosfamide | 2,500 (1900) mg/m²/day | i.v. | Day 1–3, infusion 18 h |
| Epirubicin | 100 (75) mg/m²/day | i.v. | Day 1, infusions 1 h |
| Before leukapheresis: G-CSF 5 µg/kg daily s.c., from day 5 | | | |

*"Cyclophosphamide Mob-1d"* ▶ *Protocol 13.1.4*

| | | | |
|---|---|---|---|
| Cyclophosphamide | 4000 mg/m²/day | i.v. | Day 1, infusion 1 h |

Before leukapheresis: G-CSF 5 µg/kg daily s.c., from day 5

### Therapy Protocols: High-Dose Therapy (Conditioning)

**ATTENTION:** High-dose therapy protocols must only be performed at adequately equipped transplantation centers, according to national and international guidelines.

*"BEAM"* ▶ *Protocol 14.1*

| | | | |
|---|---|---|---|
| BCNU | 300 mg/m²/day | i.v. | Day -7, infusion 1 h |
| Cytarabine | 2×200 mg/m²/day | i.v. | Day -6 to -3, infusion 1 h, |
| Etoposide phosphate | 2×100 mg/m²/day | i.v. | Day -5 to -3, bolus 15 min, |
| Melphalan | 140 mg/m²/day | i.v. | Day -2, infusion 30 min |

Day 0 stem cell transplantation

*"Melphalan"* ▶ *Protocol 14.2*

| | | | |
|---|---|---|---|
| Melphalan | 100 mg/m² | i.v. | Day -2, infusion 1 h (or 100 mg/day i.v., day -3 and day -2) |

Day 0 stem cell transplantation

*"VIC"* ▶ *Protocol 14.6*

| | | | |
|---|---|---|---|
| Etoposide phosphate | 500 mg/m²/day | i.v. | Day -4 to -2, infusion 1 h |
| Ifosfamide | 4000 mg/m²/day | i.v. | Day -4 to -2, infusion 18 h |
| Carboplatin | AUC 6 | i.v. | Day -4 to -2, infusion 18 h |

Day 0 stem cell transplantation

*"BuCy"* (autologous) ▶ *Protocol 14.4*

| | | | |
|---|---|---|---|
| Busulfan | 4 mg/kg /day | i.v. | Day -7 to -4 |
| Cyclophosphamide | 60 mg/kg/day | i.v. | Day -3 to -2, infusion 1 h |

Day 0 stem cell transplantation

### Perspectives
Progress in PBSCT is to be expected in the following areas:
- Sequential transplantation (e.g., multiple myeloma)
- Use of new hematopoietic growth factors for stimulation of recovery of platelets and neutrophils to further shorten the cytopenic phase after chemotherapy
- Improved management of side effects of induction therapy
- Generation of immunocompetent cells for the treatment of minimal residual disease

- Mobilization and high-dose protocols
- "Graft engineering", manipulation of stem cell product (elimination of tumor cells, ex vivo expansion of stem cells, dendritic cells, etc.)

**Ref:**

1. Antin JH. Long-term care after hematopoietic cell transplantation in adults. N Engl J Med 2002;347:36–42
2. Devetten M, Armitage JO. Hematopoietic cell transplantation: progress and obstacles. Ann Oncol 2007;18:1450–6
3. Gratwohl A, Baldomero H, Frauendorfer K et al. EBMT activity survey 2004 and changes in disease indication over the past 15 years. Bone Marrow Transpl 2006;37:1069–85
4. Jansen J, Hanks S, Thompson JM et al. Transplantation of hematopoietic stem cells from the peripheral blood. J Cell Mol Med 2005;9:37–50
5. Kessinger A, Sharp JG. The whys and hows of haematopoietic progenitor and stem cell mobilization. Bone Marrow Transpl 2003;31:319–29
6. Majhail NS, Ness KK, Burns LJ et al. Late effects in survivors of Hodgkin's and Non-Hodkin's lymphoma treated with autologous hematopoietic cell transplantation. Biol Blood Marrow Transpl 2007;13:1–7

**Web:**

| 1. | http://www.ebmt.org | EBMT, Eur Grp Blood Marrow Transpl |
| 2. | http://www.ibmtr.org | Blood Marrow Transpl Registry |
| 3. | http://www.asbmt.org/ | Am Soc Blood Marrow Transpl |
| 4. | http://www.bmtnet.org/ | Blood Marrow Transpl Net |
| 5. | http://www.cdc.gov/mmwr/preview/mmwrhtml/rr4910a1.htm | CDC, Guidelines |
| 6. | http://www.emedicine.com/ped/topic2593.htm | E-medicine |

## 5.3    Allogeneic Hematopoetic Stem Cell Transplantation

**J. Finke**

**Def:**    Transfer of pluripotent hemato- / lymphopoietic stem cells from healthy donors to recipients.

### Methods of Allogeneic Hematopoetic Stem Cell Transplantation (SCT)
- Bone marrow transplantation (BMT)
- Peripheral blood stem cell transplantation (PBSCT)
- Umbilical cord blood transplantation (UCBT)

**Ep:**    In 2004, 7407 allogeneic transplantations were performed in Europe (EBMT).

**Ma:**    The success of allogeneic transplantation is based on two therapeutic principles which distinguish this method from conventional chemotherapy and autologous transplantation:
- *Conditioning:* immuno- and myeloablative high-dose chemotherapy and/or total body irradiation (TBI)
- *Graft versus leukemia effect (GVL effect):* immunological reaction of donor lymphocytes from the graft against malignancy in the recipient.

While cytostatic treatment largely reduces the malignant clone, the GVL effect seems to ensure long-term reduction of the relapse rate. Complete T-cell depletion of the graft leads to increased relapse rates.

**Allogeneic Transplant Procedure**

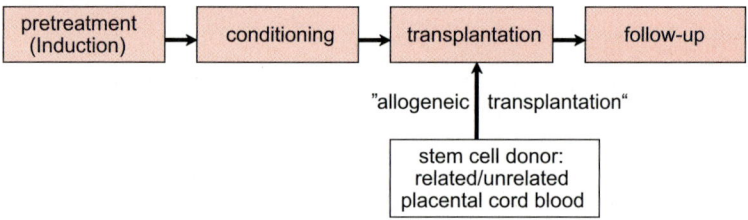

**Meth:**    ### Donor

Suitable donors are a prerequisite for allogeneic transplantation. While HLA-identical donors and recipients are preferable, HLA antigen differences to the point of haploidentity can be accepted in certain situations:
- Matched related donor (MRD)
- Volunteer unrelated donor (VUD).

### Donor Search
Allogeneic transplantation from HLA-identical siblings is preferable, however, sibling donors are available in only 25–30% of patients. Strategy:
- *Patients without related donor:* option of finding a volunteer unrelated donor; current success rate > 80%; 13 million registered voluntary donors worldwide. Blood group differences are of no importance when selecting a donor. After transplantation, the patient's blood group may be replaced by that of the donor.
- Early HLA typing of the patient, initiation of the donor search and contacting of allogeneic transplantation centers is pivotal for a successful strategy. Identification of a suitable donor may take 2–4 months. ***Initiating the donor search only when relapse has occurred is often too late.***
- *Expanding the search to the extended family:* HLA-compatible additional donors in 6% of cases.

*Donor Search Strategy*
1. HLA-Typing of the patient and close family (siblings, parents)
2. In urgent cases, parallel search for donors among members of the extended family and unrelated donors

## Selection Criteria for Related Donors
Of particular relevance are HLA alleles of the classes I A, I B and II DR.
- In patients with related donors, one allele difference in graft versus host direction (GVH direction) and three allele differences in host versus graft direction (HVG direction) are acceptable. This configuration provides for equally successful transplantation results as complete HLA identity.
- Class II DR alleles should be identified using genetic typing methods (DNA typing).
- The relevance of the class II loci DQ and DP is not yet known. When several HLA-A-, B-, and DR-identical donors are available, further selection criteria are considered (sex, age, CMV status, blood group).

## Selection Criteria for Unrelated Donors
In the typing of unrelated donors, 8 HLA antigens (two alleles each of A, B, DRB1*, DQB1*) of the patient and the prospective unrelated donor are important. Recently, the relevance of HLA-C has been emphasized, especially for graft rejection and NK cell-induced GVL effects. DP seems to be of little importance in relation to alloreactions.
- DR typing should be based on high-resolution DNA typing (4 digits), just as serological HLA-A, -B, and -C typing should be replaced by DNA methods (2 digits; recently 4 digits).
- Particularly in younger patients, minor differences may be acceptable.
- Additional HLA-DQB1* and/or HLA-DPB1* differences are at present no reason for exclusion of a donor. Allele differences in the A or B locus as well as minor DRB1* differences may also be acceptable, especially in patients with an aggressive underlying disease.
- Due to its low predictive value, mixed lymphocyte culturing (MLC) is no longer a routine procedure.
- The donor search should be coordinated by recognized immunogenetics laboratories together with a transplantation center.

## Alternatives
Options in case of unsuccessful donor search:
- Transplantation from donor after T-cell depletion
- Transplantation of umbilical cord blood (UCB): of particular importance in pediatric patients and young adults.

Cord blood banks are currently being established. So far, over 2,000 UCB transplants have been carried out worldwide. If necessary, several HLA differences may be accepted, especially in pediatric patients. The main limiting factor is the cell content of the graft in relation to the patient's body weight.

## Stem Cell Products

### Stem Cell Compartments
Hematopoietic stem cells are characterized by their expression of specific surface markers (CD34, CD133). The following hematopoetic stem cell compartments are used for transplantation:
- Bone marrow (BM) → bone marrow transplantation (BMT)
- Peripheral blood stem cells (PBSC, after stimulation with G-CSF) → peripheral blood stem cell transplantation ((PBSCT)
- Cryopreserved umbilical cord blood stem cells (UCB) → UCB transplantation (UCBT)

### Stem Cell Modification ("Graft Engineering")
Normally, the freshly collected grafts are transplanted without being manipulated or cryopreserved. However, in specific situations, the graft needs to be modified:

- T-cell depletion: prevention of graft versus host reactions
- Selection of CD34-positive cells ("stem cell selection"): reduction of immune reactions and elimination of malignant cells (autologous transplantation) ($\rightarrow$ ► Chap. 5.1)

### Bone Marrow Hematopoietic Cells

Bone marrow is collected under general anesthesia (approximately 60 min) by bilateral puncture and aspiration from multiple sites of the iliac crest.
- The bone marrow is anticoagulated and can be stored without cryopreservation for up to 1 day without significant stem cell loss (duration of transport with unrelated donor transplants).
- Potential disadvantages for the donor include blood loss, local pain and hematomas and side effects related to anesthesia.

### Cytokine-mobilized Peripheral Blood Hematopoetic Cells (PBSC)

Recently, peripheral blood stem cells have increasingly been used for allogeneic transplantation.
- Pretreatment of the donor with 5–24 µg/kg/day G-CSF s.c. for 4–6 days.
- Stem cell harvest by one or more leukaphereses.
- Depending on the rate of yield, the graft may contain more CD34$^+$ stem cells than comparable bone marrow products as well as 10 times more CD3$^+$ T-lymphocytes.
- In randomized studies, allogeneic transplantation of peripheral blood hematopoetic cells conferred an increased risk of GVHD compared with allogeneic BMT.
- Hematopoietic engraftment is faster with PBSC than with bone marrow.
- PBSC grafts allow manipulation (stem cell enrichment, selective T-cell depletion, "graft engineering"), facilitating GVHD prophylaxis and transplantation despite HLA barriers.

Co:
### Myeloablative Therapy

Successful allogeneic transplantation is ultimately "myeloablative," which is a result of both the conditioning therapy and the donor T-lymphocytes. Side effects:
- Toxic side effects of the conditioning therapy (chemotherapy, radiotherapy) depending on the therapy protocol
- Infections during the phase of bone marrow aplasia (until bone marrow reconstitution): bacterial infections, fungal infections (*Candida*, *Aspergillus*), viral infections (CMV, HSV)
- Long-term consequences: pulmonary fibrosis, bronchiolitis obliterans, gonadal insufficiency, hormonal deficiencies, cardiomyopathy, cataract, secondary neoplasia

### Graft Versus Host Disease (GVHD)

- Lymphocytes in the graft play a major role in "alloreactions," i.e., immunological reaction of transplanted immunologically active donor cells versus recipient organism $\rightarrow$ inflammatory immunological reactions in immunogenic structures, such as skin (dermatitis), intrahepatic bile ducts (cholestasis), and intestinal epithelium (enteritis); in extreme cases: destruction.
- The period of immunological adaptation and development of tolerance is divided into an acute phase (100 days after transplantation, acute GVHD) and a chronic phase (3–12 months after transplantation, chronic GVHD).
- Acute GVHD especially affects the skin, liver, and intestine.
- Chronic GVHD can potentially affect any organ. Particularly skin and mucosal dryness, generalized sicca syndrome with conjunctivitis, malabsorption syndrome, chronic cholestasis, weight loss, and increasing pulmonary obstruction may occur. In extreme cases, scleroderma-type skin symptoms and other autoimmune disorders may develop.
- GVHD prophylaxis with immunosuppressive drugs (e.g., cyclosporin A + methotrexate) is usually required in the initial weeks and months following transplantation. Unlike transplanted solid organs, an immune system developing from transplanted stem cells gradually becomes tolerant of the recipient.
- Especially in the first few months of this process, the patient is at risk of immune reactions and opportunistic infections (CMV, VZV, PCP, pneumococcal pneumonia) $\rightarrow$ close monitoring by the transplantation center in collaboration with the referring physician. A high degree of patient compliance is required.

**Th:** ## Principles of Treatment

Since different transplantation units may use center-specific protocols, consultation with experienced centers is always advisable. Variations may exist in relation to the following:
- Conditioning: based on high-dose chemotherapy with or without total body irradiation (IBI)
- Management of immunosuppression
- Stem cell graft engineering / manipulation

Furthermore, new protocols with less intensive conditioning regimens are currently being developed, for different indications and entry criteria (age). In protocols with reduced conditioning regimens, the age limit for allogeneic transplantation from related or unrelated donors has been raised from 55 years to approximately 70 years.

### Indications
See Table (p. 308)

### Pretreatment
Remission-inducing therapy (transplantation in complete remission generally leads to improved long-term outcome and cure rates)

### Conditioning Therapy and Transplantation
- Chemotherapy ± radiotherapy, high-dose or intensity-reduced (see below)
- Transplantation: transplantation of BM, PBSC, or cord blood from healthy donors via intravenous infusion; engraftment of hematopoietic stem cells in the bone marrow

### Post-Transplant Period and Long-Term Follow-Up
- Supportive administration of antibiotics, erythrocytes and platelets during the neutropenic (10–15 days) and thrombocytopenic phase (12–25 days)
- Parenteral nutrition and pain therapy in cases of severe mucositis (5–15 days). Mucositis prevention (palifermin)
- Prophylaxis and, if necessary, treatment of graft versus host disease (GVHD), (cyclosporine levels). Monitoring for clinical signs of GVHD, exanthema, diarrhea, icterus, dryness of the mouth, conjunctivitis, mucositis
- Rehabilitation, outpatient follow-up, return to work after approximately 4–9 months

### Signs of Toxicity
- Icterus, weight loss, ascites: VOD (veno-occlusive disease) → immediate hospitalization, heparin, possibly steroids
- Dyspnea, cough: bronchiolitis obliterans as chronic GVHD → high-dose steroids
- Palmoplantar erythema, dark pigmentation of the skin (busulfan, VP-16, thiotepa)
- Neuropathy, impaired vision, CNS disorders (cyclosporine, steroids)
- Hypertrichosis (cyclosporine)
- Opportunistic infections: *Pneumocystis carinii* pneumonia (PCP) → prophylaxis with cotrimoxazole; *Candida* and *Aspergillus* infections, cytomegalovirus reactivation, varicella zoster virus (VZV), bacterial infections
- With chronic GVHD and long-term immunosuppression, risk of pneumococcal sepsis / meningitis
- From 6 months post-transplantation, patients should be revaccinated with inactivated vaccines (especially tetanus, diphtheria, Pneumovax, *Haemophilus influenzae* B; later: hepatitis B, possibly polio; seasonal: influenza vaccine)

### Relapse after Transplantation
Relapse following allogeneic transplantation always constitutes a serious situation. Treatment options:
- Donor lymphocyte transfusion → specific induction of GVL with immunotherapeutic effects (CML, plasmocytoma, AML, NHL, ALL, etc.)
- Second allogeneic transplantation from a different donor

## Reduced Conditioning Prior to Allogeneic Transplantation

Terms such as "mini-transplantation," "micro-transplantation," or "non-myeloablative transplantation" have been used to describe reduced-intensity conditioning protocols which are based on dose modifications of traditional regimens (containing TBI 10–13.2 Gy or busulfan 16 mg/kg). However, these protocols represent a variation of allogeneic SCT with otherwise similar procedures and comparable immunological and infection-related problems (GVHD, opportunistic infections). Due to reduced acute toxicity, these regimens may preferably be used in patients with additional comorbidities or in older patients.

### Background
- The immunotherapeutic benefit of the GVL effect was demonstrated in patients with relapse of CML (▶ Chap. 7.3.1) after allogeneic bone marrow transplantation: the transfer of immunologically active donor lymphocytes resulted in complete remission in > 50% of these patients.
- So-called myeloablative therapy (e.g., with 10–14 Gy TBI or busulfan 16 mg/kg in combination with cyclophosphamide) is an aggressive conditioning regimen with multiple side effects limiting use to younger patients without significant comorbidity. Older patients therefore do not equally benefit from allogeneic transplantation with standard conditioning regimens.
- Dose escalation studies with radiotherapy or chemotherapy in patients with aggressive, therapy-refractory leukemias have shown that despite excessive toxicity and mortality, the risk of relapse after allogeneic transplantation was not significantly reduced.
- Recent animal experiments have shown that stable lympho-hematopoietic engraftment of donor cells can be achieved with significantly lower irradiation doses of 2 Gy, causing less side effects (so-called immunoconditioning). Parallel to the GVL effect, the treatment induces "donor chimerism," i.e., simultaneous existence of lymphatic and hematopoietic cells of the donor and the recipient.
- "Allogeneic transplantation with reduced conditioning" is aimed at utilizing the GVL effect without the disadvantages of maximum tolerable conditioning treatment. This therapeutic approach eventually constitutes a form of immunotherapy based on T-cell-mediated cytotoxicity.

### Clinical Results
- Initial clinical studies, including patients over 60 years of age, have demonstrated the feasibility of this therapeutic approach. In individual cases, post-therapeutic complete and partial remission has been described. Its applicability in patients of > 60 years of age allows curative therapeutic attempts, particularly in patients with AML, MDS, and low grade NHL.
- Donor chimerism of lymphatic and hematopoietic cells without significant myelosuppression (leuko- or thrombocytopenia) was achieved.
- Other approaches use fludarabine in combination with alkylating agents to increase tolerance prior to allogeneic transplantation. Fludarabine has a particularly toxic effect on T-cells and has added benefit in the treatment of lymphomas.
- The long-term outcome (overall survival) after reduced-intensity conditioning has not been established yet. Randomized clinical trials for individual disease entities are necessary.

### Possible Areas of Use
Treatment protocols for allogeneic transplantation with reduced conditioning are currently being developed for different disease entities and stages, giving rise to interesting prospects for a wider use of the therapeutic concept of allogeneic transplantation in patients with:
- Leukemia
- Myelodysplasia
- Multiple myeloma
- Chronic leukemias
- Lymphomas (especially low-grade NHL), multiple myeloma
- Various solid tumors

**Ref:**

1.  Appelbaum FR. Dose intensity and the toxicity and efficacy of allogeneic hematopoietic cell transplantation. Leukemia 2005;19:171–5
2.  Bertz H, Potthoff K, Finke J. Allogeneic stem-cell transplantation from related and unrelated donors in older patients with myeloid leukemia. J Clin Oncol 2003:21:1480–4
3.  Butcher BW, Collins RH. The graft-versus-lymphoma-effect: clinical review and future opportunities. Bone Marrow Transplant 2005;36:1–17
4.  Copelan EA. Hematopoietic stem-cell transplantation. N Engl J Med 2006;354:1813–26
5.  Deeg HJ. How I treat refractory acute GVHD. Blood 2007;109:4119–26
6.  Grathwohl A, Baldomero H, Frauendorfer K et al. Results of the EBMT activity survey 2005 on haematopoietic stem cell transplantation: focus on increasing use of unrelated donors. Bone Marrow Transplant 2007;39:71–87
7.  Schoemans H, Theunissen K, Maertens J et al. Adult umbilical cord blood transplantation. Bone Marrow Transplant 2006;38:83–93

**Web:**

| | | |
|---|---|---|
| 1. | http://www.ebmt.org | EBMT, Eur Grp Blood Marrow Transpl |
| 2. | http://www.asbmt.org | ASBMT, Am Soc Blood Marrow Transpl |
| 3. | http://www.bmtnet.org | Blood and Marrow Transplant Network |
| 4. | http://www.nature.com/bmt/index.html | Bone Marrow Transpl Journal |
| 5. | http://www.bmtinfonet.org | Blood and Marrow Transplant Information |
| 6. | http://www.bloodline.net | Bloodline, Hematology Education |
| 7. | http://www.marrow.org | National Marrow Donor Program |
| 8. | http://www.ibmtr.org | International Bone Marrow Transplant Registry |

**Indications for allogeneic hematopoetic stem cell transplantation in adults**

| Disease | Stage / type | Transplantation type | | Comments |
|---|---|---|---|---|
| | | Related[a] | Unrelated[b] | |
| AML | First CR, intermediate risk | + | -/(+) | Early search for potential donors |
| | First CR, high risk | + | + | |
| | First PR, second or later CR | + | + | |
| | Relapse, refractory AML or > first CR | + | + | |
| MDS | RA, RAS | + | + | With clonal markers or progressive cytopenia |
| | RAEB, RAEB-T, secondary AML, CMML | + | + | |
| ALL | First CR: high risk t(9;22), t(4;11) pre T-ALL, first PR, > first CR | + | + | Clinical trials |
| MPS | CML: chronic phase, acceleration, blast crisis | + | + | High-risk patients after failure of targeted therapies (imatinib, dasatinib) |
| | OMF, progressive | + | + | Advanced disease, refractory |
| Lymphomas | Myeloma | + | + | Frequently as tandem transplant after first remission |
| | Follicular lymphomas, stage III–IV | (+) | (+) | Advanced disease, refractory, rapid progression |
| | Mantel cell lymphoma | + | + | First PR, relapse or second CR: clinical trial |
| | Aggressive NHL | (+) | (+) | Lymphoblastic lymphomas (high risk) |
| | Hodgkin's disease | (+) | (+) | High-risk situation, relapse after autologous Tx (study protocols) |
| | CLL | (+) | (+) | High risk, rapid progression, refractory |

[a] Related allogeneic transplantation
[b] Unrelated allogeneic transplantation
+ indicated, (+) in studies only

*Tx* transplantation, *AML* acute myeloid leukemia (▶ Chap. 7.1.2), *CML* chronic myeloid leukemia, *CMML* chronic myelomonocytic leukemia, *MDS* myelodysplastic syndrome (RA, RAS, RAEB, RAEB-T) (▶ Chap. 7.1.1), *ALL* acute lymphatic leukemia (▶ Chap. 7.2), *CLL* chronic lymphatic leukemia, *MPS* myeloproliferative syndrome (▶ Chap. 7.3), *NHL* non-Hodgkin's lymphomas (▶ Chap. 7.5), *OMF* osteomyelofibrosis, *CR* complete remission, *PR* partial remission

# 5.4 Granulocyte Transfusion

H. Bertz, G. Illerhaus

**Def:** Experimental treatment procedure. Transfusion of donor granulocytes with the aim of correcting neutropenia (e.g., after chemotherapy).

The use of rhG-CSF for mobilization of donor granulocytes has been a prerequisite for successful development of granulocyte transfer. Several phase I/II studies have produced promising results in neutropenic patients with severe infections. Prospective phase III studies with comparison of granulocyte transfusion vs. standard of care are still pending.

> *Granulocyte transfusions must be carried out in accordance with transfusion guidelines and national laws.*

**Meth:** *Preparation and Storage*
- Donors and recipients must be ABO and Rh compatible (granulocyte concentrates contain erythrocytes). CMV status has to be considered
- Stimulation and mobilization of granulocytes with rhG-CSF (5 µg/kg) s.c.
- After 12 h, leukapheresis → with HAES 6% (to accelerate sedimentation) and sodium citrate (anticoagulant)
- Granulocyte yield depends on donor WBC count, leukapheresis efficiency, and volume of processed blood
- Irradiation of granulocyte concentrates with 30 Gy to avoid graft versus host reaction (large numbers of lymphocytes and stem cells in the leukapheresis sample)
- Store concentrates at room temperature, without agitation for up to 24 hrs.

*Transfusion*
- Carry out transfusion as soon after collection as possible
- Therapeutic success depends primarily on the number of transfused cells → transfusion of $\geq 1.5 \times 10^8$ granulocytes per kg body weight of recipient

**Ind:** Clinical studies in patients with severe infections not responding to anti-infective treatment, with concomitant neutropenia (< 500 neutrophils/µl) and without foreseeable bone marrow recovery.

**Ci:** *Donor*
- Pregnancy, lactation
- Severe general illness or known malignancy
- Acute and chronic infections, autoimmune diseases
- The number of maximum granulocyte donations per year must conform with national regulations

*Recipient*
- Allergic or pulmonary reaction to previous granulocyte transfusions
- No CMV-positive donor for CMV-negative recipient

**Se:** *Potential Side Effects (Donor)*
- G-CSF: bone pain, myalgia, restlessness, insomnia, headache, splenomegaly (rare) (▶ Chap. 4.3).
- Leukapheresis: anemia, thrombocytopenia
- HAES: allergic reactions, pruritus
- Sodium citrate: citrate toxicity, arrhythmia, tetany, metabolic alkalosis

*Potential Side Effects (Recipient)*
- Allergic reactions, anaphylactic shock → premedicate with antihistamines and nonsteroidal antipyretics, e.g., paracetamol

- Direct pulmonary toxicity, dyspnea, hypoxemia → monitor $O_2$ saturation
- Transfusion-induced acute pulmonary insufficiency (TRALI: transfusion-related acute lung injury) (▶ Chap. 9.8)
- Alloimmunization against HLA class I antigens and granulocyte-specific antigens → inefficiency of further transfusions, fever, respiratory symptoms, anaphylactic reactions

*Due to the risk of alloimmunization, granulocyte transfusions should be avoided prior to allogeneic bone marrow transplantation.*

**Th:**        ## Granulocyte Transfusion: Procedure

### Requirements
- Inclusion in clinical study, information and signed consent of donor and recipient
- ABO and Rh compatible donor, check CMV serology of donor and recipient (no transfusion from CMV-positive donor to CMV-negative recipient)

### Donor
- Clinical diagnosis: case history, physical examination
- Laboratory tests: full blood count with differential, blood group, hepatic and renal function parameters, coagulation parameters, serology (HAV, HBV, HCV, CMV, HIV, *Treponema pallidum*); female patients: pregnancy test where appropriate
- Cross-match (blood group testing) before each granulocyte transfusion
- ECG, optional chest x-ray, abdominal sonography (splenic enlargement)
- G-CSF 5 µg/kg s.c., 12 h before each leukapheresis
- Prior to each new leukapheresis as well as 5 and 30 days after the final donation: blood count with differential, urea and electrolytes, serum creatinine, bilirubin, ALT

### Granulocyte Sample
- Leukapheresis sample irradiated with 30 Gy
- Administer as soon as possible (within 6 h)

### Recipient
- Serological (erythrocytic) and leukocytic (lymphocyte toxicity test) compatibility must be assessed prior to each granulocyte transfusion. After administration of amphotericin B, wait at least 6 h before giving a granulocyte transfusion (pulmonary toxicity).
- Ten minutes prior to transfusion, premedication with antihistamines and antipyretics (e.g., paracetamol).
- Recommended transfusion rate: $1 \times 10^{10}$ cells per hour. Use standard filters (pore size 170–230 µm).
- Monitor blood pressure, pulse, respiratory rate, and $O_2$ saturation from the beginning until 1 h after transfusion.
- Evaluate transfusion success by measuring the post-transfusion granulocyte increase.

**Ref:**
1. Hübel K, Engert A. Granulocyte transfusion therapy for treatment of infections after cytotoxic chemotherapy. Onkologie 2003;26:73–9
2. Mousset S, Hermann S, Klein SA et al. Prophylactic and interventional granulocyte transfusion in patients with haematological malignancies and life-threatening infections during neutropenia. Ann Hematol 2005;84:234–41
3. Price TH. Granulocyte transfusion: current status. Semin Hematol 2007;44:15–23
4. Robinson SP, Marks DI. Granulocyte transfusions in the G-CSF era. Where do we stand? Bone Marrow Transplant 2004;34:839–46

**Web:**
1. http://www.aabb.org/            American Association of Blood Banks

## 5.5 Immunotherapy

### A. K. Kaskel, A. Mackensen, H. Veelken

**Def:** Specific or non-specific modulation of the immune system with the objective of immunologically mediated destruction of malignant cells.

**Meth:** Immunotherapy approaches to cancer treatment have been studied since the nineteenth century. Four different approaches can be distinguished:
- Active specific immunotherapy
- Active non-specific immunotherapy
- Passive immunotherapy
- Adoptive immunotherapy

### T-cells

The T-cellular immune response is crucial to recognize and eliminate tumor cells. T-cell subtypes include:
- CD8-positive, cytotoxic T-lymphocytes [restricted by class I MHC molecules (MHC I)]
- CD4-positive, helper T-lymphocytes [restricted by class II MHC molecules (MHC II)]

A more recent classification is based on the cytokines produced by T-lymphocytes. CD4-positive T-lymphocytes are subclassified as:
- Inflammatory Th1-cells
- Helper cells of Th2-type
- Th0-cells (intermediate type)

#### T-cell Activation: Antigen Presentation

T-lymphocytes do not recognize intact proteins, but peptides bound to MHC (major histocompatibility complex) molecules. Different types of proteins can be processed by intracellular proteases, the resulting peptides are bound to MHC molecules and expressed on the cell surface of antigen-presenting cells. Consequently, T-cell recognition is not limited to surface markers, but may include intracellular antigens, thus multiplying the diversity of T-cell target epitopes. Prerequisite for the recognition of peptides is the binding to MHC molecules:
- Peptides binding to MHC I: 7–14 amino acids
- Peptides binding to MHC II: 14–24 amino acids

The specifics of antigen recognition by T-lymphocytes are dependent on the interaction of the variable region of the T-cell receptor (TCR) molecule with the MHC–peptide complex. This binding site of the TCR is coded by a unique gene segment, which is formed by the recombination of a V-D-J segment for the β locus and a V-J segment for the α locus during T-cell differentiation. This combinatorial diversity is amplified by the random addition of nucleotides and is the basis for the diversity of the T-cell repertoire.

#### Specific recognition of tumor antigens by T-lymphocytes

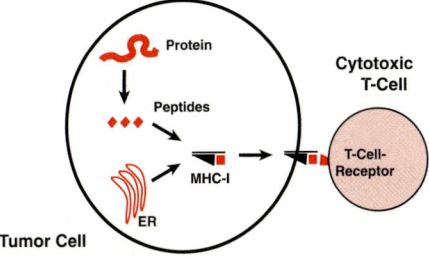

Proteins (e.g. melanoma antigens tyrosinase, MAGE 1–3, Melan-A) are processed by intracellular proteases. Resulting peptides are bound by MHC molecules and presented at the cell surface. T-cell receptor (TCR) binds to MHC-peptide-complex. ER Endoplasmatic Reticulum

311

### Costimulatory Molecules

The binding of a TCR to a specific peptide–MHC complex alone is not sufficient for activation and proliferation of naive T-cells. Additional signals are required:

- Adhesion molecules which facilitate contact with the targeted cell
- Costimulatory signal: costimulatory molecules are the antigens of the B7-family (B7-1, B7-2), which are expressed by antigen-presenting cells (APC). "Professional APCs" play a central role for the initiation of the immune response. The antigens interact with suitable ligands on T-cells (CD28, CTLA-4). If a naive T-cell meets a non-professional APC (e.g., tumor cell presenting a peptide matching a specific TCR), a second costimulatory activation signal is missing. The result is the induction of anergy, i.e., the T-cell is refractory to further stimulatory signals.

### Immune Escape Mechanisms

The immune system of a tumor patient is rarely capable of inducing regression of manifest tumors and metastases. This observation supports the hypothesis, that tumor specific antigens lead to incomplete activation of the immune system, or tumor cells "escape" immunologic toxicity through induction of immunosuppression.

Various "tumor escape" mechanisms of neoplastic cells have been described:

- Lack of expression of costimulatory molecules on tumor cells
- Loss or downregulation of MHC molecules ($\beta$2-microglobulin, HLA-A or -B) or receptors for apoptosis
- Loss of transport proteins (TAP) → reduced presentation of tumor peptides with MHC molecules
- Selection of so-called antigen-loss variants, without expression of tumor-associated antigens (MAGE, tyrosinase, gp100)
- Induction of angiogenetic or antiapoptotic factors
- Secretion of immunoinhibitory cytokines, such as TGF-$\beta$ and IL-10, by tumor cells

**The effect of costimulatory molecules**

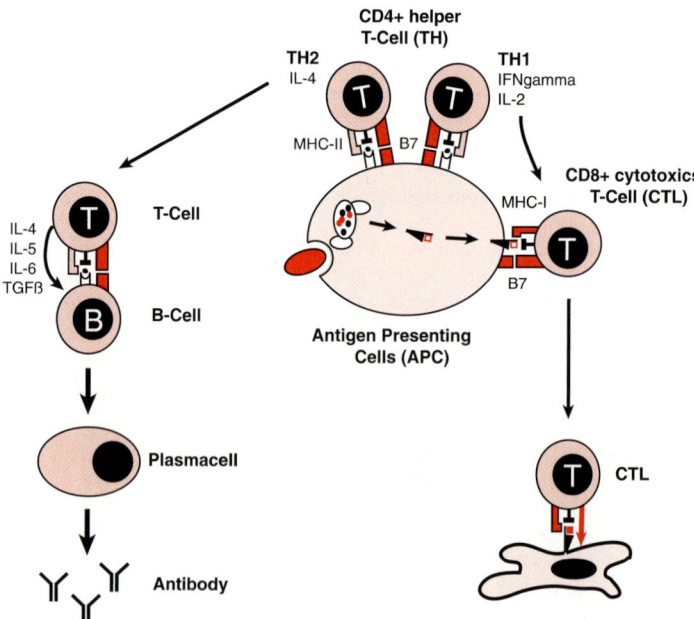

Dendritic cells or monocytes (professional antigen-presenting cells, *APC*) ingest antigenic material and disintegrate and process it to peptides. Peptides are attached to MHC-I or MHC-II molecules and transported to the cell membrane where they are presented. The TCR binds to peptide–MHC complexes, and cellular interaction is supported by adhesion molecules and costimulatory signals such as B7 (on APC) and CD28 (T-cells). Depending on the antigen and the cytokine environment, cell types preferably induced are Th2 or Th1 helper cells. Th2 cells produce cytokines (such as IL-4, -5, -6), which are particularly important for the stimulation and differentiation of B-cells to antibody-producing plasma cells. Th2 cells also interact with B-cells, which can ingest and process the same antigen complex (e.g., bacterium, tumor cells) with the help of membrane antibody molecules or the B-cell receptor – similar to dendritic cells. The interaction of B- and T-cells leads to a coordinated antigen-specific B- and T-cell immune response. Th1 cells produce interferon-γ and IL-2, which particularly promote the maturation of MHC-I–peptide complex specific cytotoxic T-cells

**Th:**

## Active Non-specific Immunotherapy

The term "active non-specific immunostimulation" relates to the administration of modifiers, which can directly modulate the immune system. "Non-specific" indicates the lack of antigen specificity. Non-specific immunity is mainly based on activated macrophages, but also NK cells and neutrophils. The following are possible biological response modifiers:
- Cytokines such as interleukin-2 and interferon
- BCG (Bacille Calmette-Guérin)
- Lipopolysaccharides, immune complexes, muramyl dipeptide

### Indications (▶ Chap. 3.4)
- Interferon α: malignant melanoma, renal cell cancer
- Interleukin-2: malignant melanoma, renal cell cancer
- BCG: bladder cancer

## Active Specific Immunotherapy

Directed activation of the antigen-specific cellular immune response by vaccination. Possible vaccines include:
- Irradiated tumor cells, without further modification
- Irradiated tumor cells + immunostimulation (e.g., BCG)
- Modified tumor cells (after transfection with cytokines or costimulatory molecules)
- Defined tumor antigens (proteins, peptides)

Tumor antigens inducing a specific T-cell response:
- Tissue- / organ-specific antigens, differentiating antigens (Melan A, tyrosinase in melanocytes/ melanoma, PSA in prostate cancer, HER2/neu in breast cancer)
- Overexpression of normal gene products (MAGE antigens in melanoma)
- Mutated cellular gene products of tumor suppressor genes or cell cycle genes (p53, cyclin)
- Viral gene products (EBNA-1 in Burkitt's lymphoma, nuclear protein E6/E7 of HPV16 in cervical carcinoma)
- Rearranged normal gene products (bcr/abl translocation in CML, immunoglobulin idiotypes in B-cell neoplasia)
- Activated protooncogene products (p21 point mutation in colon carcinoma)
- Oncofetal antigens (CEA in colon / breast cancer)

### Specific Immunotherapy with Defined Tumor Antigens
- Proteins ± adjuvant
- Immunodominant peptides ± adjuvant
- Peptide-loaded antigen-presenting cells
- Naked DNA coding for tumor-associated antigens
- Recombinant constructs in live vectors (viruses, bacteria)

### Indications
- Colon carcinoma, stage III, adjuvant therapy
- Melanoma and renal cell carcinoma, in clinical trials

## Passive Immunotherapy

Treatment with monoclonal antibodies directed against tumor antigens. Mechanisms of tumor cell lysis by monoclonal antibodies:
- Antibody-dependent cellular cytotoxicity; ADCC
- Complement-dependent cytotoxicity; CDC
- Intrinsic cytotoxic activity / induction of apoptosis
- Carrier of a cytotoxic substance (toxins, radionuclides, cytostatics)
- Antibody variants: murine antibodies, chimeric / humanized antibodies, bispecific antibodies, immunotoxins / radioconjugates

### Indications (▶ Chap. 3.5)
- B-NHL: anti-CD20 monoclonal antibody, chimeric (rituximab)
- Breast cancer: anti-HER2/neu antibody, humanized (trastuzumab)
- CLL: anti-CD52 monoclonal antibody, humanized (alemtuzumab)
- Colorectal cancer, NSCLC: VEGF monoclonal antibody (bevacizumab)
- Colorectal cancer, HNC: EGFR monoclonal antibody (cetuximab)

## Adoptive Immunotherapy

### Passive Immunotherapy with Effector Cells (Cellular Therapy)
- Donor lymphocytes in HLA-chimeric patients (graft versus leukemia effect)
- Virus-specific T-lymphocytes (CMV, EBV, HIV)
- Tumor-specific T-lymphocytes
- Antigen (peptide)-specific T-lymphocytes
- Ex vivo expanded tumor-infiltrating lymphocytes (TIL) or ex vivo expanded and activated NK cells (lymphokine-activated killer cells, LAK)
- Antigen-presenting dendritic cells

### Indications
- Adoptive transfer of donor lymphocytes in allogeneic transplantation (CML, AML, multiple myeloma)
- Adoptive transfer of virus-specific lymphocytes in allogeneic transplantation (CMV, EBV, EBV-associated lymphoproliferative disorders)
- Adoptive transfer of tumor- or antigen-specific T-lymphocytes (malignant melanoma)

**Ref:**
1. Banchereau J, Palucka A. Dendritic cells as therapeutic vaccines against cancer. Nat Rev Immunol 2005;5:296–306
2. Blattmann JN, Greenberg PD. Cancer immunotherapy: a treatment for the masses. Science 2004;305:200–5
3. Brentjens RJ, LAtouche JB, Santos E et al. Eradication of systemic B-cell tumors by genetically targeted human T lymphocytes co-stimulated by CD80 and interleukin-15. Nat Med 2003;9:279–86
4. Lake RA, Robinson BW. Immunotherapy and chemotherapy: a practical partnership. Nat Rev Cancer 2005;5:397–405
5. Mapara MY, Sykes M. Tolerance and cancer: mechanisms of tumor evasion and strategies for breaking tolerance. J Clin Oncol 2004;22:1136–51
6. Ribas A, Butterfiled LH, Glaspy JA et al. Current developments in cancer vaccines and cellular immunotherapy. J Clin Oncol 2003;21:2415–32
7. Steinmann RM, Banchereau J. Taking dendritic cells into medicine. Nature 2007;449:419–26

**Web:**
1. http://www.cancerresearch.org                         Cancer Research Institute
2. http://www.cancersupportivecare.com/immunotherapy.html Cancer Immunotherapy
3. http://www.meds.com/immunotherapy/intro.html          Immunotherapy Training
4. http://www.cancerimmunotherapy.org                     Assoc Immunother Cancer
5. http://www.meniscus.com/horizons/2-1.pdf               Cancer Immunotherapy

5.6 **Gene Therapy**

H. Veelken, F.M. Rosenthal

Def:
Treatment of a disease by expression of one / multiple specific genes in a cell or group of cells. The production of the desired gene product corrects the genetic defect or alters cellular function.

### Types
- Somatic gene therapy: expression of genes in differentiated somatic cells
- Germline therapy: expression of genes in fertilized human oocytes or embryonic stem cells

Meth:
### Gene Transfer
Adequate methods of gene transfer are a basic requirement for gene therapeutic approaches. In most cases, so-called vectors are used to transport the therapeutic gene construct into the target cells. Due to directed genetic deletions, viral vectors are usually unable to replicate after transfection of the target cell. Viral vectors are produced with the help of "packaging cells," which provide the necessary structural proteins for replication. After transfection of the genetic construct, these cells produce the required vector.

The following are important criteria for the evaluation of gene transfer methods:
- *Efficacy:* transfection quality (transient or stable), transfection efficiency, tropism (potential of organ-specific gene transfers), biological efficacy (expression of gene products)
- *Safety:* tolerance, adverse effects, immunogenicity
- Production effort, cost and compliance with GMP / GLP / GCP criteria

**Gene therapy studies: diseases, examples**

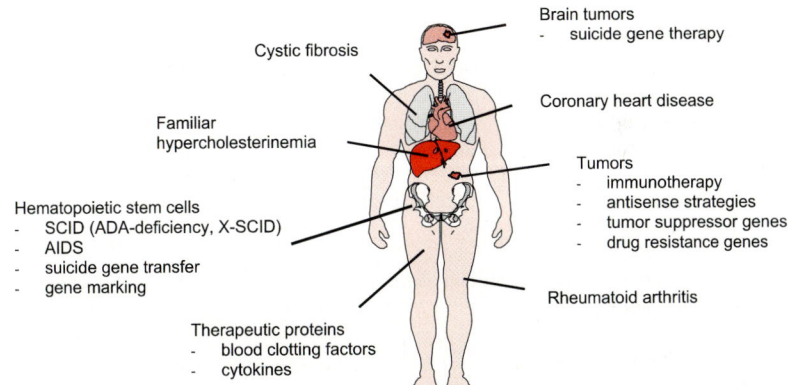

### Basics and Clinical Studies
The first somatic gene therapy was carried out in September 1990 at the NIH, USA, on a 4-year-old girl with adenosine deaminase (ADA) deficiency. Since then, more than 630 clinical gene therapy studies have been licensed worldwide and 3,500 patients have been treated. Besides monogenic hereditary diseases, gene therapy is used particularly in patients with advanced malignancy, AIDS, or multifactorial diseases such as coronary heart disease or rheumatoid arthritis.

### Strategies for Gene Therapy of Malignancies

- *Induction of specific immune responses* by transfer of immunostimulating genes (e.g., inter-leukin or interferon genes) into tumor cells, bystander cells, or immunoeffector cells
- *Transfer of tumor suppressor genes* → correction of regulation defects in tumor proliferation
- *Blockade of oncogenic effects* via antisense strategies
- *Transfer of "suicide genes"* into tumor cells: suicide genes usually encode enzymes (e.g., HSV thymidine kinase), which by means of phosphorylation convert non-toxic prodrugs (e.g., ganciclovir) into toxic substances, thus selectively killing HSV-TK-expressing cells
- *Transfer of cytostatic drug resistant genes* (MDR-1, aldehyde dehydrogenase, $O_6$-alkylgua-nine-DNA alkyltransferase, cytidine deaminase) into hematopoietic stem cells to increase the in vivo resistance of the hematopoietic system to cytostatic drugs and alleviate the hema-totoxicity of subsequent chemotherapy

Until now, mainly critically ill patients with short life expectancy were included in gene therapy studies. Therefore, the results of these studies focus primarily on safety and side effects, rather than on curative aspects. Initial data on the safety of gene therapy methods showed that close surveillance is required:

- After administration of high doses of adenoviral vectors, immune reactions to adenoviral proteins and pulmonary toxicity were detected in patients with cystic fibrosis.
- Severe adverse reactions also occurred during a clinical trial in patients with the X-chromosomal form of severe combined immunodeficiency (X-SCID), carried out in Paris. Newborn children suffering from this so far incurable disease were cured by transfer of the normal gene. However, approximately 3 years after treatment, 3 out of 11 children developed T-cell leukemia, the cause of which seemingly involved the insertion of the retroviral vector. The exact causes of this severe adverse effect are under intense medical and molecular biological investigation.
- A 17-year-old patient with a severe congenital metabolic disease died in September 2000 in the USA after infusion of high doses of genetically modified adenovirus into the liver artery.

The importance of strict adherence to the highest standards for production and quality control of gene therapy drugs as well as the conduct of controlled clinical trials was underlined by these cases.

**Th:** At present, gene therapy is used in clinical studies only (▶ Chap. 3.7). Besides legal aspects mentioned above, national and international guidelines and regulation for gene therapy products and studies have to be followed.

**Clinical Gene Therapy Studies, Germany (as of May 2005, German Register for Somatic Gene Transfer Studies)**

| *Target entities* | |
|---|---|
| Infections / parasitic diseases | 13% |
| Cardiovascular diseases | 10% |
| Malignancies | 77% |
| *Therapeutic approaches (number of trials)* | |
| Immunotherapy | 16 |
| Tumor suppressor regulation | 9 |
| Vaccination | 5 |
| Suicide gene expression | 4 |
| Regulation of angiogenesis | 3 |
| Other approaches | 9 |

A total of 46 studies with 465 patients (361 with gene transfer, 104 in control groups)

Methods of gene transfer

| Transfer method | Foreign DNA | Target cells | Transfection efficiency | Transfection | Cellular toxicity | Gene expression | Preparation | Use |
|---|---|---|---|---|---|---|---|---|
| Electroporation | 150 kb | Mitotic / resting | Stable < 0.1–1% | 1–20 copies | 20–60% survival rate | | Simple | In vitro |
| Microinjection | Unlimited | Mitotic / resting | Stable < 0.1–1%, transient up to 100% | Integration possible | 30% survival rate | | 200–400 injections/h | In vitro |
| Naked DNA | Unlimited | Especially myocytes | 10–30% of cells at injection site | Extrachromosomal | Lymphocytic infiltration | In myocytes: until cellular death | Simple, cheap | In vivo |
| Particle bombardment | 10,000 copies | Mitotic / resting | Stable < 0.01–0.1%, transient ≤ 20% | Persistence / integration? | 85–95% survival rate | 2–12 months | Simple | In vitro, in vivo |
| Lipofection (cations) | Unlimited | Mitotic / resting | Stable < 0.1–1%, transient up to 80% | Integration possible | Membranotoxic, no antigenicity | | Simple | In vitro, in vivo |
| Calcium phosphate co-precipitation | Unlimited | Mitotic / resting | Stable < 0.1% | Often multiple copies | High | | Simple | In vitro |
| Receptor-mediated | > 48 kb | Mitotic / resting | Up to 50% in vitro, very variable | Extrachromosomal, variable | High | High, transient | Labor intensive / time-consuming | In vitro, in vivo |
| Retrovirus | Approx. 8 kb | Only mitotic | Up to 100% in vitro | Stable, one copy | Non-toxic | Relatively low | Labor intensive | In vitro, in vivo |
| Adenovirus | > 8 (7–36) kb | Mitotic / resting | High | Extrachromosomal | Direct toxicity, immune reactions | High | Homolog recombination, stable | In vitro, in vivo |
| Adeno-associated virus | 4 kb | Mitotic / resting | Relatively high | Stable integration, tandem repeats | Non-toxic | | High viral stability | In vitro, in vivo |
| Herpes simplex virus | 10–100 kb, amplicon DNA: approx. 15 kb | Mitotic / resting / neurotrophic | | Extrachromosomal, multiple copies | Low | | Heat-resistant, lyophilization | CNS / PNS |

Proof-of-concept has been established for the biological or clinical efficacy of gene transfer in studies:

- Induction or amplification of tumor-specific immune responses in tumor vaccination studies
- Occasional tumor regression or stable disease after transfer of tumor suppressor genes (p53)
- Decreased incidence of GVHD after allogeneic hematopoietic transplantation due to transfer of HSV-TK suicide genes into allogeneic donor lymphocytes after administration of ganciclovir
- Correction of the immunodeficiency in X-chromosomal severe combined immunodeficiency (X-SCID)
- In patients suffering from hemophilia, factor VIII use was reduced by 50–80% after intramuscular injection of AAV vectors carrying the wildtype gene

Furthermore, genetic marking of hematopoietic stem cells showed that while contributing to long-term hematopoietic reconstitution, transplanted stem cell products can potentially contain malignant cells which act as a starting point for relapse. Although this method is a diagnostic procedure, the results of these studies are seminal for future advancement of transplantation strategies and trends in gene therapy with respect to the hematopoietic system.

The clinical use of gene therapy is still in an early stage. In addition to the safety aspects discussed above, there are numerous technical issues to be resolved:

- In vivo transfection efficiency
- Duration and degree of expression of a therapeutic gene
- Regulation of gene expression
- Organ-specific gene transfer in vivo
- Immunogenicity of vectors and therapeutic gene products
- Industrial-scale production of viral vectors

**Ref:**

1. Baum C, Düllmann J, Li Z et al. Side effects of retroviral gene transfer into hematopoietic stem cells. Blood 2003;101:2099–114
2. Eder IE, Haag P, Bartsch G et al. Gene therapy strategies in prostate cancer. Curr Gene Ther 2005;5:1–10
3. Lusky M. Good manufacturing practice production of adenoviral vectors for clinical trials. Hum Gene Ther 2005;16:281–91
4. Manilla P, Rebello T, Afable C et al. Regulatory considerations for novel gene therapy products: a review of the process leading to the first clinical lentiviral vector. Hum Gene Ther 2005;16:17–25
5. Nathawani AC, Davidoff AM, Linch DC. A review of gene therapy for haematological disorders. Br J Haematol 2005;128:3–17
6. Neff T, Beard BC, Kiem HP et al. Survival of the fittest: in vivo selection and stem cell gene therapy. Blood 2006;107:1751–60

**Web:**

| | | |
|---|---|---|
| 1. | http://www.esgct.org/ | European Society of Gene Therapy |
| 2. | http://www.asgt.org/ | American Society of Gene Therapy |
| 3. | http://www.iscgt.org.uk/ | Intl Society for Cancer Gene Therapy |
| 4. | http://www.mdanderson.org/departments/genetherapy/ | MD Anderson Gene Therapy Center |
| 5. | http://www.euregenethy.org | European Gene Therapy Network |
| 6. | http://www.cancer.gov/cancertopics/ factsheet/Therapy/gene/ | NCI, Cancernet |

## Inhibition of Angiogenesis

A. Müller, J.S. Scheele

**ef:** *Angiogenesis:* formation of new blood vessels; mostly formation of new capillaries from pre-existing blood vessels.
*Inhibition of angiogenesis:* through inhibition of endogenous angiogenic factors or administration of physiological / pharmacological angiogenesis inhibitors.

**hys:** Physiological angiogenesis is essential for the development of embryonic organs as well as the regulation of the adult vascular system:
- Embryogenesis: vasculogenesis, i.e., formation of new angioblast-derived blood vessels
- Proliferation of uterine epithelia, menstruation
- Proliferation and vascularization of muscle tissue
- Wound healing, bone growth, nerve regeneration, hair growth
- Regulation of vascular permeability → homeostasis

In adult organisms, angiogenesis is typically strictly regulated and of limited duration (local duration 1–2 weeks maximum).

### Endogenous Angiogenesis Promoters
- Angiopoietins (Ang1, Ang3, Ang4)
- Ephrines (Eph-A1, Eph-12, Eph-B2), VE-cadherin
- Fibroblast growth factors (aFGF, bFGF), hepatocyte growth factor (HGF)
- Platelet-derived growth factor (PDGF-BB)
- Transforming growth factors (TGFα, TGFβ), tumor necrosis factor alpha (TNFα)
- Interleukin 8 (IL-8)
- Integrins $\alpha_v\beta_3$, $\alpha_v\beta_5$, $\alpha_5\beta_1$
- Prostaglandins E1 (PgE1) and E2 (PgE2)
- Matrix metalloproteinases (MMPs)
- Vascular endothelial growth factors (VEGF-A, VEGF-B, VEGF-C, VEGF-D)

### Endogenous Angiogenesis Inhibitors
- Angiostatin, endostatin, protamine, vasostatin, angiopoietin 2 (Ang2)
- Thrombospondin-1
- Cartilage-derived inhibitor
- Interferons (IFNα, IFNβ)
- Interleukins (IL-4, IL-10, IL-12, IL-18)
- Platelet factor 4 (PF4)
- Prolactin fragment, SPARC fragment, osteopontin fragment, antithrombin III fragment
- Soluble VEGF receptors (sVEGF-R1, sNRP-1)
- Tissue inhibitor of metalloproteinase (TIMP), MMP inhibitors, MMP2 fragment (PEX)

**p:** **Diseases with pathological angiogenesis**

| Organ | Disease |
|---|---|
| Blood vessels | Atherosclerosis, hemangioma, hemangioendothelioma, vascular anomalies, retinopathies |
| Skin | Impaired wound healing, keloid formation, Kaposi's sarcoma, psoriasis, skin tumors, decubitus |
| Female reproductive organs | Follicular cysts, menstruation anomalies, ovarian hyperstimulation, endometriosis, tumors, preeclampsia, placental insufficiency |

**Pp:**          **Diseases with pathological angiogenesis** *(continued)*

| Organ | Disease |
|---|---|
| Skeletal system | Rheumatoid arthritis, synovitis, osteomyelitis, pannus formation, osteophyte formation, tumors, aseptic necrosis, impaired wound healing |
| Internal organs, epithelia | Hepatitis, pneumonia, glomerulonephritis, asthma, hepatic regeneration, tumors, pulmonary hypertension, diabetes |
| Eye | Vitreous body disturbances, diabetic retinopathy, choroid neovascularization |
| Endocrine organs | Thyroiditis, hyperthyroidism, pseudocysts |
| Lymphatic system | Metastasis, lymphoma, lymphedema |
| Hematopoiesis | Hematological neoplasia, AIDS |
| Other | Solid tumors |

### Angiogenic Switch

In 1970, Folkman described the transition of solid tumors from an avascular resting state to a vascularized phase with optimal tumor oxygenation and nutrition. Only in the vascularized state, i.e. after the "angiogenic switch", accelerated tumor proliferation, metastasis, and generalization can occur, as for example in prostate carcinoma, breast cancer, and renal cell carcinoma.

Similarly, increased bone marrow microvessel density has been described in proliferating hematological neoplasia, particularly in patients with leukemia (AML, ALL, CML) and myelodysplasia.

**Tumor neoangiogenesis**

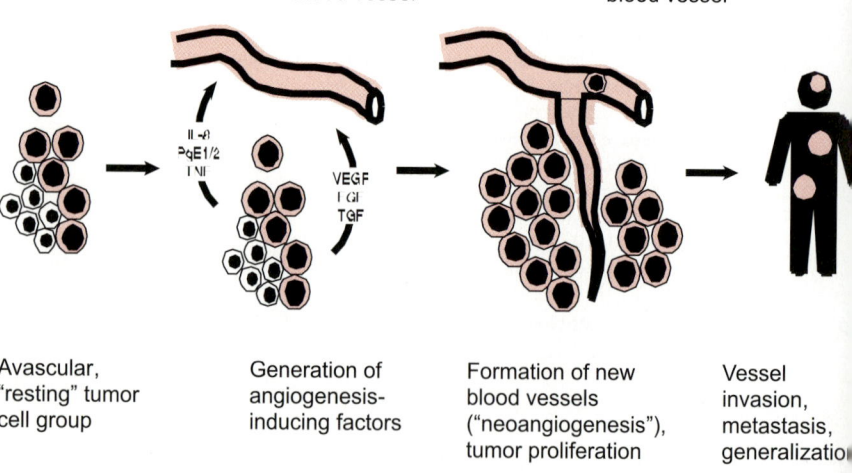

| Avascular, "resting" tumor cell group | Generation of angiogenesis-inducing factors | Formation of new blood vessels ("neoangiogenesis"), tumor proliferation | Vessel invasion, metastasis, generalization |

**Th:**          Inhibition of tumor-induced angiogenesis and the angiogenic switch of human tumors (transition from avascular state to vascularized proliferating tumor) was first demonstrated as an effective means of treatment with the VEGF-receptor antibody bevacizumab (▶ Chap. 3.5). Bevacizumab inhibits binding of VEGF to VEGF receptors (i.e. VEGF-R1 = Flt-1 and VEGF-R2 = KDR) – inhibition of tumor-induced neoangiogenesis → inhibition of tumor growth and metastasis. Th compound has been approved for treatment of metastatic colorectal cancer and non-small cell lung cancer (NSCLC). Similar approaches are followed with small molecule inhibitors of angiogenesis, e.g. sorafenib and sunitinib (▶ Chap. 3.6).

**VEGF and VEGF receptors**

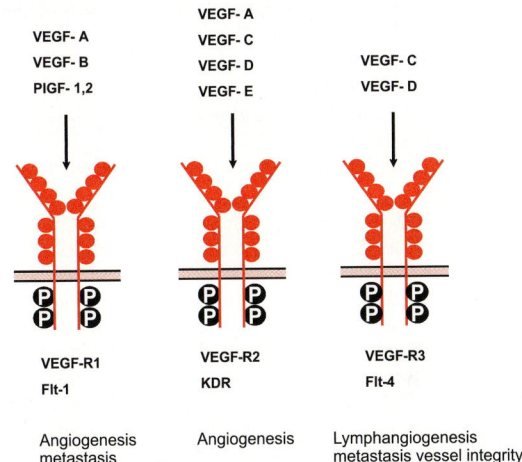

| VEGF- A | VEGF- A | |
| VEGF- B | VEGF- C | VEGF- C |
| PlGF- 1,2 | VEGF- D | VEGF- D |
| | VEGF- E | |

VEGF-R1     VEGF-R2     VEGF-R3
Flt-1         KDR         Flt-4

Angiogenesis    Angiogenesis    Lymphangiogenesis
metastasis                          metastasis vessel integrity

### Angiogenesis Inhibitors in Clinical Trials

- *Matrix metalloproteinase-inhibitors (MMPI):* CGS 27023, COL-3, BMS-275291
- *Inhibitors of endothelial cell proliferation / migration:* 2-methoxyestradiol, combretastatin A4, farnesyltransferase inhibitors, thalidomide, lenalidomide, soy isoflavone, IM862, LY317615, ZD6126, AVE8062, ABT-751, TZT-1027, AS-1404
- *Inhibitors of angiogenesis-inducing factors / tyrosine kinases:* BAY 43-9006, PTK787/ZK222584, AMG706, SU6668, Neovastat (AE-941), VEGF-Trap, ZD6474, CP-547632, aplidine
- *Endothelin / integrin antagonists:* ABT-627, vitaxin, EMD121974

**Ref:**

1. Carmeliet P. Angiogenesis in health and disease. Nature Med 2003;6:653–60
2. Fayette J, Soria JC, Armand JP et al. Use of angiogenesis inhibitors in tumour treatment. Eur J Cancer 2005;41:1109–16
3. Ferrara N, Gerber HP, LeCouter J. The biology of VEGF and its receptors. Nature Med 2003;9:669–76
4. Folkman J. Role of angiogenesis in tumor growth and metastasis. Semin Oncol 2002;6(suppl 16):15–18
5. Keyhani A, Jendiroba DB, Freireich EJ. Angiogenesis and leukemia. Leuk Res 2001;25:639–45
6. Podar K, Anderson KC. The pathophysiologic role of VEGF in hematologic malignancies: therapeutic implications. Blood 2005;105:1383–95
7. Timar J, Dome B, Fazekas K et al. Angiogenesis-dependent diseases and angiogenesis therapy. Pathol Oncol Res 2001;7:85–94
8. Tozer GM, Kanthou C, Baguley BC. Disrupting tumour blood vessels. Nat Rev Cancer 2005;5:423–35

**Web:**

1. http://www.oncolink.upenn.edu/      Oncolink
2. http://www.angio.org/      Angiogenesis Foundation
3. http://www.cancer.gov/clinicaltrials/developments/anti-angio-table    NCI, Angiogenesis Inhibitors
4. http://www.cancer.gov/cancertopics/ understandingcancer/angiogenesis    NCI, Angiogenesis Tutorial
5. http://www.angioworld.com/angiogenesis.htm    Angioworld

## 5.8     Developmental Therapeutics

### U. Martens

**Def:** Increasing understanding of the molecular mechanisms of cancer and hematologic malignancie[s] led to new strategies in the development of therapeutic agents, and this has resulted in the intro- duction of new drugs such as tyrosine kinase inhibitors in the treatment of malignant disease[s]. Promising new approaches include:

- RNA-targeted therapy
- Aurora kinase inhibition
- HSP (heat shock proteins) as targets for cancer therapeutics
- Telomerase therapeutics

### RNA Technology

#### Small RNAs

In recent years the members of the RNA family have grown rapidly. In addition to the coding mes- senger RNAs (mRNAs) and transcriptional RNAs [ribosomal RNAs (rRNAs) and transfer RNA (tRNAs)], another subfamily, called small RNAs, has been discovered, each member of which ha[s] its own particular function. Small RNAs do not code for proteins, but instead control the tran- scription and translation of protein-coding RNAs. The small RNA subfamily contains small in- terfering RNAs (siRNAs), microRNAs (miRNAs), small nucleolar RNAs (snoRNAs), and smal[l] nuclear RNAs (snRNAs). siRNAs and miRNAs have attracted much attention due to their poten- tial diagnostic and therapeutic applications in different diseases.

siRNAs and miRNAs are generated using the same pathway by processing long double stranded RNA (dsRNA) or microRNA precursors with an endonuclease known as "Dicer". Sub- sequently, the RNAs attach to an RNA-induced silencing complex (RISC) and are directed to th[e] messenger RNA (mRNA) of interest which is marked for cleavage or inhibition of translation.

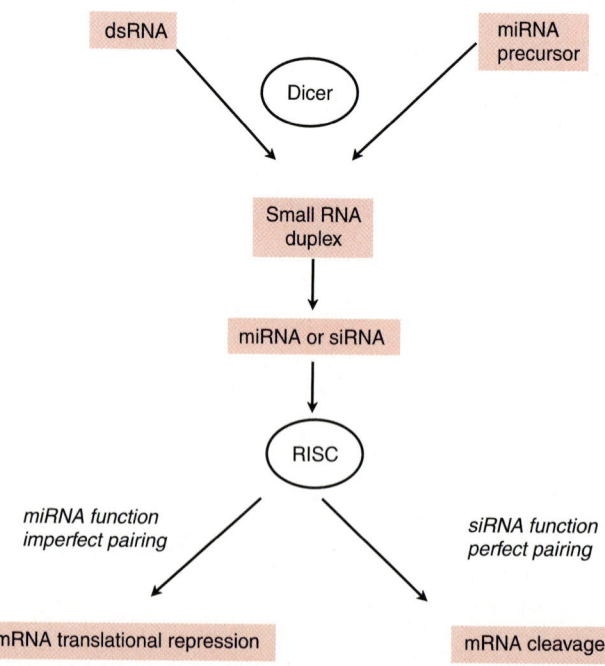

### Small Interfering RNAs (siRNAs)

**Def:** These RNAs are 21–24 nucleotides in length, double-stranded, and have 3' overhangs of 2 nucleotides. siRNAs mediate the phenomenon of RNA interference (RNAi) which is a pathway for silencing the transcript of an active gene. RNAi, discovered in 1998, is now a standard laboratory tool for knocking down gene expression.

**MOA:** Exogenous synthetic siRNAs or endogenously expressed siRNAs attach to an RNA-induced silencing complex (RISC) and are directed to the messenger RNA (mRNA) of interest which is marked for destruction.

**Th:** The highly specific silencing effect of RNAi has emerged as an attractive way to allow specific inhibition of the function of any chosen target genes, including those involved in diseases such as cancer, AIDS, and hepatitis.

- The biggest obstacle to the development of RNAi-based therapeutics is the delivery. Trigger RNAs (dsRNAs from which siRNAs are derived by the action of Dicer) can be expressed from vectors or delivered as artificial siRNAs. Inserting foreign vector sequences (gene therapy) into chromosomal DNA includes the problem of insertional activation and inactivation of cellular genes. Direct administration of siRNAs would require siRNAs that are stable and modified to be resistant to nucleases.
- Drug therapies using siRNAs are now in clinical trials for treating age-related macular degeneration and respiratory syncytial virus infection (RSV).

### MicroRNAs (miRNAs)

**Def:** MicroRNAs are short 20–22 nucleotide RNA molecules that are negative regulators of gene expression in a variety of eukaryotic organisms. miRNAs are involved in numerous cellular processes including development, differentiation, proliferation, apoptosis, and stress response. About 350 miRNAs have been identified in humans, with the total predicted to eventually reach 1,000 or more. miRNA mutations or altered expression correlate with various human cancers and indicate that miRNAs can function as tumor suppressors or oncogenes ("oncomirs").

**MicroRNAs currently associated with human cancer**

| MicroRNA | Cancer role | Cancer type | Mechanism |
|----------|-------------|-------------|-----------|
| miR-15 | Tumor suppressor | CLL | Bcl-2 inhibition |
| miR-16 | Tumor suppressor | CLL | Bcl-2 inhibition |
| miR-155 | Oncogene | Lymphoma, breast | Cooperation with myc |
| let-7 | Tumor suppressor | Lung | ras inhibition |
| miR-21 | Oncogene | Glioblastoma | Antiapoptotic |

**MOA:** Like siRNAs, miRNAs are generated from long primary precursor RNAs before being processed by the Dicer protein in the cytoplasm and incorporated as mature miRNA into the RNA-induced silencing complex (RISC). Whereas siRNAs perfectly match with the target mRNA, most miRNAs do not match the target sequence exactly, enabling them to bind to multiple mRNAs. Instead of destruction of mRNA as in RNAi interference, imprecise matching results in inhibition of translation.

**Th:** About half of the annotated human miRNAs map within fragile regions of chromosomes in cancer genomes. Expression profiling of about 200 miRNAs has been shown to be a more accurate method of classifying cancer subtypes than using the expression of protein-coding genes.

Gene therapies using miRNAs might be an effective approach to restore tumor suppressor function or to block oncogene activation.

- Administration of synthetic antisense oligonucleotides that encode sequences that are complementary to mature oncogenic miRNAs—termed anti-miRNA oligonucleotides (AMOs)—might effectively inactivate miRNAs in tumors and slow their growth.

323

- Antagomirs, a novel class of chemically engineered oligonucleotides appear to be specific and effective silencers of miRNA expression in mice when conjugated with cholesterol.

## Aurora Kinase Inhibition

**Def:**      The serine-threonine kinases Aurora A, B, and C represent a family of mitotic regulators which are essential for mitotic progression, spindle formation, centrosome maturation, chromosomal segregation, and cytokinesis. Selectively inhibiting Aurora kinase activity by RNAi or small molecules leads to chromosome segregation errors and deregulation of the spindle checkpoint associated with cell death.

**MOA:**     Aurora A localizes to centrosomes / spindle poles and is required for spindle assembly, whereas Aurora B is a chromosome passenger protein required for phosphorylation of histone H3, chromosome segregation, and cytokinesis. Elevated expression of Aurora A and B has been detected in many human cancers and overexpression of Aurora A has been shown to induce oncogenic transformation in vitro.

Tumor cells treated with Aurora kinase inhibitors show normal timing of expression of core cell cycle regulators, such as cyclins, and do not undergo arrest or delay transit through mitosis as classic antimitotic agents do. The antiproliferative effect is unique, in that tumor cells, especially those lacking functional p53 damage response, are catastrophically driven forward and out of an aberrant mitosis, which finally leads to cell death due to massive chromosomal instability.

**Th:**       Although Aurora A has received most of the attention so far in terms of a link with human cancer, Aurora B might be the more suitable anticancer drug target, because inhibition of Aurora B rapidly results in a catastrophic mitosis.
- Small molecule inhibitors in development: Hesperadin, AZD1152 (phase I), MK0457(= VX 680, inhibits also Flt-3, phase I), MLN8054 (Aurora A, phase I), JNJ-7706621 (inhibits also cyclin-dependent kinases, CDKs)
- Aurora kinases are only expressed and active as kinases during mitosis, therefore, it is assumed that non-proliferating cells would not be adversely affected by Aurora kinase inhibitors
- Reduction or abrogation of histone H3 phosphorylation could serve as biomarker
- MK0457(= VX-680) is effective against imatinib- and dasatinib-resistant bcr-abl(T315I) kinase in vitro

## HSP90 as Target for Cancer Therapeutics

**Def:**      The heat shock protein (HSP) family of proteins has emerged as a target for cancer drug discovery because it is important for mediating the action of oncogenically relevant growth factor receptors and their downstreaming signaling elements.

**MOA:**     Many HSPs form multimolecular complexes that act as chaperones binding other proteins, denoted as client proteins. HSP90 consists of two isoforms and is one of the most abundant cellular chaperone proteins. It is a cellular chaperone required for refolding of denatured proteins, cellular survival under stress conditions, and the maturation of a subset of proteins that play key roles in oncogenesis. Therefore, HSP90 does not catalyze a single reaction, but mediates the stability and function of multiple client proteins such as:
- Signaling protein kinases (e.g., PDK1, RAF-1, AKT, ZAP-70, IKK)
- Transmembrane tyrosine kinases (e.g., HER2, c-Kit, IGFR, MET)
- Mutated signaling proteins (e.g., p53, c-Kit, FLT-3, B-Raf)
- Chimeric fusion oncoprotein kinases (e.g., bcr-abl, NPM-ALK)
- Cell cycle regulatory proteins (e.g. CDK4, myc, Chk1, wee1)
- DNA repair (e.g., telomerase, DNA-PKcs)
- Steroid receptors (e.g., androgen, estrogen, progesterone receptor)

**Persp:** Natural products, including the ansamycin antibiotic geldanamycin and radiciol, that bind selectively to HSP90 and inhibit its chaperone function have been identified. However, geldanamycin is limited by its hepatotoxicity for clinical use, but a less toxic derivative 17-allylamino-17-demethoxygeldanamycin (17-AAG) has been identified.

- Due to poor chemical stability and bioavailability subsequent geldanamycin- and non-geldanamycin-based compounds are in development: KOS-953 (Tanespimycin, cremaphor-based formulation of 17-AAG, phase I/II), KOS-1022 (17-DMAG, Alvespimycin hydrochloride, orally active, phase I), CNF1010 (oil-in-water nanoemulsion of 17-AAG, phase I), CNF2024 (orally, phase I), IPI-504 (water soluble, phase I), SNX-5542 (orally active, preclinical).
- Tumors which are dependent on a given client protein are particularly sensitive to degradation of HSP90 inhibitors. The proteins observed to be most sensitive to HSP90 inhibitor-induced degradation are the HER2 and MET receptor tyrosine kinases, RAF-1 kinase, and the estrogen and androgen receptors.
- HSP90 inhibitors might be particularly effective in cancer cells in which Rb is mutationally inactivated (e.g., small cell lung cancer). Typically, HSP90 inhibition induces cell cycle arrest in G1 phase. However, in Rb-defective cells, tumor cells fail to arrest in G1 and enter a mitotic block with disordered prometaphase and unstable kinetochore assembly which is followed by apoptotic cell death.
- HSP90 inhibitors enhance the activity of cytotoxics including taxanes, anthracyclines, hormonal agents, bortezomib, trastuzumab, and radiation. There is a schedule dependence in context with an intact retinoblastoma (Rb) function due to its growth arrest in G1 phase of the cell cycle.
- Inhibitors of angiogenesis may also sensitize tumor cells to HSP90 inhibitors, because hypoxic tumor cells are under greater stress and HIF1alpha is also a client protein required for survival under these conditions.

### Telomerase Therapeutics

**Def:** Maintenance of telomeres at the ends of chromosomes is essential for unlimited cellular proliferation and confers immortality in cancer cells. Since most cancer cells are reliant on telomerase for their survival, this enzyme represents an attractive mechanism-based target for the development of new cancer therapeutics.

**Ma:** Telomeres consist of repetitive double-stranded repeats of the sequence TTAGGG associated with telomere-binding proteins. Their major function is to cap the ends of chromosomes and to provide genetic stability. Telomerase is a ribonucleoprotein enzyme, which synthesizes telomere repeats de novo. In human cells, the telomerase holoenzyme consists of a high-molecular weight complex with a template-containing RNA subunit, hTR, and protein components including the catalytic subunit human telomerase reverse transcriptase, hTERT. In addition, several additional molecules might play a role in regulating in vivo activity of telomerase such as the chaperone HSP90/p32. In most normal somatic cells telomerase activity is absent and telomere repeats are lost with cell division and with ageing. Telomere attrition beyond a certain threshold is assumed to uncap chromosome ends which subsequently induces DNA damage and onset of replicative senescence. In contrast, about 80–90% of cancer cells have detectable telomerase activity, which leads to stabilization of telomeres and unlimited growth potential.

**Persp:** Strategies targeting telomeres / telomerase in cancer cells:

- Oligonucleotide antagonists against hTR or hTERT (e.g., GRN163L, a thio-phosphoramidate oligonucleotide targeting the template region of hTR as a "template antagonist"; phase I/II). Like siRNA therapeutics (see above) there remains the issue of delivery and stability of antisense oligonucleotides.
- Small molecule inhibitors of the catalytic component hTERT (e.g., BIBR1532; preclinical); the antiproliferative effect is not induced by inhibition of the enzyme itself but through consecutive telomere dysfunction. The lag period of telomere shortening limits the widespread use of this approach.
- Heat shock protein 90 (HSP90) inhibitors which compromise telomerase assembly by targeting HSP90/p23 (phase II)

- Small molecules that stabilize the folding of the G-rich telomere strand into G-quadruple structures (e.g., BRACO19; preclinical). Such folding is incompatible with telomerase functio and may induce rapid telomere uncapping. The toxicity of such molecules is not yet clarified.
- Immunotherapy with vaccines targeting hTERT-specific epitopes on cancer cells (GV1001 PrimoVax and TeloVax trial for pancreatic cancer, phase II).
- Telomerase-directed gene therapy:
  - Suicide gene therapy: the hTERT promoter is linked to a proapoptotic gene or cytotoxi prodrug.
  - Oncolytic viral therapy: viral genes which are critical for replication are placed under con trol of the hTERT gene promoter. This results in virus vectors that are replicated only i telomerase-positive cells, and then spread to adjacent cells on cell lysis (e.g., GG5757 ad enovirus which replicates only in retinoblastoma (Rb)-defective and hTERT-positive cell preclinical).

**Ref:**

1. Bhalla KN. Heat shock protein 90 modulators in hematologic neoplasms. ASCO Educational Book 42nd Annual Meeting, 2006, pp 141–6
2. Buckingham S. The major world of microRNAs. Horizon Symposia. Understanding the RNAissance. May 2003. Nature Publishing Group
3. Carter TA et al. Inhibition of drug resistant mutants of Abl, Kit, and EGF receptor kinases. Proc Natl Acad Sci 2005;102:11011–16
4. Dorsett Y, Tuschl T. siRNAs: applications in functional genomics and potential as therapeutics. Nat Rev Drug Discov 2004;3:318–29
5. Esquela-Kerscher A, Slack FJ. Oncomirs-microRNAs with a role in cancer. Nat Rev Cancer 2006;6:259–69
6. Keen N, Taylor S. Aurora-kinase inhibitors as anticancer agents. Nat Rev Cancer 2004;4:927–36
7. Kelland LR. Overcoming the immortality of tumour cells by telomere and telomerase based cancer thera-peutics: current status and future prospects. Eur J Cancer 2005;41:971–9
8. Krutzfeldt J et al. Silencing of microRNAs in vivo with "antagomirs". Nature 2005;438:685–9
9. Shay JW, Wright WE. Telomerase therapeutics for cancer: challenges and new directions. Nat Rev Drug Discov 2006;5:577–84
10. Solit DB. Heat shock protein 90 as therapeutic target in solid tumors. ASCO Educational Book 42nd Annual Meeting, 2006, pp 136–40
11. Stevenson M. Therapeutic potential of RNA interference. New Engl J Med 2004;351:1772–7

**Web:**

1. http://www.rnaiweb.com          The RNAi Web
2. http://microrna.sanger.ac.uk/     miRBase

# Aplastic Anemia

## J. Finke, H. Bertz

**Def:** Hematopoietic (bone marrow) failure with pancytopenia (bi- or tricytopenia) of the peripheral blood. Characteristics: hypocellular bone marrow with fatty substitution; no bone marrow stromal cell defects; no malignant cells.

**ICD-10:** D61

**Ep:** Incidence worldwide: 2–6 cases per 1,000,000 population/year; much higher in China, the Far East, and South East Asia.
Age distribution: two peaks, around 20 years and 65 years.

**Pphys:**

### Pathophysiological Model

Destruction / suppression of hematopoietic stem cells or progenitor cells caused by various factors is of central importance:

- Activation of the immune system with primary or secondary (immunologically induced) bone marrow aplasia with activated cytotoxic T-cells, which cause destruction of CD34-positive progenitor cells via:
  - Direct T-cell-mediated cytotoxicity
  - Production of IFNγ and TNFβ
  - Induction of FAS receptor and antigen → apoptosis induction
- Direct DNA damage (e.g., irradiation)
- Cellular membrane damage and interference with the cellular metabolism (e.g., viral infection)
- Drug-induced: direct toxicity or hapten-mediated autoimmune reaction
- Secondary clonal expansion of hematopoiesis
- NK cells ↓ (as with other autoimmune diseases)

**Pg:**

### Genetic Factors

- Fanconi's anemia: chromosomal instability based on multiple genetic defects (Fanconi anemia genes FANC A-L). Characteristics are: progressive bone marrow aplasia, increased incidence of malignancy, and abnormalities in skin, musculature, skeletal system, and urogenital system. In > 80% of cases, manifestation is during infancy.
- Increased incidence of aplastic anemia in the presence of HLA A2, DR2, DR4, and DPw3.
- PNH association (▶ Chap. 6.4.3)
- Mutations of telomerase reverse transcriptase (TERT) gene

### Drugs (in 25% of Cases)

- Antibiotics (particularly sulfonamides, chloramphenicol), antimalarial drugs
- Thyreostatics, antidiabetics
- Antirheumatics, NSAIDs (e.g., phenylbutazone, gold)
- Diuretics (furosemide), ticlopidine, nifedipine
- Antiepileptics (e.g., carbamazepine, phenytoin)
- Cytotoxic compounds (e.g., busulfan)

### Chemical Agents

- Aromatic solvents (e.g., benzene)
- Insecticides (lindane, DDT, etc.)

### Viral / Postinfectious (5% of Cases)

- Parvovirus B19 (isolated erythropoietic aplasia, "pure red cell anemia")
- Hepatitis (non-A-B-C-G hepatitis, poor prognosis, mostly young men)
- EBV (infectious mononucleosis, rare)
- HIV

- CMV (bone marrow stromal cell invasion possible)
- Flavivirus (dengue fever)

### Radiation
- Ionizing radiation
- Thorotrast

### Other Causes
- Autoimmune diseases, associated with eosinophilic fasciitis
- Pregnancy (estrogen-mediated?)
- Thymoma
- Idiopathic (70% of cases)

**Class:**

**Classification according to number of granulocytes, platelets, and reticulocytes[a]**

| Type | Abbreviation | Granulocytes | Platelets | Reticulocytes |
|------|-------------|--------------|-----------|---------------|
| Aplastic anemia | AA | < 1,500/μl | < 50,000/μl | < 20,000/μl |
| Severe AA | SAA | < 500/μl | < 20,000/μl | < 20,000/μl |
| Very severe AA | VSAA | < 200/μl | < 20,000/μl | < 20,000/μl |

[a] At least 2 out of 3 criteria are necessary for diagnosis, hypocellular bone marrow

**NOTE:** Treatment-induced reversible hematopoietic insufficiency following chemo- or radio-therapy is not designated as aplastic anemia.

**Sy:**

Symptoms are dominated by hematopoietic failure:
- Symptoms of anemia: pallor, fatigue, reduced performance, dyspnea
- Symptoms of neutropenia: oral ulcers, gingivitis, severe infections, pneumonia
- Symptoms of thrombocytopenia: hemorrhage, petechiae (skin, mucous membranes), less commonly hematomas

**Dg:**

### Medical History, Physical Examination
- Medical history, including medication, infections
- Physical examination (hemorrhage, mucous membranes, signs of infection, splenic status etc.)

### Laboratory Tests
- Complete blood count: bi- or trilineage cytopenia, generally without pathological morphology, increased granulation, neutropenia, monocytopenia, and eosinopenia; reticulocytes ↓; in cases of thrombocytopenia: small platelets
- Ferritin, haptoglobin, Coombs' test, blood group, coagulation parameters
- ESR, total protein, electrophoresis, immunoglobulins, immunofixation, cold agglutinins, rheumatoid factor, ANA
- PNH exclusion (Ham's test, sugar water test, GPI-linked proteins, CD55, CD59)
- Vitamin $B_{12}$, folic acid (exclusion of megaloblastic anemia)
- Liver function (exclude past history of hepatitis)
- Serology (EBV, CMV, HAV, HBV, HCV, HIV, HSV, parvovirus B19)

### Bone Marrow (Aspiration, Histology, Immunohistochemistry, Iron Stain, Culture)
- Hypocellular (cellularity < 25%) with predominance of fat cells
- Lymphocytes, macrophages, and plasma cells present
- CD34-positive progenitor cells ↓; in bone marrow cultures, reduced colony formation (CFU GM, colony-forming units – granulocytes / macrophages) and LTCIC (long-term culture-initiating cells). Improved growth pattern in T-cell-depleted cultures (→ T-cell-mediated reaction?)

### Further Diagnostic Procedures

- Chest x-ray, abdominal sonography
- HLA typing (in cases of potential transplantation)
- Cytogenetics, chromosome analysis (exclusion of MDS, Fanconi's anemia)
- Increased serum levels of hematopoietic growth factors: G-CSF (granulocyte colony-stimulating factor), TPO (thrombopoietin), M-CSF, and erythropoietin; SCF (stem cell factor) not increased

**Dd:**
- Myelodysplasia with hypoplastic bone marrow (▶ Chap. 7.2)
- Primary Myelofibrosis (PM) (▶ Chap. 7.3.4)
- Vitamin $B_{12}$ deficiency, folic acid deficiency (▶ Chap. 6.4.2)
- Paroxysmal nocturnal hemoglobinuria (PNH) (▶ Chap. 6.4.3)
- Leukemias, lymphomas, solid tumors with bone marrow infiltration

**Co:**
- Development of PNH in 7% of cases (▶ Chap. 6.4.3)
- Transformation into MDS or acute leukemia in 5–12% of cases (▶ Chaps. 7.1.1, 7.1.2, 7.2)

**Th:**

### Indications for Treatment

- Severe aplastic anemia (SAA or VSAA)
- Patient at risk by complications arising from cytopenia (recurrent infections, hemorrhage, hemosiderosis)
- Prevention of alloimmunization and subsequent transfusion refractoriness

**Treatment of aplastic anemia**

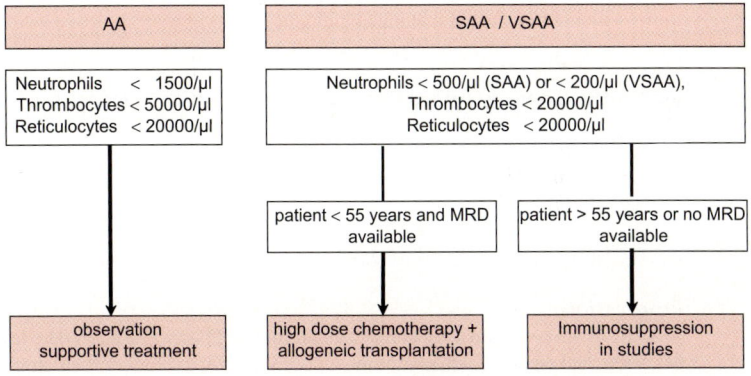

*MRD* matched related donor (HLA-identical family bone marrow or stem cell donor)

### Treatment Guidelines

1. Aplastic anemia should always be treated in a hematological center.
2. Patients under 55 years of age with HLA-identical siblings or relatives should be evaluated for matched related allogeneic bone marrow or blood stem cell transplantation.
3. In other patients, immunosuppression is carried out in the framework of clinical trials.

## Treatment Modalities

### *Supportive Measures*
- Infection prophylaxis, antibiotics, amphotericin B prophylaxis
- Oral hygiene
- Prophylaxis / therapy of hemosiderosis (desferrioxamine mesylate)
- Granulocyte transfusions (▶ Chap. 5.4)
- Suppress menses, avoid platelet aggregation inhibitors
- Blood products (CMV negative, irradiated); erythrocyte transfusions according to symptoms, platelet transfusions for counts below 5,000–10,000/μl
- Growth factors: granulocyte colony-stimulating factor (G-CSF), erythropoietic factors

*ATTENTION:* use blood products as sparingly as possible until decision on BMT / PBSCT is made (danger of alloimmunization). Do not use blood products from relatives.

### *Transplantation Types (▶ Chaps. 5.2, 5.3)*
- In patients under 55 years of age, allogeneic hematopoietic stem cell transplantation (HSCT) from HLA-identical related (family) donors in conjunction with fludarabine / cyclophospha-mide-containing protocols
- Matched unrelated donor (MUD) transplantation recommended only in patients under 15 years of age

### *Immunosuppressive Therapy*
Patients > 55 years or without suitable stem cell donor. Effective compounds:
- Antilymphocyte globulin (ALG) or antithymocyte globulin (ATG), since 1970
- Cyclosporin A (CyA), since 1980
- Methylprednisolone

Immunosuppressive therapy should only be carried out in clinical trials.

### Innovative Therapy Approaches and Treatment of Relapse

If standard treatment fails:
- Matched unrelated donor transplantation (MUD transplantation) in patients between 15 and 50 years of age
- Hematopoietic growth factors
- Treatment option without proven efficacy: androgens, used since 1954

**Prg:**      **Progression**
Aplastic anemia can precede clonal hematological diseases (e.g., PNH). Incidence over 10 years MDS 9%, leukemia 7%; after immunosuppressive therapy higher than after transplantation.

### *One-year Survival Rate with SAA*
- Untreated: 20%
- Supportive treatment: 50%
- Immunosuppressive treatment or allogeneic transplantation: 80%

### *Long-term Survival with Different Forms of Treatment*
- Patients < 25 years: 66–92%
- Patients between 25 and 39 years: 69%
- Patients > 39 years: 38%
- With immunosuppressive treatment (ATG and CyA containing): 80%
- Five-year survival after allogeneic matched related transplantation: 60–90%
- Five-year survival after MUD transplantation: 29%
- Relapse within an observation period of up to 14 years: 35%
- Immunosuppression compared with BMT: no significant difference in terms of primary response

*Relapse*
- After matched related allogeneic transplantation: 15–20%
- After immunosuppressive medication (CyA + ATG containing): 30–50%

**Ref:**

1. Bacigalupo A, Bruno B, Saracco P et al. Antilymphocyte globulin, cyclosporin, and granulocyte colony-stimulating factor for severe aplastic anemia: an update of the GITMO/EBMT Working Party. Blood 2000;95:1931–34
2. Ball SE. The modern management of severe aplastic anaemia. Br J Haematol 2000;110:41–53
3. Brodsky RA, Jones RJ. Aplastic anaemia. Lancet 2005;365:1647–56
4. Davies JK, Guinan EC. An update on the management of severe idiopathic aplastic anaemia in children. Br J Haematol 2007;136:549–64
5. Geroges GE, Storb R. Stem cell transplantation for aplastic anemia. Int J Hematol 2002;75:141–6
6. Kojima S, Hibi S, Kosaka Y et al. Immunosuppressive therapy using antithymocyte globulin, cyclosporin, and danazol with or without human granulocyte colony-stimulating factor in children with acquired aplastic anemia. Blood 2000;96:2049–54
7. Marsh JCW, Ball SE, Darbyshire P et al. British Committee for Standards in Hematology (BCSH). Guidelines for the diagnosis and management of acquired aplastic anaemia. Br J Haematol 2003;123:782–90
8. Yamaguchi H, Calado RT, Ly H et al. Mutations in TERT, the gene for telomerase reverse transcriptase, in aplastic anemia. N Engl J Med 2005;352:1413–24
9. Young NS. Immunosuppressive treatment of acquired aplastic anemia and immune-mediated bone marrow failure syndromes. Int J Hematol 2002;75:129–40

**Web:**

1. http://www.aamds.org/      AA and MDS Foundation
2. http://www.fanconi.org/      Fanconi Anemia Research Fund

## 6.2    Neutropenia and Agranulocytosis

**J. Finke, H. Bertz**

**Def:**    *Neutropenia:* Neutrophil count in the peripheral blood of adults $< 1.5 \times 10^9/l$. Limit dependent on age and race: neonates show higher neutrophil levels, while certain African and Middle Eastern populations have physiologically lower numbers of neutrophils.

*Agranulocytosis:* Neutrophil count in the peripheral blood $< 0.5 \times 10^9/l$. Usually symptomatic acquired disease with granulocytopenia and in severe cases, lymphocytopenia and monocytopenia. In adults, usually iatrogenic. Duration after discontinuation of the causative agent: 2–4 weeks.

**ICD-10:**    D70

**Ep:**    *Neutropenia:* common side effect of radio- / chemotherapy.

*Agranulocytosis:* rare occurrence, incidence of 3 cases per 1,000,000. Older patients are especially affected, male:female = 1:2. The incidence of specific forms of agranulocytosis depends on the causative agents and pathomechanisms.

**Pg:**    *Pathogenetic Mechanisms*
- Reduced production of neutrophils in the bone marrow
- Redistribution from the circulating neutrophil pool to marginal areas (endothelium, tissues)
- Peripheral destruction

*Drug-induced Forms*
- *Most common form: drug-induced toxic suppression* of granulopoiesis or direct neutrophilic damage ("delayed onset neutropenia," e.g., after radio- or chemotherapy), usually with simultaneous thrombocytopenia (▶ Chap. 6.3)
- *Drug-induced allergic reactions* with destruction of neutrophils, often caused by metabolites
- Usually, *rapid* granulocyte decrease within 1 week after exposure; in case of re-exposure, within hours. Destruction of mature granulocytes ("abrupt onset neutropenia"), acute onset with fever and chills (DD: infection). Causative agent: e.g. phenylbutazone
- In rare cases, *slow decrease*, between 1 and 12 months after the beginning of treatment, due to destruction of hematopoietic progenitor cells. Causative agent: e.g., clozapine, in patients with HLA phenotype B38 and alleles DR4 and DQw3

*Other Forms*
- *Autoimmune diseases:* T-cell-mediated inhibition of granulopoiesis (Felty's syndrome, rheumatoid arthritis) or as a result of clonal T-cell expansion in patients with T-γ-lymphoproliferative disease ("T-γ-disease")
- *Complement activation (e.g., with hemodialysis, sepsis):* expression of adhesion molecules on the surface of neutrophils → neutrophilic aggregation, capillary occlusion (esp. pulmonary capillaries)
- *Pseudoneutropenia ("shift neutropenia"):* neutrophilic redistribution (shift) from the peripheral blood into the tissues, e.g., with infections

**Class:**    *Neutropenia Caused by Congenital Granulopoietic Disorders*
- Congenital dysgenesis with familial pancytopenia
- Reticular dysgenesis with congenital aleukocytosis: agranulocytosis + lymphoid hypoplasia + thymic aplasia; unknown etiology
- Periodic neutropenia: stem cell regulation defect; neutropenic phases in 10- to 35-day intervals, compensatory monocytosis; autosomal dominant inheritance
- Kostmann's syndrome: severe agranulocytosis in children (abnormal differentiation in the promyelocytic stage), reversible by administration of G-CSF (*ATTENTION:* possibly higher risk of MDS / AML development); autosomal dominant or recessive inheritance
- X-linked agammaglobulinemia

- Schwachman-Diamond-Oski syndrome: neutropenia + pancreatic insufficiency + metaphyseal dysplasia; unknown etiology; autosomal recessive inheritance
- Neutropenia with bi- / tetraploid leukocytes: abnormal phagocytosis and chemotaxis as well as bi- and tetraploid granulocytes
- Chédiak-Higashi syndrome: albinism + neurological disorders + leukocytic granulation abnormalities; unknown etiology
- Dyskeratosis congenita: neutropenia, skin abnormalities; X-linked inheritance
- Lazy leukocyte syndrome: chemotaxis defect (actin defect); unknown etiology

### Neutropenia Caused by Acquired Disorders of Granulopoiesis
- Cytostatic treatment, immunosuppressives, azidothymidine (AZT), benzenes, ionizing radiation
- Idiosyncratic drug reactions (individual sensitivity) in 66% of cases: antibiotics (penicillin, chloramphenicol, cephalosporins, sulfonamides), sulfasalazine, nonsteroidal antirheumatics (ibuprofen, indomethacin, phenylbutazone), phenothiazine, thyreostatics, quinidine, procainamide, propafenone, ticlopidine, antihistamines, anticonvulsives, nifedipine, levamisole, tamoxifen, allopurinol, tranquilizers, neuroleptics (clozapine), gold, captopril + interferon

### Neutropenia Caused by Increased Neutrophil Destruction
- Hypersplenism
- Autoimmune neutropenia: postinfectious (mononucleosis, viral infections), AIDS, Felty's syndrome (rheumatoid arthritis + splenomegaly + neutropenia), systemic lupus erythematosus (SLE), Sjögren's syndrome, malignant lymphoma
- Neonatal isoimmune neutropenia: transplacental passage of maternal antineutrophil antibodies
- Complement activation: hemodialysis, cardiopulmonary bypass, T-γ disease

### Infections: Increased Margination / Consumption (Pseudoneutropenia)
- Bacteria: typhus, paratyphus, brucellosis, tuberculosis, tularemia
- Viruses: yellow fever, sandfly fever, infectious hepatitis, measles, influenza, chickenpox, German measles, Colorado tick fever, dengue fever, HIV, EBV
- Rickettsia: rickettsial pox, Rocky Mountain spotted fever
- Protozoa: malaria, kala-azar, recurrent fever
- Fungi: histoplasma

### Other Causes
- Bone marrow infiltration: leukemia (especially hairy cell leukemia), lymphomas, solid tumors
- Malnutrition: vitamin $B_{12}$ / folic acid deficiency, alcoholism
- T-cell-associated neutropenia (T-γ disease), myelodysplasia (MDS)
- DIDMOAD syndrome: diabetes insipidus + diabetes mellitus + optic nerve atrophy + deafness
- Metabolic disorders: hepatic cirrhosis, ketoacidosis, Gaucher's disease
- Sepsis, hypothermia, acute anaphylaxis

**Sy:**
- Initially usually asymptomatic
- General symptoms: fatigue, decreased performance, anorexia, infections

**Dg:**

### Medical History, Physical Examination
- Medical history: drug treatment, family history, infections, menstrual complaints
- Physical examination: with lymph node status, liver / spleen, signs of infection, mucositis

### Laboratory Tests
- Blood count with differential, reticulocytes
- Routine laboratory tests including vitamin $B_{12}$ and folic acid, total protein, protein electrophoresis, urinary protein (paraprotein diagnosis), copper
- Immunology: immunoglobulin assay, immunoelectrophoresis, Coombs' test, ANA, anti-DNA, rheumatoid factor, granulocyte antibodies

- Differentiation of lymphocyte subpopulations (FACS): T-cell subpopulations, NK cells, exclusion of leukemia
- Infection monitoring: blood, fecal, and urine cultures, throat swab, viral serology (including HIV)
- Cytogenetics
- Ham's test, sugar water test (exclusion of PNH)

### Histology
- Bone marrow aspiration, biopsy and culture (CFU)

### Imaging
- Abdominal sonography (spleen), chest x-ray (exclusion of infection)

**Dd:**
- Leukemia (▶ Chaps. 7.1.1, 7.1.2)
- Myelodysplasia (▶ Chap. 7.2)
- Primary Myelofibrosis (▶ Chap. 7.3.4)
- Aplastic anemia (▶ Chap. 6.1)

**Co:**
- Susceptibility to infections, fever (▶ Chap. 4.2)
- Mucositis, gastroenteritis ("neutropenic enterocolitis")

**Th:**

### Supportive Therapy
- Hygiene, anti-infectious environment, isolation
- Mucositis prophylaxis
- Selective intestinal decontamination
- Oral antimycosis (e.g., fluconazole 200 mg/day p.o.)
- Signs of infection: blood cultures, urine and stool cultures, swabs, immediate start of empirical antibiotic treatment (▶ Chap. 4.2)
- With severe infections: granulocyte transfusion (▶ Chap. 5.4)

### Treatment of Acute Agranulocytosis
- Discontinue all drugs administered within 4 weeks of onset of symptoms
- G-CSF (filgrastim, lenograstim) 5–10 µg/kg daily s.c.

### Treatment of Chronic Neutropenia
Treatment according to the assumed pathogenic causes, e.g.:
- In patients with clinically relevant recurrent infections, G-CSF may be used as long-term treatment
- Use of other hematopoietic growth factors in clinical studies: GM-CSF, IL-3, stem cell factor (SCF)
- In cases of autoimmune neutropenia:
  - Prednisolone 2 mg/kg daily p.o. (maximum 4 weeks)
  - Cyclosporin A (serum level target: 300–600 ng/ml): initial treatment over at least 4 weeks; if successful, continue for at least 3 months
  - Azathioprine 2–4 mg/kg daily
- With hypersplenism: consider splenectomy (only after pneumococcus vaccination)
- In cases of congenital neutropenia: consider allogeneic transplantation (▶ Chap. 5.3)

### Prophylaxis
With clozapine therapy and thyreostatic medication: regular weekly blood counts.

**Ref:**
1. Berliner N, Horwitz M, Loughran TP Jr. Congenital and acquired neutropenia. Hematology (ASH Educ Program) 2004:63–79
2. Boxer LA, Newburger PE. A molecular classification of congenital neutropenia syndromes. Pediatr Blood Cancer 2007;49:609–14
3. Lakshman R, Finn A. Neutrophil disorders and their management. J Clin Pathol 2001;54:7–19
4. Manny N, Zelig O. Laboratory diagnosis of autoimmune cytopenias. Curr Opin Hematol 2000;7:414–9

5.  Palmblad JE, von dem Borne AE. Idiopathic, immune, infectious and idiosyncratic neutropenias. Semin Hematol 2002;39:113–20
6.  Welte G, Zeidler C, Dale DC. Severe congenital neutropenia. Semin Hematol 2006;43:189–95

**Web:**

1.  http://www.rarediseases.org/            NORD, Rare Disorders
2.  http://www.nlm.nih.gov/medlineplus/ency/article/001295.htm  Medline Plus article
3.  http://www.mascc.org                 MASCC, Supportive Care
4.  http://www.neutropenia.ca/            Neutropenia Support Assoc
5.  http://www.emedicine.com/med/topic82.htm    E-medicine

## 6.3    Thrombocytopenia

**A.K. Kaskel, J. Heinz**

**Def:**    Decreased platelet count (< 150,000/µl), most common cause of hemorrhagic diatheses.

**ICD-10:**    D69.6

**Phys:**    *Platelet Kinetics*
- Thrombopoiesis: megakaryoblasts → megakaryocytes → platelets; regulated by thrombopoietin and other cytokines (e.g., IL-3, IL-6, IL-11)
- Directly after being released by the bone marrow, approximately one third of platelets are reversibly stored in the spleen ("pool")
- Two thirds of platelets circulate in the blood, life span 7–10 days, biological half-life 3–4 days; 15% of these platelets are spent daily to maintain hemostasis

The platelet count is influenced by:
- Nutritional status: folic acid / vitamin $B_{12}$ deficiency, alcohol abuse
- Menstrual cycle: shortly after ovulation, platelet count ↑
- Acute-phase reactions (infections, tumors) → platelet count ↑

**Pg:**    *Disorders of Thrombopoiesis*
- Infections (most common cause): e.g., CMV, EBV, HIV, mycoplasma, bacterial infection, parasites (malaria), sepsis (early symptom)
- Hematopoietic (bone marrow) deficiency: aplastic anemia, primary myelofibrosis
- Bone marrow infiltration: leukemia, lymphomas, solid tumors
- Abnormal megakaryocytic maturation: myelodysplasia, folic acid / vitamin $B_{12}$ deficiency
- Drug-induced / toxic myelosuppression: cytostatics, thiazides, alcohol, estrogens, thiamazole, gold, benzene, ionizing radiation
- Hereditary platelet disorders (rare):
  - Fanconi's anemia
  - Wiskott-Aldrich syndrome (thrombocytopenia, eczema, and immunodeficiency)
  - von Willebrand's disease type IIb
  - Thrombocytopenia with absent radii syndrome (TAR)
  - Bernard-Soulier syndrome (giant platelets and platelet dysfunction)
  - Thrombopoietin deficiency

*Increased Splenic Platelet Sequestration (Hypersplenism)*
Splenomegaly (portal hypertension, splenic infiltration with hematological neoplasia).

*Accelerated Peripheral Platelet Turnover*
- Heart valve and vascular prostheses
- Extracorporeal circulation (surface activation)
- Immune thrombocytopenia (ITP) (▶ Chap. 6.3.1)
- Microangiopathic disorders: hemolytic-uremic syndrome (HUS) , thrombotic-thrombocytopenic purpura (TTP) (▶ Chap. 6.3.3)
- Disseminated intravascular coagulation (DIC) (▶ Chap. 6.5.5)
- Disturbances in platelet and coagulation factor interaction: von Willebrand's disease type IIb, heparin-induced thrombocytopenia (HIT) (▶ Chap. 6.3.2)
- Evans' syndrome: autoimmune hemolytic anemia and thrombocytopenia

**Sy:**    *Hemorrhage*
- Petechial type of hemorrhage with small pinpoint lesions on skin / mucous membranes, occasionally epistaxis, menorrhagia
- In rare cases: hematoma / bruising / diffuse hemorrhage

**Dg:**

### Clinical Diagnosis
- Medical history (especially infections, drugs, hemorrhage)
- Clinical findings: petechial bleeding (skin, mucous membranes), lymph nodes, spleen
- In severe cases: signs of organ bleeding, anemia, hemorrhage

### Laboratory Tests
- Blood count with differential, reticulocytes, clotting studies (Quick, PTT, fibrinogen), hemolysis parameters (LDH, haptoglobin), liver function tests, CRP
- Exclusion of pseudothrombocytopenia by means of platelet count in citrated blood
- Viral serology (HIV included)
- With suspected vasculitis / SLE → immunology: antinuclear antibodies (ANA), rheumatoid factor
- With suspected HUS / TTP: screening for abnormal VWF multimers or VWF protease antibodies (▶ Chap. 6.3.3)
- With suspected Evans' syndrome (autoimmune hemolytic anemia and thrombocytopenia): Coombs' test
- Blood group
- Possibly detection of fixed thrombocytic antibodies (immune thrombocytopenia)

### Histology
Bone marrow aspiration and biopsy: megakaryocytes ↓ in case of dysfunctional thrombopoiesis, megakaryocytes normal or ↑ in cases of peripheral platelet loss. *ATTENTION:* if platelet count < 20,000/μl: risk of hemorrhage → iliac crest biopsy (no sternal puncture), apply careful pressure

### Imaging
Chest x-ray (lymphomas, infections), abdominal sonography (lymphomas, spleen)

**NOTE:** if plasmatic coagulation and blood vessels are normal, there is only a low risk of hemorrhage with a platelet count of > 10,000–20,000/μl.

**Dd:**

"Pseudothrombocytopenia": formation of platelet aggregates in EDTA blood: 0.1–2% of blood samples; cause: autoagglutinating IgG antibodies
- → In vitro platelet aggregation in the presence of the anticoagulant agent EDTA
- → False low count by automatic platelet counter
- → Repeat platelet count with citrated or heparinized blood

**Th:**

### Treatment of the Underlying Disease
- In cases of drug-induced thrombocytopenia: avoid causative agent
- Treatment of malignancies
- Treatment of immunological disorders

### Supportive Treatment
- Prevention of menstrual bleeding (e.g., lynestrenol)
- Avoid platelet aggregation inhibitors (acetyl salicylic acid)
- Platelet transfusion at signs of bleeding / acute risk of hemorrhage (*ATTENTION:* HUS / TTP)
- With thrombopathy try DDAVP (desmopressin); dosage 0.3 μg/kg body weight in 0.9% saline infusion every 8 h, maximum 3 days → repeat after 48 h

### Platelet Transfusion (▶ Chap. 4.9.1)
- Therapeutic: at signs of bleeding or acute hemorrhage (e.g., petechiae, hemorrhage of mucous membranes or epistaxis) with proven thrombocytopenia or thrombocyte dysfunction.
- Prophylactic: platelet count < 10,000–20,000/μl. With concomitant diseases (especially acute leukemia, fever, sepsis, splenomegaly) risk of hemorrhage with higher platelet counts (20,000–30,000/μl). With invasive interventions (e.g., catheter installation, punctures) the platelet count target is > 40,000–60,000/μl.

### Relative Contraindication
- Allergy to human plasma protein
- Post-transfusion purpura (PTP)
- Idiopathic thrombocytopenic purpura (ITP)
- Heparin-induced thrombocytopenia (HIT)
- Thrombotic-thrombocytopenic purpura (TTP)

To avoid alloimmunization, transfusions should be avoided in patients scheduled for allogeneic hematopoietic stem cell transplantation.

**Ref:**

1. Aster RH, Bougie DW. Drug-induced immune thrombocytopenia. N Engl J Med 2007;357:580–7
2. Bolton-Maggs PHB, Chalmers EA, Collins PW et al. A review of inherited platelet disorders with guidelines for their management on behalf of the UKHCDO. Br J Haematol 2006;135:603–33
3. Cines DB, Bussel JB, McMillan RB et al. Congenital and acquired thrombocytopenia. Hematology (ASH Educ Program) 2004:390–406
4. Deutsch VR, Tomer A. Megakaryocyte development and platelet production: Br J Haematol 2006; 134:453–66
5. Drachman JG. Inherited thrombocytopenia: when a low platelet count does not mean ITP. Blood 2004;103:390–8
6. Geddis AE, Kaushansky K. Inherited thrombocytopenias: toward a molecular understanding of disorders of platelet production. Curr Opin Pediatr 2004;16:15–22
7. George JN. Platelets. Lancet 2000;355:1531–9
8. Jelic S, Radulovic S. Chemotherapy-associated thrombocytopenia. Ann J Cancer 2006;5:371–82

**Web:**

1. http://www.pdsa.org — Platelet Disorder Support Assoc
2. http://www.med.unc.edu/isth/ — ISTH, Intl Soc Thromb Hemostasis
3. http://www.nlm.nih.gov/medlineplus/ency/article/000586.htm — MedlinePlus
4. http://www.emedicine.com/med/topic3480.htm — E-medicine
5. http://marrowfailure.cancer.gov/AMEGA.html — NCI, Marrow Failure Disorders

## 6.3.1 Immune (Idiopathic) Thrombocytopenic Purpura (ITP, Werlhof's Disease)

**A.K. Thomas, J. Heinz**

**Def:** Acquired thrombocytopenia, platelet count < 150,000/μl.

*Classic definition:* ITP = idiopathic thrombocytopenic purpura.
Diagnosis by exclusion; acquired thrombocytopenia of unknown etiology with normal to increased megakaryocyte count in the bone marrow.

*Alternative definition:* ITP = immune thrombocytopenic purpura.
Acquired thrombocytopenia caused by antithrombocytic antibodies.

**ICD-10:** D69.3

**Ep:** Incidence: 6–10 cases / 100,000 population / year. Distribution male:female = 1:2.

**Pp:** IgG-mediated immune reaction (rarely IgM) against platelet membrane antigens, e.g., GPIIb / GPIIIa (fibrinogen receptor), GPIb / IX (von Willebrand receptor), and GPIa / IIa (collagen receptor).
- Specific platelet antibodies detectable in approximately 50–70% of cases
- Macrophage binding via Fcγ I, II, and III receptors (in ITP patients: receptor polymorphism with altered binding affinity for IgG)
- Complement activation
- Complement-mediated lysis and enhancement of phagocytosis
  - → RES phagocytosis of IgG-coated platelets, esp. in spleen
  - → Biological half-life of platelets ↓↓ to a few hours
- Decreased thrombocytopoiesis (antibodies against megakaryocytes and thrombopoietic progenitor cells)
- Possibly T-cell-mediated process (in vitro, CD4+ T-cells can be activated by platelets)

**Pg:** *Etiology*
- Without known causative disease ("primary ITP")
- In conjunction with an underlying disease ("secondary ITP"): lymphoproliferative diseases, autoimmune diseases (systemic lupus erythematosus, etc.), viral diseases (e.g., HCV, HIV), bacterial infections (esp. in children), after bone marrow transplantation

*Progression*
- Children: in > 90% of cases, "acute" course: severe thrombocytopenia, usually spontaneous remission within 3 months
- Adults: in > 90% of cases, "chronic" course (thrombocytopenia > 6 months): < 5% risk of fatal hemorrhages (esp. intracranial), rarely spontaneous remission (5%), persists for more than 6 months despite adequate treatment in 35% of patients

**Path:** *Blood Count*
Thrombocytopenia with normal differential and morphology.

*Bone Marrow*
Normal or reactively increased megakaryocyte count, increased number of immature megakaryocytes. Otherwise, normal bone marrow, no abnormal cells.

**Sy:** *Hemorrhage*
- Rare with platelet count > 30,000/μl

- Petechial type of hemorrhage (skin, mucous membranes), with hematomas / bruising / epistaxis
- Complication: intracerebral hemorrhage (rare), organ bleeding, retinal bleeding, gastrointestinal bleeds

**Dg:**      The diagnosis of ITP is a diagnosis of exclusion. Therefore, the diagnostic strategies are aimed at identifying potential underlying causes of secondary thrombocytopenia.

### Clinical Diagnosis
- Medical history, family history, drug exposure, occupational hazards
- Physical examination (petechiae, bruising, mucosal bleeds)

### Laboratory Tests
- Full blood count with differential
- Virology: HCV / HIV serology in patients at risk
- Screening for platelet antibodies (50% positive)

### Histology
Bone marrow biopsy and smear in accordance with recommendations of ASH (American Society of Hematology) and BCSH (British Committee for Standards in Hematology):
- Patients over 60 years of age
- Laboratory abnormalities (neutropenia, anemia)
- Prior to splenectomy
- Poor response to primary treatment.

**Dd:**      Differential diagnosis of thrombocytopenia ▶ Chap. 6.3

**Th:**      **Indications for Treatment**

Only a small number of randomized studies have been conducted in ITP. The life expectancy of ITP patients with a platelet count > 30,000/µl is equal to that of the normal population. With higher platelet counts (30,000/µl), treatment is therefore only indicated if blood loss is expected (perioperatively, before delivery) or in the case of active hemorrhage. Recommendations of the British Committee for Standards in Hematology (BCSH) with regard to safe platelet counts in adults:
- Dental treatment: ≥ 10,000/µl
- Tooth extraction: ≥ 30,000/µl
- Minor operation: ≥ 50,000/µl
- Major operation: ≥ 80,000/µl

**Therapeutic concept for management of ITP in adults**

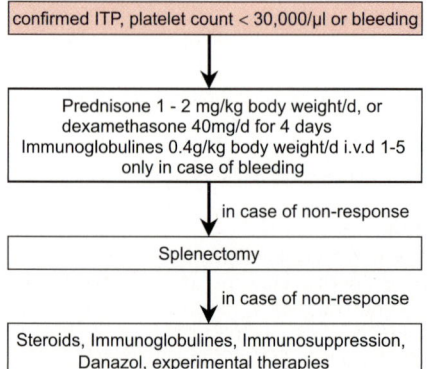

confirmed ITP, platelet count < 30,000/µl or bleeding

Prednisone 1 - 2 mg/kg body weight/d, or dexamethasone 40mg/d for 4 days
Immunoglobulines 0.4g/kg body weight/d i.v.d 1-5 only in case of bleeding

in case of non-response

Splenectomy

in case of non-response

Steroids, Immunoglobulines, Immunosuppression, Danazol, experimental therapies

## Treatment Options

### *Primary Treatment*

#### *Steroids*
- Initial response rate > 50%, long-term effect in 30% of patients, low-dose maintenance treatment is required in most cases
- Prednisolone 1–2 mg/kg daily, duration of treatment depending on response, or dexamethasone 40 mg/d for 4 days
- With durable platelet response: dose reduction of prednisolone over 6–12 weeks, monitoring of platelet counts
- If no increment to > 30,000/µl within 2–4 weeks or required steroid dose markedly above the threshold dose for Cushing's disease → change treatment to immunoglobulins or alternative immunosuppressive drugs

#### *Immunoglobulins (ivIG)*
- Initial response rate 75%, normalization of the platelet count in 50% of patients; however, only transient (up to 4 weeks)
- Standard dose: 0.4 g/kg daily i.v. days 1–5 or 1 g/kg daily i.v. day 1 + 2
- Alternative: anti-D IgG in Rh-positive patients, 75 µg/kg body weight over 2–3 days. Disadvantage: i.v. product not available in all countries, high costs

In cases of severe or life-threatening hemorrhage: combined administration of methylprednisolone 1 g daily i.v. over 3 days and immunoglobulins 0.4–1 g/kg daily over 2–4 days, platelet transfusion. Due to the short platelet half-life in ITP, the expected platelet need is approximately 2–3 times higher than in other forms of thrombocytopenia. In patients with uncomplicated ITP, platelet transfusions are, generally not indicated.

### *Secondary Treatment*

#### *Romiplostim*
Thrombopoietic agent, binds to TPO receptor and stimulates platelet production of the bone marrow. In Phase III studies in ITP, platelet responses in 80–90% of cases. Starting dose 1 µg/kg once weekly s.c., dose adjustment according to platelet counts.

#### *Splenectomy*
- Approximately 60% response rate, no known predictors of response
- Perioperatively, platelet count should be raised to > 50,000/µl (ivIG)
- Preoperative vaccination against pneumococcus, *Hemophilus influenzae*, meningococcus
- If no response, exclude accessory spleen, repeat steroids

### *Tertiary Treatment*

#### *Danazol*
- Mode of action: downregulation of Fc receptors on macrophages
- Not effective in steroid-refractory cases, but may be useful in combination with prednisolone to reduce steroid side effects

#### *Immunosuppressives*
A number of smaller studies have provided limited data on efficacy and safety of various immunosuppressives. In individual cases or in smaller groups of patients, the following substances have been used successfully: mycophenolate mofetil, azathioprine, cyclophosphamide, cyclosporin A.

### *Experimental Treatment*
- Immunoapheresis
- Rituximab (CD20 antibody)

**Px:**    Prevention of hemorrhage / trauma
- No intramuscular or intra-articular injections
- No massages
- No administration of platelet aggregation inhibitors (acetyl salicylic acid, ticlopidine, clopido-grel)
- No sports with high risk of hemorrhage
- Emergency ID card

**Ref:**
1. Andemariam B, Bussel J. New therapies for ITP. Curr Opin Hematol 2007;14:427–31
2. British Committee for Standards in Hematology (BCSH). Guidelines for the investigation and man-agement of idiopathic thrombocytopenic purpura in adults, children and pregnancy. Br J Haematol 2003;120:574–96
3. Bussel JB, Kuter DJ, George JN et al. AMG 531, a thrombopoiesis stimulating protein, for chronic ITP. N Engl J Med 2006;355:1672–81
4. Cines DB, McMillan R. Management of adult idiopathic thrombocytopenic purpura. Annu Rev Med 2005;56:425–42
5. George JN, Woolf SH, Raskob GE. Idiopathic thrombocytopenic purpura: a guideline for diagnosis and management of children and adults. American Society of Hematology. Ann Med 1998;30:38–44
6. McMillan R, Durette C. Long-term outcomes in adults with chronic ITP after splenectomy failure. Blood 2004;104:956–60
7. Portielle JEA, Westendorp RGJ, Kluin-Nelemans et al. Morbidity and mortality in adults with idiopathic thrombocytopenic purpura. Blood 2001;97:2549–54
8. Stasi R, Stipa E, Masi M et al. Long-term observation of 208 adults with chronic idiopathic thrombocyto-penic purpura. Am J Med 1995;98:436–42

**Web:**
1. http://www.pdsa.org/                                  PDSA
2. http://www.emedicine.com/EMERG/topic282.htm           E-medicine
3. http://www.emedicine.com/med/topic1151.htm            E-medicine
4. http://www.scripps.edu/itp/                           Scripps Clinic
5. http://www.itpsupport.org.uk                          ITP Support Assoc

## 6.3.2 Heparin-induced Thrombocytopenia (HIT)

A.K. Kaskel, J. Heinz

**Def:** Acquired heparin-induced thrombocytopenia

**ICD-10:** D69.5

**Ep:** Incidence of HIT type II (see below) with intravenous use of unfractioned heparin (UFH): 2–5%, with use of low-molecular-weight heparin (LMWH): < 0.5%.

**Pg:**

### Heparin-induced Thrombocytopenia (HIT) Type I
- Dose-dependent mild early-onset thrombocytopenia (platelet count 100,000–150,000/μl) in the initial 2–3 days of heparin treatment (UFH / LMWH)
- Caused by minor heparin-induced platelet aggregation, no immunological genesis
- Usually self-limiting (after 1–2 days) while heparin administration is ongoing
- Frequency of up to 30%

### Heparin-induced Thrombocytopenia (HIT) Type II
- Dose-independent late-onset thrombocytopenia, 4–20 days after start of heparin treatment (UFH / LMWH). In patients previously exposed to heparin (< 100 days), reoccurrence within hours
- Severe thrombocytopenia (platelets < 100,000/μl), median platelet count approximately 60,000/μl, rarely < 20,000/μl or decreased to < 50% of the initial count; worsening of thrombocytopenia if heparin treatment is continued
- Thromboembolic complications up to 40 days after heparin administration
- IgG antibodies mostly against the platelet factor 4 (PF4)–heparin complex
    - → Immune complex formation
    - → Platelet activation due to binding of the immune complex to the Fc receptor (Fcγ RIIA), PF4 release
    - → Platelet aggregation, endothelial cell damage, thrombin activation
    - → Thromboembolic complications ("white clot syndrome")

**Sy:** Clinical relevance: HIT type II:
- **Main symptom: thrombophilia, not hemorrhage**
- Warning signs: exanthema or necrosis at injection site
- High incidence (up to 53%) of venous and arterial thrombosis, renal dysfunction, pulmonary embolism, infarction (complications may occur weeks after discontinuation of heparin)

**Dg:**
- Exclusion of other causes of thrombocytopenia (▶ Chap. 6.3).
- Combination of a functional test (e.g., heparin-induced platelet activation, HIPA) with ELISA (detection of PF4–heparin complexes).
- *ATTENTION:* if HIT II is clinically suspected, discontinue heparin immediately and use alternatives, even without positive test. The diagnosis of HIT is based on clinical findings. Tests serve as confirmatory tools only.

**Dd:** Exclude other causes of thrombocytopenia (▶ Chap. 6.3)

**Th:** Therapeutic intervention (with HIT type II):
- Discontinue heparin treatment (UFH / LMWH). *ATTENTION:* exclude exposure to "hidden" heparin, e.g., coagulation factor products, "heparin lock" of central catheters
- Anticoagulation must be continued for at least 4 weeks, using:
    - Danaparoid sodium: heparin-free heparinoid, ATIII-mediated inhibition of factor Xa, half-life 24 h, renal elimination, monitoring via factor Xa levels, no antidote available
    - Hirudin derivatives, e.g., lepirudin: bivalent direct thrombin inhibitor, half-life 1.5 h, renal elimination, monitoring via PTT, no antidote available

- – Argatroban: direct thrombin inhibitor, interacts with the active site of thrombin. Half-live 24 min., monitored by PTT. No dose adjustment in renal failure, due to hepatic elimination.
- • In cases of existing thrombosis: coumarin overlapping with danaparoid or hirudin.
- • Avoid using LMWH (cross-reaction)

**Ref:**

1. Alving BM. How I treat heparin-induced thrombopenia and thrombosis. Blood 2003;101:31–7
2. Arepally GM, Ortel TL. Heparin-induced thrombocytopenia. N Engl J Med 2006;355:809–17
3. Keeling D, Davidson S, Watson H. British Committee for Standards in Haematology. The management of heparin-induced thrombocytopenia. Br J Haematol 2006;133:259–69
4. Newman PM, Chong BH. Heparin-induced thrombocytopenia: new evidence for the dynamic binding of purified anti-PF4-heparin antibodies to platelets and the resultant platelet activation. Blood 2000;96:182–7
5. Rice L, Attisha WK, Drexler A et al. Delayed-onset heparin-induced thrombocytopenia. Ann Intern Med 2002;136:210–5

**Web:**

1. http://www.med.unc.edu/isth/welcome          Intl Soc Thrombosis Hemostasis
2. http://www.tigc.org/eguidelines/hit05.htm     TIGC, Guidelines

**6.3.3     Thrombotic Microangiopathies (TTP-HUS)**

A.K. Kaskel, J. Heinz

**Def:**     Thrombocytopenic thrombotic microangiopathies with hemolytic anemia (microangiopathic hemolytic anemia, MAHA). Subtypes:
- *Thrombotic-thrombocytopenic purpura (TTP, Moschcowitz disease):* main symptoms are microangiopathic hemolytic anemia, thrombocytopenia, and neurological symptoms; renal dysfunction in 50% of cases
- *Hemolytic-uremic syndrome (HUS, Gasser's disease):* main symptoms are acute renal failure (renal microangiopathy, glomeruli are particularly affected) and hemolytic anemia; thrombocytopenia and neurological symptoms are less pronounced than in TTP
- *Toxic microangiopathic hemolytic anemia (toxic MAHA):* after treatment with mitomycin C or high-dose chemotherapy

It is not yet clear whether TTP and HUS are separate diseases or whether they are different manifestations of one syndrome. Due to the frequently overlapping symptoms, the more commonly used term is TTP-HUS (in adult patients). Exception: HUS in children after *E. coli* infection.

**CD-10:**     M31.1

**Ep:**     TTP: age peak 30–50 years, distribution male:female = 1:2

HUS: incidence 3–5 cases/100,000 children/year, age peak 1–5 years, distribution male:female = 1:1

**Pg:**     ***Thrombotic-Thrombocytopenic Purpura (TTP)***
- Acquired or congenital (total) dysfunction of the vWF-cleaving protease (= ADAMTS13; a disintegrin and metalloprotease with thrombospondin type-1 motifs; cleaves vWF between the amino acids 842 and 843), with unusually large von Willebrand factor multimers (UL-vWF-M), particularly in chronically recurrent TTP
- Acquired TTP: autoimmune disease with anti-vWF protease autoantibodies
- Associated with infections (HIV), pregnancy, postpartum, after allogeneic bone marrow transplantation, drugs (mitomycin C, cyclosporine, ticlopidine, clopidogrel, quinine), autoimmune diseases (SLE)

***Hemolytic-Uremic Syndrome (HUS)***
- Normal vWF protease activity.
- Commonly associated with gastrointestinal infections caused by Shiga toxin or verotoxin-producing *Escherichia coli* (serotypes OH, particularly O157:H7, O103:HU, O103:H2), rarely shigella (*Shigella dysenteriae* serotype I).
- In the absence of gastrointestinal infections, HUS is probably complement-mediated and occurs in connection with autosomal recessively inherited factor H mutations. In sporadic forms, factor H autoantibodies are thought to be involved. In this case, association with glomerulonephritis type II and involvement of autoantibodies against C3 convertase.

**Path:**     Under physiological conditions, vWF multimers are excreted by endothelial cells and deposited subendothelially. In the case of endothelial damage → complex formation of vWF multimers with thrombocytes → thrombocyte aggregation due to binding to platelet glycoproteins Ib, IX, and V as well as activated GP IIb/IIIa.

In cases of thrombotic microangiopathies, platelet aggregates or microthrombi are formed in capillaries and small vessels causing infarction, particularly in CNS and kidney.
- Thrombocytopenia due to peripheral destruction
- Anemia due to mechanical destruction of erythrocytes in partially thrombosed small vessels (fragmentocytes, LDH ↑, haptoglobin ↓↓).

**Sy:**     Symptoms according to disease subtype:
- *Microangiopathic hemolytic anemia (MAHA):* 100%; icterus, signs of acute hemolysis, pallor, reduced performance
- *Thrombocytopenia (more common in TTP):* 60–90%; petechiae, bruising, epistaxis, hemorrhage, bleeding
- *Neuropathy (more common in TTP):* 70–90%; central neurological disorders, confusion, cramps, headache, impaired vision, cerebellar ataxia, coma
- *Nephropathy (more common in HUS):* 65%; hematuria, oliguria / anuria, renal failure
- Fever: 30–50%
- In infection-associated forms: preceding watery / bloody diarrhea caused by *E. coli* / shigella, with abdominal pain, cramps
- ARDS-like pulmonary complications

**Dg:**     ### Clinical Diagnosis
- Medical history (particularly infection)
- Physical examination: type of hemorrhage, signs of infections, neuropathy, nephropathy (hematuria, oliguria, anuria), pulmonary symptoms

### Laboratory Tests
- Anemia, thrombocytopenia
- Differential blood count / smear: reticulocytosis, fragmentocytes, anisocytosis, poikilocytosis
- Signs of intravascular hemolysis: LDH ↑, haptoglobin ↓↓, bilirubin ↑
- Coombs' test negative (not antibody-mediated)
- Renal dysfunction: creatinine ↑, urea ↑, electrolytes, uric acid ↑
- Urine: proteinuria (1–2 g/24 h, up to 10 g/24 h), hematuria
- Bleeding time ↑, fibrin monomers / fibrinogen cleavage products ↑
- ELISA to detect Shiga toxin (EHEC)
- Determination of the vWF protease activity (ADAMTS13)

**Dd:**
- ITP → no hemolysis constellation
- DIC / sepsis → lack of coagulation factors
- Evans' syndrome (autoimmunohemolysis and ITP) → positive direct Coombs' test
- Glomerulonephritis → hypertension, urine results, liver / kidney function ↓, kidney biopsy
- Infections: malaria, leptospirosis, dengue fever, hantavirus infection

**Co:**
- Cardiac complications: ischemia, infarction, arrhythmia
- Brain hemorrhage (rare)

**Th:**     Thrombotic microangiopathies constitute a hematological emergency → immediate specific treatment is of vital importance. Without adequate treatment, the mortality rate is 90%.

### Plasmapheresis
- Plasma exchange via pheresis with fresh frozen plasma (FFP) initially 40 ml/kg daily
- Aim: depletion of vWF multimers and autoantibodies, substitution of vWF protease ($t\frac{1}{2} > 24$ h through FFP or as cryoprecipitate
- Success parameters: normalization of LDH and platelets, regression of neurological symptoms; once laboratory parameters have normalized, lengthening of pheresis intervals
- If symptoms persist: increase pheresis frequency to twice daily or raise volume to 80 ml/kg (in individual cases, as much as 140 ml/kg/day may be indicated → however, twice daily pheresis seems to be more effective); in addition, prednisone (1 mg/kg/day) or methylprednisolone (125 mg i.v. twice daily) and possibly vincristine or immunoglobulins
- Pheresis is often accompanied by moderate citrate toxicity (muscle cramps, tetany) → calcium replacement
- Even with adequate treatment, full reconstitution of renal function may be delayed

## Additional Treatment Options

- With suspected acquired TTP: prednisolone $3 \times 50$ mg/day i.v. or p.o. over 1 week, withdraw gradually over a period of at least 4 weeks
- Patients with acquired antibody-mediated TTP who respond insufficiently to plasmapheresis or have relapsed: additional immunosuppressive treatment, e.g., splenectomy, immunoadsorption via protein A column, possibly azathioprine or other immunosuppressives (e.g., anti-CD20 antibody rituximab ± cyclophosphamide, cyclosporine).
- Congenital vWF protease deficiency: treatment according to symptoms: replacement of vWF protease ± plasmapheresis, prophylactic platelet aggregation inhibitors may be required with platelet recovery.

*ATTENTION:* Platelet transfusion only after careful benefit-risk assessment (e.g., life-threatening hemorrhage) → possible deterioration of symptoms (increased intravascular thrombus formation).

## Supportive Treatment

- Hypovolemia: fluid replacement / hypovolemia control
- Hypertension: antihypertensive treatment → in acute cases: nitrate / beta blockers, long-term treatment: ACE inhibitors
- Dialysis as required
- Severe anemia: packed red cells

**rg:** With adequate treatment (plasmapheresis, dialysis, supportive treatment), good prognosis:
- Response rate: 80–90%, mortality 5–20%
- Relapse rate: 15–20%
- In 15–20% of cases, chronic disease-related effects: renal dysfunction, residual cerebral disorders

**Ref:**
1. Allford SL, Hunt BJ, Rose P et al. British Committee for Standards in Haematology. Guidelines on the diagnosis and management of the thrombotic microangiopathic purpura. Br J Haematol 2003;120:556–73
2. George JN. Thrombotic thrombocytopenic purpura. N Engl J Med 2006;354:1927–35
3. Ho VT, Cutler C, Carter S et al. Blood and Marrow Transplant Clinical Trials Network Toxicity Committee Consensus Summary: thrombotic microangiopathy after hematopoietic stem cell transplantation. Biol Blood Marrow Transplant 2005;11:571–5
4. Levy GG, Motto DG, Ginsburg D. ADAMTS13 turns 3. Blood 2005;106:11–17
5. Plaimauer B, Zimmermann K, Volkel D et al. Cloning, expression and functional characterization of the von Willebrand factor-cleaving protease (ADAMTS13). Blood 2002;100:3626–32
6. Richards A, Goodship JA, Goodship THJ. The genetics and pathogenesis of HUS and TTP. Curr Opin Nephrol Hypertens 2002;11:431–5
7. Sadler JE, Moake JL, Miyata T et al. Recent advances in thrombotic thrombocytopenic purpura. Hematology (ASH Educ Program) 2004;407–23
8. Tarr PI, Gordon CA, Chandler WL. Shiga-toxin-producing Escherichia coli and haemolytic uremic syndrome. Lancet 2005;365:1073–86

**Web:**
1. http://moon.ouhsc.edu/jgeorge/TTP.html — TTP-HUS Registry
2. http://www.emedicine.com/emerg/topic579.htm — TTP, E-medicine
3. http://www.emedicine.com/emerg/topic238.htm — HUS, E-medicine
4. http://www.psbc.org/bulletins/bulletin_v7_n2.pdf — Puget Sound Blood Center
5. http://www.crttp.org/ — TTP Foundation
6. http://www.nlm.nih.gov/medlineplus/ency/article/000552.htm — MedlinePlus
7. http://www.nlm.nih.gov/medlineplus/ency/article/000510.htm — MedlinePlus

## 6.4      Anemia

D.P. Berger, R. Engelhardt

**Def:**   Reduced hemoglobin concentration and hematocrit. Red blood cell (RBC) number below normal level.

**Phys:**   **Red blood cell (RBC) parameters**

| Parameter | Abbreviation | Normal value |
|---|---|---|
| Hemoglobin | Hb | ♂ 14–18 g/dl, ♀ 12–16 g/dl |
| Hematocrit | Hkt | ♂ 40–52%, ♀ 37–48% |
| Erythrocyte count | Ery | ♂ $4.3–5.7 \times 10^6$/µl, ♀ $3.9–5.3 \times 10^6$/µl |
| Mean corpuscular volume | MCV | 85–98 fl |
| Mean corpuscular hemoglobin | MCH, HbE | 28–34 pg |
| MCH concentration | MCHC | 32–37 g/dl |
| Erythrocyte diameter | | 6.8–7.3 µm |
| Reticulocyte count | Reti | 0.3–1.5% |

### Nomenclature of Red Cell Changes

*Size (Indices: Erythrocyte Diameter, MCV)*
- Macrocytosis: erythrocyte diameter ↑, MCV ↑
- Microcytosis: erythrocyte diameter ↓, MCV ↓
- Anisocytosis: pronounced variations in size of RBC

*Shape*
- Poikilocytosis: different RBC shapes in blood smear
- Elliptocytes: oval RBC
- Spherocytes: spherical cells
- Target cells: target-like appearance
- Acanthocytes: irregularly spiculated cells, "spur cells"
- Schistocytes: RBC fragments, fragmentocytes
- Dacryocytes: drop-shaped cells, "teardrop" RBC
- Drepanocytes: sickle cells (bipolar spiculated cells)

*Staining (Indices: MCH, MCHC)*
- Hypochromic: RBC staining ↓, MCH ↓
- Hyperchromic: RBC staining ↑, MCH ↑
- Polychromatic: reddish-blue-gray staining

*Cell Inclusions*
- Howell-Jolly bodies: basophilic inclusions (nuclear remnants)
- Basophil stippling: punctuate basophilic inclusions (ribosomes)
- Heinz bodies: denatured hemoglobin (special staining required)
- Cabot's rings: basophilic circular threadlike inclusions (nuclear remnants)

**Pphys:** **Erythropoiesis and classification of anemias**

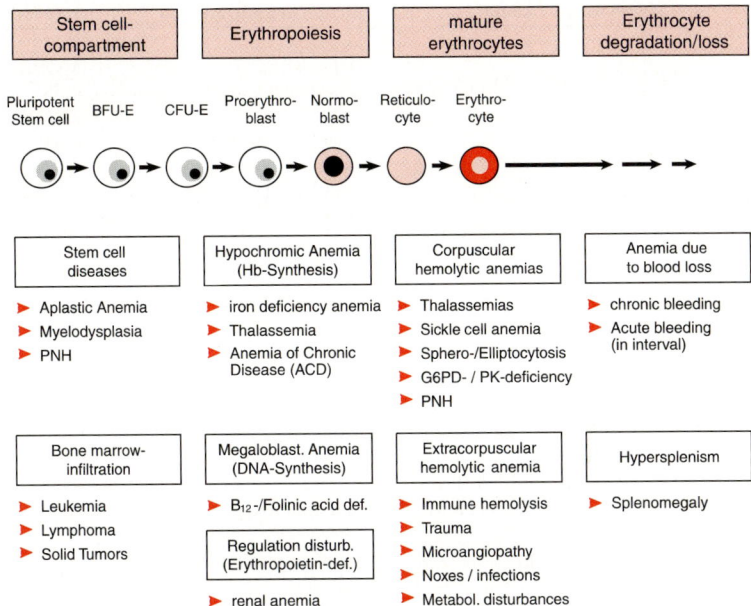

| Stem cell-compartment | Erythropoiesis | mature erythrocytes | Erythrocyte degradation/loss |

Pluripotent Stem cell — BFU-E — CFU-E — Proerythro-blast — Normo-blast — Reticulo-cyte — Erythro-cyte

| Stem cell diseases | Hypochromic Anemia (Hb-Synthesis) | Corpuscular hemolytic anemias | Anemia due to blood loss |
|---|---|---|---|
| ► Aplastic Anemia | ► iron deficiency anemia | ► Thalassemias | ► chronic bleeding |
| ► Myelodysplasia | ► Thalassemia | ► Sickle cell anemia | ► Acute bleeding (in interval) |
| ► PNH | ► Anemia of Chronic Disease (ACD) | ► Sphero-/Elliptocytosis | |
| | | ► G6PD- / PK-deficiency | |
| | | ► PNH | |

| Bone marrow-infiltration | Megaloblast. Anemia (DNA-Synthesis) | Extracorpuscular hemolytic anemia | Hypersplenism |
|---|---|---|---|
| ► Leukemia | ► $B_{12}$-/Folinic acid def. | ► Immune hemolysis | ► Splenomegaly |
| ► Lymphoma | | ► Trauma | |
| ► Solid Tumors | Regulation disturb. (Erythropoietin-def.) | ► Microangiopathy | |
| | ► renal anemia | ► Noxes / infections | |
| | | ► Metabol. disturbances | |

**Sy:**

### Symptoms of Anemia
- Pallor of skin and mucous membranes, nail beds, conjunctivae
- Weakness, tiredness, reduced performance
- Lack of concentration, headache, vertigo
- Dyspnea, tachycardia, palpitations (esp. with acute anemia)

**Dg:**

### History, Physical Examination
- Risk factors, esp. infections, drugs, bleeding (menstruation history), nutritional habits
- Physical examination including skin, mucous membranes, lymph node status, spleen / liver findings, heart (tachycardia, particularly systolic murmur), rectal examination with fecal blood test, gynecological examination

### Laboratory Tests
- Hematology: blood count, with MCV, MCH, reticulocytes, differential blood count, blood smear
- Clinical chemistry: routine tests with bilirubin, renal function parameters, total protein, protein electrophoresis, iron status (iron, ferritin, transferrin-binding capacity), parameters of hemolysis (bilirubin, LDH, haptoglobin), CRP, BSG, vitamin $B_{12}$ / folinic acid
- Coombs' test (if hemolytic anemia is suspected)
- Virus serology (including parvovirus B19)
- Blood group
- Erythropoietin level (if renal anemia is suspected)

### Histology
Bone marrow aspiration / biopsy, with iron stain (if stem cell/bone marrow disorder is suspected)

**Dd:**     **Differential diagnosis of anemia**

| Hypochromic anemia | Normochromic anemia | Hyperchromic anemia |
|---|---|---|
| MCH $\downarrow$ | MCH normal | MCH $\uparrow$ |
| Iron deficiency | Hemolysis | Megaloblastic anemia |
| Tumor | Acute blood loss | (Vitamin $B_{12}$ or folinic acid |
| Inflammation, infection | Aplastic anemia | deficiency) |
| Thalassemia | Renal anemia | Myelodysplastic syndromes |

**Th:**     *Supportive Treatment*

Substitution of packed red blood cells: restrictive indication (▶ Chap. 4.9.1).

*Guidelines for Transfusion Indication*

- Individual assessment of transfusion indication for each patient.
- In acute blood loss, consider indication when hemoglobin < 8.0 g/dl.
- With chronic anemia lower levels of hemoglobin (6–8 g/dl) are generally tolerated.
- Patients with coronary heart disease or risk of cerebral ischemia: transfusion indication a
  hemoglobin < 10 g/dl.
- Specific conditions (surgery, thalassemia major, etc.) may require RBC transfusion support.

The indication for transfusion is based on clinical symptoms. Asymptomatic blood loss does
not constitute an indication for transfusion.

**Ref:**
1.  Birgegard G, Aapro MS, Bokemeyer C et al. Cancer-related anemia: pathogenesis, prevalence and treat-
    ment. Oncology 2005;68(suppl 1):3–11
2.  Bokemeyer C, Aapro MS, Courdi A et al. EORTC guidelines for the use of erythropoietic proteins in anae-
    mic patients with cancer. Eur J Cancer 2004;40:2201–16
3.  British Committee for Standards in Hematology (BCSH). Guidelines for the clinical use of red cell transfu-
    sion. Br J Haematol 2001;113:24–31
4.  Littlewood TJ. The impact of hemoglobin levels on treatment outcomes in patients with cancer. Semin
    Oncol 2001;28(suppl 8):49–53
5.  Provan D, Weatherall D. Red cells I: inherited anaemias. Lancet 2000;355:1169–75
6.  Provan D, Weatherall D. Red cells II: acquired anemias and polycythaemia. Lancet 2000;355:1260–8
7.  Rizzo JD, Somerfield MP, Hagerty KL et al. ASH/ASCO 2007 clinical practice guideline update on the use
    of epoetin and darbepoetin. Blood 2007;111:x–y

**Web:**
1.  http://www.anemiainstitute.org/          Anemia Institute
2.  http://www.guideline.gov/               Guideline Clearinghouse
3.  http://www.nlm.nih.gov/medlineplus/anemia.html     MedlinePlus
4.  http://www.anemia.org                   Anemia Action Council

**.4.1** **Hypochromic Anemia**

**D.P. Berger, R. Engelhardt, T. Heinz**

**ef:** Anemias with decreased corpuscular hemoglobin (MCH < 28 pg) and decreased corpuscular hemoglobin concentration (MCHC < 32%):
- Iron deficiency anemia (> 90% of hypochromic anemias)
- Anemia of chronic disease (inflammation- / infection- / tumor anemia)
- Thalassemia (▶ Chap. 6.4.3)
- Rare causes: vitamin $B_6$ deficiency, lead intoxication

**d:** **Hypochromic anemia**

| Parameter | Iron deficiency anemia | Inflammation- / tumor anemia | β-Thalassemia |
|---|---|---|---|
| Serum iron | ↓ | ↓ | normal / ↑ |
| Transferrin | ↑ | ↑ | normal / ↓ |
| Serum ferritin | ↓ | ↑ | normal / ↑ |

### Iron Deficiency Anemia

**p:** Most frequent form of anemia. Proportion male:female = 1:5. About 10–20% of women in childbearing age demonstrate latent iron deficiency.

**hys:** **Iron metabolism**

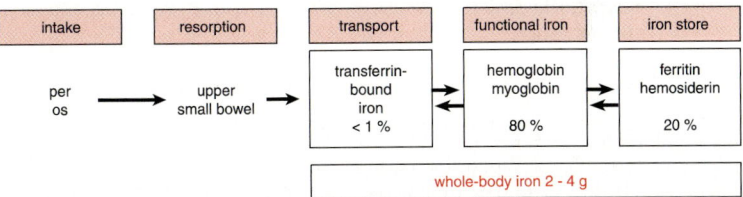

Daily iron resorption required: men 1 mg, women and adolescents 2–3 mg, pregnant women 3–4 mg. About 60–70% of body iron store bound in hemoglobin, additional 10% in myoglobin. 1 g hemoglobin contains 3.4 mg of iron.

In iron deficiency the iron need is greater than the available iron supply, resulting in hemoglobin synthesis disorders → microcytic, hypochromic erythrocytes.

#### *Parameters*
- $Ferritin_{serum}$: correlates with total iron (↓ in iron deficiency)
- $Transferrin_{serum}$: correlates with circulating iron and need (↑ in iron deficiency)

**g:** Most important cause: loss of iron due to chronic bleeding → in manifest iron deficiency evaluation of underlying cause is of central importance.

### Causes of Iron Deficiency
- Poor iron uptake: infants, small children, vegetarians, alcoholics, nutritional disorders.
- Recommended daily uptake: men 12 mg, women 15 mg, pregnancy 30 mg.
- Decreased resorption: postoperative (gastrectomy), malassimilation
- Increased need: growth, pregnancy, lactation period, during treatment of vitamin $B_{12}$ deficiency
- Blood loss: urogenital / gastrointestinal bleeding, cystitis, angiodysplasia, esophagitis, hemorrhoids
- Infection / parasites (worldwide most frequent cause of iron deficiency: hookworm infection)

**Path:**

### Peripheral Blood
Microcytic, hypochromic erythrocytes, poikilocytosis, anisocytosis, anulocytes.

### Bone Marrow
Iron stain (Prussian blue stain): storage iron not detectable (ferritin, hemosiderin).

**Sy:**

### Symptoms of Anemia
- Pallor of skin and mucous membranes, nail beds, conjunctivae
- Weakness, tiredness, reduced performance
- Lack of concentration, headache
- Exertional dyspnea, tachycardia, palpitations (DD: cardiac failure)

### Symptoms of Iron Deficiency
- Skin and nail changes: skin atrophy, spoon-shaped nails (koilonychia)
- Oral rhagades, impairment of mucous membranes, in extreme cases painful mucous membrane atrophy of tongue, pharynx, and esophagus with dysphagia (Plummer-Vinson syndrome)

**Dg:**

### History, Clinical Findings
- History, esp. infections, drugs, bleeding, nutritional habits
- Physical examination: including skin, mucous membranes, lymph node status, spleen / liver, heart (tachycardia, particularly systolic murmur), rectal examination with fecal blood test, urine dipstick
- Gynecological examination
- Endoscopy: esophago-gastro- duodenoscopy, colonoscopy, rectoscopy

### Laboratory Tests
- Hematology: blood count, MCV ↓, MCH ↓, reticulocytes, differential blood count
- Clinical chemistry: routine tests with bilirubin, renal function parameters, iron status (iron ↓, ferritin ↓, transferrin-binding capacity ↑)
- Blood group (if red cell substitution necessary)
- Iron resorption test (if resorption deficiency is suspected)

### Histology
In inconclusive cases eventually bone marrow aspiration / biopsy, including iron staining, to exclude other causes of anemia.

**Dd:**

- Anemia of chronic disease (iron ↓, ferritin normal or elevated, transferrin-binding capacity ↓)
- Thalassemia (MCV ↓↓, iron, ferritin, and transferrin-binding capacity normal)
- Hemolytic anemia (bilirubin, LDH, haptoglobin, Coombs' test)

**Th:**

Treatment of anemia with iron deficiency always requires a combined approach:
1. Treatment of the underlying cause of iron deficiency (e.g., chronic blood loss)
2. Iron substitution

### Oral Iron Substitution

- Application of ferrous II preparation, e.g., Fe(II) sulfate, fumarate, gluconate, or succinate, 100–200 mg/day p.o., for 2–6 months.
- PKIN: oral bioavailability, depending on preparation, 15–25%, better bioavailability when taken prior to food.
- SE: gastrointestinal tract symptoms (nausea, vomiting,), dark discoloration of stool (ATTENTION misdiagnosis: upper gastrointestinal bleeding).
- Treatment monitoring: after 5–7 days reticulocytes ↑, hemoglobin ↑. Most frequent cause of a treatment failure is lack of compliance, followed by combined anemia (e.g., coexisting iron deficiency and lack of vitamin $B_{12}$).

### Parenteral Iron Substitution

- Parenteral application of iron should be limited to individual cases (e.g., in malabsorption syndrome), due to severity of side effects.
- Strictly intravenous application of ferrous(III) preparations, consider premedication with steroids and antihistaminics.
- SE: thrombophlebitis, headache, flush, nausea, vomiting, fever, allergic reactions up to anaphylaxis. With paravenous injection local pain and visible iron deposits in tissue.

### Red Cell Substitution

Application of packed red blood cells is generally not indicated in iron deficiency anemia. Exceptions exist in patients with additional blood loss and clinical symptoms.

## Anemia Due to Inflammation, Infection, Tumor: Anemia of Chronic Disease (ACD)

p: Second most common form of anemia (after iron deficiency anemia).

g: Multifactorial anemia with chronic underlying disease (malignancy, inflammation, infection, collagen diseases). Pathogenetic factors:
- Cytokine-mediated (TNFα, interleukin-1, interferon γ) → erythrocyte-survival time ↓, interference with iron mobilization from reticuloendothelial iron stores (macrophages), iron uptake / utilization in normoblasts ↓, erythropoietin secretion and effect ↓, inhibition of erythroid progenitor cells, etc.
- Treatment-associated (drugs, radiation therapy, etc.)
- Consequence of underlying disease

ath: 
### Peripheral Blood
Normochromic, normocytic or hypochromic, microcytic red blood cells, poikilocytosis, anisocytosis.

y: 
### Symptoms of Anemia
- Pallor of skin and mucous membranes, nail beds, conjunctivae
- Weakness, tiredness, reduced performance, exertional dyspnea
- Lack of concentration, headache

### Symptoms of Underlying Disease
Depending on disease, generally with
- Tiredness, weakness, reduced performance
- Fever, weight loss, night sweats (B symptoms)
- Loss of appetite, myalgia, arthralgia, etc.

g: 
### History, Clinical Findings
- History: infections, drugs, exposition to hazardous substances, bleeding
- Physical examination: skin, mucous membranes, lymph node status, spleen / liver, heart (tachycardia, systolic murmur), rectal examination with fecal blood test

### Laboratory Tests

- Hematology: blood count, MCV (normal / ↓), MCH (normal / ↓), reticulocytes, differential blood count
- Clinical chemistry: renal function parameters, iron status (iron ↓, ferritin ↑, transferrin-binding capacity ↑), ESR ↑, fibrinogen ↑, CRP ↑, haptoglobin ↑ (acute-phase protein), possibly erythropoietin level
- Blood group (if red cell substitution necessary)

### Histology

In inconclusive cases consider bone marrow aspiration / biopsy, including iron staining, to exclude other causes of anemia.

**Dd:**
- Iron deficiency anemia (iron ↓, ferritin ↓, transferrin- binding capacity ↑)
- Thalassemia (MCV ↓↓, iron, ferritin, and transferrin-binding capacity normal)
- Megaloblastic anemias (vitamin $B_{12}$ / folinic acid)
- Hemolytic anemia (bilirubin, LDH, haptoglobin, Coombs' test)

**Th:**     Treatment of underlying disease

**Ref:**
1. Donovan A, Andrews NC. The molecular regulation of iron metabolism. Hematol J 2004;5:373–80
2. Goodnough LT, Skikne B, Brugnara C. Erythropoietin, iron, and erythropoiesis. Blood 2000;96:823–33
3. Littlewood TJ. The impact of hemoglobin levels on treatment outcomes in patients with cancer. Semin Oncol 2001;28(2 suppl 8):49–53
4. Means RT. Advances in the anemia of chronic disease. Int J Hematol 1999;70:7–12
5. Thomas C, Thomas L. Anemia of chronic disease: pathophysiology and laboratory diagnosis. Lab Hematol 2005;11:14–23
6. Umbreit J. Iron deficiency. Am J Hematol 2005;78:435–43
7. Weiss G, Goodnough LT. Anemia of chronic disease. N Engl J Med 2005;352:1011–23
8. Zimmermann MB, Hurrell RF. Nutritional iron deficiency. Lancet 2007;370:511–20

**Web:**
1. http://www.nlm.nih.gov/medlineplus/ency/article/000565.htm     Medline Plus
2. http://www.nlm.nih.gov/medlineplus/ency/article/000584.htm     Medline Plus
3. http://www.umm.edu/blood/aneiron.htm     Univ Maryland
4. http://www.emedicine.com/med/topic1188.htm     E-medicine

## 6.4.2    Megaloblastic Anemia

**D. P. Berger, R. Engelhardt, J. Heinz**

**Def:**  Anemia with increased erythrocyte volume (MCV > 98 fl), usually caused by lack of vitamin $B_{12}$ (cobalamin) and/or folic acid.

### Vitamin $B_{12}$ Deficiency Anemia

**Ep:**  Incidence 5–10 cases/100,000 population/year, distribution male:female = 3:2, age peak 60 years

**Phys:**  **Vitamin $B_{12}$ metabolism**

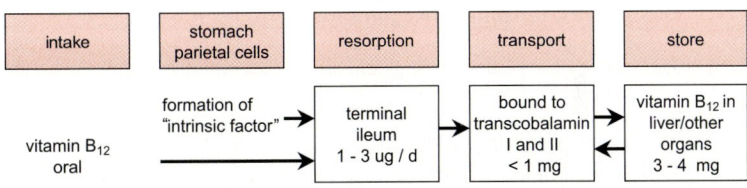

The reference nutrient intake (RNI) for vitamin $B_{12}$ is 1 µg, with maximum daily absorption in the terminal ileum of 2–3 µg. "Intrinsic factor" (glycoprotein) is a prerequisite for vitamin $B_{12}$ resorption.

#### Function of Vitamin $B_{12}$ (Cobalamin)
- Cofactor in the synthesis of succinyl CoA, methionine, and tetrahydrofolic acid
- In case of vitamin $B_{12}$ deficiency:
  - → DNA synthesis and fatty acid metabolism impaired
  - → Delayed nuclear maturation, normal cytoplasmic development
  - → Ineffective myelopoiesis, large cells with altered nucleus: plasma ratio

**Ag:**  
#### Causes of Vitamin $B_{12}$ Deficiency
- Most frequent cause: pernicious anemia (80% of cases): autoimmune atrophic gastritis with antibodies against gastric parietal cells (90% of cases) and/or antibodies against intrinsic factor (50% of cases)
  - → Achlorhydria, intrinsic factor deficiency
  - → Decreased vitamin $B_{12}$ resorption in the terminal ileum
- Insufficient vitamin $B_{12}$ uptake (strict vegetarians, alcoholics)
- Postoperatively (gastrectomy, resection of the terminal ileum, blind loop syndrome)
- Vitamin $B_{12}$ malabsorption, rare (Crohn's disease, scleroderma, amyloidosis)
- Infections / parasites (fish tapeworm, bacterial gastrointestinal infections)

**Path:**  
#### Peripheral Blood
Macrocytic hyperchromic erythrocytes, poikilocytosis, anisocytosis, hypersegmented granulocytes (right shift); in severe cases, granulocytopenia and thrombocytopenia.

### Bone Marrow

Megaloblastic changes: ineffective left-shifted erythro-, thrombo-, and granulopoiesis, pronounced erythropoiesis with increased numbers of immature erythroid precursors (erythropoietic hyperplasia with megaloblastic erythroblasts), giant band forms, immature megakaryocytes.

**Sy:**

### Anemia-related Symptoms

- Pale skin and mucous membranes, icterus (due to intramedullary hemolysis)
- Weakness, fatigue, reduced performance, dyspnea on exertion
- Difficulty concentrating, headache

### Neurological Symptoms

In advanced cases: funicular myelosis: neuropathy caused by symmetrical damage of the posterior columns of the spinal cord, the corticospinal tract and peripheral nerves; motor abnormalities mainly affecting the lower extremities; staggering gait, ataxia, spastic paresis, impaired vision, psychological disorders.

### Gastrointestinal and Other Symptoms

- Type A gastritis
- Trophic disorders of the skin and mucous membranes: Hunter's glossitis, etc.
- Sterility (gonad dysfunction), reversible

**Dg:**

### Medical History, Physical Examination

- Medical history: infections, drugs, hemorrhage, nutritional habits
- Physical examination: skin, mucous membranes, lymph node status, spleen / liver, heart (tachycardia, in some cases: systolic cardiac murmur), rectal examination and test for fecal blood, neurological examination

### Laboratory Tests

- Hematology: blood count with MCV ($\uparrow$), MCH ($\uparrow$), reticulocytes ($\downarrow$), differential blood count
- Clinical chemistry: liver and renal function tests, total protein, hemolysis parameters (bilirubin $\uparrow$, LDH $\uparrow\uparrow$, haptoglobin $\downarrow$ due to intramedullary hemolysis)
- Antibodies against gastric parietal cells and/or against intrinsic factor
- Vitamin $B_{12}$ serum level (normal: 200–900 pg/ml), folic acid serum level
- Vitamin $B_{12}$ absorption test (Schilling's test): oral administration of radioactive $B_{12}$ ± intrinsic factor, determination of urinary vitamin $B_{12}$, comparison of vitamin $B_{12}$ absorption / excretion with and without intrinsic factor
- Blood group (if red cell transfusion is necessary)

### Histology

- Gastroscopy: detection of chronic atrophic gastritis, exclusion of gastric carcinoma (incidence 3 times higher with chronic atrophic gastritis)
- Bone marrow aspiration / biopsy to confirm megaloblastic abnormalities

**Dd:**

### Other Causes of Macrocytosis

- Alcoholism (most common cause of a macrocytic blood count)
- Hepatic disorders, severe hypothyroidism
- Reticulocytosis, myelodysplasia (▶ Chap. 7.2), paraproteinemia
- Cytostatic agents (antimetabolites, anthracyclines, anthracenediones, etc.)
- Pregnancy, neonates

### Other Forms of Anemia

- Hypochromic anemia (iron deficiency anemia, anemia of chronic disease)
- Hemolytic anemia (bilirubin, LDH, haptoglobin, Coombs' test)
- Parvovirus B19, renal anemia

h:

### Vitamin B$_{12}$ Substitution

Hydroxycobalamin 1 mg i.m. → initially: 6 injections within 2–3 weeks (to replenish vitamin B$_{12}$ stores), then: one injection every 3 months. Additionally: application of ferrous II preparation and folic acid to cover increased erythropoesis during substitution phase.

ATTENTION: close monitoring during the first days of treatment: critical increase in reticulocytes and platelets possible → increased risk of thrombosis, potassium and iron deficiency.

Gastroscopy at regular intervals due to increased risk of gastric cancer.

## Folic Acid Deficiency Anemia

p:

Rare disorder

hys:

### Folic acid metabolism

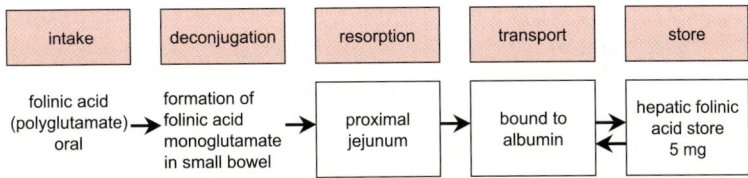

| intake | deconjugation | resorption | transport | store |
|--------|---------------|------------|-----------|-------|
| folinic acid (polyglutamate) oral | formation of folinic acid monoglutamate in small bowel | proximal jejunum | bound to albumin | hepatic folinic acid store 5 mg |

Reference nutrient intake (RNI) for folic acid: 100–200 µg, during pregnancy 400 µg.

### Function
- Folic acid is a cofactor of thymidylate synthesis (C1 transfer), i.e., DNA synthesis
- In case of folic acid deficiency:
  → Disorder of DNA synthesis
  → Delayed nuclear maturation with normal cytoplasmic development
  → Ineffective myelopoiesis, giant cells with an abnormal nucleus: plasma ratio

g:

### Causes of Folic Acid Deficiency
- Insufficient folic acid intake: nutritional deficiency, alcoholism, anorexia nervosa
- Malabsorption: gluten-induced enteropathy, tropical sprue, Crohn's disease, scleroderma, amyloidosis, postoperatively (small bowel resection, gastrectomy)
- Increased demand: pregnancy, chronic hemolytic anemia, chronic inflammatory disease, or malignancies
- Loss of folic acid: hemodialysis
- Drug-induced (with folic acid antagonists): methotrexate, trimethoprim, pyrimethamine, phenytoin, triamterene

ath:

### Peripheral Blood and Bone Marrow
See Vitamin B$_{12}$ Deficiency Anemia

y:

### Anemia-related Symptoms
- Pale skin and mucous membranes, icterus (due to intramedullary hemolysis)
- Weakness, fatigue, reduced performance, dyspnea on exertion
- Difficulty concentrating, headache

### Folic Acid Deficiency-related Symptoms
- Folic acid deficiency during pregnancy: increased incidence of neural tube defects (spina bifida, anencephaly)
- Sterility (gonadal dysfunction), reversible

**Dg:**     ***Medical History, Physical Examination***
- Case history including infections, drugs, hemorrhage
- Physical examination: skin, mucous membranes, lymph node status, spleen / liver, hear (tachycardia, in some cases: systolic cardiac murmur), rectal examination and test for feca occult blood

***Laboratory Tests***
- Hematology: blood count with MCV ($\uparrow$), MCH ($\uparrow$), reticulocytes ($\downarrow$), differential blood coun
- Clinical chemistry: liver and renal function tests, total protein, hemolysis parameters (biliru bin $\uparrow$, LDH $\uparrow$, haptoglobin $\downarrow$ due to intramedullary hemolysis)
- Vitamin $B_{12}$ level, folic acid level (normal: 6–20 ng/ml)
- Blood group (if red cell transfusion is necessary)

***Histology***
- Esophago-gastro-duodenoscopy: exclusion of gluten-sensitive enteropathy (sprue)
- Bone marrow aspiration / biopsy to confirm megaloblastic abnormalities

**Dd:**     See Vitamin $B_{12}$ Deficiency Anemia

**Th:**     ***Folic Acid Substitution***
Folic acid 5 mg daily p.o. for 4 months.

**Ref:**
1. Dharmarajan TS, Norkus EP. Approaches to vitamin $B_{12}$ deficiency. Early treatment may prevent devastat-ing complications. Postgrad Med 2001;110:99–105
2. Fenech M. The role of folic acid and vitamin $B_{12}$ in genomic stability of human cells. Mutat Res 2001;475:57–67
3. Provan D, Weatherall D. Red cells II: acquired anaemias and polycythaemia. Lancet 2000;355:1260–8
4. Toh BH, van Driel IR, Gleeson PA. Pernicious anemia. N Engl J Med 1997;337:1441–8
5. Wickramashinghe SN. The wide spectrum and unresolved issues of megaloblastic anemia. Semin Hemato 1999;36:3–18
6. Zittoun J, Zittoun R. Modern clinical testing strategies in cobalamin and folate deficiency. Semin Hematol 1999;36:35–46

**Web:**
1. http://www.nlm.nih.gov/medlineplus/ency/article/000567.htm     Medline Plus
2. http://web.indstate.edu/thcme/mwking/vitamins.html     Introduction to Vitamins
3. http://www.umm.edu/blood/aneper.htm     Univ Maryland
4. http://www.emedicine.com/MED/topic1420.htm     E-medicine
5. http://www.ashimagebank.org     ASH Image Bank

### 6.4.3 Hemolytic Anemia

**D.P. Berger, R. Engelhardt J. Heinz**

**Def:** Anemia caused by erythrocyte destruction characterized by decreased erythrocyte survival (< 120 days)

**Phys:** *Physiological Erythrocyte Turnover*
In the bone marrow, $2 \times 10^{11}$ erythrocytes are produced per day; median erythrocyte survival: 120 days; erythrocyte destruction in spleen and liver (reticuloendothelial system, RES).

**Hemoglobin degradation**

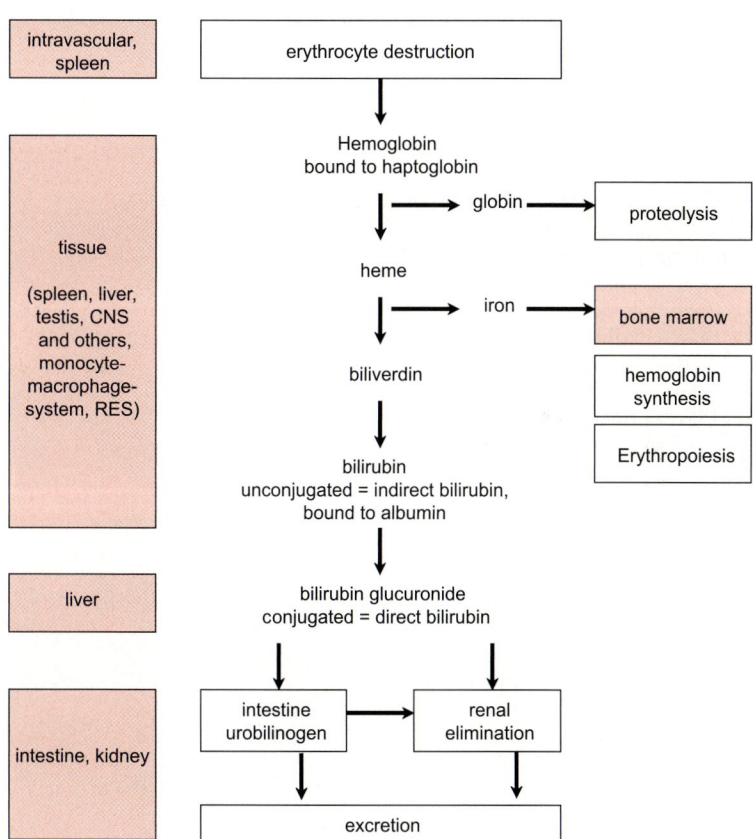

**Path:** *Peripheral Blood*
Generally, normochromic normocytic anemia with normal leukocytes and platelets; characteristic changes in cases of hereditary membrane defects (spherocytes, elliptocytes, etc.); anisocytosis, poikilocytosis, and, in some cases, fragmentocytes.

**Bone Marrow**
Erythropoietic hyperplasia, increase in erythroblasts.

Class:        ***Corpuscular Hemolytic Anemia (Erythrocyte Defects)***

*Hereditary Membrane Defects*
- Spherocytosis
- Elliptocytosis
- Stomatocytosis
- Acanthocytosis

*Hereditary Enzyme Defects*
- Glucose-6-phosphate dehydrogenase deficiency (G6PD deficiency)
- Pyruvate kinase deficiency (PK deficiency)

*Stem Cell Defects*
- Paroxysmal nocturnal hemoglobinuria (PNH)

*Defects in Hemoglobin Synthesis*
- Sickle cell anemia and other hemoglobinopathies
- Thalassemia

***Extracorpuscular Hemolytic Anemia (Extraerythrocytic Defects)***

*Autoimmune Hemolytic Anemia*
- Warm antibody autoimmune hemolytic anemia (AIHA)
- Cold antibody autoimmune hemolytic anemia (AIHA)
- Isoimmune hemolytic anemia: transfusion reactions, rhesus incompatibility

*Microangiopathic Hemolytic Anemia (MAHA)*
- Thrombotic-thrombocytopenic purpura (TTP)
- Hemolytic-uremic syndrome (HUS)

*Metabolic Disorders*
- Zieve's syndrome: hemolytic anemia + alcohol-induced hepatic disease + hyperlipidemia

*Hemolysis Due to Erythrocyte Damage*
- Traumatic hemolysis (after cardiac valve replacement, march hemoglobinuria)
- Chemically induced hemolysis (snake poison)
- Thermal hemolysis (burns)
- Infection-associated hemolysis (malaria)
- Drug-induced hemolysis

Sy:          **Anemia-related Symptoms**
- Pale skin / mucous membranes, icterus (hemolysis / bilirubin release)
- Weakness, fatigue, reduced performance
- Difficulty concentrating, headache
- Dyspnea on exertion, tachycardia, palpitations (particularly with acute hemolysis)

**Chronic Hemolysis**
Chronic hemolysis is usually associated with a lack of symptoms. Some patients can tolerate hemoglobin levels below 8 mg/dl without subjective restraints.
- Low-grade icterus
- Splenomegaly
- Bilirubin gall stones

### Acute Hemolysis ("Hemolytic Crisis")
- Fever, chills
- Headache, back pain, abdominal pain
- Icterus, hemoglobinuria

**Dg:**

### Medical History, Physical Examination
- Medical history: infections, drugs, hemorrhage, family history
- Physical examination: skin, mucous membranes, lymph node status, spleen / liver, heart (tachycardia, in some cases systolic heart murmur), rectal examination and fecal occult blood test (exclusion of hemorrhagic anemia)

### Laboratory Tests
- Hematology: blood count with MCV, MCH, reticulocytes, differential blood count, blood smear
- Clinical chemistry: electrolytes ($K^+$ ↑), liver and renal function tests, total protein, protein electrophoresis, iron status (iron ↑, ferritin ↑), hemolysis parameters (indirect bilirubin ↑, LDH ↑, haptoglobin ↓), CRP
- Coombs' test: direct (detection of erythrocyte-adherent antibodies) or indirect (detection of serum antibodies)
- Viral serology (including parvovirus B19), mycoplasma
- Blood group

### Hemolysis Parameters
- LDH ↑, HBDH ↑, serum iron ↑
- Indirect bilirubin ↑, urinary urobilinogen ↑
- Haptoglobin ↓
- Hemoglobin ↓, hematocrit ↓, erythrocyte count ↓
- Reticulocytes ↑ (with chronic hemolysis)
- Erythrocyte survival time ↓

### Histology
Consider bone marrow aspiration / biopsy, including iron stain, to exclude other causes of anemia.

**Th:**

Therapeutic options depend on the anemia subtype. Treatment components are:
- Supportive treatment: red cell transfusion (only in individual cases with symptomatic anemia, controversial in cases of autoimmune hemolytic anemia)
- Treatment of underlying disease
- Immunosuppression (in cases of autoimmune hemolytic anemia)
- Splenectomy → removal of the sequestration filter for damaged erythrocytes

ATTENTION Splenectomy
- Splenectomy can correct the decrease in erythrocyte survival, but it is not a causal therapy in the sense of a correction of the triggering hemolytic defect.
- Prior to splenectomy, MANDATORY vaccination against *Streptococcus pneumoniae*, *Neisseria meningitidis*, and *Haemophilus influenzae* because of the sepsis risk.
- After splenectomy, prevention of thromboembolic events (platelets ↑) → low-dose heparin.

## Membrane Defects

## Hereditary Spherocytosis

**Ep:**

Most common hereditary hemolytic disease; prevalence 0.02%; in most cases hereditary disease (autosomal dominant), spontaneous mutation is rare.

**Pg:**   Genetic modifications of erythrocyte membrane components: ankyrin (chromosome 8p), β-spectrin (chromosome 14q), in rare cases α-spectrin or protein 4.2.
→ Loss of membrane lipids
→ Reduced membrane stability, osmotic resistance ↓, $Na^+$ / $H_2O$ influx ↑
→ Spherical erythrocytes
→ Erythrocyte survival ↓, splenic sequestration ↑

**Sy:**
- Anemia, icterus
- Recurrent hemolytic crises (particularly after infections)
- Splenomegaly (50–95%)
- Bilirubin gall stones (20–60%)
- Aplastic crises in cases of parvovirus B19 infection

**Dg:**   ***Medical History, Physical Examination***
- Positive family history (icterus, gall stones, anemia)
- Anemia symptoms

***Laboratory Tests***
- Erythrocytes: blood smear with characteristic spherocytes, diameter < 7 μm
- Normochromic microcytic anemia, MCV → ↑, MCHC ↑
- Hemolysis parameters (LDH ↑, haptoglobin ↓, indirect bilirubin ↑)
- Osmotic resistance ↓, negative Coombs' test (exclusion of immune hemolytic anemia), reticulocytes ↑

**Th:**   In cases of severe anemia / hemolytic crises (10–15% of cases): splenectomy (not in patients under 5 years of age and preceded by splenic scintigraphy to exclude accessory spleens); consider subtotal splenectomy. Vaccination against S. pneumoniae, N. meningitidis and H. influenza mandatory.

## Hereditary Elliptocytosis

**Ep:**   Rare, higher incidence in Mediterranean countries / Africa (increased malaria resistance of elliptocytes)

**Pg:**   Heterogenic disease group with > 25% of elliptic erythrocytes; protein defects of the erythrocytic cytoskeleton (spectrin, protein 4.1R)

**Sy:**   Usually asymptomatic; only 10–30% of patients have varying degrees of anemia, icterus or hemolytic crises

**Dg:**
- Positive family history
- Blood smear with > 25% elliptocytes

**Th:**   In symptomatic patients: splenectomy

## Paroxysmal Nocturnal Hemoglobinuria

**Def:**   Acquired clonal disorder of myeloid stem cells (i.e., of the erythrocytic, granulocytic, and thrombocytic line) with somatic mutations of phosphatidylinositol-glycan A (PIG A) → defect of the "phosphatidylinositol-glycan anchor" (PIG anchor)

**Ep:**   Rare

**Pg:**

The PIG anchor fixes various proteins to the cell membrane, including three complement-regulating proteins: CD59 (membrane inhibitor of reactive lysis; MIRL), CD55 (decay accelerating factor; DAF), and "C8 binding protein" (CBP).
→ Changes in the PIG anchor lead to a decrease in the respective proteins in the cell membrane
→ Reduced resistance against activated complement factors
→ Complement-mediated lysis ↑, incidence of thromboembolic events ↑

**Sy:**

- Chronic hemolytic anemia
- Different severity levels of nocturnal hemolysis (even nocturnal hemolytic crises), with morning hemoglobinuria
- Recurrent thrombosis, particularly portal vein, liver veins (Budd-Chiari syndrome), cerebral vessels, splenic vein, skin veins (skin necrosis)
- Iron deficiency anemia due to chronic loss of iron (renal)

**Dg:**

### Medical History, Physical Examination
- Medical history: circadian occurrence of symptoms
- Physical examination: anemia signs and symptoms, urinary discoloration

### Laboratory Tests
- Normochromic normocytic anemia, in some cases with granulocytopenia and thrombocytopenia
- Hemolysis parameters (LDH ↑, haptoglobin ↓, indirect bilirubin ↑, hemoglobinuria)
- Acid hemolysis test (Ham's test) and sugar water test (sucrose test), pathological: complement-mediated lysis after addition of sugar water or acid to the blood sample
- Molecular genetic proof of the PIG defect

**Co:**

In rare cases development of aplastic anemia, myelodysplasia, or AML

**Th:**

### Supportive Approach
- Prophylactic anticoagulant therapy: phenprocoumon. *ATTENTION: avoid heparin → possible complement activation*
- Iron and folic acid supplementation
- In cases of hemolytic crisis: corticosteroids (prednisolone 50–100 mg i.v.), supportive treatment
- Blood transfusion: only washed erythrocytes to avoid administration of additional complement
- Eculizumab, antibody against complement c5, inhibits complement-mediated lysis of PNH erythrocytes

### Curative Approach
Allogeneic stem cell transplantation (▶ Chap. 5.3): only in severe cases with repeated hemolytic crises or complications (thromboembolic events, etc.)

## Enzyme Defects

### Glucose-6-phosphate Dehydrogenase Deficiency (G6PD Deficiency, Favism)

**Def:**

Hereditary disease, genetic modification of the glucose-6-phosphate dehydrogenase (> 300 mutants worldwide)

**Ep:**

One of the most common hereditary diseases worldwide, regional differences in incidence and prevalence. In Africa, Asia, and the Mediterranean region, as much as 20–60% of the population may be affected (patients are more resistant to malaria plasmodia). X-chromosomal recessive inheritance → mainly males affected. Heterozygotics have two different populations of erythrocytes and usually have less pronounced symptoms.

**Pg:**     *G6PD Deficiency*
→ Defects in the erythrocytic pentose phosphate pathway → NADPH synthesis ↓ → decreased glutathione (GSH)
→ Lysis of erythrocytes due to oxidative stress, hemolytic crises

*Triggers*
- Fava beans (*Vica fava*)
- Infections
- Drugs: primaquine, chloroquine, sulfonamides, acetylsalicylic acid, isosorbide dinitrate, anthracyclines, etc.
- Chemicals: nitrates, nitrite compounds, phenylhydrazine

**Sy:**     Hemolytic crisis with:
- Fever, chills, icterus, hemoglobinuria
- Headache, back pain, abdominal pain

**Dg:**
- Positive family history
- Decreased erythrocytic G6PD activity
- Hemolysis parameters (bilirubin ↑, LDH ↑, haptoglobin ↓), blood smear with Heinz bodies (denatured hemoglobin oxidation products)

**Th:**     Avoid exposure to triggering agents

### Pyruvate Kinase Deficiency (PK Deficiency)

**Def:**     Hereditary defect of the enzyme pyruvate kinase, i.e., the erythrocytic glycolysis.

**Ep:**     Most common hereditary glycolytic defect (Embden-Meyerhof pathway), autosomal recessive inheritance. Heterozygotic individuals are usually asymptomatic. Homozygosis (rare) leads to hemolytic anemia.

**Pg:**     Pyruvate kinase deficiency results in abnormal glycolysis:
→ ATP deficiency → abnormal $Na^+$ / $K^+$–ATPase activity in the erythrocyte membrane
→ Membrane instability, hemolysis

**Sy:**     Usually asymptomatic. In homozygotic individuals, hemolytic crises may occur.

**Dg:**
- Blood smear with acanthocytes, anisocytosis, poikilocytosis
- Hemolysis parameters, reduced erythrocytic pyruvate kinase activity

**Th:**     Symptomatic patients: splenectomy; in cases of iron overload: venesection therapy and administration of desferrioxamine.

### Hemoglobinopathies

### Sickle Cell Anemia

**Def:**     Qualitative changes in hemoglobin (hemoglobin S, HBS) with autosomal codominant inheritance and occurrence of sickle-shaped erythrocytes.

**Ep:**     Most common hemoglobinopathy (HBS); occurs in particular in Mediterranean regions, Africa, Asia, and the USA (black population). HBS carriers are more resistant to malaria plasmodia.

**Pg:** Hemoglobin S (HBS): point mutation in the β-globin locus (chromosome 11) of the hemoglobin molecule in position 6: replacement of glutamic acid by valine (β6 Glu → Val).

HBS precipitates when deoxygenated (risk factors: lack of oxygen, dehydration, fever, increased serum osmolality, stasis):
→ Sickle-shaped erythrocytes with reduced elasticity
→ Hemolysis, disturbed microcirculation, capillary occlusion

**Sy:** Heterozygotic individuals (HBAS) are usually asymptomatic. In homozygotic cases (HBSS):
- Hemolytic anemia and hemolytic crisis
- Vaso-occlusive crises: organ infarction (particularly spleen, kidney, CNS), bone infarction, pulmonary hypertension
- Abdominal pain, bone pain, cerebral disorders, in some cases with fever, tachycardia, leucocytosis
- Hepatosplenomegaly, recurrent splenic infarction → "autosplenectomy," functional asplenia

**Co:**
- Osteoporosis, growth defects due to recurrent bone infarction
- Pure red cell aplasia / aplastic crisis with parvovirus B19 infections
- Proliferative retinopathy → impaired vision
- Bilirubin gall stones
- Immunodeficiency (due to recurrent splenic infarction)

**Dg:**
- Medical history (family history), clinical examination
- Hemoglobin electrophoresis
- Sickle cell test: erythrocytes show sickle shape after addition of sodium sulfide
- Molecular genetic screening (PCR)

**Dd:** Other hemoglobinopathies: more than 450 hemoglobinopathies have been described. HB C, E, and D are the most common.

**Th:** Sickle cell anemia is treated supportively:
- Fluid replacement, at least 2,000 ml/day
- Oxygen (via nasal tube, 3–4 l/min)
- Treatment of infections, analgesia
- Red cell transfusion, in case of severe complications: exchange transfusion
- In cases of splenic infarction / hemorrhage / rupture: splenectomy
- Prophylactic pneumococcus vaccination
- Hydroxyurea

**Px:** Prevention of lack of oxygen, dehydration, and infections.

## β-Thalassemia

**Def:** Quantitative disturbance of hemoglobin synthesis due to a genetic defect in globin chain formation. Subtypes:
- β-Thalassemia: abnormal β-chain synthesis
- α-Thalassemia: abnormal α-chain synthesis (rare)

**Ep:** Regional differences in incidence: β-thalassemia in Mediterranean regions, Africa, and Asia; α-thalassemia in South East Asia and Africa.

**Pg:** Abnormal synthesis of the hemoglobin β-chain, i.e., no formation of normal adult HBA1 (αα/ββ).
→ Compensatory formation of γ- or δ-chains (HBF = αα/γγ and HBA2 = αα/δδ)
→ Ineffective erythropoiesis (free α-globin is toxic for erythroblasts) with intramedullary hemolysis
→ Hypochromic microcytic anemia, signs of hemolysis

**Sy:**    *Heterozygotic Patients: Thalassemia Minor*
Usually, no clinical symptoms; in some cases minor chronic hemolysis, anemia, and splenomegaly

*Homozygotic Patients: Thalassemia Major (Cooley's Anemia)*
- Chronic hemolysis, icterus
- Hepatosplenomegaly
- Cardiac insufficiency
- Infections

**Dg:**
- Microcytic hypochromic anemia (HB ↓, HCT ↓, MCV ↓, MCH ↓)
- $Iron_{serum}$ ↑, ferritin ↑, transferrin iron-binding capacity ↓
- Blood smear: microcytic hypochromic erythrocytes, target cells, polychromasia, isolated normoblasts
- Chronic erythropoietic bone marrow hyperplasia → expanded marrow, detectable in bone marrow scan or skull x-ray ("hair-on-end" sign)
- Hemoglobin electrophoresis: increase in HBF ($\alpha\alpha/\gamma\gamma$) and HBA2 ($\alpha\alpha/\delta\delta$)
- Molecular genetic detection of the defective globin gene (via PCR)

**Dd:**    Iron deficiency anemia (▶ Chap. 6.4.1).

**Th:**    *Supportive Approach*
- RBC transfusion
- Hemosiderosis treatment: desferrioxamine 2,000 IU/day s.c.
- Splenectomy
- Prophylaxis of infections

*Curative Approach*
In homozygotic cases / severe hemolysis: allogeneic stem cell transplantation during infancy.


## Warm Antibody Autoimmune Hemolysis (AIHA)

**Def:**    Autoimmune hemolytic anemia caused by IgG incomplete "warm" autoantibodies (incomplete antibodies: antigen-antibody binding, but no lysis or agglutination).

**Ep:**    Seventy-five percent of all autoimmune hemolytic anemias.

**Pg:**    *Formation of IgG Warm Autoantibodies*
- In non-Hodgkin's lymphoma, particularly in low-malignant NHL (CLL)
- With autoimmune diseases, e.g., systemic lupus erythematosus (SLE)
- Following infections (viral infections, rarely bacterial infections)
- Drug-induced hemolysis (various mechanisms): antibiotics, α-methyldopa, L-dopa, quinine, quinidine, x-ray contrast agents, procainamide, diclofenac
- Idiopathic (50% of cases)

*Autoimmune Hemolysis*
- Binding of incomplete antibodies to erythrocytes
- Destruction of antibody-coated erythrocytes in spleen and liver (extravascular non-complement-mediated lysis by cells of the reticuloendothelial system)

**Sy:**
- Hemolysis and hemolytic crises, with icterus, hemoglobinuria, fever, etc.
- Anemia symptoms (fatigue, weakness, reduced performance, pallor, headache, etc.)

**Dg:**    *Case History, Physical Examination*
- Case history including medication
- Physical examination including signs and symptoms of anemia

### Laboratory Tests
- Anemia (HB ↓, HCT ↓)
- Signs of hemolysis (LDH ↑, indirect bilirubin ↑, haptoglobin ↓, etc.)
- Blood group
- Exclusion of potential underlying diseases

### Coombs' Test: Detection of Incomplete Antibodies
- Direct Coombs' test: detection of incomplete antibodies bound to erythrocytes
- Indirect Coombs' test: detection of incomplete serum antibodies
- With warm antibody autoimmune hemolysis: direct Coombs' test positive, indirect Coombs' test positive or negative

**Th:** Autoimmune hemolysis can show different degrees of severity, ranging from compensated chronic hemolysis to acute life-threatening hemolytic crisis. Every case of autoimmune hemolysis must initially be treated as a hematological emergency.

### Causal Treatment
Treatment of underlying disease or discontinuation of causative drugs.

### Symptomatic Treatment
- Corticosteroids (prednisolone 100–500 mg/day i.v.), slowly taper dose after hemolysis parameters have normalized
- In cases of chronic hemolysis and poor response to corticosteroids: use alternative immunosuppressive agents, e.g., azathioprine 80 mg/m²/day, cyclophosphamide 60 mg/m²/day p.o.
- Splenectomy: in cases of treatment-refractory chronic hemolysis or refractory acute hemolytic crisis
- Transfusion of packed red cells only in cases of symptomatic anemia (e.g., cardiovascular symptoms, dyspnea, cerebral ischemia)


## Cold Agglutinin Autoimmune Hemolysis (AIHA)

**Def:** Autoimmune hemolytic anemia caused by IgM complete "cold" autoantibodies, usually targeting the I-antigen of the erythrocyte membrane (complete antibodies: capable of agglutination and lysis induction after antigen-antibody binding).

**Ep:** Fifteen percent of all autoimmune hemolytic anemias.

**Pg:**
### Secondary Formation of Polyclonal Cold Autoantibodies (Cold Agglutinin Syndrome)
- In low-malignant non-Hodgkin's lymphoma or Hodgkin's disease
- After infection (viral infections, mononucleosis / EBV infection, mycoplasma pneumoniae) → cold agglutinin titer up to 1:1,000

### Primary Formation of Monoclonal Cold Autoantibodies (Cold Agglutinin Disease)
Rare congenital disease
→ Cold agglutinin titer up to 1:256,000

### Autoimmune Hemolysis
When the intravascular temperature drops to < 20–25°C: antigen-antibody binding, agglutination and complement-mediated intravascular hemolysis.

**Sy:**
- Exposure to cold leads to hemolysis and hemolytic crisis (with icterus, hemoglobinuria, fever, etc.)
- Anemia symptoms (fatigue, weakness, reduced performance, pallor, headache, etc.)
- Acrocyanosis: painful / malperfused extremities (fingers / toes / nose)
- Splenomegaly

**Dg:**
- Medical history, physical examination
- Diagnostic clues: erythrocyte agglutination when blood is drawn and during laboratory analysis
- Anemia (HB ↓, HCT ↓), signs of hemolysis (LDH ↑, indirect bilirubin ↑, haptoglobin ↓), detection of cold autoantibodies
- Exclusion of potential underlying diseases
- Blood group

**Th:**

### Causal Approach
Treatment of the underlying disease.

### Symptomatic Approach
- Protection against cold
- With *severe acute hemolysis*: plasmapheresis (objective: removal of autoantibodies), often technically difficult (due to agglutination within the plasmapheresis system)
- With *chronic hemolysis*: immunosuppressive drugs, e.g., azathioprine, cyclophosphamide, or chlorambucil
- With symptomatic anemia (cardiovascular symptoms, dyspnea, cerebral malperfusion, etc.): transfusion of washed packed red cells (*avoid complement administration in cases of complement-mediated hemolysis*)
- Corticosteroids and splenectomy are usually ineffective

**Ref:**
1. Borgna-Pignatti C. Modern treatment of thalassaemia intermedia. Br J Haematol 2007;138:291–304
2. British Committee for Standards in Haematology. Guidelines for the diagnosis and management of hereditary spherocytosis. Br J Haematol 2004;126:455–74
3. Gallagher PG. Hereditary elliptocytosis: spectrin and protein 4.1R. Semin Hematol 2004;41:142–64
4. Gertz A. Management of cold haemolytic syndrome. Br J Haematol 2007;138:422–9
5. Hillmen P, Young NS, Schubert J et al. The complement inhibitor eculizumab in PNH. N Engl J Med 2006;355:1233–43
6. King KE, Ness PM. Treatment of autoimmune hemolytic anemia. Semin Hematol 2005;42:131–6
7. Mehta A, Mason PJ, Vulliamy TJ. Glucose-6-phosphate dehydrogenase deficiency. Baillieres Best Pract Res Clin Haematol 2000;13:21–38
8. Stuart MJ, Nagel RL. Sickle-cell disease. Lancet 2004;364:1343–60

**Web:**
1. http://www.nlm.nih.gov/medlineplus/ency/article/000571.htm    Medline Plus
2. http://www.nlm.nih.gov/medlineplus/ency/article/000534.htm    Medline Plus
3. http://www.umm.edu/blood/anehemol.htm    Univ Maryland
4. http://www.fpnotebook.com/HEM50.htm    Family Practice
5. http://www.emedicine.com/med/topic979.htm    E-medicine

## 6.4.4 Normochromic Anemia

**R. Engelhardt, J. Heinz**

**Def:** Anemia with normal corpuscular hemoglobin (MCH 27–34 pg) and normal corpuscular hemoglobin concentration (MCHC 31–36 g/dl).

**Dd:**
- Hemolytic anemia (▶ Chap. 6.4.3)
- Aplastic anemia (▶ Chap. 6.1)
- Acute posthemorrhagic anemia
- Renal anemia

### Renal Anemia

**Def:** Normochromic normocytic hyporegenerative anemia as a result of chronic renal failure.

**Ep:** Incidence: 50–60 cases/100,000 per year.

**Pg:** *Chronic Renal Failure Anemia*
- Complex pathogenesis based on renal insufficiency
- Renal erythropoietin synthesis ↓, the degree of anemia correlates with the severity of the underlying disease
- Myelosuppresion and intramedullary hemolysis due to accumulation of uremic toxins
- Concurrent chronic blood loss due to hemodialysis

**Sy:** *Anemia Symptoms*
- Pale skin and mucous membranes
- Weakness, fatigue, reduced performance, dyspnea on exertion
- Difficulty concentrating, headache

*Uremia Symptoms*
- Uremic fetor
- "Café au lait" complexion due to urochrome deposits and concurrent anemia, pruritus
- Weakness, headache

**Dg:** *Medical History, Physical Examination*
- Medical history: signs of chronic renal insufficiency
- Physical examination: skin, mucous membranes, lymph node status, spleen / liver, heart (tachycardia, systolic heart murmur), rectal examination and testing for fecal occult blood

*Laboratory Tests*
- Hematology: blood count including MCV (normal), MCH (normal), reticulocytes (↓), differential blood count
- Clinical chemistry: hepatic and renal function tests, total protein, hemolysis parameters (bilirubin, LDH, normal haptoglobin, low-grade hemolysis due to uremic toxins)
- Vitamin $B_{12}$ level, folic acid level
- Serum iron, ferritin, transferrin; in cases of chronic blood loss due to hemodialysis, iron deficiency may occur
- Erythropoietin ↓ / normal (i.e., inadequate increase given the degree of anemia)
- Blood group (if red cell transfusion is required)

**Th:** *Symptomatic Treatment*
- Erythropoiesis stimulation with darbepoetin 1.35 µg/kg body weight once weekly s.c. or i.v., adjust dose according to hemoglobin response
- Alternatively, recombinant erythropoietin, 50 IU/kg body weight three times weekly s.c. or i.v., adjust dose according to hemoglobin response

- Target hemoglobin 10–12 g/dl
- *ATTENTION*: blood pressure may rise as hematocrit increases, especially in cases of pre-existing hypertension
- Hemodialysis
- Additional iron supplementation with signs of iron deficiency (▶ Chap 6.4.1)

### Causal Treatment
- Kidney transplantation

**Ref:**

1.   Eckardt KU. Pathophysiology of renal anemia. Clin Nephrol 2000;53(1 suppl):S2–8
2.   Eschbach JW. Current concepts of anemia management in chronic renal failure: impact of NKF-DOQI. Semin Nephrol 2000;20:320–9
3.   MacDougall IC. Novel erythropoiesis stimulating protein. Semin Nephrol 2000;20:375–81
4.   Ritz E, Schwenger V. The optimal target hemoglobin. Semin Nephrol 2000;20:382–6
5.   Valderrabano F. Quality of life benefits of early anaemia treatment. Nephrol Dial Transplant 2000;15(suppl 3):23–8

**Web:**

1.   http://www.kidney.org/professionals/doqi/doqi/
     doqianemia.html                          National Kidney Foundation Guidelines
2.   http://www.anemiainstitute.org/           Anemia Institute
3.   http://www.asn-online.com/                American Society of Nephrology

## 6.5 Coagulation Disorders

J. Heinz

**Def:**  Acquired or hereditary pathological bleeding tendency due to abnormal:
- Vascular reaction → vasculopathies
- Clotting factors → coagulopathies
- Platelets

### Components of Hemostasis after Vascular Injury
- Vasoconstriction
- Platelet adhesion to endothelial lesion, aggregation, clot formation (primary hemostasis)
- Coagulation cascade, fibrinogenesis (secondary hemostasis)
- Fibrinolysis

Coagulation and fibrinolysis are physiologically balanced and are regulated by activators and inhibitors.

**Coagulation cascade**

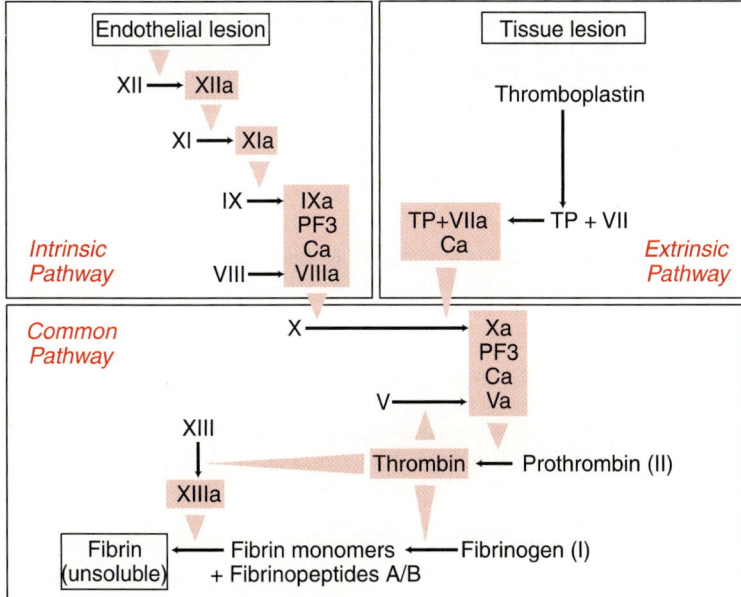

PF3 Platelet Factor 3, TP Tissue thromboplastin, Ca Calcium, I–XIII Clotting factors F I–F XIII, ⟶ chemical conversion    active factors    ▶ effect / reaction.

The distinction of an extrinsic and intrinsic system is artificial and not relevant for the physiological situation (in vivo). However, it helps to understand in vitro phenomena and clotting laboratory tests (Quick's value, PTT).

### Coagulation cascade inhibitors

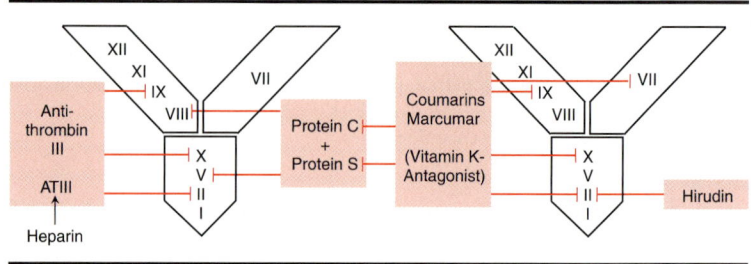

Intrinsic pathway: VIII, IX, XI, XII. Extrinsic pathway: VII. Common pathway: I, II, V, X.
⊢ Inhibition.

- *Antithrombin (AT):* prevention of excessive thrombin activation by formation of thrombin–AT complex, inhibition of IIa, IXa, Xa, XIa, XIIa; important physiological coagulation inhibitor; AT deficiency constitutes an increased risk of thrombosis (thrombophilia, ▶ Chap. 6.6)
- *Protein C:* thrombin-induced conversion into active protein C (APC); APC inhibits FVa and FVIIIa and induces the release of tPA (plasminogenic activator); protein C deficiency constitutes an increased risk of thrombosis (▶ Chap. 6.6)
- *Protein S:* cofactor of protein C
- *Heparin:* activation of physiological AT → inhibition of thrombin generation; ineffective in cases of AT deficiency. Unfractionated (UFH) and low molecular weight (LMWH) heparins
- *Hirudin:* direct thrombin inactivation, effective in cases of AT deficiency
- *Coumarin:* vitamin K antagonists; inhibition of the hepatic synthesis of the factors II, VII, IX and X as well as the proteins C and S

### Fibrinolysis cascade and fibrinolysis inhibitors

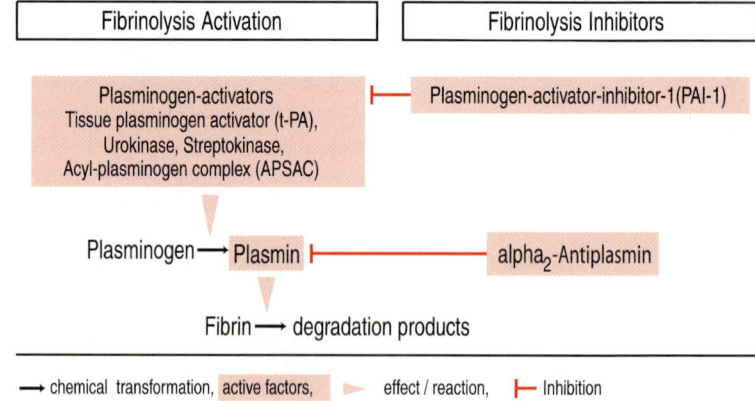

**Factors of the coagulation and fibrinolysis cascades**

| Factor | Characterization | Plasma concentration[a] | Half-life (t½) |
|---|---|---|---|
| *Clotting factors* | | | |
| I | Fibrinogen | 2.0–4.4 | 3–5 d |
| II | Prothrombin | 0.05–0.1 | 2–3 d |
| III[b] | Tissue factor, FVII activator | < 0.001 | – |
| IV[b] | $Ca^{2+}$ ions | 0.096–0.104 | – |
| V | Prothrombin activator component | 0.01 | 12 h |
| VI[b] | = FVa, prothrombin activator component | < 0.001 | – |
| VII | Proconvertin, starting point of the extrinsic system | 0.0001–0.001 | 6 h |
| VIII | Antihemophilic globulin A (AHG-A) | < 0.005 | 12–16 h |
| VIII:vWF | von Willebrand factor | 0.001–0.005 | – |
| IX | Antihemophilic globulin B (AHG-B) | 0.003–0.005 | 24 h |
| X | Stuart-Prower factor, prothrombin activator component | 0.01 | 30 h |
| XI | Rosenthal factor, thromboplastin antecedent | 0.005 | 2–3 d |
| XII | Hageman factor, start of the intrinsic system | 0.03 | – |
| XIII | Fibrin-stabilizing factor | 0.02 | 9–10 d |
| XIV | High molecular weight kininogen, activates FXII | 0.07 | – |
| XV | Prekallikrein, Fletcher factor, cofactor of FXII activation | 0.05 | – |
| *Coagulation inhibitors* | | | |
| Protein C | FV and FVIII-splitting protease | 0.003 | 6 h |
| Protein S | Protein C cofactor | 0.025 | 40 h |
| AT | Antithrombin | 0.1–0.2 | 2–4 d |
| *Fibrinolytic factors* | | | |
| Plasmino-gen | Precursor of plasmin | 0.2 | 22 d |
| t-PA | Tissue plasminogen activator | < 0.001 | 6 min |
| rt-PA | Recombinant t-PA | – | 18 min |
| SK | Streptokinase | – | 30 min |
| APSAC | Acyl-plasminogen-SK-activator complex | – | 90 min |
| UK | Urokinase | – | 5 min |
| Scu-PA | Prourokinase | < 0.001 | 7 min |
| *Fibrinolysis inhibitors* | | | |
| $α_2$-AP | $α_2$-Antiplasmin | 0.007 | 3 d |
| PAI-1 | Plasminogen activator inhibitor-1 | < 0.001 | – |

Plasma concentration in g/l
[b] Designation no longer in use
[a] activated factors, *d* day

### Inhibitors of Platelet Aggregation
- *Acetylsalicylic acid:* irreversible cyclooxygenase inhibition
- *Ticlopidine:* inhibition of fibrinogen binding by interaction with GPIIb/IIIa
- *Tirofiban hydrochloride:* GPIIb/IIIa receptor antagonist
- *Dipyridamole:* increases the level of cellular cyclic AMP (cAMP)
- *Clopidogrel:* selective inhibition of ADP binding, inhibition of ADP-mediated activation of the GPIIb/IIIa receptor complex

**Class:**

### Classification of Acquired and Congenital Coagulopathies

*Vitamin K Deficiency or Abnormal Synthesis of Vitamin K-dependent Clotting Factors* (▶ Chap. 6.5.1)
- Severe liver damage
- Antibiotic treatment, malabsorption syndrome, abnormal fat absorption, alcoholism

*Consumption Coagulopathy*
- Disseminated intravascular coagulation (DIC, ▶ Chap. 6.5.5)

*Immunocoagulopathies*
- Antibodies against clotting factors in conjunction with autoimmune diseases (e.g., lupus anti-coagulant with systemic lupus erythematosus)

*Microangiopathies*
- Thrombotic-thrombocytopenic purpura (TTP, ▶ Chap. 6.3.3)
- Hemolytic-uremic syndrome (HUS, ▶ Chap. 6.3.3)

*Hereditary Coagulopathies*
- Factor VIII deficiency (hemophilia A, ▶ Chap. 6.5.2)
- Factor IX deficiency (hemophilia B, ▶ Chap. 6.5.3)
- Von Willebrand's disease (▶ Chap. 6.5.4)
- Other clotting factor deficiencies

**Sy:**  Different coagulopathies are associated with different patterns of hemorrhage:
- *Thrombocytic abnormalities:* pinpoint hemorrhages: petechiae, purpura
- *Vascular abnormalities:* petechiae, purpura
- *Coagulopathies:* soft tissue hemorrhage, hematomas, intra-articular hemorrhage

**Dg:**

### Medical History, Physical Examination
- Medical history (including family history, bleeding, medication)
- Physical examination: type of hemorrhage

### Laboratory Tests
- Blood count including platelet count, fibrinogen
- Intrinsic pathway: PTT test (partial thromboplastin time)
- Extrinsic pathway: Quick's test (prothrombin time)
- Vascular / platelet abnormalities: platelet count, platelet function tests, bleeding time (normal: < 9 min), platelet function analysis
- Coagulation activation assessment: fibrin monomers, prothrombin fragments 1 + 2
- Assessment of fibrinolytic reactions: D-dimers (fibrin split products, signs of active fibrinolysis)
- Special tests: single factor analysis, platelet function tests, inhibitors

**Th:**  See respective coagulopathies (▶ Chaps. 6.5.1–6.5.5)

**Ref:**

1.  Baglin T, Barrowcliffe TW, Cohen A et al. Guidelines on the use and monitoring of heparin. Br J Haematol 2006;133:19–34
2.  Dahlback B. Blood coagulation. Lancet 2000;355:1627–32
3.  Falanga A. Tumor cell prothrombotic properties. Haemostasis 2001;31(suppl 1):1–4

4.  Manucci PM, Duga S, Peyvandi F. Recessively inherited coagulation disorders. Blood 2004;104:1243–52
5.  Petralia GA, Lemoine NR, Kakkar AK. Mechanisms of disease: the impact of antithrombotic therapy in cancer patients. Nat Clin Pract Oncol 2005;2:356–63

**Web:**

1.  http://www.med.unc.edu/isth/welcome                                  ISTH
2.  http://tollefsen.wustl.edu/projects/coagulation/coagulation.html      Washington Univ
3.  http://www.indstate.edu/thcme/mwking/blood-coagulation.html           Indiana State Univ
4.  http://www.nlm.nih.gov/medlineplus/ency/article/001304.htm            Medline Plus

## 6.5.1    Acquired Coagulation Disorders

**J. Heinz**

**Def:**   Coagulopathies which may occur spontaneously or as a result of an underlying disease which i not primarily related to the hemostatic system. In contrast to primary disorders, several compo nents of the hemostatic system are usually affected. Impaired synthesis and metabolic defects car be distinguished.

**ICD-10:**   D68

**Et:**   ***Causes of Acquired Bleeding Disorders***
- Vitamin K deficiency
- Liver diseases
- Uremia, nephrotic syndrome
- Malignancies (lymphoma, leukemia, myeloproliferative syndromes, solid tumors)
- Amyloidosis
- Cardiovascular disorders
- Autoimmune diseases
- Drugs (asparaginase, penicillin, cephalosporin, interferon-α)
- Pregnancy, post partum

### Vitamin K Deficiency

**Ep:**   Most common bleeding disorder

**Et:**
- Vitamin K-free diet (rare)
- Malabsorption syndrome, cholestasis, chronic pancreatitis, sprue
- Iatrogenic: antibiotic treatment (e.g., cephalosporins), coumarin treatment, parenteral nutri tion without vitamin K substitution

**Pphys:**   Vitamin K is a fat-soluble vitamin and a cofactor for synthesis of the clotting factors II, VII, IX and X as well as protein C and S. Vitamin K deficiency:
$\rightarrow$ Synthesis of prothrombin complex $\downarrow$ $\rightarrow$ bleeding tendency $\uparrow$

**Sy:**   Higher incidence of hemorrhages / hematomas

**Dg:**
- Quick's test $\downarrow$, aPTT normal or $\uparrow$
- Determination of each individual factor is not usually required

**Th:**
- *Exogenous deficiency without hemorrhage:* usually single oral dose of phytomenadione 10- 20 mg; in cases of abnormal absorption: i.v. administration. The efficacy of vitamin K substitu tion can differ considerably between individuals. Coagulation parameters (Quick's value) wi increase 6–12 h after treatment at the earliest.
- *With coumarin treatment without hemorrhage:* phytomenadione: dose according to INR (In ternational Normalized Ratio). INR within target range and no hemorrhage: dosage 2–5 mg INR too high and no hemorrhage: dosage 10–20 mg (possibly repeated).
- *Obvious hemorrhage / before emergency surgery:* administration of prothrombin complex con centrates (PPSB) 25–50 IU/kg body weight plus vitamin K 10 mg; in cases of uncontrollabl bleeding: administration of activated factor VIIa.

### Coagulation Disorders in Hepatic Diseases

**Pphys:**   The liver is the primary site of formation and elimination of coagulation factors and their inhibi tors as well as filtration $\rightarrow$ hepatic dysfunction can lead to complex hemostatic disorders:

- Impaired synthesis of clotting factors → factor deficiency (esp. factor II, V, VII, IX, X, XIII, fibrinogen, plasminogen, α2-antiplasmin, antithrombin, protein C, protein S)
- Impaired elimination of clotting factors → factor excess (e.g., VIII, von Willebrand-factor)
- Impaired thrombopoiesis / platelet function (hypersplenism, bone marrow defect due to toxic effects of alcohol, vitamin $B_{12}$ / folic acid deficiency, thrombopoietin deficiency)
- Hyperfibrinolysis
- Ascites → loss of coagulation factors (loss of coagulation factors via ascites)

Sy:
- Signs of hepatic failure
- Bleeding signs and symptoms: hematomas, mucous membrane hemorrhage, epistaxis
- Esophageal variceal bleeding (life-threatening)

Dg:
- Quick's test ↓ (earliest indication of hepatic coagulation defects: includes factor VII which is the first to decrease due to its short half life of 6 h); suitable parameter for monitoring hepatic disorders
- aPTT: may be normal or increased in advanced hepatic disorders
- Platelets ↓, fibrinogen ↓, factor V ↓, protein C ↓, protein S ↓, antithrombin ↓ (may be increased in case of cholestasis), D-dimers ↑
- Determination of separate factors usually not required

Th:

### Acute Hemorrhage
- Initial treatment with fresh frozen plasma (FFP) 10 ml/kg.
- If insufficient: antithrombin supplementation, fibrinogen supplementation (for levels below 1.0 g/l), administration of cryoprecipitate.
- Administration of platelet concentrates, desmopressin (DDAVP; 0.4 µg/kg) and antifibrinolytics (e.g., aprotinin 250,000 IU in 30 min, 2 million IU/day i.v.) may be considered. *ATTENTION*: DIC (▶ Chap. 6.5.5).
- If factor XIII concentration < 50% and FFP is without effect: administration of factor XIII concentrate.
- If initial values are unknown / emergency situations: empirical treatment with antithrombin 50 IU/kg, fibrinogen 3 g, and PPSB 50 IU/kg. In cases of severe hemorrhage, treatment with activated factor VIIa may be considered.

**Target Values in the Treatment of Hepatic Coagulation Disorders**

| Parameter | Target value range |
|---|---|
| Antithrombin | > 40% |
| Quick's value | > 40% |
| Fibrinogen | > 50–100 mg/dl |
| Platelet count | > 50,000/µl |

### Prophylaxis of Hemorrhage
Administration of antifibrinolytics (e.g., tranexamic acid 1 g three times daily), vitamin K

### Bleeding in Uremic Conditions

t:
Acute or chronic renal insufficiency

phys:
- Platelet function disorder due to accumulation of urinary toxins
- Fibrin polymerization ↓
- vWF (von Willebrand factor)-mediated platelet adhesion ↓

y:
- Signs of renal failure
- Mucous membrane hemorrhage, hematomas, gastrointestinal hemorrhage

**Dg:**
- Creatinine ↑, urea ↑, creatinine clearance ↓
- Bleeding time ↑, platelet dysfunction, in severe cases with thrombocytopenia
- vWF antigen level ↑

**Th:**
- Hemodialysis
- DDAVP (0.3 µg/kg body weight)
- In emergency situations: administration of platelet concentrates and von Willebrand factor enriched factor VIII concentrate (dose: 25 IU/kg)


## Coagulation Disorders in Malignant Diseases

**Et:**
Most frequent malignant diseases associated with bleeding disorders:
- Malignant lymphomas
- Myeloproliferative syndromes
- Multiple myeloma, monoclonal gammopathy (MGUS)
- Solid tumors (esp. prostate, ovarian, and colon carcinoma)

**Pphys:**
- Thrombocytopenia due to bone marrow infiltration
- Hepatic metastases → impaired synthesis of coagulation factors
- Functional impairment of platelets / coagulation factors
- Hyperfibrinolysis triggered by procoagulatory activity (esp. solid tumors)
- Paraprotein → increased viscosity, platelet dysfunction, inhibition of coagulation factors, and fibrin polymerization

**Sy:**
Hemorrhages of all degrees and in all locations (hematomas, mucous membrane hemorrhage, postoperative bleeding)

**Dg:**
- Platelet count usually normal
- Prolonged clinical or in vitro bleeding time (PFA 100 test)
- Platelet dysfunction after stimulation with epinephrine and / or ADP
- Quick's and aPTT usually normal (exception: inhibitor formation, severe hepatic dysfunction)
- D-dimers ↑, fibrinogen ↓ as a sign of hyperfibrinolysis

**Th:**
- Treatment of the underlying disease
- In case of thrombocytopenia and hemorrhage: administration of platelet concentrates
- In case of paraprotein-associated hemorrhage (Waldenström's macroglobulinemia or multiple myeloma): administration of DDAVP, in case of severe hyperviscosity: apheresis treatment
- Hyperfibrinolysis: antifibrinolytics (e.g., aprotinin)


## Acquired Factor VIII Inhibitor (Antigen-induced Hemophilia)

**Def:**
Antibodies to clotting factors, occurring as primary (spontaneous) or secondary (due to underlying disease) antibodies:
- Autoantibodies
  - Inhibitors to individual clotting factors (most commonly to factor VIII, antigen-induced hemophilia)
  - Antiphospholipid antibodies (▶ Chap. 6.6)
  - Monoclonal immunoglobulins, heparin-like antibodies
- Alloantibodies (inhibitors in hemophilia A / B replacement therapy)

**Ep:**
Incidence of factor VIII inhibitors 1:1,000,000

**Et:**
Acquired factor VIII inhibitors: 50% of cases occur spontaneously, secondary inhibitors in conjunction with:

- Autoimmune diseases, SLE (systemic lupus erythematodes), asthma
- Malignancies
- Drug-induced: penicillin, ampicillin, interferon-α
- Others: post partum, skin diseases, sarcoidosis, amyloidosis, GVHD

**Sy:** Spontaneous bleeding with large hematomas, mucous membrane hemorrhages, vaginal bleeding, in severe cases uncontrollable bleeding after minor injuries; high mortality of up to 25%

**Dg:**
- aPTT ↑, factor VIII ↓
- Determination of inhibitor levels according to the Bethesda method

**Th:**
### Acute Hemorrhage
- Administration of recombinant factor VIIa
- In cases of low titer inhibitors (< 5 B.U.): administration of high-dose factor VIII
- In severe cases additional administration of activated prothrombin complex concentrate, immunoadsorption therapy

### Causal Treatment
- Immunosuppressive treatment: steroids (prednisone 1 mg/kg daily for at least 4 weeks), possibly in combination with cyclophosphamide (2 mg/kg daily)
- Alternatively: i.v. immunoglobulins 1 g/kg daily for 2 days, cyclosporine, anti-CD20 antibody (rituximab)
- In cases of high titer inhibitors > 5 B.U. or severe bleeding: immunoadsorption

## Acquired von Willebrand's Syndrome

**Et:** Occurrence of von Willebrand factor inhibitors in conjunction with:
- Malignancies: lymphomas, leukemias, myeloproliferative diseases, solid tumors
- Cardiovascular diseases
- Autoimmune diseases, drugs

**Pphys:**
- Autoantibodies against von Willebrand factor
- Binding of von Willebrand factor to the surface of malignant cells
- Proteolysis of von Willebrand factor (e.g., with acute promyelocytic leukemia ▶ Chap. 7.1.2)
- High shear stress → destruction of vWF multimers (e.g., in cases of aortic stenosis)
- Impaired synthesis

**Sy:** Skin / mucous membrane hemorrhage, postoperative bleeding

**Dg:** See congenital von Willebrand's syndrome (▶ Chap. 6.5.4)

**Th:**
- Treatment of the underlying disease
- Replacement therapy with von Willebrand concentrate, inhibitor elimination

## Hemorrhagic Disorders with Asparaginase Treatment

**Et:** Asparaginase therapy of acute leukemias

**Pphys:**
- Impaired synthesis of clotting factors (esp. fibrinogen, antithrombin, protein C and S, factors II, IX, and XIII)
- Potential complication: DIC (▶ Chap. 6.5.5)

**Sy:** Hemorrhages of all degrees and in all locations (hematomas, mucous membrane hemorrhage, postoperative bleeding)

**Dg:** Levels of fibrinogen, antithrombin, D-dimers

**Th:**
- FFP 10 ml/kg (coagulation factor increase by 10–20%)
- Antithrombin concentrate: 20 IU/kg → increase by approximately 20–40%
- Fibrinogen 3 g → increase by 1 g/l

**Ref:**
1. Dahlback B. Blood coagulation and its regulation by anticoagulant pathways: genetic pathogenesis of bleeding and thrombotic diseases. J Intern Med 2005;257:209–23
2. Delgado J, Jimenez-Yuste V, Hernandez-Navarro F et al. Acquired haemophilia: review and meta-analysis focused on therapy and prognostic factors. Br J Haematol 2003;121:21–35
3. Levine JS, Branch DW, Rauch J. The antiphospholipid syndrome. N Engl J Med 2002;346:752–63
4. Li T, Chang CY, Jin DY et al. Identification of the gene for vitamin K epoxide reductase. Nature 2004;427:541–4
5. Wiestner A, Cho HJ, Asch AS et al. Rituximab in the treatment of acquired factor VIII inhibitors. Blood 2002;100:3426–8
6. Zeitler H, Ulrich-Merzenich G, Hess L et al. Treatment of acquired hemophilia by the Bonn-Malmö protocol. Blood 2005;105:2287–93

**Web:**
1. http://www.med.unc.edu/isth/welcome        Intl Soc Thrombosis Hemostasis
2. http://www.ctds.info/vitamink.html          Vitamin K Deficiency
3. http://www.emedicine.com/med/topic2385.htm  E-Medicine
4. http://www.nlm.nih.gov/medlineplus/ency/
   article/002407.htm                          Medline Plus

## 6.5.2 Factor VIII Deficiency (Hemophilia A)

O. Schmah, J. Heinz

**Def:** Hereditary bleeding disorder caused by deficiency (90% of cases) or inactivity (10%) of coagulation factor VIII (FVIII, AHG-A, antihemophilic globulin A).

**ICD-10:** D66

**Ep:** Most common hereditary coagulopathy, incidence 1 case/5,000 men/year. Women are heterozygotic carriers of the gene. Clinically apparent hemophilia in women is rare. Ratio between hemophilia A and B approximately 5:1.

**Pg:**
- Factor VIII coding gene located on the X chromosome → mainly men are affected, X-linked recessive inheritance (70% of cases) or spontaneous mutations (30%)
- Synthesis in liver, 265 kDa protein, no vitamin K dependence; half-life: 8–12 h
- Factor VIII circulates in the plasma bound to von Willebrand factor (vWF) → protection from proteolytic degradation

**Class:** Severity of FVIII deficiency

| Severity | FVIII activity | Symptoms |
|---|---|---|
| Normal | > 70% | None |
| Subhemophilia | 15–40% | No symptoms in normal life |
| Mild | 5–20% | Hematoma following trauma, discrete tendency to bleed |
| Moderate | 1–5% | Hematoma following mild trauma, tendency to bleed |
| Severe | < 1% | Spontaneous bleeding, bleeding into joints, hematuria |

**Sy:** *Increased tendency to bleed (manifestation during infancy and early childhood)*
- Extensive bleeding, hematomas
- Soft tissue bleeding, bleeding into joints (hemarthrosis)
- Gastrointestinal bleeding, hematuria

**Dg:** *Medical History, Physical Examination*
- Medical history: including family history
- Physical examination: including type of bleeding, complications

*Laboratory Tests*
- Coagulation parameters: factor VIII ↓↓, aPTT ↑, Quick's test normal (extrinsic system), normal bleeding time (verified by platelet function test)
- Genetic diagnosis: RFLP (analysis of the restriction fragment length polymorphism); most common genetic defect: intron 22 inversion

**Dd:**
- Von Willebrand's disease
- Other coagulation factor deficiencies
- Acquired factor VIII antibodies (► Chap. 6.5.1)

**Co:**
- Arthropathy → joint destruction, arthrosis, stiffening
- Retroperitoneal bleeding, psoas hemorrhage, cerebral bleeding (rare)
- Hepatitis / HIV infection due to transfusion and administration of FVIII products (especially before 1984). HIV patients on protease inhibitor treatment: bleeding risk ↑
- Pseudotumor formation / liquefaction of tissue at the hemorrhage site → surgical excision

**Th:**   Detailed recommendations see guidelines of the International Society for Thrombosis and Hemo-
stasis. The following types of treatment can be distinguished:
- Treatment on demand (spontaneous / traumatic bleeding)
- Continuous prophylactic treatment (esp. children and teenagers)
- Prophylactic treatment (before surgery, physical stress, etc.)

**ATTENTION:** Treatment must be provided as early as possible and must be sufficient with respect to dosage and treatment period.

### Mild Bleeding and FVIII > 15–40%
DDAVP, nasal spray, or intravenous administration (0.3–0.4 µg/kg in 100 ml saline over 30 min
every 12–24 h); effect occurs within 30–60 min: transient FVIII increase by factor 2–3 for up to
4 days; may also be given prior to minor surgery (e.g., tooth extraction), possibly with antifibrinolytics.

### Severe Bleeding and/or Patients with FVIII < 15%
Administration of recombinant factor VIII or plasma factor VIII. Administration of recombinant
factor products excludes the risk of viral contamination (HBV, HCV, HIV, HSV, EBV, CMV, etc.)
Coagulation factors are applied i.v. as a slow bolus injection or via continuous infusion (2–4 IU/
kg/h) with reduced factor content.

Required Amount: Dose (IU) = Desired Factor Increase (%) × 0.5 × Body Weight (kg)
Rule of Thumb: Administration of Factor VIII 1 IU/kg → Plasma FVIII ↑ by 1%

**Dosage guidelines for FVIII**

| Type of bleeding | Target FVIII activity[a] | Duration of therapy |
|---|---|---|
| Joint bleeding | 15–50% | 1–7 days |
| Extensive soft tissue bleeding, muscular bleeding | 30–50% | 2–7 days |
| Complicated bleeding (tongue, neck, forearm, calf) | 40–70% | Several weeks |
| Intracranial / gastrointestinal bleeding | 70–100% | Several weeks |
| Minor surgery | 25–40% | 3–5 days |
| Major surgery, tonsillectomy | 80–150% | 14–21 days[b] |

[a] Therapeutic factor VIII activity in plasma
[b] Or until wound healing is complete

### Monitoring of FVIII Replacement
aPTT monitoring is not sufficient, specific measurement of plasma factor VIII should be performed.
- Determine FVIII level 30–60 min after bolus was administered = confirmation of increase
  when biological half-life is reached, and prior to administration of the next dose
- 15–35% of patients develop antibodies against infused factor VIII → alloantibodies may form
  within the first 50–100 days of exposure, and may lead to treatment resistance → monitoring
  via FVII inhibitor assay

### Patients with Factor VIII Antibodies
- *Hemorrhage and low antibody titer (Bethesda titer < 5):* increase dose and frequency of FVIII
  products, close monitoring; use of porcine FVIII may be considered (no cross-reaction)
- *Hemorrhage and high antibody titer (Bethesda titer > 5):* give recombinant factor VIIa 90 µg/
  kg body weight (= 4.5 KIU/kg body weight) every 2–4 h or Factor Eight Bypassing Activity

(FEIBA) 20–100 IU/kg body weight every 8–12 h. In emergency situations: plasmapheresis or immunoadsorption

**rg:** Normal life expectancy

**x:** *Patient information and instruction are the best and most important bleeding prophylaxis*
- Early detection of signs of bleeding
- Controlled exercise and sports program to prevent bleeding into joints and to maintain mobility
- Avoid platelet aggregation inhibitors (ASS, etc.), no intramuscular injections
- Caries prophylaxis, meticulous local hemostasis during surgical procedures; no surgery without prophylactic administration of FVIII
- Hepatitis A/B vaccination is recommended
- X-linked inheritance → examine coagulation status of patient's relatives

### Special Attention when Caring for Infants
Bleeding-related arthropathy often goes unnoticed → close monitoring, permanent FVIII treatment in cases of severe hemophilia: 25–40 IU/kg 1–3 times weekly → rate of complications / arthroplasty significantly decreased.

**ef:**
1. Berntorp E. Immune tolerance induction: recombinant vs. human-derived product. Haemophilia 2001;7:109–13
2. Bolton-Maggs P, Pasi KJ. Haemophilia A and B. Lancet 2003;361:1801–9
3. Evatt BL, Farrugia A, Shapiro AD et al. Haemophilia 2002: emerging risks of treatment. Haemophilia 2002;8:221–9
4. Graw J, Brackmann HH, Oldenburg J et al. Haemophilia A: from mutation analysis to new therapies. Nat Rev Genet 2005;6:488–501
5. Kubisz P, Stasko J. Recombinant activated factor VII in patients at high risk of bleeding. Hematology 2004;9:317–32
6. Srivastava A. Dose and response in haemophilia: optimization of factor replacement therapy. Br J Haematol 2004;127:12–25
7. Van den Berg HM, Fischer K, van der Bom JG. Comparing outcomes of different treatment regimens for severe haemophilia. Haemophilia 2003;9:27–31

**Web:**
1. http://www.haemophilia-forum.org    Haemophilia Forum
2. http://www.hemophilia.org    Natl Hemophilia Foundation
3. http://www.haemophilia.org.uk    Haemophilia Society
4. http://www.wfh.org    World Fed Hemophilia
5. http://www.nlm.nih.gov/medlineplus/hemophilia.html    Medline Plus
6. http://med.unc.edu/isth/welcome    International Society of Thrombosis and Hemostasis

### 6.5.3    Factor IX Deficiency (Hemophilia B)

J. Heinz

**Def:**    Hereditary coagulopathy due to deficiency or inactivity of coagulation factor IX (FIX, Christmas factor, antihemophilic globulin B, AHG-B).

**ICD-10:**    D67

**Ep:**    Rare hereditary coagulopathy, incidence 1 case/25–30,000 men/year. Women are heterozygoti carriers of the gene.

**Pg:**
- Factor IX coding gene is located on the X chromosome → mainly men are affected X-linked recessive inheritance; hereditary forms (80% of cases) and spontaneous mutation (20%)
- Hepatic synthesis, 55 kDa protein, vitamin K-dependent, half-life 24 h

**Severity of FIX deficiency**

| Severity | FIX activity | Symptoms |
| --- | --- | --- |
| Normal | > 50% | No symptoms |
| Subhemophilia | 15–40% | No symptoms in normal life |
| Mild | 5–15% | Hematoma following trauma, discrete tendency to bleed |
| Moderate | 1–5% | Hematoma following mild trauma, tendency to bleed |
| Severe | < 1% | Spontaneous bleeding, bleeding into joints, hematuria |

**Sy:**    Increased tendency to bleed, similar to hemophilia A (clinically indistinguishable):
- Hematomas, soft tissue bleeding, bleeding into joints (hemarthrosis)
- Hematuria, gastrointestinal bleeding

**Dg:**    *Medical History, Physical Examination*
- Medical history: including family history
- Physical examination: including type of bleeding, complications

*Laboratory Tests*
Factor IX ↓↓, PTT ↑, Quick's test normal (extrinsic system), normal bleeding time (verified b platelet function test).

**Dd:**
- Von Willebrand's disease
- Other coagulation factor deficiencies

**Co:**    Arthropathy, severe bleeding, infections.

**Th:**    Detailed recommendations on aspects of hemophilia treatment see guidelines of the Internationa Society for Thrombosis and Hemostasis.

*Bleeding Management*
Administration of factor IX products, half-life 12–24 h.

Required Amount: Dose (IU) = Desired Factor Increase (%) × Body Weight (kg)
Rule of Thumb: Administration of Factor IX 1 IU / kg → Plasma IX ↑ by 2%

*Dosing Guidelines (▶ Chap. 6.5.1)*
- Mild bleeding: increase factor IX for 1–2 days by 10–30%
- Moderate bleeding: increase factor IX for 5–7 days to 30–50% of normal activity

- Severe bleeding / planned operation: increase factor IX for 3 days to > 70% , then keep at > 50% for 7 days
- In cases of emergency, fresh frozen plasma (FFP) may be used, if recombinant FIX concentrate is not available

### Monitoring of FIX Replacement
- aPTT monitoring is not sufficient, plasma factor IX should be determined (shortly after re-placement and before administration of the next dose)
- 1–4% of patients develop antibodies against infused factor, with treatment resistance → monitoring via FVII inhibitor assay

**rg:** Normal life expectancy

**x:** Patient information and instruction (▶ Chap. 6.5.2)

### Special Attention when Caring for Infants
Bleeding-related arthropathy often goes unnoticed → close monitoring, prophylactic factor IX treatment in cases of severe hemophilia in children: 25–40 IU/kg 2 times weekly → significant decrease of complication / arthropathy rate.

**Ref:**

1. Berntorp E, Astermark J, Björkman S et al. Consensus perspectives on prophylactic therapy for haemophilia: summary statement. Haemophilia 2003;9(suppl 1):1–4
2. Bolton-Maggs P, Pasi KJ. Haemophilia A and B. Lancet 2003;361:1801–9
3. Di Michele D. Inhibitor development in haemophilia B. Br J Haematol 2007;138:305–15
4. Kubisz P, Stasko J. Recombinant activated factor VII in patients at high risk of bleeding. Hematology 2004;9:317–32
5. Srivastava A. Dose and response in haemophilia: optimization of factor replacement therapy. Br J Haematol 2004;127:12–25
6. Stobart K, Iorio A, Wu JK. Clotting factor concentrates given to prevent bleeding and bleeding-related complications in people with hemophilia A or B. Cochrane Database Syst Rev 2005;CD003429
7. Van den Berg HM, Fischer K, van der Bom JG. Comparing outcomes of different treatment regimens for severe haemophilia. Haemophilia 2003;9:27–31

**Web:**

1. http://www.kcl.ac.uk/ip/petergreen/haemBdatabase.html — Hemophilia B Database
2. http://www.haemophilia-forum.org — Haemophilia Forum
3. http://www.hemophilia.org — Natl Hemophilia Foundation
4. http://www.haemophilia.org.uk — Haemophilia Society
5. http://www.wfh.org — World Fed Hemophilia
6. http://www.nlm.nih.gov/medlineplus/hemophilia.html — Medline Plus
7. http://med.unc.edu/isth/welcome — International Society of Thrombosis and Hemostasis

## 6.5.4    Von Willebrand's Disease (VWD)

O. Schmah, J. Heinz

**Def:**  Hereditary coagulopathy due to qualitative or quantitative deficiencies of the von Willebrand factor (vWF).

**ICD-10:**  D68.0

**Ep:**  Most common hereditary coagulopathy, heterozygotic gene carriers 1:100 to 1:1,000; incidence of symptomatic cases: 125 cases/1,000,000 population.

**Phys:**  Von Willebrand factor is a heterogenic multimeric plasma glycoprotein (normal serum level 10 mg/l). The vWF precursor is synthesized as a monomer in the endothelium and megakaryocytes. Active forms (vWF multimers) are found in the endothelium, platelets, and plasma. Functions:
- Mediation of platelet adhesion to vascular wall (collagen) via high-molecular vWF multimers and binding to platelet glycoprotein Ib (GPIb)
- Factor VIII carrier in plasma

**Pg:**  Hereditary defect caused by mutation in the vWF gene (chromosome 12); autosomal-dominant (subtype 1 and 2) or autosomal-recessive (subtype 2 and 3) inheritance. Consequences:
- Impaired platelet adhesion
- Reduced FVIII activity

*Rare:* acquired cases due to vWF antibodies in connection with autoimmune diseases, lymphoproliferative diseases, or after multiple transfusions ("von Willebrand syndrome," VWS). Defects in the vWF-binding glycoprotein GPIb can mimic von Willebrand's disease ("Pseudo-VWD").

**Class:**  **VWD Classification of the International Society on Thrombosis and Hemostasis ISTH (1993)**

| Type | Frequency | Definition |
|------|-----------|------------|
| 1 | 70% | Partial quantitative vWF deficiency, vWF plasma level 10–50% |
| 2 | 25–30% | Qualitative vWF deficiency, atypical binding of vWF to platelets |
| 2A | 10–15% | vWF multimers ↓↓, impaired platelet function |
| 2B | 5% | Increased affinity of vWF to platelet GPIb |
| 2M | 5–10% | Platelet function ↓↓, normal vWF multimer |
| 2N | Up to 3% | Reduced FVIII binding capacity |
| 3 | < 10% | Complete vWF deficiency, vWF level < 1% |

**Sy:**
- Type 1: mild form, bleeding time ↑, discrete tendency to bleed, epistaxis, gum bleeding, increased menstruation, bleeding after minor surgery
- Type 2: different characteristics depending on subtype; increased soft tissue bleeding, mucous membrane bleeding, gastrointestinal bleeding, hematuria; bleeding into joints less common than with hemophilia; rarely intracerebral bleeding
- Type 3: most severe form with pronounced bleeding (soft tissue bleeding, bleeding into joints and petechial type bleeding)
- ATTENTION: in all types life-threatening bleeding may occur up to 14 days after surgery.

**Dg:**  *Medical History, Physical Examination*
- Medical history (including family history)
- Physical examination including type of bleeding

## Laboratory Tests

- vWF antigen, FVIII function (FVIII:C), vWF multimers
- Ristocetin cofactor (RiCof) ↓↓, ristocetin-induced platelet aggregation (RIPA)
- Bleeding time or platelet function analysis
- Platelet count, collagen-binding assay (CBA)
- Blood group (patients with blood group O have a 25% lower vWF concentration)

## Differential Diagnosis of VWD Types

**Laboratory findings for VWD subtypes**

| Parameter | Type 1 | Type 2A | Type 2B | Type 2N | Type 3 |
|---|---|---|---|---|---|
| PTT | n | n | n | n / ↑ | ↑ |
| Bleeding time | n / ↑ | n / ↑ | n / ↑ | n | ↑ |
| Platelet count | n | n | n / ↓ | n | n |
| FVIII:C | n | n / ↓ | n | ↓ | ↓ |
| vWF antigen | n / ↓ | n / ↓ | n / ↓ | n | – |
| Multimers | n | – | – | n | – |
| RiCof | n / ↓ | n / ↓ | n / ↓ | n | – |
| RIPA | n | n | ↑ | n | – |
| CBA | ↓ | ↓ | ↓ | n | – |

*n* normal, ↑ increased, ↓ decreased, – absent, *RiCof* ristocetin cofactor, *RIPA* ristocetin-induced platelet aggregation, *CBA collagen-binding activity*

**ATTENTION:** vWF is an acute-phase protein with high intraindividual variability → findings can often be inconclusive, determination during pregnancy and acute infections is not meaningful. Retesting may be required.

## Bleeding in VWD Subtypes 1, 2A, or 2M

- Mild bleeding: vasopressin analog desmopressin (DDAVP), nasal spray or intravenously, e.g., every 12–24 h 0.3 µg/kg body weight i.v. in 100 ml saline 0.9% over 30 min → release of vWF in endothelium, increase of the vWF level by factor 3–5. Response within 30–60 min in > 80% of patients; duration of effect 8–10 h. Since not all patients respond, conduct provocation test prior to treatment; treatment must be interrupted after 3–5 days due to depletion of endogenous vWF stores.
- With menstruation, single doses of DDAVP prior to menstruation are usually sufficient; supportive estrogen therapy with subtype 1.
- Severe bleeding: similar strategy to type 2B, 2N, and 3.

## Bleeding in VWD Subtypes 2B, 2N, and 3

- Administration of high-vWF plasma products (e.g., 20–70 U/kg 2–4 times daily or 3–5 U/kg/h per infusor) until ristocetin cofactor activity > 60% for at least 72 h. ATTENTION: Recombinant FVIII products contain no vWF and are ineffective in von Willebrand's disease → use special high-vWF plasma or FVIII products.
- Platelet concentrates
- If surgery is planned: vWF antigen as well as ristocetin cofactor activity should be 60%, pre- as well as postoperatively.
- ATTENTION: With subtype 2B, DDAVP did not demonstrate a clear benefit (risk of thrombocytopenia). With subtype III, it is ineffective.

## Monitoring of Substitution

- Monitoring of vWF antigen, FVIII function (FVIII:C), ristocetin cofactor (RiCof) according to disease subtype.

- Development of vWF alloantibodies in 10–15% of cases, risk of anaphylactic reactions with repeated exposure. With neutralizing antibodies and bleeding complications factor VIIa may be given.

### Adjuvant Treatment / Preparation for Surgery

- If DDAVP has proven to be effective, give 30 min prior to surgery
- High risk of hemorrhage (e.g., tonsillectomy): raise vWF antigen and ristocetin cofactor activity up to 60%; administer high-vWF FVIII concentrate
- Intraoperative use of fibrin glue and fibrinolysis inhibitors (e.g., tranexamic acid mouthwash with dental surgery)

### During Pregnancy

- During pregnancy, hormone-induced increase in vWF and FVIII:C → with subtype 1 and 2 no further treatment required
- Peripartum: keep vWF antigen and Ristocetin cofactor activity above 50%; with cesarean section, aim for 100% pre- and postoperatively

**Ref:**

1. Battle J, Noya MS, Giangrande P et al. Advances in the therapy of von Willebrand disease. Haemophilia 2002;8:301–7
2. Ginsburg D. Molecular genetics of von Willebrand disease. Thromb Haemost 1999;82:585–91
3. Manucci PM. Treatment of von Willebrand's disease. N Engl J Med 2004;351:683–94
4. Rodeghiero F, Castaman G. Treatment of von Willebrand disease. Semin Hematol 2005;42:29–35
5. Ruggeri ZM. Developing basic and clinical research on von Willebrand factor and von Willebrand disease. Thromb Haemost 2000;84:147–9
6. Sadler JE, Mannucci PM, Berntorp E et al. Impact, diagnosis and treatment of von Willebrand disease. Thromb Haemost 2000;84:160–74
7. Schneppenheim R, Budde U. Phenotypic and genotypic diagnosis of von Willebrand disease: a 2004 update. Semin Hematol 2005;42:15–28

**Web:**

1. http://www.shef.ac.uk/vwf/                           ISTH VWF Database
2. http://www.allaboutbleeding.com/                      VWD Resource
3. http://www.nlm.nih.gov/medlineplus/ency/
   article/000544.htm                                   VWD, Medline Plus
4. http://www.hemophilia.org/bdi/bdi_types3.htm          Hemophilia Foundation
5. www.wfh.org                                           World Fed Hemophilia
6. www.hemophilia.ca/en/2.2.php                          Canadian Hemophilia Soc
7. www.emedicine.com/med/topic2392.htm                   E-Medicine

## 5.5.5 Disseminated Intravascular Coagulation (DIC)

### J. Heinz

**Def:** Systemic consumption coagulopathy due to release of coagulation activators, with intracapillary coagulation, microthrombus formation, subsequent ischemic organ damage (kidney, liver, lung) and organ failure. Diffuse tendency to bleed due to collapsed hemostasis with secondary hyperfibrinolysis.

Acute DIC is a severe life-threatening disease. Chronic DIC with continuous coagulation may occur in patients with malignant diseases.

**CD-10:** D65

**g:**
### Excessive Release of Activators of the Coagulation Cascade
- *Infections:* sepsis (gram-negative / gram-positive), malaria, rickettsia, chlamydia, mycobacteria, meningococcus (Waterhouse-Friderichsen syndrome: consumption coagulopathy with adrenocortical bleeding), viral infections
- *Solid tumors:* carcinomas of the lung, pancreas, stomach, colon, prostate, Kasabach-Merritt syndrome (hemangiomas)
- *Hematological neoplasia:* acute promyelocytic leukemia (FAB M3)
- *Obstetric complications:* placenta abruptio, amniotic fluid embolism, septic abortion, eclampsia, postpartal hemolytic-uremic syndrome
- *Hypoxia and shock:* traumatic, hemorrhagic, cardiac, septic
- *Hemolysis:* transfusion errors, toxins, paroxysmal nocturnal hemoglobinuria
- *Operations* on organs with a high thrombokinase content (prostate, pancreas, lung), extracorporeal circulation (contact activation of the endogenous coagulation system)
- *Trauma:* head injury, soft tissue damage, fat embolism
- *Others:* snake bites, heat stroke (endothelial damage), abdominal aortic aneurysms

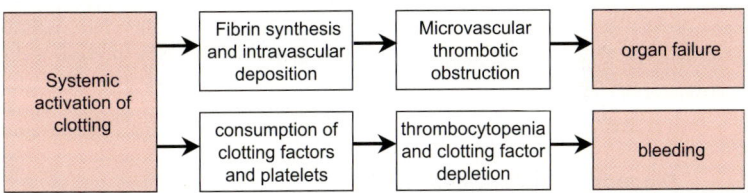

**phys:**
### Pathophysiology: Four Phases
Excessive thrombin synthesis leads to fibrin formation and subsequent intravascular coagulation with consumption of platelets and clotting factors. Inhibitory mechanisms (e.g., inhibition of FVa and FVIIIa via thrombomodulin-activated protein C) cannot compensate the thrombin formation.

| Phase | Characteristics |
|-------|-----------------|
| I | Hypercoagulability, microthrombus formation, microembolisms |
| II | Lack of coagulation factors, incipient fibrinolysis |
| III | Hemostasis collapse, severe reactive fibrinolysis |
| IV | Reconstitution |

**Sy:**    Initially (phase I and II), pathological laboratory parameters only. Only with severe consumption coagulopathy (phase III) clinically detectable symptoms:
- *Hemorrhagic diathesis with ubiquitous bleeding, 75% of cases:* skin / mucous membrane bleeding, hematomas, secondary bleeding after venipuncture / from puncture sites, pulmonary hemorrhage, gastrointestinal bleeding, renal bleeding, hematuria, adrenal bleeding / insufficiency, intracerebral bleeding
- *Multiple microthromboses with impaired organ function, 70%:* acute renal failure, impaired liver function, acute respiratory insufficiency (ARDS, "acute respiratory distress syndrome"), intradermal microvascular thrombosis → "purpura fulminans" (skin bleeding with central necrosis), cerebral small vessel ischemia (coma, epileptic seizures)
- *Shock:* tachycardia, decrease in blood pressure, edemas, organ failure
- *Chronic course:* coagulation factor synthesis ↑, thrombosis ↑ → malperfusion of larger blood vessels (embolisms, cerebral ischemia, etc.)

**Dg:**    *Case History, Physical Examination*
- Case history including risk factors
- Physical examination

### Laboratory Tests

| Phase | Description | Parameters |
|---|---|---|
| I | Activation | Rapid decrease of platelets, platelet count n / ↓, antithrombin n / ↓, FV n / ↓, FVIII n / ↓, coagulation products ↑ (soluble fibrin, prothrombin fragment F1+2, thrombin–antithrombin complex TAT) |
| II | Early consumption | Platelets ↓, antithrombin ↓, Quick ↓, coagulation factors (fibrinogen, FV) ↓, PTT ↑, TAT ↑, protein C ↓ |
| III | Late consumption | Platelets ↓↓ (< 30,000/μl), antithrombin ↓↓, Quick ↓↓, coagulation factors ↓↓ (fibrinogen, FV, and FVIII), PTT ↑↑, thrombin time ↑↑, fibrinogen degrading products / fibrin monomers +, D-dimers +++, detectable fragmentocytes |
| IV | Recovery | Decrease in coagulation products (soluble fibrin, prothrombin fragment F1+2, TAT), increase of clotting factors (fibrinogen, FV, FVIII), normalization of global clotting tests |

*n* normal, *F* factor, *TAT* thrombin-antithrombin complex, *PTT* partial thromboplastin time

### Diagnostic Key Parameters
- *Basic diagnosis:* platelets (platelet decrease often first symptom), antithrombin, D-dimers, fibrinogen, Quick's test, PTT
- *Advanced diagnosis:* fibrin monomers (soluble fibrin), prothrombin fragments F1+2, thrombin–antithrombin complex (TAT), plasmin-plasmin inhibitor complex, factor V, protein C, possibly protein S (in cases of purpura fulminans)

### DIC scoring system of the ISTH (International Society on Thrombosis and Hemostasis)

| Basic screening test | Score | | | |
|---|---|---|---|---|
| | 0 | 1 | 2 | 3 |
| Platelets | > 100/nl | 50–100/nl | <50/nl | – |
| Quick's test | INR < 1.4 | INR 1.5–2.0 | INR > 2.0 | – |
| Fibrinogen | > 100 mg/dl | ≤ 100 mg/dl | – | – |
| Fibrinogen degradation products | Normal | – | + | ++ |

*INR* international normalized ratio

A score $\geq 5$ indicates ongoing DIC; with scores $< 5$ diagnostics should be repeated every 12–24 h depending on the individual clinical condition.

**ATTENTION:**
- With tumors / infections / pregnancy, the platelet count is often increased ("reactive thrombocytosis") → normal platelet counts may already indicate DIC.
- Fibrinogen is an acute-phase protein → "normal" fibrinogen levels may already be pathologically decreased (e.g., with infections).
- With DIC, frequent monitoring is required to determine the dynamics and course of disease.

**Dd:**
- *Primary hyperfibrinolysis:* normal platelet count, normal ATIII, no fibrin monomers

**Th:** *Treatment of DIC requires a combined approach, with treatment of the underlying disease and correction of the coagulation disorder. Early diagnosis improves survival and long-term outcomes.*

### Principles of DIC Treatment
*Basic therapy*
- Antithrombin (AT) replacement if AT level $< 70\%$ (initially 1,000 IU, then 500 IU every 6 h), check level (target: 80–100%)
- Heparin: 100–300 IU/kg/day (not with AML type M3 or patients with high bleeding risk), depending on platelet count

*Organ dysfunction, bleeding*
- Fresh frozen plasma (FFP, 10 ml/kg)
- Antithrombin (AT), 500–1000 IU every 6 h
- Fibrinogen replacement with fibrinogen levels of $< 100$ mg/dl
- Platelet transfusion (target: $> 50,000/\mu l$)
- Red cell transfusion according to hemoglobin level, compensation of acidosis
- Heparin is contraindicated, no intramuscular injections
- Patients should be treated in intensive care unit
- Severe uncontrollable bleeding: administration of activated FVIIa. *ATTENTION:* potential risk of thromboembolic complications

**ATTENTION:** administration of coagulation factors can increase DIC and should be avoided. For replacement therapy, use fresh frozen plasma (FFP).

### Special Cases
- Severe sepsis: activated protein C (drotrecogin) 24 µg/kg/h over 96 h → decreases mortality from 31% to 25%. *ATTENTION:* with thrombocytopenia higher risk of hemorrhagic complications. Contraindicated after brain hemorrhage, epidural catheter, etc.
- In DIC, avoid fibrinolysis inhibitiors: → in cases of uncontrollable bleeding: use aprotinin (e.g., 250,000 units in the first half hour, followed by 2 million units/day), platelets, fibrinogen, and PPSB. In cases of life-threatening bleeding or lack of success: administer recombinant FVIIa.
- Fibrinolysis inhibitors (antifibrinolytics, e.g., tranexamic acid) may be indicated with hyperfibrinolytic conditions (prostate carcinoma, AML M3) in phase I of a DIC only.
- Low-dose heparinization is indicated in cases of: purpura fulminans, acral ischemia, venous thrombosis. For phase I, some studies favor low-molecular weight heparin (100–200 units/kg/day).

### Monitoring During Treatment
- Clinical monitoring: close monitoring of neurological, cardiovascular, respiratory and renal parameters
- Monitoring of bleeding: tachycardia, hemoglobin decrease, retroperitoneal bleeding (→ sonography), neurology
- Laboratory tests: coagulation parameters, blood count, hepatic and renal function parameters, electrolytes

**Prg:**        In cases of manifest severe DIC: 50–80% mortality

**Px:**         Administration of heparin 10,000–15,000 IU/24 h with all predisposing conditions

**Ref:**

1. Bernard GR, Vincent JH, Laterre PF, et al. Efficacy and safety of recombinant human activated protein C for severe sepsis. N Engl J Med 2001;344:699–709
2. De Cicco M. The prothrombotic state in cancer: pathogenetic mechanisms. Crit Rev Hematol Oncol 2004;50:187–96
3. Franchini M, Manzato F. Update on the treatment of disseminated intravascular coagulation. Hematology 2004;9:81–5
4. Levi M. Disseminated intravascular coagulation: what's new? Crit Care Clin 2005;21:449–67
5. Toh CH, Dennis M. DIC 2002: a review of disseminated intravascular coagulation. Hematology 2003;8:65–71
6. Warren BL, Reid A, Singer P et al. High dose antithrombin III in severe sepsis. JAMA 2001;286:1869–78
7. Yanada M, Matsushita T, Suzuki M et al. DIC in acute leukemia: clinical and laboratory features at presentation. Eur J Haematol 2006;77:282–7

**Web:**

1. http://www.med.unc.edu/isth/                                    Intl Soc Thromb Haemost
2. http://www.nlm.nih.gov/medlineplus/ency/article/000573.htm      Medline Plus
3. http://www.emedicine.com/med/topic577.htm                       E-medicine

| **6.6** | **Thromboembolism and Thrombophilia** |

### J. Heinz

**Def:** *Thrombosis:* localized intravascular aggregation of blood components → thrombus (clot) formation with consecutive vascular occlusion. Clinical symptoms differ depending on the blood vessels affected: venous or arterial thrombosis.

*Embolism:* migration of detached thrombus (clot) elements in the blood stream with consecutive vascular occlusion. Triggers: thrombotic material, tumor particles or leukemic cell thrombi, sclerotic material, fat droplets, amniotic fluid, air.

*Thrombophilia:* increased risk of occurrence of thromboembolic events, hereditary or acquired.

**ICD-10:** I82.9

**Ep:** Thrombosis incidence: 3 cases/1,000 population/year; location: > 90% in inferior vena cava or leg / pelvic veins; male:female = 1:1; particularly in patients > 50 years of age; pulmonary embolisms occur in 1–2% of all hospitalized patients.

#### Thromboembolic Events in Patients with Malignancies

- 10–30% of tumor patients experience thrombosis in the course of their disease
- Occurrence depends on tumor location and histology (common with lung cancer, gastrointestinal adenocarcinomas, pancreatic and ovarian carcinoma)
- "Idiopathic" deep vein thrombosis or pulmonary embolism in clinically "healthy" adults is due to an underlying malignancy in 6–35% of cases
- Pulmonary embolisms or venous thromboses are found in up to 50% of cancer patients at autopsy

**Pg:** **Virchow Triad:** *Major Pathomechanisms of Thrombogenesis*

- *Endothelial alterations:* vascular sclerosis, inflammation, trauma, etc.
- *Circulation disorders:* intravascular stasis, vortex formation, etc.
- *Hypercoagulability:* thrombophilia, thrombocytosis, etc.

#### Endothelial Alterations (esp. with Arterial Thrombosis)
- Arteriosclerosis
- Vascular puncture, vascular prostheses, trauma
- Vasculitis (arteritis nodosa, thromboangiitis obliterans, etc.), phlebitis

#### Circulation Disorders
- Immobilization, bed rest
- Intravascular stasis due to vascular constriction or compression: e.g., after extended periods of travel ("economy class syndrome"), varicosis, obesity, pregnancy, solid tumors, or lymphomas
- Altered blood flow due to cardiac disorders ("low output failure": cardiac insufficiency, infarction, cardiogenic shock)

#### Hypercoagulability

*Thrombocytosis*
E.g., myeloproliferative syndromes (▶ Chap. 7.3)

### Thrombophilia

- APC (activated protein C) resistance: most common cause of thrombophilia; in 95% of cases due to factor V mutations → abnormal APC binding site (mainly point mutations in the factor V gene, G1691A, "factor V Leiden") → insufficient inactivation of factor V by mutated APC. Prevalence: heterozygotic carriers 3–9% of normal population, 20–40% among patients with thrombosis. Relative thrombosis risk in heterozygotic cases approximately 3- to 7-fold, in homozygotic cases 50- to 100-fold increased. Other causes (< 5%) for APC resistance: antiphospholipid antibodies, oral contraceptives, pregnancy.
- Factor II mutation: prothrombin mutation G20120A, often associated with increased prothrombin levels. Prevalence: heterozygotic carriers 2–4% of normal population; among patients with thrombosis 5–7%. Relative risk of thromboembolisms: 2- to 4-fold increased.
- Factor VIII increase: 25% of thrombosis patients show persistent FVIII increase of unknown etiology; with significant risk for relapse thrombosis.
  ATTENTION: FVIII levels not meaningful in acute situations (acute phase protein).
- Antithrombin / protein C / protein S defects: rare hereditary disorders; AT deficiency especially is associated with a high risk of thrombosis. DD: hepatic diseases.
- Hyperhomocysteinemia: hereditary defect of cystathionine β synthetase; or acquired due to vitamin B6, B12, or folic acid deficiency.
- Antiphospholipid syndrome: most common acquired form of thrombophilia; occurs as primary or secondary (as a result of systemic lupus erythematosus SLE, collagenosis, malignancy, medication, infections) subtype. Typical triad: thrombosis (venous or arterial) + recurrent miscarriages + thrombocytopenia.

### Other Causes of Abnormal Coagulation

- *Abnormal fibrinolysis:* plasminogen deficiency, tPA deficiency (rare)
- *Hyperviscosity syndrome:* hypergammaglobulinemia with plasmocytomas, hyperglobulinemia, dehydration, leukemia
- *Trauma, burns*
- *Estrogens:* pregnancy, postpartum, contraceptives. *Contraceptives increase the thrombosis risk by factor 5, simultaneous smoking by factor 20.*

## Reasons for Increased Thrombogenesis in Patients with Malignancies

- *Vessel wall defects:* endothelial alterations due to intravascular catheters / lines, antineoplastic treatment, direct invasion of tumor tissue; cytokine-mediated activation of the endothelium → enhanced expression of tissue factor / adhesion molecules / PAI and decreased endothelial thrombomodulin expression → thrombophilic surface
- *Changes in blood flow:* immobilization, tumor-related vascular compression, stasis, hyperviscosity
- *Changes in coagulation system:* fibrinogen ↑, factor V ↑, FVIII ↑, von Willebrand factor ↑, FXII ↑, AT ↓
- *Release of procoagulating substances* ("cancer coagulants," e.g.,tissue factor = TF, FX activators) with activation of the extrinsic system via factor VII or direct FX activation; high levels of TF in promyelocytes of acute leukemia type FAB M3
- *Decrease in coagulation inhibitors* (antithrombin, protein C and S) due to chemotherapy (asparaginase)

**Path:**     ### Thrombus Types

- *White thrombus / blood platelet thrombus:* platelet aggregates occurring with endothelial defects; adherent to vascular wall
- *Coagulation thrombus:* intravascular coagulation due to stasis or decreased blood flow rate, platelet / erythrocyte / coagulation factor aggregates, only moderate adherence to vessel wall, high risk of embolism
- *Hyaline thrombus:* capillary thrombus in disseminated intravascular coagulation (DIC, ▶ Chap. 6.5.5), high content of coagulation factors

- *Tumor cell / leukemia cell thrombus:* solid tumor particles or aggregates of malignant cells in patients with leukemia (usually with cell counts of > 100,000/μl)

### Locations
- *Arterial thrombi:* aorta, coronary vessels, carotids, cerebral arteries, extremities
- *Venous thrombi:* predominantly in lower extremity veins (50%), pelvic veins (30%), vena cava inferior (10%); with iatrogenic damage of the subclavian or jugular veins (catheters)

### Embolism
- Detachment of venous thrombi results in pulmonary embolism in > 90% of cases; paradoxical arterial embolism in cases of patent foramen ovale / pulmonary hypertension
- Displacement of thrombi from the left side of the heart → arterial embolism of cerebral vessels (60%), extremity arteries (30%), renal arteries, mesenteric arteries

**Sy:**

### Deep Vein Thrombosis (DVT) of the Leg
Only < 30% of patients show classic clinical signs:
- Calf pain at dorsal flexion of the ankle (Homans' sign) or ballottement of the calf
- Tenderness when pressure is applied to the sole of the foot (Payr's sign)
- Tenderness when pressure is applied along the deep veins of the leg
- Dilation of epifascial veins
- Local swelling, hyperthermia, tightness, pain, fever

### Phlebothrombosis of the Arm (Paget-von Schroetter Syndrome)
- Swelling of the arm, hyperthermia, livid discoloration, tightness
- Pain in forearm, upper arm and/or shoulder, fever

### Phlegmasia Cerulea Dolens
- Combined venous and arterial occlusion
- Rapidly increasing swelling of the leg
- Pulseless extremity, swelling, livid discoloration, tenderness
- Severe pain

### Pulmonary Embolism
- Dyspnea, tachypnea, cough      80% of patients
- Chest pain, infradiaphragmatic pain      80%
- Tachycardia      60–70%
- Anxiety, sweating, vegetative symptoms    30–50%
- Syncope, shock      10–20%

### Arterial Occlusion: Ischemia Syndrome ("6 Ps")
Pain, pallor, pulselessness, paresthesia, paralysis (motor dysfunction), prostration

**Dg:**

### Medical History, Physical Examination
- Medical history including risk factors
- Physical examination including local signs and symptoms, cardiopulmonary signs, circulatory status

### Laboratory Tests
- *Routine laboratory analyses* including urea + electrolytes, serum creatinine, LDH
- *D-dimer:* decomposition product of cross-linked fibrin; high sensitivity with thrombosis (95–100%) but low specificity (positive D-dimers after surgery, with trauma, hemorrhage, inflammation, malignancy, and pregnancy)
- ATTENTION: if thrombosis or pulmonary embolism is suspected, further diagnostic procedures should be implemented even if D-dimers are negative.
- *Capillary / arterial blood gas analysis:* $pO_2$ ↓, $pCO_2$ ↑ (with pulmonary embolism)
- *Thrombophilia work up:*
  - *Indication:* thrombosis of unknown etiology in patients < 40 years of age; hereditary disposition; recurrence of thrombosis or embolism; unusual thrombosis location (e.g., sinus

veins, mesenteric veins); thromboembolic event despite effective anticoagulation; thrombosis during pregnancy and tendency to miscarriage and stillbirth
- *Analysis of:* fibrinogen, antithrombin, protein C, protein S, prothrombin (FII), FVIII, APC resistance, factor II mutation, antiphospholipid antibodies (lupus anticoagulants, anticardiolipin antibodies), plasminogen deficiency
- *Extended diagnostics:* homocysteine, methyltetrahydrofolate reductase (MTHFR) mutation G77T, FIX, and FXII
- In most cases, repeated tests are required. With suspected thrombophilia, patients should be referred to specialized hematology centers.

### Imaging in Cases of Suspected Thrombosis
- Sonography: CW Doppler, B-mode, duplex scan
- Only in uncertain cases: phlebography
- Possibly CT scan or MRI (esp. abdomen and pelvis)

### Imaging with Suspected Embolism
- Spiral CT
- Ventilation / perfusion lung scan
- Echocardiography revealing signs of right heart failure
- Angiography / arteriography
- ECG: signs of pulmonary embolism: sinus tachycardia, SI QIII type, incomplete right bundl branch block, P pulmonale, newly developed arrhythmia / extrasystoles

### Tumor Screening: Young Patients, Thrombosis of Unknown Etiology, Recurrent Thrombosis
- Thorough clinical examination (including lymph node status, rectal examination, fecal occul blood test, gynecological / urological examination)
- Blood count, LDH, PSA
- Chest x-ray, abdominal sonography, possibly CT abdomen / pelvis

**DD:**

### DVT of the lower extremity
- Vascular compression by tumors, aneurysms, hematomas, Baker's cyst, retroperitoneal fibrosis, vena cava compression, etc.
- Erysipelas
- Edema of different etiology (pulmonary edema, cardiac edema)
- Superficial thrombophlebitis

**Co:**

### Thrombosis-related Complications
- Venous thrombi → pulmonary embolism (in > 95% of cases due to phlebothrombosis, approximately 50% of patients with phlebothrombosis develop pulmonary embolism)
- Arterial / cardiac thrombi → cerebral malperfusion, renal infarction, extremities

### Long-term Sequelae of Lower Extremity DVT
- Post-thrombotic syndrome (after 10–15 years, in 40–60% of conventionally treated patients)
- Chronic leg ulcer (in 10% of patients)

**Th:**

## Anticoagulation

## Initial Treatment with Heparin

### Low Molecular Weight Heparin (LMWH)
- Effect: factor Xa inhibition, half-life: 100–180 min
- Dosage: enoxaparin 1 mg/kg twice daily s.c., dalteparin 100 IU/kg twice daily, or tinzaparin 175 IU/kg once daily
- Advantages of treatment with LMWH compared to UFH:

- Rapid onset of the anticoagulation effect; minimal laboratory monitoring required (platelet count during first 3 weeks, antifactor Xa levels in patients with renal failure, cachectic, or overweight patients)
- No i.v. access, outpatient treatment possible
- Low molecular weight heparin has a favorable side effect profile, hemorrhagic complications, osteoporosis, and heparin-induced thrombocytopenia are less common
- Target antifactor Xa activity: if given twice daily, 0.5–1.0 IU/ml (3–4 h postinjection); with single daily dose, 1.0–2.0 IU/ml (3–4 h postinjection); levels should be determined after steady state has been reached

### Unfractioned Heparin (UFH)
- Effect: inhibition of thrombin, factor Xa, IXa, half-life: 60 min
- Intravenous bolus: 5,000 IU i.v. in patients < 70 kg, 10,000 IU bolus > 70 kg; then continuous intravenous treatment: 30,000 IU/24 h, maximum 50,000 IU/24 h; dosage according to PTT: target PTT > 60–90 s, first PTT test after 6 h, then every 12 h; once stable, it is sufficient to check PTT once daily
- Alternatively, subcutaneous administration: 7,500–10,000 IU s.c. 3 times daily; studies have shown that with identical PTTs, intravenous and subcutaneous administration are equally effective
- Side effects: hemorrhage (in up to 10% of patients), hypersensitivity (urticaria, bronchospasm, fever, even shock), alopecia (rare), vasospasm (rare), osteoporosis (with long-term use), heparin-induced thrombocytopenia (in 2–10% of patients, ▶ Chap. 6.3.2)

### Indications
- Deep vein thrombosis of the lower extremity, thrombosis of major veins (arm veins, cerebral veins, etc.)
- Pulmonary embolism (stable circulation)
- Arterial occlusion (extremity arteries, acute myocardial infarction, etc.)

### Discontinuation of Heparin Treatment
- Adoption of coumarin: discontinuation of heparin treatment once target INR is reached (usually after 5 days); exception: in cases of extensive thrombosis (calf to pelvis), continue heparin treatment for 10–14 days, do not give coumarin before day 5.
- Absence of contraindications and patient compliance provided, LMWH treatment may be possible in an outpatient setting.

## Secondary Prophylaxis: Coumarin (Phenprocoumon)

### Effect
Vitamin K antagonism → inhibition of the hepatic synthesis of coagulation factors F II, VII, IX, X (prothrombin complex) as well as protein C and protein S.

### Indications
Introduce on first or second day of heparin treatment (exception: in case of extensive thrombosis (calf to pelvis), give oral anticoagulants only after 5 days of heparin treatment).

### Contraindications
- Patients > 65 years of age, hemorrhagic diathesis, sepsis
- Uncompensated hypertension, liver or renal insufficiency
- Surgery within last 7–10 days, arterial puncture, intramuscular injections
- CNS surgery within the last 3 months, cerebral bleeding, cerebral sclerosis, CSF puncture within the last 10 days
- Pancreatitis, endocarditis lenta, diabetic retinopathy, nephrolithiasis
- Pulmonary / gastrointestinal diseases with high risk of bleeding (tuberculosis, bronchiectasis, ulcers, colitis, esophageal varices, neoplasia)
- Pregnancy, in particular during the first 3 months

### Dosage

According to INR ("international normalized ratio").

$$INR = \frac{Patient\ Plasma\ Prothrombin\ Time\ (s)}{Normal\ Plasma\ Prothrombin\ Time\ (s)}$$

In cases of uncomplicated deep vein thrombosis and/or pulmonary embolism, the recommended INR is 2.0–3.0. A higher target INR (3.0–4.0) is recommended in cases of recurrent venous thrombosis despite adequate anticoagulation.

### Treatment Initiation

In normal weight patients ($\approx$ 70 kg), the following rule of thumb applies: current Quick value divided by 10 is the number of coumarin tablets to be given in the first 4 days. On day 1, give 3 tablets, on days 2 and 3 give 2 (or 1) tablets (slow initiation to reduce the risk of coumarin necrosis). The INR should be checked on day 4. The result determines the dosage of subsequent treatment. Heparin treatment may be discontinued once the target INR has been reached (usually after 5–6 days).

### Duration of Treatment: Depending on Thrombosis Type

The duration of anticoagulation treatment has to be determined individually for each patient based on thrombosis type, location, risk factors and comorbidities. Guideline:

| Thrombosis type and location | Duration of treatment |
| --- | --- |
| Deep vein thrombosis of the lower leg (> 2 veins, trifurcation) | 1.5–3 months |
| Arm vein thrombosis | 3 months |
| Thrombosis of the popliteal vein and/or the femoral vein | 6 months |
| Involvement of the iliac vein (pelvic vein thrombosis) | (6)–12 months |
| Pulmonary embolism with/without deep vein thrombosis of the leg | (6)–12 months |
| Recurring thrombosis | 3–4 years |
| DVT due to severe thrombophilia (AT deficiency, homozygotic FV mutation, malignancy, etc.) | Possibly life-long |
| Life-threatening pulmonary embolism or thrombosis (mesenteric, sinus veins, cerebral) | Possibly life-long |

### Secondary Prophylaxis Alternative

Patients with contraindications against coumarin may receive low molecular weight heparin as secondary prophylaxis on a long-term basis. Half the therapeutic LMWH dose is usually recommended (comparable to an INR of 2–3); start after 10–14 days of "full dose" therapeutic LMWH treatment. Cancer patients in particular benefit from treatment with low molecular weight heparin.

## Thrombolytic Therapy (Fibrinolysis Treatment)

Due to frequent occurrence of hemorrhagic complications (10–15%), increased mortality (1–2%) and limited long-term benefit (no reduction in occurrence of post-thrombotic syndrome), fibrinolysis now only plays a secondary role. An indication for treatment with fibronolytics (e.g., streptokinase, urokinase) may exist in young patients with extensive fresh thrombosis.

### Surgical Treatment

#### Surgical Thrombectomy

Surgical thrombectomy allows immediate perfusion of the blood vessel. However, endothelial injury and incomplete thrombus removal often lead to rapid reformation of thrombi. Indications:

- Phlegmasia cerulea dolens
- Fresh isolated descending pelvic vein thrombosis (not older than 1–2 days)
- Acute arterial occlusion

#### Cava Filter

Placement of a filter in the V. cava reduces the risk of severe pulmonary embolism in patients with recurrent thromboses. Indications are:

- Recurrent pulmonary embolism despite effective anticoagulation
- Contraindication against anticoagulants

### Supportive Treatment

- *Immobilization:* studies did not confirm a role for immobilization in the prevention of pulmonary embolisms.
- *In patients with severe pain or edema:* elevation and immobilization of the leg for a limited number of days.
- *Compression therapy:* compression dressings with bandages or compression stockings; contraindicated with peripheral arterial occlusive disease and phlegmasia cerulea dolens. Compression stockings should be worn for at least 2 years as secondary prophylaxis after DVT of the lower extremity. In most cases, calf compression stockings on the affected leg are sufficient.

**x:**

- Anticoagulants
- Platelet aggregation inhibitors, acetylsalicylic acid 100 mg daily p.o. (protective effect in particular with arterial occlusion and coronary heart disease)
- Elimination of risk factors (see above), early postoperative mobilization, physiotherapy, compression stockings

**Ref:**

1. Baglin IP, Cousins D, Keeling DM et al. Recommendations from the British Committee for Standards in Haematology and National Patient Safety Agency. Br J Haematol 2006;136:26–9
2. British Committee for Standards in Haematology (BCSH). Guideline. Investigation and management of heritable thrombophilia. Br J Haematol 2001;114:512–28
3. Francis CW. Prophylaxis for thromboembolism in hospitalized medical patients. N Engl Med 2007;356:1438–44
4. Klerk CPW, Smorenburg SM, Otten HM et al. The effect of low molecular weight heparin on survival in patients with advanced malignancy. J Clin Oncol 2005;23:2130–5
5. Kyrle PA, Eichinger S. Deep vein thrombosis. Lancet 2005;365:1163–74
6. Lee AYY, Rickles FR, Julian JA et al. Randomized comparison of low molecular weight heparin and coumarin derivatives on the survival of patients with cancer and venous thromboembolism. J Clin Oncol 2005;23:2123–9
7. Lopez JA, Kearon C, Lee AY. Deep venous thrombosis. Hematology (ASH Educ Program) 2004;439–56
8. Lyman GH, Khorana AA, Falanga A et al. ASCO Guideline: recommendations for venous thromboembolism prophylaxis and treatment in patients with cancer. J Clin Oncol 2007;25:5490–505

**Web:**

1. http://www.nlm.nih.gov/medlineplus/ency/article/000156.htm     Medline Plus
2. http://www.emedicine.com/emerg/topic122.htm     E-Medicine
3. http://www.med.unc.edu/isth     ISTH
4. http://www.tri-london.ac.uk/     Thrombosis Res Inst
5. http://www.tigc.org     TIGC

## 7.1    Acute Leukemias

### 7.1.1    Acute Lymphoblastic Leukemia (ALL)

**R. Wäsch, W. Digel, M. Lübbert**

**Def:**    Hematologic malignancy of lymphatic cells with transformation of a lymphoid precursor, differentiation arrest, and clonal expansion. Characteristics include: suppression of normal hematopoiesis, infiltration of extramedullary organs, and release of leukemic cells into the peripheral blood.

**ICD-10:**    C91.0

**Ep:**
- In children, 80% of acute leukemias, are ALL; incidence: 5.3 cases/100,000/year, age peak: 4 years; age-dependent distribution of the immunological subtypes: pro-B-ALL and pre-B-ALL are more common in young children, T-ALL is more common in older children
- In adults, 20% of acute leukemias are ALL; incidence: 1.1 cases/100,000/year, distribution male:female = 3:2; age peak: > 80 years (2.3 cases/100,000)

**Pg:**    *Risk Factors*
- Bone marrow damage due to ionizing radiation, environmental carcinogens, cytostatic drugs
- Immunosuppression (e.g., following renal transplantation)
- Genetic factors: increased risk associated with trisomy 21 (relative risk: 20), neurofibromatosis, Fanconi's anemia, ataxia telangiectasia syndrome, Bloom's syndrome, Li-Fraumeni syndrome; significant twin concordance (intrauterine paraplacental "transmission" has been described)

*Molecular Genetics*
- In the process of formation of immunocompetent B- and T-cells, lymphoid cells are characterized by clonal rearrangements of immunoglobulin (Ig) and T-cell receptor (TCR) genes.
- Cytogenetic and molecular genetic tests revealed clonal numerical and structural chromosomal aberrations in > 70% of patients, usually involving Ig and TCR genes.
- Genetic changes following pathological chromosome rearrangements (e.g., BCR-ABL, TEL-AML1, E2A-PBX) lead to differentiation arrest in lymphoid progenitor cells, deregulated proliferation, and clonal expansion.
- Pathologic expression patterns of genes involved in cell cycle regulation and apoptosis (Rb, p53, p16, p15, p14, p57) are due to genetic aberrations (deletion, amplification, mutation) or epigenetic deregulation (esp. promoter hypermethylation).
- Molecular genetic identification of chromosomal aberrations (clonal markers) is used for confirmation of diagnosis, identification of risk factors, and evaluation of minimal residual disease. The use of improved cytogenetic methods such as spectral karyotyping (SKY), multiplex FISH (M FISH) or DNA microarrays allows for improved identification of molecular genetic abnormalities and prognostic subtypes.

**Chromosomal aberrations in ALL**

| Chromosomal aberration | Molecular abnormality | Frequency (%) | |
|---|---|---|---|
| | | Children | Adults |
| *B-cell phenotype* | | | |
| (8;14)(q24;q32) | *c-myc* deregulation | 2 | 4 |
| t(8;22)(q24;q11) | *c-myc* deregulation | | |
| t(2;8)(p11;q24) | *c-myc* deregulation | | |

**Chromosomal aberrations in ALL** *(continued)*

| Chromosomal aberration | Molecular abnormality | Frequency (%) | |
|---|---|---|---|
| | | Children | Adults |
| *Pre-B phenotype* | | | |
| t(1;19)(q23;p13) | E2A-PBX1 fusion protein | 5 | 3 |
| t(7;19)(q22;p13) | | 1 | 1 |
| t(9;22)(q34;q11) | *bcr-abl* fusion protein | 4 | 25 |
| t(12;21) | TEL-AML1 fusion protein | 22 | 2 |
| t(1;11)(q32;q23) | MLL-AF1 fusion protein | 1 | 1 |
| t(11;19)(q23;p13) | MLL-ENL fusion protein | 1 | 1 |
| Hyperdiploidy | (> 50 chromosomes) | 25 | 6 |
| Hypodiploidy | (< 45 chromosomes) | 1 | 4 |
| *Pro-B phenotype* | | | |
| t(4;11)(q21;q23) | MLL-AF4 fusion protein | 4 | 5 |
| *T-cell phenotype* | | | |
| t(11;14)(p13p15;q11) | TCRα/δ-TtG1, zinc finger protein | 4 | 6 |
| t(11;14)(q24;q11) | TCRα/δ-TCL3, protooncogene | 1 | 1 |
| t(7;19)(q35;p13) | TCRβ lyl1, helix-loop-helix | 3 | 2 |
| Random translocations | | 28 | 41 |

Path:

### Leukemic Blasts in Blood and Bone Marrow
- Detection of leukemic blasts in the peripheral blood of > 90% of patients: immature cells, round, slightly basophilic cytoplasm, dense nuclear structure, prominent nucleoli; few segmented granulocytes
- In the bone marrow, replacement of normal hematopoiesis by a uniform blast population; usually hypercellular bone marrow, number of blasts at time of diagnosis: usually > 50%

Class:

### Morphological classification according to FAB (French-American-British Group)

| Type | Characteristics |
|---|---|
| L1 | Small-cell acute lymphoblastic leukemia, small monomorphic cells with small nucleoli |
| L2 | Polymorphocellular acute lymphoblastic leukemia, larger polymorph cells with one or more prominent nucleoli, low nucleus / cytoplasm ratio |
| L3 | Burkitt's type acute lymphoblastic leukemia, large cells with prominent, poorly structured nucleoli and basophilic cytoplasm which is often vacuolated |

*NOTE*: the clinical use of the FAB classification is generally limited (exception: subtype L3, more common in B-ALL). Immunophenotyping, cytogenetics and molecular genetics are of greater prognostic and therapeutic relevance.

### Immunophenotyping (▶ Chap 2.5)
Immunological testing of leukemic blasts for surface marker expression allows for:
- Classification of ALL cells as derived from either B-cells or T-cells
- Characterization of the differentiation grade

- Identification of morphologically / cytochemically undifferentiated blasts as acute lympho cytic leukemia
- Detection of aberrant myeloid antigen expression

**Immunophenotypes of acute lymphoblastic leukemia**

| Antigen | B-ALL subtypes | | | | T-ALL subtypes | | | |
|---------|--------|-------------|-------|-----|--------|-------|-------------|-----|
|         | Pro-B  | Com-<br>mon | Pre-B | B   | Pro-T  | Pre-T | Thy-<br>mic | T   |
| CD79a[a] | +      | +           | +     | +   | -      | -     | -           | -   |
| CD22[a]  | +      | +           | +     | +   | -      | -     | -           | -   |
| CD19[a]  | +      | +           | +     | +   | -      | -     | -           | -   |
| CD10     | -      | +           | +     | -   | -      | -     | -           | -   |
| c-IgM    | -      | -           | +     | -   | -      | -     | -           | -   |
| s-IgM    | -      | -           | -     | +   | -      | -     | -           | -   |
| TdT      | +      | +           | +     | -   | +      | +     | +           | +   |
| c-CD3    | -      | -           | -     | -   | +      | +     | +           | +   |
| s-CD3    | -      | -           | -     | -   | -      | -     | -           | +   |
| CD7      | -      | -           | -     | -   | +      | ±     | ±           | ±   |
| CD2      | -      | -           | -     | -   | -      | +[b]  | +           | +   |
| CD5      | -      | -           | -     | -   | -      | +[b]  | +           | +   |
| CD8      | -      | -           | -     | -   | -      | +[b]  | ±           | ±   |
| CD1a     | -      | -           | -     | -   | -      | -     | +           | -   |
| Frequency (%) | 11 | 51          | 10    | 4   | └—— 6 ——┘ | | └—— 18 ——┘ | |

[a] ≥ 2 of 3 positive
[b] CD2+ and/or CD5+ and/or CD8+
c cytoplasmic, s surfaces

Some forms of acute leukemia express biphenotypic markers (CD antigens, ► Chap. 2.5).

**Sy:**

### Nonspecific General Symptoms with Acute Onset
- Reduced performance, fever, night sweats, fatigue, shortness of breath
- Flu-like symptoms, anorexia, weight loss
- Bone pain

### Suppression of Normal Hematopoiesis
- Anemia → malaise, fatigue, tachycardia, pallor
- Thrombocytopenia → increased tendency to bleed, with petechiae and ecchymoses, hemato mas, epistaxis
- Granulocytopenia → skin infections, pneumonia, sepsis

### Leukemic Cell Proliferation, Organ Infiltration:     Frequency
- Hepatomegaly and/or splenomegaly:                              70%
- Lymphadenopathy:                                               60%
- CNS / meningeal involvement (meningeosis leucaemica)
  with headache, nausea, vomiting, impaired vision, CNS disorders:   < 10%
- Mediastinal involvement with lymphadenopathy:                  15%
- Infiltration of parenchymatous organs with functional impairment
  (liver, kidneys, gastrointestinal tract, testes, etc.):       < 10%
- With T-ALL: mediastinal tumors, frequent skin infiltration

Dg:

## Medical History, Physical Examination
- Medical history (risk factors, exposure)
- Physical examination: skin, mucous membranes, lymphadenopathy, hepatosplenomegaly, testes, CNS, (meningism and neurological disorders), ophthalmoscopy (fundus examination) to exclude leukemic infiltrates / hemorrhage, infection
- Siblings are potential donors for matched related allogeneic transplantation: HLA typing of both the patient and his or her relatives should be carried out as soon as possible (HLA-A, -B, -C, -DR; typing of patients with high blast count after induction of remission)

## Laboratory Tests
- Full blood count with differential and reticulocytes, cytochemistry, immunophenotyping

*ATTENTION:* A normal blood count and absence of leukemic blasts in peripheral blood do not rule out acute leukemia. In 15% of cases, the leukocyte count is normal, in 25% leukopenia

- Blood group, PT, PTT, TT, fibrinogen, ATIII, fibrinogen split products
- Routine laboratory analyses including ESR, creatinine, creatinine clearance, urea, electrolytes, AST, ALT, γGT, AP, LDH, bilirubin, total protein, electrophoresis
- Bacteriology: cultures from throat washings, feces, urine, anal and vaginal swabs
- Serology: candida, aspergillus, HSV, VZV, CMV, EBV, HBV, HIV, toxoplasmosis

## Bone Marrow and CSF (cerebrospinal fluid)
- Bone marrow smear and histology, immunocytology (CD20)
- Cytogenetics, e.g., t(9;22), t(4;11)
- Molecular diagnosis: BCR-ABL, MLL-AF4, TEL-AML1, detection of rearrangements of genes coding for light chains, heavy chains, and the TCR (see table)
- Lumbar puncture, CSF cytology (*ATTENTION: thrombocytopenia,* ▶ Chap. 10.6), possibly including molecular diagnosis

## Other Tests
- ECG, echocardiography
- Abdominal ultrasound
- X-ray: chest, paranasal sinuses, teeth, thoracic CT (T-ALL)
- Dental and possibly ENT check-up to screen for potential sources of infection

**Flow sheet of diagnosis of acute leukemia**

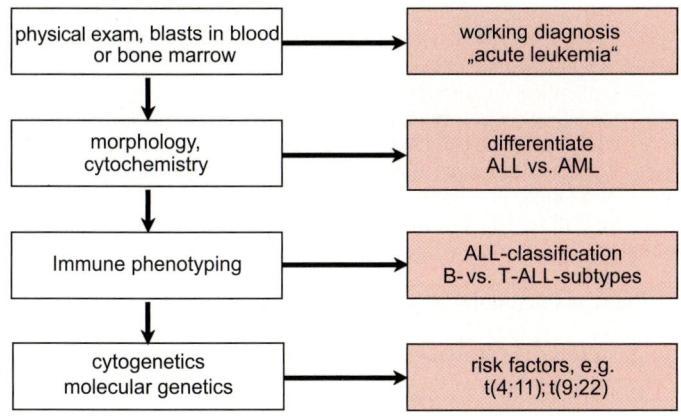

**Dd:**
- "Leukemoid reaction" due to infections or tumors
- Myelodysplastic syndrome
- Myeloproliferative syndrome, CML in blast crisis
- Acute myeloid leukemia (AML) or undifferentiated leukemia (AUL)
- Lymphoma with peripheral blood lymphocytosis, in particular high-grade NHL
- Pernicious anemia, vitamin $B_{12}$ / folic acid deficiency
- EBV infection (infectious mononucleosis with atypical lymphocytes)

The extent of bone marrow infiltration has proven to be a suitable parameter for distinguishing between ALL and lymphoblastic non-Hodgkin's lymphoma. Patients with more than 30% blasts in the bone marrow are classified as having ALL.

**Co:**
- Sepsis, other infectious complications
- Abnormal coagulation, hemorrhage, thromboembolic events, sinus vein thrombosis
- Tumor lysis syndrome, urate nephropathy (▶ Chap. 9.6)
- Leukostasis (pulmonary, cerebral)

## Treatment Concept

1. ALL is treated according to the prevalent subtype (immunophenotype), risk factors, and age. Treatment components are:
   - Systemic polychemotherapy with alternating protocols
   - Intrathecal chemotherapy
   - Prophylactic / therapeutic CNS irradiation
   - Mediastinal irradiation
   - Allogeneic stem cell transplantation

2. Large multicenter studies have led to substantial improvement of diagnosis, treatment, and prognosis of ALL. ALL patients should preferably be treated in the context of clinical trials at hematological centers.

3. Treatment of patients between 15 and 65 years according to the "Multicenter Therapy Optimization Study of Acute Lymphoblastic Leukemia in Adults or Adolescents from 15 Years of Age"—GMALL 07/2003, Prof. D. Hoelzer, Frankfurt

*ATTENTION:* The therapies specified below correspond to study protocol GMALL 07/2003. However, before treating an individual patient and for more explicit information regarding the treatment process (details on radiotherapy, dose modification, treatment intervals in case of cytopenia, etc.), the current protocol version should always be consulted. Should the patient be enrolled, contact the study coordination center regarding possible protocol changes.

4. Depending on their biological age and general performance status, older patients may be treated either according to the study or with alternative protocols (e.g., pilot study for older ALL and B-ALL patients).
5. Patients with mature B-ALL and high grade NHL (subtypes Burkitt's lymphoma, Burkitt-like lymphoma, precursor B-lymphoblastic lymphoma, large cell anaplastic lymphoma, diffuse large B-cell lymphoma) are treated according to the B-ALL / NHL protocol 2002.

## Therapy Protocol for the Treatment of ALL (GMALL 07/2003)

ALL is treated in phases—prephase, induction therapy, consolidation or intensification, re-induction, and maintenance therapy—using different treatment regimens.

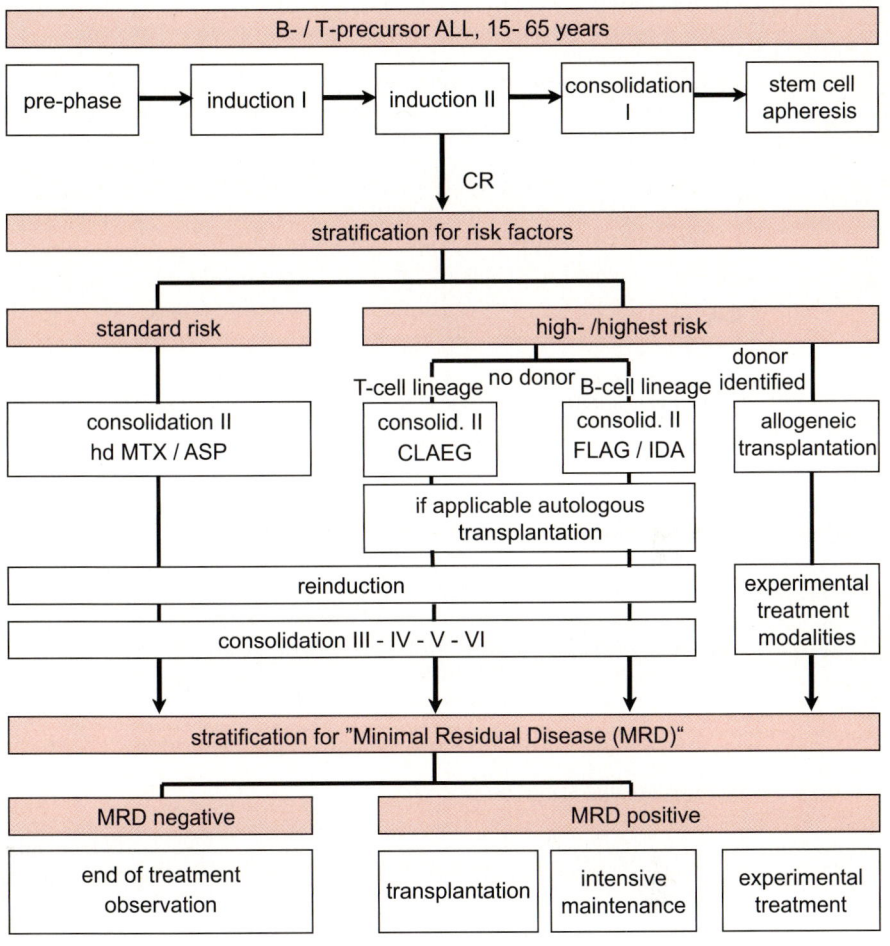

*MTX* methotrexate, *ASP* asparaginase, *FLAG* fludarabine + cytarabine + G-CSF, *IDA* idarubicin, *CR* complete remission, *CLAEG* cladribine + etoposide + cytarabine + G-CSF

## Chemotherapy

### Prephase
Objective: reduction of the initial leukemic cell load. *ATTENTION:* tumor lysis syndrome (▶ Chap. 9.6).

### Induction Therapy
- Objective: complete remission, i.e., reduction of the leukemic cell population to below the detection limit, recovery of normal hematopoiesis with normalization of blood count and bone marrow.
- Chemotherapy is based on combining dexamethasone, vincristine, anthracyclines, asparaginase, cyclophosphamide and 6-mercaptopurine in two blocks (Induction I and II).

### Consolidation I

Objective: early intensive consolidation to improve the remission quality.

### Stratification I Based on Risk Factors

ALL is not a uniform disease. Risk stratification is based on morphology, immunophenotyping, molecular genetics, and clinical parameters.

- An important prognostic factor with all subgroups is "time to complete remission".
- Patients with high-risk factors show lower remission rates (64% versus 81%) and a significantly reduced leukemia-free survival.
- The worst prognostic factor is the translocation t(9;22).

**Risk factor**

| Risk group | T-cell type | B-cell type |
|---|---|---|
| Standard risk (SR) | Thymic T-ALL T-ALL (CD1a negative) | B-Precursor ALL <br>• CR on day 26 (after Induction I) and WBC < 30,000/μl <br>• No pro B or t(4;11) positive ALL <br>• No t(9;22) / BCR-ABL-positive ALL |
| High risk (HR) | Early T or mature T-ALL (CD1a negative) | B-precursor ALL <br>• CR after day 45 or <br>• WBC > 30,000/μl <br>• Pro B or t(4;11)-positive ALL |
| Very high risk (VHR) | | B-precursor ALL t(9;22) / BCR-ABL-positive ALL |

**Risk stratification, ALL protocol**

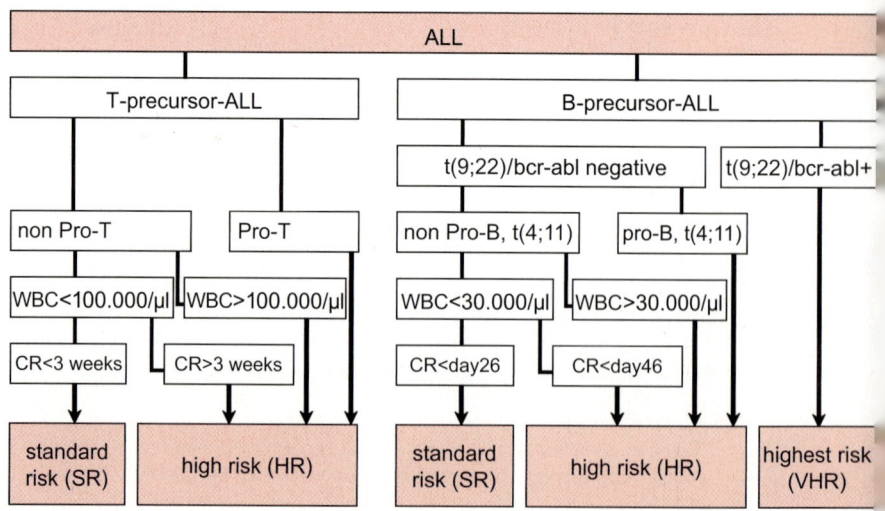

*WBC* White blood cells, *CR* complete remission

## Post-remission Therapy: Intensification

Objective: further reduction of the leukemic cell population after induction therapy and consolidation I. For standard-risk patients, consolidation treatment is based on high-dose methotrexate and asparaginase, while high and very high risk patients undergo allogeneic stem cell transplantation, provided a suitable donor (related or unrelated) is available. If no donor is available, patients with T-cell ALL are treated according to the CLAEG regimen while those with B-precursor ALL are treated according to the FLAG-Ida regimen, followed by either autologous transplantation or continuation of treatment according to the standard-risk protocol.

## Re-induction and Maintenance Therapy

Standard-risk patients receive re-induction treatment (after consolidation II). Consolidation treatment blocks are followed by maintenance treatment.

## Stratification II Based on "Minimal Residual Disease"(MRD)

Analysis of molecular genetic markers (e.g., BCR-ABL in Philadelphia chromosome-positive ALL, clonal rearrangements of Ig and TCR genes) identifies remission parameters beyond those obtained from classic bone marrow histology and allows for definition of "molecular CR" or "minimal residual disease," MRD.

- *With standard-risk patients*, an MRD-dependent decision regarding further treatment should be made after 12 months.
- *Intermediate results (after week 16):* early definition of "high risk" if MRD is $10^{-4}$ at least two times between weeks 11 and 16. Consolidation I is followed by HR / VHR treatment.
- *Low-risk MRD:* consistently $< 10^{-4}$ from day 71 until week 52 and negative by week 52.
- *High-risk MRD:* from week 16–52 at least twice $> 10^{-4}$; no drop to below $10^{-4}$ on two consecutive time points by the end of the first year of treatment.
- *Intermediate-risk MRD:* patients who cannot be clearly classified or for whom the MRD cannot be determined.

## MRD-dependent Treatment Decision

- *Low-risk MRD* from week 52: end of treatment
- *High-risk MRD* from week 16 or week 52: allogeneic SCT. Experimental therapy according to study protocols. Intensified maintenance treatment
- *Intermediate-risk MRD* from week 52: intensified maintenance treatment
- Continue to carry out MRD analyses every 4 months. Intensified maintenance treatment is similar to first year consolidation.

## Specific Therapeutic Measures

### Supportive Therapy
- Infection prevention, oral hygiene, patient care
- Prevention of tumor lysis syndrome (▶ Chap. 9.6): fluid replacement (target: urinary excretion rate > 200 ml/h), alkalinization, administration of allopurinol, rasburicase in cases of renal failure or high urea levels
- Anti-infective treatment; in case of fever, early administration of antibiotic / antimycotic drugs (▶ Chap. 4.2)
- Transfusion of red cell and platelet concentrates
- Replacement of coagulation factors; if necessary, DIC treatment
- Suppression of menstruation in premenopausal women

### Intrathecal Chemotherapy
- Lumbar puncture and prophylactic intrathecal instillation of cytostatics may only be performed if no bleeding complications are to be expected (▶ Chap. 10.6).
- Intrathecal prophylaxis with 15 mg methotrexate or (from re-induction therapy onward) combination of 15 mg methotrexate, 40 mg cytosine arabinoside, and 4 mg dexamethasone.
- In case of primary involvement of the CNS or CNS relapse: intrathecal treatment using the combination of 15 mg methotrexate, 40 mg cytosine arabinoside, and 4 mg dexamethasone,

two to three times weekly. Duration of treatment: 2 weeks beyond CSF normalization, fo[llowed] by intrathecal prophylaxis.

### Radiotherapy
- In combination with prophylactic intrathecal chemotherapy, prophylactic CNS irradiatio[n] (total dose: 24 Gy, 2 Gy/day on 5 days per week) significantly reduces the incidence of CN[S] relapse (from > 30% to < 10%).
- If CNS is involved: therapeutic CNS irradiation.
- Local irradiation: if involvement of mediastinum (usually T-ALL) or testes.

### Allogeneic Stem Cell Transplantation (SCT)
- Allogeneic SCT from an HLA-identical related ("familial") or unrelated donor is the firs[t] choice post-remission treatment with curative intention in high-risk patients (in particula[r] with $Ph^+$ t(9;22)/BCR-ABL and t(4;11), pro-T-ALL) or where CR has not been achieved i[n] time. Patients > 55 years of age or for whom the conventional conditioning treatment is con[n]traindicated, are treated with reduced intensity conditioning regimens ("non-myeloablative"[).]
- Standard-risk patients first undergo 1 year of chemotherapy. Depending on MRD results, ris[k] factor profile and the availability of a suitable donor, allogeneic SCT may be necessary.
- Relapsed patients should undergo allogeneic SCT as soon as possible, after salvage chemo[o] therapy.
- All patients without GVHD should receive donor lymphocytes on days +60, +88, and +11[6] after transplantation.

*ATTENTION:* if allogeneic BMT is planned, avoid transfusion of blood products from relate[d] donors: risk of alloimmunization.

## New Therapeutic Concepts

### Imatinib (chapter 3.6)
BCR-ABL-positive ALL constitutes the poorest prognosis with a 5-year survival rate of 0–15%[.] BCR-ABL-tyrosine kinase inhibitors (imatinib, dasatinib) represent new treatment options fo[r] this entity → response rate in monotherapy 60%, median duration of remission 2 months. Com[m]bination with chemotherapy may improve these results. The use of imatinib and dasatinib in th[e] treatment of BCR-ABL-positive ALL is the subject of current trials.

### Rituximab (Anti-CD20 Antibody Rituximab, chapter 3.5)
Rituximab is efficacious in the treatment of CD20-positive high-grade B-NHL. Efficacy and safe[ty] of rituximab in CD20-positive B-ALL and Burkitt's lymphoma are currently studied.

### Alemtuzumab (Anti-CD52 Antibody, chapter 3.5)
The therapeutic benefit of alemtuzumab in the treatment of ALL is currently tested in trials.

## Chemotherapy Regimens for Patients with B- or T-precursor ALL (Study GMALL 07/2003)

### Prephase
Objective: Prevention of tumor lysis syndrome (▶ Chap. 9.6), especially in cases of high bla[st] counts or organomegaly. Sufficient hydration and alkalinization as well as the administration [of] allopurinol and possibly rasburicase are essential.

| "ALL-Prephase" ▶ Protocol 11.1.1 | | | Study Protocol GMALL 07/2003 |
|---|---|---|---|
| Dexamethasone | 10 mg/m²/day | p.o. | Day 1–5 |
| Cyclophosphamide | 200 mg/m²/d | i.v. | Day 3–5 |

Intrathecal prophylaxis: methotrexate 15 mg i.th. day 1. With initial granulocytopenia < 500/ul G-CSF from day 1

## Induction Therapy

- Chemotherapy with several cytostatics and intrathecal methotrexate prophylaxis.
- Induction I starts directly after the prephase.
- According to study protocol GMALL 07/2003, treatment is consistent up to Consolidation I. Stratification according to risk factors is carried out only after week 16.

| "Induction I" ▶ Protocol 11.1.2 | | | Study Protocol GMALL 07/2003 |
|---|---|---|---|
| Daunorubicin | 45 mg/m²/day | i.v. | Day 6,7,13,14 |
| Vincristine | 2 mg absolute | i.v. | Day 6,13,20 |
| Pegasparaginase | 1,000 U/m²/day | i.v. | Day 20 |
| Dexamethasone | 10 mg/m²/day | p.o. | Day 6–7,13–16 |
| G-CSF | 5 µg/kg/day | s.c. | From day 6 |

Intrathecal prophylaxis: methotrexate 15 mg i.th. day 1. For patients between 55 and 65 years of age: daunorubicin 30 mg/m², pegasparaginase 500 U/m²

| "Induction II" ▶ Protocol 11.1.3 | | | Study Protocol GMALL 07/2003 |
|---|---|---|---|
| Cyclophosphamide | 1,000 mg/m²/day | i.v. | Day 26,46 |
| Cytosine arabinoside | 75 mg/m²/day | i.v. | Day 28–31,35–38,42– |
| 6-mercaptopurine | 60 mg/m²/day | p.o. | 45 |
| G-CSF | 5 µg/kg/day | s.c. | Day 26–46 |

Intrathecal prophylaxis: methotrexate 15 mg i.th. day 28,35,42 + CNS irradiation 24 Gy total, 2 Gy/day day 26–46

## Consolidation

Polychemotherapy with varying protocols. Up to Consolidation I, standard treatment for all patients, then stratification and treatment according to the risk profile.

| Consolidation I ▶ Protocol 11.1.4 | | | Study Protocol GMALL 07/2003 |
|---|---|---|---|
| Dexamethasone | 10 mg/m²/day | p.o. | Day 1–5 |
| Vindesine | 3 mg/m²/day | i.v. | Day 1 |
| Methotrexate | 1,500 mg/m²/day | i.v. | Day 1, over 24 h |
| Etoposide phosphate | 250 mg/m²/day | i.v. | Day 4,5 |
| Cytosine arabinoside | 2,000 mg/m²/day | i.v. | Day 5, over 3 h, every 12 h |
| G-CSF | 5 µg/kg/day | s.c. | Day 7–16 (until stem cell apheresis) |

Intrathecal prophylaxis: cytosine arabinoside 40 mg, methotrexate 15 mg, dexamethasone 4 mg, i.th., day 12. Vindesine max. 5 mg absolute. Patients between 55 and 65 years of age: Methotrexate 1 g/m², cytosine arabinoside 1 g/m²

Standard-risk patients are given consolidation II, re-induction I, II, consolidation III–VI, maintenance therapy.

| Consolidation II, III, VI ▶ Protocol 11.1.5 | | | Study Protocol GMALL 07/2003 |
|---|---|---|---|
| 6-Mercaptopurine | 60 mg/m²/day | p.o. | Day 1–7,15–21 |
| Methotrexate | 1,500 mg/m²/day | i.v. | Day 1,15, over 24 h |
| Pegasparaginase | 500 IU/m²/day | i.v. | Day 2,16 |

Intrathecal prophylaxis: cytosine arabinoside 40 mg, methotrexate 15 mg, dexamethasone 4 mg, i.th., day 1

| Consolidation IV ▶ Protocol 11.1.8 | | | Study Protocol GMALL 07/2003 |
|---|---|---|---|
| Cytosine arabinoside | 150 mg/m²/day | i.v. | Day 1–5 |
| Teniposide | 100 mg/m²/day | i.v. | Day 1–5 |

Intrathecal prophylaxis: cytosine arabinoside 40 mg, methotrexate 15 mg, dexamethasone 4 mg, i.th., day 1

| Consolidation V ▶ Protocol 11.1.9 | | | Study Protocol GMALL 07/2003 |
|---|---|---|---|
| Cyclophosphamide | 1,000 mg/m²/day | i.v. | Day 1, over 1 h |
| Cytosine arabinoside | 500 mg/m²/day | i.v. | Day 1, over 24 h |

Intrathecal prophylaxis: cytosine arabinoside 40 mg, methotrexate 15 mg, dexamethasone 4 mg, i.th., day 1

### Re-induction

Polychemotherapy with several cytostatics and intrathecal triple prophylaxis

| "Re-induction I" ▶ Protocol 11.1.10 | | | Study Protocol GMALL 07/2003 |
|---|---|---|---|
| Doxorubicine | 50 mg/m²/day | i.v. | Day 1,7 |
| Vindesine | 3 mg/m²/day | i.v. | Day 1,7 |
| Prednisolone | 3 × 20 mg/m²/day | p.o. | Day 1–14 |

Intrathecal prophylaxis: cytosine arabinoside 40 mg, methotrexate 15 mg, dexamethasone 4 mg i.th. day 1. Vindesine max. 5 mg absolute

| "Re-induction II" ▶ Protocol 11.1.11 | | | Study Protocol GMALL 07/2003 |
|---|---|---|---|
| Cyclophosphamide | 1,000 mg/m²/day | i.v. | Day 15 |
| Cytosine arabinoside | 75 mg/m²/day | i.v. | Day 17–20, 24–27 |
| Thioguanine | 60 mg/m²/day | p.o. | Day 15–28 |

Intrathecal prophylaxis: cytosine arabinoside 40 mg, methotrexate 15 mg, dexamethasone 4 mg i.th. day 15

## Maintenance Therapy

After re-induction, between consolidation blocks III–VI, and until further treatment decisions have been established based on the MRD risk profile, patients receive low-dose maintenance therapy.

| "Maintenance" ▶ Protocol 11.1.12 | | | Study Protocol GMALL 07/2003 |
|---|---|---|---|
| 6-Mercaptopurine | 60 mg/m²/day | p.o. | Daily |
| Methotrexate | 20 mg/m²/day | i.v./p.o. | Once weekly |

## Intensification Without Allogeneic Stem Cell Donor

High and very high risk patients without allogeneic stem cell donor recieve Consolidation II, followed by either autologous stem cell transplantation or continued treatment according to the standard-risk protocol.

| CLAEG (Consolidation II HR – T-Cell ALL – Week 16) ▶ Protocol 11.1.6 | | | |
|---|---|---|---|
| Cladribine | 0.2 mg/kg/day | i.v. | Day 1–5 |
| Etoposide, VP-16 | 60 mg/m²/day | i.v. | Day 1–5 |
| Cytosine arabinoside | 1.5 g/ m²/day | i.v. | Day 1–5 |
| G-CSF | 5 μg/kg/day | s.c. | From day 6 |

Intrathecal prophylaxis: cytosine arabinoside 40 mg, methotrexate 15 mg, dexamethasone 4 mg, i.th., day 1. Patients between 55 and 65 years of age: cytosine arabinoside 1 g/m²

| FLAG-Ida (Consolidation II HR/VHR – B-Precursor ALL – Week 16) ▶ Protocol 11.1.7 | | | |
|---|---|---|---|
| Idarubicin | 10 mg/m²/day | i.v. | Day 1,3 |
| Fludarabine | 30 mg/m²/day | i.v. | Day 1–5 |
| Cytosine arabinoside | 2,000 mg/m²/day | i.v. | Day 1–5 |
| G-CSF | 5 μg/kg/day | s.c. | From day 7 |

Intrathecal prophylaxis: cytosine arabinoside 40 mg, methotrexate 15 mg, dexamethasone 4 mg, i.th., day 1. Patients between 55 and 65 years of age: idarubicin 7 mg/m², cytosine arabinoside 1 g/m²

## Chemotherapy Regimens for Patients with B-ALL (Study GMALL-B ALL/NHL 2002/ Chemotherapy Regimens)

### Prephase

Objective: Especially with high blast counts, standard chemotherapy of B-ALL and Burkitt's lymphoma is often followed by massive cellular disintegration (tumor lysis syndrome, ▶ Chap. 9.6). The main objective of the prephase with cyclophosphamide and prednisolone is to prevent the occurrence of a tumor lysis syndrome. Sufficient hydration and alkalinization as well as the administration of allopurinol are essential.

| "B-ALL Prephase" ▶ Protocol 11.1.13 | | | Study Protocol B-ALL 2002 |
|---|---|---|---|
| Prednisolone | 3 × 20 mg/m²/day | p.o. | Day 1–5 |
| Cyclophosphamide | 200 mg/m²/day | i.v. | Day 1–5 |

### Therapy Blocks A, B, and C

Polychemotherapy with different cytostatics and intrathecal triple prophylaxis. Six therapy blocks in total, at intervals of 21 days.

| "Block A" ▶ Protocol 11.1.14 | | | Study Protocol B-ALL 2002 |
|---|---|---|---|
| Rituximab | 375 mg/m² | i.v. | Day 1 |
| Vincristine | 2 mg/day absolute | i.v. | Day 2 |
| Methotrexate | 1,500 mg/m²/day | i.v. | Day 2, infuse over 24 h |
| Ifosfamide | 800 mg/m²/day | i.v. | Day 2–6 |
| Teniposide, VM-26 | 100 mg/m²/day | i.v. | Day 5+6 |
| Cytosine arabinoside | 150 mg/m²/day | i.v. | Day 5+6 inf. over 1 h, every 12 h |
| Dexamethasone | 10 mg/m²/day | p.o. | Day 2–6 |
| G-CSF | 5 µg/kg/day | s.c. | From day 7 |

Intrathecal prophylaxis: cytosine arabinoside 40 mg, methotrexate 15 mg, dexamethasone 4 mg, i.th., day 1+5

| "Block B" ▶ Protocol 11.1.15 | | | Study Protocol B-ALL 2002 |
|---|---|---|---|
| Rituximab | 375 mg/m² | i.v. | Day 1 |
| Vincristine | 2 mg/day absolute | i.v. | Day 2 |
| Methotrexate | 1,500 mg/m²/day | i.v. | Day 2, infuse over 24 h |
| Cyclophosphamide | 200 mg/m²/day | i.v. | Day 2-6 |
| Doxorubicin | 25 mg/m²/day | i.v. | Day 5+6 |
| Dexamethasone | 10 mg/m²/day | p.o. | Day 2-6 |
| G-CSF | 5 µg/kg/day | s.c. | From day 7 |

Intrathecal prophylaxis: cytosine arabinoside 40 mg, methotrexate 15 mg, dexamethasone 4 mg, i.th., day 1+5

| "Block C" ▶ Protocol 11.1.16 | | | Study Protocol B-ALL 2002 |
|---|---|---|---|
| Rituximab | 375 mg/m² | i.v. | Day 1 |
| Vindesine | 3 mg/day absolute | i.v. | Day 2 |
| Methotrexate | 1,500 mg/m²/day | i.v. | Day 2, infuse over 24 h |
| Cytosine arabinoside | 2,000 mg/m²/day | i.v. | Day 6, inf. over 3 h, every 12 h |
| Etoposide VP-16 | 250 mg/m²/day | i.v. | Day 5+6 |
| Dexamethasone | 10 mg/m²/day | p.o. | Day 2–6 |
| G-CSF | 5 µg/kg/day | s.c. | From day 8 |

### Patients Between 15 and 55 Years of Age

- Patients with stage III–IV as well as all patients with mediastinal tumors or extranodal involvement receive 6 cycles (A1, B1, C1, A2, B2, C2).
- In patients with stage I–II, chemotherapy is discontinued after 4 cycles (A1, B1, C1, A2) if the patient has shown a definite CR after 2 cycles and there was no initial mediastinal tumor or extranodal involvement.
- Patients with treatment failure or progression after 4 cycles should discontinue the study and receive salvage therapy and stem cell transplantation.

### Patients > 55 Years of Age

- Patients > 55 years in good general condition and without contraindications may be treated according to the protocol for 15- to 55-year-olds with dose reductions for methotrexate (from 1,500 mg/m² to 500 mg/m²) and cytosine arabinoside (from 2,000 mg/m² to 1,000 mg/m²)

- For all other patients > 55 years of age, the following modifications apply:
    - No block C; instead, alternating blocks A and B (A1*, B1*, A2*, B2*, A3*, B3*)
    - Dose reduction for methotrexate (from 1,500 mg/m² to 500 mg/m²), ifosfamide (from 800 mg/m² to 400 mg/m²), vincristine (from 2 mg to 1 mg absolute), teniposide (from 100 mg/m² to 60 mg/m²), cytosine arabinoside (from 150 mg/m² to 60 mg/m²)
    - Intrathecal prophylaxis with MTX 12 mg only, instead of triple therapy

### Rituximab
In case of a 6-block therapy, 2 additional cycles of rituximab are given at intervals of 21 days. Four-block treatment involves no additional cycles of rituximab.

## Classification of Treatment Response

### Complete Remission (CR)
Normocellular bone marrow with 0% blasts (M0 marrow) or ≤ 5% blasts, ≥ 15% erythropoiesis, ≥ 25% granulopoiesis, and normal megakaryopoiesis. No blasts in the peripheral blood, organs free of leukemia cells. Sufficiently regenerated hematopoiesis with the following cell counts in the peripheral blood: granulocytes ≥ 1,500/µl, thrombocytes ≥ 100,000/µl.

### Partial Remission (PR)
Normocellular bone marrow with 6–25% blasts (M2 marrow), ≥ 10% erythropoiesis and 25% granulopoiesis. No blasts in the peripheral blood.

### Treatment Failure (F)
If one of the following criteria applies: 26–50% (M3) or > 50% (M4) blasts in the bone marrow; blasts in the peripheral blood; extramedullary leukemic infiltrates.

## Primary Refractory ALL or Relapsed ALL

### Primary Refractory ALL
No complete remission during induction therapy or remission lasting less than 6 months

### Relapse
Recurrent leukemia after complete remission (remission duration ≥ 6 months). Relapse may occur in the bone marrow and the peripheral blood or may be extramedullary (CNS, testes, skin, lymph nodes, etc.). Relapse criteria:
- Blasts in the peripheral blood
- Blasts in the bone marrow ≥ 5%
- Meningeal leukemia
- Extramedullary relapse with cytological or histological confirmation

### Salvage Therapy
- The duration of the initial remission determines the choice of treatment strategy and the likelihood of a second remission. If the remission period was less than 6 months, resistance to the cytostatics used can be assumed.
- The treatment of choice is myeloablative therapy with allogeneic stem cell transplantation (SCT) which leads to long-term remission in 10–20% of cases.
- In patients with late relapse (more than 24 months after complete remission), long-term remission may be reinstated via the initial standard ALL protocol.
- Patients with refractory lymphoblastic leukemia and good general performance status may be treated with the following high-dose therapy: cytosine arabinoside 3,000 mg/m²/day, day 1–5 i.v. and amsacrine 200 mg/m²/day, day 3–5 i.v. or, alternatively, cytosine arabinoside 3,000 mg/m²/twice daily, day 1–4 i.v. and mitoxantrone 10 mg/m²/day, day 2–6 i.v. (HAM Protocol).
- A treatment attempt with 2-chlorodeoxyadenosine is justified in cases of refractory ALL or after two or more relapses. Older patients with poor performance status may undergo cytoreduction with methotrexate and 6-mercaptopurine.
- Experimental treatment: forodesine, nelarabine

**F/U:**     Close follow-up at intervals of 1–2 months maximum. Regular monitoring of:
- Case history, clinical examination
- Blood count, bone marrow, and minimal residual disease (MRD) analysis according to the study protocol
- Signs of treatment-related toxicity (cardiotoxicity, central and peripheral neurotoxicity, bone marrow damage, secondary neoplasia, etc.)

**Prg:**     Prognosis depends on the ALL subtype and risk factors (see definition of "high risk").

| Patient group | Complete remission (%) | Five-year survival (%) |
|---|---|---|
| All patients | 70–90 | 40 |
| B-precursor ALL | 75–85 | 35 |
| Ph$^+$ / bcr-abl-positive ALL | 70–80 | 0–15 |
| Mature B-ALL | 80–85 | 55–65 |
| Mature T-ALL | 80–85 | 50 |

**Ref:**
1. Aplenc R, Lange B. Pharmacogenetic determinants of outcome in acute lymphoblastic leukemia. Br J Hematol 2004;125:421–34
2. Armstrong SA, Look AT. Molecular genetics of acute lymphoblastic leukemia. J Clin Oncol 2005;23:6306–15
3. Castor A, Nilsson L, Astrand-Grundstroem I et al. Distinct patterns of stem cell involvement in acute lymphoblastic leukemia. Nat Med 2005;11:630–7
4. Hallbook H, Hagglund H, Stockelberg D et al. Autologous and allogeneic stem cell transplantation in adult ALL. Bone Marrow Transpl 2005;35:1141–8
5. Pui CH, Evans WE. Treatment of acute lymphoblastic leukemia. N Eng J Med 2006;354:166–78
6. Ravandi F. Role of cytokines in the treatment of acute leukemias. Leukemia 2006;20:563–71
7. Rowe JM, Goldstone AH. How I treat acute lymphocytic leukemia in adults. Blood 2007;110:2268–75
8. Szczepanski T. Why and how to quantify minimal residual disease in acute lymphoblastic leukemia. Leukemia 2007;21:622–6

**Web:**
1. http://cancer.gov/cancer_information/cancer_type/leukemia     Natl Cancer Institute
2. http://www.nlm.nih.gov/medlineplus/leukemiaadultacute.html     Medline Plus
3. http://l3.leukemia-lymphoma.org/all_page?item_id=7049     Leuk Lymph Soc
4. http://www.emedicine.com/med/topic3146.htm     Emedicine
5. http://www.leukemia-net.org     Eur Leukemia Network
6. http://www.meds.com/leukemia/atlas/acute_leukemia.html     Atlas of Leukemia

## 7.1.2 Acute Myeloid Leukemia (AML)

K. Heining-Mikesch, M. Lübbert

**Def:** Group of clonal diseases with transformation of an early myeloid precursor. Different types of AML correspond to the differentiation stages of myeloid progenitor cells.

**ICD-10:** C92–C95

**Ep:** Incidence: 3–4 cases/100,000 population/year. Increasing frequency with higher age: incidence in patients > 65 years 15 cases/100,000 population/year. 3% of all malignant diseases, most frequent lethal neoplasia between 30th and 40th year of age.

**Pg:** ### Risk Factors
- Bone marrow damage: ionizing radiation, alkylating substances, topoisomerase inhibitors, benzol, cigarette smoke
- Predisposing hematological diseases: myelodysplastic syndromes, myeloproliferative syndromes, aplastic anemia, multiple myeloma, paroxysmal nocturnal hemoglobinuria → development of "secondary" AML
- Genetic factors: increased risk with trisomy 21, Fanconi's anemia, Bloom's syndrome, Li-Fraumeni syndrome

### Molecular Pathogenetic Mechanisms
- *Cytogenetics:* frequent chromosomal translocations:
  - 5–10% of cases: t(8;21), t(15;17), inv(16), t(11q23;n)
  - 2–5% of cases: t(3;5), t(3;3), t(8;16), t(6;9), t(1;3), t(9;22)
  - Numeric aberrations: deletions -5, -7, 5q-, 7q-, 20q or 12p. Trisomy +8, +13, +21
- *Molecular genetics:* oncogene activation: e.g., point mutation of c-kit, N-ras or K-ras proto-oncogenes, flt3-duplication or mutation NPM1 mutation gene rearrangements (AML1/ETO etc.)
- *Epigenetics:* hypermethylation (e.g., p15, estrogen receptor, E-cadherin); histone deacetylation of target genes of chimeric transcription factors (PML/RARA, AML1/ETO)

**Path:** ### Bone Marrow
- Expansion of myeloid precursor cells.
- Monomorphic population of "blasts": immature cells with large nucleus, prominent nucleolus, and narrow, basophilic cytoplasmic border without granulation (undifferentiated blasts) or with granulated cytoplasm (partial differentiation).
- Suppression of normal hematopoiesis.

### Peripheral Blood
- In general leukocytosis with detection of the same blast population as in the bone marrow. *ATTENTION:* leukocytosis in peripheral blood is not present in all cases ("aleukemic" presentation with leukopenia in about 10%)
- Anemia and thrombocytopenia as signs of suppression of normal hematopoiesis

### Organs
Extramedullary leukemia growth ("chloroma", "myelosarcoma", e.g., with AML FAB M2) as additional or isolated manifestation (meningeal, cutaneous, abdominal, cerebral, osseous, infiltration of soft tissue).

**Class:** The "FAB" classification of acute myeloid leukemia was developed in 1985 by the "French-American-British Cooperative Group," based in particular on morphological and cytochemical characteristics.
More recent classification models are based on recommendations of the WHO and take into account additional molecular and immunophenotypical characteristics. A double classification according to WHO and FAB should be performed.

### WHO Classification (1999, AML Definition: > 20% Blasts in Bone Marrow)

*AML with specific chromosomal translocations*
- AML with t(8;21) and AML 1/ETO rearrangement
- Acute promyelocytic leukemia with t(15;17), t(11;17) or other variant translocations
- AML with abnormal eosinophils in bone marrow and inv(16) or t(16;16) and CBFβ/MYH1 rearrangement
- AML with 11q23 translocation (MLL gene)

*AML with multilineage dysplasia*
- With preceding MDS
- Without preceding MDS

*Therapy-related AML*
- After alkylating agents
- After epipodophyllotoxins
- After radiotherapy

*Not otherwise categorized*
- AML minimally differentiated
- AML without maturation
- AML with maturation
- Acute myelomonocytic leukemia
- Acute monocytic leukemia
- Acute erythroid leukemia
- Acute basophilic leukemia
- Acute panmyelosis with myelofibrosis

*Acute biphenotypic leukemia*

### Special Entities
- Hypoplastic AML
- Smoldering leukemia

### Non specific General Symptoms Usually with Brief Medical History
- Reduced performance status, fever, night sweats, fatigue
- Loss of appetite, weight loss
- Flu-like symptoms, bone pain

### Impairment of Normal Hematopoiesis
- Anemia: weakness, fatigue, tachycardia, pallor of skin and mucous membranes
- Thrombocytopenia: increased bleeding tendency, with petechiae and ecchymoses hematoma epistaxis
- Granulocytopenia: skin infection, pneumonia, sepsis

### Leukemic Cell Proliferation, Organ Infiltration
- Hepatosplenomegaly
- Lymphoma
- Chloroma (extramedullar tumorous manifestation)
- CNS involvement with headache, nausea / vomiting, visual impairment, central nervous disturbances, polydipsia (rare)
- Disseminated intravascular coagulation (DIC), especially AML M3 (acute promyelocytic leukemia, APL), hyperfibrinolysis

FAB classification of acute myeloid leukemia (1985)

| FAB | Morphology and characteristics | Cytochemistry | | | Immuno-phenotype[a,b] | Frequency |
|---|---|---|---|---|---|---|
| | | MPO | EST | PAS | | |
| M0 | "Acute myeloid leukemia, minimally differentiated" Immature blasts, immunophenotyping required | < 3% | – | – | Myeloid | < 2% |
| M1 | "Acute myeloid leukemia without maturation" Immature blasts, immunophenotyping required | 3–10% | – | – | | 20% |
| M2 | "Acute myeloid leukemia with maturation" 3–20% promyelocytes, frequently with Auer rods Subtype "M2Baso": with basophilia | > 30% | – | – | | 30% < 2% |
| M3 | "Acute promyelocytic leukemia" > 30% promyelocytes, Auer rods often in bundle like formation, "faggots" | +++ | – | –/+ | HLA-DR- | 10% |
| | Subtype "M3v": microgranular variant: lobulated or clefted nuclei, seldom Auer rods, occasionally local azurophilic granules; morphologically resembling monocytoid blasts. Cytogenetics and molecular genetics required | ++ | – | –/+ | | |
| M4 | "Acute myelomonocytic leukemia" Similar to M2, however (pro-) monocyte fraction > 20% | + | + | – | | 30% |
| | Subtype "M4Eo": ≤ 30% abnormal eosinophils (monocytic nuclei, immature eosinophilic or basophilic granules). Cyto- / molecular genetics required | + | + | + | | |
| M5 | "Acute monoblastic leukemia" ≥ 80% of all nonerythroid cells in bone marrow monocytic. Subtype "M5a": immature monoblasts, "M5b" monoblasts with maturation, cerebriform nucleus | +/– | + | –/+ | | 10% |
| M6 | "Acute erythroleukemia" (Di Guglielmo) ≥ 50% of all nucleated cells in bone marrow are erythroid, ≥ 30% of nonerythroid cells are blasts | – | – | +/– | Glycophorin+ | < 5% |
| M7 | "Acute megakaryoblastic leukemia" Heterogeneous blast population, abnormal megakaryocytes. Frequently "dry tap," in this case immunophenotyping required | – | – | +/– | CD61+ / CD41+ | < 5% |

[a] In all types of AML: ≥ 2 of the following markers are positive: myeloperoxidase, CD13, CD33, CD65, CD117

[b] The FAB classification is based on morphological criteria and cytochemistry. With few exceptions (M0, M7) there is no strong correlation between FAB classification and immunophenotype. The listed markers correspond to frequent constellations. Immunological phenotyping ▶ Chap 2.5

MPO myeloperoxidase, EST unspecific esterase (naphthylacetatesterase), PAS periodic acid-Schiff reaction

- In particular with AML M4 / M5: skin infiltrates, gingival hyperplasia, CNS involvement
- Leukostasis (frequent with leukocytes > 100,000/µl): pulmonary symtoms (dyspnea, pulmonary leukemic infiltrates), cerebral stasis (ischemia, hemorrhage), arterial embolism

**Dg:**  **Medical History, Clinical Signs**
- History with risk factors, family history (immediate search for possible matched related blood stem cell donors)
- Physical examination: skin, mucous membranes (gingival hyperplasia), lung (infections), lymph node status, abdomen (hepato- / splenomegaly), neurological findings

**Laboratory Tests**
- Complete blood count, differential blood count (blood smear)
- Routine laboratory tests with liver and renal function parameters (uric acid), electrolytes, LDH (elevated with increased cell turnover)
- Coagulation parameters (DIC, hyperfibrinolysis)
- Microbiological diagnostics if febrile, virus serum titers
- HLA typing of patient and all siblings (search for HLA-identical family donor for possible matched related allogeneic blood stem cell transplantation)

**Histology / Cytology**
- Bone marrow aspirate and smear (morphology, cytochemistry), immunocytology, cytogenetics, molecular genetic detection of specific gene rearrangements
- Bone marrow histology (bone marrow biopsy of iliac crest)
- CSF cytology (cerebrospinal fluid) as required

**Imaging**
- Chest x-ray, abdominal ultrasound, ECG
- Echocardiography before anthracycline treatment (of possible cardiotoxicity)

**DD:**
- "Leukemoid reaction" with infections
- Myelodysplastic syndrome
- Myeloproliferative syndrome, CML in blast crisis
- Lymphoblastic leukemia or lymphoma with bone marrow involvement
- Pernicious anemia, vitamin $B_{12}$ / folic acid deficiency
- Aplastic anemia
- EBV infection (mononucleosis with atypical lymphocytes)

**Co:**
- Sepsis, other infectious complications incl. fungal and viral etiologies
- Coagulation disorders, bleeding complications / thrombosis / embolism
- Tumor lysis syndrome, urate nephropathy, electrolyte imbalances
- Leukostasis (lung, cerebral), frequently with ischemia and/or hemorrhage ($\geq$ 20% of all AML patients with leukocytes > 50,000/µl)

**Th:**  **Treatment Concept**

- Treatment of AML is conducted with curative intent and consists of systemic combination chemotherapy, resulting in transient bone marrow aplasia (myelosuppression).
- Effective antileukemic drugs are: cytosine arabinoside (AraC), anthracyclines (daunorubicin, idarubicin, aclarubicin), anthracenediones (mitoxantrone), amsacrine (m-Amsa), hydroxyurea, etoposide (VP-16), topotecan, cyclophosphamide, 6-mercaptopurin (6-MP), 6-thioguanine (6-TG), arsenic trioxide (ATO).
- In AML M3 (APL), retinoic acid derivatives (ATRA) are given with chemotherapy.

**Treatment phases**

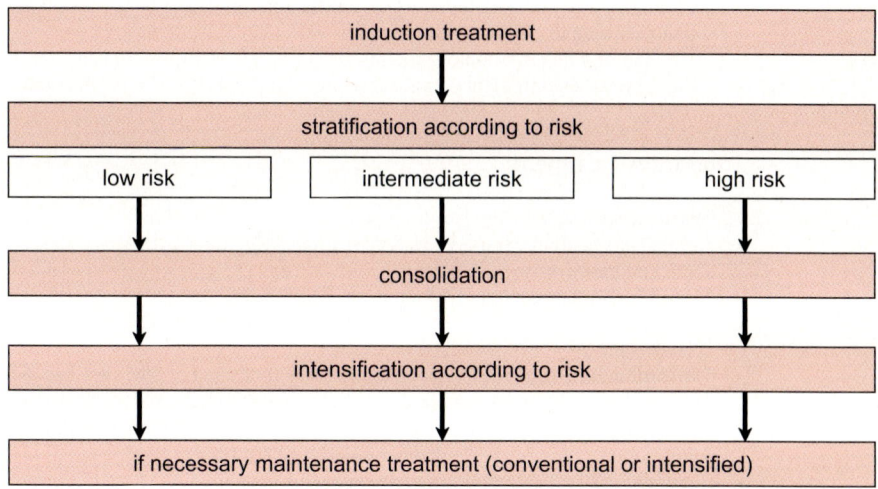

### Induction Treatment
Objective: "Induction of remission," reaching complete remission, i.e., reduction of number of leukemic cells (total number of leukemic cells at diagnosis generally between $10^{11}$–$10^{12}$) by at least 2–3 logs, normalization of blast count in bone marrow (< 5%) and peripheral blood (< 1%) (corresponds to leukemic cell number < $10^{10}$) as well as normal thrombocyte and granulocyte counts in peripheral blood. With patients up to 60 years "double induction" possible.

### Stratification
With patients up to 65 years according to response (remission) and risk groups (karyotype):
- "Good risk": t(8;21) ± loss of Y or other additional aberrations, inv(16) or del(16), t(15;17)
- "Intermediate risk": normal karyotype without flt3 mutation, no poor risk chromosomal changes
- "Poor risk": -7 or other aberrations of chromosome 7, 5q-, -5, changes in the long arm of chromosome 3, t(9;22), complex abnormalities (≥ 3 aberrations), flt3 mutation

### Consolidation
Further reduction of the malignant clone by additional chemotherapy cycles after reaching complete remission (number of cycles depending on age and performance of patients).

### Intensification
Intensification according to risk factor status, generally with related-allogeneic bone marrow transplantation (Tx). Autologous transplantation or high dose AraC in clinical trials, if no allogeneic donor available.
- Allogeneic transplantation in first remission (related or unrelated donor): with "poor risk" and "intermediate risk" karyotype.
- All other stages: no remission (refractory leukemia), relapse, second CR: allogeneic transplantation from related or unrelated donor. A CR is not a prerequisite for allogeneic transplantation, but patients with transplantation in CR have lower relapse rates.

### Maintenance Therapy (Clinical Studies)
Additional chemotherapy or immunotherapy (low-dose AraC; IL-2 in clinical studies); with APL: ATRA / 6-mercaptopurine / methotrexate.

### Acute Promyelocytic Leukemia (APL, acc. FAB: AML M3)

- In > 90% of cases detection of chromosomal aberration t(15;17) with translocation of the gene for retinoid acid receptor alpha (RAR-alpha) and formation of the fusion gene PML / RAR-alpha, resulting in differentiation arrest
- Induction of differentiation of leukemic cells with all-trans-retinoid acid (ATRA).
- With ATRA + chemotherapy (anthracycline ± AraC), long-term survival rates up to 90%.

## Supportive Treatment

- Sperm cryopreservation (prior to induction therapy, if possible)
- Prophylaxis of tumor lysis syndrome (▶ Chap. 9.6): fluid replacement, urine alkalization, allopurinol, rasburicase
- Prevention and treatment of infection (▶ Chap. 4.2)
- Substitution of red cells and platelet concentrates (in DIC and/or AML M3 keep platelets > 50,000/μl)
- Substitution of coagulation factors, if necessary treatment of DIC (▶ Chap. 6.5.5)
- In case of hyperleukocytosis / leukostasis: immediate treatment with hydroxyurea (up to 6 g/day), oxygen therapy, fluid substitution, restrictive substitution of red cells, possibly dexamethasone i.v., emergency leukapheresis may be required
- Suppression of menstruation in premenopausal females

## Chemotherapy Protocols: Induction of Remission

Patients between 18 and 60 years

| *"ICE"* ▶ *Protocol 11.2.2* | | | *Study Protocol AMLSG 7-04* |
|---|---|---|---|
| Idarubicin | 12 mg/m²/day | i.v. | Day 1, 3, 5 for 2 h |
| Etoposide / VP-16 | 100 mg/m²/day | i.v. | Day 1–3 for 1 h |
| Cytosine arabinoside, AraC | 100 mg/m²/day | i.v. | Day 1–7 for 22 h |

| *"DNR/AraC (Intergroup)"* ▶ *Protocol 11.2.4* | | | |
|---|---|---|---|
| Cytosine arabinoside | 100 mg/m²/day | i.v. | Day 1–7 for 22 h |
| Daunorubicin | 60 mg/m²/day | i.v. | Day 3–5 for 2 h |

Patients above 60 years

| *"MICE"* ▶ *Protocol 11.2.7* | | | *Study protocol AML 17 EORTC* |
|---|---|---|---|
| Mitoxantrone | 7 mg/m²/day | i.v. | Day 1, 3, 5 for 30 min |
| Etoposide | 100 mg/m²/day | i.v. | Day 1–3 for 30 min |
| Cytosine arabinoside | 100 mg/m²/day | i.v. | Day 1–7 for 22 h |

## Chemotherapy Protocols: Consolidation

Patients between 18 and 60 years

| "Consolidation" ▶ Protocol 11.2.3 | | | Study Protocol AMLSG 7-04 |
|---|---|---|---|
| Cytosine arabinoside | 3,000 mg/m² 2 ×/day | i.v. | Day 1, 3, 5, every 12 h for 3 h |
| ± ATRA (Arm B) | 15 mg/m²/day | p.o. | Day 6–21 |

| "Intermediate dose AraC (Intergroup)" ▶ Protocol 11.2.5 | | | |
|---|---|---|---|
| Cytosine arabinoside | 3,000 mg/m² 2 ×/day | i.v. | Day 1, 3, 5, every 12 h for 3 h |

Patients above 60 years

| "Mini-ICE" ▶ Protocol 11.2.8 | | | |
|---|---|---|---|
| Idarubicin | 8 mg/m²/day | i.v. | Day 1, 3, 5 for 30 min |
| Etoposide | 100 mg/m²/day | i.v. | Day 1–3, for 30 min |
| Cytosine arabinoside | 100 mg/m²/day | i.v | Day 1–7, for 22 h |

## Chemotherapy Protocols: Relapse or Primary Refractory AML

| "S-HAM" ▶ Protocol 11.2.6 | | | |
|---|---|---|---|
| Cytosine arabinoside | 1,000 mg/m² 2 ×/day | i.v. | Day 1, 2, 8, 9, every 12 h for 3 h |
| Mitoxantrone | 10 mg/m²/day | i.v. | Day 3, 4, 10, 11 |
| AraC with patients > 60 years 1,000 mg/m² | | | |

### New Treatment Approaches:
- Mylotarg (gemtuzumab ozogamicin, ▶ chapter 3.5)
- Tyrosine kinase inhibitors: PKC 412 / midostaurin, others
- Clofarabine, cloretazine
- DNA demethylating agents: 5-aza-2′-deoxycytidine (decitabine), 5-azacytidine
- Histone deacetylation inhibitors: valproic acid, depsipeptide, vorinostat
- Farnesyltransferase-inhibitors: tipifarnib, lonafarnib
- Angiogenesis inhibitors
- In Philadelphia chromosome-positive AML (Ph1+): imatinib, dasatinib
- In Flt3-ITD mutation: sorafenib

## Palliative Treatment

### Objectives
- Preservation of the patients' quality of life (if possible outpatient treatment)
- Reduction of blast counts in peripheral blood / bone marrow
- Control of general symptoms

### Therapeutic Options
- Hydroxyurea: 1,000–4,000 mg, p.o., daily
- 6-Thioguanine: 50–100 mg, p.o., daily
- 6-Mercaptopurine: 50–100 mg, p.o., daily
- Amsacrine: 100 mg, i.v., 1 × per week
- Mitoxantrone: 5 mg, i.v., 1 × per week

**Prg:**   *Prognostic Factors*
- Age (> 60 years unfavorable)
- Comorbidity
- Karyotype: good / intermediate / poor risk
  - "Good risk": t(8;21); t(15;17), inv(16)
  - "Poor risk": FAB M1, M6, M7, aberrations of chromosomes 3,5,7; t(9;22), complex karyotype (≥ 3 abnormalities)
- Leukocyte count at diagnosis (> 100,000/µl unfavorable)
- Serum LDH at diagnosis (> 400 U/l unfavorable)
- MDR 1 expression
- Karnofsky index
- Type of leukemia: unfavorable: secondary leukemia following myelodysplasia or trilineage dysplasia at diagnosis, secondary AML following radio- / chemotherapy

*Prognostic Parameters Depending on Risk Profile and Age of Patient*
- Complete remission in patients < 65 years: 60–70% of cases (range: 25–90%)
- Median duration of remission: 12–14 months
- Risk of relapse after completion of first treatment cycle: 40–90%
- Leukemia-free interval after treatment: duration reduced by 50% after each additional relapse

*Five-year Leukemia-free Survival*
- "Good risk" karyotype: 60–70%
- "Intermediate risk" karyotype: 35–45%
- "Poor risk" karyotype: 10–20%

**F/U:**   Frequent follow-up with blood counts and clinical status. Examination intervals initially monthly, after 3–6 months every 2 months, after 2 years every 3 months.

**Ad:**   **European APL-Study (APL 2006).** Prof. P. Fenaux, Hôpital Avicenne-AP-HP- Université Paris XIII, Bobigny, France
   **European Organisation for Research and Treatment of Cancer (EORTC).** Study AML17: Prof. Dr. A. Ho, Med. Klinik und Poliklinik V, Universitätsklinikum Heidelberg, Abt. Hämatologie, Int. Onkologie und Rheumatologie, Hospitalstr. 3, 69115 Heidelberg, Tel. +49-6221-568011

**Ref:**   1.   Bullinger L, Valk PJM. Gene-expression profiling in acute myeloid leukemia. J Clin Oncol 2005;23:6296–305
   2.   Craddock C, Tauro S, Moss P et al. Biology and management of relapsed acute myeloid leukemia. Br J Hematol 2005;129:18–34
   3.   Drobyski WR. The role of allogeneic transplantation in high-risk acute myelogenous leukemia. Leukemia 2004;18:1565–8
   4.   Estey H, Döhner H. Acute myeloid leukemia. Lancet 2006;368:1894–907.
   5.   Fey MF, ESMO Guidelines Task Force. Acute myeloblastic leukemia in adult patients: ESMO Clinical Recommendations for diagnosis, treatment and follow up. Ann Oncol 2007;18(suppl2):ii47–89
   6.   Milligan DW, Grimwade D, Cullis JO et al. British Committee for Standards in Haematology. Guidelines on the management of acute myeloid leukemia in adults. Br J Haematol 2006;135:450–74
   7.   Sekeres MA, Stone RM. The challenge of acute myeloid leukemia in older patients. Curr Opin Oncol 2002;14:24–30
   8.   Tallmann MS, Gilliland DG, Rowe JM. Drug therapy for acute myeloid leukemia. Blood 2005;106:1154–63
   9.   Vardiman JW, Harris NL, Brunning RD. The World Health Organization (WHO) classification of the myeloid neoplasms. Blood 2002;100:2292–302

**Web:**

| | | |
|---|---|---|
| 1. | http://www.leukemia.org/ | Leukemia Lymphoma Soc |
| 2. | http://www.marrow.org/PATIENT/aml.html | Natl Marrow Donor Prog |
| 3. | http://www.nlm.nih.gov/medlineplus/ency/article/000542.htm | Medline Plus, AML |
| 4. | http://www.nci.nih.gov/cancerinfo/pdq/treatment/adultAML/ | NCI PDQ, AML |
| 5. | http://www.emedicine.com/med/topic34.htm | E-medicine, AML |
| 6. | http://www.leukemia-net.org. | Eur Leukemia Network |

## 7.2    Myelodysplastic Syndrome (MDS)

### M. Lübbert

**Def:**  Clonal disease associated with transformation of early hematopoietic progenitor cells (stem cells) and abnormal proliferation, differentiation, and apoptosis. Usually, several cell lineages are affected.

**ICD-10:**  D46.-, C93.1 (CMML)

**Ep:**  Incidence: 3–5 cases/100,000 population/year. Incidence increasing, partly due to improved diagnostic means. MDS most commonly affects the elderly (usually > 60 years, in patients > 70 years: 20 cases/100,000/year) and is rare in children.

**Pg:**
### Primary Myelodysplastic Syndromes
Genetic and epigenetic aberrations (without known trigger factors) seem to be of pathogenetic relevance.

**Molecular abnormalities**

| Type | Frequency (%) |
|---|---|
| *Chromosomal aberrations* | |
| Frequent: numerical or structural aberrations: monosomy 7, 5q-, 7q-, 20q-; trisomy 8, 14, or 19; complex anomalies, sex chromosome loss, etc. | 40 |
| Infrequent: "AML-typical" translocations t(6;9), t(8;21), inv(16), or t(9;22), translocations t(1;3), t(5;12) | 10 |
| *Genetic aberrations* | |
| Activation of oncogenes (N-ras, less commonly K-ras, H-ras) | 10–15 |
| p53 mutations | 5–10 |
| *Epigenetic aberrations* | 40–70 |
| Hypermethylation / inactivation (e.g., p15) | 30 |
| Overexpression of bcl2 | |

### Secondary Myelodysplastic Syndromes
- After chemotherapy (esp. with alkylating agents)
- Ionizing radiation (radiotherapy, exposure to radiation)
- Benzene and other organic solvents
- Insecticides

**Path:**  Frequently bone marrow hyperplasia with varying degrees of blast proliferation, often cytopenia in the peripheral blood. Less commonly bone marrow hypoplasia ("hypoplastic MDS").

### Bone Marrow Findings
- Hypercellularity or normal cellularity (70–90% of cases), in 10% of cases hypocellular bone marrow ("hypoplastic MDS")
- Dysplastic changes in several cell lineages:
  - Dyserythropoiesis: anisocytosis / poikilocytosis, macroblasts, nuclear anomalies
  - Dysgranulopoiesis: granulation anomalies, nuclear anomalies ("pseudo-Pelger" morphology)
  - Dysmegakaryocytopoiesis: micromegakaryocytes, nuclear anomalies, giant platelets
- More than 15% of erythroid cells may be ringed sideroblasts (bone marrow iron stain, "Prussian blue"): obligatory with RARS / RCMD-RS, optional with RAEB / RAEB-T, CMML

- Blast proliferation to 5–30% of marrow cell population (RAEB, RAEB-T), up to 20% with CMML
- Proliferation of monocytic progenitors with CMML

### Peripheral Blood

- Anemia: 80–90% of cases
- Leukopenia: 20–30%
- Thrombocytopenia: 30–40%
- Impaired maturation of granulopoiesis (granulation anomalies, nuclear anomalies, "pseudo-Pelger" forms) and erythropoiesis (anisocytosis, macrocytosis)
- Leukocytosis, possibly monocytosis (CMML, see below), blasts

**Class:**  **FAB Classification (French-American-British Cooperative Group, 1982)**

### Myelodysplastic Syndromes According to FAB

| | |
|---|---|
| • RA | "Refractory Anemia" |
| • RARS | "Refractory Anemia with Ringed Sideroblasts" |
| • RAEB | "Refractory Anemia with Excess Blasts" |
| • RAEB-T[a] | "RAEB in Transformation" (to acute leukemia) |
| • CMML | "Chronic Myelomonocytic Leukemia" |

[a] According to WHO: AML

### Classification Criteria According to FAB

| Type | Blood | Bone marrow | | Special features |
|---|---|---|---|---|
| | Blasts (%) | Blasts (%) | RS > 15% | |
| RA | < 1 | < 5 | – | Usually with granulo- / thrombocytopenia |
| RARS | < 1 | < 5 | + | Ringed sideroblasts in the bone marrow |
| RAEB | < 5 | 5–20 | – / + | Usually bi- or trilineage cytopenia |
| RAEB-T[a] | > 5 | 21–30 | – / + | Blasts, possibly with Auer rods |
| CMML | < 5 | < 20 | – / + | Monocytosis > 1,000/µl in blood |

*RS* ringed sideroblasts

[a] According to WHO: AML

**WHO Classification (2001)**

| *Myelodysplastic syndromes* | |
|---|---|
| • RA / RA-RS | Refractory anemia (with / without ringed sideroblasts) |
| • RCMD / RCMD-RS | Refractory cytopenia with multilinear dysplasia (with / without ringed sideroblasts) |
| • RAEB-1 | Refractory anemia with excess blasts (5–9%) |
| • RAEB-2 | Refractory anemia with excess blasts (10–19%) |
| • 5q- | 5q- syndrome |

## WHO Classification (2001), continued

| | |
|---|---|
| • Unclassified | Myelodysplastic syndrome, nonclassifiable |
| *Myelodysplastic / myeloproliferative diseases* | |
| • CMML | Chronic myelomonocytic leukemia |
| • ACML | Atypical chronic myeloid leukemia |
| • JMML | Juvenile myelomonocytic leukemia |

**Sy:** Initially only limited symptoms; clinical diagnosis often incidental, based on blood counts done for comorbidities. Symptoms of cytopenia only occur as the disease progresses:
- Anemia → fatigue, reduced performance, tachycardia, pallor
- Thrombocytopenia → tendency to bleed, hematomas, epistaxis, petechiae
- Granulocytopenia → pneumonia, sepsis, recurrent skin infections
- Association with autoimmune diseases possible (hemolysis, arthralgia, serositis, Sweet's syndrome)

**Dg:** ### Medical History, Physical Examination
- Exposure to risk factors (occupational hazards, radiation, chemotheapy), previous changes in the blood count (retrospective)
- Clinical findings: signs of anemia, bleeding, infection

### Laboratory Tests
- Blood count: anemia, reticulocytes ↓, thrombocytopenia, leukopenia
- Blood smear: normo- or macrocytic anemia with aniso- and poikilocytosis, neutropenia, "pseudo-Pelger" cells, abnormal segmentation, granulation defects, myeloperoxidase defect, possibly blast release, monocytosis
- LDH, folic acid / vitamin $B_{12}$ level, ferritin, serum erythropoietin, haptoglobin

### Bone Marrow Tests
Aspiration (morphology, differentiation, iron stain), obligatory cytogenetic analysis, biopsy for histological examination (cellularity), optional immunocytology (blast proliferation, proliferation of monocytic progenitors)

**DD:**
- Aplastic anemia (▶ Chap. 6.1)
- Macrocytic / megaloblastic anemia in folic acid or vitamin $B_{12}$ deficiency (▶ Chap. 6.4.2)
- Bone marrow toxicity (drugs, environmental toxins)
- HIV infection, parvovirus B19, other viral infections
- Myeloproliferative syndromes (esp. CML, primary myelofibrosis ▶ Chap. 7.3.4)
- Paroxysmal nocturnal hemoglobinuria (acid hemolysis test, ▶ Chap. 6.4.3)

**Co:**
- Hemorrhagic or infectious complications
- Transformation to AML (▶ Chap. 7.1.2)
- Secondary hemosiderosis due to polytransfusions

**Th:** ### Treatment Concept

1. Treatment decisions are based on age, performance status, and comorbidity of the patient as well as the risk score (IPSS, see below).
2. Treatment with curative intent is possible in patients < 60 years and requires myeloablative therapy followed by allogeneic transplantation of hematopoietic stem cells. Allogeneic transplantation with reduced intensity conditioning represents an alternative for patients up to 70 years (biological age) and is currently investigated in clinical trials.
3. Patients from 60–70 years and older are generally treated with palliative intent, using symptomatic and supportive therapies.

4. Transformation to acute myeloid leukemia: in younger patients induction therapy similar to de novo leukemia (► Chap. 7.1.2), allogeneic transplantation (with myeloablative / non-myeloablative conditioning). Lower response rate and shorter duration of remission as compared to de novo leukemia. High complication rates, delayed hematopoietic recovery, especially thrombopoiesis.

**Treatment Pathway of Myelodysplastic Syndromes**

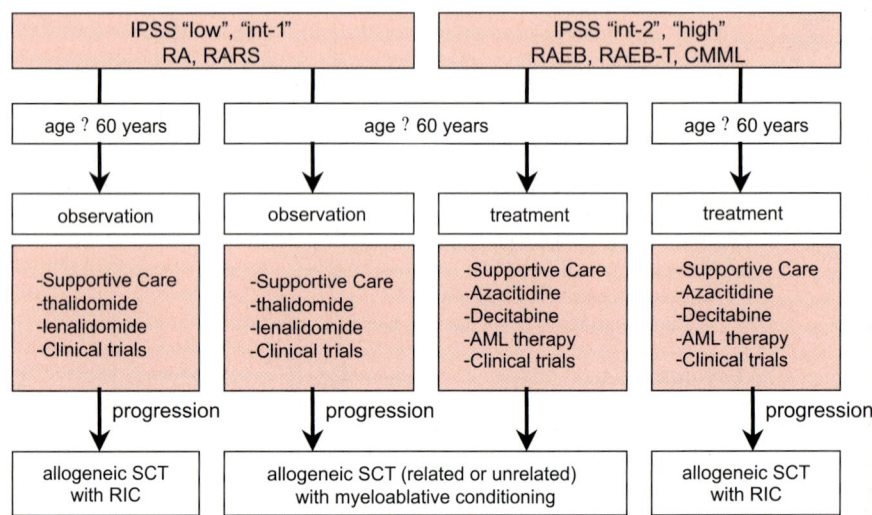

IPSS  risk score, SCT stem cell transplantation, RIC reduced intensity conditioning,
HDAC histone deacetylase-inhibitors (e.g. valproate), DNMT DNA-methyltransferase-inhibitors

## Supportive Care

- Red cell transfusion, platelet transfusion, in symptomatic patients
- Treatment of infectious complications (antibiotics, antimycotics, etc.)
- Treatment of secondary hemosiderosis with desferrioxamine mesylate, deferasirox or deferiprone
- Administration of growth factors (EPO, G-CSF) does not influence survival time, palliative use improves patients' quality of life.

## "Low-risk" MDS

- DNA methyltransferase inhibitors (decitabine, 5-azacytidine).
- Thalidomide, lenalidomide (lenalidomide treatment esp. in 5q- syndrome)
- Immunosuppressive treatment: cyclosporine, anti-thymocyte globulin (ATG), anti-lymphocyte globulin (ALG), esp. with hypoplastic MDS
- Experimental therapy: Induction of differentiation with retinoic acid or histone deacetylase inhibitors (all-trans retinoic acid, phenylbutyrate, valproic acid, SAHA / vorinostat, depsipeptide)

### "High-risk" MDS

- DNA methyltransferase inhibitors (decitabine, 5-azacytidine). 50% remission with administration of decitabine (early response of the thrombopoietic lineage), in 30% of cases trilineage response and cytogenetic remissions.
- Allogeneic transplantation with myeloablative conditioning or reduced intensity conditioning (dependent on availability of suitable donors, performance status, and age of the patient)
- Experimental therapy: induction of differentiation with retinoic acid or histone deacetylase inhibitors (all-trans retinoic acid, phenylbutyrate, valproic acid, depsipeptide)

Prg:

### *Most Common Causes of Death*
- Infections, hemorrhage
- Complications after transformation to acute myeloid leukemia

### *Prognostic Factors*
- Percentage of blasts in the bone marrow (> 10% constitutes a poor prognosis)
- Chromosomal aberrations: poor prognosis: monosomy 7 / 7q- / complex karyotype; better prognosis: normal karyotype / 5q- / 20q- / -Y as isolated aberration
- Level of cytopenia: poor prognosis: hemoglobin < 10 g/dl, platelets < 100,000/μl, neutrophils < 1,800/μl
- LDH: poor prognosis: LDH ↑

**Prognosis for myelodysplastic syndromes (according to FAB classification)**

| Type | Risk of malignant transformation[a] (%) | Survival time (median) (months) |
|------|------|------|
| RA | 10 | 37 |
| RARS | 5 | 50 |
| RAEB | 25 | 10 |
| RAEB-T | 50 | 5 |
| CMML | 20 | 22 |

[a] Median risk of developing acute leukemia within 12 months

**Risk score according to the International MDS Workshop (International Prognostic Scoring System, IPSS): individual factors**

| Prognostic factors | Score | | | | |
|------|------|------|------|------|------|
| | 0 | 0.5 | 1.0 | 1.5 | 2.0 |
| Percentage of blasts[a] | < 5% | 5–10% | – | 11–20% | 21–30% |
| Karyotype[b] | Good | Intermediate | Poor | – | – |
| Affected cell lineages[c] | 0–1 | 2–3 | – | – | – |

[a] Blasts as percentage of the bone marrow cell population

[b] Good: normal karyotype, -Y, 5q-, 20q-. Poor: complex karyotype, anomalies of chromosome 7. Intermediate: all other aberrations

[c] Number of affected cell lineages (granulo- / erythro- / thrombopoiesis)

**Risk score according to the International MDS Workshop (IPSS): risk groups**

| Risk group | Overall score | Risk of malignant transformation[a] (years) | Median survival (months) |
|---|---|---|---|
| Low risk | 0 | > 18 | 65 |
| Intermediate 1 (int 1) | 0.5–1.0 | 8 | 40 |
| Intermediate 2 (int 2) | 1.5–2.0 | 3 | 14 |
| High risk | > 2.5 | 0.5 | 5 |

[a] Median time period until development of AML

**F/U:** Symptom-oriented care in patients with long-term disease course.

**Ad:** European Organisation for Research and Treatment of Cancer (EORTC) MDS Study Group. EORTC-MDS. Theo de Witte, University Hospital Sint Radboud, Dept. of Haematology, P.O. Box 9101, 6500 HB Nijmegen, Niederlande

**Ref:**
1. Aul C, Giagounidis A, Germing U et al. A. Evaluating the prognosis of patients with myelodysplastic syndromes. Ann Hematol 2002; 81:485–97
2. Bowen D, Culligan D, Jowitt S et al. Guidelines for the diagnosis and therapy of adult myelodysplastic syndromes. Br J Hematol 2003;120:187–200
3. Corey SJ, Minden MD, Barber DL et al. MDS: the complexity of stem-cell diseases. Nat Rev Cancer 2007;7:118–29
4. Golshayan AR, Jin T, Maciejewski J et al. Efficacy of growth factors compared to other therapies for low-risk MDS. Br J Haematol 2007,137:125–32
5. Howe RB, Porwit-MacDonald A, Wanat R et al. The WHO classification of MDS does make a difference. Blood 2004;103:3265–70
6. Luger S, Sacks N. Bone marrow transplantation for myelodysplastic syndrome: who? when? and which? Bone Marrow Transpl 2002;30:199–206
7. Malcovati L, Germing U, Kuendgen A et al. Time-dependent prognostic scoring system for predicting survival and leukemic evolution in MDS. J Clin Oncol 2007;25:3503–10
8. Olney HJ, LeBeau MM. Evaluation of recurring cytogenetic abnormalities in the treatment of MDS. Leukemia Res 2007;31:427–34
9. Valent P, Horny HP, Bennet JM et al. Definitions and standards in the diagnosis and treatment of MDS: Consensus statements and report from a working conference. Leukemia Res 2007;31:727–36

**Web:**
1. http://imsdd.meb.uni-bonn.de/Cancernet/202495.html          Cancernet, NCI
2. http://www.nci.nih.gov/cancerinfo/pdq/treatment/myelodysplastic          NCI PDQ
3. http://www.mds-foundation.org/          MDS Foundation
4. http://www.emedicine.com/med/topic2695.htm          E-medicine, MDS

# 7.3 Myeloproliferative Disorders (MPD)

**C.F. Waller**

**Def:** Group of clonal hematopoietic stem cell diseases of the myeloid lineage.

**Ep:** Incidence: 2–3 cases/100,000 population/year; male:female = 1:1. The most common type is chronic myeloid leukemia.

**Class:** **Myeloproliferative Disorders (WHO, 2001)**

*Classic subtypes (Dameshek 1951)*

| | | |
|---|---|---|
| • CML | Chronic myeloid leukemia | (▶ Chap. 7.3.1) |
| • PV | Polycythemia vera | (▶ Chap. 7.3.2) |
| • ET | Essential thrombocythemia | (▶ Chap. 7.3.3) |
| • CIMF | Chronic idiopathic myelofibrosis = Primary myelofibrosis (PMF) | (▶ Chap. 7.3.4) |

*Rare subtypes*

| | |
|---|---|
| • CEL / HES | Chronic eosinophilic leukemia / hypereosinophilic syndrome |
| • CNL | Chronic neutrophilic leukemia |
| • SMCD | Systemic mast cell disease |

Overlap between individual forms of chronic myeloproliferative disorders (CMPD) and myelodysplastic syndromes (MDS) is possible. CML, polycythemia, and essential thrombocythemia may evolve into chronic myelofibrosis. All myeloproliferative disorders carry an increased risk of transformation to acute myeloid leukemia (AML).

**Clinical course / intermediate forms of the MPS subtypes**

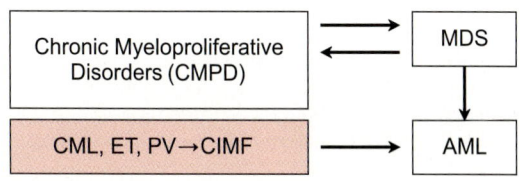

**Pg:** *Molecular Genetic Abnormalities*
- CML: Philadelphia chromosome: t(9;22), BCR / ABL oncogene
- PV, ET, CIMF: point mutation (V617F) of the tyrosine kinase JAK-2 (Janus kinase 2) on the short arm of chromosome 9 (9p), present in patients with PV (69–97%), ET (23–57%), and CIMF (43–57%). Chromosomal aberrations detectable in 10–60% of cases, including: 1q-, 5q-, 20q-, 13q-, and 12p- deletions, trisomy 8, trisomy 9
- SMCD: dysregulation of tyrosine kinase receptor: c-kit mutations (V560G, F522C, D816V)
- CNL: BCR / ABL p230 fusion gene, chromosome region 8p11

**Pp:** Malignant transformation of hematopoietic stem cells leading to myelopoietic dysregulation with hypercellular bone marrow. Clonal proliferation mainly affects granulopoiesis (CML), thrombopoiesis (essential thrombocytosis), or erythropoiesis (polycythemia vera). While one cell lineage may dominate, several lineages are usually affected.

### Common Characteristics

- Increased cell turnover → hyperuricemia
- Splenomegaly, often hepatomegaly
- Increasing bone marrow fibrosis (myelofibrosis); during late stages: extramedullary hematopoiesis
- Risk of transformation to secondary leukemia

**Characterization of individual myeloproliferative disorders**

| Disease | Hematocrit | Leukocytes | Thrombocytes | Splenomegaly | LAP index | Marrow fibrosis | Ph1-chrom. | V617F-JAK-2 |
|---------|----------|-----------|-------------|-------------|-----------|----------------|------------|-------------|
| CML | n/↓ | ↑↑↑ | ↑/n/↓ | +++ | ↓ | n/+ | +++ | − |
| PV | ↑↑ | ↑ | ↑ | + | ↑↑ | + | − | +++ |
| ET | n | n/↑ | ↑↑↑ | + | n/↑ | ± | − | + |
| CIMF | ↓ | ↑/n/↓ | ↑/n/↓ | +++ | ↑ | +++ | − | + |

*LAP* leukocyte alkaline phosphatase, *Ph1-chrom.* Philadelphia chromosome, t(9;22)
*n* normal, ↑ increased, ↓ decreased, − not detectable, ± / + / ++ / +++ detectable

**Th:** Myeloproliferative syndromes are diseases of pluripotent stem cells.

- *Curative treatment options* for patients up to 75 years of age consist of adequate conditioning protocols with subsequent allogeneic bone marrow or peripheral blood stem cell transplantation (in clinical trials).
- *New therapeutic* approaches include molecular inhibitors (targeted therapies), such as tyrosine kinase inhibitors (imatinib, ▶ Chap. 3.6) or farnesyl transferase inhibitors (in clinical trials).
- *Palliative treatment* includes supportive care, conventional chemotherapy (incl. hydroxyurea), radiotherapy, and use of cytokines (interferon α)

For the treatment of individual myeloproliferative syndromes ▶ Chaps. 7.3.1–7.3.4.

**Ref:**
1. Campell PJ, Green AR. The myeloproliferative disorders. N Engl J Med 2006;355:2452–66
2. James C, Ugo V, LeCouedic JP et al. A unique clonal JAK2 mutation leading to constitutive signalling causes polycythemia vera. Nature 2005;434:1144–48
3. Kaushansky K. On the molecular origins of the chronic myeloproliferative disorders: it all makes sense. Blood 2005;105:4187–90
4. Kralovics R, Passamonti F, Buser AS et al. A gain-of-function mutation of JAK2 in myeloproliferative disorders. N Engl J Med 2005;352:1779–90
5. Michiels JJ, De Raeve H, Hebeda K et al. WHO bone marrow features and European clinical, molecular and pathological (ECMP) criteria for the diagnosis of myeloproliferative disorders. Leukemia Res 2007;31:1031–8
6. Spivak JL, Barosi G, Tognoni G et al. Chronic myeloproliferative disorders. Hematology (ASH Educ Program) 2003:200–24

**Web:**
1. http://www.cancer.gov/cancertopics/types/myeloproliferative　　NCI PDQ
2. http://www.leukemia-lymphoma.org//all_page.adp?item_id=311829　　Leuk lymph Soc
3. http://www.mpdinfo.org　　MPD Information
4. http://www.emedicine.com/med/topic1563.htm　　E-medicine
5. http://www.pathologyoutlines.com/myeloproliferative.html　　Pathology

**7.3.1**  **Chronic Myeloid Leukemia (CML)**

W. Lange, C.F. Waller

**Def:**  Clonal hematopoietic stem cell disease. Increased proliferation of myeloid cells with full differentiation capacity.

**ICD-10:**  C92.1

**Ep:**  Incidence: 1/100,000/year; approximately 20% of all leukemias in adults. Can affect all age groups; frequency peak: 5th or 6th decade; rare in patients under 20 years. Distribution male:female = 3:2.

**Pg:**  *Risk Factors*
- Exposure to radiation (survivors of atomic bombs, after radiotherapy)
- Chemical agents: benzene, chemotherapeutic drugs, immunosuppressives

*Molecular Genetics*
Detection of a classic t(9;22) translocation in approximately 90% of all patients (altered chromosome 22 = Philadelphia chromosome); variant translocations in approximately 5% of patients. The translocation leads to formation of the BCR / ABL fusion gene, which translates to a 210-kDa protein with increased tyrosine kinase activity. Via GRB-2/SOS proteins, P210BCR/ABL interacts with P21ras and MYC, impairing their inhibitory functions in intracellular signal transduction.

*Pathophysiology*
Malignant transformation of pluripotent hematopoietic stem cells with significant increase in myeloid, monocytic, and thrombopoietic cell lineages in the bone marrow. At the time of initial diagnosis (after unknown latency period), coexistence of normal stem cells and malignant CML stem cells in the bone marrow. As the disease develops, the percentage of CML stem cells steadily increases, suppressing the normal hematopoiesis.

**Path:**  *Bone Marrow*
- Hypercellularity with distinct proliferation of myeloid progenitors and presence of all immature and mature granulocytic lineage elements
- Frequently with increase in megakaryocytes, eosinophils, and basophils
- In 10–15% of cases, detection of mild bone marrow fibrosis at time of initial diagnosis

*Peripheral Blood*
- Blood count: leukocytosis usually between 100,000 and 300,000/µl, in rare cases up to 1,000,000/µl. Thrombocytosis in up to 30% of patients. Mild normochromic, normocytic anemia may be present.
- Differential blood count: presence of all maturation stages of the myeloid lineage with emphasis on myelocytes and neutrophils; often eosinophilia and basophilia

**Class:**  Classically divided into three stages: chronic phase, accelerated phase, and blast crisis.

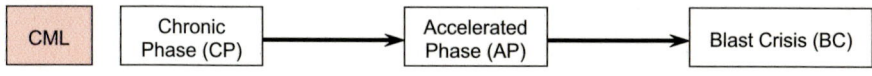

*Chronic Phase*
Initial phase, clinically stable for 3–5 years (averaging 4.5 years), no significant symptoms.
Main clinical manifestations: leukocytosis and splenomegaly. Normal hematopoiesis, blast count in bone marrow and peripheral blood < 10%.

### Acceleration

Evolves from chronic phase, normal hematopoiesis is increasingly replaced by blast population. Duration approximately 3–6 months. Increase in clinical symptoms, development of chloromas (leukemic tumors, rare) or myelofibrosis.

### Blast Crisis

Terminal phase of the disease with increasing treatment resistance and clinical picture similar to acute leukemia. Depending on cell surface marker expression, the following types are distinguished:

- Lymphoid blast crisis: 20–30% of cases
- Myeloid blast crisis: 60–70%
- Other or mixed forms: 10%

### WHO Criteria for Diagnosis of Accelerated Phase and Blast Crisis of Chronic Myelogenous Leukemia (2002)

*Accelerated phase (AP-CML)*[a]

- Peripheral blood (PB) or bone marrow (BM) blasts 10–19% of white blood cells
- PB basophils $\geq$ 20%
- Persistent thrombocytopenia (< 100,000/µl), unrelated to therapy, or persistent treatment refractory thrombocytosis (> 1.000,000/µl)
- Progressive splenomegaly and increasing WBC, unresponsive to therapy
- Additional genetic aberrations, signs of clonal evolution
- Megakaryocytic proliferation, laminar or in clusters, with reticular or collagen fibrosis and/or granulocytic dysplasia

*Blast crisis (BC-CML)*[a]

- $\geq$ 20% blasts in the PB or BM
- Extramedullary proliferation of blasts
- Large foci or clusters of BM blasts

[a] accelerated phase / blast crisis is diagnosed if at least one of the listed criteria is present

**Sy:**   Often diagnosed incidentally without any specific symptoms. As disease progresses:
- General symptoms (decreasing performance status, tendency to sweat, weight loss, fever)
- Abdominal complaints due to increasing splenomegaly
- Organ infiltration or displacement symptoms due to chloromas

**Dg:**   ### Medical History, Physical Examination
- Medical history including risk factors
- Physical examination: splenomegaly, signs of peripheral chloromas or peripheral lymphadenopathy

### Imaging / Additional Diagnostic Measures
- Abdominal ultrasound (in specific cases: abdominal CT) for diagnosis of splenomegaly and/or hepatomegaly, chloromas

### Laboratory Tests
- Full blood count with differential
- Philadelphia chromosome or bcr-abl detection using classic cytogenetics, FISH or PCR. Additional deletion on chromosome 9 detected using FISH.
- Leukocyte alkaline phosphatase, LAP $\downarrow$ (characteristic for CML: index < 10, normal: 10–100)
- Vitamin $B_{12}$ level $\uparrow$, transcobalamin III $\uparrow$

- LDH ↑, uric acid ↑ (increased cell turnover)
- Pseudohyperkalemia in patients with severe thrombocytosis
- HLA typing of the patient and his/her siblings (depending on comorbidity and age). Possible search for unrelated donors.

### Histology
Bone marrow smear and histology are only of supportive value. Definitive diagnosis is possible on the basis of the peripheral blood smear.

DD:

- Other myeloproliferative diseases (→ no Philadelphia chromosome)
- Myelodysplastic syndromes, esp. CMML (▶ Chap. 7.2)
- Leukemoid reaction to infections (reactive leukocytosis, differential blood count with shift to immature forms)

Co:

- Thrombocytosis / thrombopathy → thromboembolic events, hemorrhage
- Leukocytosis → leukemic blood clots (rare), leukostasis
- Hyperviscosity syndrome in cases of severe leukocytosis → impaired vision, priapism, confusion, respiratory symptoms, etc. → indication for immediate therapy, leukapheresis, chemotherapy with hydroxyurea
- Splenic infarction
- Infections
- Increasing myelofibrosis with a prolonged disease course

Th:

### Treatment Concept

**Pathway according to age, risk and donor situation**

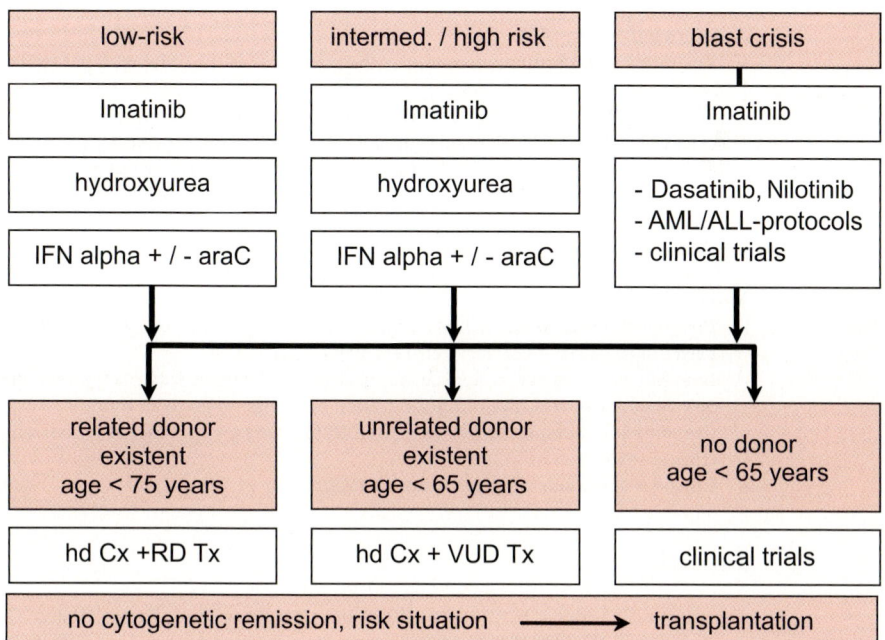

IFN interferon, araC cytosine arabinoside, hd Cx high-dose chemotherapy, Tx transplantation, RD related donor, VUD volunteer unrelated donor

## Principles of CML Therapy

Treatment decisions are based on:
- Symptoms and stage of disease
- Risk factors
- Availability of a stem cell donor
- Age and general condition of the patient

Patients of child-bearing age should be informed about the possibility of sperm or oocyte preservation prior to chemotherapy (▶ Chaps. 4.10.1, 10.2).

Classically, hydroxyurea, cytosine arabinoside, and busulfan demonstrated efficacy in the treatment of patients with CML. With the availability of new drugs (interferon IFNα, imatinib, dasatinib) and new treatment approaches (myeloablative conditioning with allogeneic stem cell transplantation), the optimal therapeutic pathway is controversial. For the time being, all CML patients should be treated within randomized controlled studies.

## Symptoms and Stage of Disease

### Chronic Phase (CP)
- *Treatment abjective:* hematological remission (normalization of blood count and spleen size, regression of CML-induced symptoms).
- *Treatment initiation:* in symptomatic patients or patients with a leukocyte count > 200,000/µl treatment should be started immediately, hydroxyurea, imatinib (400 mg/day)
- Current trials are investigating the efficacy, safety and optimal dose of imatinib, IFNα + AraC and peginterferon as first-line therapy as well as the value of early allogeneic stem cell transplantation.

### Accelerated Phase (AP)
- Treatment modification according to the symptoms of the individual patient (dosage increase or change of chemotherapy).
- With imatinib 600 mg daily, hematological response rates > 80% and cytogenetic response rates of approximately 25% were obtained, with an overall survival rate of 78% at 12 months.
- The value of combination therapies with imatinib, cytostatic drugs and IFNα as well as new molecular agents (nilotinib, dasatinib, mTOR inhibitors, aurora kinase inhibitors, farnesyl transferase inhibitors) is currently being investigated.
- Consider early allogeneic stem cell transplantation.

### Blast Crisis (BC):
- Treatment similar to acute leukemia, depending on the phenotype ("lymphoid" or "myeloid" blast crisis); AML / ALL regimens(▶ Chaps. 7.1.1, 7.1.2).
- Imatinib achieved hematological response rates in 30% of patients with lymphoid BC and in 50% of patients with myeloid BC, duration of remission up to 19 months.
- Combination therapies as well as new molecular therapy approaches are currently evaluated in clinical trials.
- Consider allogeneic stem cell transplantation.

## Risk Factors

The prognostic index ("Hasford score") of the CML Prognostic Factor Project Group has been developed with the objective to identify patients in intermediate or high risk situations, in order to allow for early initiation of aggressive interventions (e.g., allogeneic transplantation) in this patient population.

    *ATTENTION:* the prognostic index was developed for patients treated with interferons and is not yet validated for other treatment settings (e.g., imatinib therapy).

## Hasford score

Hasford score = 0.6666 × Age (years) × Multiplier[a]

$$+ 0.042 \times \text{spleen size (cm)}^{[b]} + 0.0584 \times \text{blasts (\%)}^{[c]}$$
$$+ 0.0413 \times \text{eosinophils (\%)} + 0.2039 \times \text{basophils (\%)}^{[c]}$$
$$+ 1.0956 \times \text{platelet count}^{[c]} \times \text{Multiplier}^{[d]}$$

[a] Multiplier "0" in patients < 50 years, "1" in patients > 50 years
[b] Determined by palpation; measured as "cm below the costal arc"
[c] Differential blood count
[d] Multiplier "0" with thrombocytes < 1,500,000/μl, otherwise "1"

## Risk Classification

| Risk situation | Score | Median survival (months) |
|---|---|---|
| Low risk | < 780 | 98 |
| Intermediate risk | 781–1,480 | 65 |
| High risk | > 1,480 | 42 |

## Donor Situation

Allogeneic bone marrow / stem cell transplantation is the most important curative treatment option (best results within the first year after initial diagnosis). If a related donor is available, transplantation is feasible in patients up to 70–75 years of age (adapted conditioning protocols with subsequent bone marrow or peripheral stem cell transplantation); with unrelated donors: up to 65 years → initiation of donor search at the time of diagnosis. Risks of allogeneic transplants have to be weighed against the excellent results achieved with imatinib (< 1% relapse per year after 5 years).

## Remission Criteria

### Hematological Remission
- Qualitative and quantitative normalization of the peripheral blood count
- Normalization of spleen size and clinical symptoms

### Cytogenetic Remission
Reduction of the Philadelphia chromosome-positive (Ph+) clone in the bone marrow:
- "CCR": complete cytogenetic remission: Ph+ metaphases: 0%
- "PCR": partial cytogenetic remission: Ph+ metaphases: 1–35%
- "MCR": minimal cytogenetic remission: Ph+ metaphases: 36–95%

### Molecular Remission
- "CMR": complete molecular remission: BCR / ABL mRNA not detectable by RT-PCR
- "MMR": "major" molecular remission: BCR / ABL mRNA reduced to <0.1% of baseline

## Imatinib (▶ Chap. 3.6)

- Mechanism of action: inhibition of tyrosine kinase (TK) activity of BCR / ABL → substrate phosphorylation ↓↓ → proliferation signal ↓↓
- Dose for treatment of chronic phase (CP-CML) 400 mg daily p.o., in accelerated phase (AP-CML) or blast crisis (BC-CML) 600–800 mg daily p.o.
- Treatment goal: hematological, cytogenetic, and molecular remission

- Response: CP-CML: hematological remission in > 95% of cases, cytogenetic remissions in 86% after 54 months
- Continue treatment indefinitely even if CMR has been achieved (relapse is frequent after discontinuation of imatinib)

## Treatment Objectives

| Target | Time after treatment initiation (months) |
|---|---|
| Complete hematological remission (CHR) | < 3 |
| Minimal cytogenetic remission (MCR) | 6 |
| Complete cytogenetic remission (CCR) | 12 |

## Clinical Monitoring of Imatinib Therapy

| Time points | Blood count, differential | Cytogenetics[a] Bone Marrow | PCR[b] Periph. Blood |
|---|---|---|---|
| At initial diagnosis | Weekly | Before therapy | Before therapy |
| CHR confirmed | Every 2–4 weeks | Every 3–6 months | Every 3 months |
| CCR confirmed | Every 4–6 weeks | Every 12–18 months | Every 3 months |
| CMR confirmed | Every 6 weeks | Every 12–18 months | Every 3 months |

[a] Philadelphia chromosome detection
[b] BCR-ABL analysis
CHR complete hematologic remission, CCR complete cytogenetic remission, CMR complete molecular remission

## Criteria for Failure of Imatinib Treatment
- Failure to achieve hematological remission within 3 months
- No cytogenetic remission (at least minimal cytogenetic remission, MCR) after 6 months (or cytopenia requiring discontinuation of imatinib)
- Failure to achieve cytogenetic remission (at least MCR) after 9–12 months (despite dose increase to 600 mg after 3 or 6 months, respectively)
- Progressive disease after complete hematological or cytogenetic remission (e.g., quantitative increase in BCR / ABL transcripts in the peripheral blood)
- Loss of complete hematological or cytogenetic remission: BCR / ABL mutation analysis, > 40 point mutations are known as resistance mechanisms
- New signal transduction inhibitors (nilotinib, dasatinib) seem to be more potent than imatinib → effective inhibition of BCR / ABL. Both dasatinib as well as nilotinib are approved in imatinib resistant CML

## Other Treatment Methods

### Hydroxyurea (► Chap. 3.2.1)
- Dose: 20–40 mg/kg body weight/day p.o., daily administration
- Treatment objective: leukocytes 10,000–20,000/µl
- Response: hematological remission in > 80% of cases; no cytogenetic remissions observed

### Interferon a (► Chap. 3.4)
- Dose: $5 \times 10^6$ IU/m²/day s.c., daily administration
- Treatment objective: leukocytes 2,000–5,000/µl

- Response: hematological remission in > 50% of cases, complete cytogenetic remission in 10–15% of cases
- Pegylated interferon is currently being investigated in trials

### Cytosine Arabinoside, AraC (▶ Chap. 3.2.1)
- Dose: (15–)20 mg/m² s.c., for 10 days per month, in combination with IFNα
- Treatment objective: leukocytes 2,000–5,000/µl
- Response: hematological remission in > 60% of cases, complete cytogenetic remission in approximately 40% of cases
- Continue treatment indefinitely even if complete molecular remission (CMR) has been achieved, as relapse is frequent after discontinuation

### Busulfan (Myleran)(▶ Chap. 3.2.1)
If no response to hydroxyurea and/or interferon-α, busulfan may be used with palliative treatment intent. Dose: 2–8 mg/day p.o.; decrease dose to 50% once leucocyte count ist reduced by 50%; hold dose if leukocyte count < 20,000/µl.

### Homoharringtonine
Plant alkaloid with myelosupressive activity. Continuous infusion 2,5 mg/m²/d for 14 days, followed by monthly maintenance cycles (7 days). Hematologic response > 70% of patients.

## Supportive Treatment

### Thrombocytosis
- With platelet counts > 1,000,000/µl, consider administration of thrombocyte aggregation inhibitors (acetylsalicylic acid 100–500 mg/day p.o.).
- Alternative: administration of anagrelide, a dipyridamole analog leading to reduction of platelet counts.

### Splenomegaly
In patients with severe abdominal symptoms due to splenomegaly, splenectomy may be indicated. *ATTENTION:* prior vaccination (pneumococci, meningocci and influenzae).

### Other Procedures
- Prevention and treatment of infections
- With hyperuricemia: administration of allopurinol, alkalinization
- With symptomatic anemia: blood transfusion. *ATTENTION:* avoid blood transfusions until a decision has been reached regarding allogeneic transplantation (possible alloimmunization)

### Prognostic Factors
- Chronic phase (median 4.5 years) classically followed by an accelerated phase of 6 months and a terminal blast crisis of 3 months duration. Median survival was 4.5–5 years prior to introducton of imatinib. Median survival of patients treated with imatinib has not been established yet.
- Prognostic index ("Hasford score"), see above. The relevance for imatinib-treated patients is currently being investigated.
- Five percent of patients are Philadelphia chromosome negative and do not express the bcr / abl translocation → poor prognosis.
- Other independent risk factors associated with poor prognosis: additional chromosomal aberrations, platelet count < 100,000/µl, hemoglobin < 7 g/dl, basophils > 20%.

*Survival Rates Depending on Primary Therapy*

| Therapy | 3 years[a] (%) | 5 years[a] (%) | 7 years[a] (%) |
|---|---|---|---|
| Early allogeneic transplantation | 55–75 | 50–75 | 50–65 |
| Interferon-α | | | |
| • Low risk | 95 | 75 | 40 |
| • Intermediate / high risk | 75–80 | 50 | 20 |

[a] Proportion of survivors

### Conventional Chemotherapy
- A subpopulation of patients who are in complete cytogenetic remission after interferon-α treatment has a median survival of > 9 years.
- Imatinib: CP-CML: previously untreated: hematological response rate: > 95%, cytogenetic CR 85% after 54 months, overall survival 90%.

### Transplantation
- After matched related allogeneic transplantation during chronic phase, the disease-free 5-year survival-rate is up to 75%. The transplantation-associated mortality-rate is currently approximately 10–15%. The relapse risk is also 10–15%.
- Compared to matched related allogeneic transplantation, unrelated transplantation is associated with decreased disease-free survival (transplantation-associated mortality of up to 25%). However, further improvements of HLA typing and selection of suitable donors as well as more advanced supportive treatment (including GvHD prophylaxis) have led to better results.
- The European Group for Blood and Marrow Transplantation (EBMT) has identified prognostic factors (for both related and unrelated transplantation) which can be determined prior to a planned transplantation:
  - Donor type: related / unrelated
  - Disease stage: chronic phase / acceleration / blast crisis
  - Age of the recipient: < 20 years / 20–40 years / > 40 years
  - Donor / recipient combination: female / male = unfavorable combination
  - Interval between diagnosis and transplantation < 1 year / > 1 year

Depending on the individual prognostic factors of a given patient, 5-year survival varies between 18% and 72%, transplantation-associated mortality between 20% and 73%.

**F/U:**　Follow-up includes analyses of remission status (blood smear, cytogenetics, PCR) and monitoring for side effects and long-term sequelae of treatment.

**Ref:**
1. Baccarani M, Sglio G, Goldman J et al. Evolving concepts in the management of CML: recommendations from an expert panel on behalf of the European Leukemia Net. Blood 2006;108:1809–20
2. Calabretta B, Perrotti D. The biology of CML blast crisis. Blood 2004;103:4010–22
3. Cortes C, Kantarjian HM. New targeted approaches in chronic myeloid leukemia. J Clin Oncol 2005;23:6316–24
4. Goldman J. How I treat CML in the imatinib era. Blood 2007;110:2828–37
5. Hehlmann R, Hochhaus A, Baccarani M et al. Chronic myeloid leukemia. Lancet 2007;370:342–50
6. Melo JV, Barnes DJ. CML as a model of a disease evolution in human cancer. Nat Rev Cancer 2007;7:441–53
7. Schiffer CA. BCR-ABL tyrosine kinase inhibitors for CML. N Engl J Med 2007;357:258–65
8. Simonsson B, ESMO Guidelines Working Group. CML: ESMO Clinical Recommendations for diagnosis, treatment and follow-up. Ann Oncol 2007;18(suppl.2)ii61–2
9. Ren R. Mechanisms of BCR-ABL in the pathogenesis of chronic myelogenous leukemia. Nat Rev Cancer 2005;5:172–83

**Web:**
1. www.emedicine.com/med/topic371.htm　　　　　E-medicine, CML
2. http://www.leukemia-lymphoma.org/　　　　　Leukemia Lymphoma Soc
3. http://www.nlm.nih.gov/medlineplus/ency/article/000570.htm　　MedlinePlus CML

## 7.3.2 Polycythemia Vera

**C.F. Waller, W. Lange**

**Def:** Hematopoietic stem cell disease; clonal expansion of myeloid progenitors with emphasis on erythropoiesis. Synonyms: polycythemia rubra vera, Vasquez-Osler disease.

**ICD-10:** D45

**Ep:** Rare disease. Incidence in Western Europe / North America 8–10 cases/1,000,000 population/year. Median age at diagnosis: 50–70 years. Distribution male:female = 3:2.

**Pg:** *Molecular Genetic Alterations*
- Mutation of tyrosine kinase JAK-2 (Janus kinase 2, V617F) in 65–97% of cases → erythropoietin-independent clonal proliferation of the erythropoietic lineage
- Chromosomal aberrations (13–29%), most commonly 20q-, +8, +9, del5
- Increased expression of cytokines (IGF-1, IL-3, GM-CSF, and SCF).

*Proliferation of Erythropoietic Progenitors*
- Polycythemia, hematocrit ↑↑, platelets ↑, granulocytes ↑
- Symptoms caused by increased blood volume and pathologic microcirculation (from hematocrit > 55%), thromboembolic complications due to increased blood viscosity and thrombocytosis, hemorrhages due to platelet dysfunction

**Path:** *Bone Marrow*
Initially hypercellular bone marrow with distinct proliferation of all three cell lineages (trilineary proliferation) with emphasis on erythropoiesis and megakaryopoiesis. Iron staining usually shows no stored iron. Ten percent of patients demonstrate mild reticular fibrosis at the time of initial diagnosis. With further disease progression, reticulin and collagen fibrosis in the majority of cases.

*Peripheral Blood*
Normochromic normocytic erythrocytosis, hematocrit ↑↑. Thrombocytosis in > 50% of cases. Neutrophilia and basophilia. With disease progression and increasing bone marrow fibrosis signs of extramedullary hematopoiesis.

**Sy:** The clinical course is characterized by two phases:
- Initial proliferative phase with increased erythrocyte count
- "Spent phase" with increasing cytopenia, bone marrow fibrosis, extramedullary hematopoiesis and progressive splenomegaly

Symptoms are due to increased blood viscosity, pathologic microcirculation, hypertension, and the underlying malignancy:
- Fatigue, weakness, reduced performance: 30–50% of cases
- Fever, night sweats, weight loss: 20–30%
- Dizziness, headache, tinnitus, impaired vision: 20–50%
- Vascular symptoms: transient ischemic attack (TIA), intermittent claudication, Raynaud's syndrome: 30–50%
- Bleeding from duodenal / stomach ulcers, esophageal varices, epistaxis: 30–40%
- Splenomegaly, hepatomegaly: 50–80%
- Erythema, particularly in the face (plethora), lip cyanosis: 65–85%
- Pruritus: 15–40%
- erythromelalgia ("burning feet syndrome"): 5–10%

**Dg:** *Medical History, Physical Examination*
- Physical examination: lymph node status, liver / spleen, signs of infection, signs of hemorrhage, signs of thrombosis, cardiopulmonary examination (exclusion of secondary erythrocytosis).

### Laboratory Tests
- Full blood count with differential: hematocrit ↑↑, erythrocytes ↑↑, platelets ↑, granulocytes ↑; reticulocyte count
- Routine laboratory tests including liver / renal function tests, uric acid ↑, LDH ↑, CRP, vitamin $B_{12}$ ↑ and vitamin $B_{12}$ binding capacity ↑, serum iron ↓, ferritin ↓
- Leukocyte alkaline phosphatase ↑↑
- Erythropoietin level ↓↓
- Analysis of JAK-2 mutation status (V617F)

### Histology
- Bone marrow aspiration and biopsy; with iron and fiber stain
  *NOTE:* frequently dry tap due to bone marrow fibrosis. In that case, diagnosis based on biopsy
- Cytogenetics (bone marrow): in 30% of cases abnormal karyotype, most commonly del(20q); (no Philadelphia chromosome → DD: CML)

### Imaging, Other Tests
Abdominal ultrasound, ECG, chest x-ray, echocardiography, pulmonary function, capillary blood gas analysis (exclusion of secondary polyglobulia), ocular fundus examination.

**WHO criteria for polycythemia vera diagnosis (2001)**

| *Major criteria* | |
|---|---|
| A1 | Elevated RBC mass (> 125% above mean normal predicted value), or Hb > 18.5 g/dl in men, > 16.5 g/dl in women[a] |
| A2 | No cause of secondary erythrocytosis<br>– Exclusion of familial erythrocytosis<br>– No elevation of erythropoietin level |
| A3 | Splenomegaly |
| A4 | Clonal genetic abnormality (other than Philadelphia chromosome or BCR / ABL fusion gene) in marrow cells |
| A5 | Independent erythroid colony formation in vitro |
| *Minor criteria* | |
| B1 | Thrombocytosis > 400,000/μl |
| B2 | Leucocytosis (neutrophils) > 12,000/μl |
| B3 | Bone marrow biopsy showing panmyelosis with prominent erythroid and megakaryocytic proliferation |
| B4 | Low serum erythropoietin levels |

Diagnosis of polycythemia vera established based on presence of
- Major criteria A1 + A2 + A3 or A1 + A3 +A4
- Major criteria A1 + A2 plus 2 minor criteria

[a] Or > 99th percentile of method-specific reference range for age, sex, altitude of residence

**DD:**

### Erythrocytosis
Secondary erythrocyte proliferation and hematocrit increase with:
- Dehydration, pulmonary / cardiac disease
- Sleep apnea syndrome, smoking
- Height adaptation (prolonged stay at heights of > 2,000 m)
- Hemoglobinopathies, chronic methemoglobinemia

### Erythropoietin ↑↑
Erythropoietin: 34-kDa glycoprotein, renal (90%) and hepatic (10%) synthesis
- Renal disorders
- Paraneoplastic syndromes (renal cell carcinoma, cerebellar hemangioblastoma, lung cancer pheochromocytoma, etc.) (► Chap. 8.13)

**Co:**

- Hypertension
- Hypervolemia with hyperviscosity and pathologic microcirculation (pulmonary / cerebral / renal)
- Thromboembolic events / hemorrhage (platelet dysfunction)
- Development of chronic idiopathic myelofibrosis: 9%

### Transformation to Acute Leukemia with:

- Venesection therapy: 1–2%
- Treatment with alkylating agents / $^{32}$P: 5–15%
- Hydroxyurea treatment: 5–6%

**Th:**

## Treatment Concept

- *Supportive / palliative approach:* established standard treatment approach, aimed at prevention of complications of polycythemia and thrombocytosis
- *Curative approach:* elimination of the malignant stem cell clone, in clinical trials only: myeloablative treatment and allogeneic bone marrow or stem cell transplantation in patients < 70–75 years with severe polycythemia (▶ Chaps. 5.2, 5.3). Inhibitors of mutated JAK2 in clinical development.

## Supportive / Palliative Approach

### Secondary Prophylaxis

Avoidance of risk factors for thromboembolic events (smoking, arterial hypertension, hypercholesterolemia, obesity).

### Intermittent Venesection

- Objective: hematocrit below 45% in men and < 42% in women, prevention of thrombotic and hemorrhagic complications.
- *ATTENTION:* polycythemia and prolonged venesection therapy lead to chronic iron deficiency for which iron replacement is not indicated. Lack of iron limits the pathological increased erythrocyte formation. Even in cases of clinically manifest iron deficiency (▶ Chap. 6.4.1), iron supplemention should be avoided.

### Erythrocytapheresis

Isovolemic large volume removal of red blood cells via cell separation.

- In contrast to venesection therapy, maintenance of constant plasma volume
- Better tolerated, reduced risk of thromboembolic events

### Chemotherapy

Indicated in case of increased thrombocytosis, symptomatic splenomegaly or intolerance to continued venesection therapy.

- Hydroxyurea or alkylating agents (e.g., busulfan); low-dose long-term treatment with close polycythemia monitoring
- *ATTENTION:* long-term treatment with alkylating agents increases the risk of development of acute leukemia by factor 10–15
- Hydroxyurea is treatment of first choice (lower incidence of acute leukemia)

### Radiophosphorus Therapy

- $^{32}$P, 0.1 mCi/kg, max. 5 mCi in total
- Indicated in patients > 70 years and in case of side effects / inefficacy of chemotherapy
- *ATTENTION:* transformation → increased risk of development of acute leukemia

### Interferon-α (IFNα)

Several studies have shown normalization of erythropoiesis by treatment with Interferon-α 3–5 × 10$^6$ IU s.c. 3 times weekly: CR 50–70%, PR 20–30%.

### *Symptomatic Treatment*

- Pruritus: antihistamines, H2 receptor inhibitors, possibly PUVA, cholestyramine, serotonin re-uptake inhibitors
- Hyperuricemia: allopurinol 100–300 mg/day p.o.
- Thrombocytosis: acetylsalicylic acid 100 mg/daily p.o., anagrelide 0.5–1 mg/day p.o. (▶ Chap. 6.3.3)
- Erythromelalgia: acetylsalicylic acid 100 mg/daily p.o., reduction of platelet count

**Prg:**
- Ten-year survival: 40–50% of patients
- Median survival: 9–12 years

1. Elliott MA, Tefferi A. Thrombosis and hemorrhage in polycythemia vera and essential thrombocythemia. Br J Hematol 2004;128:275–90
2. Finazzi G, Caruso V, Marchioli R et al. Acute leukemia in polycythemia vera: an analysis of 1638 patients enrolled in a prospective observational study. Blood 2005;105:2664–70
3. James C, Ugo V, Le Couedic JP et al. A unique clonal JAK2 mutation leading to constitutive signalling causes polycythemia vera. Nature 2005;434:1144–8
4. Landolfi R, Marchioli R, Kutti J et al. Efficacy and safety of low-dose aspirin in polycythemia vera. N Engl J Med 2004;350:114–24
5. Levine L, Pardanani A, Tefferi A et al. Role of JAK2 in the pathogenesis and therapy of myeloproliferative disorders. Nat Rev Cancer 2007;7:673–83.
6. McMullin MF, Bareford D, Campbell P et al. Guidelines for the diagnosis, investigation and management of polycythemia / erythrocytosis. Br J Hematol 2005;130:174–95
7. Schrader Al. Molecular basis of the diagnosis and treatment of polycythemia vera and essential thrombocythemia. Blood 2006;107:4214–22.
8. Tefferi A, Thiele J, Orazi A et al. Proposals and rationale for revision of the WHO diagnostic criteria for polycythemia vera, essential thrombocythemia, and primary myelofibrosis: recommendations from an ad hoc international expert panel. Blood 2007;110:1092–7.

**Web:**

| | | |
|---|---|---|
| 1. | http://www.emedicine.com/med/topic1864.htm | E-medicine |
| 2. | http://www.acor.org/mpd/PVFAQ.html | MPD-Net |
| 3. | http://www.nlm.nih.gov/medlineplus/ency/article/000589.htm | Medline Plus |
| 4. | http://www.aafp.org/afp/20040501/2139.html | Am Acad Family Physicians |
| 5. | http://www.MPDinfo.org | MPD Information |

**7.3.3**   **Essential Thrombocythemia**

**C.F. Waller, W. Lange**

**Def:**   Hematopoietic stem cell disease with clonal or polyclonal expansion of the thrombopoetic lineage, resulting in thrombocytosis > 600,000/µl.

**ICD-10:**   D75.2

**Ep:**   Rare disease. Incidence 1–2 cases/1,000,000/year. Median age at presentation 60–70 years. 20% of patients are < 40 years. Distribution male:female = 3:4.

**Pg:**   *Molecular Genetic Alterations*
- Autosomal dominant hereditary cases, with molecular alterations in the thrombopoietin (TPO) gene; TPO levels ↑↑.
- Mutation of the tyrosine kinase JAK-2 (Janus kinase 2, V617F) in 23–57% of sporadic cases, relevance not yet clarified. With sporadic form: TPO normal/↑.

*Clonal proliferation with emphasis on thrombopoiesis*
→ Thrombocytosis, with normal or dysfunctional platelets
→ Thromboembolic complications and hemorrhages

**Path:**   *Bone Marrow*
Pronounced proliferation of large mature megakaryocytes. Only sporadic micromegakaryocytes. No collagen fibrosis, little or no reticulin fibrosis. Positive iron stain. No signs of leukoerythroblastosis.

*Peripheral Blood*
Thrombocytosis > 600,000/µl, "giant platelets," platelet aggregates.

**Sy:**   At onset usually asymptomatic, often incidental diagnosis. Symptoms due to cell proliferation and thrombocytosis:
- Weight loss, mild fever, sweats, pruritus: 20–30%
- Cerebral, cardiac, or peripheral arterial emboli: 15–20%
- Deep vein thrombosis of the lower extremities, pulmonary emboli: 25–40%
- Hemorrhage: 25–30%
- Splenomegaly: 40–50%
- Neurological complications: 20–30%
- Skin symptoms: erythromelalgia ("burning feet syndrome"), ischemic acrocyanosis: 10%

**Dg:**   *Medical History, Physical Examination*
Physical examination: lymph node status, liver / spleen, signs of hemorrhage / thrombosis

*Laboratory Tests*
- Full blood count with differential, reticulocytes; thrombocytosis > 600,000/µl
- Routine laboratory tests including electrolytes, liver / renal function parameters, urea ↑, LDH ↑, CRP; serum $K^+$ often ↑↑ (pseudohyperkalemia due to $K^+$ release from platelets), in that case: determination of plasma $K^+$
- Leukocyte alkaline phosphatase normal / ↑ (DD: CML), serum iron, ferritin (exclusion of iron deficiency)
- Platelet function test, bleeding time
- Analysis of JAK-2 mutation status (V617F)

*Histology*
Bone marrow aspiration and biopsy with cytogenetics and molecular diagnostics (no Philadelphia chromosome or bcr / abl rearrangement detectable, DD: CML).

**Diagnostic Criteria of Essential Thrombocythemia (ET)**

*Diagnostic Criteria ("Positive Criteria")*
- Sustained platelet count > 600,000/µl
- Bone marrow with predominant proliferation of the megakaryocytic lineage with increased numbers of large mature megakaryocytes

*Exclusion Criteria ("Negative Criteria")*
- No evidence of polycythemia vera
  - Normal red cell mass, hemoglobin < 18.5 g/dl (men) and < 16.5 g/dl (women)
  - Stainable iron in bone marrow, normal serum ferritin and normal MCV
  - Iron deficiency: no increase of red cell count or hemoglobin levels with iron replacement
- No evidence of CML
  - No detectable Philadelphia chromosome and no bcr / abl fusion gene
- No evidence of chronic idiopathic myelofibrosis
  - Collagen fibrosis absent, reticulin fibrosis minimal or absent
- No evidence of myelodysplastic syndrome (MDS)
  - No typical cytogenetic aberrations for MDS (e.g., 5q-, t(3;3)(q21:q26.1)
  - No signs of granulocytic dysplasia
  - Few if any micromegakaryocytes
- No evidence that thrombocytosis is reactive due to:
  - Underlying infections nor inflammation
  - Underlying malignancies, prior splenectomy

**DD:**
- Other myeloproliferative syndromes (CML, CIMF, PV)
- Myelodysplastic syndromes (MDS)
- Secondary thrombocytosis
  - Status post splenectomy
  - Chronic iron deficiency, hemolytic anemia, blood loss
  - Acute-phase reaction in infections / tumors / vasculitis / allergic reactions, etc.

**Co:**
- Development of chronic idiopathic myelofibrosis (CIMF): 5% of patients
- Transformation into acute leukemia: 3–5% of patients

**Th:**    **Treatment Concept**

Treatment according to prognostic factors:
- *Prevention:* reduction of risk factors for thromboembolic complications (smoking, arterial hypertension, hypercholesterolemia, obesity)
- *Supportive care:* treatment of complications of thrombocytosis
- *Curative approach:* elimination of the malignant stem cell clone (high-dose chemotherapy with allogeneic stem cell transplantation); only in selected cases

**Risk Groups in Essential Thrombocythemia**

| Low risk | Age < 60 years |
|---|---|
| | + No prior thromboembolic complications |
| | + Platelet count < 1,500,000/µl |
| | + No cardiovascular risk factors |

| Intermediate risk, neither low- nor high-risk situation | |
|---|---|
| High risk | Age ≥ 60 years |
| | Or prior thromboembolic events |
| | Or platelet count > 1,500,000/μl |
| | Or cardiovascular risk factors |

### Low-risk Patients
- Low risk of occurrence of thromboembolic events (1.2–1.5% per year) as well as hemorrhagic complications (1.1% per year).
- No definite indication for cytoreductive therapy → observation.
- In case of vasomotoric symptoms / impaired microcirculation / cardiovascular risk factors → administration of acetylsalicylic acid (ASS) 100 mg/day (provided there is no history of gastrointestinal bleeding).

### Intermediate-risk Patients
- No definite indication for cytoreductive therapy → observation.
- Prophylactic administration of acetylsalicylic acid (ASS) 100 mg/day (provided there is no history of gastrointestinal bleeding).
- In clinical trials: cytoreductive therapy in cases with additional risk factors.

### High-risk Patients
- Acetylsalicylic acid (ASS) 100 mg/day.
- Cytoreductive therapy: hydroxyurea 0.5–1.5 g/day, dose adjustment according to platelet count, treatment goal is a platelet count < 400,000/μl.
- Second line: anagrelide (dipyridamole analog). Inhibits the phosphodiesterase and phospholipase A2, specific inhibition of megakaryopoiesis and thrombopoiesis (exact mode of action unknown). Side effects include headache, palpitations, tachycardia, hypotension, fluid retention, and diarrhea in up to 25% of patients, particularly during the initial 3 months of therapy. Dosage: 0.5–1 mg/day, maintenance 1–4 mg/day. Dose adjustment according to platelet counts, goal < 400,000/μl. Normalization of platelets in 94% of cases; however, increased incidence of complications (arterial thrombosis, hemorrhage, development of chronic idiopathic myelofibrosis) possible.
- Experimental treatment (clinical studies): interferon-α $3–5 \times 10^6$ IU s.c. 3 times weekly, pegylated interferon-α 50–100/μg weekly.
- In case of acute complications: thrombocytapheresis.

### ET and Pregnancy
- In approximately 45% of cases, spontaneous miscarriage during the first trimester
- Sporadic thromboembolic complications occurring in the mother
- With low-dose ASS treatment (100 mg/day), a higher rate of successful pregnancies has been reported
- Hydroxyurea and anagrelide are potentially teratogenic; careful risk vs. benefit assessment for mother and child is required

**rg:**
- Five-year survival rate: 74–93%
- Ten-year survival rate: 61–84%

**ef:**
1. Campbell PJ, Green AR. Management of polycythemia vera and essential thrombocythemia. ASH Educational Program Book 2005:201–8
2. Chim CS, Kwong YL, Lie AK et al. Long-term outcome of 231 patients with essential thrombocythemia. Arch Intern Med 2005;165:2651–8
3. Finazzi G, Harrison CN. Essential thrombocythemia. Semin Hematol 2005;42:230–8
4. Harrison CN. Essential thrombocythaemia: challenges and evidence-based management. Br J Haematol 2005;130:153–65

5.  Harrison CN, Campbell PJ, Buck G et al. Hydroxyurea compared with anagrelide in high-risk essential thrombocythemia. N Engl J Med 2005;353:33–45
6.  Schafer AI. Thrombocytosis. N Engl J Med 2004;350:1211–9
7.  Steurer M, Gastl G, Jedrzejczak WW et al. Anagrelide for thrombocytosis in myeloproliferative disorders. Cancer 2004;101:2239–46
8.  Tefferi A, Thiele J, Orazi A et al. Proposals and rationale for revision of the WHO diagnostic criteria for polycythemia vera, essential thrombocythemia, and primary myelofibrosis: recommendations from an ad hoc international expert panel. Blood 2007;110:1092–7

**Web:**

| | | |
|---|---|---|
| 1. | http://www.emedicine.com/med/topic2266.htm | E-medicine |
| 2. | http://www.mcl.tulane.edu/classware/ pathology/Krause/ET/ET.html | Tulane University |
| 3. | http://www.nlm.nih.gov/medlineplus/ency/article/000543.htm | Medline Plus |
| 4. | http://www.cancer.gov/cancertopics/types/myeloproliferative | NCL Cancer Topics |

## 7.3.4    Chronic Idiopathic Myelofibrosis (CIMF)

### C.F. Waller

**Def:**  Malignant stem cell disease with bone marrow fibrosis and subsequent cytopenia (due to replacement of hematopoetic cells). Synonyms: osteomyelofibrosis (OMF), osteomyelosclerosis, idiopathic myelofibrosis, primary myelofibrosis (PMF).

**CD-10:**  D47.1

**Ep:**  Incidence 3–15/1,000,000/year. Median age at presentation 50–70 years, higher incidence in men.

**Pg:**
- Molecular genetic changes of pluripotent hematopoietic stem cells
- Mutation of tyrosine kinase JAK-2 (Janus kinase 2, V617F) in 43–57% of cases.
- Cytogenetic changes in 30% of cases (e.g. 13q-, 20q-, +8)
- Release of growth factors (PDGF, TGFβ, EGF, TNFα, IL-1, TPO)

*Clonal myeloproliferation, atypical megakaryocytic hyperplasia*
→ Stimulation of normal fibroblasts, collagen synthesis, angiogenesis
→ Increasing reactive bone marrow fibrosis (transition of prefibrotic to fibrotic stage)
→ Suppression of normal hematopoiesis in the bone marrow, cytopenia, (anemia, neutropenia, thrombocytopenia)
→ Extramedullary hematopoiesis in spleen, liver, and other organs

**Path:**  **WHO criteria for the diagnosis of CIMF**

| *Prefibrotic stage* | |
|---|---|
| Liver / spleen | No or mild hepato- / splenomegaly |
| Peripheral blood | Mild anemia / leukocytosis / thrombocytosis, mild leukoerythroblastosis (immature myeloid and erythrocytic precursor cells), mild poikilocytosis, few dacryocytes ("teardrop" cells) |
| Bone marrow | Hypercellularity, granulopoietic and megakaryocytic proliferation with atypia, minimal reticular fibrosis |
| *Fibrotic stage* | |
| Liver / spleen | Moderate or severe hepato- / splenomegaly |
| Peripheral blood | Mild or moderate anemia, numbers of leukocytes and thrombocytes low / normal / elevated, leukoerythroblastosis, erythrocytes with prominent poikilocytosis and dacryocytosis |
| Bone marrow | Reduced cell density, reticulin and/or collagen fibrosis, expanded marrow sinus with extramedullary hematopoiesis, prominent proliferation of megakaryocytes with atypia, endophytic bone regeneration (osteosclerosis) |

**Sy:**  Initially asymptomatic, often diagnosed incidentally. As bone marrow fibrosis increases and normal hematopoiesis decreases:
- General symptoms (reduced performance status, anorexia, weight loss, fever, possibly night sweats)
- Anemia, weakness, fatigue, decreased performance, pallor
- With leukopenia: susceptibility to infection, mucositis
- With thrombocytopenia: tendency to bleed (gastrointestinal hemorrhage), petechiae
- Splenomegaly, hepatomegaly (extramedullary hematopoiesis)

**Dg:**   ***Medical History, Physical Examination***
Physical examination including lymph node status, liver / spleen, signs of infection, signs of hemorrhage.

### Laboratory Tests
- Complete blood count with differential (left shift of neutrophils, normoblasts, etc.), reticulocytes
- Routine laboratory tests including liver and renal function parameters, LDH ↑, CRP
- Alkaline leukocyte phosphatase ↑ (DD: CML)
- JAK2 mutation (V617F)

### Histology
Bone marrow smear and biopsy with cytogenetics (no Philadelphia chromosome → DD: CML). *NOTE:* often dry tap due to bone marrow fibrosis. In that case diagnosis based on biopsy.

### Imaging
- Skeletal x-ray (osteosclerosis in advanced stages of the disease)
- Distinction of normal vs. fibrotic marrow is possible with MRI

**Dd:**
- Acute myelofibrosis in acute megakaryocytic leukemia (FAB type M7, ▶ Chap. 7.1.2):
- Other myeloproliferative syndromes (CML, essential thrombocythemia, polycythemia vera rubra ▶ Chaps. 7.3.1–7.3.3.)
- Hairy cell leukemia (HCL ▶ Chap. 7.5.4)
- Aplastic anemia, bone marrow metastases
- Chronic infections (miliary tuberculosis, histoplasmosis)
- Mast cell diseases, systemic lupus erythematosus

**Co:**
- Infections (15% of patients)
- Thromboembolic events, hemorrhage (40–50% of patients)
- Hemolytic anemia (intramedullary hemolysis, hypersplenism)
- Portal hypertension (portal vein thrombosis, hepatomegaly)
- Cachexia
- Transformation into acute leukemia in 15–20% of patients

**Th:**   ***Treatment Concept***
- Supportive / palliative approach: prevention of complications of myelofibrosis and extramedullary hematopoiesis (hepato- / splenomegaly)
- Curative approach: elimination of the malignant stem cell clone (high-dose therapy and stem cell transplant, in clinical trials only)

### Supportive / Palliative Approach
- No indication for treatment in asymptomatic patients
- *With thrombocytosis:* acetylsalicylic acid, hydroxyurea, anagrelide (▶ Chap. 7.3.3)
- *With symptomatic anemia:* blood transfusions. In the event of iron overload: desferrioxamine or oral iron chelators (in clinical trials). Androgens (danazol 600 mg/day p.o., metenolon 2–5 mg/kg/day) are effective in 40% of patients. *CAUTION:* regular monitoring of liver function; contraindicated in male patients with prostate cancer
- *With symptomatic thrombocytopenia:* platelate transfusions

### Symptomatic Splenomegaly / Hypersplenism
- *Mild chemotherapy:* hydroxyurea, alternatively: chlorambucil, busulfan, or thioguanine
- *Splenic irradiation:* 0.1–0.2 Gy. *ATTENTION: severe cytopenia may occur after radiation*
- *Splenectomy:* last resort; especially in cases of symptomatic portal hypertension (esophageal variceal bleeding, ascites, etc.). Treatment alternative: TIPS (transjugular intraluminal portosystemic shunt); the spleen is the main organ of extramedullary hematopoiesis. After splenectomy, 25–50% of patients develop hepatomegaly with hepatic hematopoiesis. If splenectomy is impossible: in case of intrahepatic obstruction with portal hypertension, consider insertion of shunts / stents

### Curative Approach (Within Clinical Trials)
Myeloablative therapy with allogeneic bone marrow or stem cell transplantation in patients < 50 years. Treatment objective is the elimination of the malignant clone with regression of the bone marrow fibrosis.

### Experimental Therapies
Interferon-α, TNF-α inhibitors, thalidomide, lenalidomide are investigated in current clinical trials.

**Prg:** Independent negative risk factors (RF):
- Anemia (Hb < 10 g/dl)
- Age > 64 years
- Hypercatabolic symptoms (weight loss, pronounced fatigue, night sweats, increased temperature)
- Leukopenia (< 4,000/μl) or leukocytosis (> 30,000/μl)
- Circulating blasts ≥ 1%
- High-risk karyotype (+8, 12p-)

**Median survival according to risk categories**

| Risk categories | Risk Factors (RF) | Median survival (years) |
|---|---|---|
| Low risk | No RF | ≥ 10 |
| Intermediate risk | 1 RF | |
| High risk | ≥ 2 RF | < 3 |

**Ref:**
1. Arana-Yi C, Quintas-Cardama A, Giles F et al. Advances in the therapy of chronic idiopathic myelofibrosis. Oncologist 2006;11:929–43
2. Barosi G, Bergamaschi G, Marchetti M et al. JAK2 V617F mutational status predicts progression to large splenomegaly and leukemic transformation in primary myelofibrosis. Blood 2007;110:4030–6
3. Cervantes F. Modern management of myelofibrosis. Br J Haematol 2005;128:585–92
4. Ciurea SO, Merchant D, Mahmud N et al. Pivotal contributions of megakaryocytes to the biology of idiopathic myelofibrosis. Blood 2007;110:986–993
5. Henessy BT, Thomas DA, Giles FJ et al. New approaches in the treatment of myelofibrosis. Cancer 2005;103:32–43
6. Papageorgiou SG, Castleton A, Bloor A et al. Allogeneic stem cell transplantation as treatment for myelofibrosis. Bone Marrow Transplant 2006;38:721–7
7. Tefferi A, Thiele J, Orazi A et al. Proposals and rationale for revision of the WHO diagnostic criteria for polycythemia vera, essential thrombocythemia, and primary myelofibrosis: recommendations from an ad hoc international expert panel. Blood 2007;110:1092–7

1. http://www.myelofibrosis.net — Myelofibrosis Network
2. http://www.nlm.nih.gov/medlineplus/ency/article/000531.htm — PMF, Medline Plus
3. http://www.emedicine.com/med/topic78.htm — E-medicine

## 7.4    Hodgkin's Disease (Hodgkin's Lymphoma)

J. Heinz

**Def:**    Malignant disease of the lymphatic system, histologically characterized by a small number of tumor cells ("Hodgkin cells" and multinuclear "Reed-Sternberg cells"), as well as granulomatous tissue ("lymphogranulomatosis").

**ICD-10:**    C81

**Ep:**    Incidence: 2–4 cases/100,000 population/year. Distribution male:female = 1.4:1. Two age peaks: 20–30 years (especially nodular-sclerosing types) and > 60 years.

**Pg:**    *Etiology*

The pathogenetic causes of Hodgkin's disease remain unresolved. Under discussion are:
- Infection with EBV (Epstein-Barr virus, monoclonal EBV genome is found in Hodgkin cells)
- Retroviral infection → dysfunctional apoptosis?

**Path:**    *Histological Subtypes of Hodgkin's Lymphomas: REAL Classification*

Hodgkin's lymphoma, not further specified

Classic Hodgkin's lymphoma
- Nodular sclerosis type 1 and type 2 (NSHD), 60–80% of cases
- Mixed-cellularity type (MCHD), 15–30%
- Lymphocyte-depleted type (LDHD), < 1%
- Lymphocyte-rich classic type (LRHD), 5%
- Lymphoma with characteristics of Hodgkin's disease and anaplastic large cell lymphoma

Lymphocyte-predominant Hodgkin's lymphoma (LPHD, paragranuloma), 5%
- Nodular paragranuloma
- Nodular and diffuse paragranuloma
- Diffuse paragranuloma

Transformation of subtypes after therapy or with long disease course possible

*Location and Spread*
- Primary location: cervical > mediastinal > infradiaphragmatic
- Progression: initially lymphogenic spread into lymphatic organs or local invasion (extranodal manifestation), later hematogenic spread (liver, bone marrow)

*Histology*
The neoplastic cell population consists of Hodgkin and Reed-Sternberg cells which are largely derived from B-cells of the lymph node germinal center. Characteristics are:
- *Hodgkin cells:* mononuclear blast cells with eccentric nucleus and prominent nucleolus, not pathognomonic
- *Reed-Sternberg cells:* multinuclear giant cells with several large eosinophilic nucleoli, developing from Hodgkin cells, pathognomonic (establishing the diagnosis)
- "Colorful" histology, granulomas

### Immunohistology

- Classic Hodgkin's lymphoma: expression of CD3, CD15, CD20 +/-, CD30, LMP-1 (detection or exclusion of CMV infection)
- LPHD: CD3, CD20, CD21, Oct2, Immunoglobulin-J-chain, (CD30 and 15 negative)

### Molecular Genetic and Immunological Alterations

- Chromosomal aberrations in 35–45% of cases
- Rearrangements of immunoglobulin or T-cell receptor genes in 10–20%
- Translocation t(14;18) detectable in some Hodgkin cells
- Detection of monoclonal EBV genome in 30–50% of cases
- Reduced cellular immunity (T-cellular deficiency): increased susceptibility to infections (viral infections, fungal infections, tuberculosis), reduced response to vaccinations, negative tuberculin reaction

**Class:**

**Staging according to the Ann Arbor Classification (1971, modified German Hodgkin's Disease Study Group GHSG)**

| Stages | Definition |
|---|---|
| I | Involvement of a single lymph node region (I N) or presence of a single localized extranodal site (I E) |
| II | Lymph node involvement (II N) and/or localized extranodal sites (II E) in two or more regions on the same side of the diaphragm |
| III | Lymph node involvement (III N) and/or localized extranodal sites (III E) on both sides of the diaphragm |
| IV | Disseminated involvement of one or more extralymphatic organs with or without lymph node involvement |
| A/B | |
| A | No general symptoms |
| B | General symptoms: fever > 38°C, drenching night sweats (change of nightwear), weight loss of more than 10% in the last 6 months |

Lymphatic tissue includes: lymph nodes, spleen, thymus, lymphoid ring of the nasopharynx (Waldeyer's ring)

**Diagnostic certainty and organ involvement**

| Symbol | Characterization |
|---|---|
| CS/PS | Diagnostic certainty |
| CS | Clinical staging only (without laparotomy) |
| PS | Pathological staging following invasive diagnostic measures |
| Organ Symbol | Pattern of organ involvement |
| D | Skin |
| E | Extranodal involvement |
| H | Liver |
| L | Lung |
| M | Bone marrow |
| N | Nodes |
| O | Bone |
| P | Pleura |
| S | Spleen |

### Extranodal Involvement

Localized involvement of extralymphatic tissue (either due to direct invasion from an affected lymph node or lymphogenic / hematogenic spread). Involvement of two or more extralymphatic sites is compatible with stages II or III. Stage marked by symbol "E".

### Bulky Disease

- Massive lymph node involvement ≥ 5 cm in diameter or presence of a conglomerate tumor measuring ≥ 5 cm in one axis
- Mediastinal tumor ≥ 5 cm in diameter
- Cotswold staging system: bulk defined by tumor size ≥ 10 cm

**Sy:**

### General Symptoms

The symbol "B" is added to stages I–IV if one or more of the following general symptoms are present:

- Fever of unknow origin > 38°C (typical although rare is a periodic fever: "Pel-Ebstein fever")
- Otherwise unexplainable night sweats (requiring change of nightwear)
- Unexplained body weight loss of more than 10% over 6 months

### Lymphadenopathy

Main symptom: painless swelling of lymph nodes (on presentation in 80–90% of patients).

- Cutaneous-glandular form (especially lymph nodes of the neck region, less commonly axillary / inguinal lymph nodes, 70% of patients)
- Mediastinal form (10% of patients)
- Abdominal form (5% of patients)

### Other Symptoms

- Hepatomegaly and/or splenomegaly (20% of patients)
- Reduced performance, fatigue, anorexia, pruritus
- "Alcohol pain" of affected lymph nodes: often mentioned in literature, but rarely seen
- "Backache" resulting from enlarged retroperitoneal lymph nodes
- Symptoms of displacement / dysfunction of involved organs (neurological disorders, pulmonary involvement → respiratory insufficiency, urogenital involvement → urination problems, etc.)

**Dg:**

### Case History, Physical Examination

- Case history, including B symptoms
- Physical Examination: general condition, skin, mucous membranes and pharyngeal ring / tonsils, lymphadenopathy (size of lymphoma), hepatosplenomegaly, infections

### Laboratory Tests

- Complete blood count with differential (smear), lymphocytopenia (< 1,000/μl), eosinophilia (in 30% of cases), with bone marrow involvement anemia, granulocytopenia, thrombocytopenia
- Routine laboratory tests including electrolytes, serum creatinine, urea, liver and renal function parameters, total protein and protein electrophoresis, immunoglobulins
- ESR ↑, uric acid, LDH (raised with increased cell turnover)
- Viral serology (CMV, EBV, HIV1/2, hepatitis B and C)

### Histology

NOTE: Histological diagnosis is mandatory. If possible, avoid using inguinal lymph nodes for biopsies / diagnosis (high rate of artifacts).

- Lymph node histology
- Bone marrow smear and histology

### Imaging
- Chest x-ray, abdominal ultrasound
- CT scan of neck / thorax / abdomen (if necessary: MRI scan of chest and abdomen)
- Skeletal and/or bone marrow scan and/or PET scan
- PET (positron emission tomography): differentiation between metabolically active and inactive tissue in residual lymphomas after treatment
- Further imaging to verify suspicious findings

### Further Diagnostic Measures: Toxicity Assessment
- ECG, echocardiogram (optional: further diagnostic measures)
- Pulmonary function tests including blood gas analysis
- Hormonal status (TSH, LH, FSH, progesterone, menstrual history)

**NOTE:** A correct diagnostic process is relevant to treatment. After physical examination and chest x-ray only, 90% of patients are classified as early stage cases (stage I or II). After a comprehensive diagnostic process as described above, more than 50% of patients are classified as advanced cases (stages III–IV).

**DD:**

### Other Causes of Lymph Node Enlargement
- Non-Hodgkin's lymphoma
- Metastases from solid tumors (e.g., lung cancer, gastrointestinal tumors, head and neck cancer)
- Infections (e.g., toxoplasmosis, tuberculosis, CMV, EBV, HIV)
- Sarcoidosis
- Systemic lupus erythematosus, rheumatoid arthritis, Sjögren's syndrome

**Co:**
- Respiratory obstruction due to large mediastinal tumors, rare cases of SVC syndrome
- Neurological disorders in cases of CNS involvement (rare)
- Skeletal involvement with pathological fractures

**Th:**

## Treatment Concept

- Hodgkin's lymphoma is sensitive to chemotherapy and radiotherapy. With current treatment strategies, cure rates are 60–80% in advanced stages and as high as 90% in localized stages.
- Improved treatment concepts can only be developed in the context of randomized studies. Consequently, patients with Hodgkin's lymphoma should always be treated in the framework of clinical trials.
- The standard treatment consists of combined radiochemotherapy, adapted to disease stage, risk factors, and patient characteristics. Even in early stages, radiotherapy alone should only be used in selected cases. Advanced stages are primarily treated systemically (chemotherapy), possibly followed by radiotherapy.
- Risk factors (German Hodgkin's Disease Study Group, GHSG):
  a. Large mediastinal tumor ($\geq 1/3$ of the maximum thoracic diameter)
  b. Extranodal involvement
  c. ESR $\geq$ 50 mm/h (in the absence of B symptoms) or $\geq$ 30 mm/h (in the presence of B symptoms)
  d. Three or more affected lymph node areas
- After aggressive combined radiochemotherapy, secondary malignancies and delayed toxicity may occur. New treatment approaches aim at increased efficacy (especially in advanced stages) with simultaneous reduction of acute and delayed toxicity.
- Prior to radiotherapy and/or chemotherapy: sperm or oocyte banking (▶ Chaps. 4.10.1, 4.10.2) must be discussed with the patient and carried out if requested.

### Treatment concept of Hodgkin's lymphoma

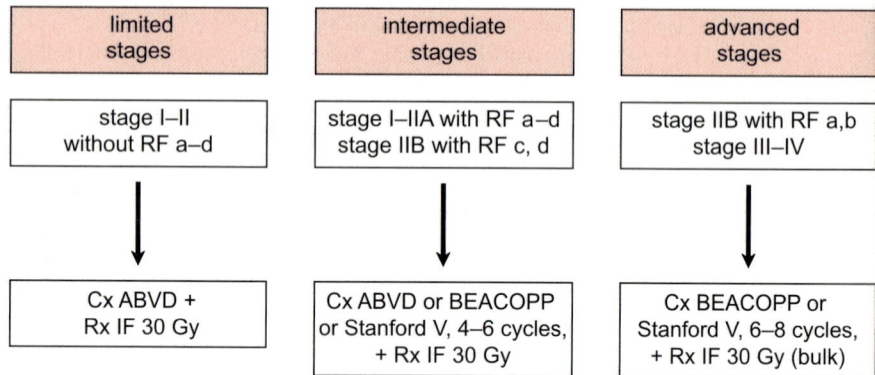

RF risk factors: *a* large mediastinal tumor, *b* extranodal involvement, *c* high ESR, *d* > 3 affected lymph node areas. *Cx* Chemotherapy, *Rx* Radiotherapy, *IF* involved field

### Principles of Radiotherapy

Treatment is based on large field techniques, ultrahard protons generated by linear accelerators or $^{60}$Co gamma rays (megavolt units). Approaches:
- *"Involved field"*: irradiation of affected lymph node areas
- *"Extended field"*: irradiation of the affected lymph node area as well as all anatomically or functionally bordering but clinically unaffected regions

### Principles of Chemotherapy

- Effective compounds include: corticosteroids, cyclophosphamide, anthracyclines (doxorubicin), bleomycin, vinca alkaloids (vincristine, vinblastine), etoposide, and procarbazine.
- In high-dose chemotherapy protocols and in the treatment of relapse, busulfan, nitrosoureas (BCNU, CCNU), cytosine arabinoside, and melphalan are also used.
- In principle, the treatment of Hodgkin's lymphoma consists of polychemotherapy with curative intention. Current therapy protocols: ABVD (▶ Protocol 11.3.1), BEACOPP Standard Dose (▶ Protocol 11.3.2), BEACOPP Escalated Dose (▶ Protocol 11.3.3), and Stanford V (▶ Protocol 11.3.4). Furthermore, accelerated application (14-day therapy intervals) on the basis of the BEACOPP protocol is currently being tested in clinical trials.

### Treatment of Relapse

In case of relapse, previously used therapy protocols are likely to be ineffective. Relapses occurring within 12 months of the primary treatment constitute a poor prognosis.

### Relapse after "Limited Stage" Treatment

With progressive disease or relapse, conventional polychemotherapy (e.g., BEACOPP Escalated Dose) or high-dose chemotherapy with autologous stem cell transplantation are conducted with curative intent. Radiotherapy only may be considered in certain cases.

### Relapse after "Intermediate Stage" or "Advanced Stage" Treatment

- Progressive disease or early relapse (≤ 1 year after completion of therapy): high-dose chemotherapy with autologous stem cell transplantation. Late relapse: high-dose chemotherapy with autologous stem cell transplantation; in selected cases conventional treatment according to the primary protocol
- After salvage therapy, lymph node regions which have not yet been irradiated should be treated with radiotherapy (30Gy)

### Second or Late Relapse

- Treatment with study protocols or alternative chemotherapy regimes (e.g. ICE, DHAP, EPOCH)
- Experimental therapy: e.g., allogeneic stem cell transplantation with reduced intensity conditioning

### Stem Cell Transplantation

The role of autologous or allogeneic stem cell transplantation has not yet been fully established.

- Some trials have demonstrated an effect of autologous stem cell transplantation independent of time of relapse (i.e., also with late relapses).
- A number of studies with allogeneic transplantation have demonstrated significantly reduced relapse rates, indicating a potential "graft-versus-Hodgkin's lymphoma" effect.
- New therapy concepts (e.g., double transplantation, use of specific antibodies, administration of EBV-specific cytotoxic T-cells) may further improve transplant outcomes.

## Chemotherapy Protocols

| ABVD ▶ Protocol 11.3.1 | | | Repeat day 29 |
|---|---|---|---|
| Doxorubicin | 25 mg/m²/day | i.v. | Day 1+15 |
| Bleomycin | 10 mg/m²/day | i.v. | Day 1+15 |
| Vinblastine | 6 mg/m²/day | i.v. | Day 1+15 |
| Dacarbazine / DTIC | 375 mg/m²/day | i.v. | Day 1+15 |

| BEACOPP-II Standard Dose ▶ Protocol 11.3.2 | | | Start next cycle on day 22 |
|---|---|---|---|
| Bleomycin | 10 mg/m²/day | i.v. | Day 8 |
| Etoposide | 100 mg/m²/day | i.v. | Day 1-3 |
| Doxorubicin | 25 mg/m²/day | i.v. | Day 1 |
| Cyclophosphamide | 650 mg/m²/day | i.v. | Day 1 |
| Vincristine | 1.4 mg/m²/day | i.v. | Day 8, max. 2 mg/day absolute |
| Procarbazine | 100 mg/m²/day | p.o. | Day 1–7 |
| Prednisolone | 40 mg/m²/day | p.o. | Day 1–14 |

| BEACOPP-II Escalated Dose ▶ Protocol 11.3.3 | | | Start next cycle on day 22 |
|---|---|---|---|
| Bleomycin | 10 mg/m²/day | i.v. | Day 8 |
| Etoposide | 200 mg/m²/day | i.v. | Day 1-3 |
| Doxorubicin | 35 mg/m²/day | i.v. | Day 1 |
| Cyclophosphamide | 1,250 mg/m²/day | i.v. | Day 1 |
| Vincristine | 1.4 mg/m²/day | i.v. | Day 8, max. 2 mg/day absolute |
| | | | Day 1–7 |
| Procarbazine | 100 mg/m²/day | p.o. | Day 1–14 |
| Prednisolone | 40 mg/m²/day | p.o. | |

| ABVD ▶ Protocol 11.3.4 | | | Start next cycle on day 29 |
|---|---|---|---|
| Doxorubicin | 25 mg/m²/day | i.v. | Day 1–10 |
| Bleomycin | 10 mg/m²/day | i.v. | Day 2 |
| Vinblastin | 6 mg/m²/day | i.v. | Day 4–7 |
| Dacarbazine/DTIC | 375 mg/m²/day | i.v. | Day 4–7 |

| *Stanford V ► Protocol 11.3.5* | | | *Start next cycle on day 29* |
|---|---|---|---|
| Mechlorethamine | 6 mg/m²/day | i.v. | Day 1 |
| Doxorubicin | 25 mg/m²/day | i.v. | Day 1,15 |
| Vinblastine | 6 mg/m²/day | i.v. | Day 1,15 |
| Etoposide Phosphate | 60 mg/m²/day | i.v. | Day 15,16 |
| Vincristine absolute | 1.4 mg/m²/day | i.v. | Day 8,22, max. 2 mg/day |
| Bleomycin | 5 U/m²/day | i.v. | Day 8,22 |
| Prednisone | 40 mg/m²/day | p.o. | Weeks 1–10 |
| Prednisone | 10 mg/m²/day | p.o. | Weeks 11–12 |

**Prg:**

### Prognostic Factors
The following criteria are associated with poor prognosis:
- Large mediastinal tumor, bulky disease (lymphomas ≥ 5 cm in diameter)
- Three or more affected lymph node areas, involvement of inguinal lymph nodes
- Extranodal involvement
- Bone marrow involvement
- ESR ≥ 50 mm/h (in the absence of B symptoms) or ≥ 30 mm/h (in the presence of B symptoms), LDH ↑ (especially with relapse therapy)
- Age > 45 years, B symptoms
- Karnofsky index < 90% (especially in relapse therapy)
- Advanced Hodgkin's lymphoma (prognostic factor index): albumin < 4 g/dl, Hb < 10.5 g/dl, male patient, age > 45 years, stage IV, leukocytosis > 15,000/µl, lymphocytopenia < 600/µl

### Five-year Survival
- Stages I and II (50% of patients): cure in > 90% of cases
- Stages III and IV: cure rates > 80%
- Adequate salvage therapy may potentially cure 20–50% of relapsed patients

**F/U:**

*Close follow-up is obligatory.* Intervals: 1st year: follow-up visits at 3, 6, 12 months after end of treatment, 2nd to 4th year: every 6 months, after 5 years: once a year (including clinical status, laboratory tests, chest x-ray, abdominal ultrasound). Objectives of follow-up include diagnosis of relapse and assessment of treatment-related toxity.

### Diagnosis of Relapse
Relapse can be treated with curative intent. The earlier a relapse is diagnosed, the better the prognosis. If a relapse is clinically suspected, thorough diagnostic work-up is required:
- Case history (B symptoms)
- Physical examination (lymphadenopathy, hepatosplenomegaly)
- Laboratory tests (ESR, LDH, blood count, liver / renal function tests)
- Imaging (chest x-ray, ultrasound, CT scan of thorax / abdomen, scintigraphy)
- New histology (bone marrow biopsy)

### Treatment-related Toxicity
- Assessment of quality of life
- Cardiac failure (LVEF ↓) after radiotherapy and anthracyclines
- Pericarditis / pericardial effusion after mediastinal irradiation
- Radiation pneumonitis / fibrosis after radiotherapy (mantle field radiation) and bleomycin
- Neurological complications after radiotherapy and vincristine
- Functional deficiencies of gonads or thyroid gland (hypothyroidism) after radiotherapy and/or chemotherapy
- Increased susceptibility to infection
- Early detection of secondary malignancy: depending on the treatment protocol used, the risk of secondary malignancy may be increased (particularly acute leukemia, lung cancer, breast cancer, gastric cancer, melanoma); after 10 years, incidence of secondary malignancy up to > 10% (with mustargen-containing radiochemotherapy) → with currently used therapy protocols: 1–2%

**Ref:**

1. Bonadonna G, Viviani S, Bonafante V et al. Survival in Hodgkin's lymphoma. Eur J Cancer 2005;41:998–1006
2. Connors JM. State-of-art therapeutics: Hodgkin's lymphoma. J Clin Oncol 2005;23:6400–8
3. Diehl V, Fuchs M. Early, intermediate and advanced Hodgkin's lymphoma: modern treatment strategies. Ann Oncol 2007;18(Suppl. 9):ix71–9
4. Ferme C, Eghbali H, Meerwaldt JH et al. Chemotherapy plus involved field radiation in early stage Hodgkin's disease. N Engl J Med 2007;357:1916–27
5. Jost L, ESMO Guidelines Working Group. Hodkin's disease: ESMO Clinical Recommendations for diagnosis, treatment and follow-up. Ann Oncol 2007;18(Suppl. 2):ii53–4
6. Lavoien JC, Connors JM, Phillips GL et al. High-dose chemotherapy and autologous stem cell transplantation for primary refractory or relapsed Hodgkin's lymphoma. Blood 2005;106:1473–8
7. Peggs KS, Hunter A, Chopra R et al. Clinical evidence of graft-versus-Hodgkin's lymphoma effect after reduced-intensity allogenic transplantation. Lancet 2005;365:1934–41
8. Re D, Küppers R, Diehl V. Molecular pathogenesis of Hodgkin's lymphoma. J Clin Oncol 2005;23:6379–86
9. Yung L, Linch D. Hodgkin's lymphoma. Lancet 2003;361:943–51

**Web:**

1. http://www.cancer.gov/cancertopics/types/hodgkinslymphoma/    NCI Cancer Topics
2. http://www.emedicine.com/MED/topic1022.htm    E-medicine
3. http://www.lymphomainfo.net/hodgkins/    Lymphoma Information Network
4. http://www.nlm.nih.gov/medlineplus/ency/article/000580.htm    Medline Plus
5. http://www.cancerbackup.org.uk/Cancertype/LymphomaHodgkins    Cancer BACKUP

## 7.5    Non-Hodgkin's Lymphomas (NHL)

J. Finke

**Def:**    Lymphoproliferative malignancies originating from the B-cell (B-NHL) or T-cell lineage (T-NHL). Depending on the clinical course, classification as high-grade (aggressive) or low-grade lymphomas is justified.

**ICD-10:**    C82–C88, C91.1

**Ep:**    Incidence 10–12 cases/100,000 population/year. Ratio low-grade:high-grade NHL = 7:3. Distribution male:female = 2:1. Age and gender distribution as well as incidence and mortality vary depending on the individual disease entity (▶ Chaps. 7.5.1–7.5.11).

**Pg:**    *Etiological Factors*
- Ionizing radiation, mutagenic compounds
- Association with viral / bacterial infections
  - Epstein–Barr virus (EBV): endemic Burkitt's lymphoma in Africa and Asia; high-grade lymphomas after immunosuppression, transplantation and in HIV infection (particularly cerebral lymphomas); Hodgkin's disease
  - HHV8: effusion-associated lymphomas
  - HTLV-1: T-lymphoblastic leukemia, in Southern Japan, Romania
  - *Helicobacter pylori*: MALT lymphomas (▶ Chap. 7.5.9)
- Immune deficiency syndromes
  - Hereditary: ataxia telangiectasia, SCID syndrome ("severe combined immunodeficiency syndrome"), "X-linked lymphoproliferative syndrome"
  - Acquired: organ and bone marrow transplantation, AIDS, Sjögren's syndrome

*Molecular Genetic Aspects*
Molecular genetic anomalies identified in the majority of patients with non-Hodgkin's lymphomas. The specific abnormalities are discussed with the individual disease entities (▶ Chaps. 7.5.1–7.5.11).

**Path:**    Clonal expansion at different stages of lymphoid differentiation. The earlier a cell is transformed during lymphatic development, the less differentiated the phenotype will be and the more aggressive its proliferative potential. All cells of a lymphoid neoplasia are characterized by identical rearrangement of the immunoglobulin heavy chain locus (B-cell lymphomas) or the T-cell receptor (T-cell lymphomas).

*Pathophysiological Process*
- Clonal expansion of lymphoid cells
  - → Lymphadenopathy, increased cell turnover, cytokine release
  - → General symptoms (fever, night sweats, weight loss)
- Organ infiltration → dysfunction and clinical symptoms, e.g.:
  - Bone marrow infiltration → anemia, thrombocytopenia, granulocytopenia
  - Splenic infiltration → splenomegaly
  - Skin infiltration (particularly T-NHL)
  - Hepatic / renal infiltration → hepatomegaly, hepatic / renal impairment
- With expansion of differentiated B-lymphocytic cells: immunoglobulin synthesis → monoclonal gammopathy

**Class:**    The WHO classification (World Health Organization, 2001) represents the international standard for the classification of lymphomas and has replaced all earlier approaches (e.g., KIEL, REAL, Working formulation). The classification is based on clinical, morphological, immunological, and molecular genetic criteria, but does not differentiate between low-grade and high-grade NHLs.

Most important objective of the WHO classification is distinction of lymphoma entities as a basis for standardized treatment. While therapy of B-cell lymphomas largely follows international standards, the optimal treatment for various T-NHL subtypes has not been established yet.

**B-cell NHL (WHO classification, 2001)**

| Lymphoma entity | ▶ Chapter |
| --- | --- |
| *Precursor B-cell lymphoma* | |
| • Precursor B-cell lymphoblastic leukemia (B-ALL) | 7.1.1 |
| • Precursor B-cell lymphoblastic lymphoma | 7.5.1 |
| *Mature B-cell lymphoma* | |
| • Chronic lymphocytic leukemia (CLL) | 7.5.2 |
| • Small lymphocytic lymphoma | |
| • B-prolymphocytic leukemia (PLL) | 7.5.3 |
| • Lymphoplasmacytic lymphoma | |
| • Follicular lymphoma (FL, grade I / II / III) | 7.5.5 |
| • Marginal zone lymphoma (extranodal / MALT, nodal, splenic) | 7.5.9 |
| • Hairy cell leukemia | 7.5.4 |
| • Plasma cell myeloma | 7.5.10 |
| • Plasmacytoma (bone, extramedullary) | 7.5.10 |
| • Mantle cell lymphoma (MCL) | 7.5.6 |
| • Diffuse large B-cell lymphoma (DLCL) | 7.5.1 |
| • Mediastinal (thymic) large B-cell lymphoma | 7.5.1 |
| • Intravascular large B-cell lymphoma | 7.5.1 |
| • Primary effusion lymphoma | 7.5.1 |
| • Burkitt's lymphoma, Burkitt's leukemia | 7.5.1 |
| *B-cell proliferation of inconclusive proliferative behavior* | |
| • Lymphomatoid granulomatosis | |
| • Post-transplantation lymphoproliferative disorder | |

**T-/NK-cell NHL (WHO classification, 2001)**

| Lymphoma entity | ▶ Chapter |
| --- | --- |
| *Precursor T-cell lymphomas* | |
| • Precursor T-cell lymphoblastic leukemia | 7.1.1 |
| • Precursor T-cell lymphoblastic lymphoma | 7.5.1 |
| • Blastic NK cell lymphoma | |
| *Mature T-cell and NK cell lymphoma* | |
| • T-cell prolymphocytic leukemia (T-PLL) | 7.5.3 |
| • T-cell large granular lymphocytic leukemia | |
| • Aggressive NK cell lymphoma (leukemia) | |
| • Adult T-cell lymphoma/leukemia | 7.5.1 |
| • Extranodal NK / T-cell lymphoma (nasal type) | 7.5.1 |
| • Enteropathic T-cell lymphoma | 7.5.1 |
| • Hepatosplenic T-cell lymphoma | 7.5.1 |

**T-/NK-cell NHL (WHO classification, 2001) *(continued)***

| Lymphoma entity | ▶ Chapter |
|---|---|
| • Subcutaneous T-cell lymphoma (panniculitis-like) | 7.5.1 |
| • Mycosis fungoides/ Sézary syndrome | 7.5.7 |
| • Primary cutaneous anaplastic large-cell lymphoma | 7.5.1 |
| • Peripheral T-cell lymphoma, not further specified | 7.5.1 |
| • Angioimmunoblastic T-cell lymphoma | 7.5.1 |
| • Anaplastic large-cell lymphoma | 7.5.1 |
| *T-cell proliferation of uncertain malignancy* | |
| • Lymphomatoid papulosis | |

**NHL Staging (Ann Arbor classification,1971)**

| Stage | Definition |
|---|---|
| I | Involvement of a single lymph node region (I) or presence of a single localized extra-nodal site (I E) |
| II | Lymph node involvement (II) and/or localized extranodal sites (II E) in two or more regions on the same side of the diaphragm |
| II$_1$ | Involvement of two neighboring lymph node regions (II$_1$) or one lymph node region with localized connection to a neighboring organ (II$_{1E}$) or two neighboring extralymphatic organs (II$_{1E}$) |
| II$_2$ | Involvement of two non-neighboring or > 2 neighboring lymph node regions (II$_2$) or of an extralymphatic organ with lymph node involvement beyond the regional lymph node (II$_{2E}$) or involvement of two non-neighboring extralymphatic organs (II$_{2E}$) |
| III | Lymph node involvement (III) and/or localized extranodal sites (III E) on both sides of the diaphragm, possibly with splenic involvement (III$_S$ or III$_{SE}$) |
| IV | Diffuse or disseminated involvement of one or more extralymphatic organs with or without lymph node involvement |
| A | No general symptoms |
| B | General symptoms: fever > 38°C, drenching night sweats (change of nightwear), weight loss of ≥ 10% in the last 6 months |

**Sy:**    *Symptoms of common lymphoma entities ▶ Chaps. 7.5.1–7.5.11.*

### Main Symptoms
- Lymphadenopathy
- Splenomegaly, hepatomegaly
- General symptoms: fever, night sweats, weight loss, anorexia
- Fatigue, reduced performance, pallor → with anemia
- Tendency to infection → with granulocytopenia, antibody deficiency syndrome, immunodeficiency
- Tendency to bleed, petechia → with thrombocytopenia
- Skin symptoms (erythema, plaque-like infiltrates), pruritus
- Signs of organ infiltration

DD:

### Differential Diagnosis of Lymphadenopathy

*Infections*
- Streptococci, staphylococci
- Toxoplasmosis
- Cat-scratch disease (*Bartonella henselae*)
- Tuberculosis, atypical mycobacteriosis
- EBV (infectious mononucleosis)
- HIV

*Autoimmune diseases*
- Rheumatoid arthritis
- Systemic lupus erythematodes
- Sjögren's syndrome

*Drug-related reactions*
- Anticonvulsives (phenytoin, carbamazepine)
- Antibiotics (penicillins, erythromycin)
- Acetylsalicylic acid, allopurinol

*Other non-cancer-associated diseases*
- Sarcoidosis
- Amyloidosis
- Silicon implants
- Vaccine reactions
- Metabolic disorders (Gaucher's disease)

*Lymphoproliferative diseases*
- Benign lymphoproliferative diseases (Kikuchi's disease, Rosai-Dorfman disease)
- Polyclonal lymphoproliferative diseases (Castleman's disease)
- Monoclonal lymphoproliferative diseases (lymphomatoid granulomatosis, lymphomatoid papulosis)

*Cancer*
- Lymphomas (Hodgkin's lymphoma, NHL), leukemia
- Metastases of solid tumors

Dg:

### Basis Principles of Lymphoma Diagnosis (▶ Chaps. 7.5.1–7.5.11)
- Medical history including B symptoms, pruritus, dynamics of lymphoma progression
- Physical examination including lymph node status and spleen
- Laboratory tests including full blood count with differential (leukemic form?), LDH ↑, ESR ↑, protein electrophoresis, immunology (monoclonal gammopathy?)
- Histology of lymph nodes, bone marrow, or affected organs; bone marrow biopsy should be carried out bilaterally (increased sensitivity).
- *NOTE: No treatment before adequate histology was obtained. If results are unclear, forward samples to a reference pathologist.*
- Immunocytology
- Imaging: diagnosis of the primary lymphoma site and metastasis, i.e., x-ray, abdominal ultrasound, CT thorax / abdomen, additional procedures (e.g., MRT, scintigraphy, as required)

Th:

*Treatment of common lymphoma entities ▶ Chaps. 7.5.1–7.5.11.*

## Basis Principles of Lymphoma Treatment

Treatment decisions have to consider the patient's age and performance status as well as histology and stage of the lymphoma. Of particular relevance are:

1. *Distinction between curative and palliative treatment intent:*
   - Curative intent (always with high-grade NHL, sometimes with low-grade lymphomas): aggressive therapy as soon as diagnosed
   - Palliative option (mainly with low-grade NHL): conservative symptom-oriented treatment to extend patient survival and improve quality of life.

2. *Distinction between localized and generalized stages of the disease:*
   - Localized stages (Ann Arbor I–II): → irradiation of low-grade lymphomas; in high-grade NHL: with curative treatment intent, aggressive systemic chemotherapy, in individual cases complementary involved field irradiation
   - Advanced stages (Ann Arbor III–IV): systemic therapy

3. *If possible, patients should always be treated within clinical trials for continuing treatment optimization.*

**Ref:**
1. Armitage JO. Staging non-Hodgkin lymphoma. CA Cancer J Clin 2005;55:368–76
2. Cheson BD, Pfister B, Juweid ME et al. Revised response criteria for malignant lymphoma. J Clin Oncol 2007;25:579–86
3. Evans LS, Hancock BW. Non-Hodgkin lymphoma. Lancet 2003;362:139–46
4. Fisher SG, Fisher RI. The epidemiology of non-Hodgkin's lymphoma. Oncogene 2004;23:6524–34
5. Jaffe ES, Harris NL, Stein H et al. (eds) Pathology and Genetics of Tumors of the Hematopoietic and Lymphoid Tissues. WHO classification of tumors, IARC Press, Lyon, 2001
6. Küppers R. Mechanisms of B-cell lymphoma pathogenesis. Nat Rev Cancer 2005;5:251–62
7. Kwee TC, Kwee RM, Nievelstein RAJ. Imaging in staging of malignant lymphoma. Blood 2008;111:504–16
8. Pals ST, De Gorter DJJ, Spaargaren M. Lymphoma dissemination: the other face of lymphocyte homing. Blood 2007;110:3102–11.
9. Rizvi MA, Evens, AM, Tallman MS et al. T-cell non-Hodgkin lymphoma. Blood 2006; 107:1255–64

**Web:**
1. http://www.lymphomainfo.net/ — Lymphoma Information Network
2. http://www.lls.org — Leukemia Lymphoma Society
3. http://www.cancer.gov/cancertopics/types/non-hodgkins-lymphoma — NCI Cancer Topics
4. http://www.nlm.nih.gov/medlineplus/lymphoma.html — MedlinePlus
5. http://www.cancerbackup.org.uk/Cancertype/Lymphomanon-Hodgkins — Cancer BACKUP
6. http://www.emedicine.com/med/topic1363.htm — E-medicine
7. http://www.lymphoma.org — Lymphoma Res Foundation

**7.5.1**    **High-grade Non-Hodgkin's Lymphoma**

J. Finke

**Def:** Lymphoid tissue neoplasia originating from the B-cell system (B-NHL) or the T-cell lineage (T-NHL). High-grade NHLs are characterized by:
- Rapid progression with generally fatal outcome if untreated
- Potentially curative treatment options even in advanced stages.

**ICD-10:** C82–C85

**Ep:** Incidence 3–5 cases/100,000 population/year, with increasing frequency. 3% of all malignant diseases. Ratio male:female = 2:1. Age peak between 40 and 80 years.

**Pg:** *Etiological Factors*
- Ionizing radiation, mutagenic compounds (cytostatics, pesticides, fungicides)
- Infections: viruses (EBV, HTLV-1 ▶ Chap. 7.5), *Helicobacter pylori* (▶ Chap. 7.5.9)
- Immunodeficiency syndromes (▶ Chap. 7.5)

**Molecular genetic alterations: translocations**

| Lymphoma type | Translocation | Affected genes |
|---|---|---|
| *B-cell type* | | |
| Burkitt's lymphoma | t(8;14), t(8;22) ,t(2;8) | myc, IgH |
| Diffuse large-cell lymphoma | t(3;14), t(3;various) | bcl-6, IgH, other |
| *T-cell type* | | |
| Anaplastic large-cell lymphoma | t(2;5) | npm-alk |

**Path:** Clonal expansion in early stages of lymphatic differentiation → undifferentiated phenotype, aggressive proliferation

*Location*
- Primarily nodal, in some cases with extralymphatic involvement: 80%
- Primarily extranodal: 20%

*Disease Stage at Diagnosis*
- Localized (stage I–II): 20%
- Advanced (stage III–IV): 80%

**Class:** *Classification*
According to the WHO classification (▶ Chap. 7.5). Correct classification is based on histology, immunohistology, cytology, immunocytology and molecular diagnostics.

The distinction between lymphoblastic lymphoma of the Burkitt's type, non-Burkitt's type and other high-grade NHLs is important for selection of adequate treatment.

**High-grade B-cell NHL: Disease Entities according to WHO classification (▶ Chap. 7.5)**

*Precursor B-cell lymphoma*
- Precursor B-cell lymphoblastic leukemia (B-ALL)
- Precursor B-cell lymphoblastic lymphoma

*Mature B-cell lymphoma*

- Follicular lymphoma (FL, grade II / III)
- Mantle cell lymphoma (MCL)
- Diffuse large B-cell lymphoma (DLBCL), centroblastic (cb), immunoblastic (ib), large cell anaplastic (lc)
- Mediastinal (thymic) large B-cell lymphoma
- Intravascular large B-cell lymphoma
- Primary effusion lymphoma
- Burkitt's lymphoma, Burkitt's leukemia

**High-grade T-cell NHL according to WHO classification (▶ Chap. 7.5)**

| | |
|---|---|
| *Precursor T-cell lymphoma* | |
| • Precursor T-cell lymphoblastic leukemia | 7.1.1 |
| • Precursor T-cell lymphoblastic lymphoma | 7.5.1 |
| *Mature T-cell and NK cell lymphoma* | |
| • Adult T-cell lymphoma/leukemia | |
| • Extranodal NK / T-cell lymphoma (nasal type) | |
| • Enteropathic T-cell lymphoma | |
| • Hepatosplenic T-cell lymphoma | |
| • Subcutaneous T-cell lymphoma (panniculitis-like) | |
| • Peripheral T-cell lymphoma, not further specified | |
| • Angioimmunoblastic T-cell lymphoma | 7.5.1 |
| • Anaplastic large-cell lymphoma | 7.5.1 |

*Staging According to the Ann Arbor System (▶ Chap. 7.5)*
- Lymphatic tissue includes: lymph nodes, spleen, thymus, Waldeyer's ring
- Extranodal involvement (E): defined as circumscribed involvement of extralymphatic tissue (either direct invasion from an affected lymph node or close anatomical proximity)
- Bulky disease: defined as lymphoma measuring ≥ 7.5 cm

Sy:     *Symptoms Usually of Rapid Onset*
- Rapidly developing lymph node enlargement
- Splenomegaly
- General symptoms: fatigue, reduced performance, pallor, susceptibility to infection
- B symptoms (fever, night sweats, weight loss)
- Dyspnea (due to anemia, pulmonary infiltration, pleural effusion, etc.)
- Abdominal symptoms due to lymphadenopathy and organ-associated complications (ileus, urinary retention)
- Possible skin infiltration
- Neurological symptoms → with involvement of the CNS / CSF spaces

**Dg:** *Medical History, Physical Examination*

- Medical history including B symptoms, performance status
- Inquire about family members to determinate the possibility of matched related allogeneic transplantation
- Physical examination: lymph node status, oral cavity, spleen / liver, jaundice, edema, signs of hemorrhage, signs of infection

*Laboratory Tests*

- Routine laboratory tests including complete blood count with differential, LDH ↑, ESR, electrolytes, $Ca^{2+}$, urea, electrolytes, serum creatinine, liver function, protein electrophoresis (gammopathy?), coagulation status with fibrinogen
- Quantitative immunoglobulin analysis, immunoelectrophoresis
- Serology: HIV, HAV, HBV, HCV, EBV, CMV, HSV, VZV, possibly HTLV1, toxoplasmosis

*Histology*

- Lymph node histology
- Bone marrow cytology, immunocytology, and histology
- In cases of involvement of paranasal sinuses, orbits, bones, bone marrow, or testes or in patients with lymphoblastic or Burkitt's leukemia: diagnostic lumbar puncture (*ATTENTION:* with prophylactic intrathecal administration of methotrexate 15 mg)
- With involvement of Waldeyer's ring: gastroscopy

*Imaging*

- Chest x-ray (PA and lateral views), abdominal ultrasound, ECG, CT thorax / abdomen / pelvis
- Optional: bone marrow scan, bone scan, PET / MRI scan before / after treatment in cases of bulky disease

*Monitoring of Toxicity, Especially Before and After High-dose Therapy*

- Pulmonary function (body plethysmography with CO-diffusion capacity) prior to administration of bleomycin, high-dose therapy, and allogeneic / autologous transplantation
- Echocardiography (determination of the ejection fraction)
- Dental status evaluation

**DD:**

- Limited stages: toxoplasmosis, EBV infection, *Bartonella henselae* (cat-scratch disease)
- Advanced stages: acute leukemia
- Hodgkin's disease

**Th:** **Treatment Concept**

1. High-grade lymphomas are always treated with curative intent.
2. Due to early dissemination, high-grade NHL must be regarded as a systemic disease, even in stages I / IE and II / IIE. Chemotherapy, possibly combined with radiotherapy, is always indicated.
3. Standard treatment consists of systemic chemotherapy combined with intrathecal chemotherapy (in case of CNS involvement) and subsequent radiotherapy ("involved field," 30–40 Gy, with bulky disease or residual lymphoma). The choice of treatment is influenced by prognostic parameters ("International Prognostic Index" IPI, "age-adjusted International Prognostic Index" aaIPI).
4. Application of the full chemotherapy dose on time (no dose delays or reductions) as per protocol is of major importance, especially for anthracyclines and alkylating agents. Dose reductions may compromise treatment outcomes.
5. With all high-grade NHL and especially with Burkitt's lymphoma: risk of tumor lysis syndrome (▶ Chap. 9.6). When therapy is initiated → prephase therapy (▶ Chap. 7.1.1), fluids therapy, alkalinization, allopurinol, if necessary rasburicase.
6. In cases of gastrointestinal involvement: risk of perforation when treatment is initiated.

**Treatment of high-grade non-Hodgkin's lymphomas**

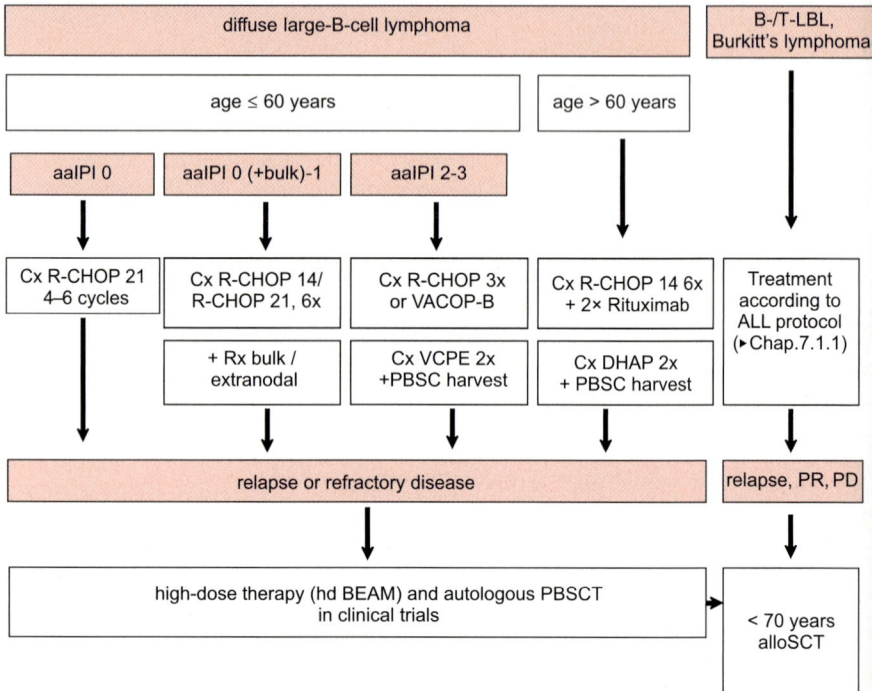

*LBL* lymphoblastic lymphoma, *aaIPI* age-adjusted International Prognostic Index (see below), *Cx* chemotherapy, *hd* high-dose, *Rx* radiation, *PBSCT* peripheral blood stem cell transplantation, *alloSCT* allogeneic stem cell transplantation, *PR* partial remission, *PD* progression

## Therapies

### Standard Therapies
- Standard treatment is chemotherapy according to the CHOP protocol → long-term survival in 40–65% of patients.
- Further improvement of survival in B-cell lymphoma has been demonstrated for dose dense chemotherapy ("CHOP14 + G-CSF"), and for combination of CHOP with rituximab ("R-CHOP," especially in patients with low-risk status).
- Patients with limited disease (stage I–II) should also receive first-line chemotherapy. Local radiotherapy may be considered in individual cases.

### Chemotherapy Guidelines
- Dose reductions should be avoided. If platelet count < 100,000/µl and leukocyte count < 2,500 µl on the scheduled day of treatment with anthracyclines or alkylating agents: delay treatment and use G-CSF. No dose delay or dose reduction with vincristine or bleomycin (VACOP-B protocol).
- Reduced pulmonary function (FEV1 < 65%, Krogh factor < 65%): methotrexate 50 mg absolute i.v. instead of bleomycin.
- With involvement of paranasal air sinuses, orbits, bones, bone marrow, or testes or in patients in a leukemic phase: CNS prophylaxis with methotrexate 15 mg i.th. absolute and intrathecal

dexamethasone 4 mg total dose at time of diagnosis and after 2, 6, and 10 weeks (6 doses in total).

- Patients with initial CSF or CNS involvement are treated twice weekly with a combination of intrathecal dexamethasone 4 mg, methotrexate 15 mg, and cytosine arabinoside (AraC) 40 mg until normalization of CSF. Initial CSF involvement does not impair the prognosis after autologous transplantation, provided full remission (CSF normalization) is achieved prior to transplantation. CSF involvement prior to the planned conditioning treatment is a reason to delay transplantation.

### Treatment of Relapse

- Patients with chemosensitive relapse of high-grade lymphoma without comorbidities should always be treated with high-dose chemotherapy and autologous transplantation. This increases long-term survival rate to 50% as compared to 10% with conventional salvage chemotherapy.
- With younger patients and available related donor, allogeneic transplantation may be considered. For patients with refractory relapse, autologous transplantation is probably of limited benefit.
- Patients not eligible for autologous transplantation (elderly, reduced performance status due to comorbidity) should be treated according to conventional rescue protocols (COP-BLAM, IMVP-16, CEPP-B, DHAP, ESHAP, COP, bendamustine, high-dose prednisolone, rituximab, etc.).

### Risk-adapted Therapy

- Specific "risk factors" impact long-term outcomes in patients with high-grade NHL.
- According to the "International Prognostic Index" (IPI), in patients up to 60 years, Ann Arbor stages III–IV, increased LDH, and Karnofsky index of < 70% constitute poor prognosis.
- Results of clinical trials suggest that for patients with 2–3 risk factors according to the age-adjusted International Prognostic Index (aaIPI), high-dose therapy with autologous transplantation in first remission after induction chemotherapy may confer a survival advantage compared to continuation of standard therapy.

### Mediastinal Lymphoma

- Patients with primary mediastinal B-cell lymphoma in particular may benefit from a more aggressive approach. Patients with residual mediastinal lymphoma after completion of chemotherapy have an increased risk of relapse.
- Patients receiving high-dose chemotherapy with autologous transplantation at an earlier stage and showing tumor bulk reduction after consolidation radiotherapy may have a better prognosis.

### Aggressive Chemotherapy for T-cell High-risk Lymphoma

Retrospective analyses demonstrated a poor prognosis for the following NHL subtypes:

- Peripheral T-cell lymphomas
- Angioimmunoblastic T-cell lymphoma (AILD)
- Intestinal T-cell lymphomas
- Hepatosplenic γ/δ lymphomas
- Subcutaneous panniculitic T-NHL
- Anaplastic large-cell lymphoma

In these cases, aggressive chemotherapy (possibly with transplantation) may improve the prognosis.

### Therapy Protocols

---

*"VACOP-B"* ▶ *Protocol 11.4.1*　　　　　　　　　　　　　*Weekly treatment, 12 weeks*

| | | | |
|---|---|---|---|
| Doxorubicin | 50 mg/m²/day | i.v. | Day 1, week 1,3,5,7,9,11 |
| Cyclophosphamide | 350 mg/m²/day | i.v. | Day 1, week 1,5,9 |
| Vincristine | 1.2 mg/m²/day | i.v. | Day 1, week 2,4,6,8,10,12, 2 mg max. |
| Bleomycin | 10 mg/m²/day | i.v. | Day 1, week 2,4,6,8,10,12 |
| Etoposide, VP-16 | 50 mg/m²/day | i.v. | Day 1, week 3,7,11 |
| Etoposide, VP-16 | 100 mg/m²/day | p.o. | Day 2+3, week 3,7,11 |
| Prednisolone | 75–100 mg absolute | p.o. | Day 1–7, week 1, Day 1,3,5,7, week 2–12 |

In cases of increased risk of CNS involvement: intrathecal therapy: cytosine arabinoside 40 mg i.th., dexamethasone 4 mg i.th., methotrexate 15 mg i.th. day 1, week 2,6,10

---

*"R-CHOP"* ▶ *Protocol 11.4.3*　　　　　　　　　　　　　　*Start next cycle on day 14*

| | | | |
|---|---|---|---|
| Rituximab | 375 mg/m²/day | i.v. | Day 0; 24-4 h prior to CHOP |
| Cyclophosphamide | 750 mg/m²/day | i.v. | Day 1 |
| Doxorubicin | 50 mg/m²/day | i.v. | Day 1 |
| Vincristine | 1.4 mg/m²/day | i.v. | Day 1, 2 mg absolute max. |
| Prednisolone | 100 mg absolute | p.o. | Day 1–5 |

---

*"CHOP14+G-CSF"* ▶ *Protocol 11.4.4*　　　　　　　　　　　*Start next cycle on day 14*

| | | | |
|---|---|---|---|
| Cyclophosphamide | 750 mg/m²/day | i.v. | Day 1 |
| Doxorubicin | 50 mg/m²/day | i.v. | Day 1 |
| Vincristine | 1.4 mg/m²/day | i.v. | Day 1, 2 mg absolute max. |
| Prednisolone | 100 mg absolute | p.o. | Day 1–5 |
| G-CSF | 5 µg/kg/day | s.c. | From day 5 |

---

*"DHAP"* ▶ *Protocol 11.4.6*　　　　　　　　　　　　*Start next cycle on day 22–day 29*

| | | | |
|---|---|---|---|
| Cisplatin | 100 mg/m²/day | i.v. | Day 1 |
| Cytosine arabinoside | 2 × 2 g/m²/day | i.v. | Day 2, over 3 h, every 12 h |
| Dexamethasone | 40 mg absolute | i.v | Day 1–4, may be given orally |
| ± Rituximab | 375 mg/m²/d | i.v. | Day 0, 24-4 h before DHAP |

---

**Prg:**　　*Risk Factors According to the "International Prognostic Index" (IPI)*
- Age > 60 years
- Performance status ECOG 2–4 or Karnofsky index ≤ 70%
- Ann Arbor Stage III–IV
- Increased LDH
- Extranodal involvement in ≥ 2 regions

*Age-adjusted International Prognostic Index (aaIPI) for Patients < 60 Years*
- Karnofsky index ≤ 70%
- Ann Arbor Stage III–IV
- Increased LDH

**Prognosis for patients with high-grade NHL according to the International Prognostic Index**

| Risk group | Number of risk factors | CR[a] (%) | Five-year survival[b] (%) | |
|---|---|---|---|---|
| | | | Relapse-free | Overall |
| Low | 0–1 | 87 | 61 | 73 |
| Low–intermediate | 2 | 67 | 34 | 51 |
| Intermediate–high | 3 | 55 | 27 | 43 |
| High | 4–5 | 44 | 18 | 26 |

[a] Complete remission rate
[b] Based on total population

Within the group of "high-grade" lymphomas, patients with immunoblastic lymphoma and peripheral T-cell lymphoma have the worst prognosis.

**F/U:** In the 1st and 2nd year after treatment, follow-up examinations every 3 months; in the 3rd year: every 6 months; then anually.

**Ref:**
1. Abramson JS, Shipp MA. Advances in the biology and therapy of diffuse large B-cell lymphoma: moving toward a molecularly targeted approach. Blood 2005;106:1164–74
2. Armitage JO. How I treat patients with diffuse large B-cell lymphoma. Blood 2007;110:29–36
3. Coiffier B, Lepage E, Brière J et al. CHOP chemotherapy plus rituximab compared with CHOP alone in elderly patients with diffuse large-B-cell lymphoma. N Engl J Med 2002;346:235–42
4. ESMO Guidelines Task Force. Relapsed large B-cell non-Hodgkin' lymphoma. ESMO Clinical Recommendations for diagnosis, treatment and follow-up. Ann Oncol 2007;18(Suppl.2):ii55–6
5. ESMO Guidelines Task Force. Newly diagnosed large B-cell non-Hodgkin's lymphoma. ESMO Clinical Recommendations for diagnosis, treatment and follow-up. Ann Oncol 2007;18(Suppl.2):ii57–8
6. Ferry JA. Burkitt's lymphoma. Oncologist 2006;11:375–83
7. Milpied N, Deconinck E, Gaillard F et al. Initial treatment of aggressive lymphoma with high-dose chemotherapy and autologous stem-cell support. N Engl J Med 2004;350:1287–95
8. Pfreundschuh M, Trümper L, Kloess M et al. Two-weekly or 3-weekly CHOP chemotherapy with or without etoposide for the treatment of young patients with good-prognosis (normal LDH) aggressive lymphomas: results of the NHL-B1 trial of the DSHNHL. Blood 2004;104:626–33
9. Seropian S, Bahceci E, Cooper DL. Allogeneic peripheral blood stem cell transplantation for high-risk non-Hodgkin's lymphoma. Bone Marrow Transpl 2003;32:763–9

**Web:**
1. http://www.lymphomainfo.net/nhl/aggressive.html — Lymphoma Info Network
2. http://www.emedicine.com/med/HEMATOLOGY.htm — E-medicine
3. http://www.cancer.gov/cancertopics/types/non-hodgkins-lymphoma — NCI, Cancer Topics
4. http://www.lymphomation.org — Lymphoma Info Portal

**7.5.2        Chronic Lymphocytic Leukemia (CLL)**

J. Burger, J. Finke

**Def:**  Low-grade leukemic lymphoma with clonal proliferation and accumulation of morphologically mature but immunologically incompetent lymphocytes of the B-cell lineage (B-CLL, < 95% of cases) or T-cell lineage (T-CLL, < 5% of cases)

**ICD-10:**  C91.10

**Ep:**  Incidence: 2–3 cases/100,000 population/year. 30% of all leukemias in western nations, 5% in Asia. Median age at diagnosis 55 years. Only 10% of patients are under 50 years of age. Gender distribution male:female = 1.7:1

**Pg:**  *Risk Factors: Unknown*
- Higher risk (factor 2–7) in relatives of patients with CLL, other lymphoproliferative, or auto-immune diseases → genetic predisposition possible
- Karyotype aberrations in up to 82% of patients, particularly deletions del 13q (55%) and del 11q (18%), trisomy 12 (15%), del 17p and del 6q. Chromosomal aberrations serve as important prognostic factors for risk-adapted therapy, especially in young patients with early stages of the disease (Rai 0–II)

*Pathogenesis*
Lymphocyte accumulation in CLL patients is not caused by accelerated cell division but by defective apoptosis. Over 90% of CLL patients show high levels of expression of the anti-apoptotic Bcl-2 protein.

*Normal Analog of B-CLL Cells: Subpopulation of Mature CD5-positive B-lymphocytes*
- Physiological occurrence in the capsular zone of lymph follicles, peripheral blood, fetal lymph nodes and fetal spleen
- Increased in association with various immunological diseases, e.g., rheumatoid arthritis, systemic lupus erythematosus, Sjögren's syndrome

*Characteristics of Neoplastic CD5-positive B-CLL Cells*
- Expression of B-cell associated surface antigens: CD19, CD20, CD21, CD23, CD24
- Expression of CD5, FMC7 negative
- Weak expression of membrane-bound immunoglobulins (IgM ± IgD), evidence of circulating IgM in 5–50% of cases
- Molecular subclassification: "naive" B-cells without mutations in the variable region of the immunoglobulin heavy chains (Ig $V_H$ genes) indicate poor prognosis. "Memory" B-cells with Ig $V_H$ mutations (approximately 60% of patients) constitute better prognosis.
- Expression of signal transduction marker zeta-associated protein 70 (ZAP-70) is associated with poor prognosis, as well as CD38+ expression.

**Path:**  *Blood Smear*
- Marked lymphocytosis with small and mature appearing lymphocytes
- Some less mature and seemingly activated cells with nucleoli ("prolymphocytes"; if > 55% prolymphocytes: prolymphocytic leukemia, ► Chap. 7.5.3)
- "Smudge cells": smear-induced lymphocyte destruction ("Gumprecht cells")
- Red blood cell alterations, including anisocytosis, poikilocytosis, and possibly hemolysis

*Bone Marrow*
- > 30% infiltration with mature lymphocyte population
- Growth: nodular (good prognosis), interstitial or diffuse (poor prognosis)
- With further progression: suppression of normal hematopoiesis

**Class:** WHO classification: mature B-cell lymphoma

**Rai staging System for CLL (1975, 1990)**

| Risk | Stage | Definition | Survival[a] (years) |
|---|---|---|---|
| Low | 0 | Lymphocytosis > 5,000/µl<br>Bone marrow infiltration > 30% | > 12.5 |
| Medium | I | Lymphocytosis + lymphadenopathy | 8.5 |
| | II | Lymphocytosis + splenomegaly and/or hepatomegaly (with or without lymphadenopathy) | 6 |
| High | III | Lymphocytosis + anemia (hemoglobin < 11 g/dl) (with or without adenopathy / organomegaly) | 1.5 |
| | IV | Lymphocytosis + thrombocytopenia (platelet count < 100,000/µl) (with or without anemia / adenopathy / organomegaly) | 1.5 |

[a] Median survival time

**Binet staging System for CLL (1981)**

| Risk | Stage | Lymphadenopathy[b] | Hemoglobin (g/dl) | Platelets (/µl) | Survival[a] (years) |
|---|---|---|---|---|---|
| Low | A | < 3 | > 10 | Normal | > 10 |
| Medium | B | ≥ 3 | > 10 | Normal | 5 |
| High | C | – | < 10 | < 100,000 | 2 |

[a] Median survival time
[b] Number of lymph node areas involved

**y:** Incidental diagnosis in 40–60% of cases during asymptomatic stages of the disease.
- Main symptom: indolent lymphadenopathy, particularly in the cervical and supraclavicular region, but also other lymph node areas (> 50% of patients)
- Fatigue, exhaustion, reduced performance
- Fever, night sweats, weight loss, pallor, tendency to bleed, infections
- Splenomegaly, in advanced cases with abdominal symptoms, hepatomegaly
- Signs of bone marrow infiltration including anemia, thrombocytopenia, and neutropenia (despite simultaneous leukocytosis due to B-CLL cells)
- Dermatological symptoms: pruritus, eczema, hemorrhage, skin infections (*Herpes zoster*, fungal infections); in advanced cases and with T-CLL: cutaneous CLL infiltrates
- Susceptibility to infection, especially pneumonia (*Streptococcus pneumoniae*, *Hemophilus influenzae*, *Pneumocystis carinii*, CMV), fungal infections (candida, aspergillus), *Herpes zoster* (VZV) and *Herpes simplex* (HSV), staphylococcal infections, legionellosis, toxoplasmosis

**g:** *Medical History, Physical Examination*
Physical examination including lymph node status, oral cavity, spleen / liver, icterus, edema, petechial bleeding, signs of infection

*Laboratory Tests*
- Full blood count with differential, reticulocytes; diagnosis is based on differential blood count and peripheral blood smear (increased number of mature lymphocytes, smudge cells)
- Routine laboratory tests including urea, electrolytes, serum creatinine, liver function tests, LDH, haptoglobin, bilirubin, c-reactive protein, thymidine kinase
- Immunology: quantitative immunoglobulin assay, immunoelectrophoresis; if patient is anemic: Coombs' test

- Recommended: surface marker analysis (FACS): immunocytochemistry for B-CLL markers CD5, CD19, CD20, CD23, light chains, ZAP-70, CD38+

### Histology
- Bone marrow aspirate and biopsy, possibly cytogenetic tests / FISH
- Lymph node histology where applicable

### Imaging
- Chest x-ray, abdominal ultrasound

## Diagnostic Criteria (National Cancer Institute Working Group, NCI WG, 1996)

- Lymphocytosis > 5,000/μl for at least 4 weeks
- Cells with κ- or λ-light chain expression, detection of pan-B-cell markers (CD19, CD20) together with CD5 and CD23 antigen expression
- Morphologically mature lymphocytes with < 55% atypical or immature lymphoid cells
- > 30% bone marrow infiltration

**DD:**
- Infection-related reactive lymphocytosis: hepatitis, cytomegalovirus, EBV, brucellosis, tuberculosis, typhoid, paratyphoid, chronic infections
- Reactive lymphocytosis in association with autoimmune diseases or allergic reactions
- Lymphadenopathy and lymphocytosis with other lymphatic diseases: immunocytoma, prolymphocytic leukemia, hairy cell leukemia, mantle cell lymphoma
- Sarcoidosis

**Co:**
- Infections: > 80% of CLL patients develop opportunistic infections; acute infections are the cause of death in 50% of cases
- Development of prolymphocytic leukemia (5–10% of patients): number of prolymphocytes ↑, therapy resistance ↑, survival period ↓
- Richter's syndrome (3–10%): transformation into high-grade non-Hodgkin's lymphoma with poor prognosis
- Secondary malignancies (8–10%): Hodgkin's disease, melanomas, CNS tumors
- Organ infiltration in advanced stages: liver, kidney, pulmonary infiltrates; parotid enlargement and infiltration of the lacrimal glands

### Immunological Disorders (10–75% of Patients)
- Positive Coombs' test: 8–35% of patients
- Autoimmune hemolytic anemia (AIHA): 10–25%
- Autoimmune thrombocytopenia: 2%
- Hypersplenism: 2%
- Hypogammaglobulinemia with susceptibility to infection: 20–60%

### Associated Disorders
- Multiple specific antibodies detectable against autoantigens: 20%
- Increased occurrence of rheumatoid arthritis, systemic lupus erythematosus, Sjögren's syndrome, thyroiditis, ulcerative colitis, vasculitis

**Th:**

### Treatment Concept

1. Conventional CLL therapy is not curative. Early treatment does not influence patient survival → generally palliative treatment in symptomatic cases only
2. *Indications for treatment:*
   - Advanced stages Rai III and IV or Binet C

- Symptomatic splenomegaly or lymphadenopathy
- Autoimmune hemolytic anemia, thrombocytopenia
- Recurrent infections
- Rapid disease progression (duplication of absolute lymphocyte counts < 6 months), rapidly progressing lymphadenopathy, transformation to high-grade NHL
- Marked B symptoms (fever, night sweats, weight loss)

3. *CLL is a systemic disease*
   → Chemotherapy is the first-line systemic treatment; in exceptional cases, local measures (radiotherapy, surgery) may be indicated to treat certain localized problems

4. *Autoimmune phenomena require immediate immunosuppressive therapy* (even in early stages of CLL): steroids (prednisolone 60–100 mg/day p.o.), alternatively: cyclophosphamide 50–100 mg/day p.o., high-dose immunoglobulins, rituximab or mycophenolate mofetil. Cases of steroid-resistant Coombs'-positive hemolytic anemia (AIHA), thrombocytopenia, or hypersplenism: splenectomy

*CAUTION: progressive autoimmune hemolytic anemia and autoimmune thrombocytopenia constitute a hematological emergency → immediate steroid administration; in steroid-resistant cases: splenectomy.*

**Treatment of CLL**

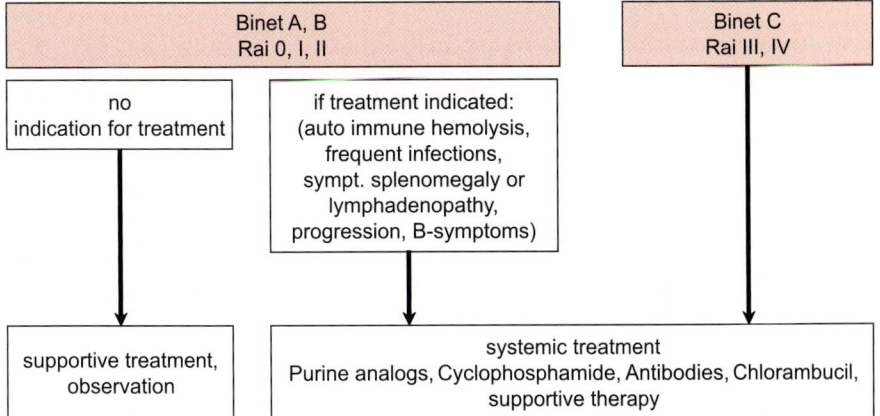

**Supportive Care**

Supportive treatment contributes to long-term survival of patients with CLL:
- Early and rigorous antibiotic / antifungal treatment with signs of infection
- Prophylactic use of immunoglobulins may be indicated in patients with recurrent infections and antibody deficiency (hypogammaglobulinemia)
- Effective CLL treatment (i.e., reduction of the malignant B-cell clone) results in normalization of hypogammaglobulinemia
- Recurrent infections are an indication for CLL treatment

**Conventional Chemotherapy**

The spectrum of treatment options has been expanded in recent years. Purine analogues (especially fludarabine), monoclonal antibodies, and combinations of chemo- and immunotherapy have become the treatment of choice in CLL patients.

### Purine Analogs

Antimetabolites with selective lymphocytotoxicity: fludarabine, pentostatin, deoxycoformycin (DCF), and 2-chlorodeoxyadenosine (2-CDA)

- Fludarabine is currently the most effective monotherapy in CLL with response rates (complete and partial remission, CR + PR) of 60–80% in first line therapy and 30–70% in pretreated patients.
- The value of purine analogs in first- and second-line therapy in CLL is established, especially in younger patients. Compared to chlorambucil, better response rates and longer disease-free periods can be achieved. However, overall survival is not prolonged significantly. Patients with del(17p) or p53 mutations show lower response rates.

### Alkylating Agents

For many CLL patients with reduced performance status and comorbidities, chlorambucil and cyclophosphamide remain an important treatment option; follow-up examination and therapy evaluation after 2–3 months; continue therapy until best response or evidence of new disease progression

### Alkylating Agents + Prednisolone

Additional administration of corticosteroids (e.g., in "Knospe" protocol) only indicated with autoimmune phenomena.

### Combination Chemotherapy

Fludarabine in combination with cyclophosphamide and/or rituximab induces a higher response rate and a longer progression-free survival compared with fludarabine monotherapy. An effect on overall survival has not been proven yet. Protocols with anthracyclines (e.g., CHOP) achieve rapid responses in lymphomas and can therefore be of particular benefit in advanced stages of the disease with symptomatic lymphadenopathy. Chemo-immunotherapies with alemtuzumab (Mab campath) are additional options.

### Antibodies

- The anti-CD52 antibody alemtuzumab has been approved for the treatment of chemotherapy resistant CLL, with response rates in fludarabine-resistant disease of up to 33%.
- The humanized monoclonal anti-CD20 antibody rituximab provides a therapeutic option which is effective in > 30% of patients, even after prior treatment.

## Therapy Protocols

| *"Chlorambucil / Prednisolone (Knospe)"* ▶ *Protocol 11.5.5* | | | *Start next cycle on day 22* |
|---|---|---|---|
| Chlorambucil | 18 mg/m²/day | p.o. | Day 1 |
| Prednisolone | 75 mg in total | p.o. | Day 1 |
| | 50 mg in total | p.o. | Day 2 |
| | 25 mg in total | p.o. | Day 3 |
| If well tolerated, the chlorambucil dose may be increased by 5 mg/m²/day per cycle | | | |

| *"Cyclophosphamide / Prednisolone"* | | | *Start next cycle on day 22* |
|---|---|---|---|
| Cyclophosphamide | 400 mg/m²/day | p.o. | Day 1–5 |
| Prednisolone | 100 mg/m²/day | p.o. | Day 1–5 |

| *"Bendamustine"* ▶ *Protocol 11.5.1* | | | *Start next cycle on day 22* |
|---|---|---|---|
| Bendamustine | 100 mg/m²/day | i.v. | Day 1–2 |

| *"Fludarabine Mono"* ▶ *Protocol 11.5.2* | | | *Start next cycle on day 29* |
|---|---|---|---|
| Fludarabine | 25 mg/m²/day | i.v. | Day 1–5 |

| *"2-CDA"* ▶ *Protocol 11.5.7* | | | *Start next cycle on day 22* |
|---|---|---|---|
| 2-CDA | 0.14 mg/kg/day | i.v. | Day 1–5, infusion over 2 h |

| *"FC"* ▶ *Protocol 11.5.3* | | | *Start next cycle on day 29* |
|---|---|---|---|
| Fludarabine | 30 mg/m²/day | i.v. | Day 1–3 |
| Cyclophosphamide | 300 mg/m²/day | i.v. | Day 1–3 |

| *"FCR"* ▶ *Protocol 11.5.4* | | | *Start next cycle on day 29* |
|---|---|---|---|
| Rituximab | 375 mg/m²/day | i.v. | Day 1 |
| Fludarabine | 30 mg/m²/day | i.v. | Day 2–4 |
| Cyclophosphamide | 300 mg/m²/day | i.v. | Day 2–3 |

| *"CHOP"* ▶ *Protocol 11.4.2* | | | *Start next cycle on day 22* |
|---|---|---|---|
| Cyclophosphamide | 750 mg/m²/day | i.v. | Day 1 |
| Doxorubicin | 50 mg/m²/day | i.v. | Day 1 |
| Vincristine | 1.4 mg/m²/day | i.v. | Day 1, max. single dose: 2 mg |
| Prednisolone | 100 mg in total | p.o. | Day 1–5 |

| *"Alemtuzumab"* ▶ *Protocol 11.5.6* | | | *Start next cycle on day 28* |
|---|---|---|---|
| Alemtuzumab | 3 mg/m²/day | s.c. | Day 1, week 1 |
| Alemtuzumab | 10 mg/m²/day | s.c. | Day 2, week 1 |
| Alemtuzumab | 30 mg/m²/day | s.c. | Day 3, week 1 |
| Alemtuzumab | 30 mg/m²/day | s.c. | Day 1, 3, 5, week 2–13 |

## Other Therapeutic Strategies

### Hematopoietic Stem Cell Transplant

High-dose chemotherapy and bone marrow or stem cell transplantation are potentially curative treatment options, particularly in younger patients.

- If an HLA-compatible donor is available, allogenic transplantation may be considered as a second- or third-line therapy for patients up to 60 or 70 years of age.
- New protocols applied in allogeneic transplantation include the use of peripheral hematopoietic stem cells of T-cell depleted donors (to avoid severe GVHD) and less toxic conditioning regimes with fludarabine. Indications for allogeneic transplantation:
  - Progressive disease/relapse < 12 months after response to purine analogs
  - Relapse < 24 months after autologous SCT
  - p53 mutation and symptomatic disease

- Autologous transplantation may be of value in some patients with early stages of the disease (e.g., Rai I, II with rapid leukocyte doubling time, > 3 enlarged lymph node areas) (only in clinical trials). *CAUTION:* pretreatment with purine analogs may render stem cell mobilization difficult.

### Splenectomy

Indicated in patients with hypersplenism (anemia, thrombocytopenia) and autoimmune hemolytic anemia. A case control study demonstrated improved post-splenectomy survival rates for Rai stage IV patients with thrombocytopenia.

**Prg:**  ### Prognostic Parameters

Parameters indicating a poor prognosis:
- Rai stages III / VI or Binet B / C
- Diffuse or interstitial type of bone marrow infiltration
- Initial blood lymphocyte count > 50,000/μl
- > 10% prolymphocytes (PL; so-called CLL / PL)
- $LDH_{serum}$ > 240 U/l, $\beta_2$-microglobulin$_{serum}$ > 3.5 mg/l, thymidine kinase$_{serum}$ > 7 U/l
- Complex cytogenetic aberrations, p53 mutation, 11q deletion
- Leukocyte doubling time < 1 year
- No Ig V gene mutations (resting B-cells)
- ZAP-70 and CD38+ Expression

**F/U:**  Three-monthly check-ups including full blood count and assessment of clinical progression; more frequent follow-up in case of complications.

**Ref:**
1. Abbott BL. Chronic lymphocytic leukemia. Oncologist 2006;11:21–30
2. Auer RL, Gribben J, Cotter FE. Emerging therapy for chronic lymphocytic leukaemia. Brit J Haematol 2007;139:635–44.
3. Catovsky D, Richards S, Matutes E et al. Assessment of fludarabine plus cyclophosphamide for patients with chronic lymphocytic leukaemia. Lancet 2007;370:230–9
4. Chiorazzi N, Rai KR, Ferrarini M. Chronic lymphocytic leukemia. N Engl J Med 2005;352:804–15
5. ESMO Guidelines Working Group. Chronic lymphocytic leukemia: ESMO Clinical Recommendations for diagnosis, treatment and follow-up. Ann Oncol 2007;18(Suppl. 2):ii49–50
6. Montserrat E, Moreno C, Esteve J et al. How I treat refractory CLL. Blood 2006; 107:1276–83
7. Linet MS, Schubauer-Berigan MK, Weisenburger DD et al. Chronic lymphocytic leukaemia: an overview of aetiology in light of recent developments in classification and pathogenesis. Brit J Haematol 2007;139:672–86.
8. Wierda WG, Kipps TJ, Keating MJ. Novel immune-based treatment strategies for chronic lymphocytic leukemia. J Clin Oncol 2005;23:6325–32

**Web:**
1. http://www.cancer.gov/cancertopics/pdq/treatment/ CLL/HealthProfessional — NCI, Cancer Topics
2. http://www.acor.org/leukemia/cll.html — CLL Links and Information
3. http://www.nlm.nih.gov/medlineplus/ency/article/000532.htm — MedlinePlus
4. http://www.emedicine.com/med/topic370.htm — E-medicine
5. http://cll.ucsd.edu/ — CLL Research Consortium

### 7.5.3 Prolymphocytic Leukemia (PLL)

J. Finke

**Def:** Low-grade leukemic lymphoma with clonal expansion of lymphocytic cells, aggressive form of chronic lymphatic leukemia. In 80% of cases B-cell prolymphocytic leukemia, in 20% T-PLL.

**ICD-10:** C91.3

**Ep:** Incidence 10% of CLL cases. Age at diagnosis in the majority of cases > 70 years, distribution male:female = 2:1.

**Pg:** *Characteristics of Neoplastic Prolymphocytes*
- B-prolymphocytic type (B-PLL) with expression of CD19, CD20, CD22; negative for CD5, CD11c, CD23, CD103; high surface immunoglobulin expression (IgM, occasionally IgD)
- T-prolymphocytic type (T-PLL) with expression of CD2, CD5, CD7; negative for CD1, TdT; in 75% of cases CD4+, in 20% CD8+

*Cytogenetics / Molecular Genetics*
Karyotypic aberrations in > 75% of patients:
- 14q+, t(11;14)(q13;q32), or inv(14) in 60% of patients
- Other aberrations: trisomy 12, 6q- deletion, translocations t(6;12)(q15;p13)

**Path:** *Blood Smear*
- Lymphocytosis with different stages of lymphocyte maturation
- > 55% prolymphocytes (immature appearing cells with prominent nucleoli)

*Bone Marrow*
- > 30% infiltration with immature lymphocyte population
- Increasing suppression of normal hematopoiesis

**Class:** *WHO classification (2001):* malignant B-cell or T-cell non-Hodgkin's lymphoma (B-PLL, T-PLL)

**Sy:** Only mild lymphadenopathy; main signs and symptoms are caused by splenomegaly and bone marrow infiltration:
- Splenomegaly, abdominal symptoms: 75–95%
- Anemia: 70%
- Thrombocytopenia: 70%
- Lymphocytosis, often > 100,000/µl: 65%
- Bruising, bleeding, petechiae
- Fatigue, reduced performance, weight loss
- With T-PLL: leukemic skin infiltration

**Dg:** *Medical History, Physical Examination*
Physical examination including splenomegaly, lymph node status, signs of hemorrhage, signs of infection, skin (infiltrates)

*Laboratory Tests*
- Complete blood count with differential, reticulocytes; blood smear shows prolymphocytes with characteristic morphology; possibly anemia and thrombocytopenia
- Routine laboratory tests including urea + electrolytes, serum creatinine, bilirubin, liver function tests, LDH, CRP
- Immunology: quantitative serum immunoglobulin levels, immunoelectrophoresis: hypogammaglobulinemia, monoclonal gammopathy
- Recommended: surface marker analysis: FACS-analysis of peripheral blood lymphocytes: CD5 negative ($\rightarrow$ DD: CLL)

### Bone Marrow Cytology and Histology
Infiltration by immature lymphocyte population, suppression of normal hematopoiesis

### Imaging
Chest x-ray, abdominal ultrasound

**Dd:**
- Splenomegaly caused by other lymphatic diseases, particularly CLL, hairy cell leukemia, immunocytoma, mantle cell lymphoma
- Acute leukemia

**Co:**    Leukostasis if leukocytosis > 200,000/µl → leukocyte reduction by cytapheresis is recommended

**Th:**

## Treatment Concept

1. The poor prognosis as compared to CLL (▶ Chap. 7.5.2) justifies a more aggressive approach. Alkylating agents with/without corticosteroids only achieve remission rates of 20%. Fludarabine, 2-chlorodeoxyadenosine (2-CDA), pentostatin, or protocols with anthracyclines (CHOP) are used in first-line therapy.
2. Alemtuzumab (monoclonal antibody to CD52) has demonstrated efficacy.
3. In cases of symptomatic splenomegaly / hypersplenism: splenectomy, splenic irradiation where applicable.
4. *ATTENTION*: In patients with high lymphocyte counts, chemotherapy may lead to tumor lysis syndrome (▶ Chap. 9.6) → adequate hydration, alkalinization, administration of allopurinol.
5. In younger patients (< 60 years): consider high-dose chemotherapy and allogeneic transplantation.

**Treatment of prolymphocytic leukemia**

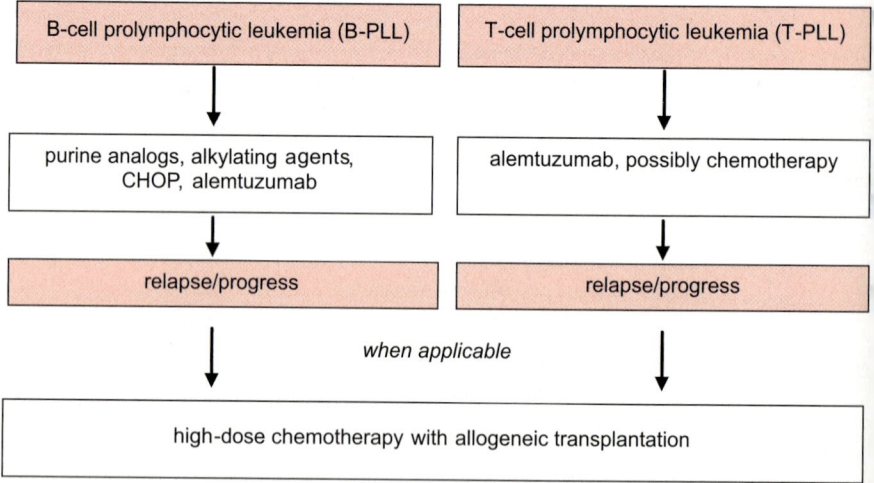

## Chemotherapy Protocols

| "2-CDA" ▶ Protocol 11.5.7 | | | | Start next cycle on day 22 |
|---|---|---|---|---|
| 2-CDA | 0.14 mg/kg/day | i.v. | Day 1–5 | |

| *"Fludarabine / Cyclophosphamide"* ▶ *Protocol 11.5.3* | | | *Start next cycle on day 29* |
|---|---|---|---|
| Fludarabine | 30 mg/m²/day | i.v. | Day 1–3 |
| Cyclophosphamide | 300 mg/m²/day | i.v. | Day 1–3 |

| *"FCR"* ▶ *Protocol 11.5.4* | | | *Start next cycle on day 28* |
|---|---|---|---|
| Rituximab | 375 mg/m²/day | i.v. | Day 1 |
| Fludarabine | 30 mg/m²/day | i.v. | Day 2–4 |
| Cyclophosphamide | 300 mg/m²/day | i.v. | Day 2–4 |

| *"CHOP"* ▶ *Protocol 11.4.2* | | | *Start next cycle on day 22* |
|---|---|---|---|
| Cyclophosphamide | 750 mg/m²/day | i.v. | Day 1 |
| Doxorubicin | 50 mg/m²/day | i.v. | Day 1 |
| Vincristine | 1.4 mg/m²/day | i.v. | Day 1, max. single dose: 2 mg |
| Prednisolone | 100 mg absolute | p.o. | Day 1–5 |

| *"Alemtuzumab"* ▶ *Protocol 11.5.6* | | | *Start next cycle on day 28* |
|---|---|---|---|
| Alemtuzumab | 3 mg/m²/day | s.c. | Day 1, week 1 |
| Alemtuzumab | 10 mg/m²/day | s.c. | Day 2, week 1 |
| Alemtuzumab | 30 mg/m²/day | s.c. | Day 3, week 1 |
| Alemtuzumab | 30 mg/m²/day | s.c. | Day 1,3,5 weeks 2–13 |

**Prg:**  Median survival: B-PLL up to 3 years, T-PLL 6–8 months

**F/U:**  Follow-up blood counts; in palliative setting: symptom-based approach

**Ref:**
1. Absi H, Hsi E, Kalaycio M. Prolymphocytic leukemia. Curr Treat Options Oncol 2005;6:197–208
2. Cao TM, Coutre SE. T-cell prolymphocytic leukemia: update and focus on alemtuzumab. Hematology 2003;8:1–6
3. Castagna L, Nozza A, Bertuzzi A et al. Allogeneic peripheral blood stem cell transplantation with re-duced intensity conditioning in primary refractory prolymphocytic leukemia. Bone Marrow Transplant 2001;28:1155–66
4. Dearden CE, Matutes E, Cazin B et al. High remission rate in T-cell prolymphocytic leukemia with CAM-PATH-1H. Blood 2001;98:1721–6
5. McCune SL, Gockerman JP, Moore JO et al. Alemtuzumab in relapsed or refractory chronic lymphocytic leukemia and prolymphocytic leukemia. Leuk Lymphoma 2002;43:1007–11
6. Montillo M, Tedeschi A, O'Brien S et al. Phase II study of cladribine and cyclophosphamide in patients with chronic lymphocytic leukemia and prolymphocytic leukemia. Cancer 2003;97:114–20
7. Shvidel L, Shtalrid M, Bassous L et al. B-cell prolymphocytic leukemia: a survey of 35 patients emphasiz-ing heterogeneity, prognostic factors and evidence for a group with an indolent course. Leuk Lymphoma 1999;33:169–79
8. Valbuena JR, Herling M, Admirand JH et al. T-cell prolymphocytic leukemia involving extramedullary sites. Am J Clin Pathol 2005;123:456–64

**Web:**
1. http://www.leukemia.org          Leukemia Lymphoma Society

### 7.5.4     Hairy Cell Leukemia (HCL)

**J. Finke**

**Def:**     Low-grade leukemic lymphoma with clonal expansion of atypical B-lymphocytes ("hairy cells"). T-cell forms have been described in a small number of cases.

**ICD-10:**     C91.4

**Ep:**     Rare form of non-Hodgkin's lymphoma; incidence 2–3 cases/1,000,000/year, most patients are > 50 years of age, distribution male:female = 4:1

**Pg:**     *Characteristics of Neoplastic "Hairy Cells"*
- Typical morphology: lymphocytic cells with fine cytoplasmic projections
- B-lymphocytic origin, expression of CD19, CD20, CD22, FMC7
- Expression of the early plasma cell antigen PCA-1 and CD11c, CD25, CD103
- Negative for CD5, CD10, CD21, CD23
- Clonal immunoglobulin rearrangements

**Path:**     *Blood Smear*
- Relative lymphocytosis with "hairy cells"
- Moderate pancytopenia

*Bone Marrow*
Bone marrow initially hypercellular, in advanced disease stages hypocellular. Focal or diffuse infiltration (> 30%) with "hairy cell" lymphocyte population. Proliferation of argyrophilic fibers (reticulin), localized bone marrow fibrosis

**Class:**     *WHO classification (1994, 1998):* mature B-NHL

**Sy:**     During the asymptomatic stages, incidental diagnosis. The main symptom is pronounced splenomegaly, not lymphadenopathy.
- Splenomegaly, "splenic tumor," abdominal symptoms: 75–95% of cases
- Hepatomegaly: 40%
- Lymphadenopathy: 5%
- Malaise, fatigue, reduced performance: 80%
- Infections: 30%
- Monocytopenia: 90%
- Thrombocytopenia: 80%
- Neutropenia: 66%
- Pancytopenia: 40%
- Hemorrhagic complications, ecchymoses: 25%

**Dg:**     *Medical History, Physical Examination*
Physical examination including splenomegaly, hepatomegaly, lymph node status, signs of hemorrhage, signs of infection

*Laboratory Tests*
- Full blood count with differential, reticulocytes: pancytopenia, characteristic leukopenia, particularly monocytopenia; diagnosis based on hairy cell morphology
- Routine laboratory tests including urea + electrolytes, serum creatinine, bilirubin, liver function tests, LDH, CRP
- Detection of tartrate-resistant acid phosphatase (TRAP) and annexin 1 (ANXA1)
- Surface marker analysis (FACS): immunocytological determination of the key markers of hairy cell leukemia: CD25+, CD11c+,FMC7+,CD103+; negative for CD5, CD10, CD23

### Bone Marrow Cytology and Histology
- Lymphocytic infiltration, "hairy cells," bone marrow fibrosis
- *NOTE*: bone marrow aspiration is often impossible (dry tap due to bone marrow fibrosis) → diagnosis based on biopsy

### Imaging
Chest x-ray, abdominal ultrasound

**Dd:**
- Splenomegaly and lymphadenopathy with other lymphatic diseases, particularly CLL, immunocytoma, prolymphocytic leukemia, mantle cell lymphoma
- Pancytopenia due to bone marrow involvement with other diseases (acute leukemia, lymphomas, myeloproliferative syndromes, solid tumors)
- Myelodysplasia or aplastic anemia

**Co:**
- Infections
- Hemorrhagic complications
- Association with polyarteritis nodosa, vasculitis, and rheumatoid arthritis

**Th:**

## Treatment Concept

- Hairy cell leukemia is a generalized disease. New systemic therapies offer treatment with curative intent.
- Chemotherapy with 2-chlorodeoxyadenosine (2-CDA) is indicated as soon as the diagnosis is established, particularly in cases associated with anemia or thrombocytopenia.
- Splenectomy used to be common practice but is now only indicated in individual cases (severe hypersplenism, ruptured spleen, etc.).

## Types of Treatment

The most effective compound is 2-chlorodeoxyadenosine (2-CDA). Also effective are deoxycoformycin (DCF, pentostatin) and interferon-α, while experience with fludarabine is limited.

### 2-Chlorodeoxyadenosine (2-CDA, Cladribine)
- Purine analog, selectively lymphocytotoxic antimetabolite; drug of choice in the treatment of hairy cell leukemia
- Side effects: transient bone marrow suppression, nausea (in rare cases: vomiting, headache, fatigue); damage to normal lymphocytes with depletion of CD4+ T-cells; *Pneumocystis carinii* prophylaxis (co-trimoxazole) recommended
- Two treatment cycles achieve durable complete remission (CR) in 95% of patients. Overall survival after 12 years: 79%. 2-CDA is also effective after treatment failure with interferon-α or deoxycoformycin (pentostatin)

### Deoxycoformycin (DCF)
- Purine analog, selectively lymphocytotoxic antimetabolite
- Alternative to 2-CDA in the treatment of hairy cell leukemia
- Side effects: transient bone marrow suppression, mild depletion of CD4+ T-cells, reversible skin rash, headaches, fatigue
- High remission rates (CR 75–90%)

### Interferon-α
- Effective therapy: remission rate (CR + PR) 80–90%, but only 5–15% complete remissions; median duration of remission 25 months
- Side effects: flu-like syndrome, gastrointestinal disorders, central nervous disorders, peripheral neuropathy
- Where required: concomitant medication with 500–1,000 mg paracetamol

### Treatment Failure

In cases of treatment failure: retreatment with purine analogs. New treatment options: rituximab (anti-CD20, monoclonal antibody, ▶ NHL), BL22 (anti-CD22, monoclonal antibody fused to *Pseudomonas* exotoxin, in clinical trials).

## Chemotherapy Protocols

| "2-CDA" ▶ Protocol 11.5.7 | | | *Start next cycle on day 22* | |
|---|---|---|---|---|
| 2-CDA | 0.14 mg/kg/day | i.v. | Day 1–5, s.c. or i.v. | |

| "Pentostatin" ▶ Protocol 11.5.8 | | | *Start next cycle on day 15, 3–5 cycles* | |
|---|---|---|---|---|
| Pentostatin | 4 mg/m²/day | i.v. | Day 1 | |

| "Interferon α" | | | *12-month therapy* | |
|---|---|---|---|---|
| Interferon α | $3 \times 10^6$ U | s.c. | 3 × weekly | |

**Prg:**
- Prior to availability of interferon-α / purine analogs: median survival 3 years
- Five-year survival after treatment with 2-CDA or pentostatin: 70–90%, after treatment with interferon-α: 20–30%

**F/U:**  Blood count, bone marrow. Initially, close monitoring, subsequently at 3-monthly intervals.

**Ref:**
1. Else M, Ruchlemer R, Osuji N et al. Long remissions in hairy cell leukemia with purine analogues. Cancer 2005;104:2442–8
2. Falini B, Tiacci E, Liso A et al. Simple diagnostic assay for hairy cell leukaemia by immunocytochemical detection of annexin A1 (ANXA1). Lancet 2004;363:1869–71
3. Goodman GR, Bethel KJ, Saven A. Hairy cell leukemia: an update. Curr Opin Hematol 2003;10:258–66
4. Jehn U, Bartl R, Dietzfelbinger H et al. An update: 12-year follow-up of patients with hairy cell leukemia following treatment with 2-chlorodeoxyadenosine. Leukemia 2004;18:1476–81
5. Tiacci E, Liso A, Piris M et al. Evolving concepts in the pathogenensis of hairy-cell leukemia. Nat Rev Cancer 2006; 6:437–48
6. Wanko SO, De Castro C. Hairy cell leukemia. Oncologist 2006;11:780–9

**Web:**
1. http://www.emedicine.com/med/topic937.htm          E-medicine
2. http://www.lls.org/          Leukemia Lymphoma Soc
3. http://www.cancer.gov/cancertopics/pdq/treatment/hairy-cell-leukemia          Cancer Topics
4. http://www.nlm.nih.gov/medlineplus/ency/article/000592.htm          MedlinePlus
5. http://www.hairycellleukemia.org          HCL Res Foundation

## 7.5.5 Follicular Lymphoma (FL)

J. Finke

**Def:** Low-grade non-Hodgkin's lymphoma; originating from follicular center of lymphoid organs. Synonyms: follicular center lymphoma (FCL), indolent lymphoma

**ICD-10:** C91

**Ep:** 15–20% of all non-Hodgkin's lymphomas, especially in western Europe and North America (low incidence rates in Asia). Median age at diagnosis 40–60 years

**Pg:** *Pathogenesis*
Originates from B cells at the center of the lymph follicle ("follicular center lymphoma")

*Molecular Changes*
t(14;18) translocation detectable in the majority of cases of FL
→ Translocation of the bcl-2 gene on chromosome 18 and the immunoglobulin heavy chain locus on chromosome 14 (detection via polymerase chain reaction, PCR)
→ bcl-2 expression ↑, inhibition of apoptosis
→ Survival advantage for FL cells, resistance to cytostatics

*Characteristics of FL Cells*
FACS analysis: FL cells negative for CD5, positive for CD19, CD20, ± CD10

**Path:** *Peripheral Blood*
- Leukemic form: centrocytes in blood smear
- With bone marrow involvement: anemia, thrombocytopenia, granulocytopenia

*Lymph Nodes*
- Lymphadenopathy
- Characteristic lymph node histology

*Bone Marrow / Organ Involvement*
At the time of diagnosis: liver, spleen, or bone marrow involvement in 80% of cases (stage IV).

**Class:** *WHO Classification (2000), REAL Classification (1994)*
Follicular lymphoma (FL), mature B-NHL, grade I–III. *NOTE:* Grade III FL is considered a high grade lymphoma, because of more aggressive course and poor prognosis (▶ Chap. 7.5.1)

*Staging*
According to Ann Arbor (1971), stages I–IV, with/without B symptoms (▶ Chap. 7.5)

**Sy:** In localized stages of disease usually asymptomatic (often incidental diagnosis)

*Advanced Disease*
- Fatigue, reduced performance, pallor (anemia)
- B symptoms (fever, night sweats, weight loss)
- Indolent lymphadenopathy
- Splenomegaly with abdominal symptoms, hepatomegaly
- Cutaneous infiltration, organ involvement (lung → respiratory disorders, CNS → neurological disorders)
- Opportunistic infections (pneumonia, *H. zoster*, *P. carinii*), antibody deficiency syndrome

**Dg:** *Medical History, Physical Examination*
- Medical history including disease course

- Physical examination including lymph node status, spleen / liver, skin, neurological status, signs of infection, signs of hemorrhage

### Laboratory Tests
- Full blood count (anemia, thrombocytopenia, granulocytopenia) with blood smear (centrocytes), reticulocytes
- Routine laboratory tests including urea + electrolytes, serum creatinine, bilirubin, liver function tests, LDH ↑, CRP
- Immunology: quantitative serum immunoglobulin levels, immunoelectrophoresis
- Surface marker expression: FACS analysis (CD5, CD10, CD19, CD20, CD22, CD23)

### Imaging
- Chest x-ray, abdominal ultrasound
- In case of localized disease (stages I / II): CT thorax/abdomen/pelvis, possibly cranial MRI to exclude a higher stage

### Histology: Mandatory for Diagnosis
- Lymph node biopsy, with histology / immunohistology
- Bone marrow biopsy and aspirate

**Histological classification (grading) of follicular lymphoma**

| Grade | Centroblasts per HPF (high power field) |
|-------|------------------------------------------|
| I | 0–5 centroblasts |
| II | 6–15 centroblasts |
| III | > 15 centroblasts |
| IIIA | > 15 centroblasts, presence of centrocytes |
| IIIB | > 15 centroblasts, without centrocytes |

**DD:**     High-grade lymphomas, CLL, Hodgkin's disease

**Co:**
- Infections
- With longer duration of disease, risk of transformation into high-grade lymphoma with poor prognosis (cumulative risk after 10 years: approximately 30%)

**Th:**     **Therapeutic approach to follicular lymphoma**

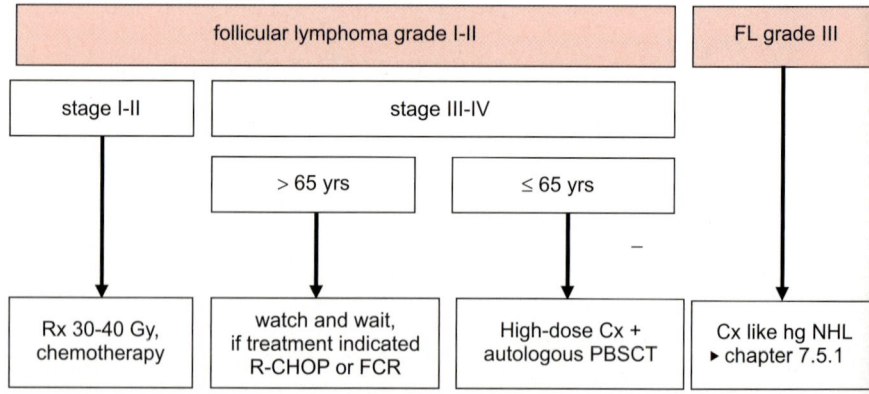

*Rx* radiotherapy, *Cx* chemotherapy, *PBSCT* peripheral blood stem cell transplantation, *FCL* follicular lymphoma, *hg NHL* high grade Non-Hodgkin's lymphoma

**Treatment Concept**

1. Treatment is stage-specific.
2. Patients with localized disease stages I–II (15–20% of patients) are primarily treated with local therapy. Extended-field radiotherapy with 30–40 Gy represents a curative treatment approach.
3. Patients with advanced disease stages III–IV (80–85%) require systemic treatment. Conventional chemotherapy is generally regarded as palliative. Rituximab in addition to chemotherapy has improved response rates and time to progression.
4. FL frequently shows slow disease progression or a stable, fluctuating and indolent course over many years (30% of patients). Treatment is indicated in case of:
   - Curative radiotherapy in early stages of disease
   - Symptomatic lymphadenopathy or splenomegaly
   - Overt B symptoms
   - Peripheral cytopenia due to bone marrow infiltration
   - Immunodeficiency with recurrent infections

**Types of Treatment**

*Ann Arbor Stages I–II*
- Extended field radiotherapy, total dose 30–40 Gy; 5-year relapse-free survival 50–75% (late relapses are possible)
- Alternatively: combined chemotherapy (4 cycles of R-CHOP) and radiotherapy (involved field) analogous to high-grade NHL (trials)
- Diagnosis of stage I after diagnostic R0 resection: "watch and wait" approach possible

*Ann Arbor Stages III–IV and Symptoms*
- Palliative chemotherapy (e.g., FCR, R-CHOP).
- Purine analogs (fludarabine, 2-chlorodeoxyadenosine) and rituximab (anti-CD20) have proven to be effective. In first line treatment, combination of fludarabine, cyclophosphamide, and rituximab (FCR protocol, 82% CR).
- *ATTENTION:* Immunosuppression → pneumocystis carinii (jiroveci) pneumonia (PCP) prophylaxis with co-trimoxazole required.
- Interferon-α as maintenance treatment has no influence on overall survival.
- The treatment of FCL°III is analogous to that of blastoid MCL and high-grade (DLCL) NHL (▶ Chap. 7.5.1).

*New Therapy Approaches*
- In cases refractory to chemotherapy, radioconjugated antibodies have demonstrated efficacy → e.g., $^{131}$I-anti-CD20 (Tositumomab) or $^{90}$Y-anti-CD20 (Ibritumomab)
- Vaccination strategies with lymphoma-specific anti-idiotypic immunoglobulins

*High-risk Situations*
In high-risk cases and patients with poor prognosis (relapse): consider high-dose therapy and autologous transplantation (PBSCT). Allogeneic transplantation protocols with reduced-intensity conditioning regimens may be useful in aggressive disease and relapse after autologous PBSCT.

### Chemotherapy Protocols

| "R-CHOP" ▶ Protocol 11.4.3 | | | *Start next cycle on day 22* |
|---|---|---|---|
| Rituximab | 375 mg/m² | i.v. | Day 0 (24–4 h prior to CHOP) |
| Cyclophosphamide | 750 mg/m²/day | i.v. | Day 1 |
| Doxorubicin | 50 mg/m²/day | i.v. | Day 1 |
| Vincristine | 1.4 mg/m²/day | i.v. | Day 1, max. single dose: 2 mg absolute |
| Prednisolone | 100 mg absolute | p.o. | Day 1–5 |

| "Fludarabine" ▶ Protocol 11.5.2 | | | *Start next cycle on day 29* |
|---|---|---|---|
| Fludarabine | 25 mg/m²/day | i.v. | Day 1–5 |

| "FCR" ▶ Protocol 11.5.4 | | | *Start next cycle on day 28* |
|---|---|---|---|
| Rituximab | 375 mg/m²/day | i.v. | Day 1 |
| Fludarabine | 30 mg/m²/day | i.v. | Day 2–4 |
| Cyclophosphamide | 300 mg/m²/day | i.v. | Day 2–4 |

| "Bendamustine" ▶ Protocol 11.5.1 | | | *Start next cycle on day 22–29* |
|---|---|---|---|
| Bendamustine | 100 mg/m²/day | i.v. | Day 1–2 |

| "Rituximab" ▶ Protocol 11.5.9 | | | |
|---|---|---|---|
| Rituximab | 375 mg/m²/day | i.v. | Day 1, 8, 15, 22 |

**Prg:**

### Survival Time

The median survival of conventionally treated FL patients (without transplantation) is approximately 8–10 years. In up to 30% of patients, transformation to high-grade lymphoma may occur within 10 years.

Risk factors according to "Follicular Lymphoma International Prognostic Index" (FL-IPI):
- Age > 60 years
- Ann Arbor stages III–IV
- Increased LDH
- Hemoglobin < 12 g/dl
- > 4 lymph node areas affected

**Prognosis according to FL-IPI**

| Risk group | Number of risk factors | Percent of patients (%) | Overall survival (%) | |
|---|---|---|---|---|
| | | | Five years | Ten years |
| Low | 0–1 | 36 | 91 | 71 |
| Intermediate | 2 | 37 | 78 | 51 |
| High | ≥ 3 | 27 | 53 | 36 |

**F/U:**
- In cases of advanced disease and palliative therapy: symptom-based approach
- Early disease stages, potentially curative radiotherapy or patient participating in trial on myeloablative radiochemotherapy: monitor closely or proceed according to study protocol

**Ref:**
1. Advani R, Rosenberg SA, Horning SJ. Stage I and II follicular non-Hodgkin's lymphoma: long-term follow-up of no initial therapy. J Clin Oncol 2005;22:1454–9
2. Bende RJ, Smit LA, Van Noessel CJM. Molecular pathways in follicular lymphoma. Leukemia 2007;21:18–29.
3. Brown J, Feng Y, Gribben JG. Long-term survival after autologous bone marrow transplantation for follicular lymphoma in first remission. Biol Blood Marrow Transpl 2007;12:1057–65.
4. ESMO Guidelines Working Group. Newly diagnosed follicular lymphoma: ESMO Clinical Recommendations for diagnosis, treatment and follow-up. Ann Oncol 2008;18(Suppl.2):ii63–4
5. Hiddemann W, Buske C, Dreyling M et al. Current management of follicular lymphomas. Br J Haematol 2006;136:191–202
6. Kaminski MS, Tuck M, Estes J et al. [131]I-tositumomab therapy as initial treatment for follicular lymphoma. N Engl J Med 2005;352:441–9
7. Solal-Celigny P, Roy P, Colombat P et al. Follicular Lymphoma International Prognostic Index. Blood 2004;104:1258–65
8. Staudt LM. A closer look at follicular lymphoma. N Engl J Med 2007;356;741–2.

**Web:**
1. www.lymphomainfo.net/nhl/follicular.html          Lymphoma Info Network
2. www.emedicine.com/med/topic1362.htm              E-medicine
3. http://www.lymphomation.org/type-follicular.htm  Lymphoma Info Portal
4. http://www.lls.org/                              Leukemia Lymphoma Soc
5. http://www.cancer.gov/cancertopics/pdq/treatment/ adult-non-hodgkins/healthprofessional          NCI, Cancer Topics

## 7.5.6    Mantle Cell Lymphoma (MCL)

J. Finke

**Def:**  Low-grade lymphoma; mantle cell lymphoma, MCL (WHO)

**ICD-10:**  C91

**Ep:**  3–5% of all non-Hodgkin's lymphomas, median age 60–70 years

**Pg:**
- Originates in the mantle zone of the lymphoid follicle ("mantle cell lymphoma")
- Characteristic translocation t(11;14)(q13;q32), involves bcl-1 and immunoglobulin locus
- Cyclin D1 synthesis ↑, Rb phosphorylation ↑, loss of cell cycle control, proliferation ↑
- FACS analysis: cells positive for CD5, CD19, CD20, CD22, negative for CD10, CD23
- Histology: detection of cyclin D1 expression (prognostically relevant)

**Path:**  *Peripheral Blood*
- Leukemic form: centrocytes in blood smear
- With bone marrow involvement: anemia, thrombocytopenia, granulocytopenia

*Lymph Nodes*
- Lymphadenopathy
- Characteristic lymph node histology

*Bone Marrow / Organ Involvement*
At the time of diagnosis: liver, spleen, or bone marrow involvement in 60% of cases.

**Class:**  *WHO Classification (2000), REAL Classification (1994)*
- Mantle cell lymphoma (MCL)

*Staging*
According to Ann Arbor (1971), stages I–IV, with/without B symptoms (▶ Chap. 7.5)

**Sy:**  During localized stages of the disease: usually asymptomatic (often incidental diagnosis).

*Advanced Disease*
- Fatigue, reduced performance, pallor (anemia)
- B symptoms (fever, night sweats, weight loss)
- Indolent lymphadenopathy
- Splenomegaly with abdominal symptoms
- Hepatomegaly
- Skin and organ involvement (lung → respiratory disorders, CNS → neurological disorders)
- Opportunistic infections (pneumonia, *H. zoster*, *P. carinii*), antibody deficiency syndrome

**Dg:**  *Medical History, Physical Examination*
- Medical history including disease course
- Physical examination including lymph node status, spleen / liver, skin, neurological status, signs of infection, signs of hemorrhage

*Laboratory Tests*
- Complete blood count (anemia, thrombocytopenia, granulocytopenia) with differential and blood smear (centrocytes), reticulocytes
- Routine laboratory tests including urea + electrolytes, serum creatinine, bilirubin, liver function tests, LDH ↑, CRP
- Immunology: quantitative serum immunoglobulin levels, immunoelectrophoresis
- Surface marker expression: FACS analysis (CD5, CD10, CD19, CD20, CD22, CD23)

### Histology: Mandatory for Diagnosis
- Lymph node biopsy, with histology / immunohistology
- Bone marrow biopsy and aspirate

### Imaging
- Chest x-ray, abdominal ultrasound
- In localized disease stages (Ann Arbor I / II): CT thorax/abdomen/pelvis, possibly cranial MRI to exclude a higher stage
- Possibly esophago-gastro-duodenoscopy (exclusion of gastrointestinal involvement, "lymphoid polyposis")

**DD:**   High-grade lymphoma, CLL, FCL

**Co:**   Infections

**Th:**   
## Treatment Concept

1. Treatment is stage-specific.
2. Patients with localized disease (stages I–II) are primarily treated with locally effective forms of therapy. Extended-field radiotherapy with 30–40 Gy represents a curative treatment option.
3. Patients with advanced disease (stages III–IV) require systemic treatment modalities. Conventional chemotherapy is to be regarded as palliative treatment.
4. MCL is characterized by poor prognosis, poor response to treatment, and rapid disease progression → initiation of therapy at time of diagnosis, particularly in patients with early stages of the disease.
5. High-dose chemotherapy with transplantation of allogeneic or autologous hematopoietic stem cells is a potentially curative treatment option in younger patients.

## Types of Treatment

### Ann Arbor Stages I–II
- Extended field radiotherapy, total dose 30–40 Gy; 5-year relapse-free survival 50–75% (late relapses are possible)
- Alternatively: combined chemotherapy (3 cycles of CHOP) and radiotherapy (involved field) analogous to high-grade NHL

### Ann Arbor Stages III–IV
Palliative chemotherapy, e.g.:
- CHOP + rituximab (R-CHOP)
- Rituximab + fludarabine + cyclophosphamide + mitoxantrone (R-FCM)

### New Therapy Approaches
- Purine analogs, (fludarabine, 2-chlorodeoxyadenosine) and rituximab (anti CD-20) have demonstrated efficacy in MCL.
- Bortezomib alone or in combination.
- In cases refractory to chemotherapy, antibodies may be effective, e.g., anti-CD20 (rituximab). Radioconjugated antibodies: $^{131}$I-anti-CD20 (tositumomab) or $^{90}$Y-anti-CD20 (ibritumomab) are currently being evaluated in clinical trials.
- The value of high-dose therapy with autologous stem cell transplantation (SCT) in first remission has been confirmed in several clinical trials. High-dose therapy with allogeneic transplantation may be a curative treatment option in selected patients. Several conditioning protocols are currently being evaluated in trials.

### Chemotherapy Protocols

| "CHOP" ▶ Protocol 11.4.2/11.4.3 | | | Start next cycle on day 22 |
|---|---|---|---|
| Cyclophosphamide | 750 mg/m²/day | i.v. | Day 1 |
| Doxorubicin | 50 mg/m²/day | i.v. | Day 1 |
| Vincristine | 1.4 mg/m²/day | i.v. | Day 1, max. single dose: 2 mg absolute |
| Prednisolone | 100 mg absolute | p.o. | Day 1–5 |
| ± Rituximab | 375 mg/m² | i.v | Day 0 (24-4 h prior to CHOP) |

| "Bendamustin" ▶ Protocol 11.5.1 | | | Start next cycle on day 22–29 |
|---|---|---|---|
| Bendamustin | 100 mg/m²/day | i.v. | Day 1–2 |

| "Fludarabine" ▶ Protocol 11.5.2 | | | Start next cycle on day 29 |
|---|---|---|---|
| Fludarabine | 25 mg/m²/day | i.v. | Day 1–5 |

| "Rituximab" ▶ Protocol 11.5.9 | | | |
|---|---|---|---|
| Rituximab | 375 mg/m²/day | i.v. | Day 1, 8, 15, 22 |

| "COP" ▶ Protocol 11.4.5 | | | Start next cycle on day 22 |
|---|---|---|---|
| Cyclophosphamide | 400 mg/m²/day | i.v | Day 1–5 |
| Vincristine | 1.4 mg/m²/day | i.v. | Day 1, max. single dose: 2 mg absolute |
| Prednisolone | 100 mg/m²/day | p.o. | Day 1–5 |

**Prg:**

### Negative Prognostic Factors
- Ann Arbor III–IV
- Splenomegaly, hepatosplenomegaly, extranodal manifestation, B symptoms
- Anemia, pathological liver function, increased LDH, increased β2-microglobulin
- Karnofsky index ≤ 70% at time of initial diagnosis
- Therapy resistance: no complete remission after initial therapy
- "International Prognostic Index" (IPI) (▶ Chap. 7.5.1)

### Survival Time
- Median survival 4 years, in advanced stages < 2 years.

**F/U:**
- In advanced disease and palliative setting: symptom-based approach

**Ref:**
1. Bertoni F, Zucca E, Cavalli F. Mantle cell lymphoma. Curr Opin Hematol 2004;11:411–8
2. Fernàndez V, Hartmann E, Ott G et al. Pathogenesis of mantle cell lymphoma: all oncogenic roads lead to dysregulation of cell cycle and DNA damage response pathways. J Clin Oncol 2005;23:6364–9
3. Hagemeister FB. Mantle cell lymphoma: non-myeloablative vs. dose-intensive therapy. Leuk Lymphoma 2003;44(suppl 3):S69–75
4. Kiss TL, Mollee P, Lazarus HM et al. Stem cell transplantation for mantle cell lymphoma: if, when and how? Bone Marrow Transplant 2005;36:655–61
5. Lenz G, Dreyling M, Hiddemann W. Mantle cell lymphoma: established therapeutic options and future directions. Ann Hematol 2004;83:71–7
6. Leonard JP, Schattner EJ, Coleman M. Biology and management of mantle cell lymphoma. Curr Opin Oncol 2001;13:342–7
7. Witzig TE. Current treatment approaches for mantle cell lymphoma. J Clin Oncol 2005;23:6409–14
8. Zelenetz AD. Mantle cell lymphoma. Ann Oncol 2006;17(suppl 4):iv12–4

**Web:**
1. http://www.lymphomainfo.net/nhl/types/mantle.html          Lymphoma Info Network
2. http://www.emedicine.com/med/topic1361.htm                 E-medicine
3. http://www.lymphomation.org/type-MCL.htm                   Lymphoma Info Portal
4. http://www.cancerbackup.org.uk/Cancertype/
   Lymphomanon-Hodgkins/TypesofNHL/Mantlecell                Cancer BACKUP

**7.5.7     Primary Cutaneous T-cell Lymphoma (CTCL)**

J. Finke

**Def:**     *Mycosis Fungoides (MF)*
Most common non-Hodgkin's T-cell lymphoma, clonal proliferation of CD4+ T-lymphocytes. Localized or generalized cutaneous manifestation, in advanced stages systemic manifestation with organ involvement.

*Sézary Syndrome (SS)*
Leukemic form of mycosis fungoides with generalized exfoliative erythroderma, organ involvement, evidence of circulating Sézary cells, and poor prognosis.

**ICD-10:**     C84

**Ep:**     Rare. Incidence of mycosis fungoides: 3–4 cases/1,000,000/year; age 30–70 years; male:female = 3:2; Sézary syndrome: 0.2 cases/1,000,000/year

70% of cutaneous lymphoma are of T-cell origin. 90% of cutaneous T-cell NHL are T-helper cell lymphomas (CD4+).

**Pg:**     *Risk Factors*
- Long-standing dermatitis
- No conclusive association to viruses, ionizing radiation, chemicals, or drugs

**Path:**     *Disease Course*
Protracted, over many years. Often manifestation of cutaneous infiltrates of uncertain significance (even retrospective) preceding diagnosis.
- Cutaneous involvement: erythrodermal, plaque-like, tumorous
- Systemic involvement: lymph nodes, organs, bone marrow

*Mycosis Fungoides*
- Mycosis cells (Lutzner cells): atypical T-cells with irregular cerebriform nuclei; phenotypically mature T-helper cells, positive for CD2, CD3, CD4, CD5, CD25
- Rearrangements of clonal T-cell-receptor genes
- Cytogenetics: chromosomal aberrations of 1p, 10q, 17p, 19 possible
- Linear infiltration at the border between dermis and epidermis with invasion of the epithelium
- Pautrier's microabscesses: intraepidermal accumulation of mycosis cells, interdigitating reticulum cells and Langerhans cells

*Sézary Syndrome*
- Sézary cells: circulating type of mycosis (Lutzner) cells in the peripheral blood
- Erythroderma with dense mycosis / Sézary cell infiltrates

**Class:**     *WHO Classification (2001)*
Mature T-cell lymphoma, mycosis fungoides / Sézary syndrome

**WHO-EORTC classification of primary cutaneous lymphomas (2005)**

| | |
|---|---:|
| *Cutaneous T-cell and NK cell lymphoma* | 75% |
| • Mycosis fungoides (MF) | |
| • MF variants (folliculotropic / pagetoid / granulomatous) | |
| • Sézary syndrome (SS) | |
| • Adult T-cell leukemia / lymphoma | |
| • Primary cutaneous CD30+ lymphoproliferative diseases | |
|    – Anaplastic large-cell lymphoma | |
|    – Lymphomatoid papulosis | |
| • Subcutaneous panniculitis-like T-cell lymphoma | |
| • Extranodal NK / T-cell lymphoma, nasal type | |
| • Primary cutaneous peripheral T-cell lymphoma | |
| *Cutaneous B-cell lymphomas* | 25% |
| • Primary cutaneous marginal zone lymphoma | |
| • Primary cutaneous follicular lymphoma | |
| • Primary cutaneous diffuse large-cell lymphoma | |
| *Progenitor neoplasia* | Rare |
| • CD4+ / CD56+ blastic NK cell lymphoma | |

**Staging according to MFCG (Mycosis Fungoides Cooperative Group)**

| Stage | Definition |
|---|---|
| *T* | *Primary Skin Lesion* |
| T0 | No clinically abnormal lesions; histology negative |
| T1 | Premycotic lesions, papules, or plaques covering < 10% of the skin surface |
| T2 | Premycotic lesions, papules, or plaques covering > 10% of the skin surface |
| T3 | One or more cutaneous tumors |
| T4 | Generalized erythroderma |
| *N* | *Involvement of Peripheral Lymph Nodes* |
| N0 | No clinically abnormal lymph nodes; histology negative |
| N1 | Clinically abnormal peripheral lymph nodes; histology negative[a] |
| N2 | No clinically abnormal lymph nodes; histology positive |
| N3 | Clinically abnormal lymph nodes; histology positive |
| *M* | *Involvement of Visceral Organs / Bone Marrow* |
| M1 | No visceral involvement |
| M2 | Visceral involvement and/or bone marrow infiltration > 40%; histology positive |
| *B* | *Leukemic Form* |
| B0 | ≤ 5% of circulating cells are atypical |
| B1 | > 5% of circulating cells are atypical |

[a] In histologically negative but clinically enlarged lymph nodes, disease may be detectable by use of sensitive techniques (e.g., detection of T-cell receptor rearrangements)

**Staging according to AJCC**

| Stage | MFCG staging | | | Median survival (years) |
|-------|--------------|------|------|-------------------------|
| IA | T1 | N0 | M0 | 8–12 |
| IB | T2 | N0 | M0 | |
| IIA | T1–2 | N1 | M0 | 4–8 |
| IIB | T3 | N0–1 | M0 | |
| III | T4 | N0–1 | M0 | 3–4 |
| IVA | All Ts | N2–3 | M0 | 2–3 |
| IVB | All Ts | All Ns | M1 | < 1 |

**Sy:**

### General Symptoms
- Fatigue, reduced performance, weight loss
- Lymphadenopathy
- Liver / spleen involvement with hepatomegaly / splenomegaly
- Organ involvement and dysfunction (lung, CNS, etc.)

### Skin Symptoms
Highly variable and fluctuating symptoms:
- "Premycotic stage": pruritus, eczematoid skin lesions, localized or generalized, alopecia, palmar / plantar keratosis
- "Plaque stage": rough infiltrating skin lesions; with facial involvement
- "Tumor stage": spontaneously disintegrating ulcerating skin tumors
- Erythroderma with exfoliation, edema, lichenification, pruritus

**Dg:**

### Medical History, Physical Examination
- Medical history including risk factors, skin lesions
- Physical examination including skin, lymph node status, spleen / liver, signs of hemorrhage, signs of infection

### Laboratory Tests
- Full blood count including differential, reticulocytes, blood smear
- Routine laboratory including electrolytes, liver / renal function tests, LDH, CRP
- Immunocytological examination via FACS analysis: CD4+ cells

### Histology
- Skin biopsy with immunohistology
- Bone marrow biopsy and aspirate, with immunocytology/ -histology
- Lymph node biopsy where required

### Imaging
Chest x-ray, abdominal ultrasound

**DD:**
- Eczematous skin diseases (psoriasis, dermatitis), contact eczema, allergic skin disorders
- Skin infiltration with other hematological neoplasia: T-ALL, T-PLL, peripheral T-cell lymphomas, T-CLL, B-cell neoplasia
- Primary skin tumors
- Lymphomatoid papulosis (LP)

**Co:**
- Infections (common cause of death with cutaneous T-cell lymphomas)
- Cytopenia

**Th:** **Treatment Concept**

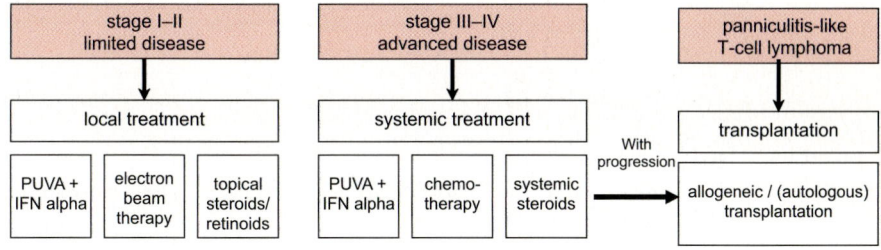

*PUVA* psoralen + UVA phototherapy, *IFN* interferon

## Types of Treatment

### Limited Stages (Stages I–II): External Treatment
- PUVA (psoralen + UVA phototherapy) + 9 MIU interferon-α s.c. 3 times weekly: complete remission (CR) in 60–90% of cases, median time to CR: 18 weeks, long-term remission in up to 25% of cases
- Radiotherapy (local or total skin irradiation) with accelerated electrons: 40–80% CR, long-term remission in 20–40% of cases
- Topical use of corticosteroids, nitrogen mustard (Mustargen), BCNU, or retinoids (isotretinoin)
- Extracorporeal photopheresis

### Advanced Stages (Stages III–IV): Systemic Treatment
- Interferon-α, e.g., 12 MIU/m²/day s.c. 3 times weekly: dose escalation if well tolerated, also effective in PUVA-resistant patients, response rate > 65%
- Interferon-α in combination with PUVA: > 60% complete remission (CR)
- Systemic application of steroids
- Systemic chemotherapy: purine analogs (fludarabine, 2-CDA, pentostatin), alkylating agents (cyclophosphamide, chlorambucil), combination chemotherapy protocols (COP, CHOP), low-dose methotrexate (+ folic acid)

### New Therapies
- Denileukin diftitox (Ontak, licensed in USA): fusion protein consisting of interleukin-2, the cytotoxic A-chain and the translocated B-chain of diphtheria toxin; target is the high-affinity IL-2 receptor (CD25, expressed in cutaneous T-cell lymphomas, non-Hodgkin's lymphomas, and Hodgkin's disease)
- Alemtuzumab: effective in the treatment of CD52-expressing CTCL
- Transplantation (autologous, allogeneic): justified in patients with subcutaneous panniculitis-like T-cell lymphoma due to the poor prognosis; induction with fludarabine-containing combinations
- Vorinostat: histone deacetylase inhibitor, 400 mg/d p.o., response rate 30%

## Chemotherapy Protocols

| *"Fludarabine"* ▶ *Protocol 11.5.2* | | | *Start next cycle on day 29* |
|---|---|---|---|
| Fludarabine | 25 mg/m²/day | i.v. | Day 1–5 |

| *"2-CDA"* ▶ *Protocol 11.5.7* | | | *Start next cycle on day 22* |
|---|---|---|---|
| 2-CDA | 0.14 mg/kg/day | i.v. | Day 1–5 |

| *"CHOP"* ▶ *Protocol 11.4.2* | | | *Start next cycle on day 22* |
|---|---|---|---|
| Cyclophosphamide | 750 mg/m²/day | i.v. | Day 1 |
| Doxorubicin | 50 mg/m²/day | i.v. | Day 1 |
| Vincristine | 1.4 mg/m²/day | i.v. | Day 1, max. single dose: 2 mg |
| Prednisolone | 100 mg absolute | p.o. | Day 1–5 |

| *"COP"* ▶ *Protocol 11.4.5* | | | *Start next cycle on day 22* |
|---|---|---|---|
| Cyclophosphamide | 400 mg/m²/day | i.v. | Day 1-5 |
| Vincristine | 1.4 mg/m²/day | i.v. | Day 1, max. single dose: 2 mg |
| Prednisolone | 100 mg/m²/day | p.o. | Day 1–5 |

**Prg:**

### Mycosis Fungoides

Good prognosis, in most cases slow progression; potential long-term survival: 20–30 years, median survival after diagnosis: 8–9 years.

### CD30-positive Primary Cutaneous T-cell Lymphoma

Local radiotherapy as needed; survival rate after 4 years: 90%.

### Lymphomatoid Papulosis (LyP)

Development of lymphomas in 80% of cases. Benign course in 20% of cases.

### Sézary Syndrome

Poor prognosis, rapid progression; clinical picture can be similar to T-cell leukemia; median survival < 18 months.

### Subcutaneous Panniculitis-like T-cell Lymphoma

Very poor prognosis.

With curative treatment intent: close follow-up; in palliative situations: symptom-based approach.

**Ref:**

1.  ESMO Guidelines Working Group. Primary cutaneous lymphomas: ESMO Clinical Recommendations for diagnosis, treatment and follow-up. Ann Oncol 2007;18(Suppl.2):ii61–2
2.  Foss F. Mycosis fungoides and the Sézary syndrome. Curr Opin Oncol 2004;16:421–8
3.  Girardi M, Heald PW, Wilson LD. The pathogenesis of mycosis fungoides. N Engl J Med 2004;350:1978–88
4.  Hwang ST, Janik JE, Jaffe ES et al. Mycosis fungoides and Sézary syndrome. Lancet 2008;371:945–57.
5.  Olsen E, Vonderheid E, Pimpinelli N et al. Revisions to the staging and classification of mycosis fungoides and Sézary syndrome: a proposal of the ISCL and the cutaneous lymphoma task force of the EORTC. Blood 2007;110:1713–22
6.  Querfeld C, Rosen ST, Guitart J et al. The spectrum of cutaneous T-cell lymphomas: new insights into biology and therapy. Curr Opin Hematol 2005;12:273–8
7.  Smith BD, Smith GL, Cooper DL et al. The cutaneous B-cell lymphoma prognostic index. J Clin Oncol 2005;23:3390–5
8.  Trautinger F, Knobler R, Willemze R et al. EORTC consensus recommendations for the treatment of mycosis fungoides / Sézary syndrome. Eur J Cancer 2006;42:1014–30

**Web:**

| | | |
|---|---|---|
| 1. | http://www.emedicine.com/MED/topic1541.htm | E-medicine |
| 2. | http://www.nci.nih.gov/cancertopics/pdq/treatment/ mycosisfungoides/HealthProfessional | NCI Cancer Topics |
| 3. | http://www.lymphomainfo.net/nhl/types/ctcl-mf.html | Lymphoma Info Network |
| 4. | http://www.clfoundation.org/ | Cutaneous Lymph Foundation |
| 5. | http://dermatlas.med.jhmi.edu/derm/ | Dermatology Atlas |

## 7.5.8 Primary Lymphoma of the Central Nervous System (CNS)

### G. Illerhaus, R. Marks, J. Finke

**Def:** Non-Hodgkin's lymphomas with primary location in the central nervous system (brain, meninges, eyes, spinal cord). Primary CNS lymphomas in immunocompetent patients are distinguished from lymphomas in the case of immunodeficiency.

**ICD-10:** C85.7

**Ep:** Incidence 2–5 cases/1,000,000 population/year; a markedly increased incidence has been observed in the last 10 years. Age peak: 45–70 years in immunocompetent patients, 30–40 years in immunodeficient patients; distribution male:female = 3:2. Primary cerebral NHL represent 4–7% of all CNS malignancies and 1–2% of all NHL.

**Pg:** *Primary CNS Lymphomas in Immunocompetent Patients*
- 50% of cases, incidence rising
- Etiological factors not clear

*Primary CNS Lymphomas in Immunodeficient Patients*
- 50% of cases, incidence rising
- Congenital / acquired immunodeficiency: congenital immunodeficiency syndrome, immunosuppressive therapy, AIDS patients (CD4+ cell count < 50/μl), allogeneic bone marrow / blood stem cell transplantation with T-cell depletion
- EBV (Epstein-Barr virus) or EBV genes or proteins (LMP-1, EBNA-2) identified in the lymphoma cells of 95% of immunodeficient patients
- Interference with apoptosis (e.g., transactivation of bcl-2 by LMP-1)

**Path:**
- Extensive meningeal involvement in up to 25% of cases; at autopsy: up to 90%
- Nodular perivascular infiltrates
- Usually B-cell lymphomas, T-cell lymphomas are rare (< 1%)
- Location: supratentorial 67–75%, infratentorial 25–33%, multiple / disseminated 20–30% of cases, ocular involvement in approximately 10–15% of cases

**Class:** **Histological classification**

| Type | Frequency (%) |
|------|---------------|
| Diffuse large-B-cell lymphoma | 80–90 |
| Burkitt's lymphoma, low-grade NHL, non-classifiable NHL | 10–20 |

**Sy:**
- Focal neurological symptoms:                          50%
- Hemiparesis:                                          35%
- Cranial nerve palsies:                                10%
- Impaired vision:                                      10%
- Personality changes:                                  36%
- B symptoms (fever, night sweats, weight loss):        12%
- Signs of increased intracranial pressure:             19%
- Fatigue, reduced performance, weight loss:            45%

**Dg:** *Medical History, Physical Examination*
- Evidence of risk factors: immunodeficiency, EBV infection
- Physical examination: neurological status, lymph node status, spleen / liver
- Ophthalmological examination to exclude ocular involvement

### Laboratory Tests
- Complete blood count with differential, reticulocytes
- Routine laboratory tests including urea + electrolytes, serum creatinine, bilirubin, liver function tests, LDH, CRP
- Serology: HIV, EBV
- Immunocytology: CD4, CD8, CD3, CD19

### Histology
- Stereotactic (or open) biopsy of CNS lesions
- Histology, immunohistology, possibly cytology, surface marker analysis
- CSF examination (with immunocytology) → lymphoma diagnosed in 30%
- Bone marrow biopsy and aspirate if systemic disease is suspected or to exclude primary extra-cerebral lymphomas

### Imaging
- Cranial MRI, cranial PET
- CT chest / abdomen / pelvis to exclude systemic disease

Cerebral masses ALWAYS require a histological examination. 4% are primary cerebral NHL which may be curable. Avoid administration of steroids prior to biopsy (otherwise lymphoma diagnosis may be more difficult).

Dd:

Systemic hematologic malignancies with secondary cerebral involvement (high-grade NHL, low-grade NHL, acute leukemias, etc.).

Th:

### Treatment Concept

1. Radiotherapy alone achieves high response rates, but almost all patients (> 80%) develop cerebral relapses. Combined treatment approaches are necessary to achieve long-term remissions.
2. High-dose methotrexate at doses exceeding 3500 mg/m$^2$ is the most effective treatment of CNS lymphoma. Study protocols demonstrate sufficiently cytotoxic CSF levels with doses of up to 8,000 mg/m$^2$. Other active compounds with penetrance into CSF: nitrosoureas (BCNU, CCNU), procarbazine, temozolomide, high-dose AraC, thiotepa, high-dose busulfan, topotecan.
3. New therapeutic approaches combine various types of treatment (intrathecal chemotherapy, systemic chemotherapy, radiotherapy, and steroids) achieving response rates (CR + PR) of 80–90%, with median survival of 29–62 months and 5-year survival of 20–44%.
4. The main complication with combined therapies is leukoencephalopathy (30% of all patients, 40–80% in patients > 60 years). Risk factors:
   - Combination of intrathecal methotrexate and radiotherapy
   - Chemotherapy after radiotherapy
   - Age > 60 years
   A key objective of new study protocols is the reduction of treatment toxicity without decreasing efficacy.
5. Primary ocular lymphomas are essentially treated like primary cerebral lymphomas.
6. High-dose chemotherapy and autologous stem cell transplantation with or without whole brain radiotherapy (WBRT) may be effective for younger patients. Five year overall survival rates of up to 69% in combination with WBRT were reported.

## Chemotherapy Protocols

As treatment of CNS lymphoma should be performed in clinical trials, our approach is outlined as an example of a clinical trial protocol.

---

*"Freiburg Protocol", Phase II Study* ▶ *Protocol 11.6.2*

*Initial therapy*

| | | | |
|---|---|---|---|
| Rituximab | 375 mg/m² | i.v. | Day 0 (pretherapy day -6) |
| Methotrexate, MTX | 8,000 mg/m²/day | i.v. | Day 1, infuse over 4 h |
| | | | Leucovorin rescue |
| | | | Start next cycle on day 10/11 |

—4 cycles, intensification (see below) if no CR or PR after 2 cycles

*Intensified chemotherapy: (after HD-MTX as first-line treatment, progressive disease or relapse after MTX-containing / conventional chemotherapy)*

| | | | |
|---|---|---|---|
| Rituximab | 375 mg/m² | i.v. | Day 0 |
| Cytosine arabino-side, AraC | 3,000 mg/m²/day | i.v. | Day 1, 2 |
| Thiotepa | 40 mg/m²/day | i.v. | Day 1 |

—2 cycles, stem cell mobilization after cycle 1 with G-CSF (day 5–10), leukapheresis

*High-dose therapy*

| | | | |
|---|---|---|---|
| Rituximab | 375 mg/m² | i.v. | Day -7 |
| BCNU | 400 mg/m²/day | i.v. | Day -6 |
| Thiotepa | 2 × 5 mg/kg/day | i.v. | Day -5, -4 |
| Autologous stem cell transplantation | | | Day 0 |

Patients with residual tumor: → whole brain radiotherapy 45 Gy (1.5 Gy/day)

Leucovorin rescue, 15 mg/m², initiate 24 h after start of MTX, every 6 h

---

*"R-MCP"* ▶ *Protocol 11.6.1*                    *Start next cycle on day 45, 3 cycles*

| | | | |
|---|---|---|---|
| Rituximab | 375 mg/m² | i.v. | Day 1, 15, 29 (pretreatment day -6) |
| Methotrexate | 3,000 mg/m²/day | i.v. | Day 1, 15, 30, infuse over 4 h |
| | | | Leucovorin rescue |
| Lomustine | 110 mg/m²/day | p.o. | Day 1 |
| Procarbazine | 60 mg/m²/day | p.o. | Day 1–10 |

Leucovorin rescue, 15 mg/m², initiate 24 h after start of MTX, every 6 h
If residual tumor after 3 cycles: whole brain radiotherapy 45 Gy (WBRT)

---

**Prg:**    ***Negative Prognostic Factors:***
- Age > 60 years
- Performance status 2–4 or Karnofsky scale < 70%
- Elevated LDH
- Elevated CSF protein
- Involvement of deep regions of the brain (basal ganglia, periventricular, brain stem, cerebellum)

| Treatment modality | Median survival (months) | Five-year survival (%) |
|---|---|---|
| Surgery | 3–4 | 0 |
| Radiotherapy | 12–22 | 3–7 |
| Chemotherapy | 23–37 | 20–60 |
| Combined radiochemotherapy | 29–62 | 20–44 |

**F/U:** Patients treated with curative intent should be monitored closely (neurological status, cranial MRI). In palliative situations: symptom-based approach.

**Ref:**

1. Abrey LE, Batchelor TT, Ferreri AJ et al. Report of an international workshop to standardize baseline evaluation and response criteria for primary CNS lymphoma. J Clin Oncol 2005;23:5034–43
2. Batchelor T, Loeffler JS. Primary CNS lymphoma. J Clin Oncol 2006;24:1281–8
3. Bessell EM, Hoang-Xuan K, Ferreri AJM et al. Primary central nervous system lymphoma – Biological aspects and controversies in management. Eur J Cancer 2007;43:1141–52.
4. DeAngelis LM, Hormigo A. Treatment of primary central nervous system lymphoma. Semin Oncol 2004;31:684–92
5. Grimm SA, Pulido JS, Jahnke K et al. Primary intraocular lymphoma: an IPCNSLCG Report. Ann Oncol 2007;18:1851–5.
6. Nguyen PL, Chakravarti A, Finkelstein DM et al. Results of whole-brain radiation as salvage of methotrexate failure for immunocompetent patients with primary CNS lymphoma. J Clin Oncol 2005;23:1507–13
7. Omuro AM, DeAngelis LM, Yahalom J et al. Chemoradiotherapy for primary CNS lymphoma: an intent-to-treat analysis with complete follow-up. Neurology 2005;64:69–74
8. Poortmans PMP, Kluin-Nelemans HC, Haaxma-Reiche H et al. High-dose methotrexate-based chemotherapy followed by consolidating radiotherapy in non-AIDS-related primary central nervous system lymphoma. J Clin Oncol 2003;21:4483–8
9. Illerhaus G, Marks R, Ihorst G et al. High-dose chemotherapy with autologous stem-cell transplantation and hyperfractionated radiotherapy as first-line treatment of primary CNS lymphoma. J Clin Oncol 2006;24:3865–70

**Web:**

1. http://www.cancer.gov/cancertopics/pdq/treatment/ primary-CNS-lymphoma/HealthProfessional — NCI Cancer Topics
2. http://www.emedicine.com/neuro/topic519.htm — E-medicine
3. http://www.lymphomation.org/type-cns.htm — Lymphoma Info Portal
4. http://www.cns-lymphoma.de — Freiburg Protocol

## 7.5.9          Marginal Zone Lymphoma (MZL)

A. Spyridonidis, J. Finke

**Def:** Group of lymphomas originating from marginal zone B-cells of secondary lymph follicles. Subtypes:
- B-cell lymphomas of the mucosa-associated lymphoid tissue (MALT), particularly gastric MALT NHL
- Splenic MZL with/without villous lymphocytes
- Nodal MZL with/without monocytic B-cells

**ICD-10:** C85.7

**Ep:** Most common form of primary extranodal non-Hodgkin's lymphomas, 2–3% of all NHL. Age peak: 50–70 years, male:female = 1:1.

**Pg:** *Etiological Factors*
- Chronic inflammatory disorders (antigen contact):
    - *Helicobacter pylori* → gastric MALT lymphoma
    - *Borrelia burgdorferi* (Lyme's disease) → cutaneous MALT lymphoma
    - *Campylobacter jejuni* → small bowel lymphoma, JPSID
- Autoimmune diseases: Hashimoto's thyroiditis, Sjögren's syndrome
- Molecular genetic changes, e.g., trisomy 3, t(11;18), t(1;14)

*Pathogenetic Model*
- MALT lymphomas originate from B-cells of the marginal zone of the mucosa-associated lymphoid tissue, e.g., Peyer's patches of the terminal ileum.
- MALT lymphomas are most commonly located in the stomach which physiologically has no organized MALT tissue. Gastric polyclonal B-lymphoid tissue with MALT characteristics is only formed following chronic antigen stimulation, especially in *Helicobacter pylori* (HP) infection → *H. pylori* detectable in 90% of gastric MALT lymphoma cases.
- Clonal expansion and genetic alterations with simultaneous T-cell activation result in the formation of a monoclonal lymphatic B-cell population which typically infiltrates the epithelium (lymphoepithelial lesions):
    - → Early MALT lymphoma: antigen-dependent proliferation. Responds to *H. pylori* eradication therapy.
    - → Transformation into high-grade MALT: additional genetic mutations [t(1;14), t(11;18)] lead to proliferation independent of antigens. Clinical course similar to aggressive lymphomas.

**Path:** *Primary Location*
- Gastrointestinal tract, esp. stomach: 80%
- Other: lung, eyes (orbit, lacrimal gland, conjunctivae, eyelids), breast, bladder, salivary gland, thyroid gland, kidneys, liver, skin: 20%

*Spread*
- Initial proliferation confined to the original tissue, often multifocal
- In approximately 30% of cases: spread to other MALT organs (tonsils, gastrointestinal tract)
- With increasing progression: lymph node involvement, bone marrow infiltration

*Immunophenotype of malignant MZL-cells*
Positive for B-cell antigens and surface immunoglobulins (usually IgM, less frequently IgG or IgA), negative for CD5, CD10, CD23, bcl-1/cyclin D1.

**Class:** *WHO classification:* extranodal marginal zone lymphoma (EMZL) of the MALT type, mature B-NHL.

**Staging of gastric MALT lymphomas**

| Stage | Definition |
|---|---|
| I | Unilocular or multilocular gastric lymphoma without lymph node involvement<br>I 1: limited to the mucosa and submucosa<br>I 2: involvement of the muscularis propria, subserosa, and/or serosa |
| II | Gastric lymphoma of any depth of infiltration with lymph node involvement<br>II 1: invasion of regional lymph nodes (perigastric to celiac trunk)<br>II 2: infradiaphragmatic lymph node involvement beyond the regional lymph nodes |
| IIE | Gastric lymphoma with local invasion of adjacent organs / tissues with/without lymph node involvement<br>IIE 1: invasion of regional lymph nodes<br>IIE 2: infradiaphragmatic lymph node involvement beyond the regional lymph nodes |
| III | Not defined |
| IV | Discontinuous / disseminated invasion of extragastric organs with/without lymph node involvement (including supradiaphragmatic lymph nodes) |
| CS | Clinical staging |
| PS | Pathological staging (after surgery) |

**Sy:**
- Anorexia, nausea / vomiting, weight loss
- Abdominal pain, feeling of pressure / space-occupying lesion in the epigastric area
- Gastrointestinal bleeding

**Dg:**
*Medical History, Physical Examination*
- Medical history including gastrointestinal symptoms
- Physical examination including lymph node status, abdomen (spleen, liver, tumorous lesions), oral / pharyngeal cavity (examination by an ENT specialist)

*Laboratory Tests*
- Complete blood count with differential, reticulocytes
- Routine laboratory tests including urea + electrolytes, serum creatinine, uric acid, AST, ALT, γGT, bilirubin, alkaline phosphatase, LDH, total protein, protein electrophoresis, CRP, β2 microglobulin
- Immunoelectrophoresis, quantitative immunoglobulin assay
- Anemic patients: iron, ferritin, vitamin $B_{12}$, folic acid
- Infection serology (PCR)

*Histology*
- Endoscopic biopsy (esophago-gastro-duodenoscopy): multiple superficial and deep biopsies from invaded and apparently "normal" areas ("mapping") → test for *H. pylori* (*H. pylori* is only detectable in intact epithelium)
- Bone marrow aspirate and biopsy

*Imaging*
- Endoscopy and endosonography (depth of infiltration, perigastric lymphomas)
- Chest x-ray, ultrasound abdomen / neck
- CT thorax / abdomen / pelvis
- In individual cases: contrast x-ray, colonoscopy

**DD:**
- Reactive lymphatic hyperplasia / chronic inflammatory infiltrates (no lymphoepithelial lesions, polyclonal IgH gene rearrangements)
- Other gastrointestinal lymphomas, e.g., mantle cell lymphoma (centrocytic NHL) → in the gastrointestinal tract: lymphomatous polyposis

- Burkitt's lymphoma and other high-grade lymphomas
- Enteropathy-associated T-cell lymphoma (EATL) in patients with celiac disease (sprue): most common gastrointestinal T-cell lymphoma, aggressive course

**Th:**

### Treatment Concept

1. Stage I: *H. pylori*-positive low-grade gastric MALT lymphomas respond well to the elimination of the chronic antigen stimulus (i.e., *H. pylori* eradication). Therapy protocols for eradication: omeprazole 40 mg 3 times daily p.o. (days 1–14) + amoxicillin 750 mg 3 times daily p.o. (days 1–14) + metronidazole 400 mg twice daily p.o. (days 1–14), or omeprazole 40 mg 3 times daily p.o. (days 1–14) + amoxicillin 750 mg 3 times daily p.o. (days 1–14) + clarithromycin 500 mg 3 times daily p.o. (days 1–14).
   → *Helicobacter* eradication in > 90% of cases, complete NHL remission in approximately 80% of cases after 3 months (sometimes up to 1 year); in < 10% relapse after full remission.
   → Close endoscopic / endosonographic monitoring.
   → If lymphoma persists, treatment as for stage II disease.
   Stage I: other locations: treatment option with antibiotics (doxycycline; with *C. jejuni*: erythromycin), local radiotherapy.
2. In stage II, radiotherapy is usually indicated (surgery only in cases of emergency). Alternatively or in cases where radiotherapy is contraindicated: chemotherapy.
3. Stage IV: advanced MZL/MALT lymphoma should be treated similar to other types of indolent lymphoma. An interdisciplinary approach with chemotherapy and radiation is indicated.

**NOTE:** Effective systemic treatment may cause complications, e.g., gastrointestinal bleeding or perforation.

4. Standard treatment of all stages of diffuse large-cell B-NHL of the stomach with or without MALT-type EMZL component consists of chemotherapy (e.g., 6 cycles of CHOP or R-CHOP) with curative intent. Subsequent involved-field radiotherapy may be indicated.
5. Surgery is only indicated in cases of emergency (e.g., perforation or acute gastrointestinal hemorrhage.)

**Treatment of gastic MALT lymphoma**

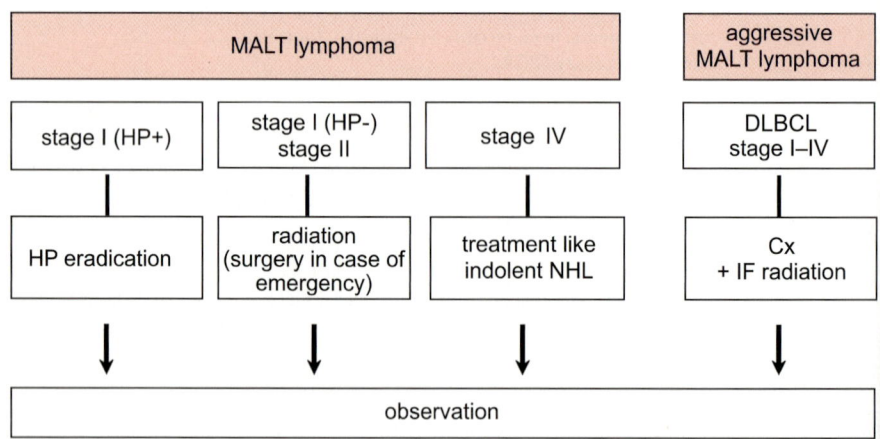

*Cx* chemotherapy, *HP Helicobacter pylori*, *IF* involved field, *DLBCL* difuse large B-cell lymphoma

## Chemotherapy Protocols

| *"Chlorambucil"* ▶ *Protocol 11.5.5* | | | *Start next cycle on day 22* |
|---|---|---|---|
| Chlorambucil | 18 mg/m²/day | p.o. | Day 1 |
| Dose increase of 5 mg/m²/day per cycle if well tolerated | | | |

| *"CHOP±R"* ▶ *Protocol 11.4.2 / 11.4.3* | | | *Start next cycle on day 22* |
|---|---|---|---|
| Cyclophosphamide | 750 mg/m²/day | i.v. | Day 1 |
| Doxorubicin | 50 mg/m²/day | i.v. | Day 1 |
| Vincristine | 1.4 mg/m²/day | i.v. | Day 1, max. 2 mg absolute |
| Prednisolone | 100 mg absolute | p.o. | Day 1–5 |
| ± Rituximab | 375 mg/m²/day | i.v. | Day 0, 24-4 h prior to CHOP |

| *"COP"* ▶ *Protocol 11.4.5* | | | *Start next cycle on day 22* |
|---|---|---|---|
| Cyclophosphamide | 400 mg/m²/day | i.v. | Day 1–5 |
| Vincristine | 1.4 mg/m²/day | i.v. | Day 1, max. 2 mg absolute |
| Prednisolone | 100 mg/m²/day | p.o. | Day 1–5 |

**Prg:**
- Localized low-grade disease (stage I–II): 10-year survival 80–90%
- High-grade gastric lymphomas have a prognosis similar to nodal NHL (▶ Chap. 7.5.1).

**F/U:** Patients treated with curative intent should be closely monitored (endoscopy, endosonography, repeated biopsies). Follow-up examinations initially every 3 months, and every 6–12 months once remission has occurred. In palliative situations: symptom-based approach.

**Ref:**
1. Bertoni F, Zucca E. State-of-the-art therapeutics: marginal-zone lymphoma. J Clin Oncol 2005;23:6415–20
2. Cohen SM, Petryk M, Varma M et al. Non-Hodgkin's Lymhoma of Mucosa-Associated Lymphoid Tissue. Oncolist 2006;11:1100–17
3. ESMO Guidelines Working Group. Gastric marginal zone lymphoma of mucosa-associated lymphoid tissue type: ESMO Clinical Recommendations for diagnosis, treatment and follow-up. Ann Oncol 2007;18(Suppl.2):ii59–60
4. Farinha P, Gascoyne R. Molecular pathogenesis of mucosa-associated lymphoid tissue lymphoma. J Clin Oncologist 2005;26:6370–8
5. Ferrucci PF, Zucca E. Primary gastric lymphoma pathogenesis and treatment: what has changes over the past 10 years? Br J Haematol 2006;136:521–38
6. Isaacson PG, Du MQ. MALT lymphoma: from morphology to molecules. Nat Rev Cancer 2004;4:644-53
7. Schmidt WP, Schmitz N, Sonnen R. Conservative management of gastric lymphoma: the treatment option of choice. Leuk Lymphoma 2004;45:1847–52

**Web:**
1. http://www.ielsg.org — Intl Extranodal Lymphoma SG
2. http://www.lymphomainfo.net/nhl/types/malt.html — Lymphoma Info Network
3. http://www.lymphomation.org/type-extranodal.htm — Lymphoma Info Portal
4. http://www.emedicine.com/med/topic3204.htm — E-medicine

## 7.5.10     Multiple Myeloma

R. Wäsch, C.I. Müller, J. Finke, M. Engelhardt

**Def:**     Clonal expansion of terminally differentiated B-lymphocytes (plasma cells); characterized by monoclonal immunoglobulins ("paraprotein"), osteolysis, renal dysfunction, and immunodeficiency.

**ICD-10:**     C90.0

**Ep:**     Incidence 3–5 cases/100,000/year; > 60 years: 8 cases/100,000/year. Median age at diagnosis 65 years, male:female = 3:2.

**Pg:**     *Risk Factors*

Pathogenetic factors have not yet been fully determined. Potential factors are:
- Ionizing radiation
- Chronic antigen exposition, viruses (KSHV: Kaposi sarcoma-associated herpes virus)
- Chemicals: heavy metals, organic solvents, benzene

*Molecular / Genetic Abnormalities*

Chromosome aberrations detectable in > 50% of cases. Particularly affected are chromosomes 14 [immunoglobulin locus, t(11;14), t(4;14)], 13 (del 13q14), 11 (bcl-1, cyclin D), or 8 (c-myc).

**Path:**     *Characteristics of Myeloma Cells*
- Production of monoclonal immunoglobulins ("paraprotein"): IgG, IgA, IgD (IgM ▶ Chap. 7.5.11, immunocytoma)
- Low proliferation index
- Expression of CD38, CD138, aberrant CD56, CD126, CD221, κ or λ
- Expression of interleukin 6 (IL-6) and IL-6 receptor
- Expression of osteoclast-activating factors (IL-1β, TNFβ, IL-6) → osteolysis
- In 1–5% "non-secretory" multiple myeloma → no paraprotein secretion

*Blood Smear*
- Advanced disease: anemia, thrombocytopenia, granulocytopenia
- Erythrocyte "coating" by immunoglobulins and adhesion → pseudohemagglutination
- Rarely blood lymphocytosis (plasma cell leukemia) and presence of circulating malignant plasma cells (< 5% of cases).

*Bone Marrow*
- Clonal plasma cell expansion (eccentric nucleus with perinuclear halo)
- Diffuse or focal growth ("plasma cell nests")

**Class:**     *Types of Myeloma*

Classification based on type of paraprotein

| Type | Frequency |
|------|-----------|
| IgG myeloma | 55% |
| IgA myeloma | 25% |
| IgD, IgE, IgM myeloma | Rare |
| κ- / λ-light chain myeloma (Bence-Jones myeloma) | 20% |
| Non-secretory myeloma | < 1–5% |

**Benign and malignant forms**

- Monoclonal gammopathy of undetermined significance (MGUS)
- Indolent myeloma
- "Smoldering" myeloma
- POEMS syndrome (Polyneuropathy, Organomegaly, Endocrinopathy, Monoclonal protein, Skin changes)
- Plasma cell leukemia
- Solitary myeloma, extramedullary myeloma = plasmacytoma

**Classification based on the Durie and Salmon Staging System (1975)**

| Stage | Definition | Median survival (years) |
|---|---|---|
| I | Hemoglobin > 10 g/dl<br>$Ca^{2+}$ < 12 mg/dl (normal)<br>Either none or only a single osteolytic lesion<br>Low M-gradient (paraprotein): IgG < 5 g/dl, IgA < 3 g/dl or light chains (Bence-Jones protein) in urine < 4 g/24 h | > 5 |
| II | Neither stage I nor stage III | 2.5–4 |
| III | Hemoglobin < 8.5 g/dl<br>$Ca^{2+}$ > 12 mg/dl<br>≥ 2 osteolytic lesions<br>High paraprotein synthesis: IgG > 7 g/dl, IgA > 5 g/dl or light chains (Bence-Jones protein) in urine > 12 g/24 h | 1–2 |
| A | $Creatinine_{serum}$ < 2 mg/dl | |
| B | $Creatinine_{serum}$ > 2 mg/dl | < 1 |

**Classification based on the International Staging System (ISS)**

| Stage | Definition | Median survival (years) |
|---|---|---|
| I | β2-MG < 3.5 mg/l, albumin ≥ 3.5 g/dl | > 5 |
| II | neither stage I<br>nor stage III | 3.7 |
| III | β2-MG ≥ 5.5 mg/l | 2.4 |

*β2-MG* β2-microglobulin

In early stages, usually asymptomatic or diagnosed incidentally. Advanced stages are characterized by symptoms caused by osteolysis, paraprotein synthesis, and bone marrow infiltration:

- Osteolysis, bone pain, spontaneous fractures: 70% of patients
- Anemia, pallor, fatigue, reduced performance status: 40–60%
- Renal failure, oliguria, anuria: 20–50%
- Thrombocytopenia, hemorrhages (petechial type): 15%
- Granulocytopenia, antibody deficiency, susceptibility to infection: 15%
- Cardiac failure (amyloidosis): 10%
- Impaired vision, seizures, peripheral neuropathy: 5–10%
- Hyperviscosity syndrome, perfusion abnormalities: < 5%
- Weight loss, fever, night sweats: < 5%

**Dg:**    ### Medical History, Physical Examination
- Medical history including physical height, signs of compression fractures / destruction of the vertebral bodies, carpal tunnel syndrome, amyloidosis
- Physical examination including skin, lymph node status, spleen / liver, signs of bleeding, signs of infection

### Laboratory Tests
- Complete blood count with differential
- Routine laboratory tests including electrolytes, $Ca^{2+}$, serum creatinine, urea, uric acid, bilirubin, albumin, LDH, CRP, ESR ↑, β2-microglobulin ↑
- Total serum protein ↑, serum protein electrophoresis, immunofixation, detection of monoclonal paraprotein ("M-gradient")
- Urinary protein, urinary protein electrophoresis (M-gradient), detection of urinary light chains ("Bence-Jones proteinuria") in 60% of cases
- Detection of serum light chains (recently available assay), serum analysis more sensitive than urinary analysis)
- Quantitative immunoglobulin level determination, immunoelectrophoresis, serum viscosity (if necessary)

### Histology
- Bone marrow cytology, histology, and cytogenetics
- In cases of suspected amyloidosis: mucous membrane biopsy, echocardiography

### Imaging
- X-ray (lateral skull, lateral spine, humerus, pelvis, femur): osteolysis or diffuse osteoporosis of the axial skeleton, multiple osteolytic skull lesions (punched-out skull)
- Suspected risk of fracture due to osteolysis (spinal column): CT / MRI / PET
- *NOTE*: bone scans do not provide diagnostic evidence of multiple myeloma / osteolysis. Avoid iodine-containing contrast media due to potential nephrotoxicity.

### Multiple Myeloma: Diagnostic Criteria

*Main criteria:*

1. Histological evidence of multiple myeloma in tissue biopsy

2. Bone marrow: > 30% plasma cells

3. Monoclonal paraprotein in serum: IgG > 35 g/l, IgA > 20 g/l, urine: κ- or λ-light chains (Bence-Jones proteins) > 1 g/24 h

*Secondary criteria:*

A. Bone marrow: 10–30% plasma cells

B. Detection of monoclonal paraprotein (quantitatively less than "main criterion")

C. Osteolytic bone lesions

D. Antibody deficiency: IgM < 0.5 g/l, IgA < 1 g/l, IgG < 6 g/l

*Diagnosis of "multiple myeloma" requires at least:*

- 1 main criterion + 1 secondary criterion: 1+B, 1+C, 1+D, 2+B, 2+C, 2+D, 3+A, 3+C, 3+D
- 3 secondary criteria: A+B+C, A+B+D

### Monoclonal Gammopathy of Undetermined Significance (MGUS): Diagnostic Criteria

- Bone marrow: < 10% plasma cells
- Monoclonal paraprotein in serum < 30 g/l
- No impairment of organ functions associated with multiple myeloma, no osteolysis
- No evidence of B-cell proliferation or light-chain disease

### "Smoldering" Multiple Myeloma (SMM): Diagnostic Criteria

- Bone marrow: > 10% plasma cells
- Monoclonal paraprotein in serum > 30 g/l
- Smoldering disease course with few symptoms

d:
- CLL, B-NHL (including Waldenström's disease)
- Chronic inflammatory disease
- Other causes of osteolysis, osteoporosis, bone marrow infiltration by other tumors

o:
- Pathological fractures
- Antibody deficiency syndrome → recurrent infections
- Hyperviscosity syndrome → malperfusion of the lung, CNS, and kidney
- Hypercalcemia → fatigue, lethargy, confusion, nausea, vomiting, polyuria, polydipsia, constipation, muscle weakness, cardiac arrhythmia
- Secondary amyloidosis (deposition of monoclonal proteins, especially light chains) → cardiac failure, impaired renal function, polyneuropathy
- Renal dysfunction / acute renal failure due to: paraprotein deposition (particularly light chains), amyloidosis, hyperviscosity, infections, hypercalcemia, hyperuricemia, tumor infiltration; glomerulonephritis, nephrotic syndrome
- Polyneuropathy: mainly IgM antibodies against myelin-associated glycoprotein (MAG)
- Bleeding due to autoantibodies against coagulation factors, cold agglutinins (IgM), hemolysins

## Amyloidosis

### Definition
Localized or generalized extracellular deposition of abnormal fibrillar proteins (amyloid). Impairment of organ function by amyloid deposits.
- Generalized amyloidosis: immunoglobulin-associated amyloidosis (AL) with plasma cell diseases; amyloid A (acute phase protein) amyloidosis (AA) with chronic inflammatory diseases; various types of familial amyloidosis (AF).
- Localized amyloidosis: in Alzheimer's disease, diabetes mellitus type II, or medullary carcinoma of the thyroid.

### Clinical Symptoms
Amyloid deposition in various organs with consecutive organ dysfunction.

### Treatment Options
- Melphalan + prednisolone p.o.,
- high-dose dexamethasone + interferon-α,
- high-dose melphalan and autologous stem cell transplantation.

## Treatment of multiple myeloma

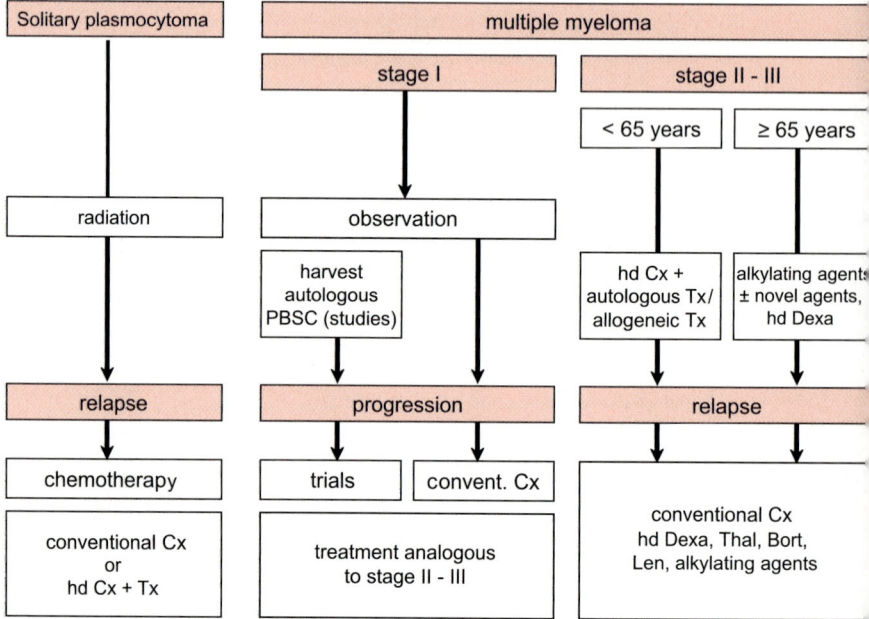

*Cx* chemotherapy, *hd* high-dose, *Tx* transplantation, *Dexa* dexamethasone, *Thal* thalidomide, *Bort* bortezomib, *PBSC* peripheral blood stem cells, *Len* lenalidomide

## Treatment Concept

1. Conventional therapies do not provide a curative treatment option for multiple myeloma. Therapy is adjusted to disease stage and age of the patient. In patients < 70–75 years high-dose chemotherapy with autologous transplantation should be considered.
2. Therapy is not indicated in initial stages, which may stay asymptomatic for several years. Indications for chemotherapy include CRAB = C: hypercalcemia, R: renal insufficiency, A: anemia, B: bone disease; in particular:
   - Myeloma-induced renal insufficiency (stages IB, IIB, IIIB, Bence-Jones proteinuria)
   - Stage II with rapid disease progression
   - Stage III
   - Anemia < 10 g/dl
   - Osteolysis, osteonecrosis with compression fractures
   - Symptomatic hyperviscosity
   - Amyloidosis
   - Recurrent bacterial infections (> 2 episodes/month)

## Conventional Chemotherapy

### Durie and Salmon Stage I and MGUS
No treatment (early intervention with alkylating agents increases the risk of secondary MDS/AML; a later start of treatment does not impair therapeutic outcome and prognosis).

### Durie and Salmon Stage II / III

- The alkylating agents melphalan and cyclophosphamide in combination with prednisolone are effective forms of treatment. Melphalan is toxic to stem cells and, when high-dose chemotherapy is considered, should not be given prior to stem cell mobilization / harvest.
- In older patients, standard treatment is melphalan + prednisolone (MP, Alexanian) given every 4–6 weeks, with response evaluation after 3 cycles. Response rate: 40%, median remission duration: 2 years, median overall survival 3 years. Novel agents, such as thalidomide, lenalidomide, and bortezomib are studied with oral melphalan and prednisone for first line therapy. Maintenance therapy does not influence survival. *ATTENTION:* no alkylating agents during radiotherapy.
- In younger patients high-dose therapy with autologous transplantation is generally recommended. For initial cytoreduction VAD, IEV, or high-dose dexamethasone are used.
- High-dose dexamethasone ± anthracyclines or VAD should preferably be used as an induction therapy prior to stem cell mobilization.
- New therapy approaches (bortezomib, thalidomide, and lenalidomide) have been approved based on single agent studies and are evaluated as combined treatment in clinical trials.

## Chemotherapy Protocols

| *"MP" (Alexanian)* ▶ Protocol 11.7.1 | | | *Start next cycle on day 29 (-d43)* |
|---|---|---|---|
| Melphalan | 8 mg/m²/day | p.o. | Days 1–4, fasting |
| | or 15 mg/m²/day | i.v. | Day 1 |
| Prednisolone | 60 mg/m²/day | p.o. | Days 1–4, postprandial |
| Melphalan dose increase by 20% per cycle according to response / side effects | | | |

| *"VAD"* ▶ Protocol 11.7.3 | | | *Start next cycle on day 43* |
|---|---|---|---|
| Vincristine | 0.4 mg absolute | c.i.v. | Days 1–4, continuous 24 h infusion |
| Doxorubicin | 9 mg/m²/day | c.i.v. | Days 1-4, continuous 24 h infusion |
| Dexamethasone | 40 mg absolute | p.o. | First cycle: days 1–4, 9–12, 17–20 |
| | | | Subsequent cycles: days 1–4, 17–20 |
| Continuous intravenous infusion of vincristine and doxorubicin only via central venous line | | | |

| *"hd DEXA"* ▶ Protocol 11.7.2 | | | *Start next cycle on day 36* |
|---|---|---|---|
| Dexamethasone | 40 mg absolute | p.o. | First cycle: days 1–4, 9–12, 17–20 |
| | | | Subsequent cycles: days 1–4, 17–20 |
| ATTENTION: Infections → Bactrim prophylaxis; steroids cause side effects esp. in older patients → monitor blood glucose, blood pressure, stomach ulcers, psychoses | | | |

| *"IEV"* ▶ Protocol 13.1.6 < 60 | | | *Start next cycle on day 22* |
|---|---|---|---|
| Epirubicin | 100 mg/m²/day | i.v. | Day 1 |
| Etoposide phosphate | 150 mg/m²/day | i.v. | Days 1–3 |
| Ifosfamide | 2,500 mg/m²/day | i.v. | Days 1–3 |

### New Therapeutic Approaches

Bortezomib: proteasome inhibitor, monotherapy response (CR + PR) 35% in relapsed / refractory patients; with dexamethasone and given as first-line therapy up to 85–90%. Main side effects thrombocytopenia, polyneuropathy (protocols 11.7.7, 11.7.8)

Thalidomide 100–200 mg/day p.o.: antiproliferative and anti-angiogenic effect, inhibition of IL-6. Response rate: 30% in relapsed / refractory patients, in combination with dexamethasone 60%. Main side effects are fatigue, polyneuropathy, constipation, thromboembolic events, and skin changes. Prophylaxis with low-dose heparin is recommended to lower the thromboembolic risk. *ATTENTION:* Do not use during pregnancy. (protocols 11.7.6, 11.7.10)

Lenalidomide: thalidomide analog with reduced toxicity.
Others: VEGF inhibitiors, arsenic trioxide, TNFα inhibitors

### High-dose Chemotherapy with Autologous Stem Cell Transplantation (PBSCT)

- Single autologous transplantation leads to increased remission rates and prolonged overall survival (5-year survival: 30–50%), but is usually not curative.
- The potential of repeated high-dose chemotherapy with autologous PBSCT is subject of current trials.
- High-dose chemotherapy: melphalan: for patients ≤ 70 years: 200 mg/m² i.v., for patients > 70 years or impaired organ function: 140 mg/m² i.v.

### High-dose Chemotherapy with Allogeneic Stem Cell Transplantation (PBSCT)

- For selected patients (up to 60–70 years), allogeneic PBSCT represents a potentially curative option (possibly active in 20–30% of multiple myeloma patients).
- The benefit of a graft-versus-myeloma effect has been demonstrated. Allogeneic transplantation should be conducted early in the course of the disease. At a later stage, higher relapse rates are to be expected, due to the development of resistance.
- Current studies are investigating the potential of allogeneic transplantation after autologous transplantation in high-risk patients (13q14 deletion) and the role of different maintenance approaches as performed after autologous PBSCT.

### Radiotherapy

#### Treatment of Bone Plasmacytoma
Radiotherapy ≥ 45 Gy. Additional radiotherapy only in cases of persistent paraprotein or relapse. Median survival 10 years. Complete disappearance of paraprotein (may take several months) constitutes an excellent prognosis: median survival 20 years, 75% relapse-free.

#### Primary Extraosseous Plasmacytoma
- Typical locations: nasopharynx, paranasal air sinuses, lung, spleen, kidneys, stomach
- 35 Gy radiotherapy; 10-year survival > 70%

### Supportive Treatment

Early administration of supportive care measures can reduce the rate of complications and markedly improve quality of life in myeloma patients:
- Pain control in patients with osteolysis / diffuse osteoporosis: analgesics (▶ Chap. 4.5), palliative radiotherapy
- Symptomatic osteolysis / risk of fracture: local radiotherapy (15–20 Gy), orthopedic treatment; after pathological fracture: surgical stabilization + radiotherapy

- Treatment of hypercalcemia (▶ Chap. 9.5): 0.9% saline 2,000–3,000 ml daily, zoledronate 4 mg or pamidronate 60–90 mg i.v., prednisolone 100 mg i.v.; if necessary: calcitonin, dialysis, furosemide. *ATTENTION:* bisphosphonate-induced osteonecrosis
- Treatment of infections: early use of antibiotics / antimycotics (▶ Chap. 4.2); in cases of recurrent infections and antibody deficiency syndrome: immunoglobulins (10 g)
- Hyperviscosity syndrome: plasmapheresis
- Bisphosphonates, e.g., zoledronate, ibandronate, pamidronate: osteoclast inhibitors significantly reduce the rate of bone complications; prophylactic administration once diagnosis has been established: e.g., zoledronate 4 mg i.v., pamidronate 60–90 mg i.v., once a month for 1 year, then every 3 months; with stable or no bone lesions cessation of bisphosphonates to avoid osteonecrosis of the jaw.
- Hyperuricemia: urinary alkalinization, allopurinol, possibly rasburicase (▶ Chap. 9.6)

*ATTENTION:* Nephrotoxic drugs, such as nonsteroidal antiinflammatories, aminoglycosides, or contrast media are contraindicated.

## Treatment Evaluation: Classification of Response (EBMT Criteria)

### Complete Remission (CR)
Serum or urine: monoclonal paraprotein (immunofixation and routine electrophoresis) remains undetectable for at least 6 weeks. Bone marrow (BM): < 5% plasma cells, nonexpanding static osteolytic lesions. Complete regression of soft tissue manifestations.

### Partial Remission (PR)
Serum: > 50% reduction of paraprotein levels for at least 6 weeks. Urine: > 90% reduction of light chains in the 24-h urine or < 200 mg/24 h for at least 6 weeks. Stable osteolytic lesions. Nonsecretory myeloma: > 50% reduction of the number of plasma cells in the BM for at least 6 weeks.

### Minimal Response (MR)
Serum: 25–49% reduction of paraprotein levels for at least 6 weeks. Urine: 50–89% reduction of light chains in the 24-h urine for at least 6 weeks. Nonsecretory myeloma: 25–49% reduction of the number of plasma cells in the BM for at least 6 weeks.

### No Change (NC)
Criteria for PR or MR not fulfilled. Readings: stable plateau ± 25% for at least 3 months.

### Progressive Disease (PD)
Increase of M-protein in serum and/or urine; > 25% increase in the concentration of light chains. BM: > 25% increase in the number of plasma cells or 10% absolute BM infiltration. New osteolytic lesions or expansion of existing lesions. New soft tissue manifestations or increase in size of existing lesions.

**Prg:**

### Prognostic Factors
Factors associated with poor prognosis:
- Advanced disease (higher number of atypical plasma cells, thrombocytopenia, anemia, renal impairment)
- β2-microglobulin ↑, CRP ↑, albumin ↓
- Cytogenetic aberrations: del 13, t(4;14), t(14;16), p53 deletion
- Age > 70 years
- Plasma cell leukemia

### Survival
- Median survival: 3–5 years, 5-year survival: 25–30%
- Median survival depends on disease stage (see above): stage I: > 5 years, stage II: 2.5–4 years, stage III: 1–2 years

**F/U:**
- MGUS and multiple myeloma patients: follow-up every 3 months, with blood count, total protein and paraprotein levels. Approximately 25% of MGUS patients develop multiple myeloma within 15 years, however, the risk/year remains low at 1%.
- Palliative therapy: symptom-based approach

**Ref:**
1. Bensinger W. Stem-cell transplantation for multiple myeloma in the era of novel drugs. J Clin Oncol 2008;26:480–92
2. Bladé J. Monoclonal Gammopathy of undetermined significance. N Engl J Med 2006;355:2765–70
3. Dimopoulos M, Spencer A, Attal M et al. Lenalidomide plus dexamethasone for relapsed or refractory multiple myeloma. N Engl J Med 2007;357:2123–32
4. ESMO Guidelines Working Group. Multiple myeloma: ESMO Clinical Recommendations for diagnosis, treatment and follow-up. Ann Oncol 2007;18(Suppl. 2):ii44–6
5. Gonzalez D, van der Burg M, García-Sanz M et al. Immunoglobulin gene rearrangements and the pathogenesis of multiple myeloma. Blood 2007;110:3112–21
6. Katzel JA, Hari P, Vesole DH. Multiple Myeloma: Charging Toward a Bright Future. CA Cancer J Clin 2007;57:301–18
7. Kyle RA, Rajkumar SV. Multiple myeloma. Blod 2008;111:2962–72
8. Kumar SK, Rajkumar SV, Dispenzieri A et al. Improved survival in multiple myeloma and the impact of novel therapies. Blood 2008;111:2516–20
9. Wechalekar AD, Hawkins PN, Gillmore JD. Perspectives in treatment of AL amyloidosis. Br J Haematol 2008;140:365–77

**Web:**

| | | |
|---|---|---|
| 1. | http://www.myelom.net | Leukemia, University of Bonn |
| 2. | http://www.multiplemyeloma.org/ | Mult Myeloma Res Foundation |
| 3. | http://www.nlm.nih.gov/medlineplus/multiplemyeloma.html | Medline Plus |
| 4. | http://www.myeloma.org/ | Intl Myeloma Foundation |
| 5. | http://www.emedicine.com/med/topic1521.htm | E-medicine |

**7.5.11**     **Immunocytoma (Waldenström's Macroglobulinemia)**

C.I. Müller, R. Wäsch, J. Finke, M. Engelhardt

**Def:**     Low-grade non-Hodgkin's lymphoma with clonal expansion of terminally differentiated B-lymphocytes (plasma cells); characteristic formation of monoclonal immunoglobulins ("IgM paraprotein").
*Synonyms:* immunocytoma = Waldenström's macroglobulinemia

**Ep:**     Incidence: 2–3 cases/1,000,000/year; median age: 63 years; male:female= 1:1

**Pg:**     *Risk Factors*
Pathogenetic factors are not finally determined. Potential factors are:
- Exposure to solvents
- Genetic disposition (family clusters, occurrence in identical twins)

**Path:**     *Characteristics of Immunocytoma Cells*
- Release of monoclonal IgM immunoglobulin ("IgM paraprotein"), monoclonal surface and cytoplasmic IgM
- Coexpression of IgD (rare)
- Marker profile: CD19+, CD20+, CD21+, CD22+, CD24+, CD79a+; CD5-, CD10-, CD23-
- Cytogenetics: in 50% of cases t(9;14)(p13;q32)

*Peripheral Blood*
- Pancytopenia may occur in advanced stages of the disease

*Bone Marrow*
- Diffuse infiltration of small and partly plasmacytoid lymphocytes (cells with basophilic cytoplasm, but lymphocyte-like nuclei) and plasma cells
- Occasionally, mast cells and "Dutcher bodies" [periodic acid-Schiff (PAS)-positive intracytoplasmic and intranuclear IgM inclusions] are observed

**Class:**     *WHO classification (2001):* mature B-NHL

**Sy:**     *Tumor Infiltration*
- Anemia, fatigue, reduced performance status, B symptoms
- Lymphadenopathy, hepatomegaly, splenomegaly
- Organ infiltration (gastrointestinal tract, lung, kidneys, meninges)

*Circulating IgM paraprotein (Macroglobulin)*
- Hyperviscosity syndrome: fatigue, bleeding of mucous membranes, impaired vision, neurological disorders, cardiovascular complications
- Cryoglobulinemia (in 10–20% of patients): Raynaud's phenomenon, purpura, glomerulonephritis (in < 5% of cases)
- Cold agglutinin disease (in approximately 10% of cases, IgM acts as cold-active antibody and reacts with erythrocyte antigens): acrocyanosis, Raynaud's phenomenon, recurrent or chronic hemolytic crises
- Autoantibodies against coagulation factors: hemorrhages

*IgM Deposition in Organs*
- Polyneuropathy (demyelination, cryoglobulinemia, amyloid deposits)
- Renal dysfunction: hypercalcemia, Bence-Jones proteinuria (less common than in multiple myeloma patients), immune-mediated glomerulonephritis
- Amyloidosis of the heart, kidneys, liver, lung, skin, and mucous membranes
  - Skin deposits: flesh-colored papules, urticaria (Schnitzler's syndrome)
  - Intestinal deposits: diarrhea, malabsorption

**Dg:**     *Medical History, Physical Examination*
- Medical history including carpal tunnel syndrome, amyloidosis
- Physical examination including skin, lymph node status, spleen / liver, signs of bleeding, signs of infection

*Laboratory Tests*
- Complete blood count with differential
- Routine laboratory tests including electrolytes, $Ca^{2+}$, serum creatinine, urea, uric acid, bilirubin, albumin, LDH, CRP, ESR ↑, β2-microglobulin ↑
- Total serum protein ↑, serum protein electrophoresis, immunofixation, detection of monoclonal paraprotein ("M-gradient")
- Urinary protein, urinary protein electrophoresis ("M-gradient"), immunofixation, detection of urinary light chains ("Bence-Jones proteinuria") in 60% of cases
- Detection of serum light chains (serum analysis more sensitive than urinary test)
- Quantitative immunoglobulin levels, immunoelectrophoresis, serum viscosity

*Histology*
- Bone marrow cytology, histology, and cytogenetics
- In cases of suspected amyloidosis: mucous membrane biopsy, echocardiography

*Imaging*
- Chest x-ray
- Abdominal ultrasound

**Dd:**     Monoclonal gammopathy of undetermined significance (MGUS) of the IgM type

**Th:**     **Treatment Concept**

1. In asymptomatic patients: observe until disease progression
2. Treatment is indicated in cases of: anemia, B symptoms, hyperviscosity syndrome, significant hepatosplenomegaly and/or lymphadenopathy, complications due to increased IgM levels

*Primary Treatment*
- Alkylating agents, e.g., chlorambucil ± corticosteroids (especially in cases of immunohemolytic anemia, cold agglutinin disease, cryoglobulinemia; ► Chap. 7.5.2, protocol 11.5.5)
  *NOTE:* with long-term treatment, increased risk of MDS or secondary leukemia
- Purine analogs: rapid cytoreduction first-line treatment in cases of serious complications, such as hyperviscosity, pancytopenia, peripheral neuropathy. 2-CDA / cladribine (75% CR and PR) or fludarabine (response in 33%). Side effects: myelosuppression, immunosuppression (especially CD4+ and CD8+ lymphocytes ↓, monocytes ↓)

*Secondary Treatment*
- After prior treatment with alkylating agents: fludarabine, fludarabine + cyclophosphamide (FC), rituximab (R), FC-R, 2-CDA, CHOP, high-dose dexamethasone, doxorubicin, IFN-α, splenectomy

*Other Therapy Approaches*
- With hyperviscosity syndrome: plasmapheresis
- Rituximab (anti-CD20): 23% partial remission (PR) in first-line therapy
- In younger patients: high-dose chemotherapy with autologous stem cell transplantation (PBSCT) or, if unsuccessful, allogeneic PBSCT in clinical studies

## Treatment Evaluation

- Complete remission (CR): immunofixation completely negative for paraprotein, complete remission of lymphadenopathy and splenomegaly; < 20% of lymphocytes in the bone marrow
- Partial remission (PR): 50% reduction in monoclonal IgM for at least 2 months and 50% decrease in tumor infiltrates in all affected regions

**Prg:**  Median survival: 5 years, 20% > 10 years

### Prognostic Factors

- Main risk factors: age > 70 years, cryoglobulinemia, weight loss, anemia (Hb < 9 g/dl)
- Other risk factors include: thrombocytopenia, neutropenia, hypoalbuminemia, male gender

**Ref:**

1. Chen CI. Treatment for Waldenström's macroglobulinemia. Ann Oncol 2004;15:550–8
2. Dimopoulos MA, Kyle RA, Anagnostopoulos A et al. Diagnosis and management of Waldenström's macroglobulinemia. J Clin Oncol 2005;23:1564–77
3. Fonseca R, Hayman S. Waldenström macroglobulinaemia. Br J Haematol 2007;138:700–20
4. Johnson SA, Birchall J, Luckie C et al. Guidelines on the management of Waldenström macroglobulinemia. Br J Haematol 2006;132:683–97
5. Kyle RA, Treon SP, Alexanian R et al. Prognostic markers and criteria to initiate therapy in Waldenström's macroglobulinemia. Semin Oncol 2003;30:116–20
6. Treon SP, Gertz MA, Dimopoulos M et al. Update on treatment recommendations from the Third International Workshop on Waldenström's macroglobulinemia. Blood 2006; 207:3442–6

**Web:**

1. http://www.iwmf.com — Intl Waldenström Foundation
2. http://www.nlm.nih.gov/medlineplus/ency/article/000588.htm — Medline Plus
3. http://www.emedicine.com/med/topic2395.htm — E-medicine

## 7.6    Langerhans Cell Histiocytosis (LCH)

### M. Stockschläder

**Def:**    Dendritic cell disease with variable biological behavior and clinical course. Clonal proliferation of CD1a+ histiocytes. It is not yet certain whether Langerhans cell histiocytosis (LCH) is a neoplastic disease, a disorder of immune dysregulation, or a reactive state with characteristics of both.

*Synonyms:* histiocytosis X, eosinophilic granuloma, Hand-Schueller-Christian disease, Abt-Letterer-Siwe syndrome

**ICD-10:**    D76.0

**Ep:**    Incidence: 1–2 cases/1,000,000/year, mean age at diagnosis 35±15 years

**Pg:**    Etiology unknown. Sporadic occurrence, most cases in childhood. Autocrine and paracrine secretion of cytokines by LCH cells and T-lymphocytes is a key process in the pathogenesis of Langerhans cell histiocytosis (fibrosis, necrosis, and osteolysis). TNF-$\alpha$, IL-1$\beta$, and prostaglandin E2 trigger osteolytic activity, weight loss, and fever. Aberrant (co-)expression of chemokine receptors (e.g., CCR6, CCR7) leads to tropism of LCH cells to skin, bones, and lymphatic tissues.

Cytokine expression patterns:
- LCH cells: IL-1$\alpha$, IL-10, GM-CSF, INF$\gamma$
- T-cells: IL-2, IL-3, IL-4, IL-5, TNF-$\alpha$; GM-CSF, INF$\gamma$
- Macrophages: IL-3, IL-7, IL-10, GM-CSF, INF$\gamma$
- Eosinophilic granulocytes: IL-3, IL-5, IL-7, IL-10, GM-CSF, INF$\gamma$

Phenotype and function of the LCH cells contribute to the clinical presentation and disease course.
- Immature LCH cells: expression of CD1a, CD14, CD40, CD68, CD107 (Langerin). CD83- CD86-, and DC lamp negative $\rightarrow$ bone lesions and chronic disease
- Mature LCH cells: CD86 positive, DC lamp positive, CD14 negative $\rightarrow$ isolated skin lesions and self-limiting disease

**Path:**    *Histology*
- Destructive granulomatous lesions; histiocyte morphology and phenotype (positive for CD1a Langerin, MHC class II, S100, Fc receptor) similar to dendritic antigen-presenting Langerhans cells of the epidermis and other organs
- Compared to normal Langerhans cells, LCH cells are positive for PNA ("peanut agglutinin") PLAP ("placental alkaline phosphatase"), interferon-gamma receptor (IFN$\gamma$ Rc) and CD31
- Electron microscopic identification of Birbeck granules which are specific to Langerhans cells

*Organ Involvement*
- Skeleton (skull > long bones > flat bones > vertebral bodies)
- CNS, pituitary gland
- Skin (inguinal, axillary, scalp)
- Cervical lymph nodes, lung

*Disease Course*
Acute, subacute, chronic / stable disease as well as progressive or recurrent disease can be distinguished. Spontaneous regression has been described.

**Class:**

### Staging According to the Histiocyte Society

"Single System Disease"
- Involvement of only one region: monostotic bone involvement, isolated skin lesions, solitary lymph node involvement.
- Multilocular disease; polyostotic bone involvement, multifocal bone involvement, multiple lymph node involvement

"Multisystem disease"
- "Low risk group": disseminated disease (involvement of multiple organs) without involvement of risk organs
- "High risk group": disseminated disease with involvement of risk organs (hematopoietic system, lung, liver, spleen)

**y:**

Symptoms vary depending on stage and course of the disease:
- General symptoms: weight loss (11%), fever (10%), localized pain (especially with bone involvement, 34%), thoracic pain
- Gingival hypertrophy
- Skin rashes, genital ulcerations
- Polyuria, polydipsia
- Impairment of balance and memory

**g:**

### Medical History, Physical Examination
- Medical history including smoking habits, polydipsia, polyuria
- Physical examination including lung, lymph nodes, neurology, ENT, gynecology

### Laboratory Tests
- Routine laboratory tests: complete blood count with differential, LDH, alkaline phosphatase, total protein, electrolytes, liver / renal function tests, CRP, urine osmolality
- Immunophenotype: CD1a, CD68, CD207, S100 (100% positive), PLAP (80% positive)
- Endocrine function parameters

### Histology / Cytology
- Biopsy of affected tissue
- Bone marrow aspirate and biopsy

### Imaging
- Ultrasound upper abdomen
- Chest x-ray, skeletal x-rays
- Bone scan

### Other Diagnostic Procedures
- Pulmonary function tests (including diffusion capacity and CO transfer), bronchoscopy, bronchoalveolar lavage
- Gastroduodenoscopy, liver biopsy
- Cranial MRI, dental x-ray
- Audiogram

**d:**

### Histiocytic Diseases
- Non-Langerhans cell histiocytosis (NLCH)
    - Primary hemophagocytic lymphohistiocytosis (HLH)
    - Reticuloendotheliosis with eosinophilia (Omenn's syndrome)
    - Sinus histiocytosis with massive lymphadenopathy (SHML, Rosai-Dorfman disease)
    - Hashimoto-Pritzker syndrome (congenital self-limiting cutaneous reticulohistiocytosis)
- Malignant histiocytic diseases
    - Monocyte- or macrophage-related histiocytic sarcoma (MMHS)
    - Dendritic cell-related histiocytic sarcoma

- Lymphomas (non-Hodgkin's lymphomas, Hodgkin's disease)
- Skin diseases
  - Seborrheic eczema
  - Juvenile xanthogranuloma
  - Xanthoma disseminatum (factor XIIIa positive, CD68 positive)
- Pulmonary diseases
  - Sarcoidosis
  - Idiopathic pulmonary fibrosis
  - Chronic eosinophilic pneumonia
  - Hypersensitivity pneumonitis

**Co:**   In patients with chronic progressive and recurrent disease:
- Orthopedic disorders, fractures
- Neurological disorders, impaired hearing, pituitary disorders
- Chronically impaired pulmonary and hepatic function
- Secondary malignancies

**Th:**   **Treatment Concept**

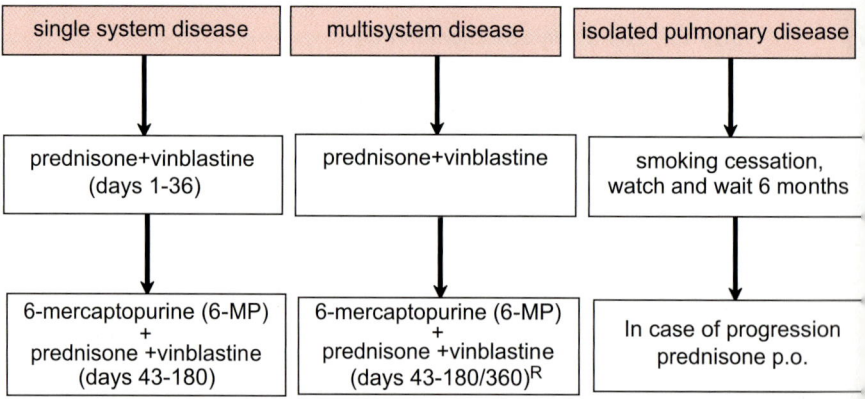

*Prednisone+vinblastine:* prednisone 1 mg/kg/day p.o. (max 60 mg) d 1–28, taper over a 2 week-period + vinblastine 6 mg/m² (max 10 mg) i.v. d1, 8,15,22,29,36; *6-MP+prednisone+vinblastine* starting day 43 after initial treatment: 6-MP 30 mg/m²/day (50 mg max) p.o. + prednisone 1 mg/kg/day (60 mg max) p.o. d 1–5 every 3 weeks + vinblastine 6 mg/m² (10 mg max) i.v. d 1 every 3 weeks; Prednisone for isolated pulmonary disease 1 mg/kg/d (max 60 mg) for 1 month, 0.5 mg/kg/d for 1 month, 0.25 mg/kg/d for 2 months, 0.125 mg/kg/d for 2 months. R=Randomisation

### Localized Disease ("Single System Disease")

- Isolated bone lesions: intralesional corticosteroid injection or curettage; lesions in specific locations or secondary disease: radiotherapy (4–8 Gy)
- Isolated lymph node involvement: surgical resection ± systemic steroids (prednisolone 1 mg/kg/day, days 1–7, p.o.)
- Nodular skin manifestation: surgical removal
- Disseminated skin lesions: topical steroids; in severe cases, nitrogen mustard solution ± systemic steroids (prednisolone 1–2 mg/kg/day, days 1–7, p.o.); refractory disease: PUVA therapy (methoxypsoralen + UV-A phototherapy)
- Refractory cases: corticosteroids ± vinblastine
- Involvement of pituitary gland: radiotherapy, DDAVP

### Salvage Therapy
- Late relapse: repeat initial therapy
- 2-Chlorodeoxyadenosine (2-CDA): response rate 75%
- matched related allogeneic transplantation or immunomodulation / suppression
- lung / liver transplantation
- Clinical trial, e.g., protocol LCH-S-2005

**rg:**

### Prognostic Factors
- Disseminated or localized disease
- Involvement of high-risk organs (bone marrow, liver, spleen, lung)
- Response to treatment
- IL-2 receptor serum levels

### Five-year Progression-free Survival
- Localized LCH: 100%
- Isolated lung involvement: 85%
- Disseminated LCH: 90%

**U:**

Follow-up including blood count, liver function tests, protein, coagulation parameters, chest x-ray, and skeletal x-rays.

**ef:**

1. Aricò M. Langerhans cell histiocytosis in adults: more questions than answers? Eur J Cancer 2004;40:1467–73
2. Gadner H, Grois N, Pötschger U et al. Improved outcome in multisystem Langerhans cell histiocytosis is associated with therapy intensification. Blood 2008;111:2556–62
3. Geissmann F, Lepelletier Y, Fraitag S et al. Differentiation of Langerhans cells in Langerhans cell histiocytosis. Blood 2001;97:1241–8
4. Götz G, Fichter J. Langerhans cell histiocytosis in 58 adults. Eur J Med Res 2004;9:510–4
5. Steiner M, Matthes-Martin S, Attarbaschi A et al. Improved outcome of treatment-resistant high-risk Langerhans cell histiocytosis after allogeneic stem cell transplantation with reduced-intensity conditioning. Bone Marrow Transplant 2005;36:215–25
6. Stockschlaeder M, Sucker C. Adult Langerhans cell histiocytosis. Eur J Haematol 2006;76:363–8
7. Vassallo R, Ryu JH, Colby TV et al. Pulmonary Langerhans cell histiocytosis. N Engl J Med 2000;342:1969–78

**Web:**

1. http://www.histio.org — Histiocytosis Assoc America
2. http://www.histio.org/society — Histiocyte Society
3. http://www.nlm.nih.gov/medlineplus/ency/article/000068.htm — Medline Plus
4. http://www.emedicine.com/PED/topic1997.htm — E-medicine

# 7.7     Mastocytosis

**A. Spyridonidis, J. Finke**

**Def:**     Heterogeneous group of diseases characterized by pathological accumulation of mast cells in skin (cutaneous mastocytosis) and/or in various organs (systemic mastocytosis).

*Synonyms:* Nettleship's disease, urticaria pigmentosa, lymphadenopathic mastocytosis with eosinophilia

**ICD-10:**     Q82.2 (cutaneous), C96.2 (systemic)

**Ep:**     Incidence: 2 cases/300,000/year, 75% of cases in children, 25% in adults (30th–50th year of life).

**Pg:**     *Mast Cells (MC)*
- Originating from pluripotent hematopoietic stem cells in bone marrow, maturation in peripheral tissues. Stem cell factor (SCF) controls development, differentiation, and maturation of mast cells. MC of all development stages express the SCF receptor (c-kit, CD117).
- Confined to connective tissue, particularly in areas with direct environmental contact. Characteristics include metachromatic granules containing mediators and cytokines (histamine, chymase, tryptase, heparin, leukotrienes, prostaglandin D2, PAF, TNFα, interleukins, GM-CSF, G-CSF) → release following stimulation.
- The physiological role of mast cells has not been been finally elucidated; potential functions include infection defense, immune regulation, and allergic type I reaction.

*Mastocytosis in Childhood*
- Reactive, polyclonal proliferation of mast cells, 80% of patients < age of 2, 20% between 2 and 15 years, mostly with spontaneous remission.
- In childhood usually cutaneous manifestation; systemic involvement is rare.
- No activating c-kit mutations detectable. Secretion of SCF by keratinocytes or mast cells has been described.

*Adult Mastocytosis*
- Clonal disease, usually systemic mastocytosis, pure cutaneous forms are rare. Chronic course, spontaneous remissions are uncommon.
- *Systemic mastocytosis (SM):* in > 80% initial manifestation as indolent mastocytosis, over several years in 30% evolution into aggressive mastocytosis, particularly in cases without cutaneous involvement. In 20–40% development of associated hematologic neoplasms (AHN). Mast cell leukemia may present as secondary disease or de novo, but is extremely rare.
- *Cutaneous mastocytosis (CM):* transformation into systemic mastocytosis possible (5–10%), incidence of AHN is low.
- Detection of identical c-kit mutations in mast cells of bone marrow and affected organs: e.g. point mutations of the cytoplasmic kinase domain (A816V) or the juxtamembrane region (V 560 G). Activating point mutations of the c-kit receptor may lead to continuous stimulation of proliferation and apoptosis inhibition in mast cells.

**Path:**     Cytological differentiation of mast cells:
- Typical MC: round, centrally located nucleus, strongly granulated cytoplasm
- Atypical MC type I: spindle formed, eccentrically located nucleus, hypogranular
- Atypical MC type II: bi- / polylobulated / blastic nucleus, strongly hypogranulated

*Immune Cytology (FACS)*
- Normal mast cells: positive for CD117 (c-kit), CD45, CD33, CD11c, negative for CD2, CD25, CD34
- Neoplastic mast cells: frequently aberrant expression of CD2 and/or CD25

### Peripheral Blood

Normal mast cells do not circulate in peripheral blood → detection of CD117+ / CD34- mast cells is always pathological, > 10% mast cells in blood are diagnostic for mast cell leukemia.

### Bone Marrow

- In normal adult bone marrow mast cells represent < 0.1% of all nucleated cells.
- Bone marrow mast cell proliferation is detectable in > 90% (indolent SM) up to 100% (aggressive SM) of cases with systemic mastocytosis.
- Aspirate: in indolent systemic mastocytosis up to 1% mast cells in bone marrow, in aggressive SM > 5%, in mast cell leukemia > 20%. Accumulation of mast cells mostly focal, detection of dense mast cell infiltrates, and/or detection of mast cells with cytological atypias is a diagnostic sign.
- Biopsy: detection of dense infiltrates (> 10–15 mast cells) is diagnostic. Mast cells in systemic mastocytosis frequently dysplastic / hypogranulated → immune histochemical staining for mast cell-specific tryptase and/or CD117.
- ATTENTION: bone marrow aspiration frequently difficult or impossible because of fibrosis; biopsy may be of limited diagnostic value due to focal infiltration pattern.

### Organ Involvement

In systemic mastocytosis involvement of skin (50–90%), spleen (50–70%), lymph nodes, (20–70%), liver, and other organs (CNS, lung, kidney, muscles).

**Class:** **Revised classification of mastocytoses (Vienna Consensus Meeting 2000)**

| Form | Incidence |
|---|---|
| *Cutaneous mastocytosis (CM)* | |
| • Urticaria pigmentosa (UP) | Children, adults |
| • Diffuse cutaneous ("erythrodermic") mastocytosis | Children |
| • Mastocytoma of skin | Children |
| • Teleangiectasia macularis eruptiva perstans (TMEP) | Adults |
| *Systemic mastocytosis (SM)* | |
| • Indolent SM (variant: "smoldering" mastocytosis) | Adults |
| • SM with associated hematological neoplasia (AHN) | Adults |
| • Aggressive SM | Rare |
| • Mast cell leukemia (MCL) | Rare |
| • Mast cell sarcoma | Rare |
| *Special form* | |
| • SM with eosinophilia (FIP1L1-PDGFRα positive) | Rare |

**Subtypes of systemic mastocytosis**

| Subtype | Skin involvement | BM mast cells | c-kit mutation | Blood | Organ involvement |
|---|---|---|---|---|---|
| Indolent SM | > 90% | 1–5% | + | Normal | – |
| "Smoldering" SM | +/- | > 5% | +/- | Normal | + |
| Aggressive SM | < 50% | > 5% cellularity ↑ | +/- | Normal / pathological | +/- |
| Mast cell leukemia | – | > 20% | +/- | > 10% MC | + |

*BM* bone marrow, *MC* mast cells, *SM* systemic mastocytosis, + present, - absent

**Sy:**    Characteristic are: flush attacks, anaphylactic reactions, pruritus, abdominal pain, nausea, vomiting, diarrhea, dyspnea.

*Symptoms related to:*
- Uncontrolled proliferation of mast cells → organ infiltration → changes in blood count, malabsorption, weight loss, bleeding, spleen enlargement, hypersplenism, hepatomegaly, ascites, osteoporosis, osteolytic lesions, depression, concentration disorders, CNS changes
- Release of mast cell mediators → pruritus, flush, diarrhea, abdominal pain, peptic ulcers, recurrent syncopes, shock, dyspnea, headache
- Associated hematologic neoplasia

**Dg:**    ### History, Physical Examination
- Medical history: esp. flush, syncopes, GI symptoms, bleeding, fever / night sweats / weight loss (B symptoms)
- Physical examination: skin (reddish-brown spots / macules, most common on trunk, "Darier's sign": urticaria and erythema upon mechanical irritation, e.g., after rubbing the skin with a spatula), lymphadenopathy, hepatomegaly, splenomegaly, hemorrhagic signs

### Laboratory Tests
- Blood count with differential (frequently eosinophilia), LDH, PTT, liver / renal function parameters, total protein
- *Tryptase*$_{serum}$: normal values 1–15 ng/ml, > 20 ng/ml indicative of SM. In pure cutaneous mastocytosis serum tryptase is generally not elevated. *NOTE:* false increased levels after anaphylactic events (normalization within 12–14 h) and in hematological neoplasia (AML, MDS, MPS)
- *Histamine in 24-h urine:* determination of main metabolite methyl-histamine in 24-h urine, normally 5–35 µg/l, increased levels correlate with mast cell load. In pure cutaneous mastocytosis histamine$_{urine}$ is generally not increased. *NOTE:* elevated levels following anaphylactic events or in bacteriuria (decarboxylation of histidine to histamine). Before urine collection avoid food with high histamine content (cheese, red wine)
- Mutation analysis of c-kit gene: detection of c-kit point mutation at codon 816 (others: V560G, Gly 839 Glut) in bone marrow, blood or other organs. Detection of FIP1-PDGFRα fusion by FISH or PCR

### Cytology, Histology
- Cell surface antigen expression in peripheral blood (FACS): CD117, CD34
- Bone marrow aspiration and biopsy, esp. when systemic mastocytosis is suspected. In children a bone marrow biopsy is not necessary, in adults with urticaria pigmentosa mandatory
- Histology from involved tissue

### Imaging Studies, Additional Diagnostic Procedures
- Abdominal ultrasound
- X-ray chest / skeleton, bone scan

### Diagnostic Criteria of Systemic Mastocytosis

*Major criterion:*
- Multifocal, dense mast cell infiltrates (> 10–15 mast cells) in bone marrow or organ biopsy

*Minor criteria:*
- Cytological atypias in > 25% of all mast cells
- Detection of A816V c-kit mutation in bone marrow or organs
- Aberrant expression of CD2 or CD25 in CD117+ mast cells
- Serum tryptase > 20 ng/ml

*Diagnosis:*
- 1 major + 1 minor criterion or 3 minor criteria present

**DD:**
- Reactive mastocytosis: in parasitic infections, neoplasia, aplastic anemia, lymphoma
- Allergic / anaphylactic reaction
- Pheochromocytoma, carcinoid, VIPoma, osteoporosis, malabsorption, Zollinger-Ellison syndrome
- Myeloproliferative syndromes, acute basophilic leukemia, hypereosinophil syndrome, NHL, tryptase-positive AML, AML with c-kit mutation

**Th:**
### Treatment Concept
- There is no curative treatment available. In cutaneous mastocytosis or indolent systemic mastocytosis, symptomatic treatment. In aggressive forms, antineoplastic therapy.
- In mast cell leukemia, immediate initiation of antineoplastic therapy, treatment according to AML protocols. Achievement of complete remission possible, however, duration of remission usually short.

*ATTENTION:* with effective treatment risk of mast cell degranulation → release of mast cell mediators → complications up to lethal shock.

### Symptomatic Treatment
- Avoidance of unspecific mast cell degranulation, emergency set (epinephrine)
- Pruritus, urticaria, flush: H1 receptor blockers, mast cell stabilizers (ketotifen), topical steroids if applicable or psoralen–UV-A (PUVA) treatment. Acetylsalicylic acid (ASS) 1,000–1,500 mg/day (*ATTENTION:* ASS may lead to mast cell degranulation)
- Mastocytoma: surgical removal
- Gastrointestinal symptoms, peptic ulcers, diarrhea, malabsorption: H2 receptor blockers, disodium cromolyn, corticosteriods
- Osteoporosis: bisphosphonates

### Antineoplastic Treatment
- IFNα 4 MIU/day, 3 × per week up to 3 MIU/day s.c. ± steroids. Initiation of treatment under inpatient conditions recommended
- 2-CDA and hydroxyurea are effective cytostatics
- In mast cell leukemia: polychemotherapy analogous to AML protocols. Experimental: allogeneic bone marrow transplantation
- Imatinib seems to be effective in patients who do not have the A816V mutation and in systemic mastocytosis with eosinophilia and FIPIL1-PDGFRα

**Prg:**
- Cutaneous mastocytosis: normal life expectancy
- Indolent systemic mastocytosis: median survival > 10 years
- Aggressive systemic mastocytosis: median survival 1–2 years
- Mast cell leukemia: median survival < 9 months

*Negative prognostic factors:* age, missing skin involvement, elevated LDH, elevated alkaline phosphatase, changes in blood count.

**F/U:**
Close monitoring to detect progression to more aggressive forms of hematological neoplasia, with physical examination, blood count with differential, LDH, tryptase$_{serum}$, histamine$_{24\text{-h urine}}$.
- Cutaneous mastocytosis, indolent systemic mastocytosis: annual follow-up
- "Smouldering" / aggressive forms: follow-up at least every 6 months

**Ref:**
1. Akin C, Metcalfe DD. Systemic mastocytosis. Annu Rev Med 2004;55:419–32
2. Kirshenbaum AS, Goff JP, Semere T et al. Demonstration that human mast cells arise from a progenitor cell population that is CD34+ ,c-kit+ , and expresses aminopeptidase N (CD13). Blood 1999;94:2333–42
3. Ma Y, Zeng S, Metcalfe DD et al. The c-KIT mutation causing human mastocytosis is resistant to STI571 and other KIT kinase inhibitors. Blood 1002;99:1741 4
4. Metcalfe DD, Akin C. Mastocytosis: molecular mechanisms and clinical disease heterogeneity. Leuk Res 2001;25:577–82

5.  Pardanani A, Ketterling RP, Brockman SR et al. CHIC2 deletion, a surrogate for FIP1L1-PDGFRA fusion, occurs in systemic mastocytosis associated with eosinophilia and predicts response to imatinib mesylate therapy. Blood 2003;102:3093–6

6.  Tefferi A, Li CY, Butterfield JH et al. Treatment of systemic mast cell disease with cladribine. N Engl J Med 2001;344:307–9

7.  Valent P, Akin C, Sperr WR et al. Mastocytosis: pathology, genetics, and current options for therapy. Leuk Lymphoma 2005;46:35–48

8.  Yavuz AS, Lipsky PE, Yavuz S et al. Evidence for the involvement of a hematopoietic progenitor cell in systemic mastocytosis from single-cell analysis of mutations in the c-kit gene. Blood 2002;100:661–5

**Web:**

1.  http://www.tmsforacure.org/                          Mastocytosis Society
2.  http://www.niaid.nih.gov/factsheets/masto.htm        Mastocytosis Fact Sheet
3.  http://www.emedicine.com/med/topic1401.htm           E-medicine
4.  http://www.mastokids.org/                            Mastocytosis Kids

## 8.1    Head and Neck Tumors

**M. Daskalakis, K. Henne, H. Henß**

**Def:**    Heterogenic group of malignant tumors of the mouth, nose, and upper respiratory tract.

**ICD-10:**    C00–14, C30–32

**Ep:**    Incidence: 25–30 cases/100,000 population/year, approximately 3–6% of all newly diagnosed malignancies; geographic variation depending on regional risk factors such as alcohol and nicotine intake; betel chewing. Ratio male:female = 4:1; age peak: 60 years.

**Pg:**    *Risk Factors*
- Alcohol and nicotine abuse (particularly in combination, > 85% of patients)
- Tobacco chewing, betel nut chewing, consumption of salt-cured meat and fish
- Poor oral hygiene, chronic inflammation
- Noxious chemicals: propanol, wood dust (adenocarcinomas), occupational disease in the textile industry
- Radiation: Radium (clock industry), Thorotrast, preoperative radiotherapy (e.g., in Hodgkin's disease)
- Viruses: nasopharyngeal carcinoma is associated with EBV (endemically occurring in East Asia); squamous cell carcinoma is associated with HPV (human papilloma virus), particularly HPV-16

*Molecular Genetics*
- Frequent changes in chromosome 11 (particularly 11q13)
- Mutated tumor suppressor genes: p16 (80%), p53 (50%); proto-oncogenes: cyclin D1 (30%), p63 (30%)

**Path:**    *Histology*

| Type | Frequency |
| --- | --- |
| Squamous cell carcinoma | > 90% |
| Adenocarcinoma, particularly tumors of the salivary glands / nasopharynx | 5% |
| Other: sarcomas, lymphomas, multiple myeloma, melanoma, acoustic neurinoma | Rare |
| Special forms: | |
| • Transitional epithelial carcinoma (paranasal air sinuses) | |
| • Undifferentiated carcinoma of the nasopharyngeal type | |
| • Lymphoepithelial tumors of the nasopharynx (Schmincke-Regaud) | |
| • Mucoepidermoid carcinoma | |

*Locations*
- Oral cavity, tongue
- Oropharynx, nasopharynx (including the paranasal air sinuses)
- Hypopharynx, larynx

*Spread Pattern*
- Initially, direct invasion of adjacent structures
- Primary lymphogenic spread into regional lymph nodes
- Distant metastases in advanced disease stages

Class: | TNM Staging of Head and Neck Tumors

| TNM | Characteristics |
|------|-----------------|
| **T** | **Primary Tumor** <br> *Lip, oral cavity, salivary glands, pharynx, paranasal sinuses* |
| TX | Primary tumor cannot be assessed |
| T0 | No evidence of primary tumor |
| Tis | Carcinoma in situ |
| T1 | Tumor size ≤ 2 cm |
| T2 | Tumor size 2–4 cm |
| T3 | Tumor size > 4 cm |
| T4 | Infiltration of adjacent structures (soft tissue of the neck, skin, skeleton) |
| | *Hypopharynx carcinoma* |
| T1 | Solitary tumor |
| T2 | Extending into adjacent region without laryngeal fixation |
| T3 | Extending into adjacent region with laryngeal fixation |
| T4 | Infiltration of adjacent structures (soft tissue of the neck, skin, skeleton) |
| | *Laryngeal carcinoma* |
| T1 | Tumor restricted to one (T1a) or both (T1b) vocal cords, normal vocal cord mobility |
| T2 | Extending into the glottic, supraglottic, and/or subglottic regions |
| T3 | Extending within the laryngeal region with fixation of the vocal cords |
| T4 | Tumor extending beyond the laryngeal region, with or without infiltration of adjacent structures |
| **N** | **Lymph Node Involvement** |
| NX | Regional lymph nodes cannot be assessed |
| N0 | No involvement of lymph nodes |
| N1 | Involvement of one ipsilateral lymph node, < 3 cm in diameter |
| N2 | Extended lymph node involvement |
| | A  Involvement of one ipsilateral lymph node, 3–6 cm in diameter |
| | B  Involvement of several ipsilateral lymph nodes, ≤ 6 cm in diameter |
| | C  Bilateral / contralateral lymph node involvement, ≤ 6 cm in diameter |
| N3 | Lymph node involvement, > 6 cm in diameter |
| **M** | **Distant Metastasis** |
| MX | Distant metastasis cannot be assessed |
| M0 | No distant metastasis |
| M1 | Distant metastasis |

**Staging according to AJCC**

| Stage | TNM system | | | Five-year survival (%) |
|---|---|---|---|---|
| 0 | Tis | N0 | M0 | 95–100 |
| I | T1 | N0 | M0 | 75–90 |
| II | T2 | N0 | M0 | 40–70 |
| III | T3 | N0 | M0 | 20–50 |
| | T1–3 | N1 | M0 | |
| IV | T4 | N0–1 | M0 | 10–30 |
| | Any T | N2–3 | M0 | |
| | Any T | Any N | M1 | |

**Sy:**  Few patients display early symptoms. Patients with poor social status may only be seen in advanced stages of disease:
- General symptoms: fatigue, lassitude, weight loss
- Hoarseness, dysphagia, "lump feeling"
- Tumor and/or enlarged lymph nodes, unilateral tonsillar enlargement
- Ulceration and necrosis of mucous membranes
- Local pain, headache, toothache
- Leukoplakia (in 5–10% of cases with in situ carcinoma)

**Dg:**

### Medical History, Physical Examination
- Medical history including risk factors (alcohol / nicotine abuse, work environment)
- Physical examination and local diagnostics (including endoscopy)

### Laboratory Tests
- Routine laboratory tests including blood count, liver / renal function parameters
- Tumor markers: SCC (low sensitivity, only useful for assessment of disease progression)
- Molecular staging: EBV-DNA, HPV-DNA, possibly p16, p53, cyclin D1, p63

### Histology
- Panendoscopy under general anesthesia, with biopsies
- Bronchoscopy / esophagoscopy (where applicable) to rule out simultaneous primary tumors

### Imaging
- Ultrasound of the neck / abdomen (including lymph nodes)
- CT / MRI of the neck and base of the skull
- Chest x-ray (pulmonary metastases, secondary tumors)
- PET, bone scan, lymphoscintigraphy (where applicable)

10–15% of all patients with head and neck tumors present with a simultaneous second primary tumor (respiratory tract, upper gastrointestinal tract). Most common location: esophagus.

**Co:**
- Hemorrhage, venous / lymphatic obstruction, venous congestion
- Airway obstruction
- Loss of hearing (mainly unilateral) due to nerve damage / serous otitis
- Impaired vision (cranial nerve damage)

h:

## Treatment Concept

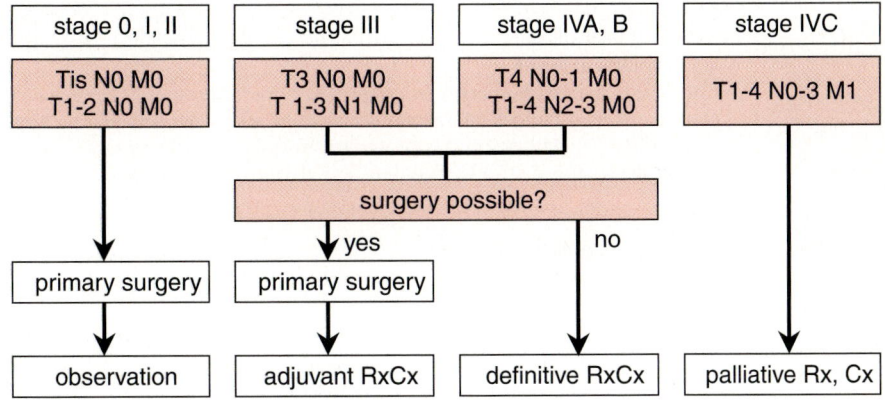

RxCx radiochemotherapy, Rx radiotherapy, Cx chemotherapy

## Surgical Treatment

### Indications
- Primary treatment is surgery
- Stage I and II (T1–3): surgical treatment with curative intent
- Advanced tumors (T4): palliative indication (pain, hemorrhage, dysphagia, etc.)
- Local relapse or regional lymph node recurrence after primary radiotherapy / surgery

### Procedures
- Full resection (RO, with resection margins histologically free of tumor) is the most important prerequisite for curative treatment. Cosmetic aspects are secondary, but organ preservation and maintenance of physiologic function are important treatment objectives.
- Where applicable, preservation of function / reconstructive surgery; en bloc resection of suspicious or involved lymph nodes (radical or partial neck dissection)

### Adverse Effects of Surgical Treatment
- Cosmetic and/or functional impairment
- Loss of speech, dysphagia, aspiration pneumonia
- Plexus damage after neck dissection

## Radiotherapy

### Indications
- Resectable tumors: adjuvant (postoperative) radiochemotherapy with curative intention in case of:
    - Histological evidence of lymphangiosis carcinomatosa
    - Resectable tumors in stage III–IV
- Locally unresectable tumors: definitive radiochemotherapy with curative intention
- Laryngeal carcinomas T1–2 N0 M0 or carcinomas of the tongue T1–2 N0 M0 → improved preservation of physiological organ function compared to surgical approach
- Schmincke-Regaud tumor and carcinoma of the nasopharyngeal region: primary radiochemotherapy as radical resection is impossible
- Palliative radiotherapy with symptomatic indication (tumor-related complications), especially with postoperative relapse

### Procedures

- Radiation treatment of tumor and regional lymph nodes with at least 60 Gy (exception: NC tumors → 50 Gy); boost to the region of the primary tumor 66–70 Gy (75 Gy maximum); boost application: percutaneous (small field) or interstitial using brachytherapy (afterloading) treatment intensification via hyperfractionated accelerated radiotherapy (2–3 sessions per day at intervals of at least 6 h)
- Combined chemoradiotherapy has improved tumor outcomes as compared to radiotherapy alone; combined radiochemotherapy seems to be associated with shorter treatment, reduced risk of distant metastases, and improved survival. Cisplatin, carboplatin, or combination chemotherapy (cisplatin + 5-FU, platinum-derivative + taxane) are used.

### Adverse Effects of Radiotherapy

- Dental disorders (potentially irreversible), xerostomia, mucositis
- Loss of taste
- Hypoparathyroidism
- Skin atrophy, subcutaneous induration, fibrosis

## Chemotherapy

### Indications

- In combination with radiotherapy (see above)
- Palliative chemotherapy in patients with relapse after surgery and radiotherapy

### Procedures

- With relapse after surgery and radiotherapy: indication for palliative chemotherapy should be carefully evaluated; consider the often severely reduced performance status and concomitant diseases (hepatic dysfunction, etc.); after prior radiotherapy: increased risk of mucositis → dose reduction in the first cycle; response rate: 40–50%
- Combination therapies including cisplatin and/or methotrexate are more effective than single drug treatment; most effective compounds: cisplatin, carboplatin, methotrexate, 5-fluorouracil, epirubicin, ifosfamide, bleomycin, paclitaxel and docetaxel
- In previously untreated tumors, primary chemotherapy is often highly effective (response rate 80–90%); however, relapses are frequent, even after complete remission.
- The impact of adjuvant chemotherapy has not been established yet; use in clinical trials only

### New Compounds / Therapies

- Pemetrexed (antifolate analog): monotherapy response rate: 20–30%; use in combination therapies is currently being investigated
- Cetuximab: EGF-R1 inhibitor, monoclonal antibody, effective in combination with radiotherapy and as monotherapy

## Chemotherapy Protocols Head and Neck Tumors

| "5-FU / Carboplatin" ▶ Protocol 12.1.1 | | | Start next cycle on day 22–29 |
|---|---|---|---|
| 5-Fluorouracil | 1,000 mg/m²/day | i.v. | Day 1–5 |
| Carboplatin | AUC 6 | i.v. | Day 1 |

| *"EMB"* ▶ *Protocol 12.1.2* | | | *Start next cycle on day 22* |
|---|---|---|---|
| Epirubicin[a] | 50 mg/m²/day | i.v. | Day 1 |
| Methotrexate | 40 mg/m²/day | i.v. | Day 11, 18 |
| Bleomycin | 10 mg/m²/day | i.v. | Day 4, 11, 18 |
| [a]Alternatively: cisplatin 50 mg/m²/day i.v., day 4 | | | |

| *"Docetaxel / Cisplatin"* | | | *Start next cycle on day 22* |
|---|---|---|---|
| Docetaxel | 175–280 mg/m²/day | i.v. | Day 1 |
| Cisplatin | 75 mg/m²/day | i.v. | Day 1 |

| *"Methotrexate Monotherapy"* | | | *Weekly* |
|---|---|---|---|
| Methotrexate | 40–60 mg/m²/day | p.o. | Day 1, if difficulty swallowing: i.v. |

**Prg:**

### Prognostic Factors
- Tumor stage (especially lymph node involvement) and histology
- Location: tonsillar carcinoma and laryngeal carcinoma have a better prognosis, hypopharyngeal carcinoma: poor prognosis
- Continuous drinking and smoking (especially smoking): poor prognosis

### Five-year Survival Depending on Tumor Stage
See above (p. 530)

**F/U:**

Patients treated with curative intent: initially follow-up every 3 months (medical history, clinical examination, local findings, endoscopy, ultrasound, chest x-ray). It is particularly important to monitor for potential second primary tumors (bronchoscopy, esophagoscopy).

In palliative situations: symptom-based approach.

**Px:**

### Primary Prevention
- Avoid alcohol and nicotine abuse
- Elimination of noxious chemicals (workplace safety)

### Secondary Prevention
- In patients with alcohol and nicotine abuse, "field cancerization" occurs. A total of 20–30% of all patients with head and neck tumors develop a second primary tumor (head and neck region, bronchial carcinoma, esophageal carcinoma) within 2–3 years. According to recent studies, daily administration of isotretinoin (13-cis retinoic acid) 1 mg/kg/day p.o. significantly lowers the risk of development of a second primary tumor. However, isotretinoin prophylaxis did not impact overall survival.
- Other agents are currently tested for potential chemoprevention: vitamin A, β-carotin, etretinate, selenium, interferon-α.

**Ref:**

1. Bernier J, Domenge C, Ozsahin M et al. Postoperative irradiation with or without concomitant chemotherapy for locally advanced head and neck cancer. N Engl J Med 2004;350:1945–52

2. Bonner JA, Harari PM, Giralt J et al. Radiotherapy plus cetuximab for squamous cell carcinoma of the head and neck. N Engl J Med 2006;354:567–78

3. Colevas AD. Chemotherapy options for patients with metastatic or recurrent squamous cell carcinoma of the head and neck. J Clin Oncol 2006;24:2644–52

4. Cooper JS, Pajak TF, Forastiere AA et al. Postoperative concurrent radiotherapy and chemotherapy for high-risk squamous cell carcinoma of the head and neck. N Engl J Med 2004;350:1937–44

5. ESMO Guidelines Working Group. Squamous cell carcinoma of the head and neck: ESMO Clinical Recommendations for diagnosis, treatment and follow-up. Ann Oncol 2007;18(Suppl 2):ii65–6

6. Le Tourneau C, Faivre A, Siu LL. Molecular targeted therapy of head and neck cancer: Review and clinical development challenges. Eur J Cancer 2007;43:2457–66

7. Posner MR, Hershock DM, Blajman CR et al. Cisplatin and fluorouracil alone or with docetaxel in head and neck cancer. N Engl J Med 2007;357:1705–15

8. Salama JK, Seiwert TY, Vokes EE. Chemoradiotherapy for locally advanced head and neck cancer. J Clin Oncol 2007;25:4118–26

9. Seiwert TY, Cohen EEW. State-of-the-art management of locally advanced head and neck cancer. Br J Cancer 2005;92:1341–8

1. http://www.nlm.nih.gov/medlineplus/headandneckcancer.html    Medline Plus
2. http://www.cochrane-ent.org    Cochrane HNO
3. http://www.cancer.gov/cancertopics/types/head-and-neck    NCI, Cancertopics
4. http://www.cancerbackup.org.uk/Cancertype/Headneck    Cancer BACKUP
5. http://www.emedicine.com/plastic/topic376.htm    E-medicine

## 8.2 Tumors of the Respiratory System

### 8.2.1 Lung Cancer

**U. Martens, W. Digel**

**Def:** Malignant pulmonary tumors, originating from:
- Surface epithelium of bronchi or bronchioli → non-small cell lung cancer, NSCLC
- Neuroectodermal cells / APUD ("amine precursor uptake and decarboxylation") system → small cell lung cancer, SCLC

**ICD-10:** C34.-

**Ep:** Incidence: 25% of all carcinomas worldwide; most common tumor in men, second most common tumor in women. More than 25% of all tumor-associated deaths are lung cancer related; ratio male:female = 3:1; age peak: 55–60 years.

**Pg:** *Smoking*
The main risk factor is smoking (especially for small cell lung cancer and squamous cell carcinoma). Other carcinogens are secondary. The relative risk of developing lung cancer is 30 times higher in smokers than in non-smokers. Only 5–10% of all patients with lung cancer are non-smokers. Relevant factors include:
- Number of cigarettes and duration of smoking habit ("pack years" = number of cigarette packs per day × total number of years)
- Age when taking up smoking
- Way of smoking (inhalation)
- Contact with cocarcinogens (industrial carcinogens, asbestos, etc.)

*Industrial Carcinogens*
Industrial carcinogens are responsible for a maximum of 8% of lung cancer-related deaths:
- Radionuclides such as uranium, radon in miners, radon derivatives (especially small cell lung cancer)
- Asbestos, especially with heavy smoking; asbestos fibers include: actinolite, amosite, anthophyllite, chrysotile, crocidolite, and tremolite
- Arsenic compounds: arsenic trioxide, arsenic pentoxide, arsenic acid and derivatives
- Beryllium and beryllium compounds
- Chromium compounds: especially chromium (VI) compounds, calcium / zinc chromate
- Nickel and nickel compounds: nickel sulfide / oxide / carbonate
- Polycyclic aromatic hydrocarbons (PAH): benzopyrene, dibenzanthracene, benzofluoranthene, indenopyrene, chrysene, PVC dust
- Halogenated ethers: dichloromethyl ether, dichlorodiethyl sulfide (Lost, mustard gas), acryl nitrite

*Fibrosis / Scars*
- Scars ("scar carcinoma"), cavitary lesions after tuberculosis ("cavitary carcinoma")

*Genetic Predisposition*
- Risk in relatives of lung cancer patients increased by factor 2–4
- Molecular genetic abnormalities: 3p21 deletion (chromosome 3), mutations of tumor suppressor genes p53 and Rb, altered oncogene expression (myc in small cell lung cancer; K-ras, Her2/neu in adenocarcinomas)
- In East Asia, 40% of lung cancer cases occur in never smokers and are associated with increased incidence of EGFR mutations

Sequence: epithelial metaplasia → dysplasia → carcinoma in situ → invasive carcinoma

**Path:**    **Histopathological classification (WHO 2001)**

| Type | Frequency (%) |
|------|---------------|
| *Small Cell Lung Cancer* | *20–25* |
| • Oat cell carcinoma | |
| • Combined oat cell carcinoma (with non-small cell components) | |
| *Non-small Cell Lung Cancer* | *75–80* |
| *Squamous Cell Carcinoma (Epidermoid)* | *35–40* |
| • Variant: spindle cell carcinoma | |
| *Adenocarcinoma* | *25–30* |
| • Acinar cell adenocarcinoma | |
| • Papillary adenocarcinoma | |
| • Bronchioloalveolar carcinoma | |
| *Large Cell Lung Cancer* | *5–10* |
| • Giant cell carcinoma | |
| • Clear cell carcinoma | |
| *Other* | 5 |
| • Adenoid cystic carcinoma | |
| • Adenosquamous carcinoma | |
| • Mucoepidermoid carcinoma | |
| • Mixed tumors | |

**Macroscopic forms**

| Type | Frequency (%) |
|------|---------------|
| *Central Lung Cancer*<br>Near hilus, mostly small cell or squamous cell carcinomas | 70 |
| *Peripheral Lung Cancer*<br>Distant to the hilus, nodular structure, frequently large cell lung cancer or adenocarcinomas | 25 |
| *Diffuse Lung Disease*<br>Alveolar cell carcinoma | 3 |
| *Pancoast's Tumor* | 2 |

**Metastatic spread and histological type**

| Location | Frequency of metastases (%) | | | |
|----------|------------------------------|---|---|---|
| | Squamous cell carcinoma | Large cell lung cancer | Adenocarcinoma | Small cell lung cancer |
| Mediastinal nodes | 30 | 40 | 40 | 95 |
| Liver | 30 | 30 | 45 | 50 |
| Brain | 20 | 30 | 30 | 40 |
| Bone | 25 | 40 | 40 | 35 |
| Bone marrow | 5 | not known | 5 | 30 |

**Class:**    **TNM Staging of Lung Cancer**

| $T$ | *Primary Tumor* |
|---|---|
| T0 | No evidence of primary tumor |
| TX | Primary tumor cannot be evaluated or has been detected by positive cytology |
| Tis | Carcinoma in situ |
| T1 | Tumor < 3 cm in diameter, not located in the main bronchus |
| T2 | Tumor > 3 cm, involvement of the main bronchus, 2 cm or more from the carina, invasion of the visceral pleura, partial atelectasis or obstructive pneumonia |
| T3 | Direct invasion of chest wall, diaphragm, mediastinal pleura, or parietal pericardium or involvement of the main bronchus < 2 cm from the carina or complete atelectasis or obstructive pneumonia |
| T4 | Direct invasion of mediastinum, heart, large blood vessels, trachea, esophagus, vertebral bodies or carina, or malignant pleural or pericardial effusion |
| $N$ | *Lymph Node Involvement* |
| N0 | Regional lymph nodes without metastases |
| NX | Regional lymph nodes cannot be assessed |
| N1 | Metastasis to ipsilateral peribronchial and/or hilar lymph nodes |
| N2 | Metastasis to ipsilateral mediastinal and/or subcarinal lymph nodes |
| N3 | Metastasis to contralateral mediastinal or hilar lymph nodes or to supraclavicular lymph nodes |
| $M$ | *Distant Metastasis* |
| M0 | No distant metastasis |
| MX | Distant metastasis cannot be assessed |
| M1 | Distant metastasis |

**Staging according to AJCC (2006)**

| Stage | TNM system | | |
|---|---|---|---|
| 0 | Tis | N0 | M0 |
| IA | T1 | N0 | M0 |
| IB | T2 | N0 | M0 |
| IIA | T1 | N1 | M0 |
| IIB | T2 | N1 | M0 |
| | T3 | N0 | M0 |
| IIIA | T1–3 | N2 | M0 |
| | T3 | N1 | M0 |
| IIIB | T1–3 | N3 | M0 |
| | T4 | N0–3 | M0 |
| IV | T1–4 | N0–3 | M1 |

**Staging of small cell lung cancer**

| Stage | Characteristics |
|---|---|
| *Limited Disease* | *Primary tumor limited to one hemithorax* |
| | ± Ipsilateral hilar lymph nodes |
| | ± Ipsilateral supraclavicular lymph nodes |
| | ± Ipsilateral and/or contralateral mediastinal lymph nodes |
| | ± Ipsilateral atelectasis |
| | ± Ipsilateral small pleural effusion without malignant cells |
| | ± Recurrent nerve and/or phrenic nerve palsy |
| *Extensive Disease* | *Any tumor spread exceeding the definition of "limited disease"* |
| | • ED I: thoracic spread (including chest wall, supraclavicular region, pleural effusion, mediastinal vessels) |
| | • ED II: metastases to the contralateral lung and/or other hematogenic metastases |

**Sy:**  Symptoms primarily depend on tumor location, size, and metastasis. Early symptoms are non-specific.

### Early Symptoms
- Fatigue, reduced performance, anorexia, weight loss
- Cough, hemoptysis, stridor, dyspnea
- Chronic pneumonia
- Paraneoplastic syndromes

### Late Symptoms
- Recurrent nerve palsy, phrenic nerve palsy
- Pleural effusion
- Chest pain

**Dg:**

### Medical History, Physical Examination
- Medical history including smoking habits, risk factors
- Physical examination (lungs, signs of metastasis, neurology, etc.)

### Laboratory Tests
- Routine laboratory tests: full blood count with differential, LDH, alkaline phosphatase, total protein, $Na^+$, $Ca^{++}$, liver and renal function tests, uric acid, inflammatory parameters
- Tumor markers: non-small cell lung cancer: CYFRA 21-1, CEA; small cell lung cancer: NSE
  NOTE: only suitable for disease monitoring, not for initial diagnosis.

### Histology / Cytology
- Bronchoscopy with cytology, lavage, biopsy
- Mediastinoscopy
- Possibly thoracotomy to obtain histology sample

### Other Diagnostic Procedures, Exclusion of Distant Metastases
- Imaging: chest x-ray (PA and lateral views), thoracic CT scan
- Preoperatively: lung function tests, perfusion scan, ECG
- Thoracic MRI scan (with Pancoast's tumors or suspected spinal infiltration)
- Bone scan (exclusion of metastases)
- Abdominal ultrasound, abdominal CT scan (exclusion of metastases)
- Bone marrow biopsy, cranial MRI scan

**Dd:**

*Differential Diagnosis of Intrapulmonary Masses*

*Malignant Tumors*

| | |
|---|---|
| • Lung cancer | 40–50% of cases |
| • Metastases | 10% of cases; lymphangitis carcinomatosis or hematogenous metastasis (▶ Chap. 8.12.3) |
| • Carcinoid | Originating from the APUD system (▶ Chap. 8.7.2) |
| • Cylindroma | Adenoid cystic carcinoma, poor prognosis |

*Benign Tumors*

| | |
|---|---|
| • Bronchial adenoma | |
| • Chondroma | Benign hamartoma |
| • Other benign tumors | Neurinoma, lipoma, fibroma, osteoma, etc. |

*Other*

| | |
|---|---|
| • Infections | Tuberculosis, actinomycosis, pneumonia |
| • Sarcoidosis | |

The nature of treatment-resistant coughs and sneezes or pulmonary nodules must be clarified. In patients over 40 years, they are highly suspicious of a carcinoma. Isolated pulmonary nodules are malignant in 50% of cases.

**Co:**

### Pancoast's Syndrome

Apical pleural dome / lung cancer with infiltration of the chest wall:
- Destruction of the first rib and thoracic vertebral body
- Damage to cervical nerve roots, cervical sympathetic chain, and brachial plexus → plexus / intercostal neuralgia, Horner syndrome (miosis, ptosis, enophthalmus)
- Upper extremity edema (lymphedema, venous congestion)

### Paraneoplastic Syndromes (▶ chapter 8.13)

Mainly in small cell lung cancer, rarely with non-small cell lung cancer

### Paraneoplastic Endocrinopathies

- SIADH syndrome (inadequate ADH secretion)
- Cushing's syndrome (ectopic ACTH production)
- Hypercalcemia (due to production of PTH-RP (parathormone-related peptide) or cytokines such as IL-1, IL-6, TNFα)
- Gynecomastia

### Paraneoplastic Hypercoagulability

Increased susceptibility to thrombosis

### Paraneoplastic Osteopathies, Myopathies, and Neuropathies

- Hypertrophic osteoarthropathy
- Marie-Bamberger syndrome (hypertrophic osteoarthropathy + drumstick fingers)
- Lambert-Eaton syndrome (myasthenia-type syndrome with weakness of the proximal extremity muscles)
- Polymyositis, dermatomyositis

### Superior Vena Cava Syndrome

▶ Chap. 9.2

**Th:**

Lung cancer is treated according to histology and tumor spread as well as age and performance status of the patient.

## Small Cell Lung Cancer

### Treatment Concept

1. Small cell lung cancer is characterized by early metastasis and should be managed as a systemic disease from diagnosis onwards. Surgical treatment with adjuvant chemotherapy only in early stages (T1 N0 M0).
2. Small cell lung cancer is sensitive to chemotherapy. Especially in limited disease, chemotherapy should be conducted with curative intent. However, relapses are frequent, and the long-term survival rate is approximately 10%. In extensive disease, chemotherapy must be considered a palliative treatment.
3. Combined chemoradiotherapy is a standard in limited disease. Combined approaches, e.g., concurrent or sequential chemoradiotherapy, achieve better survival rates but are associated with increased systemic toxicity. High-dose chemotherapy should only be considered in clinical studies.
4. Small cell lung cancer is sensitive to radiotherapy. In patients with small cell lung cancer in complete remission, isolated radiation of the head significantly improves overall survival and disease-free survival.

**Treatment of small cell lung cancer**

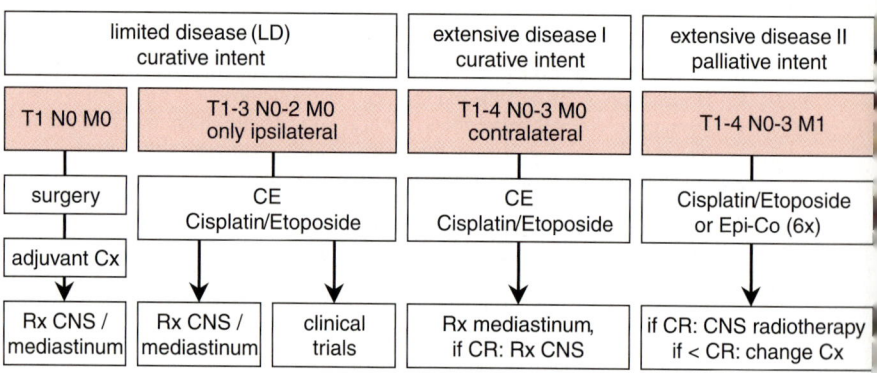

*Cx* chemotherapy, *Rx* radiotherapy, *Epi-Co* epirubicin+ cyclophosphamide+ vincristine, *CR* complete remission

### Chemotherapy Protocols for Small Cell Lung Cancer

| "Cisplatin/ Etoposide" ▶ Protocol 12.2.1 | | | Start next cycle on day 29 |
|---|---|---|---|
| Cisplatin | 75 mg/m²/day | i.v. | Day 1 |
| Etoposide | 100 mg/m²/day | i.v. | Days 1–3 |

| "EpiCO" ▶ Protocol 12.2.2 | | | Start next cycle on day 22 |
|---|---|---|---|
| Epirubicin | 70 mg/m²/day | i.v. | Day 1 |
| Cyclophosphamide | 1,000 mg/m²/day | i.v. | Day 1 |
| Vincristine | 2 mg | i.v. | Day 1 |

| *"Carboplatin/Etoposide"* ▶ Protocol 12.2.4 | | | *Start next cycle on day 22* |
|---|---|---|---|
| Carboplatin | AUC 6 | i.v. | Day 1 |
| Etoposide | 120 mg/m²/day | i.v. | Days 1–3 |


| *"VIPE"* ▶ Protocol 13.1.2 | | | *Start next cycle on day 22* |
|---|---|---|---|
| Etoposide | 500 mg/m²/day | i.v. | Day 1 |
| Ifosfamide | 4,000 mg/m²/day | i.v. | Day 1 |
| Cisplatin | 50 mg/m²/day | i.v. | Day 1 |
| Epirubicin | 50 mg/m²/day | i.v. | Day 1 |


| *"Paclitaxel weekly"* ▶ Protocol 12.2.3 | | | *Weekly* |
|---|---|---|---|
| Paclitaxel | 80 mg/m²/day | i.v. | Day 1 |


| *"Topotecan mono"* ▶ Protocol 12.2.5 | | | *Start next cycle on day 22* |
|---|---|---|---|
| Topotecan | 1.5 mg/m²/day | i.v. | Days 1–5 |

### Second-line Therapies

- Trofosfamide p.o., etoposide (VP16) monotherapy p.o.
- Cis-/carboplatin-containing chemotherapy protocols
- Newer drugs: topotecan, irinotecan; also used in combination therapies, e.g., topotecan / cisplatin in trials

## Non-small Cell Lung Cancer

### Treatment Concept

1. The treatment of choice in non-small cell lung cancer is surgery. Standard procedures include lobectomy, bilobectomy, pneumonectomy, and wedge resection, always with systematic lymph node dissection. At the time of diagnosis, 25–30% of patients (stages I and II) are operable with curative intent.
2. In locally advanced disease (stages IIIA and B), the treatment of choice is combined radiochemotherapy, if possible in clinical trials, with the aim to achieve resectability.
3. Inoperable stages of the disease (stage IV) are treated palliatively. Polychemotherapy is one option after diagnosis. Patients with advanced disease may benefit substantially from supportive and/or palliative therapeutic measures (radiotherapy, chemotherapy, laser treatment, stent insertion, pain control, high-calorie diet).
4. Primary radiotherapy is indicated particularly in patients functionally inoperable due to age or concomitant diseases. Preoperative radiation is recommended for Pancoast's tumors. Patients with mediastinal metastases (pN2) may receive postoperative radiotherapy. Radiotherapy is applied in the form of megavolt irradiation with a target dose of 60 Gy. Side effects include esophagitis, pneumonitis, pulmonary fibrosis (< 5% of cases) and, less commonly, cardiac damage.
5. "Targeted therapies": EGFR inhibitors (erlotinib in the 2nd / 3rd line treatments) and angiogenesis inhibitors (bevacizumab in 1st line setting) improve response rates and survival.

### Treatment of non-small cell lung cancer

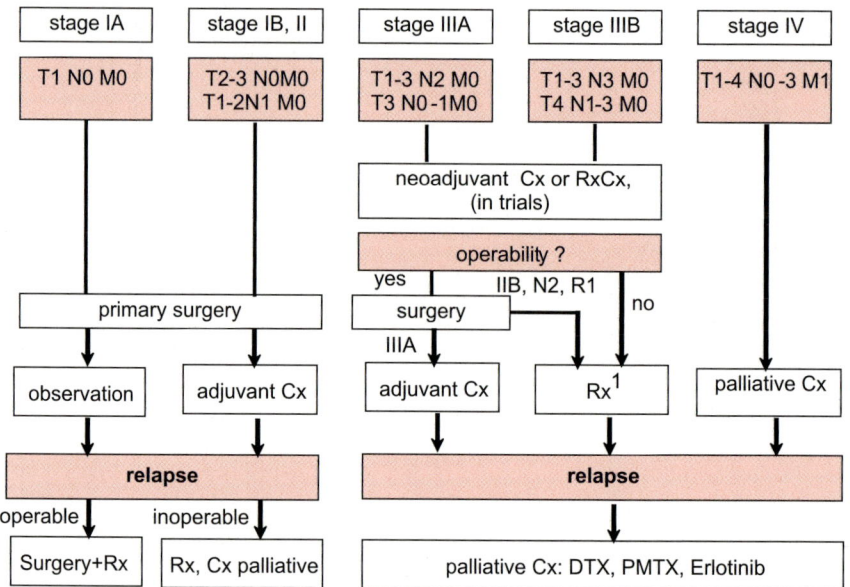

*RxCx* combined radiochemotherapy, *Rx* radiotherapy, *Cx* chemotherapy, *DTX* docetaxel, *PMTX* pemetrexed, *EGFR* epidermal growth factor receptor
[1]If no prior neoadjuvant combined radiochemotherapy

## Neoadjuvant Approach with Stage IIIA and IIIB Disease

Patients with locally advanced disease are treated with combined radiochemotherapy, with the goal to achieve resectability. Indicated in patients with:
- Good performance status (Karnofsky scale > 70)
- Biological age < 65 years
- Minimal weight loss (< 5% of the original weight)

Locally advanced stages of the disease where surgical treatment is not an option are treated with chemotherapy and radiotherapy.

## Chemotherapy Protocols for Non-small Cell Lung Cancer

### Adjuvant Chemotherapy Stage IB

| "Paclitaxel / Carboplatin" ▶ Protocol 12.2.8 | | | Start next cycle on day 22 |
|---|---|---|---|
| Paclitaxel | 100 mg/m²/day | i.v. | Day 1, 8 15, over 3 h |
| Carboplatin | AUC | i.v. | Day 1 |
| For dose calculation according to AUC ▶ Chap. 3.2.1 | | | |

### Adjuvant Chemotherapy Stage IIA–IIIA

| "Cisplatin / Vinorelbine" ▶ Protocol 12.2.11 | | | Start next cycle on day 22 |
|---|---|---|---|
| Vinorelbine | 30 mg/m²/day | i.v. | Days 1, 8 |
| Cisplatin | 80 mg/m²/day | i.v. | Day 1 |

### Palliative Chemotherapy Stage IV

| "Gemcitabine / Cisplatin" ▶ Protocol 12.2.9 | | | Start next cycle on day 22 |
|---|---|---|---|
| Gemcitabine | 1,000 mg/m²/day | i.v. | Days 1, 8 |
| Cisplatin | 70 mg/m²/day | i.v. | Day 1 |

| "Vinorelbine / Carboplatin" ▶ Protocol 12.2.7 | | | Start next cycle on day 22 |
|---|---|---|---|
| Vinorelbine | 25 mg/m²/day | i.v. | Days 1, 8, 15 |
| Carboplatin | AUC 6 | i.v. | Day 1 |

| "Docetaxel/Cisplatin" | | | Start next cycle on day 22 |
|---|---|---|---|
| Docetaxel | 75 mg/m²/day | i.v. | Day 1 |
| Cisplatin | 75 mg/m²/day | i.v. | Day 1 |

### Second-line Therapies

| "Docetaxel" ▶ Protocol 12.2.10 | | | Start next cycle on day 22 |
|---|---|---|---|
| Docetaxel | 75 mg/m²/day | i.v. | Day 1 |

| "Pemetrexed" ▶ Protocol 12.2.12 | | | Start next cycle on day 22 |
|---|---|---|---|
| Pemetrexed | 500 mg/m²/day | i.v. | Day 1 |

### New Compounds
"Targeted Therapies"(▶ Chap. 3.6).
In recent clinical trials inhibitors of EGFR (erlotinib) and angiogenesis (bevacizumab) were evaluated. Targeted therapies succeed in increasing response and overall survival.
- Bevacizumab: monoclonal antibody against VEGF (vascular endothelial growth factor). Used in combination with carboplatin / paclitaxel with advanced NSCLC. *NOTE:* occurrence of severe bleedings, hemoptysis
- EGFR inhibitors: erlotinib: effective especially in tumors positive for mutated EGFR (10% of all patients with NSCLC)

### Palliative Therapies

Even in advanced stages of lung cancer, palliative treatment may significantly improve the patient's quality of life. Procedures:

- Bronchoscopy with secretion clearance
- Drainage in cases of postobstructive pneumonia with abscess formation
- Laser coagulation or endobronchial blocking in cases of hemorrhage
- Laser treatment, usually in the form of bronchoscopic endoluminal treatment, possibly combined with photosensitizers ("photodynamic therapy"); alternatively: use of cryoprobes or high-frequency diathermy
- Endoluminal high-dose radiotherapy
- Implantation of endoprostheses or stents in cases of respiratory obstruction, aerodigestive fistulas, or postobstructive pneumonia
- Pain control: analgesics (▶ Chap. 4.5), bisphosphonates in case of bone metastases (▶ Chap. 4.7)
- Palliative chemotherapy or radiotherapy

**Prg:**     *Prognostic Factors*

- Histology, tumor stage (resectability)
- Age and performance status of the patient, weight loss
- Lactate dehydrogenase (LDH)

*Small Cell Lung Cancer*

Poor overall prognosis; survival without treatment: 2–8 weeks; median survival after treatment 8–12 months; long-term survival: 5–10% in total, < 1% in patients with "extensive disease."

*Non-Small Cell Lung Cancer*

Long-term survival is only achievable in patients with resectable tumors or localized disease which can be treated with combined therapy. At presentation, 50% of all patients are in inoperable stages of the disease. After surgery with curative intent, 25% of patients are long-term disease-free.

*Five-year Survival in Non-small Cell Lung Cancer:*

- Stage I–IIA:     55–67%
- Stage IIB:     38–39%
- Stage IIIA:     23–25%
- Stage IIIB:     3–7%
- Stage IV:     1%

**F/U:**     Patients treated with curative intent should initially undergo follow-up (medical history, physical examination, laboratory tests, chest x-ray, abdominal ultrasound) every 3 months. After 2 years every 6 months, after 5 years: every 12 months.

In palliative situations: symptom-based approach.

**Px:**     *Prophylactic Measures*

- Abstinence from smoking
- Ban on asbestos, occupational health and safety measures

**Ref:**

1. Blackstock AW, Govindan R. Definitive chemoradiation for the treatment of locally advanced NSCLC. J Clin Oncol 2007;25:4146–52
2. ESMO Guidelines Working Group. NSCLC: ESMO Clinical Recommendations for diagnosis, treatment and follow-up. Ann Oncol 2007;18(suppl 2):ii30–1
3. ESMO Guidelines Working Group. SCLC: ESMO Clinical Recommendations for diagnosis, treatment and follow-up. Ann Oncol 2007;18(Suppl.2):ii32–3
4. Jackman DM, Johnson BE. Small-cell lung cancer. Lancet 2005;366:1385–96
5. Lally BE, Urbanic JJ, Blackstock AW et al. SCLC: have we made any progress over the last 25 years? Oncologist 2007;12:1096–104

6.  Pfister DG, Johnson DH, Azzoli CG et al. ASCO treatment of unresectable non-small-cell lung cancer guideline: Update 2003. J Clin Oncol 2004;22:330–53

7.  Pfister KMW, Evans WK, Azzoli CG et al. Cancer Care Ontario and ASCO adjuvant chemotherapy and adjuvant radiation therapy for stages I-IIIA resectable NSCLC Guideline. J Clin Oncol 2007;25:5506–18

8.  Ramalingam S, Belani C. Systemic chemotherapy for advanced NSCLC: recent advances and future directions. Oncologist 2008;13:5–13

9.  Sandler A, Gray R, Perry MC et al. Paclitaxel-carboplatin alone or with bevacizumab for NSCLC. N Engl J Med 2006;355:2542–50

**Web:**

1.  http://www.nlm.nih.gov/medlineplus/lungcancer.html  MedlinePlus
2.  http://www.cancer.gov/cancertopics/types/lung  NCI, CancerNet
3.  http://www.emedicine.com/med/topic1333.htm  E-medicine
4.  http://www.lungcanceronline.org/  Lung Cancer Online
5.  http://www.lungcancer.org/  Lung Cancer Focus

## 8.2.2     Mesotheliomas

### H. Henß, W. Digel

| | |
|---|---|
| **Def:** | Tumors of mesenchymal origin originating primarily from pleura (pleural mesothelioma), peritoneum (peritoneal mesothelioma, rare), or pericardium (pericardial mesothelioma, rare). |
| **ICD-10:** | C45.0 |
| **Ep:** | Incidence 1/100,000 population/year; 0.2% of all malignant tumors; increasing incidence in industrial nations; ratio male:female = 2:1; age peak: 50–60 years. |

**Pg:**

### Etiology
- *Main etiological factor: asbestos* → environmental carcinogen, long latency period between exposure and manifestation (up to > 20 years); high prevalence in certain regions (Anatolia) due to extensive asbestos use or exposure to asbestos-related substances. *70–80% of patients show evidence of exposure to asbestos. Pleural mesothelioma is recognized as an occupational disease of workers in the asbestos industry.*
- Previous radiotherapy (e.g., Hodgkin's disease, Thorotrast exposure)
- Possibly genetic factors (hereditary occurrence)
- Smoking (not confirmed)

**Path:**

### Histological Types
- Epithelial (mesothelial mesothelioma)
- Sarcomatous
- Mixed

### Invasion / Spread
Sheet-like pleural involvement, extensive pleural nodules; frequent lymph node involvement and invasion of the mediastinum; often invasive growth, e.g., into diaphragm or chest wall; distant metastases in approximately 50% of patients with advanced disease.

### Molecular Diagnosis
Deletion of chromosome 22 (del22) or structural rearrangements of chromosome 1p, 3p, 6q, or 9p.

**Class:**     **TNM staging of Pleural Mesothelioma (UICC 2002)**

| T | Primary Tumor |
|---|---|
| TX | Primary tumor cannot be assessed |
| T0 | No evidence of primary tumor |
| T1 | Tumor limited to the ipsilateral parietal and/or visceral pleura |
| T2 | Invasion of ipsilateral lungs, endothoracic fascia, diaphragm, or pericardium |
| T3 | Invasion of ipsilateral chest wall, ribs, mediastinum |
| T4 | Direct invasion of contralateral pleura, lungs, peritoneum, abdominal organs, or structures of the neck |
| **N** | **Lymph Node Involvement** |
| NX | Regional lymph nodes cannot be assessed |
| N0 | No regional lymph node metastases |
| N1 | Metastasis to ipsilateral peribronchial and/or hilar lymph nodes |
| N2 | Metastasis to ipsilateral mediastinal and/or subcarinal lymph nodes |
| N3 | Metastasis to contralateral hilar and/or mediastinal lymph nodes or to supraclavicular lymph nodes |

**Class:** TNM Staging of Pleural Mesothelioma (UICC 2002) *(continued)*

| M | Distant Metastasis |
|---|---|
| MX | Distant metastasis cannot be assessed |
| M0 | No distant metastasis |
| M1 | Distant metastasis |

AJCC Staging of Pleural Mesothelioma

| Stage | TNM system | | |
|---|---|---|---|
| I | T1 | N0 | M0 |
| II | T2 | N0 | M0 |
| III | T1–2 | N1–2 | M0 |
| | T3 | N0–2 | M0 |
| IV | T4 | Any N | M0 |
| | Any T | N3 | M0 |
| | Any T | Any N | M1 |

**Sy:** Often non-specific and slowly worsening. For pleural mesothelioma:
- Dyspnea (pleural effusion)
- Chest pain
- Weight loss, fatigue, reduced performance

**Dg:** *Medical History, Physical Examination*
- Medical history, particularly exposure to asbestos
- Physical examination including chest percussion and auscultation

*Laboratory Tests*
- Blood count, liver / renal function test
- Serum marker SMRP ("serum mesothelin-related protein"), CA 125, CA 15-3 suitable for monitoring of the disease course

*Cytology / Histology of Pleural Mesothelioma*
- Bronchoscopy / bronchial lavage (detection of asbestos particles)
- Biopsy via thoracoscopy or thoracotomy (cytological analysis of the pleural effusion often difficult to interpret → frequent false-negative results)

*Imaging*
- Chest x-ray, thoracic CT scan, MRI (where applicable)
- Ultrasound: pleural effusion
- Possibly PET (staging, detection of vital mesothelioma residual disease after therapy)

**Th:** Treatment Options in Pleural Mesothelioma

*Supportive Treatment*
Pain control (possibly blockade / inactivation of intercostal nerves)

*Surgical Treatment*
Surgical mesothelioma resection is treatment of choice, although it is seldom curative. If possible, pleuro-pneumonectomy or radical extrapleural pleuro-pneumonectomy is carried out. Simple

pleurectomy is a palliative procedure. Extensive reduction of the tumor load ("debulking") appears to improve prognosis.

### Radiotherapy
Palliative radiotherapy is indicated to control pain, however, radiotherapy does not seem to prolong survival.

### Chemotherapy
The benefit of chemotherapy in the treatment of pleural mesothelioma is under discussion:
- Effective drugs: pemetrexed, cisplatin, gemcitabine
- Drugs with limited efficacy: doxorubicin, ifosfamide, cyclophosphamide, mitomycin C, methotrexate, oxaliplatin, paclitaxel, and vinorelbine
- In clinical trials: imatinib

### Immunotherapy
Clinical trials have shown limited efficacy of interferon-α, interferon-γ, or IL-2 if given intrapleurally or systemically.

### Multimodal Therapies
The combination of pleuro-pneumonectomy with postoperative radiotherapy and chemotherapy is currently being investigated in clinical studies. Prolonged median survival and higher 5-year survival rates have been reported.

## Chemotherapy Protocols in Pleural Mesothelioma

| "Vinorelbine" | | | Start next cycle on day 29 |
|---|---|---|---|
| Vinorelbine | 25 mg/m²/day | i.v. | Days 1, 8, 15 |

| "Pemetrexed / Cisplatin" ▶ Protocol 12.3.2 | | | Start next cycle on day 22 |
|---|---|---|---|
| Pemetrexed | 500 mg/m²/day | i.v. | Day 1 |
| Cisplatin | 75 mg/m²/day | i.v. | Day 1 |

| "Paclitaxel / Carboplatin / RT" ▶ Protocol 12.3.1 | | | Start next cycle on day 29 |
|---|---|---|---|
| Paclitaxel | 200 mg/m²/day | i.v. | Days 1, 22 |
| Paclitaxel | 50 mg/m²/day | i.v. | Day 43 |
| Carboplatin | AUC 6mg/mlxmin | | Days 1, 22 |
| Radiotherapy | 30–54 Gy | | Start day 43 |

| "Gemcitabine / Cisplatin" ▶ Protocol 12.2.9 | | | Start next cycle on day 22 |
|---|---|---|---|
| Gemcitabine | 1,000 mg/m²/day | i.v. | Days 1, 8 |
| Cisplatin | 70 mg/m²/day | i.v. | Day 1 |

**Prg:**     *Prognostic Factors*
- Tumor size / stage (involvement of regional lymph nodes → poor prognosis)
- Histology (epithelial histology favorable; sarcomatous histology less favorable)
- Age, performance status (older age or reduced performance status less favorable)
- Gender (men: less favorable prognosis)
- Extent of tumor resection (better prognosis if minimal residual disease)
- Leukocytosis: poor prognosis

*Median Survival*

Without treatment: 4–18 months

**Px:**     Ban on asbestos and asbestos-related substances, occupational health and safety measures.

**Ref:**
1. Bofetta P. Epidemiology of peritoneal mesothelioma: a review. Ann Oncol 2007;18:985–90
2. Ceresoli GL, Betta GP, Castagneto B et al. Malignant pleural mesothelioma. Ann Oncol 2006;17(suppl 2): ii13–6
3. ESMO Guidelines Working Group. Malignant pleural mesothelioma: ESMO Clinical Recommendations for diagnosis, treatment and follow-up. Ann Oncol 2007;18(Suppl. 2):ii34–5
4. Hassan R, Alexander R, Antman K et al. Current treatment options and biology of peritoneal mesothelioma. Ann Oncol 2006;17:1615–9
5. Robinson BWS, Lake RA. Advances in malignant mesothelioma. N Engl J Med 2005;353:1591–603
6. Vogelzang NJ, Rusthoven JJ, Symanowski J et al. Phase III study of pemetrexed in combination with cisplatin versus cisplatin alone in patients with malignant pleural mesothelioma. J Clin Oncol 2003;21:2636–44
7. Zucali PA, Giaccone G. Biology and management of malignant pleural mesothelioma. Eur J Cancer 2006;42:2706–14

**Web:**
| | | |
|---|---|---|
| 1. | http://www.cancer.gov/cancertopics/types/malignantmesothelioma | NCI, Cancer Topics |
| 2. | http://www.emedicine.com/MED/topic1457.htm | E-medicine |
| 3. | http://www.mesolink.org | Mesothelioma Info |
| 4. | http://www.mesotheliomanews.com | Mesothelioma News |

### 8.2.3     Mediastinal Tumors

**R. Engelhardt, W. Digel**

**Def:**     Malignant neoplasms of the mediastinum.

**ICD-10:**     C38.

**Path:**     The mediastinum is located in the thorax between the pericardium, spine, and pleural cavities and consists of six compartments. Due to the multitude of anatomical structures involved, ontogenetically different tumors may arise. The most common mediastinal tumor types are thymoma, lymphoma, and carcinoids as well as mesenchymal and neurogenic tumors.

**Location and histology of the most common mediastinal tumors**

| Compartment | Posterior | Axial | Anterior |
|---|---|---|---|
| Upper | Thyroid tumors<br>Neurogenic tumors | Thyroid tumors | Thyroid tumors<br>Lymphoma<br>Teratoma<br>Thymoma |
| Middle | Neurogenic tumors | Bronchogenic cysts | Teratoma<br>Thymoma |
| Lower | Neurogenic tumors | Bronchogenic cysts | Lipoma<br>Pleuropericardial cysts<br>Thymoma |

### Thymoma

**Def:**     Lymphoepithelial neoplasms originating from epithelial cells of the thymus with malignant lymphoid cells components.

**Ep:**     Incidence 0.2–0.4 cases/100,000 population/year; ratio male:female = 1:1; age peak: 50 years. Thymomas are the most common neoplasms of the anterior upper mediastinum (20–30% of cases) and account for 0.2–1.5% of all malignant tumors. 5% of thymomas are of ectopic origin and arise from the lung, trachea, or neck.

**Pg:**     Pathogenetic mechanisms are not fully elucidated. In lymphoepithelial thymomas, Epstein-Barr virus (EBV) DNA has been detected.

**Path:**     Differentiation between benign (completely encapsulated) thymomas, malignant thymomas and thymic carcinomas.

**Pathological classification according to Levine and Rosai**

| | |
|---|---|
| *Benign Thymoma* | No capsular invasion, cytologically benign |
| *Malignant Thymoma* | |
| • Category 1 | Capsular invasion or metastasis |
| • Category 2 | No capsular invasion, no metastasis, cytologically malignant |
| *Thymic Carcinoma* | Locally aggressive with tendency to local relapse, capsular invasion, and metastasis |

**Class:** TNM staging has not been established. A clinically relevant classification has been described by Masaoka.

**Thymoma staging according to Masaoka**

| | |
|---|---|
| I | Macroscopically: completely encapsulated tumor, microscopically: no capsular invasion |
| II | Macroscopic invasion into surrounding fatty tissue or mediastinal pleura or microscopic invasion into capsule |
| III | Macroscopic invasion into neighboring organs (lung, pericardium, large vessels) |
| IV | A: pleural and/or pericardial tumor dissemination |
| | B: lymphogenic and/or hematogenic metastases |

**Sy:** Symptoms arise due to local expansion as well as compression and infiltration of adjacent structures. Early symptoms are non-specific.
- Cough, hoarseness, stridor
- Difficulty swallowing, dysphagia
- Fatigue, reduced performance, anorexia
- Paraneoplastic symptoms (myasthenia), (▶ Chap. 8.13)

**Dg:** *Medical History, Physical Examination*
- Medical history including systemic diseases
- Physical examination: superior vena cava compression, stridor (tracheal compression)

*Laboratory Tests*
- Routine laboratory tests, including blood count and hepatic / renal function parameters
- 5-HIES in urine, vanillylmandelic acid in urine, catecholamine excretion (exclusion of neurogenic tumors, pheochromocytoma)
- AFP, β-HCG (exclusion of germ cell tumors)
- Immunoglobulins (exclusion of hypogammaglobulinemia)
- Mestinon test (exclusion of myasthenia)

*Imaging*
- Chest x-ray (PA and lateral views), thoracic CT scan
- Angiography, bronchoscopy, esophagoscopy

**DD:**
- Carcinomas originating from the thymus without thymus-specific differentiation (squamous cell carcinomas, small cell carcinomas, etc.)
- Metastases of other primary tumors
- Castleman's syndrome: benign and potentially extensive mediastinal lymph node enlargement
- Pericardial, pleuropericardial, and gastroenteric cysts
- Thymic hyperplasia, e.g., after chemotherapy in children or adolescents

**Co:** More than 70% of thymomas are associated with systemic diseases, particularly immunological disorders and endocrine diseases:
- Myasthenia gravis: 30–50% of cases
- Hypogammaglobulinemia: 5–10% of cases
- Erythropoietic aplasia: 5% of cases
- Autoimmune diseases: systemic lupus erythematosus (SLE), polymyositis, thyroiditis, rheumatoid arthritis, colitis ulcerosa
- Endocrine disorders: hyperthyroidism, Addison's disease, panhypopituitarism

**Th:**     **Treatment Concept**

1.  In localized stages I and II, radical resection with curative intent is most effective with respect to progression-free survival and overall survival.
2.  In locally advanced thymoma (stage III), indication for radical resection depends on whether R0 resection (resection with tumor-free margins) is possible. Debulking is of questionable benefit. If R0 resection seems impossible, neoadjuvant chemotherapy should be considered.
3.  In advanced metastatic stages of the disease, chemotherapy is indicated. Radiotherapy is applied in case of local tumor-induced symptoms.

**Thymoma therapy**

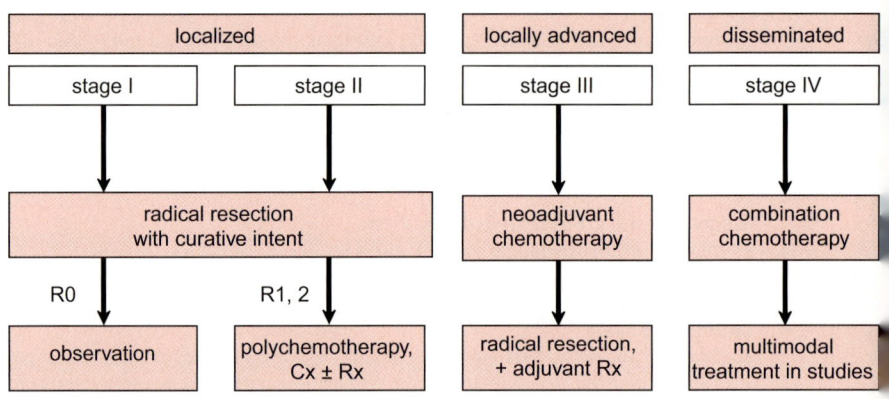

*Cx* chemotherapy, *Rx* radiotherapy

## Treatment Modalities

### Chemotherapy
*   All histological subtypes of thymoma are considered sensitive to chemotherapy. Best results are obtained with platinum-containing chemotherapy. In inoperable cases or cases of incomplete resection in stages II and III, combination chemotherapy with curative intent is indicated.
*   In advanced stages III and IVa, chemotherapy (e.g., VIP-E ▶ Protocol 13.1.2) should be part of a multimodal therapy concept with the objective of long-term remission.

### Radiotherapy
*   Thymomas are considered radiosensitive (in particular the lymphatic tissue components).
*   Primary radiotherapy alone is only indicated where surgery or chemotherapy are impossible.
*   Adjuvant radiotherapy is indicated in stages II and III.

**F/U:**     Close follow-up in patients treated with curative intent; follow-up frequency in first 2 years: every 3 months, then every 6 months (up to 5 years).

**Prg:**     Survival rates depend on disease stage and resectability. Median 5-year survival:
*   Stage I:     89–95%
*   Stage II:    71–85%
*   Stage III:  70–80%
*   Stage IV:   50–60%

## Thymic Carcinoma

**Path:** Thymic carcinomas are aggressive epithelial tumors of the thymus with a marked tendency to local invasion. Thymic carcinomas metastasize primarily via lymphatic vessels into mediastinal, cervical, and axillary lymph nodes. In advanced disease hematogenic spread into bones, lung, and liver.

**Th:** A multimodal approach is critical to achieve remission.
- Due to early invasion of mediastinal structures, complete resection is often impossible.
- Platinum-based combination chemotherapy can sometimes lead to complete remission. In unresectable tumors, neoadjuvant platinum-containing chemotherapy, e.g., according to the VIPE, PAC, or ADOC protocol should be used.
- Adjuvant radiotherapy has not demonstrated clinical benefit in recent studies.

| "PAC" ▶ Protocol 12.4.1 | | | Start next cycle on day 22 |
|---|---|---|---|
| Doxorubicin | 50 mg/m²/day | i.v. | Day 1 |
| Cisplatin | 50 mg/m²/day | i.v. | Day 1 |
| Cyclophosphamide | 500 mg/m²/day | i.v. | Day 1 |

**Prg:** Poor; 5-year survival: 35%

## Lymphomas (▶ Chap. 7.5)

**Path:** In the mediastinum, all types of malignant lymphoma may occur. The most important types of mediastinal lymphoma are:
- Hodgkin's disease
- Mediastinal B-cell lymphoma (primarily large-cell sclerosing lymphomas)
- Lymphoblastic lymphoma of the T-cell type
- Acute T-cell leukemia

**Th:** Treatment and prognosis of mediastinal lymphomas follow the general principles of lymphoma therapy (▶ Chap. 7.5).

## Germ Cell Tumors (▶ Chap. 8.5.2)

**Ep:** Ectopic mediastinal germ cell tumors most commonly occur in patients between 20 and 40 years of age.

**Sy:** Symptoms depend on histology, expansion, and proliferation rate of the tumor:
- *Mature teratoma:* often asymptomatic
- *Malignant teratoma:* due to compression and invasion of mediastinal structures, symptoms usually occur at an early stage (cough, hoarseness, dyspnea, stridor, difficulty swallowing, etc.)
- *Seminoma:* symptomatic only at later stages
- *Non-seminomatous germ cell tumors:* invasive behaviour; in over 90% of cases, symptoms due to invasion and compression of mediastinal structures; increase in tumor markers AFP and β-HCG; increased incidence of other malignant tumors, e.g., AML, MDS, essential thrombocythemia, carcinomas, sarcomas

**Th:** Mediastinal germ cell tumors are treated like germ cell tumors in other locations (▶ Chap. 8.5.2).
- *Mature teratoma:* surgical resection
- *Malignant teratoma:* surgical resection, combination chemotherapy, e.g., PEB protocol
- *Seminoma:* resection, radiotherapy, combination chemotherapy
- *Non-seminomatous germ cell tumors:* resection, radiotherapy, combination chemotherapy

### Thymus Carcinoid

**Path:** Rare tumor of the APUDoma group (▶ Chap. 8.7.2); in 25% of cases, associated with multiple endocrine neoplasm type I (MEN 1 syndrome, ▶ Chap. 8.7.3); symptoms due to local invasion and compression of mediastinal structures; frequently paraneoplastic syndromes due to ACTH secretion; early metastasis into lymph nodes, skeletal system, lung, liver.

**Th:** Resection. Radiotherapy and chemotherapy offer no therapeutic benefit.
In octreotide-binding tumors: treatment with radioactive or native octreotide.

### Mesenchymal Tumors of the Mediastinum

**Path:** *Thymic Lipoma*
Histologically consisting of mature fatty cells and thymic tissue. CT scan: typical density of fatty tissue. Standard treatment is surgical resection.

*Mediastinal Lipoma*
Lipomas can occur throughout the entire mediastinum. Liposarcomas are rare and occur mainly in the posterior mediastinum. Primary treatment is resection. Malignant liposarcomas are treated like soft tissue sarcomas in other locations (▶ Chap. 8.9.1)

*Vascular Tumors*
Tumors of the vascular system include hemangioma, hemangioendothelioma, and hemangiopericytoma. Approximately 30% of all vascular tumors are malignant. Treatment consists of resection or embolization.

*Neurogenic Tumors*
Neurogenic tumors are derived from structures of the autonomic or peripheral nervous system and are usually benign and asymptomatic. Neurofibromas can occur in von Recklinghausen's disease. Treatment: resection; with malignant neurogenic tumors, consider neoadjuvant chemotherapy.

**Ref:**
1. De Jong WK, Blaauwgeers JLG, Schaapveld M et al. Thymic epithelial tumors: A population-based study of the incidence, diagnostic procedures and therapy. Eur J Cancer 2008;44:123–30
2. Giaccone G. Treatment of malignant thymoma. Curr Opin Oncol 2005;17:140–6
3. Riedel RF, Burfeind WR. Thymoma: benign appearance, malignant potential. Oncologist 2006;11:887–94

**Web:**
1. http://www.cancer.gov/cancertopics/types/thymoma/      NCI, Cancer Topics
2. http://www.emedicine.com/med/topic2752.htm      E-medicine
3. http://www.acor.org/cnet/62708.html      ACOR

# 8.3 · Gastrointestinal Tumors

## 8.3.1 Esophageal Carcinoma

R. Engelhardt, F. Otto

**Def:** Malignant tumor of the esophagus.

**ICD-10:** C15.-

**Ep:** Incidence: 6 cases/100,000/year in Europe; large geographical differences (high incidence in China, Iran, South Africa); ratio male:female = 6:1; age peak: sixth decade; significant increase in the number of esophageal adenocarcinomas since 1980.

**Pg:** *Risk Factors*
- Alcohol (hard liquor) and heavy smoking
- Nitrosamines
- Achalasia
- Vitamin and iron deficiency (Plummer-Vinson syndrome)
- Palmoplantar keratosis
- Caustic injury → squamous cell carcinomas
- Barrett's syndrome in chronic reflux esophagitis → adenocarcinomas
- Obesity → adenocarcinomas of the lower third of the esophagus

**Path:** Since 1997, steady increase (approximately 10% per year) in esophageal adenocarcinomas. In men under 50 years of age, adenocarcinomas have become the most common type of esophageal carcinoma.

| Histology | Frequency (%) |
|---|---|
| • Squamous cell carcinoma, mainly in the middle and upper third of the esophagus | 70 |
| • Adenocarcinoma, mainly in the lower third of the esophagus | 25–30 |
| • Other (anaplastic or small cell carcinoma, cylindroma, carcinoid, leiomyosarcoma) | < 5 |

*Growth Pattern*
- Polypoid growth: 60%
- Diffuse infiltrating growth: 15%
- Ulcerous growth: 25%

*Location*
- Upper third of the esophagus: 15%
- Middle third of the esophagus: 45–50%
- Lower third of the esophagus: 35–40 %

**Class:** **TNM Staging of Esophageal Cancer (2002)**

| T | Primary Tumor |
|---|---|
| TX | Primary tumor cannot be assessed |
| T0 | No evidence of primary tumor |
| Tis | Carcinoma in situ |
| T1 | Tumor limited to lamina propria and submucosa |
| T2 | Tumor invades the muscularis mucosae |

**Class:**       **TNM Staging of Esophageal Cancer (2002)** *(continued)*

| | |
|---|---|
| T3 | Tumor invades the adventitia |
| T4 | Tumor invades adjacent extraesophageal structures |
| **N** | ***Lymph Node Involvement*** |
| NX | Regional lymph nodes cannot be assessed |
| N0 | Regional lymph nodes without metastases |
| N1 | Metastasis to regional lymph nodes (cervical esophagus: cervical lymph nodes, supraclavicular and thoracic esophagus: mediastinal, perigastric lymph nodes) |
| **M** | ***Distant Metastasis*** |
| M0 | No distant metastasis |
| M1 | Distant metastasis (including tumors of the thoracic esophagus with abdominal or cervical lymph node metastasis) |
| | A: metastases in celiac (tumor in lower esophagus) or cervical lymph nodes (tumor in upper esophagus) |
| | B: non-regional lymph node metastases (tumor in middle third of the esophagus) or other distant metastases |

**Staging according to AJCC (2002)**

| Stage | TNM system | | | Five-year survival (%) |
|---|---|---|---|---|
| 0 | Tis | N0 | M0 | 80 |
| I | pT1 | N0 | M0 | 67 |
| IIA | pT2–3 | N0 | M0 | 43 |
| IIB | pT1–2 | N1 | M0 | 26 |
| III | pT3 | N1 | M0 | 16 |
| | pT4 | Any N | M0 | |
| IVA | Any pT | Any N | M1A | 3 |
| IVB | Any pT | Any N | M1B | 3 |

**Sy:**       Symptoms usually only in advanced stages of the disease:
- Dysphagia, regurgitation
- Retrosternal pain
- Weight loss, fatigue
- Mediastinal infiltration: hoarseness
- Tracheo- or bronchoesophageal fistulas: cough, dyspnea

**Dg:**       ***Medical History, Physical Examination***
- Medical history, particularly dysphagia, risk factors
- Physical examination including body weight

***Laboratory Tests***
- Routine laboratory tests including blood count, liver and renal function tests
- Possibly tumor markers: CEA, SCC, only suitable for monitoring (not for confirmation of diagnosis)

***Imaging***
- Chest x-ray
- Contrast-based x-ray (if aspiration risk: with water-soluble contrast medium)
- Abdominal ultrasound, endosonography
- Thoracic and abdominal CT scan (to facilitate staging), PET (where applicable)

### Histology
- Esophago-/gastro-/duodenoscopy (with biopsy)
- Laryngoscopy, bronchoscopy, colonoscopy (to explore feasibility of a possible colon conduit)

*NOTE:* frequent occurrence of second primary tumors in the bronchial tree or ENT region

All cases of symptomatic dysphagia require immediate attention (endoscopy, histology).

**DD:**
- Esophageal diverticulum, hiatus hernia
- Abnormal esophageal motility (hypercontractile esophagus, etc.)

**Co:**
- Esophagotracheal fistulas → risk of aspiration
- Esophagomediastinal fistulas → risk of mediastinitis
- Recurrent hemorrhage

**Th:**

## Treatment Concept

1. Multimodal therapy concepts combining surgery, chemotherapy, and radiotherapy are probably superior to single modality approaches. Treatment should be adapted to tumor stage and performance status.
2. *ATTENTION:* no PEG tube prior to surgery (stomach required as conduit), no stent implantation prior to radiotherapy (risk of perforation).
3. Even in palliative situations, supportive therapies (dilatation, tube or stent implantation, insertion of a PEG tube) can significantly improve quality of life.

### Multimodal Treatment of Esophageal Carcinoma (squamous cell/adenocarcinoma)

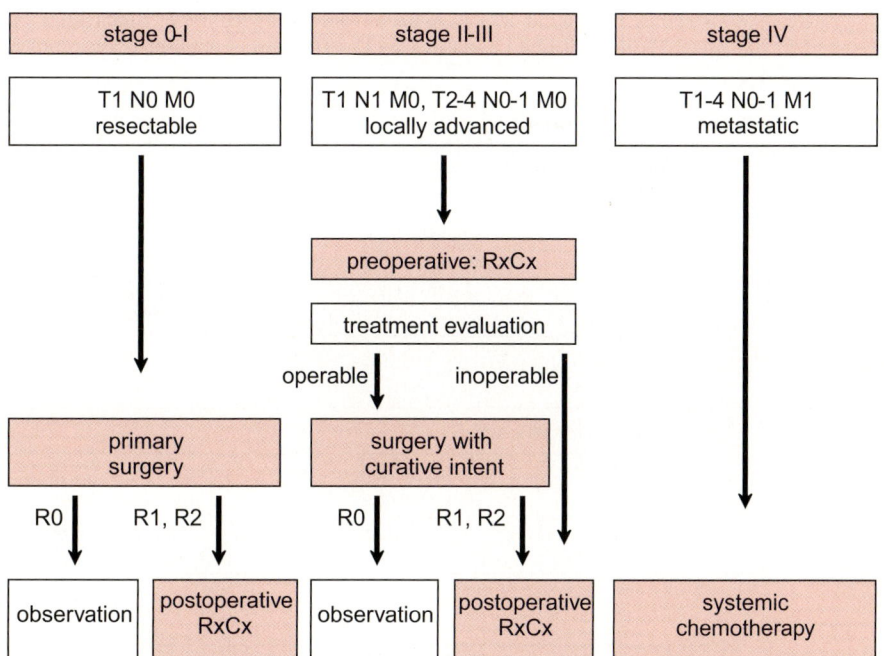

*RxCx* radiochemotherapy, *R0* tumor-free after resection, *R1, R2* residual tumor

### Surgical Treatment
- In stages I–II, complete tumor resection (R0) with curative intent is the standard of care. However, resection alone with curative intent only achieves median survival times of 12–15 months.
- Surgery-associated mortality has decreased. In experienced centers, it is well below 5%.
- In patients with Barrett's disease and high-grade dysplasia, early resection should be considered, as 50% of cases progress to esophageal adenocarcinoma. Endoscopic mucosa resection (EMR) may be an alternative to surgical resection for T1 tumors limited to the mucosal layer.

### Radiotherapy
- Preoperative radiotherapy does not confer a statistically significant survival advantage.
- Postoperative radiotherapy can reduce local relapse rates, but does not improve median survival. Comparative studies (radiotherapy versus combined radiochemotherapy) have shown combined treatment to be significantly more effective.

### Chemotherapy and Multimodal Strategies
- The most effective single drugs in the treatment of squamous cell carcinomas are cisplatin, 5-FU, bleomycin, paclitaxel, mitomycin, vinorelbine, and methotrexate. Most effective in the treatment of adenocarcinomas are 5-FU, paclitaxel, mitomycin, and cisplatin.
- Studies have shown that extended 5-FU / cisplatin combination chemotherapy with concomitant radiotherapy (50–60 Gy) leads to significantly improved survival; complete histological remission can be achieved in 20–30% of cases. However, without subsequent surgical treatment, high local relapse rates are observed.
- Neoadjuvant chemotherapy with cisplatin and 5-FU can improve the survival rate in patients with resectable esophageal carcinoma.
- Postoperative adjuvant radiochemotherapy should only be performed in studies.
- Radiochemotherapy without surgery should be restricted to patients with inoperable T4 tumors or cases with a significantly increased surgical risk. Also in this setting, comparative studies have shown combined radiochemotherapy to be superior to radiotherapy only.
- Response rates of 30–50% have been reported for the use of combination chemotherapy in stage IV of the disease (cisplatin + 5-FU, + taxane or + topoisomerase inhibitor).

### Chemotherapy Protocols

| "RxCx I," 5-FU / Cisplatin (Naunheim) ▶ Protocol 12.5.1 | | | |
|---|---|---|---|
| 5-Fluorouracil | 500 mg/m²/day | i.v. | Days 1–5, 8–12, 15–19, 22–26 |
| Cisplatin | 20 mg/m²/day | i.v. | Days 1–5, 22–26 |
| Radiotherapy | 1.8 Gy/day | | Days 1–5, 8–12, 15–19, 22–26 (total dose: 36 Gy) |

| "RxCx II," Radiochemotherapy II | | | |
|---|---|---|---|
| 5-Fluorouracil | 500 mg/m²/day | i.v. | Days 1–5, 8–12, 15–19 |
| Cisplatin | 20 mg/m²/day | i.v. | Days 1–5 |
| Radiotherapy | 1.8 Gy/day | | Days 1–5, 8–12, 15–19 (total dose: 27 Gy) |

| "5FU / Carboplatin" ▶ Protocol 12.1.1 | | | Start next cycle between days 22–29 |
|---|---|---|---|
| 5-Fluorouracil | 1,000 mg/m²/day | i.v. | Days 1–5 |
| Carboplatin | AUC 6 | i.v. | Day 1 |

| *"Paclitaxel / 5FU / Leucovorin"* | | | *Start next cycle on day 29* |
|---|---|---|---|
| Paclitaxel | 175 mg/m²/day | i.v. | Day 1 |
| 5-Fluorouracil | 350 mg/m²/day | i.v. | Days 1–3 |
| Leucovorin | 300 mg | i.v. | Days 1–3 |

**Prg:** Prognosis is generally poor:
- Overall 5-year survival: 5–10%
- Resection with curative intent is only possible in one third of cases, 5-year survival of these patients: 10–25%
- Five-year survival according to AJCC stages (see above)

**F/U:** Treatment with curative intent: close monitoring (initially every 3 months)
Palliative treatment: symptom-based approach

**Ref:**
1. Cunningham D, Starling N, Rao S et al. Capecitabine and oxaliplatin for advanced esophagogastric cancer. N Engl J Med 2008;358:36–46
2. ESMO Guidelines Working Group. Esophageal cancer: ESMO Clinical Recommendations for diagnosis, treatment and follow-up. Ann Oncol 2007;18(Suppl. 2):ii15–6
3. Heitmiller RF. Epidemiology, diagnosis, and staging of esophageal cancer. Cancer Treat Res 2001;105:375–86
4. Kleinberg L, Forastiere AA. Chemoradiation in the management of esophageal cancer. J Clin Oncol 2007;25:4110–7
5. Koshy M, Esiashvilli N, Landry JC et al. Multiple management modalities in esophageal cancer: epidemiology, presentation and progression, work-up, and surgical approaches. Oncologist 2004;9:137–46
6. MRC Oesophageal Cancer Working Party. Surgical resection with or without chemotherapy in oesophageal cancer. Lancet 2002;359:1727–33
7. Souza RF, Spechler SJ. Concepts in the prevention of adenocarcinoma of the distal esophagus and proximal stomach. CA Cancer J Clin 2005;55:334–51
8. Tew WP, Kelsen DP, Ilson DH. Targeted therapies for esophageal cancer. Oncologist 2005;10:590–601
9. Van Meerten E, Van der Gaast A. Systemic treatment for oesophageal cancer. Eur J Cancer 2005;41:664–72

**Web:**
1. http://www.nlm.nih.gov/medlineplus/esophagealcancer.html — Medline Plus
2. http://www.cancer.gov/cancertopics/types/esophageal/ — NCI, Cancer Topics
3. http://www.emedicine.com/MED/topic741.htm — E-medicine
4. http://www.cancerbackup.org.uk/Cancertype/Gulletoesophagus — Cancer BACKUP
5. http://www.cancerlinksusa.com/esophageal.htm — Cancerlinks

## 8.3.2      Gastric Cancer

**R. Engelhardt, F. Otto**

**Def:**      Malignant tumors of the stomach

**ICD-10:**      C16.-

**Ep:**      Incidence: 35–40 cases/100,000 population/year; in western industrial nations, incidence has been steadily decreasing over recent years; significant regional differences: high incidence in South East Asia, Finland, Chile. Ratio male:female = 3:2; age peak: 55–65 years.

**Pg:**      *Exogenous Risk Factors*
- High nitrate content in smoked or salt-cured food products
- Alcohol abuse, nicotine abuse
- *Helicobacter pylori* infection

*Endogenous Risk Factors*
- Chronic atrophic gastritis type A, pernicious anemia, achlorhydria
- Recurrent stomach ulcers
- Blood group A
- Adenomatous gastric polyps (carcinoma incidence: up to 20%)
- Ménétrier's syndrome (carcinoma incidence: up to 10%)
- After partial gastrectomy (especially after Billroth II)
- Hereditary syndromes: familial adenomatous polyposis (FAP), hereditary non-polyposis colorectal cancer (HNPCC)

**Path:**      Histology (WHO 1977)

| Type | Frequency (%) |
| --- | --- |
| *Adenocarcinoma* | 95 |
| • Papillary | |
| • Tubular | |
| • Mucinous | |
| • Signet-ring cell carcinoma | |
| *Adenosquamous Carcinoma* | 4 |
| *Other* | Rare |
| • Squamous cell carcinoma | |
| • Undifferentiated carcinoma | |

*Histological Classification According to Lauren (1965)*
- Intestinal type: polypous growth, well-defined, good prognosis
- Diffuse type: infiltrating growth, poor prognosis
- Mixed type: similar clinical behavior to diffuse type carcinomas

*Location*
- Antrum and pylorus:     50–80%
- Fundus and corpus:      20–30%
- Cardia:                        0–20%
- Solitary carcinoma:       80–90%
- Multicentric carcinoma:  10–20%

### Growth Pattern
- Type I: polypoid
- Type II: flat
- Type III: excavated

### Metastasis
- Regional lymph nodes (i.e., perigastric lymph nodes, lymph nodes along the left gastric, common hepatic, splenic, and celiac arteries)
- Direct infiltration of neighbouring organs (esophagus, duodenum, spleen, pancreas, diaphragm), peritoneal carcinosis, ascites
- Distant metastases: liver → lung → skeletal system
- Krukenberg's tumors: metastases to the ovaries
- Invasion of distant lymph node regions (e.g., para-aortic lymph nodes) is regarded as distant metastasis (TNM classification: M1)
- Virchow's lymph node: metastases to the lymph node at the junction of the thoracic duct and the left subclavian artery (TNM classification: M1)

### Early Gastric Cancer
- Defined as "gastric cancer restricted to the mucosa or submucosa," i.e., tumor stage Tis or T1
- Truly invasive carcinoma, lymph node metastasis is possible
- Surgical treatment similar to other gastric carcinomas
- Compared with advanced carcinoma: favorable prognosis after curative surgery

**Class:**   **TNM Staging of Gastric Cancer (AJCC 2002)**

| *T* | *Primary Tumor* |
|---|---|
| TX | Primary tumor cannot be assessed |
| T0 | No evidence of primary tumor |
| Tis | Carcinoma in situ, no invasion of lamina propria mucosae |
| T1 | Invasion of lamina propria mucosae and/or submucosa |
| T2 | Invasion of muscularis propria or subserosa |
| T2a | Invasion of muscularis propria |
| T2b | Invasion of subserosa |
| T3 | Invasion of serosa, no metastasis to neighbouring organs |
| T4 | Metastasis to neighbouring organs (transverse colon, liver, pancreas, diaphragm, spleen, abdominal wall, kidney, adrenal gland, small intestine, retroperitoneum) |
| *N* | *Lymph Node Involvement* |
| NX | Regional lymph nodes cannot be assessed |
| N0 | Regional lymph nodes without metastases[a] |
| N1 | Metastasis to 1–6 regional lymph nodes |
| N2 | Metastasis to 7–15 regional lymph nodes |
| N3 | Metastasis to more than 15 regional lymph nodes |
| *M* | *Distant Metastasis* |
| MX | Distant metastasis cannot be assessed |
| M0 | No distant metastasis |
| M1 | Distant metastasis[b] |

[a] Regional lymph nodes are the perigastric lymph nodes along the lesser and greater curvature, the lymph nodes along the left gastric, common hepatic, splenic, and celiac artery and the hepatoduodenal lymph nodes. N0 classification should be based on histological analysis of at least 15 lymph nodes

[b] Metastases to the para-aortic, retropancreatic, hepatoduodenal, mesenteric, or extra-abdominal lymph nodes: M1

**Staging according to AJCC (2002)**

| Stage | TNM system | | | Frequency (%) | Five-year survival (%) |
|-------|------------|------|------|---------------|------------------------|
| 0 | Tis | N0 | M0 | 5 | 90–100 |
| IA | T1 | N0 | M0 | 5 | 60–70 |
| IB | T1 | N1 | M0 | | |
| | T2 | N0 | M0 | | |
| II | T1 | N2 | M0 | 20 | 20–25 |
| | T2 | N1 | M0 | | |
| | T3 | N0 | M0 | | |
| IIIA | T2 | N2 | M0 | 40 | 5–10 |
| | T3 | N1 | M0 | | |
| | T4 | N0 | M0 | | |
| IIIB | T3 | N2 | M0 | | |
| IV | T1–3 | N3 | M0 | 30 | < 1 |
| | T4 | N1–3 | M0 | | |
| | Any T | Any N | M1 | | |

**Sy:**

Early symptoms are rare. In advanced stages of the disease:
- General symptoms: weight loss, fatigue, anorexia, reduced performance
- Dysphagia, abdominal fullness, nausea
- Halitosis
- Epigastric pain
- Hemorrhage, hematemesis, melena
- Aversion to certain foods

**Dg:**

### Medical History, Physical Examination
- Medical history, particularly risk factors
- Physical examination: palpable tumor in the upper abdomen, enlarged lymph nodes (especially in the left supraclavicular region: Virchow's lymph node)

### Laboratory Tests
- Routine laboratory tests, LDH, blood count, liver and renal function tests
- Possibly tumor markers: CEA, CA 72-4, CA 19-9, CA 50 (suitable for monitoring of the disease course, not for confirmation of initial diagnosis)

### Imaging
- Abdominal ultrasound, chest x-ray
- Abdominal CT scan
- For suspected bone metastasis: bone scan

### Histology
- Endoscopy with histology → multiple biopsies (> 5)
- Endosonography with assessment of depth of invasion and regional lymph nodes
- Laparoscopy to rule out peritoneal carcinosis

**Dd:**

- Peptic ulcer disease, reflux disease, Ménétrier's syndrome
- Functional dyspepsia (diagnosis by exclusion)
- Diseases of the liver, bile ducts, or pancreas
- Other neoplastic lesions of the stomach: gastrointestinal stromal tumor, GIST, non-Hodgkin's lymphoma, sarcoma, carcinoids, adenoma, polyps, leiomyoma, metastases of other primary tumors

**Co:**
- Anemia caused by acute or chronic hemorrhage
- Pyloric stenosis
- Contained or free perforation, with peritonitis
- Malignant ascites, in case of peritoneal carcinosis
- Biliary obstruction: icterus
- Paraneoplastic syndromes (acanthosis nigricans, thromboses, myositis)

**Th:**

### Treatment Concept

1. Treatment according to tumor stage and performance status.
2. In stage IA, surgical treatment (if necessary, subtotal gastrectomy with lymphadenectomy) seems to be sufficient. In patients with stage II – IV disease without distant metastases, multimodal approaches are superior to surgery alone.
3. In palliative situations, supportive treatment (bougienage, tube or stent implantation, insertion of a PEG tube, long-term parenteral nutrition) can significantly improve quality of life.

**Treatment of gastric cancer**

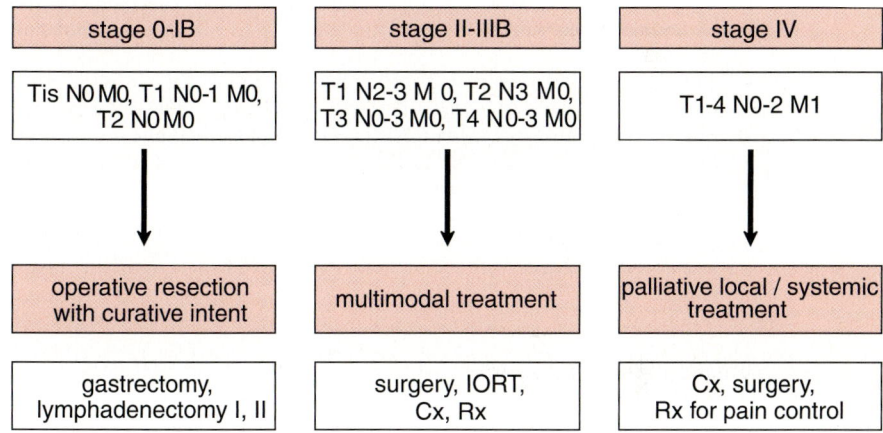

*Cx* chemotherapy, *Rx* radiotherapy, *IORT* intraoperative radiotherapy

### Surgical Treatment

- Every resectable tumor should be surgically removed (in the absence of distant metastases).
- The choice of surgical technique is based on tumor location and stage, Lauren classification, and intraoperative histological analysis; decision for or against gastrectomy depending on the individual risk potential. Safety margins of at least 5 cm (intestinal type) or 8 cm (diffuse type) must be observed.
- Standard surgical procedure with curative intent is gastrectomy with omentectomy and lymphadenectomy (compartment I and II). In case of gastric cardia carcinomas, the distal esophagus is also resected. Subtotal distal gastrectomy is only carried out in patients with small intestinal-type tumors in the distal third of the stomach.
- Views differ on the benefits of concomitant splenectomy. With respect to overall survival, total gastrectomy is not always superior to subtotal gastrectomy.
- Palliative resection or bypass in case of symptomatic indication (necrosis, hemorrhage, or obstruction).

### Radiotherapy

The treatment benefit of radiotherapy in patients with gastric cancer is limited due to:
- The required radiation dose (minimum of 60–70 Gy)
- High radiosensitivity of the surrounding tissues (intestine, liver, lung, kidneys)
- Mobility of the stomach → changes in position and topography

Radiotherapy is therefore mainly indicated as:
- Adjuvant radiochemotherapy in stages IB – IV N0 after surgical resection with curative intent, especially if no systematic lymphadectomy was performed.
- Intraoperative radiotherapy (IORT, single dose of 25 Gy); advantages: direct application, limited side effects; in clinical trials.

Palliative radiotherapy is indicated in case of:
- Pain, obstruction
- Symptomatic metastasis

### Chemotherapy

- Gastric cancer is chemosensitive. Effective single drugs achieving response rates of up to 25% are taxanes, 5-fluorouracil, doxorubicin, mitomycin C, methotrexate, cisplatin, oxaliplatin and nitrosoureas.
- Perioperative chemotherapy with 5-FU + cisplatin with or without epirubicin results in significantly increased survival in stages II – IV (in the abscence of distant metastases).
- Adjuvant chemotherapy based on 5-FU does not confer a definite survival advantage.
- In localized disease stages (up to IIIB), inoperable patients can reach an operable stage by application of neoadjuvant chemotherapy ("down staging"). In 20% of cases, neoadjuvant chemotherapy allows for R0 resection with long-term survival.
- In advanced stages of the disease, randomized studies have demonstrated a survival advantage in patients treated with chemotherapy compared to patients of the "best supportive care" group.

### Chemotherapy Protocols

| "DCF" ▶ Protocol 12.6.3 | | | Start next cycle on day 22 |
|---|---|---|---|
| Docetaxel | 75 mg/m²/day | i.v. | Day 1 |
| Cisplatin | 75 mg/m²/day | i.v. | Day 1 |
| 5-Fluorouracil | 2400 mg/m²/day | i.v. | Day 1 |

| "ECF" ▶ Protocol 12.6.2 | | | Start next cycle on day 22 |
|---|---|---|---|
| Epirubicin | 50 mg/m²/day | i.v. | Day 1 |
| Cisplatin | 60 mg/m²/day | i.v. | Day 1 |
| 5-Fluorouracil | 200 mg/m²/day | i.v. | Days 1–21 |

### New Therapy Options

New potentially effective drugs:
- Cytostatics: pemetrexed, raltitrexed, irinotecan, capecitabine
- Angiogenesis inhibitors (bevacizumab) and EGFR inhibitors (cetuximab)

**Prg:** ### *Prognostic Factors*
- Disease stage (tumor size and lymph node involvement)
- Type according to Lauren (diffuse type less favorable than intestinal type)
- Type of initial surgical treatment

### *Five-year Survival*
- According to AJCC stages (see above)
- Early carcinoma (Tis / T1 N0 M0): 95%
- Advanced stages (T2–4 N0–3 M0–1): 25–40%

**F/U:**
- Treatment with curative intent: initially close monitoring (every 3 months) with medical history, physical examination, laboratory tests (e.g., ESR, blood count, LDH, AST, ALT, alkaline phosphatase, $\gamma$GT, protein, iron), tumor markers, chest x-ray, and abdominal ultrasound
- After gastrectomy: vitamin $B_{12}$ and iron supplements
- After 2 years: follow-up every 6 months, then every 12 months
- After local therapy in cases of early gastric cancer: gastroscopy every 6 months for 3 years
- Palliative treatment: symptom-based approach

**Px:** Effective treatment of chronic *Helicobacter pylori* infections and administration of antioxidants (ascorbic acid, $\beta$-carotene) seem to lower the incidence of gastric cancer in high-risk populations.

**Ref:**
1. Ajani JA. Evolving chemotherapy for gastric cancer. Oncologist 2005;10(Suppl. 3):49–58
2. Cunningham D, Allum WH, Stenning SP et al. Perioperative chemotherapy versus surgery alone for resectable gastroesophageal cancer. N Engl J Med 2006;355:11–20
3. De Vita F, Giuliani F, Galzia G. et al. Neo-adjuvant and adjuvant chemotherapy of gastric cancer. Ann Oncol 2007;18(Suppl. 6):vi120–3
4. ESMO Guidelines Working Party. Gastric cancer: ESMO Clinical Recommendations for diagnosis, treatment and follow-up. Ann Oncol 2007;18(Suppl. 2):ii17–8
5. Hejna M, Wöhrer S, Schmidinger M et al. Postoperative chemotherapy for gastric cancer. Oncologist 2006;11:136–45
6. Jansen EPM, Boot H, Verheij M et al. Optimal locoregional treatment in gastric cancer. J Clin Oncol 2005;20:4509–17
7. Lim L, Michael M, Mann GB et al. Adjuvant therapy in gastric cancer. J Clin Oncol 2005;23:6220–32
8. Matysiak-Budnik T, Mégraud F. Helicobacter pylori infection and gastric cancer. Eur J Cancer 2006;42:708–16
9. Tabernero J, Macarulla T, Ramos FJ et al. Novel targeted therapies in the treatment of gastric and esophagus cancer. Ann Oncol 2005;16:1740–8

**Web:**
1. http://www.nlm.nih.gov/medlineplus/stomachcancer.html — Medline Plus
2. http://www.cancer.gov/cancertopics/types/stomach/ — NCI, Cancer Topics
3. http://www.emedicine.com/MED/topic845.htm — E-medicine
4. http://www.medicinenet.com/stomach_cancer/article.htm — Medicine Net

### 8.3.3 Cancer of the Small Intestine

**B. Deschler, R. Engelhardt, F. Otto**

**Def:** Malignant epithelial tumor of the small intestine.

**ICD-10:** C17

**Ep:** Incidence: 1 case/100,000 population/year; approximately 1% of all tumors of the gastrointestinal tract; age peak: 60–70 years; approximately 25% of patients have second primary tumors of the colon, endometrium, breast, or prostate.

**Pg:** *Risk Factors*
- Raw meat, salt-cured foods
- Congenital or acquired immunodeficiency
- Diseases with reduced intestinal passage time
- Crohn's disease (usually small bowel carcinoma located in the ileum)
- Peutz-Jeghers syndrome
- Adult celiac disease

**Path:** *Histology*
- Adenocarcinoma: 45% of cases
- Carcinoid: 29%
- Lymphoma: 15%
- Sarcoma: 10%

*Location*
- Proximal: mainly adenocarcinomas (65% periampullary)
- Distal: mainly carcinoids, sarcomas, lymphomas

**Class:** **TNM Staging (2002)**

| T | Primary Tumor |
|---|---|
| TX | Primary tumor cannot be assessed |
| T0 | No evidence of primary tumor |
| Tis | Carcinoma in situ |
| T1 | Invasion of lamina propria or submucosa |
| T2 | Invasion of muscularis propria |
| T3 | Invasion of subserosa or nonperitonealized perimuscular tissue ($< 2$ cm) |
| T4 | Perforation of the visceral peritoneum or invasion of adjacent organs including other loops of small intestine |
| N | Lymph Node Involvement |
| NX | Regional lymph nodes cannot be assessed |
| N0 | Regional lymph nodes without metastases |
| N1 | Regional lymph node metastasis |
| M | Distant Metastasis |
| MX | Distant metastasis cannot be assessed |
| M0 | No distant metastasis |
| M1 | Distant metastasis |

**AJCC Staging (2002)**

| AJCC Stage | TNM system | | |
|---|---|---|---|
| 0 | Tis | N0 | M0 |
| I | T1–2 | N0 | M0 |
| II | T3–4 | N0 | M0 |
| III | Any T | N1 | M0 |
| IV | Any T | Any N | M1 |

**Sy:** Early symptoms are non-specific. In advanced stages of the disease:
- Abdominal pain
- Small bowel obstruction / ileus
- Hemorrhage
- Weight loss
- Icterus (periampullary tumors)

**Dg:** *Medical History, Physical Examination*
- Medical history, particularly intestinal disorders (Crohn's disease)
- Physical examination

*Laboratory Tests*
- Routine laboratory tests, blood count, liver and renal function tests

*Imaging*
- Abdominal x-ray
- Barium contrast x-ray (upper gastrointestinal series with short bowel follow-through and enteroclysis)
- Abdominal CT scan
- Abdominal ultrasound (exclusion of hepatic metastases)
- Chest x-ray (exclusion of pulmonary metastases)
- Capsular endoscopy

**Dd:**
- Malignant tumors: neuroendocrine tumors, lymphoma, sarcoma
- Benign tumors: adenoma, leiomyoma, fibroma, lipoma
- Metastases: melanoma, breast cancer, lung cancer, renal cell carcinoma

**Co:**
- Perforation, peritonitis
- Subileus, ileus
- Hemorrhage (acute / chronic)
- Icterus with obstruction of bile ducts (periampullary tumors)

**Th:** **Surgical Treatment**

Standard treatment of small bowel cancer is surgery. Techniques:
- Partial resection of the small intestine
- Duodenal carcinoma: pancreaticoduodenectomy or a more conservative approach with intra-operative histological analysis of the margins of the resected tissue
- Palliative surgical treatment in case of inoperable tumors or complications

### Chemotherapy

Due to the rareness of small bowel cancer, a standard of care has not been established.
- Neoadjuvant radiochemotherapy may be beneficial in treatment of duodenal carcinomas
- Adjuvant chemotherapy may be beneficial in stage III of the disease
- Palliative chemotherapy similar to colorectal cancer

### Chemotherapy Protocols for Small Bowel Cancer

| *5-FU / Leucovorin (Mayo) adjuvant ▶ Protocol 12.7.5* | | | *Start next cycle on day 29* |
|---|---|---|---|
| 5-Fluorouracil | 425 mg/m²/day | i.v. | Days 1–5 |
| Leucovorin | 20 mg/m²/day | i.v. | Days 1–5 |

| *5-FU + Irinotecan (FOLFIRI) palliative ▶ Protocol 12.7.1* | | | *Start next cycle on day 29* |
|---|---|---|---|
| Irinotecan | 180 mg/m²/day | i.v. | Days 1, 15, over 2 h |
| Folinic acid | 400 mg/m²/day | i.v. | Days 1, 15, over 30 min |
| 5-Fluorouracil | 400 mg/m²/day | i.v. | Days 1, 15, bolus injection |
| 5-Fluorouracil | 2,400 mg/m²/day | i.v. | Days 1, 15 |

| *5-FU + Oxaliplatin (FOLFOX6) palliative ▶ Protocol 12.7.7* | | | *Start next cycle on day 29* |
|---|---|---|---|
| Oxaliplatin | 100 mg/m²/day | i.v. | Days 1, 15, over 2 h |
| Folinic acid | 400 mg/m²/day | i.v. | Days 1, 15, over 30 min |
| 5-Fluorouracil | 400 mg/m²/day | i.v. | Days 1, 15, bolus injection |
| 5-Fluorouracil | 2,400 mg/m²/day | i.v. | Days 1, 15 |

In 75% of cases, cancer of the small bowel is only diagnosed in advanced stages of disease (III and IV) → prognosis is generally poor.

### Five-year Survival Depending on Tumor Stage (Duodenal Carcinoma)
- Stage I:        100%
- Stage II:       52%
- Stage III:      45%
- Stage IV:       0%

**F/U:**  Treatment with curative intent: initial monitoring every 3 months (medical history, physical examination, endoscopy, ultrasound, chest x-ray).
Palliative situations: symptom-based approach.

**Ref:**

1.  Barnes G, Romero L, Hess KR et al. Primary adenocarcinoma of the duodenum: management and survival in 67 patients. Ann Surg Oncol 1994;1:73–7
2.  Delaunoit T, Neczyporenko F, Limburg PJ et al. Pathogenesis and risk factors of small bowel adenocarcinoma: a colorectal cancer sibling? Am J Gastroenterol 2005;100:703–10

3. North JH, Pack MS. Malignant tumors of the small intestine: a review of 144 cases. Am J Surg 2000;66:46–51
4. Stang A, Stegmaier C, Eisinger B et al. Descriptive epidemiology of small intestinal malignancies: the German Cancer Registry experience. Br J Cancer 1999;80:1440–4
5. Wheeler JMD, Warren BF, Mortensen NJ et al. An insight into the genetic pathway of the small intestine. Gut 2002;50:218–23

**Web:**

| | | |
|---|---|---|
| 1. | http://www.cancer.gov/cancertopics/pdq/treatment/smallintestine/healthprofessional/ | NCI Cancer Topics |
| 2. | http://www.emedicine.com/med/topic2652.htm | E-medicine |
| 3. | http://www.csmc.edu/pf_5626.html | Cedars Sinai |
| 4. | http://www.thedoctorsdoctor.com/diseases/small_bowel_adenocarcinoma.htm | Doctor's Doctor |
| 5. | http://gastroresource.com/gitextbook/en/Chapter7/7-24.htm | Gastroenterology Resource |

## 8.3.4     Colorectal Cancer

B. Deschler, F. Otto

**Def:**     Malignant epithelial tumors of the colon and rectum.

**ICD-10:**     C18–C20

**Ep:**     Incidence: 30–40 cases/100,000 population/year in Europe, geographical differences; approximately 15% of all solid tumors; second most common cancer in men, third most common cancer in women; ratio male:female = 1:1; age peak: 50–70 years; rarely occurs before the age of 40 years.

**Pg:**     *Risk Factors*
- Family history of colorectal cancer (especially first-degree relatives)
- Colorectal adenomas (especially villous adenoma, adenomas > 20 mm)
- Chronic inflammatory intestinal disorders (ulcerative colitis, especially if associated with primary sclerosing cholangitis, Colitis Crohn)
- Dietary factors: low-fiber diet, fat consumption
- Nitrosamines, asbestos
- Long-standing drinking or smoking
- Obesity, lack of exercise
- Previous malignancy (ovarian / endometrial / breast cancer)

*Hereditary Syndromes Associated with Increased Risk of Colorectal Cancer:*
- Hereditary non-polyposis colorectal cancer (HNPCC); 5–10% of all colorectal carcinomas, Lynch syndrome I: multiple predominantly early-onset proximal colon carcinomas; Lynch syndrome II (hereditary adenocarcinomatosis): multiple colon carcinomas and adenocarcinomas of other organs (ovaries, pancreas, breast, bile ducts, stomach, etc.)
- Familial adenomatous polyposis (FAP): incidence 1:8,000 population, autosomal-dominant inheritance, gene located on chromosome 5q; polyposis of the entire colon, carcinoma risk > 95%; rare variants: Turcot's syndrome, Gardner's syndrome
- Hamartomatous polyposis (familial juvenile polyposis, Peutz-Jeghers syndrome)

*Molecular Genetics*
Multistep carcinogenesis (Vogelstein 1988): progression from normal mucosa to carcinoma, with several successive steps of dysplasia and specific molecular genetic changes ("adenoma-carcinoma sequence"):
- Oncogene activation (K-ras)
- Inactivation / deletion of tumor suppressor genes: APC gene ("adenomatous polyposis coli" in familial adenomatous polyposis, DCC gene ("deleted in colorectal carcinoma"), p53 gene mutations, etc.
- Germline mutations in HNPCC in 1 of 6 DNA mismatch repair genes (MMR): hMSH2, hMLH1, hPMS1, hPMS2, hMSH6, hMLH3
- Detection of microsatellite instability (MSI): sign for mismatch repair defect.

**Path:**     *Histology*
- Adenocarcinoma: 90–95% of cases, in 2–5% multiple synchronous primary tumors
- Carcinoid: 2–7%
- Other (sarcomas, hematological neoplasia, etc.): rare

*Location of Colon Carcinomas*
- Cecum / ascending colon:          25%
- Transverse / descending colon:     25%
- Sigmoid colon:                    50%

*Metastasis of Colon Cancer: Sequence*
Regional lymph nodes → liver → lung → other organs

### Rectal Cancer: Three Routes of Metastatic Spread Depending on Location

| Location | Distance from anal margin (cm) | Route of metastasis |
|---|---|---|
| Low | 0–4 | Para-aortic and inguinal lymph nodes, pelvic wall |
| Middle | 4–8 | Para-aortic lymph nodes and pelvic wall |
| High | 8–16 | Para-aortic lymph nodes |

**Class:**

### TNM Staging of Colorectal Tumors (2002)

| | |
|---|---|
| *T* | *Primary Tumor* |
| TX | Primary tumor cannot be assessed |
| T0 | No evidence of primary tumor |
| Tis | Carcinoma in situ |
| T1 | Invasion of submucosa |
| T2 | Invasion of muscularis propria |
| T3 | Invasion of subserosa or non-peritonealized pericolic / perirectal tissue |
| T4 | Perforation of the visceral peritoneum or invasion of adjacent organs and other colorectal segments |
| *N* | *Lymph Node Involvement* |
| NX | Regional lymph nodes cannot be assessed |
| N0 | Regional lymph nodes without metastases |
| N1 | Metastasis to 1–3 regional lymph nodes |
| N2 | Metastasis to ≥ 4 regional lymph nodes |
| *M* | *Distant Metastasis* |
| MX | Distant metastasis cannot be assessed |
| M0 | No distant metastasis |
| M1 | Distant metastasis |

### AJCC Staging (2002)

| Stage | TNM system | | |
|---|---|---|---|
| 0 | Tis | N0 | M0 |
| I | T1–2 | N0 | M0 |
| IIA | T3 | N0 | M0 |
| IIB | T4 | N0 | M0 |
| IIIA | T1–2 | N1 | M0 |
| IIIB | T3–4 | N1 | M0 |
| IIIC | Any T | N2 | M0 |
| IV | Any T | Any N | M1 |

**Sy:**

Early symptoms uncommon; in advanced stages of the disease:
- General symptoms: fatigue, lassitude, weight loss
- Irregular bowel movements: constipation, diarrhea, "paradoxical diarrhea" (alternating constipation and diarrhea), pencil-like stools
- Hemorrhage, blood in stool (visible or occult), pain

**Dg:** **_Medical History, Physical Examination_**
- Medical history, especially family history, risk factors
- Physical examination including rectal examination

**_Laboratory Tests_**
- Routine laboratory tests, including blood count, hepatic / renal function parameters
- Tumor markers: CEA, CA 19-9

**_Histology_**
- Endoscopy with histology (colonoscopy)

**_Imaging_**
- Abdominal ultrasound (exclusion of hepatic metastases)
- Chest x-ray (exclusion of pulmonary metastases)
- Abdominal CT or MRI scan
- Contrast enema with water-soluble contrast medium (risk of fistula, perforation, or ileus)

Irregular stools always require immediate attention and adequate diagnostic procedures (endoscopy, histology).

**Co:**
- Hemorrhage
- Intestinal obstruction, subileus, ileus
- Perforation, fistulas

**Th:** **Treatment Concept of Colon Cancer**

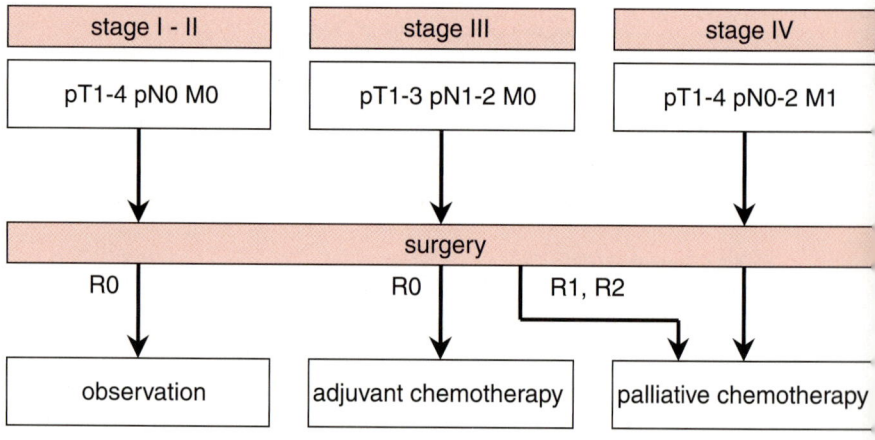

| stage I - II | stage III | stage IV |
|---|---|---|
| pT1-4 pN0 M0 | pT1-3 pN1-2 M0 | pT1-4 pN0-2 M1 |

surgery

| R0 | R0 | R1, R2 |
|---|---|---|
| observation | adjuvant chemotherapy | palliative chemotherapy |

**Surgery: Colon Cancer**

Colon cancer is primarily treated surgically (90% of cases). Techniques:
- Curative intent: en bloc resection of the tumor, mesentery and regional lymph nodes (curative in approximately 50% of patients)
- Resection of hepatic or pulmonary metastases with curative intent (metastases limited to one organ system, maximum 5 metastases in both hepatic lobes or if > 5 metastases, operable by hemihepatectomy): 5-year survival rates of 20–40%
- Palliative resection of the primary tumor in cases of advanced metastatic disease to avoid local complications
- In case of inoperable hepatic metastases: consider local intervention (cryosurgical ablation or radiofrequency ablation)

## Postoperative Care and Chemotherapy: Colon Cancer

- Stage I: surgical treatment with curative intent, close monitoring, no need for adjuvant treatment
- Stage II: benefit of adjuvant chemotherapy not established; studies have demonstrated reduced risk of relapse, however, in meta-analysis only marginal survival advantage; treatment in clinical trials
- Stage III: postoperative adjuvant chemotherapy (5-FU + leucovorin or capecitabine or FOLFOX for 6 months) to reduce relapse rates and improve survival rates
- Stage IV: chemotherapy has only palliative effect but leads to improved overall survival and quality of life
- Bevacizumab may prolong survival if added to first line chemotherapy
- If tumors are refractory to irinotecan, combination of irinotecan and cetuximab can improve response
- Combination chemotherapy with 5-FU / leucovorin and irinotecan or oxaliplatin is more effective in palliative care than 5-FU / leucovorin alone
- Efficacy of adjuvant chemotherapy following resection of metastases is not established

## Treatment Concept for Rectal Cancer

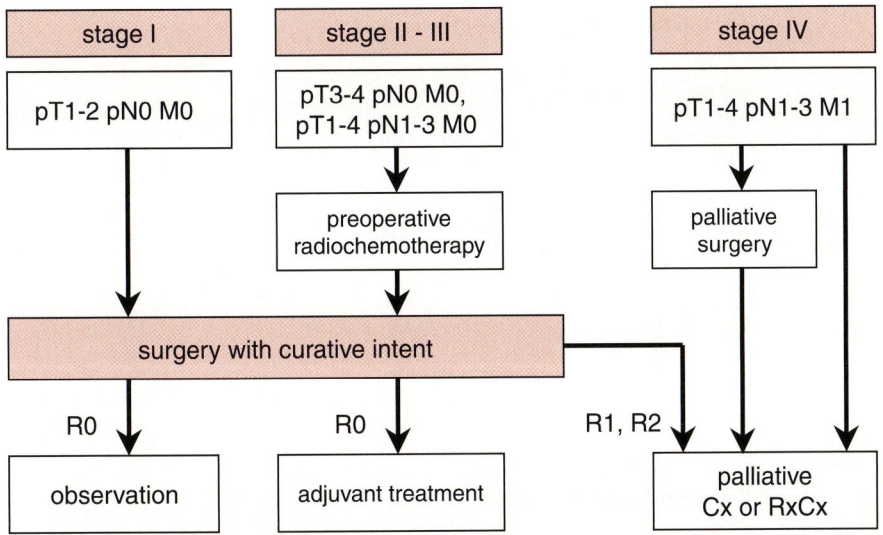

*Cx* chemotherapy, *RxCx* radiochemotherapy

## Surgery: Rectal Cancer

Rectal cancer is primarily treated surgically. Techniques:
- Objectives of surgery include complete tumor resection and preservation of continence, especially with tumors of the upper and middle third of the rectum (85%).
- Only with tumors of the lower third: abdominoperineal excision of the rectum with permanent colostomy (15%).
- Solitary hepatic / pulmonary metastases: resection with curative intent.
- Stage T4 N1–2 M0 (R0 resection not possible): neoadjuvant radiochemotherapy to achieve resectability ("down staging"); with T3–4 tumors in the lower rectum: neoadjuvant radioche-

motherapy aimed at continence-preserving surgery; even with resectable tumors, neoadjuvant radiotherapy leads to a reduction in local relapse rates and may confer a survival advantage.
- Palliative resection of the primary tumor in advanced, metastatic disease to avoid local complications.

## Postoperative Care and Chemotherapy: Rectal Cancer

- Stage I: surgical treatment with curative intent, close monitoring; no indication for adjuvant therapy outside of clinical trials
- Stages II and III: postoperative adjuvant radiochemotherapy may contribute to reduced relapse rates and improved survival (standard treatment: radiotherapy + continuous 5-FU infusion)
- Stage IV: with limited hepatic metastasis, surgical approach → 5-year survival: 20–40%; the benefit of adjuvant chemotherapy after resection of metastases has been established
- Nonresectable hepatic metastases: long-term tumor control by cryosurgery or radiofrequency ablation (RFA) possible, especially in patients without lymph node involvement and after R0 resection (negative margins after removal of the primary tumor)
- Palliative situations: chemotherapy protocols similar to advanced colon cancer

## Chemotherapy Protocols for Colorectal Cancer

### Colorectal Cancer, Adjuvant Treatment

| "FOLFOX4" ▶ Protocol 12.7.6 | | | Start next cycle on day 15 |
|---|---|---|---|
| Oxaliplatin | 85 mg/m²/day | i.v. | Day 1, over 2 h |
| Folinic acid | 200 mg/m²/day | i.v. | Days 1, 2, over 2 h |
| 5-Fluorouracil | 400 mg/m²/day | i.v. | Days 1, 2, bolus injection |
| 5-Fluorouracil | 600 mg/m²/day | c.i.v. | Days 1–2, for 24 h |

| "5-FU / Leucovorin (Mayo)" ▶ Protocol 12.7.5 | | | Start next cycle on day 29 |
|---|---|---|---|
| 5-Fluorouracil | 425 mg/m²/day | i.v. | Days 1–5 |
| Leucovorin | 20 mg/m²/day | i.v. | Days 1–5 |

### Colorectal Cancer, Palliative Treatment

| "FOLFIRI" ▶ Protocol 12.7.1 | | | Start next cycle on day 29 |
|---|---|---|---|
| Irinotecan | 180 mg/m²/day | i.v. | Days 1, 15, over 2 h |
| Folinic acid | 400 mg/m²/day | i.v. | Days 1, 15, over 30 min |
| 5-Fluorouracil | 400 mg/m²/day | i.v. | Days 1, 15, bolus injection |
| 5-Fluorouracil | 2,400 mg/m²/day | c.i.v. | Days 1, 15 |

| "FOLFIRI+Bevacizumab" ▶ Protocol 12.7.2 | | | Start next cycle on day 29 |
|---|---|---|---|
| Bevacizumab | 5 mg/kg | i.v. | Days 1, 15, over 30 min |
| Irinotecan | 180 mg/m²/day | i.v. | Days 1, 15, over 2 h |
| Folinic acid | 400 mg/m²/day | i.v. | Days 1, 15, over 30 min |
| 5-Fluorouracil | 400 mg/m²/day | i.v. | Days 1, 15, bolus injection |
| 5-Fluorouracil | 2,400 mg/m²/day | i.v. | Days 1, 15 |

| *"Irinotecan+Cetuximab"* ▶ Protocol 12.7.3 | | | *Start next cycle on day 29* |
|---|---|---|---|
| Cetuximab | 250 mg/m²/day | i.v. | Days 1, 8, over 1 h |
| | Loading dose 40 mg/m²/day | i.v. | First application only, over 2h |
| Irinotecan | 180 mg/m²/day | i.v. | Day 1, over 1 h |

| *"FOLFOX6"* ▶ Protocol 12.7.7 | | | *Start next cycle on day 29* |
|---|---|---|---|
| Oxaliplatin | 100 mg/m²/day | i.v. | Days 1, 15, over 2 h |
| Folinic acid | 400 mg/m²/day | i.v. | Days 1, 15, over 30 min |
| 5-Fluorouracil | 400 mg/m²/day | i.v. | Days 1, 15, bolus injection |
| 5-Fluorouracil | 2,400 mg/m²/day | i.v. | Days 1, 15 |

| *Capecitabine* ▶ Protocol 12.7.9 | | | *Start next cycle on day 22* |
|---|---|---|---|
| Capecitabine | 2,500 mg/m² | p.o. | Days 1–14 |

### Neoadjuvant Radiochemotherapy: Rectal Cancer

| *5-FU+Radiotherapy neoadjuvant* | | | |
|---|---|---|---|
| 5-Fluorouracil | 1,000 mg/m²/day | i.v. | Days 1–5, week 1 and 5 |
| Radiotherapy | 50 Gy | | Weeks 1–6 |

### Adjuvant Radiochemotherapy: Rectal Cancer

| *5-FU+Radiotherapy adjuvant* | | | |
|---|---|---|---|
| 5-Fluorouracil | 500 mg/m²/day | i.v. | Days 1–3 (weeks 1, 5, 9) |
| | | | Days 1–5 (weeks 13, 17, 21) |
| Radiotherapy | 45 Gy small pelvis | | Weeks 1–6 |
| | 5.4 Gy tumor / lymph nodes | | |

### New Therapies

Monoclonal antibodies (▶ Chap. 3.5), "targeted therapy" (▶ Chap. 3.6), and inhibitors are effective, especially:

- Bevacizumab → inhibitor of angiogenesis
- Cetuximab → EGF-receptor inhibitor

### Prognostic Factors

- Age (under 40 years: poor prognosis)
- Gender (women have better prognosis)
- Tumor location (rectum or sigmoid: less favorable)

### Five-year Survival

- Stage I:      90–95%
- Stage II:     60–80%
- Stage III:    30–50%
- Stage IV:     < 10%

**F/U:**  Patients treated with curative intent: initial follow-up every 3 months: medical history, physical examination, laboratory tests including CEA, CA 19-9, endoscopy, ultrasound, chest x-ray, abdominal CT scan for high risk cases
Palliative situations: symptom-based approach.

**Px:**  Screening from the age of 50 years (earlier in high-risk groups):
- Rectal examination
- Fecal occult blood tests
- Colonoscopy every 10 years
- High-risk groups: regular colonoscopy every 1–3 years
- Avoid risk factors (obesity, nicotine abuse, lack of physical exercise)

**Ref:**
1. Benson AB, Schrag D, Somerfield MR et al. ASCO recommendations on adjuvant chemotherapy or stage II colon cancer. J Clin Oncol 2004;22:3408–19
2. Board RE, Valle J. Metastatic colorectal cancer. Drugs 2007;67:1851–67
3. Desch CE, Benson AB, Somerfield MR et al. Colorectal cancer surveillance: 2005 update of an ASCO Practice Guideline. J Clin Oncol 2005;23:8512–9
4. ESMO Guidelines Working Group. Colon cancer: ESMO Clinical Recommendations for diagnosis, treatment and follow-up. Ann Oncol 2007;18(suppl 2):ii21–2
5. ESMO Guidelines Working Group. Rectal cancer: ESMO Clinical Recommendations for diagnosis, treatment and follow-up. Ann Oncol 2007;18(suppl 2):ii23–4
6. ESMO Guidelines Working Group. Advanced colorectal cancer: ESMO Clinical Recommendations for diagnosis, treatment and follow-up. Ann Oncol 2007;18(suppl 2):ii25–6
7. Jackson C, Cunningham D. Where to position monoclonal antibodies in first-line treatment of advanced colorectal cancer. Eur J Cancer 2008;44:652–62
8. Meyerhardt JA, Mayer RJ. Systemic therapy for colorectal cancer. N Engl J Med 2005;352:476–87
9. Wolpin BM, Meyerhardt JA, Mamon HJ et al. Adjuvant treatment of colorectal cancer. CA Cancer J Clin 2007;57:168–85

**Web:**
1. http://www.nlm.nih.gov/medlineplus/colorectalcancer.html          MedlinePlus
2. http://cancernet.nci.nih.gov/cancertopics/types/colon-and-rectal   NCI Cancernet
3. http://www.emedicine.com/med/topic413.htm                          E-medicine
4. http://www.emedicine.com/med/topic1994.htm                         E-medicine
5. http://www.nccn.org/professionals/physician_gls/PDF/colon.pdf      NCCN Guideline
6. http://www.nccn.org/professionals/physician_gls/PDF/rectal.pdf     NCCN Guideline

**3.3.5**    **Anal Carcinoma**

**D.P. Berger, R. Engelhardt, F. Otto**

**Def:**    Malignant tumors of the anal canal or the anal margins.

**ICD-10:**    C21.-

**Ep:**    Rare disease; incidence 1/100,000 population/year; < 2% of all colorectal tumors; ratio male:female = 1:3; age peak: 50–60 years

**Pg:**

### Risk Factors
- High incidence in homosexual men and HIV-positive individuals
- Viral infections, condylomata accuminata (human papilloma virus HPV-16, herpes virus)
- Preoperative radiotherapy (e.g., with cervical carcinoma), smoking

**Path:**

### Histology
- Squamous cell carcinoma: 70–75% of cases
- Transitional cell carcinoma (cloacogenic carcinoma of the anal margin): 20–25%
- Adenocarcinoma: 5–7%
- Basal cell carcinoma: 2–4%
- Other (small cell carcinoma, melanoma, etc.): 5%

### Metastasis
- Direct spread: infiltration of the anal sphincter as well as vagina, bladder, urethra, and prostate
- Lymphatic spread of tumors located above the dentate line → pararectal lymph nodes → mesenteric lymph nodes
- Lymphatic spread of tumors located below the dentate line → inguinal lymph nodes → iliac lymph nodes
- Hematogenic spread: occurs if tumor located below the dentate line (→ particularly into liver, lung, skeletal system) but generally rare: at the time of diagnosis: < 20% of patients

**Class:**    **TNM Staging of Anal Carcinoma (2002)**

| *T* | *Primary Tumor* |
|---|---|
| TX | Primary tumor cannot be assessed |
| T0 | No evidence of primary tumor |
| Tis | Carcinoma in situ |
| T1 | Tumor measuring < 2 cm |
| T2 | Tumor measuring 2–5 cm |
| T3 | Tumor measuring > 5 cm |
| T4 | Tumor of any size with invasion of adjacent organs (e.g., vagina, urethra, bladder) |
| *N* | *Lymph Node Involvement* |
| NX | Regional lymph nodes cannot be assessed |
| N0 | Regional lymph nodes without metastases |
| N1 | Metastasis to perirectal lymph nodes |
| N2 | Unilateral metastasis to inguinal and/or iliac lymph nodes |
| N3 | Metastasis to perirectal and inguinal lymph nodes and/or bilateral metastasis to inguinal / iliac lymph nodes |

**Class:**     **TNM Staging of Anal Carcinoma (2002)** *(continued)*

| M | Distant Metastasis |
|---|---|
| MX | Distant metastasis cannot be assessed |
| M0 | No distant metastasis |
| M1 | Distant metastasis |

Tumors located distal to the anocutaneous line (with involvement of the perianal skin) are classified like skin tumors

**AJCC Staging (2002)**

| Stage | TNM system | | |
|---|---|---|---|
| 0 | Tis | N0 | M0 |
| I | T1 | N0 | M0 |
| II | T2–3 | N0 | M0 |
| IIIA | T1–3 | N1 | M0 |
| | T4 | N0 | M0 |
| IIIB | T4 | N1 | M0 |
| | Any T | N2-3 | M0 |
| IV | Any T | Any N | M1 |

**Staging according to Nigro (1987)**

| Stage | Criteria |
|---|---|
| 0 | No residual tumor after local excision |
| IA | Tumor < 2 cm, without lymph node involvement |
| IB | Tumor < 2 cm, with lymph node involvement |
| IIA | Tumor 2–5 cm, without lymph node involvement |
| IIB | Tumor 2–5 cm, with lymph node involvement |
| IIIA | Tumor > 5 cm, without lymph node involvement |
| IIIB | Tumor > 5 cm, with lymph node involvement |
| IV | Distant metastases |

**Sy:**     Depending on tumor location, anal carcinoma can be detected at an early stage. However, symptoms usually only occur in more advanced disease stages:
* Itchiness, foreign body sensation, pain
* General symptoms: fatigue, lassitude, weight loss
* Irregular bowel movement, incontinence
* Peranal hemorrhage, visible blood in stools

**Dg:**     *Medical History, Physical Examination*
* Medical history including risk factors
* Physical examination including digital anorectal examination, lymph node status

*Laboratory Tests*
* Blood Count, hepatic / renal function parameters

*Histology*
* Rectoscopy with histology

### Imaging
- Endorectal ultrasound (tumor size)
- Barium enema with water-soluble contrast medium (risk of fistulas or perforation)
- Abdominal and pelvic CT / MRI scan
- Abdominal ultrasound (hepatic metastases?)

### Other
- Gynecological examination (infiltration?)

**Dd:**

- Benign anal lesions (hemorrhoids, perianal thrombosis, fistulas / abscesses, hypertrophic anal papillae, Bowen's disease)
- Other malignancies (adenocarcinoma / small cell carcinoma / basal cell carcinoma, melanoma)

**Th:**

## Treatment Concept

1. Approximately 50% of patients (particularly in early stages of the disease: Tis / T1 N0 M0) can be cured by surgical resection with full preservation of continence. Potential undesirable consequences of surgery include anal sphincter dysfunction and local infection. Abdomino-perineal resection of the rectum is only performed if multimodal therapy concepts remain unsuccessful.
2. Anal carcinomas are radiosensitive. Doses of > 60 Gy are required. Side effects of radiotherapy include proctitis, cystitis, and fibrosis.
3. Multimodal therapy concepts combining surgery, chemotherapy, and radiotherapy achieve 5-year survival rates of > 70%. The required radiation doses are generally lower resulting in reduced rates of acute and chronic side effects. Radiotherapy combined with 5-FU has been proven to be effective (longer colostomy-free and disease-free survival if mitomycin C is added). The efficacy of a combination of radiotherapy and continuous 5-FU infusion plus cisplatin is currently being evaluated in trials.

**Treatment of Anal Carcinoma**

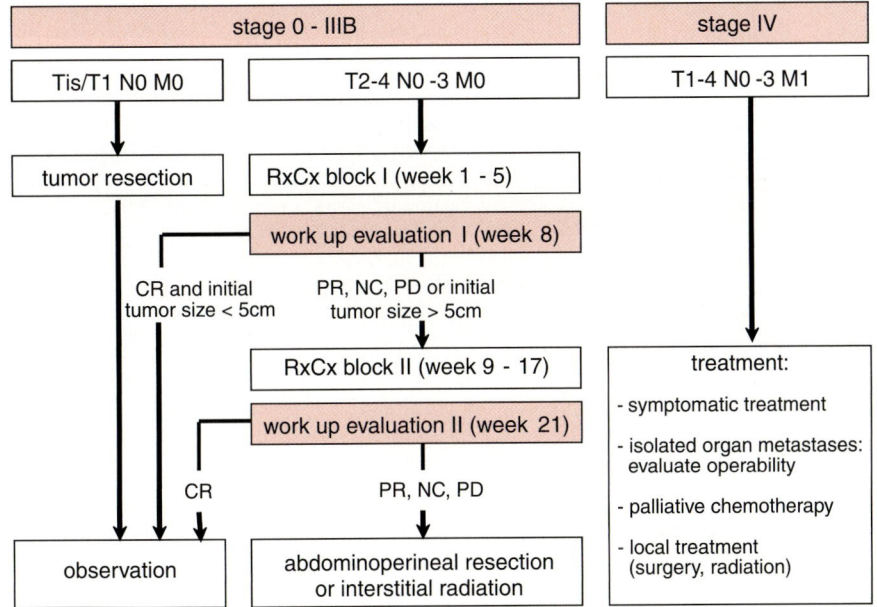

*RxCx* radiochemotherapy, *CR* complete remission, *PR* partial remission, *NC* no change, *PD* progression

## Therapy Protocols

| "Radiochemotherapy I" ► Protocol 12.7.10 | | | | |
|---|---|---|---|---|
| Mitomycin C | 15 mg/m²/day | i.v. | Day 1 | Week 1 |
| 5-Fluorouracil | 1,000 mg/m²/day | i.v. | Days 1–4 | Weeks 1 + 5 |
| Radiotherapy | 2 Gy/day | | Days 1–5 | Weeks 1–3 |

| "Radiochemotherapy II" ► Protocol 12.7.10 | | | | |
|---|---|---|---|---|
| 5-Fluorouracil | 1,000 mg/m²/day | i.v. | Days 1–4 | Weeks 10, 14, 18 |
| Cisplatin | 100 mg/m²/day | i.v. | Day 1 | Weeks 10, 14, 18 |
| Radiotherapy | 2 Gy/day | | Days 1–5 | Weeks 10 + 11 |

**Prg:**    With an adequate multimodal therapy concept, anal carcinomas can be treated with curative intent.

### Prognostic Factors
- Location (anal canal versus perianal area)
- Tumor size
- Degree of differentiation (highly differentiated tumors: less favorable)

### Five-year Survival
- Tumors without lymph node involvement (N0) or distant metastasis (M0): 60–90%
- Tumors with lymph node involvement: < 50%
- Anal carcinomas, purely surgical treatment: 50%
- Anal carcinomas, multimodal therapy: > 70%

**F/U:**    Patients treated with curative intent: initial follow-up every 3 months (with rectoscopy, endosonography, imaging). After 2 years: follow-up every 6 months, after 5 years: every 12 months. Palliative situations: symptom-based approach.

**Px:**    Early detection via tumor screening. In clinical trials: HPV vaccination.

**Ref:**
1. Clark MA, Hartley A, Geh JI. Cancer of the anal canal. Lancet Oncol 2004;5:149–57
2. Einstein MH, Kadish AS. Anogenital neoplasia in AIDS. Curr Opin Oncol 2004;16:455–62
3. Rousseau DL, Thomas CR, Petrelli NJ et al. Squamous cell carcinoma of the anal canal. Surg Oncol 2005;14:121–32
4. Steinbrook R. The potential of human papillomavirus vaccines. N Engl J Med 2006;354:1109–12
5. Uronis HE, Bendell JC. Anal Cancer. Oncologist 2007;12:524–34

**Web:**
1. http://www.nlm.nih.gov/medlineplus/analcancer.html          MedlinePlus
2. http://www.nccn.org/professionals/physician_gls/PDF/anal.pdf          NCCN Guideline

**8.3.6**  **Pancreatic Carcinoma**

**R. Engelhardt, F. Otto**

**Def:** Malignant tumors of the pancreas; mainly adenocarcinoma of the pancreatic duct epithelium.

**CD-10:** C25.-

**Ep:** Incidence: 10 cases/100,000 population/year; 2–3% of all malignant tumors; ratio male:female = 4:3; age peak: 60–80 years.

**Pg:**
### Risk Factors
- Smoking
- Chronic pancreatitis / cholecystitis
- Toxic chemicals: 2-naphthylamine, benzidine, DDT
- Hereditary recurrent pancreatitis (rare)
- Hereditary predisposition (e.g., Peutz-Jeghers syndrome)

### Molecular Genetic Abnormalities
Mutations of the oncogenes K-ras, p53, p16, and smad 4.

**Path:**
### Histology

| Type | Frequency (%) |
|---|---|
| *Tumors of the Exocrine Pancreas* | 95 |
| • Adenocarcinoma deriving from the epithelium of the pancreatic duct → ductal carcinoma | 80 |
| • Adenocarcinoma deriving from the acinar epithelium → acinar carcinoma | 10 |
| • Papillary carcinoma | < 5 |
| • Adenosquamous carcinoma | < 5 |
| • Undifferentiated carcinoma | < 5 |
| • Other | Rare |
| *Tumors of the Endocrine Pancreas* | 5 |
| • Insulinoma | |
| • Glucagonoma | |
| • Gastrinoma | |
| • Carcinoids | |
| • VIPoma | |
| *Other* | Rare |
| • Lymphomas, sarcoma, etc. | |

### Location
- Head of pancreas: 70%
- Body of pancreas: 20%
- Tail of pancreas: 10%

**Metastasis**
- Early lymphogenic and hematogenic spread (regional lymph nodes, liver, peritoneum, lung, skeletal system, CNS)
- Direct invasion of adjacent structures

**Class:** TNM Staging of Pancreatic Cancer (2002)

| | |
|---|---|
| **T** | **Primary Tumor** |
| TX | Primary tumor cannot be assessed |
| T0 | No evidence of primary tumor |
| Tis | Carcinoma in situ |
| T1 | Tumor limited to pancreas, $\leq 2$ cm |
| T2 | Tumor limited to pancreas, $> 2$ cm |
| T3 | Tumor extends beyond the pancreas |
| T4 | Invasion of the celiac trunk or the superior mesenteric artery |
| **N** | **Lymph Node Involvement** |
| NX | Regional lymph nodes cannot be assessed |
| N0 | Regional lymph nodes without metastases |
| N1 | Metastasis to regional lymph nodes |
| **M** | **Distant Metastasis** |
| MX | Distant metastasis cannot be assessed |
| M0 | No distant metastasis |
| M1 | Distant metastasis |

AJCC Staging (2002)

| Stage | TNM system | | |
|---|---|---|---|
| 0 | Tis | N0 | M0 |
| IA | T1 | N0 | M0 |
| IB | T2 | N0 | M0 |
| IIA | T3 | N0 | M0 |
| IIB | T1–3 | N1 | M0 |
| III | T4 | Any N | M0 |
| IV | Any T | Any N | M1 |

**Sy:** No specific symptoms in early stages. In later stages of disease:
- General symptoms: fatigue, anorexia
- Weight loss (80% of patients)
- Pain, usually belt-like, in upper abdomen and back
- Icterus (50% of patients; painless icterus is indicative of malignant obstruction of the bile duct)
- "Courvoisier's sign": enlarged gallbladder forms palpable non-tender resistance in the area of the costal arch due to malignant obstruction of the bile duct
- Ascites

**Dg:**

### Medical History, Physical Examination
- Medical history including pain (belt-like pain in the upper abdomen), smoking, alcohol abuse, family history
- Physical examination: palpable tumor in the upper abdomen, icterus, ascites, splenomegaly, Courvoisier's sign

### Laboratory Tests
- Amylase, lipase, blood glucose, $Ca^{2+}$, alkaline phosphatase, γGT, bilirubin, LDH
- Tumor markers: CEA, CA 19-9, CA 125 (monitoring of disease course)

### Histology
- Needle biopsy (ultrasound or CT guided) or laparoscopy (biopsies of hepatic metastases, lymph node metastases, peritoneal carcinosis); 80–90% sensitivity
- Endoscopic retrograde cholangiopancreaticography (ERCP) with cytology of the pancreatic secretion (possibly simultaneous stent placement)
- *NOTE: If a laparotomy is planned for the purpose of tumor resection or palliative surgical treatment, preoperative histological analysis is unnecessary and can be carried out intraoperatively instead.* If no laparotomy is planned (palliative situation), the diagnosis must be verified by histology or cytology before starting chemo- or radiotherapy.

### Imaging
- Ultrasound, possibly endosonography
- Chest x-ray
- Spiral CT or MRI of the abdomen
- Angiographic procedures: celiac angiography, splenoportography, angio MRI
- PET scan to exclude metastases
- With suspected gastric / duodenal invasion: gastrointestinal passage / gastroduodenoscopy
- Laparoscopy to exclude peritoneal carcinosis

**Dd:**

Chronic pancreatitis

**Co:**

- Concomitant pancreatitis
- Hypercoagulability → thromboses, thrombophlebitis, embolism
- Splenomegaly with obstruction of splenic vein
- Pancreatic failure → steatorrhea, pathological glucose tolerance / diabetes mellitus
- Subileus / ileus

**Th:**

### Treatment Concept

1. Pancreatic carcinomas are usually diagnosed in advanced stages of the disease; lymph node involvement (N+) in 90% of cases. Only tumors diagnosed early (T1–2 N0 M0) are surgically resectable with curative intent. Multimodal treatment concepts (clinical trials) should be considered.
2. Adjuvant chemotherapy may achieve a reduction in the local relapse rate with an overall survival advantage.
3. Neoadjuvant radiochemotherapy seems to be justified both for patients with resectable tumors (where it may possibly reduce the rate of R1 resections) and in patients with operable T1 and T2 tumors who often (50–90%) have lymph node metastases. Due to postoperative complications, adjuvant therapy is not possible in 30% of patients.
4. Even in palliative situations, supportive treatment can significantly improve quality of life.

### Treatment of pancreatic carcinoma

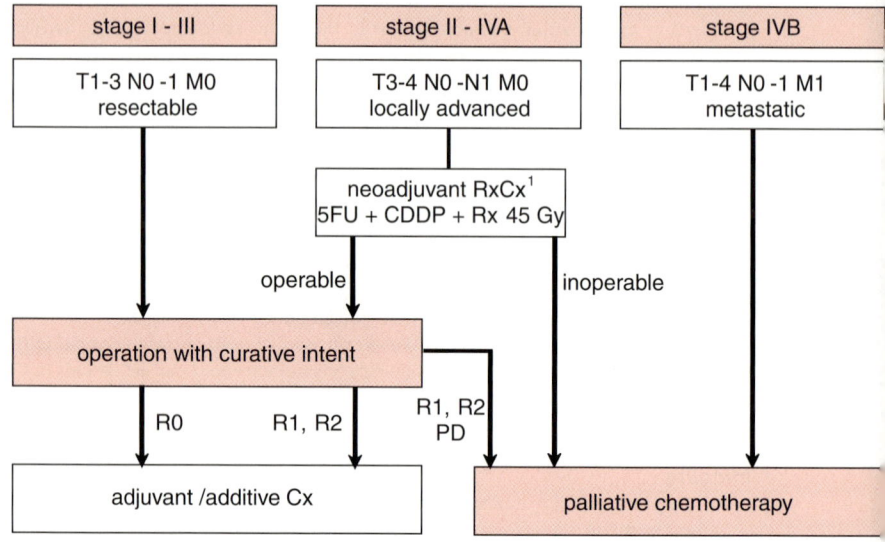

*5-FU* 5-fluorouracil, *CDDP* cisplatin, *Rx* radiotherapy, *Cx* chemotherapy, *RxCx* combined radiochemotherapy
PD progressive disease
[1]In clinical trials

## Treatment Modalities

### Surgery
- Surgical treatment with curative intent is feasible in stages T1–3 N0–1 M0. The goal is complete tumor resection with tumor-free surgical margins including the regional lymphatic drainage system (R0 resection).
- Risk and success of surgical treatment depend largely on experience of surgeon and institution. Therefore, patients should ideally be treated at specialized centers.
- Only 10–20% of all pancreatic carcinomas are operable with curative intent. The surgery-related mortality rate is approximately 5%.

### Contraindications for Surgical Treatment
- Distant metastasis (including metastasis to non-regional lymph nodes)
- Extensive deep retroperitoneal infiltration
- Extensive infiltration into the mesenteric root of the small intestine
- *NOTE*: local infiltration of the portal vein, the superior mesenteric vein, the stomach, the spleen, or the colon is not a contraindication for surgical treatment.

### Surgical Techniques
- Papillary / pancreatic head carcinoma: partial pancreaticoduodenectomy with ≥ 2 cm safety margins → "Whipple's operation" or papilla-preserving operation with similar long-term prognosis
- Pancreatic head and body carcinoma: subtotal or total pancreaticoduodenectomy
- Pancreatic tail carcinoma: left hemipancreatectomy
- Pancreatic tail and corpus carcinoma: subtotal left pancreatectomy
- Extensive infiltration: total pancreatectomy
- Palliative surgical treatment in nonresectable cases: biliodigestive anastomosis; with duodenal stenosis, possibly antecolic gastroenterostomy
- *ATTENTION*: pancreatectomized patients require life-long replacement therapy with insulin, pancreatic enzymes, and fat-soluble vitamins (vitamins A, D, E, K)

### Radiotherapy
- Palliative treatment with inoperable tumors
- Palliative indications for radiotherapy: pain, symptomatic carcinomas
- Combined radiochemotherapy or intraoperative radiotherapy (IORT) in clinical trials

### Chemotherapy
- Pancreatic carcinomas are resistant to the majority of cytostatic drugs.
- The antimetabolite gemcitabine achieves remission rates of 5–10%. 5-Fluorouracil is less effective with response rates < 5%. Other potentially effective compounds: anthracyclines (doxorubicin, epirubicin), docetaxel, irinotecan, oxaliplatin.
- Combination chemotherapy (e.g., gemcitabine + capecitabine) may lead to a survival advantage over monotherapy.
- Adjuvant chemotherapy with 5-FU or gemcitabine seems to positively affect survival.

### Supportive / Palliative Treatment
- Pain control (▶ Chap. 4.5):
  - Systemic treatment: WHO analgesic ladder
  - Inactivation of the celiac ganglion via CT-guided alcohol instillation, splanchnicectomy
- Enteral nutrition via duodenal feeding tube or PEG, alternatively: parenteral nutrition
- Icterus: percutaneous transhepatic drainage (PTD), endoscopic stent placement, or biliodigestive anastomosis

### Multimodal Therapy Concepts
For the treatment of pancreatic carcinomas of stage T1–3 N0–1 M0 or T3–4 N1 M0, multimodal treatment concepts are currently being evaluated in clinical trials:
- Neoadjuvant radiochemotherapy + surgery
- Surgery + intraoperative radiotherapy (IORT), tumor dose 20–30 Gy
- Surgery + adjuvant chemotherapy
- Surgery + IORT + postoperative radiochemotherapy with percutaneous completion of the radiation dose (up to a total of 60 Gy) and simultaneous chemotherapy (e.g., 5-fluorouracil + cisplatin)

## Chemotherapy Protocols: Pancreatic Carcinoma

| "Gemcitabine" ▶ Protocol 12.8.1 | | | Start next cycle on day 29 |
|---|---|---|---|
| Gemcitabine | 1,000 mg/m²/day | i.v. | Days 1, 8, 15 |

| Combined Radiochemotherapy | | | |
|---|---|---|---|
| Cisplatin | 15 mg/m²/day | i.v. | Days 1–5, 22–26 |
| 5-Fluorouracil | 200 mg/m²/day | c.i.v. | Days 1–5, 8–11, 15–19, 22–26, 29–33 |
| Radiotherapy | 45 Gy | | 1.8 Gy/day |

**Prg:**

| Stage | Five-year survival (%) | Median survival (months) |
|---|---|---|
| T1 N0 M0, surgery with curative intent | 20–30 | 12–18 |
| T1–3 NX M0, after surgery | 5 | 4–6 |
| TX NX M1 | < 1 | 3 |

**F/U:**     Mainly symptom-based follow-up; in patients treated with curative intent: abdominal ultrasound every 3 months; relapse pattern: primarily local or in the form of hepatic metastases.

**Ref:**
1.  Cardenes Hr, Chiorean EG, De Witt J et al. Locally advanced pancreatic cancer. Oncologist 2006;11:612–23
2.  Chua YJ, Cunningham D. Adjuvant treatment for resectable pancreatic cancer. J Clin Oncol 2005;23:4532–7
3.  ESMO Guidelines Working Group. Pancreatic cancer: ESMO Clinical Recommendations for diagnosis, treatment and follow-up. Ann Oncol 2007;18(Suppl. 2):ii19–20
4.  Neoptolemos JP, Stocken DD, Friess H et al. A randomized trial of chemoradiotherapy and chemotherapy after resection of pancreatic cancer. N Engl J Med 2004;350:1200–10
5.  Sultana A, Tudur Smith C, Cunningham D et al. Meta-analyses of chemotherapy for locally advanced and metastatic pancreatic cancer. J Clin Oncol 2007;25:2607–15
6.  Verslype C, Van Cutsem E, Dicato M et al. The management of pancreatic cancer. Ann Oncol 2007;18(Suppl. 7):vii1–vii10
7.  Willett CG, Czito BG, Bendell JC et al. Locally advanced pancreatic cancer. J Clin Oncol 2005;23:4538–44
8.  Yang GY, Wagner TD, Fuss M et al. Multimodality approaches for pancreatic cancer. CA Cancer J Clin 2005;55:352–67

**Web:**
1.  http://www.nlm.nih.gov/medlineplus/pancreaticcancer.html          MedlinePlus
2.  http://www.emedicine.com/MED/topic1712.htm          E-medicine
3.  http://www.cancer.org/docroot/CRI/CRI_2_3x.asp?dt=34          Am Cancer Soc
4.  http://www.path.jhu.edu/pancreas          Johns Hopkins Univ

**8.3.7**     **Hepatocellular Carcinoma (HCC)**

H.-P. Allgaier, R. Engelhardt, F. Otto

**Def:**     Primary carcinoma of liver cells.

**ICD-10:**     C22.

**Ep:**     Incidence: 2–4 cases/100,000/year in Europe; ratio male:female = 3:1; age peak: between 50 and 70 years; marked geographical differences: most common malignancy in South East Asia and parts of Africa (due to high incidence of chronic HBV infections); recent studies have shown HCC incidence in industrial nations to be rising (HCV-associated).

**Pg:**     *Risk Factors*
- Chronic hepatitis B or C, HCC risk increased by a factor of 140 in carriers of the Hbs antigen
- Hepatic cirrhosis (due to toxic effect of alcohol or other causes), 80% of cases
- Aflatoxin-contaminated foods (particularly aflatoxin B1, *Aspergillus flavus*)
- Metabolic disorders: hemochromatosis, tyrosinemia, Wilson's disease, α1-antitrypsin deficiency
- Smoking, alcohol
- Toxins: toluene, dimethylnitrosamine, anabolic steroids

*Molecular Genetic Abnormalities*
- Mutation of the p53 tumor suppressor gene
- HBV infections: modulation of p53 expression and function by the viral gene X

*Development*
Adenomatous hyperplasia → atypical hyperplasia → hepatocellular carcinoma

**Path:**     *Histology*
Tumor cells derived from hepatocytes. Distinction of highly differentiated, moderately differentiated, and undifferentiated HCC. In 5% of cases, mixed HCC and cholangiocarcinoma (CCC) tumors.
Special type: fibrolamellar HCC in younger patients without underlying hepatic disease → favorable prognosis.

*Manifestation / Metastasis*
- Majority of cases with multilocular hepatic invasion / intrahepatic metastasis
- Invasion into portal vein (35%), hepatic vein (15%), or abdominal organs (15%)
- Extrahepatic metastasis at presentation is rare; as disease progresses, metastasis to regional lymph nodes, lung, and bone

**Class:**     Beside the TNM / AJCC staging system, further classifications are in use which include functional parameters such as liver function, albumin, bilirubin, tumor markers.
The CLIP score (Cancer of the Liver Italian Program) is reliable in predicting the prognosis of HCC patients. In addition to information on liver function (Child-Pugh stage), it takes into account data regarding tumor morphology (number of lesions, tumor behaviour) as well as AFP serum levels and the presence of malignant infiltration of the portal vein. All required data are obtained during the baseline diagnostic procedures.

**TNM Staging of HCC (2002)**

| *T* | *Primary Tumor* |
|-----|-----------------|
| TX | Primary tumor cannot be assessed |
| T0 | No evidence of primary tumor |
| T1 | Solitary tumor < 2 cm without vascular invasion |

**TNM Staging of HCC (2002)** *(continued)*

| | |
|---|---|
| T2 | Solitary tumor < 2 cm with vascular invasion or<br>Solitary tumor > 2 cm without vascular invasion or<br>Multiple tumors < 2 cm in one hepatic lobe without vascular invasion |
| T3 | Solitary tumor > 2 cm with vascular invasion or<br>Multiple tumors > 2 cm in one hepatic lobe with/without vascular invasion or<br>Multiple tumors < 2 cm in one hepatic lobe with vascular invasion |
| T4 | Multiple tumors in more than one hepatic lobe or<br>Involvement of a major branch of the portal or hepatic vein or<br>Direct invasion of adjacent organs |
| ***N*** | ***Lymph Node Involvement*** |
| NX | Regional lymph nodes cannot be assessed |
| N0 | Regional lymph nodes without metastases |
| N1 | Metastasis to regional lymph nodes |
| ***M*** | ***Distant Metastasis*** |
| MX | Distant metastasis cannot be assessed |
| M0 | No distant metastasis |
| M1 | Distant metastasis |

**AJCC Staging (2002)**

| Stage | TNM system | | |
|---|---|---|---|
| I | T1 | N0 | M0 |
| II | T2 | N0 | M0 |
| III | T1–2 | N1 | M0 |
| | T3 | Any N | M0 |
| IVA | T4 | Any N | M0 |
| IVB | Any T | Any N | M1 |

**Staging according to Okuda**

| Criteria | Positive | Negative |
|---|---|---|
| Tumor size | > 50% of liver | < 50% of liver |
| Ascites | Present | None |
| Bilirubin | > 51 µmol/l | < 51 µmol/l |
| Albumin | < 30 g/l | > 30 g/l |

| | |
|---|---|
| Stage I | Negative for all criteria |
| Stage II | 1–2 criteria positive |
| Stage III | 3–4 criteria positive |

**Staging according to CLIP**

| Parameter | Points | | |
|---|---|---|---|
| | **0** | **1** | **2** |
| Child-Pugh stage | A | B | C |
| HCC morphology | Solitary and extended ≤ 50% | Multiple and extended ≤ 50% | Infiltrating or extended > 50% |
| AFP (ng/ml) | < 400 | ≥ 400 | Not defined |
| Portal vein thrombosis | No | Yes | Not defined |

| CLIP score | Median survival (months) | One-year survival (%) | Two-year survival (%) |
|---|---|---|---|
| 0 | 36 | 84 | 65 |
| 1 | 22 | 66 | 45 |
| 2 | 9 | 45 | 17 |
| 3 | 7 | 36 | 12 |
| 4–6 | 3 | 9 | 0 |

**Sy:**

*Mostly in advanced stages of the disease:*
- Abdominal discomfort, pain in the upper abdomen
- Pain in right shoulder due to diaphragm irritation
- Weight loss, fatigue, reduced performance
- Icterus, hepatomegaly, liver dysfunction
- Ascites, intra-abdominal bleeding (hematoperitoneum as primary manifestation), gastrointestinal hemorrhage (portal vein thrombosis)

**Dg:**

### Medical History, Physical Examination
- Medical history including hepatitis, liver cirrhosis
- Physical examination: hepatomegaly, ascites, palpable tumor, signs of hepatic cirrhosis (hard nodular liver)

### Laboratory Tests
- Routine laboratory tests: full blood count, LDH, total protein, electrophoresis, coagulation, liver / renal function tests, inflammation parameters
- Tumor markers: α1-fetoprotein (AFP, increased in 50–80% of cases), CEA, des-γ-carboxy prothrombin (increased sensitivity if combined with AFP)

### Histology
- Histological analysis of fine-needle biopsy (ultrasound or CT guided)
- In cases of diffuse hepatic invasion: blind liver biopsy
- In rare cases, laparoscopic liver biopsy

### Imaging
- B-flow and color Doppler ultrasound (portal vein infiltration and/or thrombosis?)
- Multidetector spiral CT (non-contrast, early arterial, and portal-venous phases) or abdominal MRI
- Chest x-ray or thoracic CT scan (exclusion of pulmonary metastases)
- Bone scan (exclusion of metastases)
- Optional: Lipiodol angiography (with subsequent CT scan after 10–14 days) or angio-CT

**DD:**    **Differential diagnosis of intrahepatic lesions**

*Malignant Tumors*

| | |
|---|---|
| • Metastases | Common malignant hepatic lesions (90%) |
| • Hepatocellular carcinomas | "HCC" |
| • Cholangiocarcinomas | "CCC," rare |
| • Angiosarcomas | Noxious agents: vinyl chloride, arsenic, ionizing radiation |
| • Hepatoblastomas | Embryonic tumors occurring in children |

*Benign Tumors*

| | |
|---|---|
| • Hemangiomas | Most common benign liver tumors |
| • Hepatocellular adenomas | Women >> Men, risk factor: oral contraceptives |
| • Bile duct adenomas | Rare |
| • Focal nodular hyperplasia | "FNH," mainly women |

*Cystic Disorders*

| | |
|---|---|
| • Solitary hepatic cysts | Common |
| • Dysontogenetic cysts | Rare, hereditary |
| • Cystic echinococcosis | Caused by dog tapeworm (*Echinococcus granulosus*) |
| • Alveolar echinococcosis | Caused by fox tapeworm (*Echinococcus multilocularis*) |
| • Liver abscess | Pyogenic, amoebae |

**Co:**    ***Paraneoplastic Syndromes***
- Hypoglycemia, hypercalcemia
- Polycythemia
- Carcinoid syndrome
- Polymyositis

**Th:**    **Treatment Concept**

1. First-line treatment is surgical resection of affected liver tissue. However, tumor resection with curative intent is only possible in <20% of cases, due to hepatic failure (more than 80% of patients have hepatic cirrhosis), multicentricity, age, or concomitant diseases. In individual cases, potentially curative orthotopic liver transplant (OLTx).
2. Patients with inoperable but localized disease without distant metastases are treated with locally effective palliative therapeutic measures:
   - Transarterial chemoperfusion without (TAC) or with (TACE) subsequent embolization of the blood supply to the tumor
   - Percutaneous ethanol injection (PEI)
   - Thermoablative coagulation with high-frequency (HFTA) microwaves or laser
3. Patients with advanced HCC and contraindications for local treatment (e.g., portal vein thrombosis, therapy-refractory ascites) or distant metastases may benefit from palliative systemic treatment. Sorafenib improves survival in patients with hepatocellular carcinoma and Child-Pugh A cirrhosis of the liver.

**Treatment of HCC**

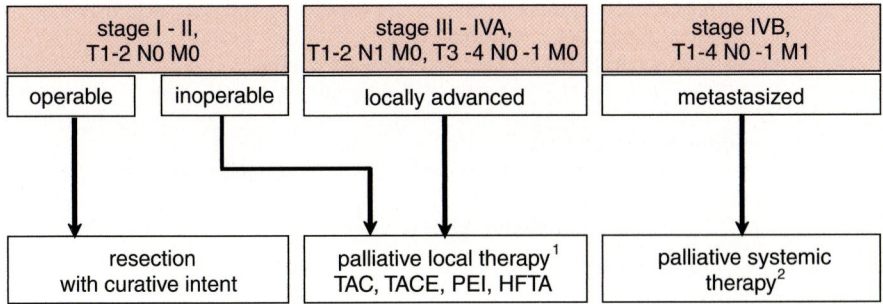

[1] *TAC* transarterial chemoperfusion, *TACE* transarterial chemoperfusion with embolization, *PEI* percutaneous
ethanol instillation, *HFTA* high-frequency thermoablation
[2] Pain control, drainage of abdominal ascites, etc.

## Treatment Modalities

### Surgery
Resection is indicated only in cases of localized tumors and with satisfactory hepatic functional
reserve. Surgical techniques:
- Resection of one or more liver segments; with sufficient functional reserve, extended hemi-
  hepatectomy may be possible
- Orthotopic liver transplant (OLTx): HCC stage I–II (AJCC), fibrolamellar carcinoma, hepa-
  toblastoma. Patients with advanced tumors, esp. with distant metastases, do not qualify for
  OLTx

### Regional Chemotherapy I: Transarterial Chemoperfusion (TAC)
TAC via transfemoral access: direct infusion of cytostatic drugs (doxorubicin, cisplatin, mitomycin C) into the hepatic artery; carrier substance Lipiodol prolongs retention due to selective affinity to HCC.
→ Response rates up to 50%, however, a survival benefit has not been established.

### Regional Chemotherapy II: TAC with Subsequent Embolization (TACE)
Direct intra-arterial administration of cytostatic drugs and subsequent vascular embolization
with microspheres, gelatin foam, Lipiodol, or starch compounds; potential side effects: nausea,
infection, icterus, abdominal pain, encephalopathy; contraindicated in patients with portal vein
thrombosis.
→ Recent randomized trials have demonstrated a survival advantage in patients treated with
   TACE

### Percutaneous Ethanol Instillation (PEI)
Used in inoperable liver cell carcinomas; alternative to use of ethanol: acetic acid; limited by the
number of lesions (≤ 3) and the size of individual lesions (≤ 5 cm). Side effects: abdominal pain,
hemorrhage, infection; needs to be repeated several times.
→ In some cases, good local tumor control; no randomized studies.

### Thermoablative Treatment
Minimally invasive ultrasound or MRI-guided percutaneous insertion of special probes into the
tumor. Advantage compared to other procedures: single treatment is usually sufficient.
→ A current randomized controlled trial has demonstrated significantly improved local relapse-
   free survival in patients treated with HFTA over patients with PEI

### Systemic Chemotherapy

Palliative approach; response rates 15–20%. Cytostatic drugs with efficacy in HCC: doxorubicin, epirubicin, mitoxantrone, mitomycin C. Systemic chemotherapy has not demonstrated a survival benefit; in some cases, considerable toxicity.

Recently, sorafenib has been shown to prolong survival.

NOTE: systemic cytostatic treatment is often limited due to impaired liver function (cirrhosis).

### Hormone Therapy

- Controlled trials with tamoxifen did not result in improved survival.
- A pilot study with octreotide (somatostatin analog) was able to demonstrate prolonged survival in patients with advanced-stage HCC.

### Multimodal Therapy Concepts

Combined therapies are being tested in clinical trials.

**Prg:**    Generally poor prognosis; most patients die due to progressive liver failure.

### Median Survival

- Without treatment: 2–6 months
- Inoperable HCC: 6–10 months
- Surgical treatment in stage I: 36 months
- Surgical treatment in stage II: 20 months

### Prognostic Factors

- Tumor stage according to CLIP, AJCC, or Okuda (multiple tumors, diffuse growth, vascular invasion, lymph node metastasis: poor prognosis)
- Liver function (Child-Pugh classification)

**F/U:**    Symptom-based follow-up.

**Px:**    Prophylactic measures concentrate on risk groups (patients with hepatic cirrhosis or viral hepatitis) or high-risk populations (countries with high prevalence of HBV infections):

- HBV vaccination
- Treatment of chronic hepatitis C with interferon-α
- AFP monitoring, abdominal ultrasound, if necessary: abdominal CT scan every 6 months

**Ref:**
1. Blum HE. Hepatocellular carcinoma: therapy and prevention. World J Gastroenterol 2005;11:7391–400
2. Greten TF, Papendorf F, Bleck JS et al. Survival rate in patients with hepatocellular carcinoma. Br J Cancer 2005;92:1862–8
3. Hertl M, Cosimi AB. Liver transplantation for malignancy. Oncologist 2004;10:269–81
4. Llovet JM, Burroughs A, Bruix J. Hepatocellular carcinoma. Lancet 2003;362:1907–17
5. Mann CD, Neal CP, Garcea G et al. Prognostic molecular markers in hepatocellular carcinoma. Eur J Cancer 2007;43:979–92
6. Nowak AK, Chow PKH, Findlay M. Systemic therapy for advanced hepatocellular carcinoma. Eur J Cancer 2004;40:1474–84
7. Zhu AX. Systematic therapy of advanced hepatocellular carcinoma: how hopeful should we be? Oncologist 2006;11:790–800

**Web:**
1. http://www.nlm.nih.gov/medlineplus/livercancer.html    MedlinePlus
2. http://www.emedicine.com/MED/topic2664.htm    E-medicine
3. http://www.livercancer.com/    Liver Cancer Network
4. http://www.livertumor.org/    Liver Tumor Portal
5. http://www.cnn.com/HEALTH/library/DS/00399.html    CNN Health

## 8.3.8 Tumors of the Gallbladder and Bile Duct

**J. Harder, H. Henß, F. Otto**

| | |
|---|---|
| **Def:** | Malignant epithelial neoplasia of the biliary system. |
| **ICD-10:** | C23, C24 |
| **Ep:** | Incidence: 1–3 cases/100,000/year; ratio male:female = 1:3; age peak: 60–80 years. |

**Pg:**

### Risk Factors
- Primary sclerosing cholangitis (PSC) and ulcerative colitis
- Gallbladder polyps > 1 cm, bile duct adenomas
- "Porcelain gallbladder," gallstones, hepaticolithiasis
- Choledochal cysts, Caroli's disease
- Long common channel of the common bile duct and pancreatic duct
- Chronic carriers of *Salmonella typhi*
- Leaches (*Opisthorchis viverrini, Clonorchis sinensis*)
- Smoking

**Path:**

### Histology

*Adenocarcinoma: >90%*
- Papillary adenocarcinoma
- Intestinal-type adenocarcinoma
- Mucinous adenocarcinoma
- Clear cell adenocarcinoma

*Other: < 10%*
- Squamous cell carcinoma
- Small cell (oat cell) carcinoma
- Sarcoma
- Undifferentiated carcinoma

### Classification According to Location
- Intrahepatic (peripheral) cholangiocarcinomas (20–25%)
- Perihilar "Klatskin's" tumors (40–50%)
- Gallbladder carcinomas
- Distal extrahepatic bile duct carcinomas
- Periampullary carcinomas or carcinomas of the ampulla of Vater

**Class:**

### TNM Staging of Gallbladder Carcinoma (2002)

| T | Primary Tumor |
|---|---|
| TX | Primary tumor cannot be assessed |
| T0 | No evidence of primary tumor |
| Tis | Carcinoma in situ |
| T1 | Invasion of mucosa (T1a) or muscularis (T1b) |
| T2 | Invasion of perimuscular tissue but not beyond the serosa or the liver |
| T3 | Invasion beyond the serosa or into a neighboring organ |
| T4 | Invasion of the main branch of the portal vein or the hepatic artery and/or two or more neighboring organs |

**Class:**      **TNM Staging of Gallbladder Carcinoma (2002)** *(continued)*

| N | Lymph Node Involvement |
|---|---|
| NX | Regional lymph nodes cannot be assessed |
| N0 | Regional lymph nodes without metastases |
| N1 | Metastasis in cystic duct, pericholedochal and/or hilar (hepatoduodenal ligament) lymph nodes |
| **M** | **Distant Metastasis** |
| MX | Distant metastasis cannot be assessed |
| M0 | No distant metastasis |
| M1 | Distant metastasis |

### Metastasis

Pericholedochal lymph nodes → cholecystic lymph nodes → retroportal / posterosuperior / pancreaticoduodenal / interaortocaval lymph nodes

### AJCC Staging of Gallbladder Carcinoma (2002)

| Stage | TNM-system | | |
|---|---|---|---|
| 0 | Tis | N0 | M0 |
| IA | T1 | N0 | M0 |
| IB | T2 | N0 | M0 |
| IIA | T3 | N0 | M0 |
| IIB | T1–3 | N1 | M0 |
| III | T4 | N0–1 | M0 |
| IV | T1–4 | N0–2 | M1 |

### Staging of perihilar (Klatskin's) tumors according to Bismuth

| Stage | Characterization |
|---|---|
| I | Perihilar tumor not reaching the bifurcation of the hepatic duct |
| II | Perihilar tumor reaching the bifurcation of the hepatic duct |
| IIIa | Perihilar tumor extends into right secondary intrahepatic duct |
| IIIb | Perihilar tumor extends into left secondary intrahepatic duct |
| IV | Involvement of the secondary intrahepatic ducts on both sides |

For staging of intrahepatic cholangiocarcinomas, ► Chap. 8.3.7

**Sy:**      *Main Symptom*
- Icterus

*Late Symptoms*
- Hepatomegaly: abdominal pain
- Nausea, vomiting, weight loss
- Obstruction distal to the cystic duct: palpable gallbladder (Courvoisier's sign)

**Dg:**

### Medical History, Physical Examination
- Medical history including risk factors
- Physical examination including palpation of the upper abdomen

### Laboratory Tests
- Routine laboratory tests including blood count, hepatic / renal function parameters
- Tumor markers: CA 19-9, CEA, CA 125

### Imaging
- Ultrasound, endosonography
- With icterus: endoscopic retrograde cholangiography (ERC) with stent insertion
- Percutaneous transhepatic cholangiography and drainage (PTCD) if ERC unsuccessful or with centrally located tumors
- MRI or MRCP (magnetic resonance cholangio-pancreatography)
- Primary sclerosing cholangitis (PSC): PET scan
- Endoscopy of the stomach, duodenum, or colon if suspected invasion
- Laparoscopy prior to surgical resection

### Histology
- Biopsy in conjunction with ERC
- In some cases, incidental diagnosis during cholecystectomy → diagnosis based on surgical specimen

**Dd:**
- Intrahepatic lesion of other origin
- Cholecystitis, cholangitis, choledocholithiasis

**Co:**
- Obstruction of the common bile duct

**Th:**

### Treatment Concept

1. Gallbladder / cholangiocarcinomas are primarily treated surgically (complete resection feasible in approximately 30–40% of cases).
2. In inoperable cases, palliative treatment may significantly improve quality of life.
3. Benefit of chemotherapy or combined radiochemotherapy is uncertain → use in clinical studies.
4. With incidental diagnosis (cholecystectomy specimen): often early stages → thorough diagnosis (exclusion of metastases), close monitoring.

### Surgical Treatment

#### Gallbladder Carcinoma
- Carcinoma in situ, mucosal carcinoma, T1b tumor: removal of gallbladder is sufficient; resection of the gallbladder bed with safety margin of ≥ 3 cm; if necessary, segmental hepatectomy
- T2 tumor: partial hepatectomy (segments IVb and V) with lymphadenectomy along the hepatoduodenal ligament
- T3 tumor: additional resection of the choledochal duct; hemihepatectomy sometimes required

#### Intrahepatic / Perihilar Cholangiocarcinomas
- Resection of one or more liver segments or hemihepatectomy depending on location

#### Endoscopic Interventional Therapy
- Non-resectable tumors with bile duct obstruction: endoscopic stent implantation → drainage improves quality of life
- Experimental method: photodynamic therapy

## Chemotherapy

Palliative treatment in patients with advanced disease; if possible, in clinical trials. Therapies:
- 5-FU / leucovorin (▶ Protocol 12.7.1)
- Combination chemotherapy with cisplatin + 5-FU + leucovorin
- Other effective cytostatic drugs: gemcitabine, oxaliplatin, irinotecan

| *"Gemcitabine / Oxaliplatin"* ▶ Protocol 12.9.1 | | | *Start next cycle on day 29* |
|---|---|---|---|
| Gemcitabine | 1,000 mg/m²/day | i.v. | Days 1, 8, 15 |
| Oxaliplatin | 100 mg/m²/day | i.v. | Days 1, 15 |

| *"Gemcitabine mono"* ▶ Protocol 12.8.1 | | | *Start next cycle on day 29* |
|---|---|---|---|
| Gemcitabine | 1,000 mg/m²/day | i.v. | Days 1, 8, 15 |

**Prg:**    *Five-year Survival: Resectable Tumors*
- Gallbladder carcinomas:          2–10%
- Tumors of the distal choledochus:    30%
- Tumors of the hepatic fork:       10–20%

**F/U:**    Symptom-based follow-up.

**Ref:**
1. Anderson CD, Pinson CW, Berlin J et al. Diagnosis and treatment of cholangiocarcinoma. Oncologist 2004;9:43–57
2. Brugge WR. Endoscopic techniques to diagnose and manage biliary tumors. J Clin Oncol 2005;23:4561–5
3. De Groen PC, Gores GJ, LaRusso NF et al. Biliary tract cancers. N Engl J Med 1999;341:1368–78
4. Khan SA, Thomas HC, Davidson BR et al. Cholangiocarcinoma. Lancet 2005;366:1303–14
5. Patel T. Cholangiocarcinoma. Nat Clin Pract Gastroenterol Hepatol 2006;3:33–42
6. Randi G, Franceschi S, La Vecchia C. Gallbladder cancer worldwide: geographic distribution and risk factors. Int J Cancer 2006;118:1591–602
7. Wistuba II, Gazdar AF. Gallbladder cancer: lessons from a rare tumor. Nature Rev Cancer 2004;4:695–706

**Web:**
1. http://www.cancer.gov/cancertopics/types/gallbladder          Cancer Topics
2. http://www.nlm.nih.gov/medlineplus/ency/article/000291.htm     Medline Plus
3. http://www.emedicine.com/med/topic343.htm                      E-medicine
4. http://www.nccn.org/professionals/physian_gls/PDF/hepatobiliary.pdf   NCCN Guideline

## 8.4 Tumors of the Female Reproductive System

### 8.4.1 Breast Cancer

**D. Behringer, C.F. Waller, M. Trepel**

**Def:** Malignant tumor of the mammary gland.

**ICD-10:** C50.-

**Ep:** Age dependent annual incidence: 5/100,000 women at age 25, 150/100,000 at age 50, and > 200/100,000 at age 75. Mortality rate 30/100,000 women/year. Most common malignant tumor in women (25% of all cancers in women). Cumulative risk of a woman developing breast cancer is 12%, the risk of dying of it is 4–6% (USA). Annual incidence in men ≤ 1/100,000.

**Pg:** *Risk Factors*
70–80% of breast cancer cases occur in patients without risk factors. In patients who have recovered from breast cancer, the risk of developing a second breast cancer is 1%/year.

| Risk factors | Relative risk (RR) |
|---|---|
| Disease in a first-degree relative | 2–3[a] |
| Early menarche, late menopause, nulliparous women | Increased[a] |
| First pregnancy at > 24 years | 2[b] |
| First pregnancy at > 30 years | 4[b] |
| Nulliparous women | 2[a] |
| Age > 50 years | 2[a] |
| Previous cancer in one breast | 3[a] |

[a] Compared to total population
[b] Compared to women aged 18 years at first pregnancy

*Hormones (Estrogen Therapy / Oral Contraceptives)*
- If oral contraceptives are used for > 10 years, the relative risk is increased fourfold.
- Women using oral contraceptives for > 4 years prior to their first completed pregnancy have a relative risk of 1.7 for developing breast cancer.

*Tumor Suppressor Genes*
Germline mutations of oncogenes pose an increased risk (< 10% of breast cancer patients):
- BRCA1, BRCA2
- p53 (Li-Fraumeni syndrome)

*Other Risk Factors*
- Alcohol abuse
- Exposure to radiation
- Atypical lobular ductal hyperplasia
- Benign diseases of the breast (minimal risk increase, unless histological detection of atypical behaviour)

**Path:**          *Histopathological Classification*

| Type | Percentage of cases |
|---|:---:|
| *Carcinoma in situ*[a] | 15–20 |
| • Ductal type (DCIS) | 14–19 |
| • Lobular type (LCIS) | 1 |
| *Invasive Carcinoma* | 80–85 |
| • Invasive ductal carcinoma | > 70 |
| • Invasive lobular carcinoma | 10 |
| • Medullary carcinoma (associated with better prognosis when node negative) | 5 |
| *Miscellaneous* | < 5 |
| • Mucinous carcinoma (associated with better prognosis when node negative) | |
| • Scirrhous carcinoma | |
| • Papillary carcinoma (associated with better prognosis when node negative) | |
| • Inflammatory carcinoma (poor prognosis) | |
| • Paget's disease | |
| • Comedocarcinoma | |
| • Undifferentiated carcinoma | |
| • Metaplastic carcinoma (squamous cell) | |

[a] Not crossing basal membrane, no stromal invasion; apparent incidence increase of in situ carcinomas from 1% (30 years ago) to 15–20% of all tumors due to mammography screening

### Receptors / Important Histochemical Markers
- Estrogen and progesterone receptors
- HER2/neu receptors

### Location of the Primary Tumor
- Nipple: 14%
- Upper outer quadrant: 50%
- Upper inner quadrant: 15%
- Lower outer quadrant: 12%
- Lower inner quadrant: 6%
- Multicentric: 3%

### Metastatic Spread
- Regional lymph nodes (stage N1–N3a)
- Supraclavicular lymph nodes (stage N3c)
- Bone
- Lung
- Pleura
- Liver
- CNS
- Ovaries
- Skin

**Class:**     **TNM Staging of Breast Cancer**

| | |
|---|---|
| *T* | *Primary Tumor* |
| TX | Primary tumor cannot be assessed |
| T0 | No evidence of primary tumor |
| Tis | Carcinoma in situ: |
| | Tis (DCIS): ductal carcinoma in situ |
| | Tis (LCIS): lobular carcinoma in situ |
| | Tis (Paget): Paget's disease of the nipple with no tumor |
| T1 | Tumor ≤ 2 cm in greatest dimension |
| T1mic | Microinvasion ≤ 0.1 cm |
| T1a | Tumor > 0.1 ≤ 0.5 cm |
| T1b | Tumor > 0.5–1 cm |
| T1c | Tumor > 1–2 cm |
| T2 | Tumor > 2 cm and ≤ 5 cm |
| T3 | Tumor > 5 cm |
| T4 | Direct extension to chest wall or skin (ribs, intercostal, serratus anterior muscle) |
| T4a | Infiltration of chest wall |
| T4b | Edema (including peau d'orange), ulceration of skin, satellite skin nodules |
| T4c | Infiltration of chest wall and skin |
| T4d | Inflammatory carcinoma (diffuse infiltration) |
| *N* | *Clinical Lymph Node Involvement* |
| NX | Regional lymph nodes cannot be assessed |
| N0 | No regional lymph node metastasis |
| N1 | Ipsilateral axillary node(s), movable |
| N2 | Ipsilateral axillary node(s), fixed, or clinically apparent internal mammary lymph nodes |
| N2a | Axillary lymph node metastasis, fixed to one another or to other structures |
| N2b | Metastasis only in clinically apparent internal mammary lymph nodes[a] |
| N3 | Metastasis in: |
| N3a | Infraclavicular lymph node(s) |
| N3b | Internal mammary and axillary lymph nodes |
| N3c | Supraclavicular lymph node(s) |
| *pN* | *Pathological (Histologically Assessed) Lymph Node Involvement* |
| pNX | Regional lymph nodes cannot be assessed |
| pN0 | No regional lymph node metastasis |
| pN1mic | Micrometastases (> 0.2 mm and ≤ 2 mm) |
| pN1a | 1–3 axillary lymph node metastases, including at least one > 2 mm |
| pN1b | Internal mammary lymph nodes with microscopic metastasis, not clinically apparent[b] |

[a] By clinical examination or imaging (except lymphoscintigraphy)
[b] Detected by sentinel lymph node biopsy
[c] Optional nomenclature

**Class:**     **TNM Staging of Breast Cancer** *(continued)*

| | |
|---|---|
| pN1c | Metastasis in 1–3 axillary lymph nodes and internal mammary lymph nodes, not clinically apparent[b] |
| pN2a | 4–9 axillary lymph nodes, including at least one measuring > 2 mm |
| pN2b | Lymph nodes ipsilateral to internal mammary artery, clinically apparent in absence of axillary lymph node metastasis |
| pN3a | Metastasis in ≥ 10 axillary lymph nodes (at least one > 2 mm) or in infraclavicular lymph nodes |
| pN3b | Metastasis in clinically apparent internal mammary lymph nodes in the presence of positive axillary lymph node(s) or metastasis in > 3 axillary lymph nodes and in internal mammary lymph nodes not clinically apparent[b] |
| pN3c | Metastasis in supraclavicular lymph node(s) |
| **M** | **Distant Metastasis** |
| MX | Distant metastasis cannot be assessed |
| M0 | No distant metastasis |
| M1 | Distant metastasis |
| M1(i)[c] | Isolated epithelial tumor cells in the bone marrow |

[a] By clinical examination or imaging (except lymphoscintigraphy)
[b] Detected by sentinel lymph node biopsy
[c] Optional nomenclature

**Class:**     **AJCC Staging**

| Stage | TNM system | | |
|---|---|---|---|
| 0 | Tis | N0 | M0 |
| I | T1 | N0 | M0 |
| IIA | T0–1 | N1 | M0 |
| | T2 | N0 | M0 |
| IIB | T2 | N1 | M0 |
| | T3 | N0 | M0 |
| IIIA | T0-2 | N2 | M0 |
| | T3 | N2 | M0 |
| IIIB | T4 | N1–2 | M0 |
| | Any T | N3 | M0 |
| IV | Any T | Any N | M1 |

**Sy:**

### Main Symptoms
- Hard, nontender mass in the breast or axilla (in 70% of cases)
- Serous or sanguinous nipple discharge
- Nipple eczema

### Locally Advanced Tumors
- Protruding or inverted nipple
- Skin ulceration

**Dg:**

In more than 80% of cases, breast cancer is diagnosed by palpation of a suspicious mass (importance of self-examination). The number of breast cancer diagnoses in asymptomatic patients by mammography screening is increasing (studies have shown that the use of mammography in cancer screening results in reduced mortality rates). Nipple discharge is often caused by benign lesions. However, any discharge must be followed. Sanguinous secretion is the result of a malignant lesion in approximately 10–20% of cases.

### Medical History, Physical Examination
- Medical history including family history, risk factors
- Examination of both breasts (inspection, palpation)
- Lymph node examination, particularly axillary, parasternal, and supraclavicular nodes

### Laboratory Tests
- Routine laboratory tests including complete blood count, liver and renal function tests, alkaline phosphatase
- Tumor markers: CEA, CA 15-3, suitable for disease monitoring (not reliable for screening). *NOTE:* CA 15-3 is not specific for breast cancer, 20–50% of patients with benign breast disease have increased CA 15-3 levels.

### Histology
- Minimally invasive breast biopsy (high-speed punch biopsy, stereotactic vacuum biopsy) for preoperative diagnosis.
- More reliable: excision (where applicable: marking under local anesthesia) with frozen section analysis and collection of additional material for further diagnostics.

### Imaging
- Breast ultrasound
- Bilateral mammography (preoperatively) for detection of synchronous tumors
- MRI (especially for mammographically dense breast tissue, after breast-preserving surgery, and silicone implants)
- Chest x-ray, abdominal ultrasound, bone scan

### Prognostic Factors
Analysis of various established prognostic parameters as part of routine diagnosis is of key importance for appropriate treatment planning:
- *Tumor size, histology, grading, and stage*
- *Lymph nodes:*
  - Number of involved axillary lymph nodes (pathological classification requires the excision of > 10 lymph nodes; may be dispensable if sentinel lymph node is negative).
  - Location of involved lymph nodes (level I, II, or III)
  - Histological assessment of: invasion of lymphatic or blood vessels, fixation to surrounding structures, penetration of the lymph node capsule
- *Receptors:* estrogen and progesterone receptor expression (immunohistochemical and biochemical receptor status tests are equally valid)
- *HER2/neu* overexpression level (score 0 through 3)

### Other Prognostic Indices

The prognostic relevance of the following parameters is uncertain:

- Detection of epithelial tumor cells in the bone marrow [M1(i)]
- Proliferation markers: Ki-67, thymidine kinase (high expression levels associated with poor prognosis)
- Ploidy (euploidy implies better prognosis)
- Expression level of p53, cathepsin D
- Tumor-associated proteolysis factors: urokinase-type plasminogen activator (uPA), plasminogen activator inhibitor type 1 (PAI-1)
- Response to neoadjuvant chemotherapy (no response = poor prognosis)

**Dd:**

### Differential Diagnosis of Breast Lesions

- Breast cancer
- Lymphoma
- Mastopathy
- Benign tumors (fibroadenoma, fibroma, lipoma, etc.)
- Abscess, mastitis
- Cyst

## Carcinoma in situ (CIS)

## Treatment Concept

1. Treatment goal: curative.
2. Treatment strategy according to histological type of the CIS.
3. Frozen section examination alone is not sufficient for the assessment of noninvasive carcinoma.
4. Classification of in situ carcinomas according to current histopathological criteria does not comprehensively describe biological behaviour. Based on additional criteria (e.g., nuclear grading, necrosis, cell polarity, histoarchitecture) a prognostic index (Van Nuys Prognostic Index, VNPI) has been defined for treatment stratification in clinical trials.

### Ductal Carcinoma in situ (DCIS)

- Total gross tumor removal ± radiotherapy or mastectomy; axillary dissection is not routinely recommended, considering low risk of axillary involvement (0.5%).
- For widespread DCIS, sentinel node biopsy is recommended.
- Tamoxifen has been proven to be effective in the adjuvant treatment of receptor-positive DCIS.

### Lobular Carcinoma in situ (LCIS)

- Frequently incidental diagnosis, premenopausal, bilateral
- Local excision
- Increased risk (25%) of an ipsilateral or contralateral invasive, mostly ductal tumor; independent of the initial extent of the disease
- Close monitoring as with high-risk patients
- Alternatively: bilateral subcutaneous mastectomy (due to multicentric growth) ± deep axillary dissection. Benefit of radiotherapy not established.

### Invasive Carcinoma, Adjuvant Situation (Stage I–III)

### Treatment Concept

1. Therapeutic intent: curative, justifying combined intensive treatment strategies.
2. The choice of treatment is based on risk classification according to tumor size, axillary lymph node involvement, tumor grading, hormone receptor and HER2/neu expression, and patient age.
3. Treatment in clinical trials represents an ideal opportunity for treatment optimization.
4. Treatment is always interdisciplinary, including surgery, radiotherapy, chemotherapy, immunotherapy, and hormone therapy. General guidelines for adjuvant treatment are defined at regular time intervals in international consensus conferences (e.g., St. Gallen Recommendations, 2007).

### Surgery

Standard local treatment is complete tumor removal by breast-conserving surgery followed by radiotherapy or, alternatively, mastectomy.

#### Contraindications for Breast-conserving Surgery
- Incomplete tumor removal (despite secondary resection)
- Intraductal carcinoma in situ and around the tumor (extensive intraductal component > 25% of the tumor tissue)
- Multifocal or multicentric carcinoma, skin lymphangiosis

#### Axillary Lymph Node Dissection
- Obligatory dissection of level I and II (removal of > 10 lymph nodes) to facilitate prognosis evaluation and treatment planning and to reduce local relapse rate
- Removal of only primary draining lymph node ("sentinel node") as standard procedure in defined situations (clinically no node involvement and specifically trained surgeon)

**Risk groups for patients with breast cancer stage I–III (Treatment Recommendations, St. Gallen, 2007)**

| Risk group | Hormone-responsive | Hormone-resistant |
|---|---|---|
| Low risk | ER and/or PR positive and N0 and pT1 and G1 and age ≥ 35 years and L0, V0 and HER2/neu negative | Not applicable |
| Intermediate risk | ER and/or PR positive and N0 and L0, V0 and HER2/neu negative and pT > 1 or G2–3    or age < 35 years    or N+ (1–3 LN) | ER and PR negative |
| High risk | N+ (> 3 LN) or N+ (1–3 LN) and L1 or V1 or HER2/neu positive | ER and PR negative |

*ER* estrogen receptor, *PR* progesterone receptor, *LN* lymph nodes, *N0 / N+* lymph nodes tumor free / lymph nodes affected, *L0 / L1* no / detectable lymph vessel invasion, *V0 /V1* no / detectable venous blood vessel invasion, *G1–3* grades 1–3

**Adjuvant systemic therapy for patients with operable breast cancer (Treatment Recommendations, St. Gallen, 2007)**

| Risk Category | Endocrine responsive | Uncertain endocrine responsiveness | Endocrine non-responsive |
|---|---|---|---|
| • Low risk | ET | ET | n.a. [a] |
| • Intermediate risk | ET alone, or CT → ET (CT + ET)[b] if Her2+: additional Trastuzumab | CT → ET (CT + ET)[b] if Her2+: additional Trastuzumab | CT if Her2+: additional Trastuzumab |
| • High risk | CT→ET (CT + ET)[b] if Her2+: additional Trastuzumab | CT → ET (CT + ET)[b] if Her2+: additional Trastuzumab | CT if Her2+: additional Trastuzumab |

*ET* endocrine therapy, *CT* chemotherapy

[a] If ER/PR negative, classify as intermediate or high risk

[b] For tamoxifen, sequential endocrine therapy after chemotherapy is clearly preferable, for aromatase inhibitors or GnRH analogues no data available from randomized studies comparing sequential versus simultaneous application

## Adjuvant Chemotherapy

- Adjuvant chemotherapy prolongs relapse-free survival as well as overall survival.
- Anthracycline-containing triple combination protocols (e.g., FEC 6 cycles), are standard chemotherapies and confer improved survival compared to the classic CMF regimen, particularly in HER2/neu-positive breast cancers. The CMF regimen, which has less side effects, should only be used in patients with low-risk situation or contraindications for anthracyclines.
- The additional use of taxanes in adjuvant therapy improves both disease-free survival and overall survival, especially in node-positive and/or hormone receptor-negative groups.
- Additional administration of trastuzumab in patients with HER2/neu overexpression (score 3 or FISH positive) prolongs disease-free and overall survival. Trastuzumab is used sequentially to anthracycline-containing therapy and/or parallel to taxane treatment, followed by trastuzumab monotherapy for 1 year.

## Postoperative Radiotherapy

- Mandatory in addition to breast-conserving surgery; focal dose 45–50 Gy.
- After mastectomy, radiotherapy is recommended in cases of subtotal tumor removal or involvement of ≥ 3 lymph nodes.
- Also to be considered in presence of other unfavorable prognostic factors (age < 35 years, metastasis to the pectoral fascia, 1–3 lymph nodes, grade G3, no hormone receptors, multicentricity, peritumoral vascular invasion).
- Start of radiotherapy is recommended after completion of chemotherapy.

## Hormone Therapy (▶ Chap. 3.3)

- Standard adjuvant treatment (low-risk constellation) is tamoxifen at 20 mg/day for 5 years or, for postmeopausal women, tamoxifen for 2–3 years followed by aromatase inhibitors or aromatase inhibitors upfront.

- In postmenopausal patients, extended adjuvant hormone therapy with aromatase inhibitors (5 years tamoxifen + ≥ 2 years letrozole) or the early switch to aromatase inhibitors (exemestane after 2–3 years tamoxifen) is superior to tamoxifen therapy only.
- First-line administration of aromatase inhibitors is recommended in high-risk situations, esp. in cases with HER2/neu overexpression, PR negative, or contraindications for tamoxifen.
- Endocrine treatment is initiated after completion of chemotherapy.
- Ovarian function suppression (GnRH analogs for 2 years) is performed in premenopausal patients with hormone-sensitive disease.

## Special Situations

### Inflammatory Breast Cancer
Generally poor prognosis → aggressive multimodal approach:
- Neoadjuvant chemotherapy anthracycline- and taxane-based.
- Mastectomy and axillary node dissection
- Radiotherapy to the chest wall and axilla
- Adjuvant hormone therapy

### Neoadjuvant Therapy
Neoadjuvant chemotherapy should be considered in locally advanced and inoperable disease as well as in inflammatory breast cancer. Furthermore, primary systemic chemotherapy is an alternative for patients with mastectomy indication and who wish to obtain breast-conserving surgery. In addition, chemotherapy sensitivity can be evaluated by tumor response and serves as a prognostic marker.

## Advanced Breast Cancer (Stage IV)

## Treatment Concept

1. Therapeutic intent: palliative.
2. Metastatic breast cancer is a systemic disease. Therefore, treatment is primarily systemic in most cases.
3. The most important individual factor determining the therapeutic approach is the dynamics of the disease. Other factors are the individual situation of the patient, comorbidity, age, sites of metastasis, and local treatment options.

### Treatment strategy for advanced breast cancer

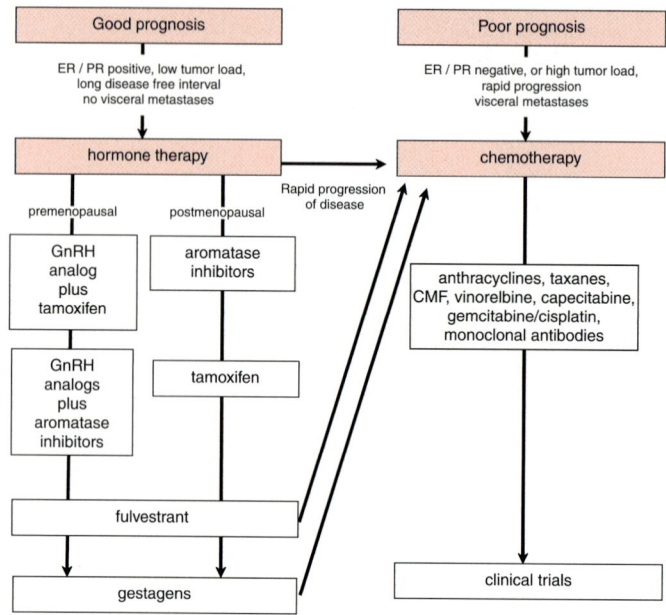

*ER* estrogen receptor, *PR* progesterone receptor, *CMF* cyclophosphamide + methotrexate + 5-fluorouracil

## Hormone Therapy

Hormone therapy is less toxic than chemotherapy, therefore it is usually the first-line treatment in patients with favorable prognostic criteria:

- Positive estrogen and/or progesterone receptors (no endocrine therapy in receptor negative patients)
- Long disease-free interval (> 2 years)
- Low tumor mass, metastasis confined to bone and soft tissue
- Late premenopausal or late postmenopausal situation (younger or perimenopausal women respond poorly to hormone therapy)
- Previous response to hormone therapy

Approximately 30–60% of patients respond well to hormone therapy within 8 weeks. First remission usually lasts 9–18 months; subsequent remissions tend to be shorter. In approximately 20% of cases, the receptor status changes during the course of the disease. Women who have previously benefited from hormone therapy often respond well to a second endocrine therapy after disease progression (objective response rate to second-line hormone therapy in women with positive receptor status: 10–30%).

### Premenopausal (at Time of Treatment)
Ablative hormone therapy: treatment with GnRH analogs is preferable to surgical oophorectomy. Ablative hormone therapy combined with tamoxifen or aromatase inhibitors appears to be advantageous.

### Postmenopausal (at Time of Treatment)
Third generation aromatase inhibitors are more effective than tamoxifen and are therefore the first-line treatment of choice in patients with advanced breast cancer and positive receptor status

In patients with breast cancer recurrence who received aromatase inhibitors as adjuvant treatment, tamoxifen is a good treatment alternative.

*Possible hormone therapy sequence in premenopausal women: 1 → 1+2 → 1+3 → 1+4*
*Possible hormone therapy sequence in postmenopausal women: 3 → 2a → 2b → 4*

| Therapy | Compounds | Dose |
|---|---|---|
| 1. GnRH analogs | Goserelin | 3.6 mg s.c. once monthly |
| 2. Antiestrogens | Tamoxifen[a] | 20 mg p.o. daily |
| | Fulvestrant[b] | 250 mg i.m. once monthly |
| 3. Aromatase inhibitors | Anastrozole[c] | 1 mg p.o. daily |
| | Exemestane[d] | 25 mg p.o. daily |
| | Letrozole[c] | 2.5 mg p.o. daily |
| | Formestane[d] | 250 mg i.m. every 2 weeks |
| 4. Gestagens | Medroxyprogesterone acetate | 300–500 mg p.o. daily |
| | Megestrol acetate | 160 mg p.o. daily |

[a] With intrinsic estrogen activity, side effects include nausea, thrombosis risk↑, endometrial carcinoma risk ↑ (twofold); severe hot flushes (can be treated with clonidine)
[b] No intrinsic estrogen activity, approved for postmenopausal women with hormone receptor-positive advanced breast cancer; equally effective as anastrozole
[c] Reversible aromatase inactivation (nonsteroidal inhibitor), not necessarily cross-resistant to Formestane
[d] Irreversible aromatase inactivation (steroidal inhibitor), not necessarily cross-resistant to Letrozole

## Chemotherapy

### Choice of Protocol
- The intensity of the required chemotherapy depends on the dynamics of the disease, as characterized by parameters such as tumor size, impaired organ function, weight loss, or overall performance status (Karnofsky performance scale).
- Treatment response can be expected after 1–3 months. The response rate (CR and PR) for first-line treatment is 50–80%. If more than 12 months have passed between the end of therapy and relapse or progression, the chemotherapy response rate for pretreated subjects is similar to chemotherapy-naive patients. With shorter intervals, lower response rates are to be expected.
- In patients showing adequate response, conventional chemotherapy should be continued for 6–12 months. The maximum length of treatment depends on the clinical course and is most often limited by treatment failure. Combination chemotherapy is usually associated with higher toxicity and higher response rates compared to sequential monotherapy.
- If two different chemotherapies fail to obtain a satisfactory response, it is unlikely that a third chemotherapy will produce a result positive enough to justify side effects.
- There is no official consensus as to which chemotherapies should be applied in which order in advanced breast cancer. We prefer the following sequence (with frequent exceptions according to previous treatment and the limitations mentioned above): anthracycline-containing regimen → taxane-containing regimen → CMF → gemcitabine and cis- or carboplatin → capecitabine → vinorelbine.

### Targeted Therapies (▶ Chaps. 3.5, 3.6)
Various targeted therapy approaches are effective in advanced breast cancer:
- Trastuzumab: humanized monoclonal antibody against the extracellular domain of the EGF receptor type 2 ("epidermal growth factor receptor 2," HER2/neu) which is overexpressed in 20–30% of all breast cancers. Effective as monotherapy in tumors with high HER2/neu expression (score 3 or FISH positive) and considerably enhances efficacy of chemotherapy. Due to potential cardiotoxicity, combination with (regular, nonliposomal) anthracyclines must be avoided.

- Bevacizumab: humanized monoclonal antibody against vascular endothelial growth factor. Inhibition of tumor angiogenesis and normalization of blood vessel pathology in tumor vasculature. Bevacizumab has little effect as monotherapy in advanced breast cancer but doubles the response rate of capecitabine and taxane chemotherapy.
- Further growth regulation inhibitors and angiogenesis inhibitors are currently tested in clinical trials.

## Chemotherapy Protocols: Breast Cancer

| *"CMF"* ▶ *Protocol 12.10.1* | | | *Start next cycle on day 29* |
|---|---|---|---|
| Cyclophosphamide | 100 mg/m²/day | p.o. | Days 1–14 |
| If oral intolerability | 600 mg /m²/day | i.v. | Day 1, 8 |
| Methotrexate | 40 mg/m²/day | i.v. | Day 1, 8 |
| 5-Fluorouracil | 600 mg/m²/day | i.v. | Day 1, 8 |

| *"FAC" (FEC¹)* ▶ *Protocol 12.10.2* | | | *Start next cycle on day 22* |
|---|---|---|---|
| 5-Fluorouracil | 500 mg/m²/day | i.v. | Day 1 |
| Doxorubicin (epirubicin¹) | 50 (50–100) mg/m²/day | i.v. | Day 1 |
| Cyclophosphamide | 500 mg/m²/day | i.v. | Day 1 |

¹In adjuvant setting, 100 mg/m² epirubicin are more effective than 50 mg/m²

| *"AC" ("EC")* ▶ *Protocol 12.10.3* | | | *Start next cycle on day 22* |
|---|---|---|---|
| Doxorubicin (epirubicin) | 60 (90) mg/m²/day | i.v. | Day 1 |
| Cyclophosphamide | 600 mg/m²/day | i.v. | Day 1 |

| *"Epirubicin mono"* ▶ *Protocol 12.10.5* | | | *Repeat weekly* |
|---|---|---|---|
| Epirubicin | 20 mg/m²/day | i.v. | Day 1 |

| *"Paclitaxel / Trastuzumab"* ▶ *Protocol 12.10.9* | | | *Repeat weekly* |
|---|---|---|---|
| Paclitaxel | 100 mg/m²/day | i.v. | Day 1 for 3 h |
| Trastuzumab | 2–4 mg/kg/day | i.v. | Days 1, 8, 15 |

| *"Vinorelbin"* ▶ *Protocol 12.10.7* | | | *Repeat weekly* |
|---|---|---|---|
| Vinorelbine | 30 mg/m²/day | i.v. | Day 1 |

| *"Docetaxel* ▶ *Protocol 12.10.4* | | | *Start next cycle on day 22* |
|---|---|---|---|
| Docetaxel | 100 mg/m²/day | i.v. | Day 1 for 90 min |

| "EP" ► Protocol 12.10.6 | | | Start next cycle on day 22 |
|---|---|---|---|
| Paclitaxel | 175 mg/m²/day | i.v. | Day 1, for 3 h |
| Epirubicin | 60 mg/m²/day | i.v. | Day 1 |

| "Liposomal Doxorubicin" ► Protocol 12.10.8 | | | Start next cycle on day 22 |
|---|---|---|---|
| Liposomal Doxorubicin | 50 mg/m²/day | i.v. | Day 1, 1 h infusion |

| "EC + Paclitaxel" ► Protocol 12.10.10 | | | Start next cycle on day 22 |
|---|---|---|---|
| Epirubicin | 90 mg/m²/day | i.v. | Day 1, bolus 15 min |
| Cyclophosphamide | 600 mg/m²/day | i.v. | Day 1, 1 h infusion |
| Paclitaxel | 175 mg/m²/day | i.v. | Day 1, 3 h infusion |

## Special Situations

### CNS Metastases
Radiotherapy is the first-line treatment with high response rates and often a lasting effect. In case of a single metastasis, neurosurgical intervention or stereotactic radiotherapy should be considered.

### Pleural Effusions (► Chap. 4.8.1)
Pleural effusions are not always a consequence of systemic disease progression. Local treatment ► Chaps. 4.8.1 and 10.1.

### Bone Metastases (► Chap. 8.12.5)
- Localized symptomatic bone involvement or risk of fracture: radiotherapy
- Multiple metastases, particularly when associated with bone pain → chemotherapy; if pain control is insufficient, combination with radiotherapy possible
- *Bisphosphonates:* reduction of pain (unclear mode of action) and fracture risk; possible antitumoral effect; e.g., zoledronate 4 mg every 4 weeks, pamidronate 60–90 mg over 2–3 h i.v. every 3–4 weeks or clodronate p.o. (► Chap. 4.7)

### Male Breast Cancer
Rare (< 1% of all cases of breast cancer). Treatment strategies are based on those for female breast cancer. Since male breast tumors express estrogen receptors (in > 80%) and progesterone receptors (in > 70%), hormonal treatment is of particular importance. This usually involves treatment with aromatase inhibitors or tamoxifen. Men seem to tolerate tamoxifen less well than women.

### Five-year Survival Based on AJCC Staging
- Stage I:    85%
- Stage II:   66%
- Stage III:  41%
- Stage IV:   10%

The treatment strategy for breast cancer patients with known genetic anomalies (BRCA1 and BRCA2 mutations) is similar to sporadic disease cases. There is evidence that the prognosis is the same for both groups.

Prg:

**Px:**

### Screening

- Self-examination at monthly intervals (however, there is no evidence that self-examination lowers breast cancer-related mortality).
- Basic mammography from age 40 (high-risk groups: from age 25) through 49 annually. Biannual mammography thereafter.
- High-risk patients (patients with disease in first-degree relatives): annual mammography.

### Primary Prevention

Bilateral prophylactic mastectomy and/or oophorectomy is an option for high-risk patients which can effectively lower the risk of breast cancer and should be discussed as part of the genetic counseling process. Current prospective studies are testing possible protective effects of tamoxifen and retinoids (e.g. fenretinide).

**F/U:**

Frequent follow-up focusing on the site of initial disease and the contralateral breast is mandatory since local relapse and secondary tumors in the contralateral breast can be treated with curative intent if discovered in time.

- Annual bilateral mammography (during the first year, follow-up every 3 to 6 months is recommended)
- Regular self-examination and clinical follow-up by the treating physician
- Laboratory tests and other diagnostic procedures to detect or exclude systemic tumor spread are only indicated in patients with clinical symptoms.

With palliative intention, treatment and follow-up are based on clinical symptoms.

**Ref:**

1. Beslija S, Bonneterre J, Burstein H et al. Second consensus on medical treatment of metastatic breast cancer. Ann Oncol 2007;18:215–25
2. Cinierie S, Orlando L, Fedele P et al. Adjuvant strategies in breast cancer: new prospectives, questions and reflections at the end of 2007 St Gallen International Expert Consensus Conference. Ann Oncol 2007;18(Suppl. 6):vi63–5
3. ESMO Guidelines Working Group. Primary breast cancer: ESMO Clinical Recommendations for diagnosis, treatment and follow-up. Ann Oncol 2007;18(Suppl. 2):ii5–8
4. ESMO Guidelines Working Group. Recurrent or metastatic breast cancer: ESMO Clinical Recommendations for diagnosis, treatment and follow-up. Ann Oncol 2007;18(Suppl. 2):ii9–11
5. Goldhirsch A, Wood WC, Gelber RD et al. Progress and promise: highlights of the international expert consensus on the pimary therapy of early breast cancer 2007. Ann Oncol 2007;18:1133–44
6. Kaufmann M, von Minckwitz G, Bear HD et al. Recommendations from an international expert panel on the use of neoadjuvant (primary) systemic treatment of operable breast cancer: new perspectives 2006. Ann Oncol 2007;18:1927–34
7. Khatcheressian JL, Wolff AC, Smith TJ et al. ASCO 2006 update of the breast follow-up and management guidelines in the adjuvant setting. J Clin Oncol 2007;24:5091–7
8. Perry N, Broeders M, De Wolf C et al. European guidelines for quality assurance in breast cancer screening and diagnosis. Ann Oncol 2008;19:614–22
9. Von Minckwitz G. Evidence-based treatment of metastatic breast cancer – 2006 recommendations by the AGO Breast Commission. Eur J Cancer 2006;42:2897–908

**Web:**

| | | |
|---|---|---|
| 1. | http://www.cancer.gov/cancerinfo/types/breast | NCI Cancer Topics |
| 2. | http://www.nlm.nih.gov/medlineplus/breastcancer.html | MedlinePlus |
| 3. | http://www.nccn.org/professionals/physician_gls/PDF/breast.pdf | NCCN Guideline |
| 4. | http://www.emedicine.com/med/topic2808.htm | E-medicine |

**8.4.2**     **Malignant Ovarian Tumors**

I.B. Runnebaum, R. Wäsch, C.F. Waller

**Def:**     Malignant neoplasia of the ovaries; approximately 65–70% of all ovarian tumors are carcinomas, i.e., of epithelial origin; other ovarian neoplasia include malignant germ cell tumors, stromal tumors, and borderline tumors (▶ Chaps. 8.4.3–8.4.5).

**ICD-10:**     C56.-

**Ep:**     Incidence: 15/100,000/year; regional differences: higher incidence in industrial nations; occurring from 40 years of age, age peak: 60 years.

**Pg:**     *Risk Factors*
- Factors associated with *prolonged and continuous ovulation* increase the risk: early menarche, late menopause, nulliparity
- Ovulation-suppressing factors *lower* the risk: birth, breastfeeding, oral contraception. Postmenopausal estrogen replacement therapy seems to have no influence.
- *Family history:* history of ovarian cancer in first-degree relatives (relative risk: 2.0)
- *Genetic factors:* hereditary breast- and ovarian carcinoma syndrome (BRCA1, BRCA2), Lynch II syndrome (hereditary nonpolyposis colorectal cancer syndrome, HNPCC), Li-Fraumeni syndrome (p53), each with autosomal-dominant inheritance
- *Regional differences:* increased risk in industrial nations
- *Ionizing radiation*

*Molecular Genetics*
- *Oncogene expression:* in up to 25% of patients alterations of the oncogenes HER2/neu, c-myc, ras
- *Loss / alteration of tumor suppressor genes:* p53, BRCA1, BRCA2, PTEN, BRCA2, DNA mismatch repair genes MLH1 and MSH2

**Path:**     *Histology (WHO 2002)*

| Type | Frequency (%) |
|---|---|
| *Malignant Epithelial Tumors* | 60–65 |
| •   Serous | 40 |
| •   Mucinous | 20 |
| •   Endometrioid | 4 |
| •   Mesonephric (clear cell) | 2 |
| •   Brenner tumor | Rare |
| •   Mixed types | Rare |
| •   Undifferentiated, unclassified | 4 |
| *Stromal Tumors* | 5–10 |
| •   Granulosa cell tumor (▶ Chap. 8.4.4) | 5 |
| •   Sertoli / Leydig cell tumor (▶ Chap. 8.4.5) | 2 |
| •   Thecoma | Rare |
| •   Androblastoma | Rare |
| •   Unclassified | Rare |

| Type | Frequency (%) |
|---|---|
| *Germ Cell Tumors* (▶ Chap. 8.4.3) | 10–15 |
| • Dysgerminoma | 1 |
| • Teratoma | 3 |
| • Endodermal sinus tumors ("yolk sac tumors") | 1 |
| • Embryonic carcinoma, choriocarcinoma, polyembryoma | Rare |
| • Mixed germ cell tumors | Rare |
| *Borderline Tumors* | 5–7 |
| • "Tumors of low malignant potential," non-invasive | |
| *Other* | 8–12 |
| • Lipid cell tumor | |
| • Gonadoblastoma | |
| • Mesenchymal tumor (sarcoma, fibroma, etc.) | |
| • Lymphoma | |
| • Metastases | |

### "Borderline Tumors"
- Noninvasive tumors with increased proliferation, increased mitotic rate, and cellular / nuclear atypia; in some cases primary multifocal occurrence
- Main prognostic factor: evidence of invasive intraperitoneal implants
- Surgical treatment with good prognosis: 5-year survival with stage I 99%, with stage II–III 77%, relapse rate 7–10%

### Patterns of Spread
- Local spread: intraperitoneal
- Peritoneal carcinosis: intraperitoneal spread after rupture of the ovarian capsule
- Lymphatic metastasis: para-aortic lymph nodes, in rare cases retrograde invasion of inguinal / femoral lymph nodes
- Hematogenic metastasis to liver, lung, CNS, in rare cases bone involvement

**Class:**    **TNM Staging of Ovarian Cancer (2002)**

| *T* | *Primary Tumor* |
|---|---|
| TX | Primary tumor cannot be assessed |
| T0 | No evidence of primary tumor |
| T1 | Tumor limited to ovaries<br>A: limited to one ovary, capsule intact<br>B: limited to both ovaries, capsule intact<br>C: rupture of capsule, tumor cells on ovarian surface |
| T2 | Tumor extending into the pelvis<br>A: invasion of the uterus and/or the fallopian tubes<br>B: invasion of other pelvic organs<br>C: tumor cells in ascites / peritoneal lavage |
| T3 | Metastasis beyond the pelvis, peritoneal involvement<br>A: microscopic detection<br>B: tumor size ≤ 2 cm<br>C: tumor size > 2 cm |

**Class:**

**TNM Staging of Ovarian Cancer (2002)** *(continued)*

| N | Lymph Node Involvement |
|---|---|
| NX | Regional lymph nodes cannot be assessed |
| N0 | Regional lymph nodes without metastases |
| N1 | Metastasis to regional lymph nodes |
| **M** | **Distant Metastasis** |
| MX | Distant metastasis cannot be assessed |
| M0 | No distant metastasis |
| M1 | Distant metastasis (except peritoneal metastases) |
| **G** | **Differentiation** |
| GX | Differentiation cannot be assessed |
| GB | Borderline tumor |
| G1 | Well differentiated |
| G2 | Moderately differentiated |
| G3 | Poorly differentiated |
| G4 | Undifferentiated |

**FIGO Staging**

| FIGO stage | TNM stage | | | Frequency (%) | Five-year survival |
|---|---|---|---|---|---|
| | **T** | **N** | **M** | | |
| I | T1 | N0 | M0 | 15 | 80 |
| II | T2 | N0 | M0 | 15 | 60 |
| III | T3 | N0 | M0 | 65 | 30 |
| IV | Any T | Any N | M1 | 5 | 5 |

**Sy:**

Ovarian carcinomas tend to be asymptomatic at early stages and are often discovered at a late stage (on presentation 70% FIGO stage III and IV). Characteristic symptoms of locally and/or systemically advanced disease:
- Abdominal pain, feeling of pressure
- Weight loss, loss of appetite, reduced performance
- Ascites, pleural effusion, dyspnea
- Genital bleeding, in premenopausal women abnormal menstruation
- Subileus, ileus, increased urinary frequency

**Dg:**

### Medical History, Physical Examination
- Medical history including risk factors (see above)
- Physical and gynecological examination, obligatory: rectal and vaginal examination, assessment of the pouch of Douglas

### Laboratory Tests
- Routine laboratory tests including blood counts, LDH, liver / renal function
- *Tumor markers:* in epithelial tumors: CA 125 (sensitivity 50–90%), in germ cell tumors: β-HCG, AFP; suitable for monitoring of the disease course, *not suitable for diagnosis or screening* (▶ Chap. 2.4)

### Histology
- Examination of ascites or pleural effusion fluid (sensitivity 50%). *ATTENTION:* abdominal wall metastases, fine-needle biopsy of the ovarian tumor is *contraindicated* due to potential risk of tumor spread and bleeding
- Laparotomy, laparoscopy: only if low malignancy is suspected

### Imaging
- Abdominal and transvaginal ultrasound
- Chest x-ray, intravenous pyelogram, abdominal CT / MRI
- Preoperatively: cystoscopy, rectoscopy

**Dd:**

### Differential Diagnosis of Ovarian Lesions

| | |
|---|---|
| Benign cysts | Mostly ≤ 5 cm, cycle dependent, possibly biopsy, ultrasound |
| Endometriosis | Cyclical bleeding and pain |
| Extrauterine pregnancy | 5–8 weeks after last menstruation, β-HCG ↑, ultrasound, possibly laparoscopy |
| Inflammation | Adnexitis, pyosalpinx, tubo-ovarian abscess, diverticulitis (CRP ↑, ESR ↑, leukocytosis, fever) |
| Benign tumors | E.g., cystadenoma |
| Uterine tumors | E.g., leiomyoma (imaging) |
| Ovarian tumors | E.g., carcinoma, stromal cell tumor, germ cell tumor |
| Metastases | E.g., breast cancer, gastric cancer, endometrial cancer, colorectal cancer, bladder carcinoma |
| Artifacts | Full bladder, scybala |

**Co:**
- *Torsion:* severe and usually unilateral peritoneal pain, peritonism, shock
- *Rupture of cystic tumors:* transient peritonism, normal temperature, usually negative pelvic examination (collapsed tumor); consecutive peritoneal spread; special case: rupture of benign mucinous cystomas can result in the implantation of mucous-producing cells in the entire abdomen → "jelly belly," peritoneal pseudomyxoma
- *Hemorrhage*
- *Meigs' syndrome:* ascites + pleural effusion (unilateral or bilateral)

### Paraneoplastic Syndromes (► Chap. 8.13)
- Hirsutism / virilization with androgen-producing tumors (androblastomas)
- Bleeding disorders with estrogen-producing tumors
- Cushing's syndrome
- Hypercalcemia ("parathyroid hormone-related protein," PTH-RP)
- Neurological disorders: polyneuropathy, dementia, cerebellar ataxia

**Th:**

### Treatment Concept

1. Ovarian cancer is treated multimodally by surgery and chemotherapy, preferably at specialized centers.
2. Primary surgery usually serves a therapeutic (tumor resection) and diagnostic (surgical staging) purpose; and has to be conducted according to quality criteria (FIGO standards). In early stages of the disease, complete surgical staging confers a survival advantage. Maximum—ideally complete—tumor resection is the prerequisite for successful subsequent systemic treatment.
3. Most effective drugs: platinum derivates (cisplatin, carboplatin) and taxanes (paclitaxel).
4. Treatment of other malignant ovarian tumors: see chapter on germ cell cancer (► Chap. 8.4.3) and chapters on stromal cell tumors (► Chaps. 8.4.4, 8.4.5).

**Treatment of epithelial ovarian tumors**

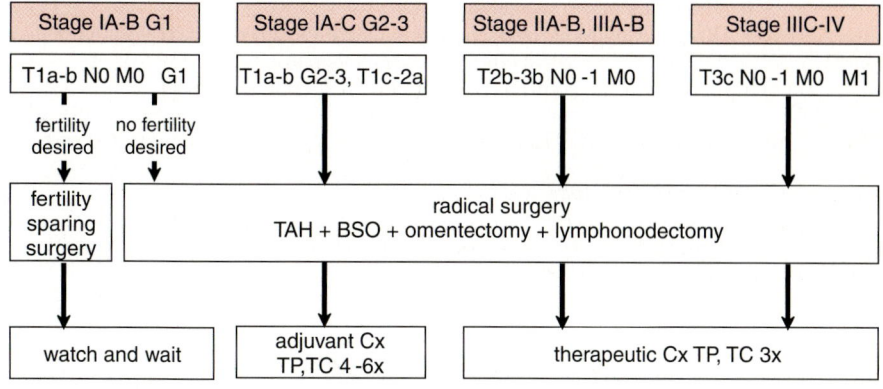

OP surgery, *TAH* total abdominal hysterectomy, *BSO* bilateral salpingo-oophorectomy, *Cx* chemotherapy, *TP* paclitaxel + cisplatin, *TC* paclitaxel + carboplatin

## Surgical Treatment

- *Standard surgery: radical surgery / staging according to FIGO standards (vertical midline laparotomy):* total abdominal hysterectomy (TAH), bilateral salpingo-oophorectomy (BSO), appendectomy, pelvic and para-aortic lymphadenectomy, omentectomy, peritoneal biopsies or resection, peritoneal lavage or ascites sample, smear of the diaphragmatic domes; if required, retroperitoneal lymphadenectomy, resection of involved parts of the intestine.
- *Stage Ia:* preservation of the ovary in premenopausal women wanting children ("fertility-preserving surgery").
- *Stages III and IV:* if complete tumor resection is not possible, surgical reduction of all tumors so that maximum diameter of remaining implants is < 1 cm , "second look" surgery: no improvement of prognosis if prior surgery was according to state-of-the-art criteria (high diligence).
- *Relapse:* relapse surgery only in late relapses (relapse-free interval after primary therapy > 12 months) and possibility to achieve macroscopic tumor-free results.

## Chemotherapy: Epithelial Tumors

### Initial Treatment ("First Line")

- Platinum and taxane-containing therapy protocols are superior to all other therapies.
- *Adjuvant chemotherapy:* early-stage disease with high risk of relapse: stage IA/B with G2/3 tumor or clear cell tumor, stages IC, IIA; chemotherapy with paclitaxel / carboplatin regimen, 4–6 cycles.
- *"Therapeutic" chemotherapy:* after surgical reduction of tumor mass and stages IIB–IV; chemotherapy with paclitaxel /carboplatin regimen (patients with neurological symptoms: docetaxel / carboplatin) > 6 cycles.
- *Intraperitoneal "first-line" therapy:* in advanced stage (III–IV); intraperitoneal administration of cisplatin and paclitaxel (i.p.) combined with paclitaxel intravenous (i.v.). Randomized trials demonstrated improved overall survival: 50 months (i.v. standard chemotherapy) compared to 66 months (combined i.p. + i.v. chemotherapy). *ATTENTION:* high rate of side effects.
- *Trials:* the efficacy of platinum-containing combinations or sequential therapies with other compounds such as gemcitabine, topotecan, docetaxel is currently beeing evaluated in trials.

### Salvage Therapy: Platinum-sensitive Relapse ("Second Line")

Patients with relapse-free intervals of > 12 months should undergo further surgery to completely remove tumor before chemotherapy.

- Repeated adjuvant treatment with standard therapy paclitaxel + platinum derivative or platinum- or taxane-containing combination therapy
- Alternative: monotherapy with PEGylated liposomal doxorubicin
- Response is defined by complete remission (CR), partial remission (PR), or reduction of the tumor marker CA 125 to < 50% of baseline after 2 cycles of standard therapy

### Platinum-refractory Relapse ("Third Line")

Secondary relapse or refractory to platinum-containing salvage therapy. Options include combination chemotherapy (in line with studies) or monotherapy with taxanes, topotecan, etoposide, gemcitabine, vinorelbine, ifosfamide, oxaliplatin. For example:

- Topotecan 1.0–1.5 mg/m²/day on days 1–5
- Ifosfamide 1.0–1.2 g/m²/day i.v. days 1–5 + Uromitexan 1,500 mg/m²/day i.v. days 1–5 every 21 days
- Paclitaxel 175 mg/m²/day i.v. on day 1 (every 3 weeks) or 80–100 mg/m²/day i.v. on day 1 (weekly)
- Etoposide 50 mg/m²/day p.o. on days 1–21 every 29 days, 3 cycles
- Tamoxifen 20 mg twice daily p.o., regularly

### Intraperitoneal Chemotherapy

Intraperitoneal instillation of cytostatics in palliative situations with malignant ascites / peritoneal carcinosis:

- Advantage: high local dose with few systemic side effects
- Compounds used: 5-FU, cisplatin, etoposide, etc.
- Combination of intraperitoneal and intravenous chemotherapy to reduce toxicity (see above)

## Chemotherapy Protocols

| "Paclitaxel / Carboplatin" ▶ Protocol 12.11.1 | | | Start next cycle on day 29 |
|---|---|---|---|
| Paclitaxel | 175 mg/m²/day | i.v. | Day 1, for 3 h |
| Carboplatin | AUC 6 | i.v. | Day 1 |

| "Paclitaxel / Cisplatin" | | | Start next cycle on day 22 |
|---|---|---|---|
| Paclitaxel | 185 mg/m²/day | i.v. | Day 1, for 3 h |
| Cisplatin | 75 mg/m²/day | i.v. | Day 1 |

| "Paclitaxel weekly" ▶ Protocol 12.2.3 | | | Repeat weekly |
|---|---|---|---|
| Paclitaxel | 80 mg/m²/day | i.v. | Day 1, for 3 h |

| "Intraperitoneal Cisplatin / Paclitaxel" | | | Start next cycle on day 22 |
|---|---|---|---|
| Paclitaxel | 135 mg/m²/day | c.i.v. | Day 1, for 24 h |
| Cisplatin | 100 mg/m²/day | i.p. | Day 2 |
| Paclitaxel | 60 mg/m²/day | i.p. | Day 8 |

### Experimental Therapies

Current studies include new chemotherapeutic drugs, molecular therapies ("targeted therapies") as well as immuno- and gene therapeutic approaches. Concepts:

- Tumor cell transfection with p53, BRCA1 (tumor suppressor genes) or HSV-TK ("cytotoxic suicide gene," herpes simplex virus thymidine kinase)
- Intraperitoneal instillation of IL-2
- HER2/neu antibodies, bispecific monoclonal antibodies or antibody conjugates with toxins, cytostatics, or radioisotopes, anti-idiotype CA 125 antibody
- Tyrosine kinase inhibitors, farnesyl transferase inhibitors, anti-angiogenic factors

**Prg:**

### Prognostic Factors

- Tumor staging, histology, grading
- Size of the residual tumor after surgery, postoperative tumor marker profile
- Malignant ascites or tumor cells in peritoneal lavage
- Age, Karnofsky scale
- Proliferation index (percentage of S-phases), ploidy

### Five-year Survival

According to FIGO stages, see above. Germ cell tumors (▶ Chap. 8.4.3), stromal cell tumors (▶ Chap. 8.4.4, 8.4.5).

**F/U:**

Patients treated with curative intent should be closely monitored. Follow-up: first 3 years: every 3 months, year 4: every 6 months, then annual

- *Objectives:* management of treatment-related side effects, relapse diagnosis, quality of life, psychosocial care
- *Methods:* medical history, physical and gynecological examination, transvaginal ultrasound; CA 125, complex diagnostic procedures (CT, MRI) only with clinically suspected relapse
- Hormone replacement therapy (HRT) with estrogens may confer improved quality of life; HRT does not increase relapse risk
- After organ-preserving surgery in early stages of the disease: gynecological examination with transvaginal ultrasound and CA 125 level in 2-monthly intervals

**Px:**

Women with hereditary or genetic risk factors:

- Screening every 6 months: rectal and gynecological examination with transvaginal ultrasound, CA 125
- Diagnostic laparoscopy in case of suspicious ovarian lesions

Primary prevention approaches: oral contraception over 5 years reduces the risk of ovarian cancer by 50%, tube ligation by 67%, hysterectomy by 37%; prophylactic bilateral adnexectomy (salpingo-oophorectomy) in BRCA1/2 mutation carriers reduces the risk of ovarian cancer by 96% and the risk of breast cancer by 50%.

**Ref:**

1. Cadron I, Leunen K, Van Gorp T et al. Management of borderline ovarian neoplasms. J Clin Oncol 2007;25:2928–37
2. Cannistra SA. Cancer of the ovary. N Engl J Med 2004;351:2519–29
3. Collaborative Group on Epidemiological Studies of Ovarian Cancer. Ovarian cancer and oral contraceptives. Lancet 2008;317:303–14
4. DuBois A, Quinn M, Thigpen T et al. 2004 consensus statements on the management of ovarian cancer: final document of the 3rd International Gynecologic Cancer Intergroup Ovarian Cancer Consensus Conference. Ann Oncol 2005;16(suppl 8):viii7–12
5. ESMO Guideline Working Group. Epithelial ovarian carcinoma: ESMO Clinical Recommendations for diagnosis, treatment and follow-up. Ann Oncol 2007;18(suppl 2):ii12–4
6. Rao G, Crispens M, Rothenberg ML. Intraperitoneal chemotherapy for ovarian cancer: overview and perspective. J Clin Oncol 2007;25:2867–72
7. Rose PG, Nerenstone S, Brady MF et al. Secondary surgical cytoreduction for advanced ovarian carcinoma. N Engl J Med 2004;351:2489–97

**Web:**

| | | |
|---|---|---|
| 1. | http://www.cancer.gov/cancertopics/types/ovarian/ | NCI Cancer Topics |
| 2. | http://www.nlm.nih.gov/medlineplus/ovariancancer.html | MedlinePlus |
| 3. | http://www.nccn.org/professionals/physician_gls/PDF/ovarian.pdf | NCCN Guideline |
| 4. | http://www.emedicine.com/med/topic1698.htm | E-medicine |
| 5. | http://www.cnn.com/HEALTH/library/DS/00293.html | CNN Health |

### 8.4.3 Malignant Germ Cell Tumors in Women

I.B. Runnebaum, C.F. Waller

**Def:** Malignant neoplasms of the ovaries originating from primordial germ cells (primitive pluripotent germ cells). Germ cell tumors are classified as dysgerminomas, choriocarcinomas (non-pregnancy-related), and teratomas.

**ICD-10:** C56: dysgerminoma
C58: choriocarcinoma
C80: malignant teratoma
C36.9: benign teratoma

**Ep:** Approximately 20–25% of ovarian neoplasms are germ cell tumors. Only 3–5% of germ cell tumors in women are malignant; median age at diagnosis 16–20 years. Approximately 70% of all ovarian tumors in women between 10 and 30 years are germ cell tumors.

**Pg:** Risk increased in Y-chromosome-positive women:
- Klinefelter's syndrome (karyotype 47XXY or variants)
- Women with pure (46XY) or mixed gonadal dysgenesis
- Complete androgen insensitivity (testicular feminization, 46XY)

**Path:** *Histological Classification of Malignant Germ Cell Tumors in Women*

| Type | Frequency (%) |
|---|---|
| *Primitive Germ Cell Tumors* | 50–70 |
| •   Dysgerminoma | 30–50 |
| •   Endodermal sinus tumor | 10 |
| •   Embryonic carcinoma | 2 |
| •   Polyembryoma | Rare |
| •   Choriocarcinoma (non-pregnancy-related) | 1 |
| •   Mixed forms | 6 |
| *Teratomas* | 30–40 |
| •   Immature solid teratoma | Rare |
| •   Immature cystic teratoma | 30–35 |
| •   Immature mixed teratoma (solid / cystic elements) | Rare |
| •   Mature solid teratoma | Rare |
| •   Mature cystic teratoma (dermoid cyst) with/without transformation | Rare |
| *Monodermal Tumors* | Rare |
| •   Struma ovarii (benign / malignant) | |
| •   Carcinoid | |
| *Germ Cell – Sex Cord Stromal Tumors* | Rare |
| •   Gonadoblastoma | |
| •   Mixed germ cell – sex cord stromal tumors | |

#### Tumor Types
- *Dysgerminoma* is morphologically similar to seminoma in men. With presence of syncytiotrophoblastic giant cells: β-HCG ↑, PLAP ↑ (placental alkaline phosphatase).
- *Embryonic carcinomas* are histologically similar to those of the male testis.

- *Choriocarcinomas* originate from extraembryonic trophoblastic structures. They consist of chorionic cells and frequently contain other malignant germ cell elements. Distinction of two groups: pregnancy-related choriocarcinomas (trophoblastic tumors, ▶ Chap. 8.4.6) and non-pregnancy-related choriocarcinomas (classified as germ cell tumors). Choriocarcinoma is characterized by frequent metastasis and early hematogenous spread.
- *Teratomas* consist of immature to highly differentiated tissue emerging in atypical locations. Immature teratomas include ectodermal, mesodermal, and endodermal elements. Classification and grading describe the percentage of neural elements, degree of differentiation, and presence of embryonic tissue. Mature teratomas are cystic in approximately 95% of cases, with mature tissue of ecto-, meso-, or endodermal origin. Monodermal tumors are rare.
- *Mixed germ cell tumors* contain components of at least two different malignant ovarian germ cell neoplasias. Mixed tumors consisting of dysgerminomas and endodermal sinus tumors are frequently observed. Teratocarcinomas contain tissues from all three germinal layers together with elements of embryonic carcinoma.

### Pattern of Spread
Compared to epithelial ovarian cancer, higher incidence of metastasis:
- *Dysgerminoma:* in 10–15% of cases, involvement of the contralateral ovary at the time of initial diagnosis
- *Local:* infiltration (e.g., polyembryoma), spread to peritoneal cavity
- *Lymphatic:* para-aortic lymph nodes, retroperitoneal lymph nodes (dysgerminoma)
- *Hematogenous:* placenta, lung, brain, liver, bone

**Class:**  Staging according to the classification of malignant epithelial tumors of the ovaries (▶ Chap. 8.4.2)

**Sy:**  On presentation: often stage I, i.e., tumor restricted to ovary. Symptoms are frequently due to rapid growth, esp. with embryonic carcinoma, dysgerminoma, and endodermal sinus tumor. Approximately 15–20% of dysgerminomas are diagnosed during pregnancy or postpartum.
- Extended abdomen, ascites, abdominal pain, fullness
- Estrogen- / androgen secretion → premature puberty (e.g., embryonic carcinoma), oligomenorrhea, amenorrhea
- Pregnancy-like symptoms
- Uterine hemorrhage (e.g., choriocarcinoma)

**Dg:**  ### Medical History, Physical Examination
- Medical history including family history
- Physical examination; gynecological examination often limited due to young age of patients; rectal examination to assess the pouch of Douglas and the internal genitalia

### Laboratory Tests
- Routine laboratory tests including complete blood count, LDH, renal / liver function tests
- Possibly chromosome analysis (particularly in premenarche)
- Tumor markers (▶ Chap. 2.4), β-HCG, AFP, placental alkaline phosphatase (PLAP)

**Tumor markers of germ cell tumors in women**

| Tumor type | βHCG | AFP | LDH |
|---|---|---|---|
| Dysgerminoma | + | – | ++ |
| Immature teratoma | – | + | + |
| Embryonic carcinoma | ++ | ++ | + |
| Endodermal sinus tumor | + | ++ | + |

*AFP* α1 fetoprotein, *βHCG* human chorionic gonadotropin β (chorion elements), *LDH* lactate dehydrogenase.
– negative, + increased, ++ high

### Imaging
- Ultrasound (transvaginal, abdominal), chest x-ray
- MRI abdomen / pelvis with contrast medium, possibly CT abdomen / pelvis in advanced stages of the disease

### Histology
- Analysis of ascites or pleural effusion
- Laparotomy, laparoscopy, only if malignancy is unlikely

**Dd:** ### Extraovarian
- Ectopic pregnancy, hydrosalpinx
- Tubo-ovarian abscess, diverticulitis, or appendicitis-related abscess

### Ovarian
- Benign cysts (cycle-dependent), corpus luteum cyst, endometriosis
- Benign / malignant tumors, metastases from solid tumors

**Co:** Torsion, rupture with hemoperitoneum, hemorrhage

**Th:** Treatment usually involves a combination of surgery (resection) and chemotherapy, similar to epithelial ovarian cancer (▶ Chap. 8.4.2). Except for early stage dysgerminomas (stage IA) and malignant early stage teratoma (stage IA, highly differentiated), postoperative chemotherapy is indicated. Treatment of choriocarcinoma ▶ Chap. 8.4.6.

### Surgical Treatment
- Staging laparotomy with longitudinal incision; thorough exploration of the abdomen, oophorectomy, possibly contralateral ovarian biopsy, multiple peritoneal biopsies, infracolic omentectomy, pelvic / para-aortic lymphadenectomy.
- Based on careful surgical staging, unilateral adnexectomy is possible in patients with stage I disease (preservation of contralateral adnexa).
- With metastasized disease: removal of all visible and palpable tumor tissue.
- Preservation of fertility possible in most patients.

### Radiotherapy
- Dysgerminomas stage IA: close monitoring (relapse rate 15–25%). Due to high rate of contralateral dysgerminomas and frequent loss of fertility, adjuvant radiotherapy is not applied anymore. Patients with more advanced stages of the disease are treated with adjuvant platinum-based chemotherapy.
- In cases of incompletely resected dysgerminomas, local radiotherapy (25–30 Gy) may be beneficial. However, due to a high local relapse rate of approximately 40%, combination chemotherapy is used increasingly.
- Palliative situations: possibly local radiotherapy.

### Chemotherapy
- *Adjuvant situation:* all patients with malignant dysgerminomas (except stage IA) and choriocarcinoma should receive adjuvant platinum-containing chemotherapy. Standard treatment: PEB (cisplatin, etoposide, and bleomycin), 3 cycles, alternatively: PVB or VAC. The value of adjuvant chemotherapy in immature teratomas is uncertain; in stage II / III, adjuvant chemotherapy is nonetheless recommended.
- *Advanced stages:* in cases of incomplete resection or relapse, at least 3–4 cycles of a cisplatin-based chemotherapy should be given (PEB protocol). Alternatively, cisplatin can be replaced by carboplatin (e.g., in cases of impaired renal function). In case of disease progression or early relapse → administration of VAC (response rate > 30%). High-dose chemotherapy only in clinical trials.

| "PEB" ▶ Protocol 12.11.3 | | | Start next cycle on day 22 |
|---|---|---|---|
| Cisplatin | 20 mg/m²/day | i.v. | Days 1–5 |
| Etoposide | 100 mg/m²/day | i.v. | Days 1–5 |
| Bleomycin | 30 mg/day | i.v. | Days 1, 8, 15 |

| "PEI" ▶ Protocol 12.11.4 | | | Start next cycle on day 22 |
|---|---|---|---|
| Cisplatin | 20 mg/m²/day | i.v. | Days 1–5 |
| Etoposide | 100 mg/m²/day | i.v. | Days 1–5 |
| Ifosfamide | 1,200 mg/m²/day | i.v. | Days 1–5 |

| "VAC" | | | Start next cycle on day 22 |
|---|---|---|---|
| Vincristine | 1.5 mg/m²/day | i.v. | Day 1 |
| Dactinomycin | 350 µg/m²/day | i.v. | Days 1–5 |
| Cyclophosphamide | 150 mg/m²/day | i.v. | Days 1–5 |

**Prg:** As with testicular germ cell tumors, the overall prognosis for patients with malignant germ cell tumors of the ovaries has dramatically improved since the introduction of cisplatin-based combination chemotherapy → due to the high chemosensitivity of these tumors, curative intent even in advanced stages of the disease.
- Five-year survival: > 90% (even after fertility-preserving surgery)
- Unfavorable prognostic factors include large primary tumor, distant metastases, young age at presentation, and high mitotic rate (histological analysis)

**Ref:**
1. Gershenson DM. Management of ovarian germ cell tumors. J Clin Oncol 2007;25:2938–43
2. Lai CH, Chang TC, Hsueh S et al. Outcome and prognostic factors in ovarian germ cell malignancies. Gynecol Oncol 2005;96:784–91
3. Lu KH, Gershenson DM. Update on the management of ovarian germ cell tumors. J Reprod Med 2005;50:417–25
4. Schmoll HJ, Souchon R, Krege S et al. European consensus on diagnosis and treatment of germ cell cancer: a report of the European Germ Cell Cancer Consensus Group (EGCCCG). Ann Oncol 2004;15:1377–99
5. Zanetta G, Bonazzi C, Cantu M et al. Survival and reproductive function after treatment of malignant germ cell ovarian tumors. J Clin Oncol 2001;19:1015–20

**Web:**
1. http://www.cancer.gov/cancertopics/pdq/treatment/ ovarian-germ-cell/HealthProfessional      NCI Cancer Topics
2. http://www.emedicine.com/med/topic601.htm      E-medicine

## 8.4.4     Granulosa Cell Tumors of the Ovary

**I.B. Runnebaum, C.F. Waller**

**Def:**     Malignant stromal tumors of the ovary originating from gonad-specific stromal tissue or undifferentiated mesenchymal tissue:
- "Female" differentiation: granulosa cell tumors
- "Male" differentiation: Sertoli-Leydig cell tumors
- Mixed differentiation: gynandroblastomas

**ICD-10:**     C56 (ovarian cancer)

**Ep:**     Incidence: 1 case/100,000 population/year; age peak: 50–54 years; most common malignant stromal tumor; < 5% of all malignant ovarian tumors; 80% endocrine active, mainly estrogen secretion. At diagnosis: 85% of cases in adults, 15% in children.

**Path:**     Large tumors, with cysts and hemorrhages, in 95% of cases unilateral; usually no metastasis; often diagnosed in stage I; distant metastases are rare (liver, lung, skeleton).

### Histology
- Small granulosa cells with "coffee-bean" grooved nucleus; characteristic "Call-Exner bodies" in 30–60% of cases (cystic formations surrounded by granulosa cells)
- Immunohistochemical markers: inhibin α, CD99, cytokeratins (CK), EMA

**Class:**     **Classification of ovarian stromal tumors according to WHO**

- *Granulosa Cell Tumors:* adult form, juvenile form
- *Sertoli-Leydig Cell Tumors:* highly / moderately / poorly differentiated
- *Gynandroblastomas*
- *Fibroma / Thecoma:* thecoma, fibroma, fibrosarcoma
- *Sclerosing Stromal Tumors*
- *Sex Cord Stromal Tumors* with annular tubules
- *Unclassified Tumors:* lipid cell tumors, hilar cell tumors

For clinical classification, see ovarian carcinoma according to FIGO (▶ Chap. 8.4.2)

**Sy:**
- Abdominal pain
- Uterine hemorrhage, postmenopausal bleeding, vaginal bleeding in older women
- Infertility, precocious pseudopuberty (juvenile estrogen-producing tumor), in rare cases virilization
- Ascites in advanced stages
- In approximately 10% of cases: ruptured tumor, hemoperitoneum, possibly acute abdomen

**Dg:**     ***Medical History, Physical Examination***
- Medical history: indications for estrogen-producing tumors
- Physical examination: palpable pelvic tumors; firm elastic, smooth surface

### Laboratory Tests
- Routine laboratory, liver / renal function parameters, tumor marker CA 125
- Hormone status: estradiol ↑, possibly DHEA-S, testosterone, gonadotropins (FSH, LH), inhibin

### Imaging
- Ultrasound (transvaginal and abdominal)
- Possibly pelvic and abdominal MRI (adrenal glands?)

**Co:**
- Tumor rupture, intra-abdominal bleeding, acute abdomen
- Due to tumor-related estrogen production → precocious pseudopuberty, abnormal uterine hemorrhage, infertility, endometrial hyperplasia (50%), endometrial carcinoma (5–10%)

**Th:** Primary surgical excision of tumor. Chemotherapy is indicated in patients with advanced disease (FIGO II–IV), relapse, or adjuvant after R1/R2 resection. Younger women: fertility-preserving surgery, older women: hysterectomy, due to risk of simultaneous endometrial carcinomas.

### Surgical Treatment
- *Complete tumor resection with surgical staging:* total tumor excision by oophorectomy (AT-TENTION: cysts may rupture), frozen section analysis, exploration of the abdomen, intraperitoneal cytology sampling. If frozen section analysis reveals malignancy → multiple peritoneal biopsies, infracolic omentectomy, hysterectomy, contralateral adnexectomy, pelvic and para-aortic lymphadenectomy.
- *Patients with FIGO IA and wishing to preserve fertility:* preservation of uterus and contralateral adnexa possible. In case of tumors with higher malignant potential: radical surgery at later stage is advisable; if uterus is preserved: hysteroscopy (HSC) and abrasion to exclude endometrial hyperplasia or endometrial carcinoma.
- Relapse after a period of > 12 months → repeat surgery (if applicable, several times)

### Radiotherapy
Since stromal tumors are radiosensitive, patients with inoperable but limited disease can be treated with radiotherapy. Benefit of adjuvant radiotherapy following complete tumor resection not yet established.

### Chemotherapy
- Due to the rare occurrence of the tumor, no randomized chemotherapy trials have been conducted. Generally, treatment approach similar to ovarian carcinomas. Cisplatin-containing protocols are effective, usually 6–8 cycles.
- *Stage I:* no definite benefit of adjuvant chemotherapy after radical surgery; chemotherapy advisable in case of large tumors, high mitotic rates, or rupture.
- *Stage II–IV, relapse, R1/R2 resection:* chemotherapy is indicated, usually cisplatin-containing protocols.
- Inoperable cases: primary systemic chemotherapy is indicated, possibly additional radiotherapy.
- Endocrine therapies with GnRH analogs, medroxyprogesterone acetate (MPA), or tamoxifen have no definite long-term effect, even in relapsed patients.
- Drugs currently evaluated in clinical trials: paclitaxel.

### Chemotherapy Protocols

| "PEB" ▶ Protocol 12.11.3 | | | Start next cycle on day 22 |
|---|---|---|---|
| Cisplatin | 20 mg/m²/day | i.v. | Days 1–5 |
| Etoposide | 100 mg/m²/day | i.v. | Days 1–5 |
| Bleomycin | 30 mg/day | i.v. | Days 1, 8, 15 |

| "PVB" | | | Start next cycle on day 22 |
|---|---|---|---|
| Cisplatin | 20 mg/m²/day | i.v. | Days 1–5 for 1 h |
| Vinblastine | 0.2 mg/kg/day | i.v. | Days 1+2 bolus |
| Bleomycin | 30 mg | i.v. | Days 1, 8, 15 |

| "PAC" | | | Start next cycle on day 22 |
|---|---|---|---|
| Doxorubicin | 50 mg/m²/day | i.v. | Day 1 |
| Cisplatin | 50 mg/m²/day | i.v. | Day 1 |
| Cyclophosphamide | 500 mg/m²/day | i.v. | Day 1 |

**Prg:** Due to early diagnosis (on presentation often stage I) curative treatment approach; however, late relapses may occur even after long-term relapse-free interval. Prognostically relevant:
- Disease stage, tumor size > 15 cm, ruptured tumor, lymph node status
- Differentiation grade, mitotic frequency
- Poor prognosis: ruptured tumor
- Poor prognosis: age > 40 years

**Ref:**
1. Colombo N, Parma G, Zanagnolo V et al. Management of ovarian stromal tumors. J Clin Oncol 2007;25:2944–51
2. Schumer ST, Cannistra SA. Granulosa cell tumor of the ovary. J Clin Oncol 2003;21:1180–9
3. Uygun K, Aydiner A, Saip P et al. Clinical parameters and treatment results in recurrent granulosa cell tumor of the ovary. Gynecol Oncol 2003;88:400–3

**Web:**
1. http://www.emedicine.com/med/topic928.htm          E-medicine

## 8.4.5    Sertoli-Leydig Cell Tumors

**I.B. Runnebaum, C.F. Waller**

**Def:** Malignant stromal tumors of the ovary originating from gonad-specific stromal tissue and containing both Sertoli and Leydig cells. Androgenic hormone production is characteristic.

**ICD-10:** C56 (ovarian carcinoma)

**Ep:** Rare disease, 0.2% of all ovarian carcinomas, 97% of the tumors are diagnosed in stage I, age at diagnosis 20–30 years.

**Path:** Macroscopic tumors usually 5–15 cm in diameter and solid; characteristics of clinically malignant Sertoli-Leydig tumors (< 20% of cases) are:
- Large tumors (> 15 cm), high mitotic index, tumor rupture
- Poor histological differentiation
- Extraovarian spread (intraperitoneal metastasis, retroperitoneal lymph node involvement)

### Histology
- Highly differentiated tumors with mainly tubular appearance
- Moderately or poorly differentiated tumors frequently with heterogeneous histology (retiform / cystic / glandular / mesenchymal components)
- Immunohistochemistry: positive for testosterone, AFP (mainly Leydig cells)

**Class:** Staging as in epithelial ovarian carcinoma (▶ Chap. 8.4.2)

**Sy:**
- Menstruation changes
- Virilization, androgenic symptom complex: amenorrhea, deep voice, hirsutism, breast atrophy, enlarged clitoris, disappearance of feminine contours, temporary hair loss
- Non-specific signs of a tumor of the lower abdomen: pain, fatigue, abdominal distension, acute abdomen

**Dg:**
### Medical History, Physical Examination
- Medical history, seemingly healthy young women

### Laboratory Tests
- Serum testosterone ↑, often AFP ↑, androstenedione / DHEA-S normal or slightly increased; in some cases inhibin ↑

### Imaging
- Transvaginal and abdominal ultrasound, abdominal / pelvic CT
- Chest x-ray, possibly CT of thorax

**Co:** Metastasis to intraperitoneal and retroperitoneal lymph nodes, lung, liver, skeleton

**Th:** First-line therapy: surgical tumor resection; fertility preservation possible in patients with stage I disease; higher stages or relapse: individualized approach to treatment

### Surgical Treatment
- *Standard:* oophorectomy (*ATTENTION:* tumor may rupture), frozen section analysis, exploration of the abdomen, intraperitoneal biopsy for cytology, if frozen section analysis reveals malignancy → multiple peritoneal biopsies, infracolic omentectomy, hysterectomy and contralateral adnexectomy, pelvic and para-aortic lymphadenectomy.
- Patients with FIGO Ia and wanting children: preservation of uterus and contralateral adnexa possible; highly malignant tumors (G3, heterogeneous components): radical surgery after completed family planning.
- Relapse after a period of > 12 months: repeat surgery.

### Radiotherapy
Benefit of radiotherapy is uncertain.

### Chemotherapy
- Undifferentiated tumors (G3) or R1/R2 resection of advanced tumor stages and inoperable cases (e.g., due to poor performance status): chemotherapy is indicated.
- Not necessary with highly and well-differentiated tumors and complete tumor resection (relapse rate without chemotherapy 20%).

### Chemotherapy Protocols

| "PEB" ▶ Protocol 12.11.3 | | | Start next cycle on day 22 |
|---|---|---|---|
| Cisplatin | 20 mg/m²/day | i.v. | Days 1–5 |
| Etoposide | 100 mg/m²/day | i.v. | Days 1–5 |
| Bleomycin | 30 mg/day | i.v. | Days 1, 8, 15 |

| "PVB" | | | Start next cycle on day 22 |
|---|---|---|---|
| Cisplatin | 20 mg/m²/day | i.v. | Days 1–5 for 1 h |
| Vinblastine | 0.2 mg/kg/day | i.v. | Days 1+2 bolus |
| Bleomycin | 30 mg | i.v. | Days 1, 8, 15 |

| "PAC" ▶ Protocol 12.4.1 | | | Start next cycle on day 22 |
|---|---|---|---|
| Doxorubicin | 50 mg/m²/day | i.v. | Day 1 |
| Cisplatin | 50 mg/m²/day | i.v. | Day 1 |
| Cyclophosphamide | 500 mg/m²/day | i.v. | Day 1 |

**Prg:** After surgical tumor resection: regression of androgen-induced and tumor-related symptoms, restoration of menstruation after approximately 3 months, no fertility impairment, complete disappearance of signs of androgenization in only 50% of cases

**Ref:**
1. Gheorghisan-Galateanu A, Fica S, Terzea DC et al. Sertoli-Leydig cell tumor: a rare androgen-secreting ovarian tumor in postmenopausal women. J Cell Mol Med 2003;7:461–71
2. Schneider DT, Calaminus G, Wessalowksi R et al. Ovarian sex cord-stromal tumors in children and adolescents. J Clin Oncol 2003;12:2357–63
3. Young RH, Scully RE. Ovarian Sertoli-Leydig cell tumors. A clinicopathological analysis of 207 cases. Am J Surg Pathol 1985;8:543–69

**Web:**
1. http://www.nccn.org/      NCCN Guidelines

## 8.4.6    Malignant Trophoblastic Tumors

### C.F. Waller, I.B. Runnebaum

**Def:**    Malignant neoplasia as a result of abnormal proliferation of the trophoblast (nutritional layer of the early embryo) occurring during pregnancy.

**Types of malignant trophoblastic tumors**

| Type | Incidence |
|------|-----------|
| Hydatidiform mole | 1 case / 1,000 pregnancies |
| Invasive mole | 1 case / 15,000 pregnancies |
| Choriocarcinoma | 1 case / 30,000 pregnancies |
| Trophoblastic tumors of the placenta | Rare |

**ICD-10:**    D39.2: hydatidiform mole
C58: choriocarcinoma

**Ep:**    Rare disease. Incidence of hydatidiform moles: approximately 1/1,000 pregnancies in Germany and the USA, approximately 1/500 pregnancies in Asia and South America; approximately 15% develop into an invasive mole and approximately 2–3% into choriocarcinoma.

**Pg:**    *Risk Factors*
- Nulliparity
- Pregnancy at a very young (< 15 years) or advanced age (> 50 years)
- Presence of enlarged theca lutein cysts
- Abnormally high βHCG serum concentration during pregnancy
- Previous malignant trophoblastic tumors

**Path:**    *Complete and partial hydatidiform moles* differ in terms of morphology, histology, karyotype, and clinical signs. Partial moles contain embryonic tissue, complete moles do not.

| Characteristics | Complete moles | Partial moles |
|-----------------|----------------|---------------|
| Karyotype | Normal | Triploidy |
| Embryonal tissue | – | + |
| Trophoblastic proliferation | Circumferential, marked | Focal, minimal |
| Trophoblastic atypia | + | – |
| Immunocytochemistry | HCG, rarely PLAP | PLAP, rarely HCG |

*HCG* human chorionic gonadotropin, *PLAP* placental alkaline phosphatase

*Choriocarcinomas* are a malignant variation of trophoblastic hyperplasia characterized by lack of chorionic villi and invasion of the myometrium.

*Trophoblastic tumors of the placenta* mainly consist of cytotrophoblastic cells without chorionic villi.

*Hematogenous Metastasis*
- Invasive mole: lung, vagina
- Choriocarcinoma: lung, brain, liver, pelvis, vagina, spleen, intestine, kidneys

**Class:**  **TNM staging of trophoblastic tumors**

| | |
|---|---|
| *T* | *Primary Tumor* |
| TX | Primary tumor cannot be assessed |
| T0 | No evidence of primary tumor |
| T1 | Tumor confined to uterus |
| T2 | Tumor extends to other genital structures: vagina, ovary, tube, broad ligament, fallopian tube by metastasis or direct extension |
| *N* | *Lymph Nodes* |
| NX | Regional lymph nodes cannot be assessed |
| N0 | Regional lymph nodes without metastasis |
| *N1* | Metastasis to regional lymph nodes |
| *M* | *Metastasis* |
| MX | Metastasis cannot be assessed |
| M0 | No distant metastasis |
| M1 | Distant metastasis |
| | A Metastasis to lung |
| | B Other distant metastasis |

**Prognostic index of malignant trophoblastic tumors according to WHO**

| Prognostic factors | Points | | | |
|---|---|---|---|---|
| | 0 | 1 | 2 | 4 |
| Age (years) | < 40 | ≥ 40 | – | – |
| Previous pregnancy | Mole | Abortion | Term | – |
| Cx delay[a] (months) | < 4 | 4–6 | 7–12 | > 12 |
| βHCG before therapy (IU/ml) | $< 10^3$ | $\geq 10^3$ | $\geq 10^4$ | $\geq 10^5$ |
| Largest tumor | < 3 cm | 3–5 cm | > 5 cm | – |
| Location of metastases | Lung | Spleen, kidney | GI tract | CNS, liver |
| Number of metastases | – | 1–4 | 5–8 | > 8 |
| Ineffective chemotherapy | – | – | 1 drug | ≥ 2 drugs |

[a]Interval between end of pregnancy and start of chemotherapy (Cx)

The prognostic score is formed by the sum of points for the individual prognostic factors:
- Low risk situation: < 8 points
- High risk situation: ≥ 8 points

**FIGO / AJCC Staging of trophoblastic tumors**

| TNM classification | | FIGO | Prognostic score | | | |
|---|---|---|---|---|---|---|
| T1 | M0 | I | IA | Low risk | IB | High risk |
| T2 | M0 | II | IIA | Low risk | IIB | High risk |
| Any T | M1A | III | IIIA | Low risk | IIIB | High risk |
| Any T | M1B | IV | IVA | Low risk | IVB | High risk |

**Sy:**        Due to regular ultrasound examinations and monitoring of βHCG serum levels, trophoblastic tumors are usually discovered at an early stage. Symptoms of a molar pregnancy often occur late:
- Vaginal bleeding, in some cases with hydropic vesicles before the 20th week of pregnancy
- Discrepancy between uterine size and gestation period
- Hyperemesis gravidarum, anemia, hyperthyroidism

**Dg:**        *Medical History, Physical Examination*
- Medical history
- Physical examination, gynecological examination, rectal examination, assessment of the pouch of Douglas

*Laboratory Tests*
- Routine laboratory tests including LDH, complete blood count, liver and renal function, thyroid function
- Tumor markers: βHCG (human chorionic gonadotropin, elevated levels, persistence past the 14th week of pregnancy), serum PLAP (placental alkaline phosphatase)

*Imaging*
- Ultrasound (transvaginal and abdominal)
- Chest x-ray, thoracic CT scan, abdominal CT scan
- Abdominal and pelvic MRI, cranial MRI

*Histology*
- Analysis of ascites or pleural effusion
- Suction curettage, hysterectomy (see surgical treatment)

**Th:**        Curative treatment intent → initiation of therapy at diagnosis. Multimodal treatment approach:

*Surgical Treatment*
Surgical resection is first-line therapy in localized disease stages:
- *Hydatidiform moles:* uterus evacuation via suction curettage; in exceptional cases, primary simple hysterectomy (provided patient does not wish to preserve fertility)
- *Malignant trophoblastic tumors or substantial persistent uterine hemorrhage:* hysterectomy, possibly adjuvant chemotherapy
- *Chemoresistant pulmonary metastases:* resection

*Radiotherapy*
- Cerebral metastases: radiotherapy (30 Gy) is indicated, possibly in combination with chemotherapy

*Chemotherapy*
Primary treatment of persistent hydatidiform moles, invasive moles, and choriocarcinomas:
- *Adjuvant situation:* indications for postoperative chemotherapy: βHCG persistence > 12 weeks after hydatidiform mole; invasive moles; non-metastasizing malignant trophoblastic tumors. The most commonly used drugs are methotrexate (MTX, with leucovorin rescue) and Actinomycin D.
- *Advanced stages:* in high-risk situations and cases of relapse: polychemotherapy with MAC or EMA / CO with curative intent (see below).

*Chemotherapy Protocols*

*Low Risk*

| *"MTX Monotherapy"* | | | *Start next cycle on days 12–14* |
|---|---|---|---|
| MTX | 0.4–0.6 mg/kg | i.m.. | Days 1–5, bolus |

| *"MTX plus Leucovorin"* | | | |
|---|---|---|---|
| MTX | 1 mg/kg | i.m. / i.v. | Days 1, 3, 5, 7, bolus |
| Leucovorin | 0.1 mg/kg | | 24 h after MTX |

| *"Actinomycin D Monotherapy"* | | | *Start next cycle on day 15* |
|---|---|---|---|
| Actinomycin D | 1.25 mg/m$^2$ | i.v. | Days 1–5, bolus |

### High Risk or Refractory Disease: Combination Chemotherapy

| *"EMA / CO"* | | | |
|---|---|---|---|
| Etoposide | 100 mg/m$^2$ | i.v. | Days 1, 2, 1 h – infusion |
| Methotrexate | 300 mg/m$^2$ | i.v | Day 1, 12 h – infusion |
| Dactinomycin | 0.5 mg | i.v. | Days 1, 2, bolus |
| Leucovorin | 15 mg | p.o. | Days 2, 3, twice daily |
| Cyclophosphamide | 600 mg/m$^2$ | i.v. | Day 8, infusion |
| Vincristine | 1 mg/m$^2$ | i.v. | Day 8, bolus |

High-risk patients: usually 4 cycles

| *"EMA"* | | | |
|---|---|---|---|
| Etoposide | 100 mg/m$^2$ | i.v. | Days 1, 2, 1 h – infusion |
| Methotrexate | 300 mg/m$^2$ | i.v | Day 1, 12 h – infusion |
| Dactinomycin | 0.5 mg | i.v. | Days 1, 2, bolus |

| *"MAC"* | | | *Start next cycle on day 22* |
|---|---|---|---|
| Methotrexate | 0.3 mg/kg | i.v. | Days 1–5, bolus |
| Dactinomycin | 8–10 µg/kg | i.v | Days 1–5, bolus |
| Cyclophosphamide or | 3 mg/kg | i.v. | Days 1–5, bolus |
| Chlorambucil | 0.2 mg/kg | | |

**Prg:** Patients with malignant trophoblastic tumors have a favorable overall prognosis. Even patients with advanced disease can be cured in 85–100% of cases.

Prognostic factors for malignant trophoblastic tumors (WHO; see above) can predict the likelihood of response to chemotherapy, and improve treatment planning.

**Ref:**
1. Altieri A, Franceschi S, Ferlay J et al. Epidemiology and aetiology of gestational trophoblastic diseases. Lancet Oncol 2003;4:670–8
2. Carney ME. Treatment of low risk gestational trophoblastic disease. Clin Obstet Gynecol 2003;46:579–92
3. Dainty LA, Winter WE, Maxwell GL. The clinical behavior of placental site trophoblastic tumor and contemporary methods of management. Clin Obstet Gynecol 2003;46:607–11
4. Ngan HY, Bender H, Benedet JL et al. Gestational trophoblastic neoplasia, FIGO 2000 staging and classification. Int J Gynaecol Obstet 2003;83(suppl 1):175–7
5. Smith HO, Kohorn E, Cole LA. Choriocarcinoma and gestational trophoblastic disease. Obstet Gynecol Clin North Am 2005;32:661–84

6.    Soper JT, Mutch DG, Schink JC et al. Diagnosis and treatment of gestational trophoblastic disease: ACOG Practice Bulletin No. 53. Gynecol Oncol 2004;93:575–85

7.    Wright JD, Mutch DG. Treatment of high-risk gestational trophoblastic tumors. Clin Obstet Gynecol 2003;46:593–606

**Web:**    1.    http://www.nlm.nih.gov/medlineplus/ency/article/001496.htm        MedlinePlus

2.    http://www.emedicine.com/MED/topic866.htm        E-medicine

3.    http://cancerweb.ncl.ac.uk/cancernet/201163.html        CancerWeb

4.    http://www.fpnotebook.com/OB65.htm        FP Notebook

## 8.4.7 Cervical Cancer

**I.B. Runnebaum, C. Weissenberger, C.F. Waller**

**Def:** Malignant tumors of the uterine cervix.

**ICD-10:** C53

**Ep:** Approximately 15 cases/100,000 women/year; two age groups: 35–50 years and 65–75 years; average age: 50 years, with carcinoma in situ (CIS): approximately 35 years; 25% of patients are younger than 43 years. Second most common female cancer representing 5% of all carcinomas in women. Socioeconomic factors and cultural background play an important role (incidence worldwide between 2 and 90 new cases/100,000 women/year).

Since the introduction of cervical cancer screening, incidence of cervical cancer has gradually decreased. More preinvasive cervical lesions are discovered due to improved screening programs → in Germany approximately 300,000 cases of cervical intraepithelial neoplasia (CIN) per year (incidence approximately 1%).

**Pg:** In >95% of cervical carcinomas, human papilloma virus DNA (particularly HPV 16, 18, 31, 45, 51, 52, 56) can be detected.
- → Interaction of the viral oncoproteins E6 and E7 with the tumor suppressor proteins p53 and pRb
- → Loss of cell cycle control, modulation of cytokines / cyclin E / cyclin A / c-fos / c-jun
- → Abnormal apoptosis, immortalization

### Risk Factors
- HPV infection (sexual intercourse)
- Promiscuous behavior, first sexual contact at early age (cohabitation at < 15 years)
- Poor sexual hygiene (circumcision in men possibly protective)
- Immune deficiency, immunosuppression, HIV
- Smoking, multiparity, contraceptives

**Path:** ### Cervical Intraepithelial Neoplasia (CIN)
Cervical dysplasia most commonly develops at the border between squamous epithelium and columnar epithelium (transformation zone).

- CIN I: mild dysplasia
- CIN II: moderate dysplasia
- CIN III: severe dysplasia, carcinoma in situ

### Growth Pattern
- CIN → superficial carcinoma of the cervix → invasive carcinoma
- Growth of invasive carcinoma: ulcers of the ectocervix, exophytic tumors, or endocervical tumors
- Further local tumor expansion into vaginal cavity or paravaginal tissue / parametrium
- Possibly infiltration of the urinary bladder and/or the rectum

### Metastasis Pattern
- Lymphatic: pelvic → para-aortic → supraclavicular lymph nodes
- Hematogenous: liver, lung, bones

*Invasive Carcinoma of the Cervix Uteri: Histology*

| Type | Frequency (%) |
|---|---|
| *Squamous Cell Carcinoma* | 60–80 |
| • Keratinizing / non-keratinizing | |
| • Large cell / small cell | |
| • Verrucous / condylomatous / papillary / lymphoepitheliomatous | |
| *Adenocarcinoma* | 10–15 |
| • Mucinous, endocervical | |
| • Intestinal / signet ring cell type | |
| • Endometrioid ± squamous cell metaplasia (adenoacanthoma) | |
| • Clear cell / serous type | |
| • Mesonephric carcinoma | |
| • Highly differentiated villous-glandular adenocarcinoma | |
| *Other Epithelial Tumors* | Rare |
| • Adenosquamous / adenoid-cystic / adenoid-basal carcinoma | |
| • Mucoepidermoid carcinoma | |
| • "Glassy cell" carcinoma | |
| • Carcinoid-like tumor | |
| • Neuroendocrine carcinoma | |
| • Small cell / undifferentiated carcinoma | |

**Class:**     **TNM staging of cervical cancer (2004)**

| | |
|---|---|
| ***T*** | ***Primary Tumor*** |
| TX | Primary tumor cannot be assessed |
| T0 | No evidence of primary tumor |
| Tis | Carcinoma in situ, intraepithelial neoplasia (CIN) |
| T1 | Tumor confined to uterus |
| | A1: stromal invasion ≤ 3 mm in depth and ≤ 7 mm in width |
| | A2: stromal invasion 3–5 mm in depth and ≤ 7 mm in width |
| | B1: tumor limited to cervix, > T1A2 and ≤ 4 cm |
| | B2: tumor limited to cervix and > 4 cm ("bulky T1B") |
| T2 | Cervical carcinoma invades beyond uterus |
| | A: without parametrial invasion |
| | B: with parametrial invasion |
| T3 | Tumor extends to pelvic wall / lower vagina / ureter |
| | A: tumor extends to lower third of the vagina |
| | B: tumor extends to pelvic wall / hydronephrosis / kidney dysfunction |
| T4 | Tumor invades mucosa of bladder / rectum, or extension beyond true pelvis |
| ***N*** | ***Lymph Node Involvement*** |
| NX | Regional lymph nodes cannot be assessed |
| N0 | No regional lymph node metastasis |
| N1 | Regional lymph node metastasis |

**Class:**

**TNM staging of cervical cancer (2004)** *(continued)*

| M | Distant Metastasis |
|---|---|
| MX | Distant metastasis cannot be assessed |
| M0 | No distant metastasis |
| M1 | Distant metastasis |

**FIGO Staging (1998)**

| Stage | TNM classification | | | Survival rates (%) | | |
|---|---|---|---|---|---|---|
| | T | N | M | 1 year | 2 years | 5 years |
| 0 | Tis | N0 | M0 | 100 | 99 | 98 |
| IA1 | T1A1 | N0 | M0 | 98 | 97 | 95 |
| IA2 | T1A2 | N0 | M0 | 98 | 95 | 93 |
| IB1 | T1B1 | N0 | M0 | 99 | 97 | 90 |
| IB2 | T1B2 | N0 | M0 | 96 | 91 | 80 |
| IIA | T2A | N0 | M0 | 96 | 89 | 76 |
| IIB | T2B | N0 | M0 | 95 | 86 | 74 |
| IIIA | T3A | N0 | M0 | 86 | 67 | 51 |
| IIIB | T3B | N0 | M0 | 80 | 64 | 46 |
| IVA | T4 | N0 | M0 | 64 | 46 | 30 |
| | Any T | N1 | M0 | | | |
| IVB | Any T | Any N | M1 | 49 | 32 | 22 |

According to FIGO guidelines, staging of stage IA cervical cancer is based on biopsy, while staging of tumors ≥ stage IB is based on clinical assessment:
- Speculum examination, bimanual rectovaginal palpation (possibly under anesthesia)
- Cystoscopy, rectoscopy
- Intravenous pyelogram, chest x-ray, lymph node status

**Sy:**

### Early Symptoms
- Vaginal discharge with traces of blood
- Metrorrhagia, bleeding upon contact

### Late Symptoms
- Fatigue, reduced performance, weight loss
- Hydronephrosis, flank pain
- Edema of lower extremities, pelvic vein thrombosis
- Pain (spreading to inside of the thigh)

**Dg:**

### Medical History, Physical Examination
- Medical history including risk factors
- Physical examination including speculum examination and bimanual rectovaginal palpation

### Laboratory Tests
- Complete blood count, electrolytes, coagulation status (preoperatively), liver / renal function tests
- Tumor markers: SCC (squamous cell carcinoma), CEA, CA 125 (adenocarcinoma) → to monitor disease course

### Imaging
- Chest x-ray
- Intravenous pyelography, ultrasound
- Cystoscopy / rectoscopy, colon barium enema in stages IIB–IVA
- From stage IB2: pelvic MRI / abdominal CT

### Cytology / Histology
- Cervical cytology screening: cervical smear from transformation zone; cytological classification according to Papanicolaou ("PAP I–V"); thin preparation with similar sensitivity.
- HPV identification in cervical smear combined with cytology potentially increases sensitivity of cytological analysis; negative HPV test constitutes low risk of cervical cancer.
- Colposcopy: without staining, or with application of acetic acid wash (3%), Lugol's iodine
- Colposcopic biopsy (punch biopsy) or cone biopsy with endocervical curettage
- With endocervical processes: cervical curettage, possibly with hysteroscopy

**Dd:**
- Cervical polyps, cervical erosion, hyperkeratosis
- Metastases of extragenital tumors

**Th:**

### Treatment Concept

1. Localized stages (CIN III, stage IA to IIA): standard treatment is surgical resection. Radiotherapy alone is as effective as surgical treatment alone. A combination of both is usually futile (more side effects without increased therapeutic benefit). The benefit of adjuvant simple hysterectomy in stage IB2 has not been established. Patients with contraindications to surgery receive primary radiotherapy, usually intracavitary contact radiotherapy (brachytherapy) + external radiotherapy.
2. Regionally advanced stages (IIB, III, IV): radiotherapy, possibly with simultaneous chemotherapy. In patients treated with curative intent, radiotherapy should be combined with a radiosensitizer such as cisplatin. In some patients with stage IIIA disease primary surgical treatment may be considered.
3. Distant metastases (stage IVB): palliative chemotherapy possible; effective compounds include cisplatin, carboplatin, alkylating agents (ifosfamide, cyclophosphamide), anthracyclines (doxorubicin, epirubicin), irinotecan, and paclitaxel. In case of vaginal bleeding, pain in true pelvis, or urinary obstruction by tumor masses: local palliative radiotherapy.

**Treatment of cervical cancer**

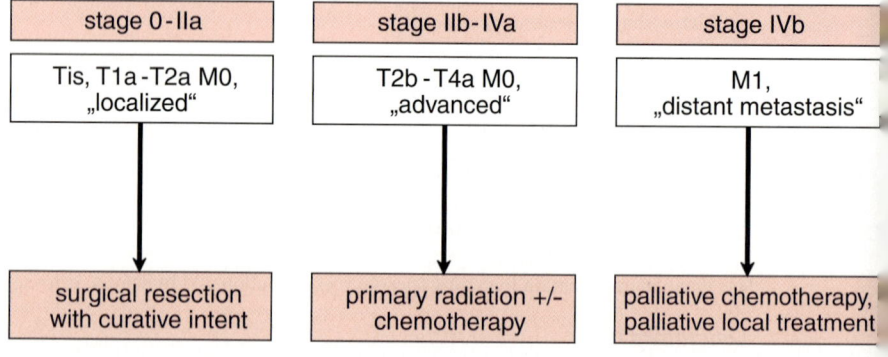

| stage 0-IIa | stage IIb-IVa | stage IVb |
|---|---|---|
| Tis, T1a-T2a M0, „localized" | T2b-T4a M0, „advanced" | M1, „distant metastasis" |
| surgical resection with curative intent | primary radiation +/- chemotherapy | palliative chemotherapy, palliative local treatment |

## Preinvasive Lesions of the Cervix and Carcinoma in situ

### Local Surgical Treatment
- Surgical cone biopsy
- LEEP (loop electrosurgical excision procedure)
- LLETZ (large loop excision of the transformation zone)


## Invasive Carcinoma

### Stage IA1 (No Lymph Vessel Invasion)
- To preserve fertility: cone biopsy with complete cervical curettage (after full explanation to patient)
- In patients without lymph vessel invasion not wanting children: simple hysterectomy (Piver-Rutledge I) recommended
- Prospective studies demonstrated comparable outcomes for primary surgical treatment and primary radiotherapy in patients with stage I tumors.

### Stage IA1 (With Lymph Vessel Invasion), IA2, IB1, IIA, Early IIB
- Studies have shown that cervical cancer patients with stage IA2 disease (diagnosis based on cone biopsy, excised fully) have a low risk of lymph node metastasis and a 5-year survival rate > 90%. Lymph vessel invasion correlates significantly with the presence of pelvic and paraaortic lymph node metastases.
- First step during surgery: laparoscopic pelvic and lower paraaortic lymphadenectomy with intraoperative frozen section analysis (lymphadenectomy prior to hysterectomy). Next step depending on frozen section analysis.
- No pelvic or paraaortic lymph node metastases: radical surgery according to Wertheim (Piver-Rutledge II–III). Due to increased morbidity and lack of clinical benefit, preoperative and postoperative radiotherapy is not recommended.
- Involvement of pelvic or paraaortic lymph nodes: no hysterectomy but irradiation of the primary tumor. Depending on the histological lymph node status, paraaortic extension of the radiation field; even with enlarged pelvic and/or paraaortic lymph nodes, debulking is recommended to assist radiotherapy of the pelvic wall. Percutaneous radiation dose: 45–55 Gy; possibly simultaneous chemotherapy (cisplatin as "radiosensitizer"). At the end of percutaneous radiotherapy: brachytherapy (afterloading) with radium or iridium; total dose at the center of the tumor: 85–100 Gy.

### Stages IIB, III, IV
- Primary radiotherapy
- Possibly with simultaneous chemotherapy (cisplatin as "radiosensitizer")

### Stage IVB (Distant Metastasis)
- In patients with primary distant metastasis (stage IVB): chemotherapy with palliative intent is indicated; response rate approximately 40%, response duration 3–4 months
- Combination chemotherapy does not seem to improve overall survival compared to cisplatin single agent therapy; combination chemotherapies should only be used in clinical trials

### Treatment of Relapse
Primary therapy of local or regional relapse of cervix carcinoma is surgery, possibly in combination with chemotherapy. Treatment options depend on tumor location:
- Local relapse after (sole) surgical treatment → combined radiochemotherapy (40% cure)
- Relapse in deeper structures of the vagina after radiotherapy → colpectomy or second radiation field caudally (brachytherapy)
- Central relapse (limited to the true pelvis without affecting the pelvic wall) → radical and complete surgery, usually requiring exenteration (curative in 30–60% of cases)
- Pelvic wall relapse within previous radiation field → surgery, possibly in combination with interstitial radiotherapy; surgical resection combined with intraoperative radiotherapy (IORT) of the tumor bed in clinical studies

- Paraaortic metastases → selective surgical resection (3-year DFS in 20–30% of cases); para-aortic high lymph node relapses are best diagnosed by MRI and PET scan, possibly also CT and ultrasound of the urinary tract
- If relapsed disease or lymph node metastases cannot be treated surgically or by radiotherapy (or with distant metastases): palliative chemotherapy according to symptoms

## Chemotherapy Protocols

| *Cisplatin "mono" (radiochemotherapy)* | | | |
|---|---|---|---|
| Cisplatin | 40 mg/m²/day | i.v. | Days 1, 22, 43 |

| *Cisplatin "mono"* | | *Start next cycle on day 22* | |
|---|---|---|---|
| Cisplatin | 50–75 mg/m²/day | i.v. | Day 1 |

| *BIP (Buxton)* | | *Start next cycle on day 22* | |
|---|---|---|---|
| Bleomycin | 30 mg/day | i.v. | Day 1 |
| Ifosfamide | 5 g/m²/day | i.v. | Day 1 |
| Cisplatin | 50 mg/m²/day | i.v. | Day 1 |

| *Carboplatin / Ifosfamide* | | *Start next cycle on day 29* | |
|---|---|---|---|
| Carboplatin | 300 mg/m²/day | i.v. | Day 1 |
| Ifosfamide | 5 g/m²/day | i.v. | Day 1 |

| *Paclitaxel / Cisplatin* | | *Start next cycle on day 29* | |
|---|---|---|---|
| Paclitaxel | 135–170 mg/m²/day | i.v. | Day 1 |
| Cisplatin | 75 mg/m²/day | i.v. | Day 1 |

Prg:      ***Prognostic Factors***
- Stage, histology, vascular invasion
- Lymph vessel invasion in the area of the tumor, lymph node metastasis
- Lymphocytic stromal reaction
- Expression of CD44, VEGF, factor VIII
- Infections: HIV

Px:      ***Prevention***
- Education about human papilloma virus (HPV), cervical carcinoma and risk factors for acqui-sition of HPV infection; especially young women / girls
- Primary prevention: prevention of HPV infection (use of condoms, hygiene)
- Secondary prevention: laboratory tests to detect HPV infections, definition of risk groups, monitoring of precancerous lesions

- HPV vaccination: randomized, placebo-controlled clinical studies demonstrated a decreased incidence of HPV 16 infections and HPV-related CIN in vaccinated subjects versus controls. Administration of effective vaccines as primary prophylaxis as well as secondary prevention
- We recommend immunization with HPV vaccine, as suggested by current guidelines in girls and women 9–26 years of age. Quadrivalent HPV 0/11/16/18 L1 VL0 vaccine is administered in 3 doses at 0, 2, and 6 months. The duration of immunity is yet unknown.

**Ref:**

1. Bosch FX, Castellsagué X, De Sanjosé. HPV and cervical cancer: screening or vaccination? Br J Cancer 2008;98:15–21
2. Joura EA, Leodolter S, Hernandez-Avila M et al. Efficacy of a quadrivalent prohylactic human papillomavirus (types 6,11,16 and 18) L1virus-like-particle vaccine against high-grade vulval and vaginal lesions: a combined analysis of three randomised clinical trials. Lancet 2007;369:2161–70
3. Long HC. Management of metastatic cervical cancer. J Clin Oncol 2007;25:2966–74
4. Mayrand MH, Duarte-Franco E, Rodrigues I et al. Human papillomavirus DNA versus Papanicolaou screening tests for cervical cancer. N Engl J Med 2007;1579–88
5. Monk BJ, Tewari KS, Koh WJ. Multimodality therapy for locally advanced cervical carcinoma. J Clin Oncol 2007;25:2952–65
6. Saslow D, Castle PE, Cox JT et al. ASCO Guideline for human papillomavirus (HPV) vaccine use to prevent cervical cancer and its precursors. CA Cancer J Clin 2007;57:7–28
7. Schiffman M, Castle PE, Jeronimo J et al. Human papillomavirus and cervical cancer. Lancet 2007;370:890–907
8. Stanley M. Prophylactic HPV vaccines: prospects for eliminating ano-genital cancer. Br J Cancer 2007;96:1320–3
9. Woodman CBJ, Collins SI, Young LS. The natural history of cervical HPV infection: unresolved issues. Nat Rev Cancer 2007;7:11–22

**Web:**

1. http://www.nlm.nih.gov/medlineplus/cervicalcancer.html     MedlinePlus
2. http://www.cancer.gov/cancerinfo/types/cervical     NCI Cancer Topics
3. http://www.emedicine.com/med/topic324.htm     E-medicine

**8.4.8    Endometrial Carcinoma**

C.F. Waller, I.B. Runnebaum

**Def:**    Malignant epithelial tumor, usually with glandular differentiation, arising in the endometrium Potential to invade myometrium and spread to distant sites.

**ICD-10:**    C54

**Ep:**    Incidence: 18/100,000 women/year, age peak 65–70 years; incidence increasing but low mortality

**Pg:**    *Risk Factors*
- Obesity; often associated with diabetes mellitus, arterial hypertension
- Early menarche, late menopause, nulliparity
- Polycystic ovarian syndrome (PCOS)
- Atypical adenomatous endometrial hyperplasia
- Estrogen-producing tumors
- Estrogen therapy ("unopposed," i.e., without progesterone)
- Tamoxifen therapy, pelvic radiotherapy

*Genetic Factors*
- Familial predisposition: HNPCC (hereditary non-polyposis colorectal cancer; Lynch II syndrome): high risk of extraintestinal tumors, e.g., endometrial carcinomas, in 43% of affected women
- Other aberrations: K-ras and PTEN mutations, rarely p53 mutations

**Path:**    *Histological Classification of Endometrial Carcinomas*

| Type | Frequency (%) |
| --- | --- |
| *Adenocarcinoma* | |
| • Endometrioid / villo-glandular / secretory / ciliated cell | 60–80 |
| • Clear cell | 5–10 |
| • Serous / serous-papillary (poor prognosis) | 1-5 |
| • Mucinous /squamous | <2 |
| *Other* | 20–40 |
| • Squamous cell carcinoma | 20 |
| • Mixed types (adenoacanthomas, adenosquamous carcinoma) | <10 |
| • Undifferentiated carcinoma | <10 |

*Endometrial Hyperplasia*
- Simple hyperplasia: glandular-cystic, no atypia
- Complex hyperplasia: adenomatous hyperplasia grade I and II, low- to medium-grade hyperplasia without atypia
- Simple *atypical* hyperplasia: precancerous lesion, carcinoma risk 5–10%
- Complex *atypical* hyperplasia: precancerous lesion, carcinoma risk 30%

*Metastatic Spread*
- Local: peritoneal space
- Lymphatic: pelvic and para-aortic lymph nodes
- Hematogenous: lung, liver, bones

**Class:**     **TNM staging of endometrial carcinoma[a]**

| | |
|---|---|
| *T* | *Primary Tumor* |
| TX | Primary tumor cannot be assessed |
| T0 | No evidence of primary tumor |
| Tis | Carcinoma in situ |
| T1 | Tumor confined to corpus uteri |
| | A: tumor limited to endometrium |
| | B: tumor invades ≤ 50% of myometrium |
| | C: tumor invades > 50% of myometrium |
| T2 | Tumor invades cervix but does not extend beyond uterus |
| | A: endocervical glandular involvement |
| | B: cervical stromal invasion |
| T3 | Tumor infiltration beyond uterus |
| | A: tumor involves serosa and/or adnexa |
| | B: vaginal involvement |
| T4 | Tumor invades bladder and/or bowel |
| *N* | *Regional Lymph Nodes* |
| NX | Regional lymph nodes cannot be assessed |
| N0 | No regional lymph node metastasis |
| N1 | Metastasis to regional lymph nodes (pelvic, para-aortic) |
| *M* | *Distant Metastasis* |
| MX | Distant metastasis cannot be assessed |
| M0 | No distant metastasis |
| M1 | Distant metastasis (excluding vagina, pelvic serosa, adnexa) including intraabdominal lymph nodes without paraaortic and/or inguinal lymph nodes |
| *G* | *Differentiation Grade* |
| G1 | ≤ 5% solid tumor components |
| G2 | 6–50% solid tumor components |
| G3 | > 50% solid tumor components |

[a] Exact classification requires surgical staging with hysterectomy and salpingo-oophorectomy

**FIGO Staging and prognosis of endometrial carcinoma (1998)**

| FIGO stage | TNM classification | | | Overall survival (%) | | |
|---|---|---|---|---|---|---|
| | T | N | M | 1 year | 2 years | 3 years |
| 0 | Tis | N0 | M0 | > 98 | > 95 | > 90 |
| IA | T1a | N0 | M0 | 98 | 96 | 90 |
| IB | T1b | N0 | M0 | 98 | 96 | 90 |
| IC | T1c | N0 | M0 | 96 | 91 | 81 |
| IIA | T2a | N0 | M0 | 95 | 89 | 80 |
| IIB | T2b | N0 | M0 | 95 | 88 | 72 |
| IIIA | T3a | N0 | M0 | 88 | 77 | 63 |
| IIIB | T3b | N0 | M0 | 77 | 62 | 39 |

**FIGO Staging and prognosis of endometrial carcinoma (1998)** (*continued*)

| FIGO stage | TNM classification | | | Overall survival (%) | | |
|---|---|---|---|---|---|---|
| | T | N | M | 1 year | 2 years | 3 years |
| IIIC | T1-3 | N1 | M0 | 87 | 70 | 51 |
| IVA | T4 | Any N | M0 | 51 | 40 | 20 |
| IVB | Any T | Any N | M1 | 48 | 32 | 17 |

**Sy:**  Early symptoms are menorrhagia, metrorrhagia, postmenopausal bleeding.

**Dg:**  *Medical History, Physical Examination*
- Medical history including risk factors
- Physical examination including gynecological examination, lymph node status

*Laboratory Tests*
- Complete blood count, ESR, electrolytes, liver / renal function tests, coagulation status, urinary status
- Tumor markers CA 125 and CEA (monitoring of disease course with adenocarcinomas)

*Histology*
- Histological confirmation of diagnosis by endometrial biopsy, hysteroscopy, or fractionated curettage (abrasion)

*Imaging*
- Ultrasound (transvaginal and abdominal), chest x-ray
- MRI abdomen, possibly abdominal CT
- Cystoscopy, rectoscopy (if suspected tumor infiltration)
- Intravenous pyelography (if invasion of parametrium suspected)

**Dd:**
- Glandular-cystic endometrial hyperplasia, endometrial polyps
- Hormone-induced dysfunctional uterine hemorrhage
- Uterine myoma, endometriosis, internal adenomyosis

**Th:**  **Treatment Concept**

1. Surgery is the first-line treatment of choice in stages I–III and is performed with curative intent.
2. In stage IIIB with vaginal involvement and stage IVA, surgery alone is usually not curative — combination with radiotherapy, possibly chemotherapy.
3. Palliative chemotherapy is used in cases of stage IVB disease and metastasis.

**Surgical Treatment**

*Technique*
Hysterectomy, bilateral adnexectomy, frozen section analysis (histology, grading, depth of myometrial invasion, lymphangitis carcinomatosa, cervical involvement, adnexal infiltration).

*Lymphadenectomy (Pelvic and Paraaortic Lymph Nodes)*
Decision to carry out lymphadenectomy (pelvic and paraaortic lymph nodes) is based on the following risk factors: stage IC–IVA, G2–3, tumor size > 2 cm, clear cell and serous adenocarcinomas, adenocarcinoma with squamous cell differentiation, malignant Müllerian mixed tumor.

### Surgical Treatment According to Disease Stage
- *Stage I:* abdominal hysterectomy, bilateral adnexectomy, lymphadenectomy (pelvic, paraaortic) according to risk factors
- *Stage II:* extended radical hysterectomy (Wertheim), bilateral adnexectomy, lymphadenectomy (pelvic and paraaortic)
- *Stage III:* hysterectomy, bilateral adnexectomy, lymphadenectomy (pelvic, paraaortic), omentectomy, colpectomy (partial or complete)
- *Stage IVA:* anterior and/or posterior exenteration, alternatively (with contraindications to surgery) percutaneous irradiation of the true pelvis
- *Stage IVB:* multimodal therapy, combination of hysterectomy, surgical tumor reduction and radiotherapy as well as chemotherapy

## Radiotherapy

### Primary Radiotherapy
- Even in inoperable cases, radiotherapy at an early stage with curative intent
- *Stages I–III:* combination of brachytherapy and percutaneous radiotherapy
- Stage IVA: primary percutaneous radiotherapy if surgical treatment not applicable

### Adjuvant Radiotherapy
The benefit of adjuvant radiotherapy has not been established.

### Intravaginal Brachytherapy
Postoperative brachytherapy prolongs relapse-free interval (incidence of local relapse reduced in stage I from 7% to 2%) but not overall survival.

### Radiotherapy According to Disease Stage
- *Stages IA–IB:* only with unfavorable prognostic factors (G2, G3, clear cell and serous adenocarcinoma, adenocarcinoma with squamous cell differentiation, malignant Müllerian mixed tumor)
- *Stage IC:* brachytherapy; in combination with percutaneous radiotherapy unless lymphadenectomy; with lymph node involvement: postoperative radiotherapy, benefits of percutaneous radiotherapy not established. *ATTENTION:* high risk of intestinal complications and lymphedema
- *Stages IIA, IIB, III:* adjuvant radiotherapy depending on surgical radicality and overall tumor expansion
- Stage IVa: total tumor resection prior to brachytherapy, alternatively combination of brachytherapy and percutaneous radiotherapy

## Systemic Treatment

### Endocrine Therapy
- Endocrine therapy with medroxyprogesterone acetate (MPA) is first-line treatment of metastatic endometrial carcinomas with progesterone receptor expression (after surgical resection of the primary lesion); response rate 90%, possible long-term remission; response rate in receptor-negative metastases: 5–10%; dose: medroxyprogesterone acetate (MPA) 100–300 mg/day p.o.
- Endometrial hyperplasia (without atypia) or simple atypical hyperplasia are also treated with gestagens (MPA); after 3 months, examination with abrasion and hysteroscopy

### Chemotherapy
- *Adjuvant chemotherapy:* indicated with clear cell and serous-papillary endometrial carcinomas (cisplatin, paclitaxel or PAC protocol)
- *Palliative chemotherapy:* with metastatic endometrial carcinomas without progesterone receptor expression; initial response is followed by rapid development of resistance to chemotherapy
- In stage III or IV disease with residual tumors < 2 cm following resection, chemotherapy with doxorubicin and cisplatin is superior to external beam radiotherapy

## Chemotherapy Protocols

### Postoperative

| "PAC" ▶ Protocol 12.4.1 | | | *Start next cycle on day 22* |
|---|---|---|---|
| Cisplatin | 50 mg/m²/day | i.v. | Day 1 |
| Doxorubicin | 50 mg/m²/day | i.v. | Day 1 |
| Cyclophosphamide | 500 mg/m²/day | i.v. | Day 1 |

### Palliative

| "AC" ▶ Protocol 12.10.3 | | | *Start next cycle on day 22* |
|---|---|---|---|
| Doxorubicin | 60 mg/m²/day | i.v. | Day 1 |
| Cyclophosphamide | 600 mg/m²/day | i.v. | Day 6 |

| "Doxorubicin mono" | | | *Start next cycle on day 22* |
|---|---|---|---|
| Doxorubicin | 50 mg/m²/day | i.v. | Day 1 |

| "Doxorubicin + Cisplatin" | | | *Start next cycle on day 21; 7 cycles* |
|---|---|---|---|
| Doxorubicin | 60 mg/m²/day | i.v. | Day 1 |
| Cisplatin | 50 mg/m² | i.v. | Day 1 |

### Relapse

70–80% of relapses occur within the first 2–3 years after treatment; if discovered at an early stage and particularly with vaginal relapse → repeated surgery combined with radiotherapy (unless previous radiotherapy). Hormone therapy if surgical treatment not possible; response to gestagen therapy dependent on receptor status. Chemotherapy, if neither surgical treatment nor radiotherapy are applicable.

**Prg:**

### Prognostic Factors
- Stage, histology, grading, depth of endometrial invasion
- Lymphangitis carcinomatosa
- Lymph node metastasis, extrauterine manifestation
- Hormone receptor status, p53 expression, HER2/neu (c-erbB2) expression

**Ref:**

1. Amant F, Moermann P, Timmermann D et al. Endometrial cancer. Lancet 2005;366:491–505
2. Carey MS, Gawlik C, Fung-Kee-Fung M et al. Systematic review of systemic therapy for advanced or recurrent endometrial cancer. Gynecol Oncol 2006;101:158–67
3. Fleming GF. Systemic chemotherapy for uterine carcinoma: metastatic and adjuvant. J Clin Oncol 2007;25:2983–90
4. Hecht JL, Mutter Gl. Molecular and pathologic aspects of endometrial carcinogenesis. J Clin Oncol 2006;24:4783–91
5. Humber CE, Tierney JF, Symonds RP et al. Chemotherapy for advanced, recurrent or metastatic endometrial cancer: a systematic review of Cochrane collaboration. Ann Oncol 2007;18:409–20
6. Markman M. Hormonal therapy of endometrial cancer. Eur J Cancer 2005;41:673–5

7.  Million Women Study Collaborators. Endometrial cancer and hormone-replacement therapy in the Million Women Study. Lancet 2005;365:1543–51
8.  Polyzos NP, Pavlidis N, Paraskevaidis E et al. Randomized evidence on chemotherapy and hormonal therapy regimens for advanced endometrial cancer. Eur J Cancer 2006;42:319–26

**Web:**

1.  http://www.nlm.nih.gov/medlineplus/uterinecancer.html          MedlinePlus
2.  http://www.cancer.gov/cancertopics/types/endometrial          NCI Cancer Topics
3.  http://www.mayoclinic.com/health/endometrial-cancer/DS00306          Mayo Clinic
4.  http://www.emedicine.com/MED/topic2832.htm          E-medicine

## 8.4.9    Uterine Sarcoma

**C.F. Waller, I.B. Runnebaum**

**Def:**    Malignant mesenchymal tumor of the uterus arising from the endometrial lining of the uterus or the myometrium.

**ICD-10:**    C55

**Ep:**    Rare, incidence 1–2 cases/100,000 women/year; age peak 55–60 years; high mortality rate due to aggressive growth and rapid hematogenous and lymphatic metastasis.

**Pg:**    Not yet resolved; previous pelvic radiotherapy constitutes a risk factor; in rare cases, malignant transformation of leiomyomas (0.7%).

**Path:**    ***Histopathological Classification of Mesenchymal Tumors of the Uterus***
- Mixed epithelial stromal cell sarcomas (adenosarcomas, carcinosarcomas, malignant mixed Müllerian tumors, MMT), 50% of cases
- Leiomyosarcoma (LMS, originating from uterine muscle), 35% of cases
- Endometrial stromal cell sarcomas (ESS), 10% of cases

**Class:**    Exact classification requires surgical staging; staging according to the FIGO classification of endometrial cancer (▶ Chap. 8.4.8).

**FIGO Staging of Uterine Sarcoma (1988)**

| Stage | Characterization |
|-------|------------------|
| I | Tumor limited to body of the uterus |
| II | Infiltration of the cervix |
| III | Tumor limited to true pelvis |
| IV | Extrapelvic distant metastases |

***Metastatic Spread***
- Local: peritoneal metastasis
- Lymphatic: pelvic → paraaortic → mediastinal lymph nodes
- Hematogenous: lung, liver, bone, CNS

**Sy:**
- Early symptoms: abnormal vaginal bleeding
- Pain, vaginal discharge, pelvic pressure

**Dg:**    ***Medical History, Physical Examination***
- Physical examination including gynecological examination, lymph node status

***Laboratory Tests***
- Complete blood count, electrolytes, liver / renal function tests, coagulation tests, urinanalysis
- Tumor markers: increased CA 125 in patients with malignant mixed Müllerian tumor

***Histology***
- Fractionated curettage for confirmation of diagnosis in carcinosarcomas. Purely mesenchymal tumors (leiomyosarcomas) in early stages are usually diagnosed incidentally after hysterectomy

### Imaging
- Transvaginal and abdominal ultrasound
- Chest x-ray, thoracic CT, abdominal MRI
- Cystoscopy, proctosigmoidoscopy (if suspected tumor infiltration)
- Intravenous pyelography (urinary obstruction, anatomical anomalies of the kidneys and the urinary tract)

**Th:** Due to low incidence of the disease, no specific systemic treatment concept has yet been established.

### Surgical Treatment
- *Objectives:* complete tumor resection, surgical staging
- *Technique:* hysterectomy, bilateral extirpation of the adnexa, pelvic and paraaortic lymphadenectomy (in cases of extrauterine tumor manifestation: lymphadenectomy of any conspicuous lymph nodes)

### Radiotherapy
Palliative indication only; pelvic radiotherapy, 50–60 Gy; efficacy of adjuvant radiotherapy not yet established.

### Chemotherapy
Palliative indication only; efficacy of adjuvant chemotherapy not established.
- *Carcinosarcomas:* combination chemotherapy with ifosfamide, cisplatin, and doxorubicin, or monotherapy with paclitaxel
- *LMS:* palliative therapy with doxorubicin (response rate 30–40%) or with combination of gemcitabine + docetaxel (response rate approximately 50%)

### Relapse
Mainly local relapses followed by lung metastases and abdominal manifestations; with local relapse: where applicable, repeat surgery and/or radiotherapy or palliative chemotherapy. MMT and ESS: ifosfamide monotherapy (or combination ifosfamide + carboplatin), however: no proven survival advantage of combination therapy.

### Chemotherapy Protocols

| *"Ifosfamide + Cisplatin"* | | | *Start next cycle on days 22–29* |
|---|---|---|---|
| Cisplatin | 20 mg/m$^2$/day | i.v. | Days 1–5 |
| Ifosfamide | 1,500 mg/m$^2$ | i.v. | Days 1–5 |

| *"CAV"* | | | *Start next cycle on day 29* |
|---|---|---|---|
| Cisplatin | 50 mg/m$^2$/day | i.v. | Day 1 |
| Doxorubicin | 50 mg/m$^2$/day | i.v. | Day 1 |
| Etoposide, VP-16 | 100 mg/m$^2$/day | i.v. | Days 1, 2 |

| *"Gemcitabine + Docetaxel"* | | | *Start next cycle on day 22* |
|---|---|---|---|
| Gemcitabine | 900 mg/m$^2$/day | i.v. | Days 1+8 |
| Docetaxel | 100 mg/m$^2$/day | i.v. | Day 8 |

| *"Doxorubicin mono"* | | | Start next cycle on day 22 |
|---|---|---|---|
| Doxorubicin | 50 mg/m²/day | i.v. | Day 1 |


| *"Ifosfamide mono"* | | | Start next cycle on day 29 |
|---|---|---|---|
| Ifosfamide | 1,500 mg/m²/day | i.v. | Days 1–5 |


| *"Paclitaxel mono"* | | | Start next cycle on day 22 |
|---|---|---|---|
| Paclitaxel | 175 mg/m²/day | i.v. | Day 1 |

**Prg:**

### Prognostic Factors
- Stage, histology, grading, mitotic rate (leiomyosarcomas)

### Five-year Survival
- Leiomyosarcoma: 15–25%
- Endometrial stromal cell sarcoma (high-grade): 0–50%
- Endometrial stromal cell sarcoma (low-grade, stage I): 98%
- Adenosarcoma: 25%
- Malignant mixed Müllerian tumor: 40–50%

**Ref:**

1. Curtin JP, Blessing JA, Soper JT et al. Paclitaxel in the treatment of carcinosarcoma of the uterus: a gynecologic oncology group study. Gynecol Oncol 2001;83:268–70
2. Kempson RL, Hendrickson MR. Smooth muscle, endometrial stromal, and mixed Mullerian tumors of the uterus. Mod Pathol 2000;13:328–42
3. Nordal RN, Kjorstad KE, Stenwig AE et al. Leiomyosarcoma (LMS) and endometrial stromal sarcoma (ESS) of the uterus. Int J Gynecol Cancer 1993;3:110–15
4. Sutton GP, Brunetto VL, Kilgore L et al. A phase III trial of ifosfamide with or without cisplatin in carcinosarcoma of the uterus. Gynecol Oncol 2000;79:147–53
5. Toyoshima M, Akahira J, Matsunaga G et al. Clinical experience with combination paclitaxel and carboplatin therapy for advanced or recurrent carcinosarcoma of the uterus. Gynecol Oncol 2004;94:774–8
6. Van Rijswijk REN, Vermorken JB, Reed N et al. Cisplatin, doxorubicin and ifosfamide in carcinosarcoma of the female genital tract. Eur J Cancer 2003;39:481–7
7. Yamada SD, Burger RA, Brewster WR et al. Pathologic variables and adjuvant therapy as predictors of recurrence and survival for patients with surgically evaluated carcinosarcoma of the uterus. Cancer 2000;88:2782–6

**Web:**

1. http://www.cancer.org/docroot/cri/cri_2_3x.asp?dt=63      Am Cancer Soc
2. http://www.cancer.gov/cancertopics/types/uterinesarcoma      NCI Cancer Topics

## 8.4.10    Vaginal Cancer

### C.F. Waller, K. Henne, I.B. Runnebaum

**Def:** Malignant tumors of the vagina, usually squamous cell carcinomas.

**ICD-10:** C52

**Ep:** Incidence of vaginal cancer: 4 cases/100,000 women/year; decreasing. Median age at presentation: 60–65 years; incidence of VAIN (vaginal intraepithelial neoplasia) 2/100,000 women/year.

**Pg:**
### Risk Factors
- Vaginal intraepithelial neoplasia (VAIN): incidence increasing, median age decreasing; low malignant potential; rarely transformation into vaginal cancer (< 5%)
- History of cervical neoplasia (approximately 30% of patients): frequently following radiation treatment; possibly association with HPV infection
- Low socioeconomic status
- Long-term mechanical irritation, e.g., vaginal diaphragm
- *Special case:* vaginal clear cell adenocarcinoma: young women (15–25 years): approximately 60% of cases correlated to diethylstilbestrol (DES) exposure in the first trimester of pregnancy of the patient's mother

**Path:**
### Histology

| Type | Frequency (%) |
|---|---|
| Squamous cell cancer | >80 |
| Adenocarcinoma | 5–10 |
| Melanoma | 3 |
| Sarcoma | 3 |

### Location
Squamous cell carcinoma: mainly located in the proximal third of the vagina (52%) and the anterior vaginal wall (58%), ulcerating endo- or exophytic tumors

### Metastasic Spread
- Vaginal metastasis due to cervical cancer, vulvar cancer, endometrial cancer or infiltration "per continuitatem" from the rectum or bladder: per definition not classified as vaginal cancer
- Squamous cell carcinomas: usually local invasion, lymphatic or hematogenous metastasis
- Regional lymph node involvement: upper parts of the vagina: obturatory and internal iliac lymph nodes (involvement similar to cervical cancer), lower parts of vagina: inguinal and external iliac lymph nodes (similar to vulvar cancer)
- Adenocarcinoma: metastases to pelvic lymph nodes
- Hematogenous metastasis: lung, liver, bone

**Class:**
### TNM staging of Vaginal Cancer (2002)

| *T* | *Primary Tumor* |
|---|---|
| TX | Primary tumor cannot be assessed |
| T0 | No evidence of primary tumor |
| Tis | Carcinoma in situ, intraepithelial neoplasia (VAIN) |
| T1 | Tumor confined to the vaginal wall |

**Class:**   TNM staging of Vaginal Cancer ( 2002) *(continued)*

| | |
|---|---|
| T2 | Infiltration of submucosa and parametrium |
| T3 | Infiltration of the pelvic wall |
| T4 | Tumor invades mucosa of bladder / rectum, tumor invades beyond the pelvis |
| *N* | *Lymph Node Involvement* |
| NX | Regional lymph nodes cannot be assessed |
| N0 | Regional lymph nodes without metastases |
| N1 | Metastasis to regional lymph nodes |
| *M* | *Distant Metastasis* |
| MX | Distant metastasis cannot be assessed |
| M0 | No distant metastasis |
| M1 | Distant metastasis |

**FIGO Staging and prognosis of vaginal carcinoma (1998)**

| Stage | TNM classification | | | Survival rates (%) | | |
|---|---|---|---|---|---|---|
| | T | N | M | 1 year | 2 years | 3 years |
| 0 | Tis | N0 | M0 | 100 | 100 | 63 |
| I | T1 | N0 | M0 | 92 | 88 | 73 |
| II | T2 | N0 | M0 | 78 | 64 | 51 |
| III | T3 | N0 | M0 | 63 | 40 | 33 |
| | T1–3 | N1 | M0 | | | |
| IVA | T4 | Any N | M0 | 48 | 31 | 20 |
| IVB | Any T | Any N | M1 | 33 | 0 | 0 |

**Sy:**   80–90% of patients with invasive carcinoma show typical symptoms:
- Irregular vaginal bleeding (50–60%), often postcoital
- Pain in perineum, bladder, or rectum
- Vaginal discharge, palpable tumor

**Dg:**   *Medical History, Physical Examination*
- Medical history including social background
- Physical examination: local inspection (vulva, urethra, introitus, vagina, ectocervix, perineum, anus); palpation of rectum, groins, lymph node status

*Laboratory Tests*
- Routine laboratory tests including LDH, urinary status
- Tumor markers: SCC (only to monitor the disease course)

*Imaging*
- Pelvic / abdominal ultrasound, chest x-ray, intravenous pyelogram
- Optional: abdominal / pelvic CT or MRI; if applicable, vaginal or rectal ultrasound
- In case of bone pain: bone scan, conventional skeletal x-ray

*Histology*
- *Always biopsy* (depth of invasion is most important prognostic criterion): deep punch biopsy preferable (particularly in cases of Paget's disease)

**Th:**      **Vaginal Intraepithelial Neoplasia (VAIN)**

### Therapy Options
- *Surgical treatment:* local excision, partial / total colpectomy, $CO_2$ laser ablation
- *Topical administration of 5-FU*
- *Intracavitary radiotherapy*

Factors determining choice of treatment: previous treatment, multifocal spread, performance status, risk of anesthesia. Relapse risk: approximately 20%, independent of treatment.

### Invasive Vaginal Carcinoma

### Treatment Concept
Standard treatment is surgery, in cases of advanced disease: radiochemotherapy. Doses of > 60 Gy are required despite likelihood of local complications (especially skin ulcers); individualized concepts according to location, size, and clinical stage of the tumor. Important factors:
- Invasion of bladder, urethra, and rectum
- Anatomical facts which may necessitate exenteration to allow wide resection
- Psychosexual factors

### Stage I
- Proximal vagina, < 2 cm in diameter: radical hysterectomy with partial resection of the vagina and bilateral pelvic lymphadenectomy; alternatively: intracavitary radiotherapy
- Median / distal vagina: radiotherapy

### Stage I (> 2 cm in diameter) and Stages II–IV
- External radiotherapy with/without intravaginal or interstitial radiotherapy with/without chemotherapy (5-FU + cisplatin) as radiosensitizer
- Alternatively in stage II patients: radical colpectomy or pelvic exenteration in combination with radiotherapy

**Prg:**      Most important factor: clinical tumor stage (size, depth of invasion, lymph node involvement) at presentation. Survival rates depending on FIGO stages (see above).

**Px:**      **Early Prevention / Screening**
- Primary prevention: gynecological examination from 30 years of age
- Other screening methods: only indicated with risk factors (see above): inspection, vulvo- / vaginoscopy, cytology, confirmation of diagnosis by punch biopsy or excision of tissue samples (high-risk groups)

**Ref:**
1. Creasman WT. Vaginal cancers. Curr Opin Obstet Gynecol. 2005:17:71–6
2. Grigsby PW. Vaginal cancer. Curr Treat Options Oncol 2002;3:125–30

**Web:**
1. http://www.nlm.nih.gov/medlineplus/vaginalcancer.html      MedlinePlus
2. http://www.cancer.gov/cancertopics/types/vaginal      NCI Cancer Topics

## 8.4.11    Vulvar Cancer

**I.B. Runnebaum, K. Henne, C.F. Waller**

**Def:**   Malignant tumors of the vulva, usually squamous cell carcinomas.

**ICD-10:**   C51.-

**Ep:**   Incidence of vulvar cancer 1–2/100,000 women/year; median age at presentation: 60–80 years. Incidence of vulvar intraepithelial neoplasia (VIN) 7/100,000 women/year.

**Pg:**

### Risk Factors
- HPV infection ("human papilloma virus"), usually HPV-16, HPV-18
- Chronic infections, lichen sclerosis
- Immune deficiencies, immunosuppression, HIV infections
- Genetic defects, e.g., p53 mutations

### Vulvar Intraepithelial Neoplasia (VIN)
Precancerous lesion of the vulva with intraepithelial neoplasia, mainly affecting labia minora; particularly in younger patients (40–60 years), incidence increasing; human papilloma virus (HPV) present in 80–90% of cases; staging according to extent of dysplasia.

| Grade of VIN | Dysplasia |
|---|---|
| I | Mild dysplasia |
| II | Moderate dysplasia |
| III | Severe dysplasia, carcinoma in situ (CIS), substitution of squamous epithelium with atypical cells, usually multifocal |

### Vulvar Carcinomas and HPV Infection
- HPV-positive tumors: women between 35 and 55 years of age; often multifocal disease; commonly associated with VIN. Risk factors similar to cervical cancer: smoking, number of sexual partners, first intercourse at an early age, low socioeconomic status; often in combination with cervical and anal cancer
- HPV-negative tumors: average age 65–85 years; usually unifocal; associated with vulvar infections, lichen sclerosis

**Path:**

### Histology of Invasive Vulvar Carcinomas

| Type | Frequency (%) |
|---|---|
| *Keratinized Squamous Cell Carcinoma* | > 90 |
| • Highly differentiated | 70 |
| • Moderately differentiated | 20 |
| • Anaplasia | 10 |
| *Other Tumors* | |
| • Verrucous carcinoma | 5 |
| • Basal cell carcinoma, transitional cell carcinoma | Rare |
| • Malignant melanoma, sarcoma | Rare |

### Spread

- Often multicentric, polypous, or ulcerating
- Most common location: labia majora > labia minora
- Local spread with invasion of adjacent organs
- Mainly lymphatic metastasis to superficial inguinal and pelvic lymph nodes
- Hematogenous metastasis: lung, liver, bones

**Class:**

**TNM staging of Vulvar Cancer (2002)**

| | |
|---|---|
| **T** | **Primary Tumor** |
| TX | Primary tumor cannot be assessed |
| T0 | No evidence of primary tumor |
| Tis | Carcinoma in situ |
| T1 | Tumor confined to vulva/perineum, ≤ 2 cm in greatest dimension |
| | A: stromal invasion ≤ 1 mm |
| | B: stromal invasion > 1 mm |
| T2 | Tumor confined to vulva/perineum, size > 2 cm in greatest dimension |
| T3 | Tumor invades lower urethra, vagina, or anus |
| T4 | Tumor invades bladder mucosa, rectal mucosa, upper urethra, or is fixed to pubic bone |
| **N** | **Lymph Node Involvement** |
| NX | Regional lymph nodes cannot be assessed |
| N0 | No regional lymph node metastasis |
| N1 | Unilateral regional lymph node metastasis |
| N2 | Bilateral regional lymph node metastasis |
| **M** | **Distant Metastasis** |
| MX | Distant metastasis cannot be assessed |
| M0 | No distant metastasis |
| M1 | Distant metastasis (including pelvic lymph nodes) |

**FIGO Staging and Prognosis of Vulvar Carcinoma (1998)**

| Stage | TNM classification | | | Survival rates (%) | | |
|---|---|---|---|---|---|---|
| | T | N | M | 1 year | 2 years | 3 years |
| 0 | Tis | N0 | M0 | > 98 | > 95 | > 92 |
| IA | T1A | N0 | M0 | 97 | 92 | 77 |
| IB | T1B | N0 | M0 | | | |
| II | T2 | N0 | M0 | 88 | 77 | 55 |
| III | T3 | N0 | M0 | 66 | 47 | 31 |
| | T1–3 | N1 | M0 | | | |
| IVA | T1–3 | N2 | M0 | 40 | 17 | |
| | T4 | Any N | M0 | | | |
| IVB | Any T | Any N | M1 | | | |

**Sy:** Approximately 50% of patients with invasive carcinoma are asymptomatic. Typical symptoms:
- Vulvar pruritus or burning sensation
- Visible lesions around the vulva
- In advanced stages: bleeding, palpable tumor, foul smelling discharge

**Dg:** *Medical History, Physical Examination*
1. Medical history including social background
2. Physical examination: local inspection (vulva, urethra, introitus, vagina, ectocervix, perineum, anus); rectal examination, groins, lymph node status

*Laboratory Tests*
- Routine laboratory tests including LDH, urinanalysis
- Tumor marker: SCC (only for monitoring of the disease course)

*Imaging*
- Pelvic / abdominal ultrasound, chest x-ray, intravenous pyelography
- Optional: abdominal / pelvic CT or MRI; if applicable, vaginal or rectal ultrasound
- In case of bone pain: bone scan, conventional skeletal x-ray

*Endoscopy*
- Cystoscopy / urethroscopy and rectoscopy
- Colposcopy (including 3% acetic acid or 1% toluidine blue staining)
- Cervical cytology, endocervical curettage

*Histology*
- Always biopsy (depth of invasion is most important prognostic criterion): deep punch biopsy, particularly in cases of Paget's disease (as often occult adenocarcinomas)

**Th:** **Vulvar Intraepithelial Neoplasia (VIN)**

*Therapy Options*
- Local excision
- "Skinning" vulvectomy in case of multifocal or large confluent lesions
- Laser ablation, particularly with VIN I–II (low morbidity, outpatient surgery, good esthetic results)
- Topical administration of 5-FU (> 50% treatment failure; indicated in immunodeficient patients) or imiquimod (81% response)
- Paget's disease: wide excision or simple vulvectomy (exclusion of invasive adenocarcinoma by surgery and subsequent histological assessment)

**Invasive Vulvar Carcinomas**

Standard treatment: surgery; in advanced stages radiochemotherapy. Radiotherapy doses > 60 Gy are required despite likelihood of local complications (especially skin ulcers).

*FIGO Stage IA (< 1 mm Invasion)*
- Standard treatment: radical local excision (wide excision, 1–2 cm safety margin)
- Low risk of inguinal lymph node metastases (< 1%) → no lymphadenectomy

*FIGO Stage IB (> 1 mm Invasion)*
- Standard treatment: radical local excision (wide excision) or radical vulvectomy with bilateral femoral and inguinal lymphadenectomy (risk of inguinal lymph node metastases ≥ 8%) in case of superficial central lesions
- Ipsilateral lymphadenectomy in case of lateral lesions (> 2 cm from clitoris, urethra, or posterior commissure); if one positive lymph node → contralateral lymphadenectomy, if ≥ 2 positive lymph nodes → pelvic lymphadenectomy via extraperitoneal lymphadenectomy

### FIGO Stage II
- Modified radical vulvectomy with bilateral femoral and inguinal lymphadenectomy ("triple incision technique")
- Adjuvant radiotherapy if positive inguinal lymph nodes (microscopically > 2 involved lymph nodes or clinically > 1 involved lymph node), penetration through the capsule or R1 or R2 resection

### FIGO Stage III/IV
- Radical vulvectomy with bilateral femoral and inguinal lymphadenectomy, if necessary with resection of involved neighboring organs or exenteration
- Due to high morbidity rates, downstaging with neoadjuvant combined radiochemotherapy (e.g., with 5-FU, cisplatin, MTX or mitomycin C) prior to surgery becomes increasingly important

### Relapse
- Local relapse: repeat surgery, possibly combined with radiotherapy
- Regional or systemic relapse: radiotherapy, chemotherapy

**Prg:** Most important factor: clinical tumor stage (size, depth of invasion, lymph node involvement) at presentation, also: tumor ploidy. Survival rates of FIGO stages: see above.

**Px:**
### Early Prevention / Screening
- Gynecological examination: in women from 30 years of age
- Other screening methods: only indicated with risk factors (see above): inspection, vulvo- / vaginoscopy, cytology, confirmation of diagnosis by punch biopsy or excision (high-risk groups)

**Ref:**
1. Coleman RL, Santoso JT. Vulvar carcinoma. Curr Treat Options Oncol 2000;1:177–90
2. Fonseca-Moutinho JA. Recurrent vulvar cancer. Clin Obstet Gynecol 2005;48:879–83
3. Geisler JP, Manahan KJ, Buller RE. Neoadjuvant chemotherapy in vulvar cancer: avoiding primary exenteration. Gynecol Oncol 2006;100:53–7
4. Hakim AA, Terada KY. Sentinel node dissection in vulvar cancer. Curr Treat Options Oncol 2006;7:85–91
5. Montana GS. Carcinoma of the vulva: combined modality treatment. Curr Treat Options Oncol 2004;5:85–95
6. Rouzier R, Haddad B, Atallah D et al. Surgery for vulvar cancer. Clin Obstet Gynecol 2005;48:869–78
7. Tyring SK. Vulvar squamous cell carcinoma: guidelines for early diagnosis and treatment. Am J Obstet Gynecol 2003;189(3 suppl):S17–23
8. Van Seters M, Van Beurden M, Ten Kate FBW et al. Treatment of vulvar intraepithelial neoplasia with topical imiquimod. N Engl J Med 2008;358:1465–73

**Web:**
1. http://www.nlm.nih.gov/medlineplus/vulvarcancer.html       MedlinePlus
2. http://www.cancer.gov/cancertopics/types/vulvar       NCI Cancer Topics
3. http://www.cancer.org/docroot/cri/cri_2_3x.asp?dt=45       Am Cancer Soc
4. http://www.emedicine.com/med/topic3296.htm       E-medicine

## 8.5     Tumors of the Male Reproductive System

## 8.5.1     Testicular Tumors

**C.F. Waller**

**Def:**     Malignancies of the testicles

**ICD-10:**     C62.

**Ep:**     Incidence: 7 cases/100,000 men/year; 1% of all malignancies in men; most common malignant tumor in men aged 20–40 years; age peak: 20–25 and 55–65 years; in approximately 2% of cases bilateral primary testicular tumors

**Pg:**     *Risk Factors*
- Mal- / undescended testicles, often bilaterally (40 times higher risk). *ATTENTION:* in case of one maldescended testis, the *contralateral normally descended* testis is also at increased risk of malignant transformation
- Cryptorchidism (risk increase by 10–40%, in 60% seminomas)
- Orchitis, trauma, ionizing radiation
- Family history (4–10 times increased risk if father or brother are affected)
- After contralateral testicular tumor

*Genetic Defects*
- *Structural aberrations:* inversions, duplications, deletions; Inv(12p) in > 80% of tumors, dupl(12p) in 20%; rare: del(12q12-24), del(6q14-q25), del(7q11-q36)
- *Numerical aberrations:* mono- and trisomy, particularly of chromosomes 4, 5, 8, 9, 11, 13, 18, 21

**Path:**     *Histology*
- Testicular tumors mostly originate from testicular cell populations (seminomatous and non-seminomatous); seminomatous tumors occur mainly in patients over 30 years of age
- Other types of tumors (lymphoma, metastases, etc.) occur mainly in older patients (> 60 years)

**Histological Classification**

| Type | Frequency (%) |
| --- | --- |
| *Seminomatous Germ Cell Tumors* | 40–50 |
| • Classic or typical seminoma | 35–40 |
| • Anaplastic seminoma | 3–5 |
| • Spermatocytic seminoma | 3–5 |
| • Seminoma with giant cells | < 1 |
| *Non-seminomatous Germ Cell Tumors* | 50–60 |
| • Intermediate malignant teratoma | 20–25 |
| • Embryonal carcinoma | 15–20 |
| • Other mixed tumors (some with seminoma tissue) | 8 |
| • Differentiated teratoma | 3 |
| • Choriocarcinoma | 3 |
| • Yolk sac tumor (endodermal sinus tumor) | 3 |
| *Other Testicular Tumors* | Rare |
| • Sertoli cell tumor, Leydig cell tumor | |
| • Malignant mesothelioma of the tunica vaginalis | |

### Metastatic Spread

- Regional lymph nodes: abdominal, para-aortic, paracaval and parapelvic; following scrotal or inguinal surgery also inguinal lymph node involvement
- Spread via retroperitoneal lymph nodes → to hilar lymph nodes
- In 10% of cases, hematogenous metastasis: lung, liver, skeleton, CNS

**Class:**      **TNM staging of Testicular Tumors (2002)**

| | |
|---|---|
| *T* | *Primary Tumor* |
| pTX | Primary tumor cannot be assessed (or if no radical orchiectomy is performed) |
| pT0 | No evidence of primary tumor (e.g., histological scar in testis) |
| pTis | Intratubular germ cell neoplasia (carcinoma in situ) |
| pT1 | Tumor limited to the testis and epididymis without vascular / lymphatic invasion; tumor may invade tunica albuginea, but not tunica vaginalis |
| pT2 | Tumor limited to testis and epididymis with vascular or lymphatic tumor invasion, or tumor extending through tunica albuginea with involvement of tunica vaginalis |
| pT3 | Tumor invades the spermatic cord with or without vascular / lymphatic invasion |
| pT4 | Tumor invades the scrotum with or without vascular / lymphatic invasion |
| *N* | *Clinical Lymph Node Involvement* |
| NX | Regional lymph nodes cannot be assessed |
| N0 | No regional lymph node metastasis |
| N1 | Regional lymph node metastasis ≤ 2 cm in diameter, and ≤ 5 positive nodes, none > 2 cm |
| N2 | Regional lymph node metastasis > 2 cm but ≤ 5cm in diameter, or multiple lymph nodes > 2 cm but ≤ 5 cm |
| N3 | Regional lymph node metastasis > 5 cm in diameter |
| *pN* | *Pathological Lymph Node Involvement* |
| pNX | Regional lymph nodes cannot be assessed |
| pN0 | No regional lymph node metastasis |
| pN1 | Lymph node metastasis ≤ 2 cm in diameter, and ≤ 5 positive nodes, none > 2 cm |
| pN2 | Lymph node metastasis > 2 cm but ≤ 5 cm in diameter, or > 5 positive nodes, non > 5 cm in diameter |
| pN3 | Lymph node metastasis > 5 cm in diameter |
| *M* | *Distant Metastasis* |
| MX | Distant metastasis cannot be assessed |
| M0 | No distant metastasis |
| M1 | Distant metastasis |
| | a: Non-regional lymph nodes or pulmonary metastasis |
| | b: Distant metastasis other than to non-regional lymph nodes and lungs |
| *S* | *Serum Tumor Markers* |
| SX | Marker studies not performed |
| S0 | Marker levels within normal limits |
| S1 | LDH ≤ 1.5 × normal and β-HCG < 5,000 mIU/ml and AFP < 1,000 ng/ml |
| S2 | LDH 1.5–10 × normal or β-HCG 5,000–50,000 mIU/ml or AFP 1,000–10,000 ng/ml |
| S3 | LDH > 10 × normal or β-HCG > 50,000 mIU/ml or AFP > 10,000 ng/ml |

**AJCC Staging (2002)**

| Stage | TNM system | | | |
|-------|-----------|-----|-----|-----|
| 0 | pTis | N0 | M0 | S0, SX |
| I | pT1–4 | N0 | M0 | SX |
| IA | T1 | N0 | M0 | S0 |
| IB | T2–4 | N0 | M0 | S0 |
| IS | Any T | N0 | M0 | S1–3 |
| II | Any pT / T | N1–3 | M0 | SX |
| IIA | Any pT / T | N1 | M0 | S0–1 |
| IIB | Any pT / T | N2 | M0 | S0–1 |
| IIC | Any pT / T | N3 | M0 | S0–1 |
| III | Any pT / T | Any N | M1 | SX |
| IIIA | Any pT / T | Any N | M1–1a | S0–1 |
| IIIB | Any pT / T | N1–3 | M0–1a | S2 |
| IIIC | Any pT / T | N1–3 | M0–1a | S3 |
| | | | M1b | Any S |

**Risk categories for advanced germ cell tumors (International Germ Cell Cancer Collaborative Group, IGCCCG, 1997)**

| Prognosis group | Frequency / characterization | Prognosis / markers |
|-----------------|------------------------------|---------------------|
| *"Good risk"* | | |
| *NSGCT* | *56% of NSGCT patients* | *Five-year PFS 98%, OS 92%* |
| | Testicular / retroperitoneal primary tumor | AFP < 1,000 ng/ml |
| | No extrapulmonary visceral metastases | HCG < 5,000 mIU/ml |
| | | LDH < 1.5 × normal |
| *Seminoma* | *90% of seminoma patients* | *Five-year PFS 82%, OS 86%* |
| | Any primary location | Normal AFP |
| | No extrapulmonary visceral metastases | Any HCG, any LDH |
| *"Intermediate"* | | |
| *NSGCT* | *28% of NSGCT patients* | *Five-year PFS 75%, OS 80%* |
| | Testicular / retroperitoneal primary tumor | AFP 1,000–10,000 ng/ml |
| | No extrapulmonary visceral metastases | HCG 5,000–50,000 mIU/ml |
| | | LDH 1.5–10 × normal |
| *Seminoma* | *10% of seminoma patients* | *Five-year PFS 67%, OS 72%* |
| | Any primary location | Normal AFP |
| | Extrapulmonary visceral metastases | Any HCG, any LDH |
| *"High risk"* | | |
| *NSGCT* | *16% of NSGCT patients* | *Five-year PFS 41%, OS 48%* |
| | Mediastinal primary tumor | AFP > 10,000 ng/ml |
| | Extrapulmonary visceral metastases | HCG > 50,000 mIU/ml |
| | | LDH > 10 × normal |

*NSGCT* non-seminomatous germ cell tumors, *PFS* progression-free survival, *OS* overall survival

**Sy:**     *Caused by local invasion, hormone secretion, and metastases:*
- Painless swelling of the testis
- Pain in the scrotum, inguinal region, or lower abdomen (30–50%)
- Infertility (3%)
- Feeling of heaviness in the scrotum or change in the consistency of a testicle
- Gynecomastia (10%)
- Lumbar back pain, gastrointestinal discomfort (due to metastases)

**Dg:**     ### Medical History, Physical Examination
- Medical history including family history, maldescended testis
- Physical examination: local examination of the testis, lymphadenopathy, gynecomastia

### Laboratory Tests
- Routine laboratory tests, LDH, HBDH, alkaline phosphatase, renal function tests, urinary status
- Total testosterone, LH, FSH, possibly spermiogram / cryopreservation of sperm

### Imaging
- Mandatory: abdominal ultrasound including both testicles, chest x-ray, CT abdomen / pelvis, thoracic CT; patients allergic to contrast medium: MRI abdomen / pelvis
- Optional: MRI brain (if CNS involvement suspected), bone scan (if bone metastases suspected)
- Monitoring of disease course: PET (with seminomas; at the earliest 3–6 weeks after chemotherapy)

### Histology
- Bioptic or surgical histology of the affected testicle
- Contralateral testicular biopsy → diagnosis / exclusion of contralateral testicular intraepithelial neoplasia (TIN) or carcinoma in situ (Cis)

### Tumor Marker
AFP (α1 fetoprotein), ßHCG (human chorionic gonadotropin β), LDH; with seminomas: PLAP (placental alkaline phosphatase) optional. Determination:
- Prior to surgery: once
- After surgery: days 1, 5, 22
- During chemotherapy: before each chemotherapy cycle
- After chemotherapy: 3–4 weeks after the last cycle
- Follow up: at each check-up

**Tumor markers in different testicular tumor types**

| Tumor type | AFP | ßHCG | LDH |
|---|---|---|---|
| Seminoma | – | ± | + |
| Teratoma | + | ± | + |
| Embryonal carcinoma | + | ± | + |
| Choriocarcinoma | – | ++ | + |
| Yolk sac tumor | ++ | – | + |

*AFP* α1 fetoprotein, produced by yolk sac components, normal serum level < 15 ng/ml (1,200 U = 1 ng)
*ßHCG* human chorionic gonadotropin β, produced by chorionic cells, normal serum level in men < 5 U/l
*LDH* lactate dehydrogenase, – negative, ± not always detectable, + increased, ++ severely increased

During the initial 7–10 days after chemotherapy tumor marker levels may increase, which is usually followed by an exponential drop. Serum half-life: β-HCG 18–24 h, AFP 3–6 days.

**DD:**
- Hydrocele, varicocele, spermatocele, epididymitis, orchitis
- Inguinal hernia, hematoma, testicular torsion

**Co:**
- Hemorrhage, infarction, torsion

**Th:**

### Treatment Concept

1. Treatment of testicular cancer is dependent on the tumor type (seminomatous versus non-seminomatous), stage, risk group (IGCCCG classification), and the patient's performance status.
2. Sperm preservation: with patients wanting children, sperm should be preserved prior to treatment. All patients have to be educated about sperm preservation options and risks (e.g., treatment delay).
3. *Testicular Intraepithelial Neoplasia (TIN)*
   With TIN: increased risk of testicular cancer (in 70% of cases within 7 years). Therapy guidelines for TIN:
   - Patients with one testis (e.g., after orchiectomy of contralateral testis in cases of testicular tumor) and wanting children, sufficient residual spermiogenesis and good compliance: watch and wait.
   - Metastatic disease and planned chemotherapy: no primary radiotherapy of the TIN (increased toxicity for Leydig cells). Approximately 6 months after completion of chemotherapy: rebiopsy of the affected testicle → if TIN persists: radiotherapy (20 Gy)
   - Intact contralateral testicle: unilateral orchiectomy of the affected testicle

### Seminomatous Testicular Cancer

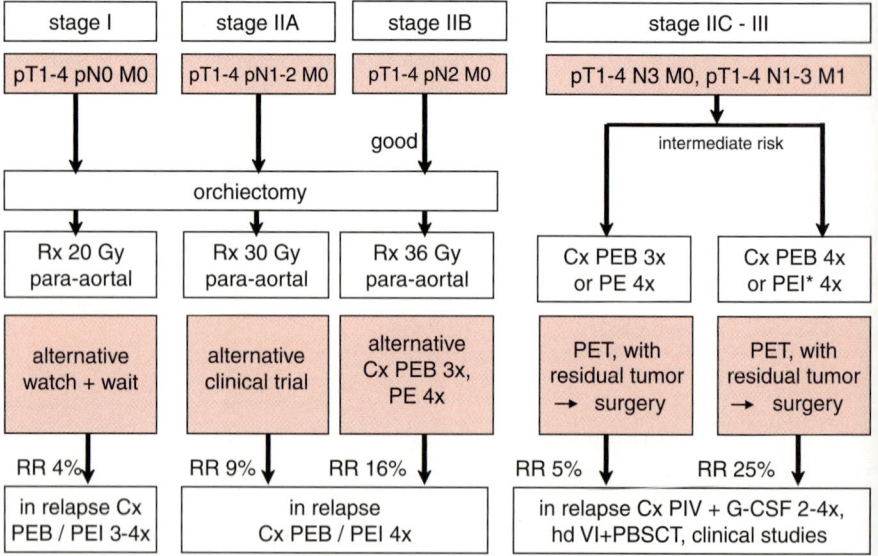

*Cx* chemotherapy, *Rx* radiotherapy, *RR* relapse risk, *PEB* cisplatin + etoposide + bleomycin, *PEI* cisplatin + etoposide + ifosfamide, *PET* positron emission tomography, *PBSCT* peripheral blood stem cell transplantation, hd high dose, *PIV* cisplatin ifosfamide + efoposide

### Treatment according to Disease Stage

- Stage I–IIB: high cure rates after surgical treatment and radiotherapy.
- Stage IIC–III: patients with extensive abdominal lymph node involvement (> 5 cm), invasion of the mediastinum, or visceral distant metastases require primary chemotherapy.
- Patients with increased AFP levels are treated like patients with non-seminomatous testicular cancer. Patients with increased HCG or LDH levels are treated according to the guidelines below.
- With residual tumor: PET scan after 4 weeks; negative PET scan: repeat PET scan after 6–8 weeks; with signs of proliferation: biopsy, possibly surgery. Detection of vital tumor cells: salvage chemotherapy.

## Non-seminomatous Germ Cell Tumors

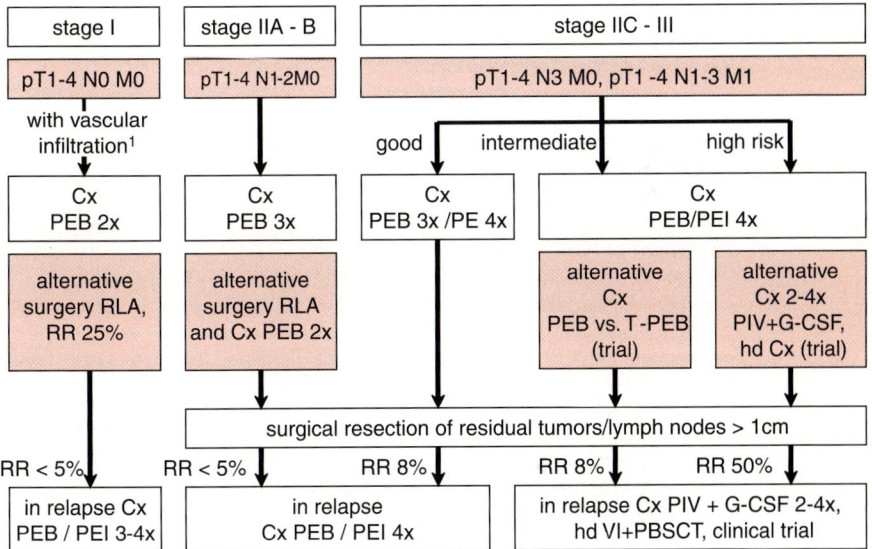

*Cx* chemotherapy, *hd Cx* high-dose chemotherapy, *RLA* retroperitoneal lymphadenectomy, *Rx* radiotherapy, *RR* relapse risk, *hd PIV* high-dose carboplatin + ifosfamide + etoposide, *PBSCT* peripheral blood stem cell transplantation, *PEB* cisplatin + etoposide + bleomycin, *PEI* cisplatin + etoposide + ifosfamide, *PIV* cisplatin + ifosfamide + etoposide

[1] Without vascular infiltration: watch and wait, relapse risk 15–20%; alternatively: surgery: RLA, relapse risk 7–10%

### Monitoring of Disease Course

- Documentation of treatment response via imaging and tumor marker analysis; in rare cases tumor marker levels decrease without visible tumor regression ("growing teratoma syndrome") → if possible, early surgical resection
- If tumor marker levels increase after two chemotherapy cycles: salvage therapy or high-dose chemotherapy (only at specialized centers)

### Indications for High-dose Chemotherapy

- Primary treatment in patients with non-seminomatous testicular cancer and poor prognosis (in clinical trials)

- Salvage therapy (in clinical trials) in relapsed patients who responded well to the initial cisplatin-containing therapy or primary treatment in cases of incomplete response (tumor marker levels rising again)
- Treatment of cisplatin-refractory tumors (clinical trials)

### Secondary Surgical Treatment: Resection of Residual Non-seminomatous Germ Cell Tumors

- *Marker-negative after chemotherapy*: all patients should undergo secondary surgery to remove any residual tumor tissue (including all lymph nodes ≥ 1 cm in diameter). Patients with residual viable tumors (except mature teratomas) should receive 2 additional cycles of cisplatin-based chemotherapy (*ATTENTION*: cumulative bleomycin dose). In borderline cases: reevaluation after 6–8 weeks with CT and PET.
- *Marker-positive after chemotherapy*: some patients with persistent tumor markers after cisplatin-based chemotherapy seem to benefit from surgical resection. However, surgery should only be performed after at least two different cisplatin-containing protocols have been used. Patients with normal β-HCG and only one tumor site have the best prognosis.

### Resection of Recurrent Tumors

- Recurrent tumors (documented by imaging) in the area of previously involved lymph nodes in patients with normal or slightly increased tumor markers frequently consist of mature teratoma tissue and should be surgically resected.
- With viable undifferentiated tumors: 2 additional cycles of cisplatin-containing chemotherapy (standard protocol).

### Treatment of Patients with CNS Metastases

- CNS metastases in approximately 10% of patients with advanced disease
- Long-term survival in approximately 35% of cases (with primary cerebral metastases: 30–40%, metastases occurring during treatment or in relapsed patients: 2–5%)
- Common causes of death: systemic tumor progression (20–25% of cases) or intracerebral metastasis (40–45%)
- Good prognosis if single metastasis identified at presentation
- Treatment with curative intent: combination of chemotherapy (4 cycles of platinum-containing chemotherapy) and cerebral radiotherapy (36 Gy, boost to the metastatic region up to 45 Gy); with single metastasis: surgical resection depending on the extent of the systemic disease

### Treatment of Primary Mediastinal Non-seminomatous Germ Cell Tumors

▶ Chap. 8.5.2

### Chemotherapy Protocols: Testicular Cancer

| "PEB, Induction Therapy" ▶ Protocol 12.11.3 | | | Start next cycle on day 22 |
|---|---|---|---|
| Cisplatin | 20 mg/m²/day | i.v. | Days 1–5 |
| Etoposide | 100 mg/m²/day | i.v. | Days 1–5 |
| Bleomycin | 30 mg/day | i.v. | Days 1, 8, 15 |

| "PE" | | | Start next cycle on day 22 |
|---|---|---|---|
| Cisplatin | 20 mg/m²/day | i.v. | Days 1–5 |
| Etoposide | 100 mg/m²/day | i.v. | Days 1–5 |

| *"PEI"* ▶ *Protocol 12.11.4* | | | *Start next cycle on day 22* |
|---|---|---|---|
| Cisplatin | 20 mg/m²/day | i.v. | Days 1–5 |
| Etoposide | 100 mg/m²/day | i.v. | Days 1–5 |
| Ifosfamide | 1,200 mg/m²/day | i.v. | Days 1–5 |

| *"PIV + Pegfilgrastim"* ▶ *Protocol 12.11.5* | | | *Start next cycle on day 29* |
|---|---|---|---|
| Cisplatin | 25 mg/m²/day | i.v. | Days 1–5 |
| Ifosfamide | 1,200 mg/m²/day | i.v. | Days 1–5 |
| Etoposide | 150 mg/m²/day | i.v. | Days 1–5 |
| Pegfilgrastim | 6 mg | s.c. | Day 6 |

| *"VIC high-dose"* ▶ *Protocol 14.6* | | | |
|---|---|---|---|
| Etoposide | 500 mg/m²/day | i.v. | Day -4 to day -2 |
| Ifosfamide | 4,000 mg/m²/day | i.v. | Day -4 to day -2/-3 |
| Carboplatin | AUC 6 | i.v. | Day -4 to day -2/-3 |
| G-CSF | 300–480 µg | s.c. | Day 9 until neutrophil recovery |

**F/U:**

### Curative Treatment Intent

- Close monitoring according to recommendations; after end of therapy: follow-up every 3 months; from 4th year: every 6 months; from 5th year: annually. With high-risk situation: shorter intervals.
- Follow-up visits include physical examination, tumor marker levels, imaging, optional: serum testosterone and FSH levels, ultrasound of contralateral testis.

### Palliative Treatment

- Symptom-based approach.

**Px:** Men should regularly examine their testicles. Any swelling is suspicious and must be followed up.

**Ref:**

1. Albers P, Albrecht W, Algaba F et al. Guidelines on testicular cancer. Eur Urol 2005;48:885–94
2. Dearnaley D, Huddart R, Horwich A. Managing testicular cancer. BMJ 2001;322:1583–8
3. De Wit R, Fizazi K. Controversies in the management of clinical stages I testis cancer. J Clin Oncol 2006;24:5482–92
4. ESMO Guidelines Working Group. Testicular seminoma: ESMO Clinical Recommendation for diagnosis, treatment and follow-up. Ann Oncol 2007;18(suppl 2):ii40–1
5. ESMO Guidelines Working Group. Mixed or non-seminomatous germ-cell tumors: ESMO Clinical Recommendation for diagnosis, treatment and follow-up. Ann Oncol 2007;18(suppl 2):ii42–3
6. Horwich A, Shipley J, Huddart R. Testicular germ-cell cancer. Lancet 2006;367:754–65
7. MacVicar GR, Pienta KJ. Testicular cancer. Curr Opin Oncol 2004;16:253–6
8. Schmoll HJ, Souchon R, Krege S et al. European consensus on diagnosis and treatment of germ cell cancer: a report of the European Germ Cell Cancer Consensus Group (EGCCCG). Ann Oncol 2004;15:1377–99
9. Van Dijk MR, Steyerberg EW, Habbema JDF. Survival of non-seminomatous germ cell cancer patients according to the IGCC classification: An update based on meta-analysis. Eur J Cancer 2006;42:820–6

**Web:**

1. http://tcrc.acor.org/ — Testicular Cancer Resource Center
2. http://www.nlm.nih.gov/medlineplus/testicularcancer.html — MedlinePlus
3. http://www.cancer.gov/cancertopics/types/testicular/ — NCI Cancer Topics
4. http://www.nccn.org/professionals/physician_gls/PDF/testicular.pdf — NCCN Guideline
5. http://www.emedicine.com/med/topic3232.htm — E-medicine

## 8.5.2    Extragonadal Germ Cell Tumors

### A. Spyridonidis, C.F. Waller

**Def:**    Germ cell tumors located in mediastinum, retroperitoneum, pineal region, coccygeal region, less frequently in prostate, liver, esophagus, stomach.

**ICD-10:**    According to location

**Ep:**    Germ cell tumors show a primary extragonadal location in 5–10% of cases in adults and in 82% of pediatric cases. Age peak: 20–40 years; distribution male:female = 12:1 (exception: benign teratoma: male:female = 1:1)

**Pg:**    *Pathogenesis*
Possible pathogenetic factors:
- Prenatal migration of primordial germ cells from yolk sac to midline structures (coccygeal region, retroperitoneum, mediastinum, head)
- Dislocation of residual totipotent cells from blastula or morula stage
- Retroperitoneal germ cell tumors: metastasis from regressed testicular tumor (primary tumor not detectable)

*Genetic Predisposition*
- Frequent detection of isochromosome 12p
- Non-seminomatous mediastinal germ cell tumors: increased incidence in patients with Klinefelter's syndrome (47, XXY) (20% of cases)
- Predisposition (in approximately 20% of cases) for hematological neoplasia, e.g., acute leukemia (AML, FAB M7), myelodysplastic syndrome, malignant histiocytosis; isochromosome 12p present in leukemic blasts
- Retroperitoneal germ cell tumors: increased risk of in situ (CIS) testicular carcinoma (40%)

**Path:**    *Histology*
Extragonadal germ cell tumors are histologically similar to gonadal germ cell tumors. Differentiation between pure seminomas and non-seminomatous tumors bears therapeutic and prognostic relevance. Approximately 20% of all germ cell tumors are mixed tumors.

### Histological Types of Extragonadal Germ Cell Tumors

*Benign germ cell tumors*
- Mature teratomas (potentially malignant if containing > 50% immature tissue)

*Malignant germ cell tumors*
- Seminomas (intracranial seminomas = "germinomas"), 20–24%
- Non-seminomatous germ cell tumors (immature teratoma, embryonic carcinoma, teratocarcinoma, choriocarcinoma, yolk sac tumor)
- Mixed tumors (including seminoma-containing tumors)

### Location in Children (≤ 15 Years of Age)
- Coccygeal region: 27% of cases
- Intracranial: 15%
- Retroperitoneum: 4%
- Mediastinum: 3%

Teratomas are often already present at birth; age peak for highly malignant non-seminomatous tumors: 1–5 years; seminomas mainly in children > 7 years.

### Location in Adults (> 15 Years of Age)
- Mediastinum: 50–70% of cases
- Retroperitoneum: 20–30%
- Intracranial: 2–10%
- Coccygeal region: rare

Origin of mediastinal and retroperitoneal malignant germ cell tumors is often non-seminomatous (76%). Seminomas frequently occur intracranially (65%, "germinomas"); age peak: 20–30 years.

**Sy:**   Symptoms depending on tumor location:
- *Mediastinal germ cell tumors:* symptoms only in late stages: cough, chest pain, dyspnea, superior vena cava syndrome; 50% of mediastinal tumors are diagnosed incidentally
- *Retroperitoneal germ cell tumors:* symptoms often only in late stages: abdominal pressure, flank pain / backache, organ displacement symptoms (constipation, dysfunctional voiding, abdominal distension); often incidental diagnosis
- *Pineal tumors:* signs of increased intracranial pressure, headaches, reduced visual field, ataxia, lethargy, nausea, Parinaud's syndrome (vertical gaze palsy, nystagmus), diploidy; signs of pituitary failure (e.g., diabetes insipidus) with invasive tumors or suprasellar location
- *Coccygeal region:* pain, sciatica, rectal compression, compression of the urinary bladder, voiding and defecation disorders
- General symptoms (fever, night sweats, weight loss, anorexia, reduced performance) with malignant and rapidly progressive tumors, gynecomastia if β-HCG increased

**Dg:**   ### Medical History, Physical Examination
- Medical history including course and dynamics of the disease
- Physical examination including neurological symptoms, palpation of testis

### Laboratory Tests
- Routine laboratory tests including complete blood count with differential, liver and renal function tests, LDH
- Serum tumor markers: α1-fetoprotein (AFP), β-human chorionic gonadotropin (β-HCG); with seminoma: possibly placental alkaline phosphatase (PLAP) (*NOTE:* false-positive levels with smoking) and NSE. Pure seminomas never secrete AFP → AFP ↑ levels are always indicative of a non-seminomatous or mixed tumor; mixed tumors are treated like non-seminomatous tumors
- Pituitary hormones with suspected intracranial germ cell tumors

### Imaging
- Abdominal and testicular ultrasound (obligatory, especially with retroperitoneal germ cell tumors)
- Chest x-ray, thoracic / abdominal CT
- MRI brain and spinal cord (mandatory with intracranial tumors)
- PET scan (in clinical studies)

### Histology
Histology obligatory; access depending on location; fine-needle biopsy possible, some centers prefer open biopsy to avoid sampling errors in case of heterologous tumors
- Mediastinal tumors: mediastinoscopy
- Intracranial tumors: modern stereotactic techniques have minimized mortality of the procedure as well as incidence of metastatic seeding. CSF analysis (cytology, AFP, β-HCG) is mandatory
- Uni- or bilateral testicular carcinoma in situ (CIS, synonym: TIN, testicular intraepithelial neoplasia) in 30% of all cases of extragonadal germ cell tumors. As patients with extragonadal tumors are treated with platinum-based therapy (curative for TIN), testicular biopsy is not necessary in case of normal ultrasound findings

**Dd:**

- *Anterior mediastinum:* thymoma, lymphomas, mesenchymal tumors, endocrine tumors, cysts
- *Retroperitoneal tumors:* tumors of the adrenal glands, mesenchymal tumors, lymphomas, lymph node metastases; most primary retroperitoneal germ cell tumors manifest themselves along the midline; in contrast, lymph node metastases to the left or the right are indicative of an occult primary ipsilateral tumor
- *Pineal region:* glioma, pineoblastoma, pineocytoma, cysts

**Th:** Interdisciplinary treatment approach.

## Mediastinal / Retroperitoneal Germ Cell Tumors

### Seminomatous Extragonadal Germ Cell Tumors

Retroperitoneal tumors < 5 cm are primarily treated by radiotherapy; all others: cisplatin-containing chemotherapy (e.g., 3–4 cycles of PEB or PEI) followed by surgical resection of residual tumor tissue (▶ Chap. 8.5.1)

### Non-seminomatous Extragonadal Germ Cell Tumors

- Treatment like high-risk testicular tumors (▶ Chap. 8.5.1): early intensification with high-dose chemotherapy and resection of residual tumor (esp. with mediastinal tumors) → 5-year survival 75%
- Poor prognosis: relapsed tumors; 3-year survival after salvage high-dose chemotherapy of retroperitoneal tumors 48%; mediastinal tumors 14%

### Teratomas

- Primary surgery
- With large tumors: neoadjuvant chemotherapy to reduce tumor size followed by resection with curative intent
- Benign teratomas: tumor resection, chemotherapy and radiotherapy not indicated

## Intracranial Germ Cell Tumors

- Treatment according to existing pediatric protocols (e.g. SIOP CNS GCT 96)
- *Germinomas* (intracranial seminomas): radiotherapy, 24 Gy craniospinal + 16 Gy tumor bed or 2 cycles of PEI + 40 Gy focal radiotherapy
- *Non-germinomas* (yolk sac tumors, choriocarcinomas, embryonic carcinomas): 4 cycles of PEI, possibly resection of residual tumor followed by radiotherapy
- *Teratomas:* primary surgery; with large tumors, neoadjuvant chemotherapy followed by surgery

## Chemotherapy Protocols

| *"PEB"* ▶ Protocol 12.11.3 | | | *Start next cycle on day 22* |
|---|---|---|---|
| Cisplatin | 20 mg/m²/day | i.v. | Days 1–5 |
| Etoposide | 100 mg/m²/day | i.v. | Days 1–5 |
| Bleomycin | 30 mg/day | i.v. | Days 1, 8, 15 |

| *"PEI"* ▶ Protocol 12.11.4 | | | *Start next cycle on day 22* |
|---|---|---|---|
| Cisplatin | 20 mg/m²/day | i.v. | Days 1–5 |
| Etoposide | 100 mg/m²/day | i.v. | Days 1–5 |
| Ifosfamide | 1,200 mg/m²/day | i.v. | Days 1–5 |

**Prg:**    The prognostic classification of testicular germ cell tumors does not apply to extragonadal tumors. Prognosis of extragonadal germ cell tumors:

- Extragonadal seminomatous tumors carry a favorable prognosis similar to testicular seminomas.
- Extragonadal non-seminomatous germ cell tumors carry a poor prognosis compared to testicular non-seminomatous tumors. The prognostic score of Hartmann is used.

**Prognostic score for extragonadal non-seminomatous tumors (Hartmann 2002)**

| Prognostic factors | Score |
|---|---|
| Mediastinal tumor | 2 |
| βHCG ↑ | 1 |
| Metastasis to lung | 1 |
| Metastasis to liver | 1 |
| CNS Metastasis | 2 |

| Prognosis (sum) | Five-year survival (%) |
|---|---|
| Intermediate low (0–1) | 52 |
| Intermediate high (2–3) | 47 |
| Poor (> 3) | 11 |

**F/U:**    Patients treated with curative intent should be closely monitored including physical examination, tumor marker assays, and imaging. In palliative situations: symptom-based approach.

**Ref:**

1.  Bokemeyer C, Nichols CR, Droz JP et al. Extragonadal germ cell tumors of the mediastinum and retroperitoneum: results from an international analysis. J Clin Oncol 2002;20:1864–73
2.  De Giorgi U, Demirer T, Wandt H et al. Second-line high-dose chemotherapy in patients with mediastinal and retroperitoneal primary non-seminomatous germ cell tumors. Ann Oncol 2005;16:146–51
3.  Göbel U, Schneider DT, Calaminus G et al. Germ-cell tumors in childhood and adolescence. Ann Oncol 2000;11:263–71
4.  Hartmann JT, Nichols CR, Droz JP et al. Prognostic variables for response and outcome in patients with extragonadal germ-cell tumors. Ann Oncol 2002;13:1017–28
5.  Schmoll HJ, Souchon R, Krege S et al. European consensus on the diagnosis and treatment of germ cell cancer: a report of the European Germ Cell Cancer Consensus Group (EGCCCG). Ann Oncol 2004;15:1377–99

**Web:**

| | | |
|---|---|---|
| 1. | http://tcrc.acor.org/egc.html | Testicular Cancer Resource Center |
| 2. | http://www.cancer.gov/cancertopics/types/extragonadal-germ-cell/ | NCI Cancer Topics |
| 3. | http://www.emedicine.com/MED/topic759.htm | E-medicine |

### 8.5.3 Prostate Cancer

**W. Schultze-Seemann, C.F. Waller**

**Def:** Malignant, usually hormone-dependent neoplasia of the prostate.

**ICD-10:** C61

**Ep:** Incidence: 60 cases/100,000/year in Europe; 30% of all carcinomas in men, most common malignancy in men; median age: 69 years; incidence increasing with age from 0.02% (50 years) to 1.5% (80 years); latent prostate carcinoma discovered at autopsy: 10% at 50 years of age, 70% at 80 years of age.

**Pg:**

*Risk Factors*
- Age, high-fat diet, obesity
- Geographical differences: highest risk in USA, Canada, and Sweden; lowest risk in Asia
- Increased risk with disease in a first-degree relative
- Occupational risks: chemical industry (cadmium)

*Molecular Genetic Mechanisms*
There are no known characteristic chromosomal abnormalities. In some cases mutation of the RNAse L gene (HPC1 locus, chromosome 1), mutations of the tumor suppressor genes PTEN and p53, as well as susceptibility loci for prostate cancer on chromosomes 1, 8, 20, 17, and X have been described. A possible role of retroviral infections and polymorphic androgen and vitamin D receptors in the carcinogenesis of prostate cancer is under discussion.

**Path:**

*Histology*

| Type | Frequency (%) |
|---|---|
| *Adenocarcinoma* | > 95 |
| *Other* | < 5 |

- Sarcoma, small cell carcinoma, squamous cell carcinoma
- Metastases (bladder carcinomas, melanomas, etc.)

*Location*
- Mostly originating in the peripheral zone of the prostate; multifocal in 35% of cases

*Manifestation / Spread*
- *Low-grade* prostate cancer: slow localized growth; in some cases, no metastasis for many years
- *Direct* spread via vessels and nerves
- *Direct* invasion of adjacent structures: rectum, bladder, etc.
- *Lymphatic* metastasis to regional lymph nodes (obturator group)
- *Hematogenous:* most common: bone metastases, mainly osteoplastic metastases, rarely osteolytic lesions; spread to lumbar spine and pelvis via periprostatic veins → lumbar pain often the first symptom of prostate cancer; rarely: metastases to liver, CNS, lung. and soft tissue

*Types*
- *Latent carcinoma:* incidental diagnosis at autopsy
- *Incidental carcinoma:* incidental diagnosis based on histological analysis of tissue derived from transurethral resection or adenoma resection due to benign prostate abnormalities
- *Occult carcinoma:* metastatic prostate cancer without clinical symptoms
- *Clinical carcinoma:* all other cases

**Class:**    **TNM Staging of Prostate Cancer**

| | |
|---|---|
| *T* | *Primary Tumor* |
| TX | Primary tumor cannot be assessed |
| T0 | No evidence of primary tumor |
| T1 | Clinically inapparent tumor not visible by imaging |
| | a: incidental histological finding of tumor cells in ≤ 5% of resected tissue |
| | b: incidental histological finding of tumor cells in > 5% of resected tissue |
| | c: Tumor identified by needle biopsy (e.g., with PSA ↑) |
| T2 | Palpable tumor confined within prostate (including apex and capsule) |
| | a: Tumor involves ≤ 50% of a lobe |
| | b: Tumor involves > 50% of a lobe |
| | c: Tumor involves both lobes |
| T3 | Tumor extends through the prostatic capsule |
| | a: Unilateral or bilateral extracapsular extension |
| | b: Tumor invades seminal vesicle(s) |
| T4 | Tumor is fixed or invades adjacent structures (other than seminal vesicles): bladder neck, external sphincter, rectum levator muscles, pelvic wall |
| *N* | *Lymph Node Involvement* |
| NX | Regional lymph nodes cannot be assessed |
| N0 | Regional lymph nodes without metastases |
| N1 | Metastases in regional lymph nodes |
| *M* | *Distant Metastasis* |
| MX | Distant metastasis cannot be assessed |
| M0 | No distant metastasis |
| M1 | Distant metastasis |
| | A: Non-regional lymph nodes |
| | B: Bone |
| | C: Other sites |

**Grade of differentiation and Gleason score (2002)**

| Grade | Gleason score[a] | Differentiation |
|---|---|---|
| GX | | Grade of differentiation cannot be assessed |
| G1 | 2–4 | Well differentiated, slight anaplasia |
| G2 | 5–6 | Moderately differentiated, moderate anaplasia |
| G3–4 | 7–10 | Poorly differentiated / undifferentiated, marked anaplasia |

[a] Gleason score: analysis of tumor histology: sum of all values of two predominant histological types, added and assessed independently of each other. Grade 1: highly differentiated, grade 5: undifferentiated

**AJCC Staging of Prostate Cancer**

| Stage | TNM system | | | Differentiation |
|-------|------------|------|------|-----------------|
| I | T1a | N0 | M0 | G1 |
| II | T1a | N0 | M0 | G2–4 |
| | T1b–c | N0 | M0 | Any G |
| | T2 | N0 | M0 | Any G |
| III | T3 | N0 | M0 | Any G |
| IV | T4 | N0 | M0 | Any G |
| | Any T | N1 | M0 | Any G |
| | Any T | Any N | M1 | Any G |

**Sy:** Symptoms identical to benign prostatic hyperplasia (BPH); early stages usually asymptomatic. Advanced stages:
- *Pollakiuria*, compelling urinary urgency, nocturia, incontinence, dysuria, hematuria; sudden onset and rapid deterioration of symptoms in men ≥ 50 years are highly suspicious of prostate cancer
- Bone pain caused by distant metastasis (lumbar spine syndrome is often first symptom)
- Advanced tumor stages: lymphedema of the lower extremities, venous congestion due to pelvic lymphomas; paraplegia, incontinence with thoracic / lumbar spine metastasis

**Dg:** ### Medical History, Physical Examination
- Medical history including family history and dysuria
- Physical examination: digital rectal examination is most important and efficient diagnostic procedure → solid, hard masses with irregular edges are characteristic for prostate carcinoma, sensitivity: 50%; less with tumors ≤ 1.5 cm; lymph node status (inguinal lymph nodes)

### Laboratory Tests
- Full blood count, liver and renal function tests, alkaline phosphatase, $Ca^{2+}$, phosphate, urinary status

### Tumor Marker: Prostate-specific Antigen (PSA)
- Tissue-specific marker for prostate changes; any PSA increase must be evaluated; sensitivity: 75%; in conjunction with rectal examination and rectal ultrasound best screening method for prostate cancer.
- Normal PSA level increases with age (due to increased prostate volume, inflammatory and ischemic processes). Upper normal level in men up to 49 years: 2.5 ng/ml, 50–59 years: 3.5 ng/ml, 60–69 years: 4.5 ng/ml, 70–79: 6.5 ng/ml.
- For better differentiation between benign prostatic hyperplasia (BPH) and carcinoma: PSA density, PSA velocity, and age-specific reference values; PSA density: amount of PSA per unit volume of prostate tissue determined by transrectal ultrasound.
- Sequential PSA assays increase the specificity by 90% and the sensitivity by 70%; > 0.7 ng/ml increase per year measured with the same assay is a positive predictor of cancer, provided the initial value was < 4 ng/ml; with higher initial values (PSA > 4 ng/ml): increases by 0.4 ng/ml per year positively predictive; PSA velocity (or PSA doubling time) is a promising method for early detection of locoregional tumors
- With known prostate cancer: PSA suitable for monitoring the disease course; often increases years before occurrence of clinically relevant relapse

**Prostate Cancer Screening**

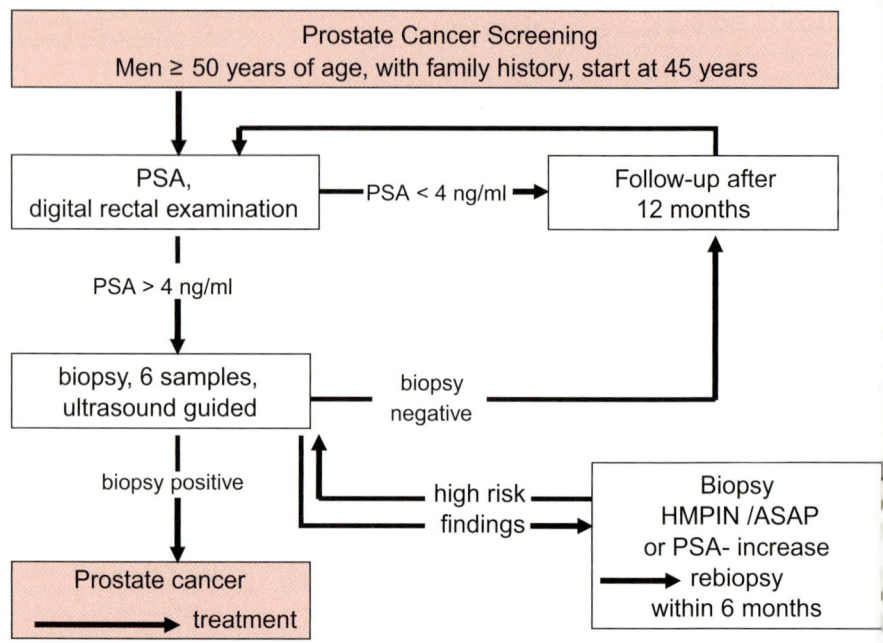

*PSA* prostate cancer antigen, *HMPIN* highly malignant prostatic intraepithelial neoplasia, *ASAP* atypical small acinary proliferation

### Histological Analysis
- Fine-needle aspiration or biopsy (TRU-Cut 18G): 95% transrectal, 5% transperineal; indicated if increased PSA, bone metastases, or unexplained voiding abnormalities; standard diagnostic procedure for prostate cancer; sensitivity high but dependent on experience of the performing physician.
- Transurethral resection (TURP): standard treatment for benign prostatic hyperplasia; occasionally, incidental diagnosis of early prostate cancer.

### Imaging
- Transrectal ultrasound (TRUS): sensitivity 80–85%, specificity 85%; ultrasound-guided biopsy / fine-needle aspiration (obligatory); not suitable for screening due to low specificity
- Abdominal ultrasound, abdominal and pelvic MRI, chest x-ray
- Bone scan and monitoring of suspicious lesions by conventional x-ray
- Experimental: [11]choline PET-CT scan, especially with PSA rise after prostate resection

**DD:**
- Benign prostatic hyperplasia (BPH): by far the most common differential diagnosis from the age of 30 years onwards, prevalence in 80-year-old patients: 80%; palpable masses often cannot be distinguished from prostate cancer
- Chronic and granulomatous prostatitis due to bacteria (tuberculosis), fungi, or protozoa
- Rare: prostatic calculi, amyloidosis, benign adenomas

**Co:**
- Macrohematuria
- Anuria, hydronephrosis, renal failure
- Coagulation disorders (disseminated intravascular coagulation DIC, hyperfibrinolysis)
- Paraneoplastic neuromuscular disorders
- Bone marrow infiltration with anemia, thrombocytopenia, leukopenia

**Th:**    **Treatment Concept**

1. Prostate cancer is primarily treated by surgery.
2. Inoperable patients (reduced performance status, age): good results with radiotherapy or radioisotope therapy.
3. Hormone therapy is used in the majority of patients, as adjuvant or palliative treatment.
4. Survival of > 15 years is usually achievable, even with untreated prostate cancer. Clinical trials and established treatment vary substantially with regard to aggressiveness. For every patient, individual risk-benefit should be assessed, taking into consideration age and performance status of the patient as well as aggressiveness of the procedure.

**Treatment of prostate cancer**

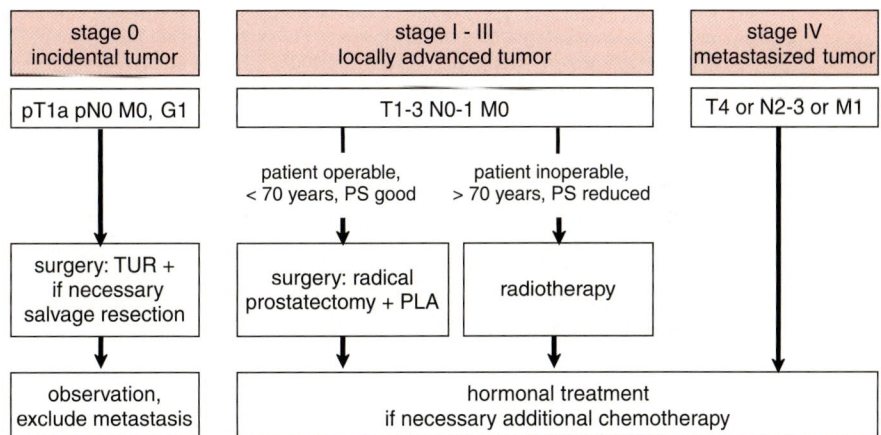

*TUR* transurethral resection, *PLA* pelvic lymphadenectomy, *PS* performance score

### Surgical Treatment

#### Indications
- Age ≤ 75 years, good performance status
- Primary tumor and lymph nodes radically resectable, i.e., stage I–III
- Stage IV, T4 N0 M0, intrapelvic lymph node involvement but still operable

#### Contraindications
- Age > 75 years, life expectancy < 10 years

#### Radical Prostatovesiculectomy
For exact pathological staging: pelvic lymphadenectomy prior to prostatectomy (not if PSA < 10 ng/ml or Gleason score < 7).

#### Complications
- Radical prostatovesiculectomy: incontinence grade III < 1%, stress incontinence 3–10%; impaired potency or postoperative impotence in ≥ 40% of patients (T2 tumor 50%, T3 tumor 80–100%) depending on the experience of the surgeon
- Lymphadenectomy: lymphocele, lymphedema
- Pulmonary embolism, wound infection

### Radiotherapy

*Indications*
- Stage I–III: with localized tumor radiotherapy should only be used if surgical treatment contraindicated
- Stage IV, T4 N0 M0, or intrapelvic lymph node involvement and surgical treatment contraindicated
- Palliative radiotherapy: pain, bone metastases, obstruction, etc.

*Techniques*
- Percutaneous radiotherapy including the draining lymph nodes (50 Gy), focal boost up to total dose of > 70 Gy (duration approximately 7 weeks)
- Three-dimensional conformal high-dose radiotherapy and intensity-modulated radiotherapy (IMRT) are standard radiotherapy techniques sparing normal tissues
- Combined interstitial / external beam radiotherapy
- In stage I–III, local treatment as an alternative to external beam radiotherapy: interstitial therapy with $I^{128}$ or $Pd^{103}$ seeds (permanent / periodic) with / without external beam radiotherapy; afterloading with $Ir^{192}$ in combination with external beam radiotherapy

*Complications*
- Impotency in 30–70% of cases, other radiation-associated complications: cystitis, proctitis, dysuria, development of fistulas
- In 10–30%, persistent tumor rate (symptomatic improvement) persistent prostatic enlargement (fibrosis) in 80% of patients

### Radioisotope Therapy

*Indications*
- Bone pain due to advanced metastasis

*Techniques*
- Severe bone pain: intravenous administration of $^{89}Sr$, $^{153}Sm$ or $^{186}Re$ (palliative); individual dose adjustment according to changes in blood count, with diffuse metastasis, or use of other myelosuppressive therapies (chemotherapy)
- $^{89}Sr$ treatment may be repeated after 12 weeks, $^{153}Sm$ or $^{186}Re$ treatment repeated after 4–6 weeks

*Complications*
- Local treatment: impotency, cystitis, proctitis, dysuria, fistulas
- Systemic administration of radioisotopes: blood count changes (cytopenia)

### Hormone Therapy (▶ Chap. 3.3)

*Indications*
- Stage IV with advanced primary tumor, lymph node involvement or distant metastases, inoperable situation
- Adjuvant hormone therapy is a palliative treatment; effect on long-term survival not established
- Treatment should be initiated with evidence of metastasis; with PSA increase, or with detection of new tumor manifestation (N+, M+) in patients in complete remission after surgery or radiotherapy

## Approach

**Principles of hormone therapy**

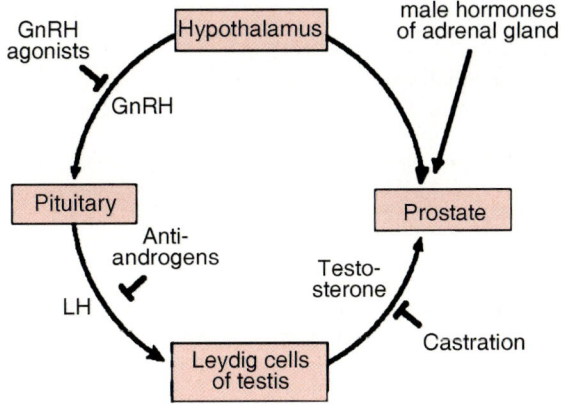

*Standard treatment:* combined treatment with antiandrogens and LHRH agonists → complete androgen deprivation (hormonal castration) in patients with minimal disease confers survival advantage; current data show no disadvantages to intermittent hormone blockade; combination treatment has been shown to slightly yet significantly prolong overall survival compared with LHRH agonists alone; treatment should be started with a 7- to 10-day antiandrogen monotherapy to suppress "flare" phenomenon.

- *Agents:* goserelin or leuprorelin implants for 1 or 3 months of treatment; antiandrogens: flutamide 3 × 250 mg/day; bicalutamide 50–150 mg/day
- Alternatively: orchiectomy (surgical castration; more cost effective)
- Response with symptomatic improvement approximately 80% for all therapies
- Effective for 15–18 months, then usually tumor resistance

### Treatment of Progressive Disease During Hormone Therapy

- After orchiectomy or monotherapy with LHRH agonists: addition of antiandrogen (especially if testosterone level identified)
- After combined androgen blockade: discontinue antiandrogen (possibility of antiandrogen withdrawal response in 25% of cases); then possibly change to alternative antiandrogen (e.g., from flutamide to bicalutamide)
- Where applicable: treatment attempt with ketoconazole 3 × 200 mg (blockade of testicular and adrenal androgen synthesis) + hydrocortisone (5–10% of circulating androgens are produced by the adrenal glands)

### Other Agents with Endocrine Activity

Diethylstilbestrol (DES), stilbestrol, chlorotrianisene (TACE), and megestrol acetate are hormonally active and may be used as alternative treatment in case of failure of the initial hormone therapy. Whether any of these compounds confers prolonged survival is uncertain.

### Chemotherapy

### Indication

- In case of failure of hormone therapy

### Approach

- Effective compounds (up to 20% response): docetaxel, paclitaxel, estramustine phosphate, mitoxantrone, cyclophosphamide, 5-fluorouracil, anthracyclines, dacarbazine, cisplatin, hydroxyurea, and melphalan.
- Combination chemotherapy is not superior to monotherapy; a multicenter, randomized trail demonstrated a survival advantage of a combination of docetaxel and prednisolone versus mitoxantrone and prednisolone.
- The use of adjuvant / neoadjuvant chemotherapy is currently tested in clinical trials
- In 70% of cases, symptomatic improvement after failure of hormone therapy; in 20–30% of patients objective remissions
- Estramustine phosphate: combination molecule consisting of 17β-estradiol and alkylating agent → antigonadotropic and cytotoxic effect; dosage: initially 280 mg 3 times daily p.o., maintenance 280 mg twice daily p.o.

### Chemotherapy Protocols

| "Docetaxel/ Prednisolone" ▶ Protocol 12.12.2 | | | Start next cycle on day 22 |
| --- | --- | --- | --- |
| Docetaxel | 75 mg/m²/day | i.v. | Day 1 |
| Prednisolone | 10 mg/day | p.o. | Days 1–21 |

| "Docetaxel + Estramustine" | | | Start next cycle on day 21 |
| --- | --- | --- | --- |
| Docetaxel | 70 mg/m² | i.v. | Day 2 |
| Estramustine | 280 mg/m² | i.v. | Days 1–5 and 7–11 |

| "Mitoxantrone / Prednisolone" | | | Start next cycle on day 22 |
| --- | --- | --- | --- |
| Mitoxantrone | 12 mg/m²/day | i.v. | Day 1 |
| Prednisolone | 10 mg/day | i.v. | Days 1–21 |

| "Doxorubicin Monotherapy" ▶ Protocol 12.12.1 | | | Start next cycle on day 29 |
| --- | --- | --- | --- |
| Doxorubicin | 20 mg/m²/day | i.v. | Days 1, 8, 15, 22 |

### Experimental Therapies

- Hyperthermia / thermotherapy
- "Molecular therapies": targeted therapies

### Supportive Therapy

- Bone metastases → use of bisphosphonates (zoledronate, pamidronate, etidronate, bondronate, etc.)
- Adequate pain control by analgesic treatment (if applicable, radioisotopes: [153]Sm, [89]Sr, [186]Re)

Prg:
### Prognostic Factors

- Tumor stage
- Grade of differentiation: 5-year survival: G1 60%, G2 35%, G3 15%, G4 5%

### Ten-year Survival According to AJCC Stages
- Stage I:     85%
- Stage II:    72%
- Stage III:   55%
- Stage IV:    30%

**F/U:** Patients treated with curative intent should be monitored closely including PSA screening; follow-up: initially: every 3 months, after 2 years: every 6 months, after 5 years: annually.
Palliative situation: symptom-based approach.

**Px:** Screening: PSA, rectal examination from the age of 45 up to life expectancy < 10 years.

**Ref:**
1. Antonarakis ES, Blackford AL, Garrett-MayerE et al. Survival in men with nonmetastatic prostate cancer treated with hormone therapy. J Clin Oncol 2007;25:4998–5008
2. Basch EM, Somerfield MR, Beer TM et al. ASCO Endorsement of the Cancer Care Ontario Practice Guideline on nonhormonal therapy for men with metastatic hormone-refactory (castration-resistant) prostate cancer. J Clin Oncol 2007;25:5313–8
3. ESMO Guidelines Working Group. Prostate cancer: ESMO Clinical Recommendations for diagnosis, treatment and follow-up. Ann Oncol 2007;18(suppl 2):ii36–7
4. Lilja H, Ulmert D, Vickers AJ. Prostate-specific antigen and prostate cancer: prediction, detection and monitoring. Nat Rev Cancer 2008;8:268–78
5. Loblaw DA, Virgo KS, Nam R et al. Initial hormonal management of androgen-sensitive metastatic, recurrent or progressive prostate cancer: 2006 Update of an ASCO Practice Guideline. J Clin Oncol 2007;25:1596–605
6. Nelson WG, De Marzo AM, Isaacs WB. Prostate cancer. N Engl J Med 2003;349:366–81
7. Speight JL, Roach M. Radiotherapy in the management of clinically localized prostate cancer: evolving standards, consensus, controversies and new directions. J Clin Oncol 2005;23:8176–85
8. Taichman RS, Loberg RD, Mehra R et al. The evolving biology and treatment of prostate cancer. J Clin Invest 2007;117:2351–61
9. Walsh PC, DeWeese Tl, Eisenberger MA. Localized Prostate Cancer. N Engl J Med 2007;357:2696–705

**Web:**
1. http://www.nlm.nih.gov/medlineplus/prostatecancer.html — MedlinePlus
2. http://www.cancer.gov/cancertopics/types/prostate — NCI Cancer Topics
3. http://www.cdc.gov/CANCER/prostate/prostate.htm — Ctr Disease Control
4. http://www.nccn.org/professionals/physician_gls/PDF/prostate.pdf — NCCN Guideline
5. http://www.emedicine.com/med/UROLOGY.htm — E-medicine

### 8.5.4    Penile Cancer

**C.F. Waller, K. Henne, W. Schultze-Seemann**

**Def:**    Malignant neoplasia of the penis.

**ICD-10:**    C60.9: penile carcinoma

**Ep:**    Incidence: 1–2 cases/100,000 men/year; after 50 years of age: 9 cases/100,000 men/year; median age: 50–70 years; < 1% of all male cancers in Europe and the USA, higher incidence in parts of Africa and South America (up to 10% of all male cancers).

**Pg:**    *Risk Factors*
- Age, smoking
- Chronic irritation (e.g., phimosis), poor hygiene, smegma retention
- Sexual promiscuity, recurrent balanoposthitis
- HPV infection: particularly with genotypes 16 and 18 (rarely 31, 35, and 39); HPV detected in 27–71% of patients with penile cancer (▶ Chaps. 8.4.7, 8.4.11)
- PUVA therapy
- Occupational risk (chimney sweeper)

*Precancerous Lesions of the Penis*
A number of penile lesions have the potential of malignant transformation. The exact role of these lesions in the development of penile cancer is uncertain.
- Balanitis xerotica obliterans, balanitis plasmacellularis of Zoon
- Erythroplasia of Queyrat, leukoplakia
- Bowen's disease
- Buschke-Löwenstein giant condyloma (verrucous carcinoma)

**Path:**    *Histology*

| Type | Frequency (%) |
| --- | --- |
| Squamous cell carcinoma | > 93 |
| Basal cell carcinoma | 4 |
| Carcinoma in situ | 1 |
| Melanoma | 1 |
| Sarcoma | 1 |
| Malignant hemangioendothelioma | rare |
| Kaposi's sarcoma (especially in HIV patients) | rare |
| Metastases | rare |

*Spread / Metastasis*
- Primary tumor location is usually the glans penis; frequently long delays in diagnosis (variability of the clinical picture, partly with concurrent phimosis, hesitant behavior of most men)
- Lymphatic metastasis: primarily via superficial and deep inguinal lymph nodes → iliac lymph nodes → pelvic lymph nodes
- Hematogenous metastasis: rare; affected organs include lung, liver, bones, and brain

**Class:**      **TNM Staging of penile cancer**

| | |
|---|---|
| *T* | *Primary Tumor* |
| TX | Primary tumor cannot be assessed |
| T0 | No evidence of primary tumor |
| Tis | Carcinoma in situ |
| Ta | Noninvasive verrucous carcinoma |
| T1 | Tumor invades subepithelial connective tissue |
| T2 | Tumor invades corpus spongiosum |
| T3 | Tumor invades urethra or prostate |
| T4 | Tumor invades contiguous structures |
| *N* | *Regional Lymph Node Involvement* |
| NX | Regional lymph nodes cannot be assessed |
| N0 | No regional lymph node metastasiss |
| N1 | Metastasis to a single superficial inguinal lymph node |
| N2 | Metastasis to multiple or bilateral superficial inguinal lymph nodes |
| N3 | Metastasis to deep iliac or pelvic lymph nodes |
| *M* | *Distant Metastasis* |
| MX | Distant metastasis cannot be assessed |
| M0 | No distant metastasis |
| M1 | Distant metastasis |

**AJCC Staging (2002)**

| Stage | TNM classification | | |
|---|---|---|---|
| 0 | Tis-a | N0 | M0 |
| I | T1 | N0 | M0 |
| II | T1 | N1 | M0 |
| | T2 | N0–1 | M0 |
| III | T1–2 | N2 | M0 |
| | T3 | N0–2 | M0 |
| IV | T4 | Any N | M0 |
| | Any T | N3 | M0 |
| | Any T | Any N | M1 |

**Staging according to Jackson**

| | |
|---|---|
| Stage 0 (A) | Tumor limited to glans / prepuce |
| Stage I (B) | Tumor invades shaft of penis |
| Stage III (C) | Tumor with operable inguinal lymph nodes |
| Stage IV (D) | Tumor invades contiguous structures, inoperable inguinal lymph nodes, or distant metastasis |

**Sy:**
- Exophytic masses of the penis (47%)
- Pain, ulcers (35%)
- Inflammatory changes of the penis (17%)
- Burning or stabbing sensation under the prepuce
- Enlarged inguinal lymph nodes (20–60% of men have palpable lymph nodes → in 50% lymph node metastases, and in 50% infection)
- In some cases: weight loss, fatigue
- Late symptoms: bleeding, urethral fistula or obstruction, weight loss, fatigue

**Dg:**    ### Medical History, Physical Examination
- Medical history including social background
- Physical examination: genitalia, lymph node status

### Laboratory Tests
- Routine laboratory tests (including LDH), urinary status

### Imaging
- Pelvic ultrasound including inguinal region / abdomen, chest x-ray
- MRI pelvis, CT abdomen / pelvis
- Bone pain: bone scan, conventional skeletal x-ray

### Endoscopy
- Possibly cystoscopy / urethroscopy

### Histology
- Obligatory: biopsy for histological analysis

**Th:**    ## Carcinoma in situ

Treatment consists of local surgical excision, laser treatment, topical 5-FU, cryotherapy, and radiotherapy.

## Invasive Penile Carcinoma

### Surgical Treatment
- *Standard approach:* radical surgical resection. Local tumor stage and involvement of regional lymph nodes determine extent of resection.
- *Stage T1 (localized):* wide excision with a free proximal margin of 2 cm (smaller margins result in local relapse rates of up to 32%).
- *Stage T2-3:* total penectomy.
- *Stage T4:* wide en bloc resection of the primary lesion and any involved sections of the abdominal wall as well as bilateral inguinal lymphadenectomy.

### Inguinal Lymph Nodes
- *Bilateral inguinal lymphadenectomy:* should be performed in patients with persistent lymph node enlargement after 4–6 weeks of adequate antibiotic treatment. Earlier tumor stages (T1, 2) without palpable lymph nodes: watch and wait. In locally advanced stages (T3, 4), "prophylactic" bilateral lymph node dissection probably does improve overall survival.
- Only 20% of men with occult lymph node metastases can be treated with curative intent (cure rate approximately 88%), while 80% of men probably do not benefit from prophylactic lymphadenectomy (no lymph node metastasis). The procedure is associated with a mortality rate of < 1% and complications such as lymphedema, pulmonary embolism, infection, etc.
- Modified inguinal lymphadenectomy and selective lymphadenectomy can be carried out in certain patients. The value of sentinel lymph node biopsy is uncertain.

### Radiotherapy

May be used in earlier stages of the disease as an organ-preserving form of treatment. Local relapse rate of approximately 10–20%. With locally nonresectable tumors or relapses, and in cases where lymphadenectomy is impossible, palliative percutaneous radiotherapy should be considered.

### Adjuvant Treatment

The value of adjuvant radiotherapy or chemotherapy following surgical resection is uncertain.

### Treatment of Relapse and Advanced Disease

- Local relapse is common after penis-preserving treatment; salvage therapy: complete penectomy and, if necessary, total anterior exenteration. Prophylactic or therapeutic bilateral inguinal lymphadenectomy should be considered.
- Conservative (non-surgical) approach: neoadjuvant chemotherapy, radiochemotherapy, or intra-arterial chemotherapy.
- The treatment of metastic penile cancer requires a combination of local therapy and systemic chemotherapy. Active drugs include bleomycin, MTX, 5-FU, cisplatin, and cyclophosphamide alone or in combination. Other compounds such as ifosfamide, docetaxel, paclitaxel, gemcitabine, or vinorelbine, which have been successfully used in squamous cell carcinomas of the cervix and of the head and neck, have not yet been tested in randomized studies in penile cancer.

**Px:**

### Primary Prevention

Circumcision in neonates reduces the risk of penile HPV infection, contributing to the prevention of penile cancer as well as cervical cancer (in female partner).

**Prg:**

Most important prognostic factor is clinical tumor stage (size, depth of infiltration, involvement of regional lymph nodes) at presentation. Patients with positive lymph nodes have a significantly reduced 5-year survival (27% versus 66% if lymph node negative).

**Ref:**

1. Castellsague X, Bosch FX, Munoz N et al. Male circumcision, penile human papillomavirus infection, and cervical cancer in female partners. N Engl J Med 2002;346:1105–12
2. Culkin DJ, Beer TM. Advanced penile carcinoma. J Urol 2003;170(2 Pt 1):359–65
3. McDougal WS. Advances in the treatment of carcinoma of the penis. Urology 2005;66(suppl 5):114–17
4. Misra S, Chaturvedi A, Misra NC. Penile carcinoma: a challenge for the developing world. Lancet Oncol 2004;5:240–7
5. Mosconi AM, Roila F, Gatta G et al. Cancer of the penis. Crit Rev Oncol Hematol 2005;53:165–77
6. Rippentrop JM, Joslyn SA, Konety BR. Squamous cell carcinoma of the penis: evaluation of data from the surveillance, epidemiology, and end results program. Cancer 2004;101:1357–63
7. Sanchez-Ortiz RF, Pettaway CA. The role of lymphadenectomy in penile cancer. Urol Oncol 2004;22:236–44
8. Solsona E, Algaba F, Horenblas S et al. European Association of Urology Guidelines on Penile Cancer. Eur Urol 2004;46:1–8

**Web:**

1. http://www.nlm.nih.gov/medlineplus/ency/article/001276.htm     MedlinePlus
2. http://www.nci.nih.gov/cancertopics/pdq/treatment/penile/ HealthProfessional     NCI Cancer Topics
3. http://www.emedicine.com/MED/topic3046.htm     E-medicine

## 8.6          Tumors of the Urinary Tract

### 8.6.1          Renal Cell Carcinoma

#### K.G. Schrenk, C.F. Waller

**Def:**          Malignant neoplasia of the kidney arising from the epithelium of the renal tubules. Synonym: hypernephroma.

**ICD-10:**          C64.

**Ep:**          Incidence: 15–22 cases/100,000/year, 2% of all malignant tumors; distribution male:female = 2:1; age peak: 50–70 years.

**Pg:**

*Risk Factors*
- Nicotine abuse, obesity, hypertension
- Chronic hemodialysis
- Ionizing radiation, exposure to cadmium, trichloroethylene
- Nephropathy associated with analgesic abuse

*Hereditary Forms*
- von Hippel-Lindau syndrome: 35% of all renal cell carcinomas, multifocal, bilateral
- Hereditary clear cell / papillary / chromophilic renal cell carcinoma
- Tuberous sclerosis
- Renal carcinoma with hereditary cystic kidney disease

*Molecular Genetic Abnormalities*
- Chromosome aberrations: deletion 3p- (VHL gene), translocation t(3;8) (FHIT gene) and t(3;11), trisomy 7, t(X;1)(p11;q21) (TFE3 and PRCC genes), various monosomies and trisomies
- In 80% of sporadic renal cell carcinomas: VHL gene aberrations (on chromosome 3p25). VHL mutations lead to dysregulation of HIFs (hypoxia-inducible factors) with simultaneous over-expression of VEGF (vascular endothelial growth factor). VEGF overexpression in > 70% of cases → angiogenesis, tumor vascularization ↑, metastasis ↑
- Oncogene aberrations: c-myc, c-fms, c-erbB, c-met

**Path:**

*Histology*
- Adenocarcinomas (> 95%) derived from tubular cells
- Other histological types rarely occur in adults

**Renal tumor types in adults**

| Histology | Frequency (%) | Genetic aberrations |
|---|---|---|
| *Adenocarcinomas* | 95 | |
| Clear cell carcinomas | 70–75 | 3p-, +7, +5, +10 |
| Chromophilic (papillary) carcinomas | 12 | +7, +17, -4, t(X;1), -Y |
| Chromophobic carcinomas | 5 | -1,-2,-6,-10,-13,-17,-21 |
| Bellini duct carcinomas | 1 | - |
| Spindle cell carcinomas | 1 | |
| Nonclassifiable carcinomas | 3–5 | |
| *Other* | | |
| Nephroblastomas, sarcomas, lymphomas | *Rare* | |
| Hemangiopericytomas, angiomyolipomas | | |

### Metastatic Spread
- In 30% of cases distant metastases at diagnosis
- Tumors < 3 cm in diameter usually without metastasis
- Hematogenic metastasis (lung / liver / bone / CNS) > lymphatic (pelvic / paraaortal) > local
- Regional lymph nodes: paraaortic, paracaval, renal hilum

### Metastatic Pattern
- Lung and mediastinum:     55%
- Regional lymph nodes:     34%
- Liver:     33%
- Bone:     32%
- Adrenal gland:     19%
- Kidney (contralateral):     11%
- CNS:     6%

**Class:**     TNM Staging of renal cell carcinoma ( 2002)

| | |
|---|---|
| *T* | *Primary Tumor* |
| TX | Primary tumor cannot be assessed |
| T0 | No evidence of primary tumor |
| T1 | Tumor ≤ 7 cm, confined to kidney |
| | a: Tumor ≤ 4 cm in greatest dimension; confined to kidney |
| | b: Tumor > 4 cm but < 7 cm in greatest dimension; confined to kidney |
| T2 | Tumor > 7 cm, confined to kidney |
| T3 | Tumor extends into major veins or invades adrenal gland or perinephric tissues |
| | a: Tumor invades adrenal gland or perinephric tissues |
| | b: Invasion into renal vein(s) or vena cava below the diaphragm |
| | c: Invasion into vena cava above the diaphragm or vena cava wall |
| T4 | Tumor invades beyond Gerota's fascia, infiltration of neighboring organs |
| *N* | *Lymph Node Involvement* |
| NX | Regional lymph nodes cannot be assessed |
| N0 | No regional lymph node metastasis |
| N1 | Metastasis in a single regional lymph node |
| N2 | Metastasis in more than one regional lymph node |
| *M* | *Distant Metastasis* |
| MX | Distant metastasis cannot be assessed |
| M0 | No distant metastasis |
| M1 | Distant metastasis |

### AJCC Staging of renal cell carcinoma (2002)

| Stage | TNM system | | | Frequency (%) |
|---|---|---|---|---|
| I | T1 | N0 | M0 | 40–45 |
| II | T2 | N0 | M0 | 10–20 |
| III | T1–2 | N1 | M0 | 20 |
| | T3 | N0–1 | M0 | |
| IV | T4 | Any N | M0 | 20–30 |
| | Any T | Any N | M1 | |

**Sy:** No early symptoms. In advanced stages:
- Hematuria:                                              60%
- Flank pain:                                             40%
- Palpable abdominal mass:                                45%
- Classic triad (hematuria + flank pain + tumor):        10%
- Weight loss:                                            35%
- Anemia:                                                 20%

*ATTENTION:* 60% of renal cell carcinomas are diagnosed incidentally through ultrasound examinations.

**Dg:**     *Medical History, Physical Examination*
- Medical history including family history, exposure to risk factors
- Physical examination: abdominal tumor, abdominal flow murmur

*Laboratory Tests*
- Routine laboratory tests including complete blood count, liver and renal function tests, LDH, alkaline phosphatase, ESR, urinary tests (hematuria, in some cases proteinuria)
- To monitor disease course in advanced stages: possibly serum levels of pyruvate kinase isoenzyme TUM2

*Imaging*
- Abdominal ultrasound, abdominal CT, MRI
- Intravenous pyelography, possibly isotopic nephrogram if reduced renal function of the affected or contralateral kidney
- Chest x-ray, possibly thoracic CT
- Cranial MRI (if CNS involvement suspected)
- Bone scan (if metastases suspected clinically)
- Doppler sonography / echocardiography to detect intravascular thrombi or tumor thrombi
- Prior to surgery: possibly angiogram

*Histology*
Diagnosis based on imaging is highly reliable. Histological analysis is usually carried out during curative surgery. Due to risk of tumor cell spread, fine-needle biopsy (ultrasound- or CT-guided) only in exceptional cases:
- Patients for whom primary surgery is not an option
- Patients with metastatic tumors where treatment concept requires histological diagnosis (consider biopsy of metastasis)

**Dd:**     *Differential Diagnosis of Lesions in the Renal Area*
- Renal cyst, renal echinococcosis, renal infarction
- Benign renal cortical adenoma, angiomyolipoma (benign)
- Nephroblastoma (Wilms' tumor), renal sarcoma

**Co:**     *Consequences of Vascular Invasion*
Varicocele, edema of the leg (due to invasion of the renal vein or inferior vena cava)

*Paraneoplastic Syndromes due to Tumor-associated Cytokine or Hormone Production*
- Fever, thrombocytosis, ESR ↑ (interleukins, esp. IL-6)
- Hypertension (renin), erythrocytosis (erythropoietin)
- Hypercalcemia (parathyroid hormone-related protein, PTH-RP)
- Amyloidosis
- Stauffer's syndrome (focal liver necrosis, enzyme increase, fever, weight loss)
- Non-metastatic elevation of alkaline phosphatase

**Th:** **Treatment Concept**

1. Renal cell carcinomas are primarily treated by surgery:
   - *Standard treatment:* radical tumor nephrectomy, (en bloc resection of the tumor, affected kidney, fatty tissue and Gerota's fascia, removal of any tumor thrombi in the renal vein and the vena cava; possibly ipsilateral adrenalectomy)
   - Views differ on the importance of lymphadenectomy
   - Organ-preserving surgical techniques in patients with single kidney, dysfunctional contra-lateral kidney, bilateral tumors, small tumors (T1a, < 4 cm) incidentally diagnosed during ultrasound examination
   - Single soft tissue metastases are surgically removed with curative intent. Multiple metastases or inoperability define a palliative approach
   - New therapeutic approaches (laparoscopic cryotherapy, radiofrequency ablation)
2. Preoperative or postoperative radiotherapy of the renal bed is not indicated. In certain cases, radiotherapy may be used as palliative treatment (pain, bone metastases).
3. Cytostatic treatment yields poor response rates (< 10–15%) and is only recommended in clinical trials.
4. Overall, 20% of metastatic renal cell carcinomas respond to immunotherapy with cytokines (interferon-α, interleukin-2, etc.). The effect is most likely due to a T-cell-mediated immune response (cytotoxic T-cells, CTL) against tumor antigens (RAGE and mutated HLA-A2 molecules). In patients with advanced metastatic renal cell cancer, immunotherapy with interferon after tumor nephrectomy has led to improved survival.
5. Targeted therapies (▶ Chaps. 3.5, 3.6):
   - Angiogenesis inhibition: e.g., VEGF antibodies (bevacizumab) or multikinase inhibitors (sorafenib, sunitinib)
   - EGFR inhibitors (gefitinib, erlotinib)
   - M-TOR inhibitors (temsirolismus); other antibodies (e.g., G250)

**Therapy of renal cell carcinoma**

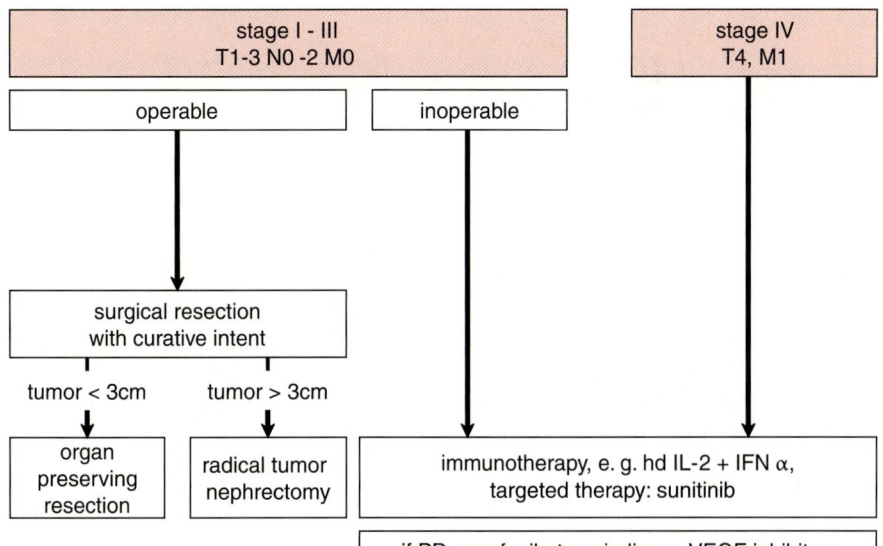

*hd IL-2* high-dose interleukin-2, *IFN* interferon-α, *PD* progressive disease

### Inoperable Metastatic Renal Cell Carcinoma

#### First-line Therapy
- High-dose interleukin-2 + interferon-α for selected patients: good performance status, low tumor volume or predominant lung metastasis. *ATTENTION*: side effects, particularly capillary leak syndrome.
- Interferon-α monotherapy: interferon-α 10 MIU s.c. 3 times weekly

#### Second-line Therapies
- Targeted therapies: sunitinib, sorafenib, VEGF inhibitors, temsirolismus
- Vaccination with autologous / allogeneic tumor material: genetically modified or with dendritic cells (several studies)
- Clinical trials (vaccination, others)

### Therapy Protocol Renal Cell Carcinoma

| "hd IL-2 / IFNα / 5-FU" | | | Start next cycle after 8 weeks |
|---|---|---|---|
| Interferon α | 5 MIU | s.c. | Day 1, weeks 1 + 4 |
| | 5 MIU | s.c. | Days 1, 3, 5, weeks 2 + 3 |
| | 10 MIU | s.c. | Days 1, 3, 5, weeks 5–8 |
| Interleukin-2 | 10 MIU/m² | s.c. 2 ×/day | Days 3–5, weeks 1 + 4 |
| | 5 MIU/m² | s.c. 2 ×/day | Day 1, 3, 5, weeks 2 + 3 |
| 5-Fluorouracil | 1,000 mg/m² | i.v. | Day 1, weeks 5–8 |

**Prg:**

#### Spontaneous Course of Metastatic Disease
- Spontaneous remission:                0.3%
- One-year survival:                     25%
- Three-year survival:                    4%
- Five-year survival:                     2%

#### Disease Course with Standard Treatment

| Stage | Five-year survival (%) | Ten-year survival (%) |
|---|---|---|
| T1, T2 | 80 | 45 |
| T3a | 60 | 25 |
| T3b–c | 50 | 15 |
| T4 | 10 | 3 |

#### Factors Associated with Poor Prognosis in Cases of Advanced Disease
- Karnofsky scale < 80%
- Serum $Ca^{2+}$ > 10 mg/dl (2.5 mmol/l), LDH ↑
- Hb < normal

**F/U:**   Patients treated with curative intent should be monitored closely, including abdominal ultrasound, chest x-rays, and if required CT / MRI. Follow-up initially every 3 months, after 2 years: every 6 months, after 5 years: once a year.
Palliative situations: symptom-based approach.

**Ref:**

1.  Costa LJ, Drabkin HA, Renal cell carcinoma: new developments in molecular biology and potential for targeted therapies. Oncologist 2007;12:1404–15
2.  Cohen HT, McGovern FJ. Renal-cell carcinoma. N Engl J Med 2005;353:2477–90
3.  Escudier B, Eisen T, Stadler WM et al. Sorafenib in advanced clear-cell renal-cell carcinoma. N Engl J Med 2007;356:125–34
4.  Garcia JA, Rini Bl. Recent progress in the management of advanced renal cell carcinoma. CA Cancer J Clin 2007;57:112–25
5.  Hudes G, Carducci M, Tomczak P et al. Temsirolismus, interferon alfa, or both for advanced renal-cell carcinoma. N Engl J Med 2007;356:2271–81
6.  Lam JS, Breda A, Belldegrun AS et al. Evolving principles of surgical management and prognostic factors for outcome in renal cell carcinoma. J Clin Oncol 2006;24:5565–75
7.  Motzer RJ, Hutson TE, Tomczak P et al. Sunitinib versus interferon alfa in metastatic renal-cell carcinoma. N Engl J Med 2007;356:115–24
8.  Pavlovich CP, Schmidt LS. Searching for the hereditary causes of renal cell carcinoma. Nat Rev Cancer 2004;4:381–93
9.  Yang JC, Childs R. Immunotherapy for renal cell cancer. J Clin Oncol 2006;24:5576–83

**Web:**

1.  http://www.cancer.gov/cancertopics/types/kidney     NCI Cancer Topics
2.  http://www.nlm.nih.gov/medlineplus/kidneycancer.html     Medline Plus
3.  http://www.emedicine.com/MED/topic2002.htm     E-medicine
4.  http://www.nccn.org/professionals/physician_gls/PDF/kidney.pdf     NCCN Guideline

## 8.6.2    Tumors of the Renal Pelvis, Ureter, and Bladder

**W. Schultze-Seemann, C.F. Waller**

**Def:**   Malignant neoplasms of the urinary tract, usually transitional cell cancer (urothelial carcinoma).

**ICD-10:**   C67.

**Ep:**
- *Urinary bladder cancer:* incidence 25 cases/100,000/year in Europe, distribution male:female = 3:1; 3% of all malignant solid tumors; age peak 60–70 years.
- *Cancer of the renal pelvis / ureter:* incidence 0.7 cases/100,000/year; distribution male:female = 5:2; ratio renal pelvis cancer:ureteral cancer = 3:1; age peak 50–70 years.

**Pg:**   *Risk Factors*
- Smoking (relative risk 2.0–10.0)
- Aromatic amines: 2-naphthylamine, benzidine, 4-aminobiphenyl, orthotolidine
- Drugs: alkylating agents (cyclophosphamide), analgesics (phenacetin)
- Chronic urinary infections, schistosomiasis (40% squamous cell cancer)
- Ionizing radiation, radiotherapy
- Family history of bladder carcinoma (relative risk 1.45)

*Occupational Risk Factors*
- Dye (anilin) industry, rubber industry, coal industry, aluminum industry
- Textile / dyeing industry, printing industry

*Molecular Genetic Abnormalities*
No characteristic aberrations have been identified. Deletions of chromosomes 3p / 8p / 9p21 / 11p / 17p / mutations in the tumor suppressor genes Rb and p53, as well as aberrations in the oncogenes H-ras, c-myc, and HER2/neu are frequently observed.

**Path:**   *Histology*

| Type | Frequency (%) |
|---|---|
| Transitional cell carcinoma | 90 |
| Squamous cell carcinoma | 6–8 |
| Adenocarcinoma | 2–3 |
| Sarcoma, carcinoid, lymphoma, small cell cancer | < 1 |

*"Field Cancerization"*
Cancer of the bladder, renal pelvis, and ureter is often a panurothelial disease. Common carcinogenetic mechanisms (polychronotropism) result in multiple preneoplastic changes. Primary multilocular carcinoma develops in 30–50% of cases. In addition to invasive carcinoma, there are usually large areas of intraurothelial lesions (carcinoma in situ, CIS). Over 50% of patients with untreated CIS develop an invasive carcinoma within 5 years.

*Manifestation / Spread*
- At presentation: 80% superficial carcinomas, 20% invasive tumors
- Regional lymphatic metastasis (lymph nodes of the pelvis minor) or retroperitoneal lymph node involvement (ureter or renal pelvis carcinomas)
- Hematogenous metastasis: lung, liver, skeletal system, CNS
- Direct invasion of adjacent structures: rectum, prostate, etc.

**Class:** **TNM staging of bladder cancer (2002)**

| *T* | *Primary Tumor* |
|---|---|
| TX | Primary tumor cannot be assessed |
| T0 | No evidence of primary tumor |
| Ta | Noninvasive papillary carcinoma |
| Tis | Carcinoma in situ: "flat tumor" |
| T1 | Invasion of the subepithelial connective tissue (lamina propria) |
| T2 | Tumor invades muscle |
| | a: Superficial muscle (inner half) |
| | b: Deep muscle (outer half) |
| T3 | Tumor invades perivesical tissue |
| | a: Microscopically |
| | b: Macroscopically (extravesical mass) |
| T4 | Tumor invades any of the following: prostate, uterus, vagina, pelvic wall, abdominal wall |
| | a: Tumor invades prostate, uterus, or vagina |
| | b: Tumor invades pelvic wall or abdominal wall |
| *N* | *Lymph Node Involvement* |
| NX | Regional lymph nodes cannot be assessed |
| N0 | No metastasis in regional lymph nodes |
| N1 | Metastasis in a single lymph node, ≤ 2 cm |
| N2 | Lymph node metastasis > 2 cm to ≤ 5 cm |
| N3 | Lymph node metastasis > 5 cm |
| *M* | *Distant Metastases* |
| MX | Distant metastasis cannot be assessed |
| M0 | No distant metastasis |
| M1 | Distant metastasis |

**Grade of differentiation (WHO) and correlation with infiltration / metastasis**

| Grade | Differentiation | Frequency (%) | Infiltration (%) | Metastasis (%) |
|---|---|---|---|---|
| G1 | Well differentiated | 25 | 19 | < 10 |
| G2 | Moderately differentiated | 50 | 40–60 | 30 |
| G3–G4 | Poorly differentiated | 25 | 80–90 | 80 |

**AJCC and Jewett-Marshall Staging of Bladder Carcinoma**

| AJCC | Jewett-Marshall | TNM system | | |
|------|----------------|-----------|------|------|
| 0is | Cis | Tis | N0 | M0 |
| 0a | 0 | Ta | N0 | M0 |
| I | A | T1 | N0 | M0 |
| II | B1 | T2a | N0 | M0 |
| | B2 | T2b | N0 | M0 |
| III | C | T3 | N0 | M0 |
| | D1 | T4a | N0 | M0 |
| IV | | T4b | N0 | M0 |
| | | Any T | N1–3 | M0 |
| | D2–3 | Any T | Any N | M1 |

**Sy:**
- Painless hematuria, micro- or macroscopic, 75–90% of patients, may occur early
- Dysuria, frequent voiding, 25% of cases
- Tumors of the bladder: pain in the pelvis / kidney area
- Carcinomas of the renal pelvis or ureter: flank pain

**Dg:**
### Medical History, Physical Examination
- Medical history including family history, occupation, risk factors
- Physical examination

### Laboratory Tests
- Routine laboratory tests, including liver / renal function tests, LDH, alkaline phosphatase
- Urinary nuclear matrix protein 22 (NMP22)

### Histology
- Urine cytology, lavage cytology
- Cystoscopy with collection of multiple biopsies, possibly photodynamic examination
- Transurethral tumor resection (TUR-B)

### Imaging
- Abdominal ultrasound, chest x-ray
- Ureterorenoscopy, possibly intravenous pyelography
- CT / MRI abdomen and pelvis, thoracic CT
- Bone scan in cases of invasive carcinoma or bone pain

**DD:**
- Interstitial cystitis (cystoscopy and histology, follow up)
- Benign lesion of the urinary bladder or renal pelvis
- Endometriosis, bladder stones (histology, cystoscopy)
- Renal cell cancer, solid tumor metastases

**Co:**
- Gross hematuria, hydronephrosis, renal failure, fistula
- Coagulopathies (disseminated intravascular coagulation (DIC), hyperfibrinolysis)
- Paraneoplastic neuromuscular syndromes

**Th:**     **Treatment concept of urinary bladder carcinoma**

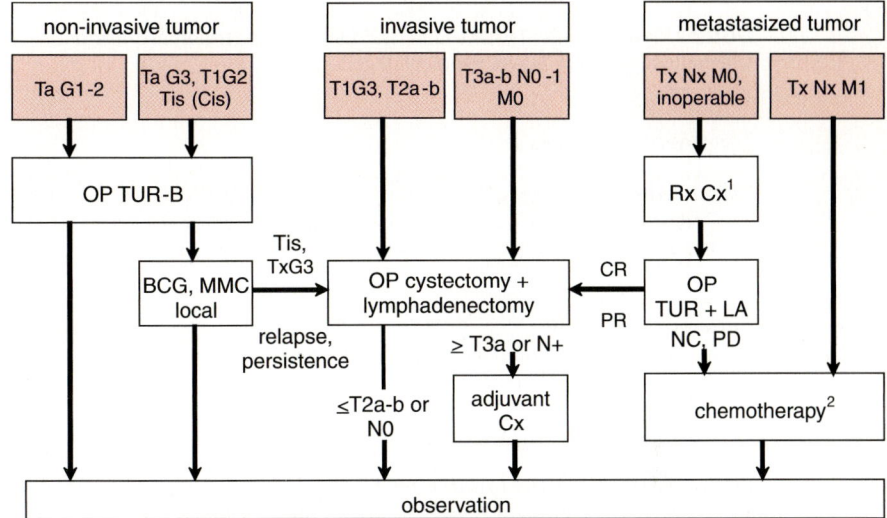

*TUR* transurethral resection (*B* bladder), *OP* surgery, *LA* lymphadenectomy, *Cx* chemotherapy, *RxCx* combined radiochemotherapy, *BCG* bacillus Calmette-Guérin, *MMC* mitomycin C, *CR* complete remission, *PR* partial remission, *NC* no change, *PD* progressive disease
[1] Cisplatin + 5-FU + radiotherapy
[2] Systemic chemotherapy (e.g., gemcitabine + cisplatin, MVAC)

### Non-invasive Tumors (Ta / T1 N0 M0, Tis)

- Transurethral resection (TUR-B) with curative intent, always followed by additional resection; alternatively: laser therapy
- Adjuvant intravesical therapy: when risk factors (multiple tumors, poorly differentiated tumor, recurrent tumor) are present
- No adjuvant therapy with Ta G1 tumors or small isolated Ta tumors
- Experimental: photodynamic therapy
- Recurrent / persistent tumor after intravesical therapy / high-risk situation: consider radical cystectomy + lymphadenectomy; with multiple tumors also ureterectomy / urethrectomy

#### Special Case: T1 G3 Tumor
Alternative treatment approach due to high-risk situation:
- Usually, radical cystectomy + lymphadenectomy
- Alternatively: TUR + secondary resection + adjuvant intravesical therapy; after 6 weeks: follow-up examination and histological analysis (with single focal tumor, without carcinoma in situ)

### Invasive Tumors / Metastasis

#### Invasive Operable Tumors (cT2–3b N0 M0)
- Radical cystectomy + lymphadenectomy
- If applicable, intraoperative radiotherapy (IORT; experimental)
- High-risk situation (T3b, lymph node involvement, poorly differentiated tumor): adjuvant chemotherapy (GC or MVAC protocol)

### Invasive Inoperable Tumors or Lymphatic Metastasis (cT4 Nx M0, cTx N1–3 M0)

With lymph node involvement or T4 tumors without distant metastasis: neoadjuvant radiochemo-therapy to achieve secondary operability.

### Distant Metastasis (cT1–4 N1–3 M1): Palliative Treatment Situation

Chemotherapy, GC or MVAC protocol (6 cycles)

## Treatment Modalities

### Transurethral Resection (TUR)

- Obligatory diagnostic TUR at presentation and for staging purposes
- Therapeutic TUR: treatment of local disease (Ta N0 M0, T1 N0 M0) with curative intent, always secondary resection after 10 days

### Intravesical Therapy

- Intravesical instillation treatment with administration of biological response modifiers: BCG (bacillus Calmette-Guérin, attenuated *Mycobacterium bovis* strain), or intravesical chemotherapy (monotherapy with epirubicin, doxorubicin, mitomycin C).
- Administration for 6–8 weeks of treatment; then biopsy, close cytological monitoring

### Radical Cystectomy and Lymphadenectomy

- Males: resection of bladder, prostate, and seminal vesicles
- Females: resection of bladder, uterus (not obligatory with T2a/b tumors)
- Urinary conduit
  - *Incontinent:* ureter / skin fistula, conduit (ileal or colon conduit)
  - *Continent:* ileal neobladder, catheterizable pouches, ureterosigmoidostomy (quality of life similar to that of healthy individuals)
- Complications: approximately 1% mortality, impotency (males), infection, fistulas, incontinence (females), hypercontinence (self-catheterization, especially women)

### Radiotherapy

- Local radiotherapy including regional lymph nodes in inoperable cases or older patients (stages T2–T4); total dose 50–60 Gy; significantly lower 5-year survival rates (20–40%) than with radical cystectomy; long-term consequences: dysfunctional contracted bladder, hemorrhagic cystitis, proctitis
- Palliative radiotherapy: local symptoms (bone metastases, uretral obstruction)
- Combined radiochemotherapy (e.g., 5-FU / cisplatin): inoperable cases or older patients (stages T2–T4); better 5-year survival rates (45–55%) than with radiotherapy alone.

### Chemotherapy

- Adjuvant and neoadjuvant chemotherapy in clinical trials
- Palliative chemotherapy in metastatic disease (symptomatic patients)

## Chemotherapy Protocols

| *"GC"* ▶ *Protocol 12.2.9* | | | *Start next cycle on day 29* |
|---|---|---|---|
| Cisplatin[1] | 70 mg/m²/day | i.v. | Day 1 |
| Gemcitabine | 1,000 mg/m²/day | i.v. | Days 1 + 8 + 15 |

[1] In older patients or with limited renal function: cisplatin 35mg/m²/day i.v. days 1 + 2

| "MVAC" ▶ Protocol 12.13.2 | | | Start next cycle on day 29 |
|---|---|---|---|
| Methotrexate | 30 mg/m²/day | i.v. | Days 1, 15, 22 |
| Vinblastine | 3 mg/m²/day | i.v. | Days 2, 15, 22 |
| Doxorubicin | 30 mg/m²/day | i.v. | Day 2 |
| Cisplatin | 70 mg/m²/day | i.v. | Day 2 |

| "MPC Salvage" | | | Start next cycle on day 22 |
|---|---|---|---|
| Methotrexate | 30 mg/m²/day | i.v. | Day 1 |
| Paclitaxel | 200 mg/m²/day | i.v. | Day 1, for 3 h |
| Cisplatin | 70 mg/m²/day | i.v. | Day 1 |

| "PC Salvage" | | | Start next cycle on day 22 |
|---|---|---|---|
| Paclitaxel | 175 mg/m²/day | i.v. | Day 1, for 3 h |
| Carboplatin | AUC: 6 | i.v. | Day 1 |

| "DC Salvage" | | | Start next cycle on day 22 |
|---|---|---|---|
| Docetaxel | 75 mg/m²/day | i.v. | Day 1 |
| Cisplatin | 75 mg/m²/day | i.v. | Day 1 |

| "Combined Radiochemotherapy"[1] | | | Start next cycle on day 22 |
|---|---|---|---|
| Cisplatin | 15 mg/m²/day | i.v. | Days 1–5, weeks 1 and 4 |
| 5-Fluorouracil | 350 mg/m²/day | i.v. | Days 1–5, weeks 1–5 |
| Radiotherapy[2] | 1.8 Gy/day | | Days 1–5, weeks 1–6 |

[1] Complete protocol: 2 cycles of chemotherapy with the GC protocol, then combined radiochemotherapy

[2] Total dose: 54Gy

## Treatment of Renal Pelvis Cancer and Ureter Cancer

### Localized Disease

#### Standard: Surgical Treatment

Complete surgical resection is the only curative treatment of urothelial carcinoma of the renal pelvis and the ureter. Methods:

- Radical surgery (nephroureterectomy) including excision of parts of the bladder with mucosa and regional lymphadenectomy; complete ureterectomy is recommended, due to high incidence of multiple ipsilateral lesions in the ureter and relapse in the residual ureter (20%)
- Alternatively: organ-preserving treatment (e.g., patients with single kidney, reduced renal function, Balkan nephropathy, bilateral tumors); local excision of renal pelvic lesions with or without partial nephrectomy or ureterectomy, or ureterectomy with ileum replacement
- Endoscopic approach: in patients with early stage low-grade tumors; long-term outcome not established

### Adjuvant Therapy
- Therapeutic benefit not established in clinical trials
- *Radiotherapy:* may be considered in case of high-grade tumors to prevent local relapse (poorly differentiated tumors, stages III–IV, lymph node involvement)
- *Adjuvant chemotherapy:* benefit in patients with renal pelvis and ureter carcinomas not certain.

## Advanced Stages

Palliative chemotherapy, e.g., with gemcitabine / cisplatin or MVAC or taxane (similar to treatment of bladder cancer).

**Prg:**

### Prognostic Factors
- Stage, grading (high relapse risk with poorly differentiated tumors)
- Multicentric tumor
- Vascular invasion
- p53 aberrations

### Five-year survival rate

| Stage | Urinary bladder carcinoma (%) | Renal pelvis / ureter carcinomas (%) |
|---|---|---|
| 0 | 50–90 | > 95 |
| I | 50–90 | > 95 |
| II | 40–80 | 90–95 |
| III | 2–40 | 40–70 |
| IV | < 10 | 0–40 |

**F/U:**   Patients treated with curative intent should be monitored closely including (uretero-) cystoscopy + histological analysis (alternatively: urinary cytology), abdominal ultrasound, chest x-rays; follow-up: initially every 3 months, after 2 years: every 6 months, after 5 years: once a year. MRI / CT abdomen / pelvis initially every 6 months, from 3rd year: every 12 months.
Palliative situations: symptom-based approach.

**Px:**   Occupational health and safety: no exposure to aromatic amines. Avoid tobacco.

**Ref:**
1. Advanced Bladder Cancer (ABC) Meta-analysis Collaboration. Adjuvant chemotherapy for invasive bladder cancer. Cochrane Database Syst Rev. 2006;(2):CD006018
2. Amiel GE, Lerner SP. Combining surgery and chemotherapy for invasive bladder cancer. Expert Rev Anticancer Ther 2006;6:281–91
3. Bamias A, Tiliakos I, Karali MD et al. Systemic chemotherapy in inoperable or metastatic bladder cancer. Ann Oncol 2006;17:553–61
4. Borden LS Jr, Clark PE, Hall MC. Bladder cancer. Curr Opin Oncol 2005;17:275–80
5. ESMO Guidelines Working Group. Invasive bladder cancer: ESMO Clinical Recommendations for diagnosis, treatment and follow-up. Ann Oncol 2007;18(suppl 2):ii38–9
6. Garcia JA, Dreicer R. Systemic chemotherapy for advanced bladder cancer: update and controversies. J Clin Oncol 2006;24:5545–51
7. Habuchi T, Marberger M, Droller MJ et al. Prognostic markers for bladder cancer: International Consensus Panel on bladder tumor markers. Urology 2005;66(6 suppl 1):64–74
8. Rödel C, Weiss C, Sauer R. Trimodality treatment and selective organ preservation for bladder cancer. J Clin Oncol 2006;24:5536–44
9. Wolff EM, Liang G, Jones PA. Mechanisms of disease: genetic and epigenetic alterations that drive bladder cancer. Nat Clin Pract Urol 2005;2:502–10

**Web:**

| | | |
|---|---|---|
| 1. | http://www.cancer.gov/cancertopics/types/bladder | NCI Cancer Topics |
| 2. | http://www.nlm.nih.gov/medlineplus/bladdercancer.html | MedlinePlus |
| 3. | http://www.emedicine.com/MED/topic2344.htm | E-medicine |
| 4. | http://www.nccn.org/professionals/physician_gls/PDF/bladder.pdf | NCCN Guideline |

# 8.7      Tumors of the Endocrine System

## 8.7.1      Thyroid Cancer

**R. Engelhardt, H. Henß**

**Def:**      Malignant tumors of the thyroid gland derived from thyrocytes or C-cells.

**ICD-10:**      C73

**Ep:**      Incidence 2–3 cases/100,000 population/year, distribution male:female = 1:2; age peak 25–65 years.

**Pg:**      *Risk Factors*
- Ionizing radiation, e.g., radiotherapy in children and teenagers, radioactivity
- Iodine deficiency

*Hereditary Neoplastic Syndromes*
Familial neoplastic syndromes are commonly associated with thyroid cancer:
- Multiple endocrine neoplasia type 2 (MEN 2): mutation of the RET protooncogene → medullary thyroid cancer, endocrine neoplasia (▶ Chap. 8.7.3)
- Familial adenomatous polyposis (FAP): mutation of the APC gene → differentiated thyroid carcinoma, intestinal adenomas
- Peutz-Jeghers syndrome → differentiated thyroid carcinoma
- Cowden's disease: mutation of the PTEN tumor suppressor gene → thyroid cancer, breast cancer, skin cancer

**Path:**      *Histological Types*

| Tumor type | Frequency (%) |
|---|---|
| *Differentiated Carcinomas* | 80–90 |
| • Papillary carcinoma | 60–70 |
| • Follicular carcinoma | 10–20 |
| *Undifferentiated (Anaplastic) Carcinomas* | 5–10 |
| *Medullary Carcinomas (C-cell Carcinomas)* | 5–10 |
| *Other* | 5 |
| • Sarcomas, lymphomas, teratomas, etc. | rare |
| • Metastases from extrathyroid tumors | |

*Papillary Carcinoma*
- Mainly local and lymphatic spread; distant metastasis in young patients (< 40 years) rare; favorable prognosis (esp. patients < 40 years)
- Primary tumor often small, multiple tumors in 50% of cases → negative scan
- Iodine metabolizing, thyroglobulin synthesis (tumor marker)

*Follicular Carcinoma*
- Mainly hematogenous metastases (lung, bone)
- Iodine metabolizing, thyroglobulin synthesis (tumor marker)
- Special form: Hürthle cell tumor: more aggressive, oxyphilic galectin-3-expressing tumor cells

*Undifferentiated Anaplastic Carcinoma*
- Mainly older patients, age peak 60–70 years
- Early hematogenous and lymphatic metastasis, usually palliative treatment
- No iodine metabolism, no thyroglobulin synthesis

### Medullary Carcinoma

- Carcinoma arising from the C-cells of the thyroid gland, sporadic or hereditary (20–25%, esp. in connection with MEN 2 syndromes)
- Initially locoregional metastasis (at presentation: 50% of cases), later hematogenous metastasis; > 90% of patients with MEN 2 bilateral, multiple tumors
- No iodine metabolism
- Tumor markers calcitonin, CEA
- In 35% of cases calcitonin-induced diarrhea

### MEN2 Syndromes

- "MEN" syndrome (multiple endocrine neoplasia): hereditary neoplastic syndrome with neoplastic transformation of various endocrine tissues
- MEN 2 syndrome: germline mutations of the RET protooncogene on chromosome 10q11.2, autosomal-dominant inheritance; MEN 2A syndrome (multiple endocrine neoplasia type 2A): mutations in exons 10–14, MEN 2B: mutations in exon 16
- MEN 2A: medullary thyroid carcinoma + pheochromocytoma + primary hyperparathyroidism
- MEN 2B: medullary thyroid carcinoma + pheochromocytoma + marfanoid habitus + ganglioneuromatosis of the mucous membranes
- Aberrations of the RET protooncogene in 20–25% of all medullary thyroid carcinomas

**Class:**     **TNM staging of tyroid cancer (2002)**

| | |
|---|---|
| *T* | **Primary Tumor** |
| TX | Primary tumor cannot be assessed |
| T0 | No evidence of primary tumor |
| T1 | Tumor ≤ 2 cm, limited to thyroid |
| T2 | Tumor > 2 to 4 cm, limited to thyroid |
| T3 | Tumor > 4 cm, limited to thyroid |
| T4 | Tumor of any size extending beyond the thyroid capsule |
| | a: Invasion of subcutaneous soft tissues, larynx, trachea, esophagus, recurrent laryngeal nerve |
| | b: Invasion of the prevertebral fascia or encases carotid artery or mediastinal vessels |
| *N* | **Lymph Node Involvement**[a] |
| NX | Regional lymph nodes cannot be assessed |
| N0 | No regional lymph node metastasis |
| N1 | Regional lymph node metastasis |
| | a: Metastasis to level VI (pretracheal, paratracheal, and prelaryngeal / Delphian lymph nodes) |
| | b: Metastasis to unilateral or bilateral cervical or superior mediastinal lymph nodes |
| *M* | **Distant Metastasis** |
| MX | Distant metastasis cannot be assessed |
| M0 | No distant metastasis |
| M1 | Distant metastasis |
| *R* | **Residual Tumor** |
| RX | Presence of residual tumor cannot be assessed |
| R0 | No residual tumor |
| R1 | Microscopic residual tumor |
| R2 | Macroscopic residual tumor |

[a] Regional lymph nodes: central, lateral, and mediastinal compartment

**Sy:**
- Palpable nodules of thyroid → solid, hard, possibly fixed
- Hard nodular goiter with or without palpable tumor
- Pain around the neck / ears / occiput, dysphagia
- Hoarseness (recurrent laryngeal nerve palsy)
- Miosis, ptosis, enophthalmus (Horner's syndrome)
- In rare cases: clinical picture of thyroiditis (inflammation, tenderness, warm)
- Advanced disease: dysphagia, stridor, superior vena cava syndrome

**Dg:**

### Medical History, Physical Examination
- Medical history including risk factors and family history
- Physical examination, ENT examination including vocal cord mobility

### Laboratory Tests
- Routine laboratory tests including serum calcium
- Tumor markers: thyroglobulin (differentiated carcinomas), calcitonin / CEA (medullary carcinoma) → *used particularly for monitoring following surgery*
- Thyroid function: TSH, T3 / FT3, T4 / FT4
- Pentagastrin test for medullary carcinoma of the thyroid: measuring serum calcitonin after stimulation with pentagastrin
- Medullary carcinoma of thyroid: screening for mutations of the RET protooncogene (possibly including family members)

### Histology
- Fine-needle biopsy: *preoperative test*, indicated due to high incidence of goiter in endemic areas (iodine-deficient areas)
- *NOTE:* negative result does not exclude carcinoma (particularly for follicular tumors)
- Unclear situations or inconsistency with negative cytology but suspicious symptoms: always histological analysis (either biopsy or diagnostic extirpation of cervical lymph nodes)

### Imaging
- Ultrasound examination of the thyroid, neck region and abdomen
- Chest x-ray, possibly thoracic CT
- Thyroid scintigraphy (assessment of endocrine activity, exclusion of metastasis)
- Cervical CT / MRI, esophageal barium study, tracheal imaging (if organ invasion suspected)
- ATTENTION: avoid iodine-containing contrast agents (reduced efficacy of postoperative radioactive iodine therapy)
- Medullary and undifferentiated thyroid carcinomas: further diagnostics to rule out distant metastasis

**Dd:**
- Nodular goiter
- Thyroid adenoma

**Th:**

### Treatment Concept

1. Treatment of differentiated thyroid carcinoma is always multimodal (surgery, radioactive iodine therapy, external beam radiotherapy, suppressive hormone therapy).
2. Medullary and anaplastic carcinomas, including local relapse, are primarily treated surgically. Other therapies are only of palliative value. Quality of surgery is of central importance (centers of excellence).
3. Radioactive iodine therapy is used in tumors participating in iodine metabolism (follicular and papillary carcinomas), with curative potential even in cases with distant metastases. Radioiodine therapy is not indicated in undifferentiated tumors and medullary carcinoma (here, possibly palliative external beam radiotherapy). *NOTE:* no thyroid hormone replacement therapy (L-thyroxine) 4 weeks prior to radioactive iodine therapy.
4. Chemotherapy is used with palliative intention in patients with systemically advanced i.e., metastatic disease

## Surgical Treatment

### Techniques
Standard procedure is total thyroidectomy with central lymph node dissection (i.e., removal of perithyroidal, prelaryngeal, and pretracheal lymph nodes).

### Indications
- Papillary carcinoma > 1 cm in greatest diameter (from T2) or multiple papillary carcinoma of any size
- Follicular carcinoma
- Medullary carcinoma (C-cell carcinoma)
- Undifferentiated carcinoma limited to the thyroid

### Surgical Techniques Without Lymph Node Dissection (Only in Exceptional Cases):
- Lobectomy / hemithyroidectomy: single papillary carcinoma < 1 cm (pT1a)
- Incidental diagnosis of isolated papillary thyroid carcinoma < 1 cm (pT1a) during bilateral subtotal resection of the thyroid: no additional surgery required if R0 resection without evidence of lymph node involvement

### Certain Situations Require Advanced Surgery:
- Lateral cervical lymph node involvement → lateral neck dissection
- Sporadic medullary carcinoma → unilateral lymph node dissection
- Familial medullary carcinoma → bilateral lymph node dissection
- Mediastinal lymph node involvement → mediastinal lymph node dissection
- Invasion of adjacent structures → multivisceral surgery

### Risks Associated with Surgery
- Hypoparathyroidism (10–15% of patients)
- Recurrent laryngeal nerve palsy

## Radioactive Iodine Therapy

### Technique
Administration of 1–3 GBq $^{131}$I (beta radiation, focal dose: > 300 Gy). Objectives:
- Ablation of any residual thyroid tissue
- Exclusion or detection and treatment of "hot" metastases

### Indications
- All cases of papillary and follicular thyroid carcinoma following thyroidectomy with or without lateral lymph node dissection
- *Not indicated* in papillary thyroid carcinoma (stage pT1a) after limited radical surgery, medullary carcinoma, and undifferentiated carcinoma

## External Beam Radiotherapy

### Technique
Reference dose: 50–60 Gy to the area of regional lymph drainage pathways, 60–70 Gy around the primary tumor ("thyroid bed").

### Indications
- Following thyroidectomy of undifferentiated carcinoma limited to the thyroid (adjuvant, questionable survival benefit)
- Differentiated thyroid carcinoma stage pT4 pN0–1, R0–2 GI–III
- After R1 or R2 resection of differentiated thyroid carcinoma and contraindication for secondary surgery and/or radioactive iodine therapy

- Adjuvant external beam radiotherapy after R0 resection and adequate radioactive iodine therapy of differentiated carcinomas is usually not indicated

## Chemotherapy

### Indications
Palliative situations, especially with diffusely metastatic and rapidly progressive disease, after all surgical and radio-oncological treatment options have been exhausted.

### Studies
Current interdisciplinary study concepts including chemotherapy are used particularly in undifferentiated carcinomas extending beyond the thyroid or metastatic tumors. Treatment concepts involve surgery as well as preoperative and/or postoperative radiochemotherapy.

### Chemotherapy Protocols

| *"Doxorubicin mono"* | | | *Start next cycle on day 22* | |
|---|---|---|---|---|
| Doxorubicin | 60–75 mg/m²/day | i.v. | Day 1 | |

| *"Cisplatin mono"* | | | *Start next cycle on day 22* | |
|---|---|---|---|---|
| Cisplatin | 75 mg/m²/day | i.v. | Day 1 | |

| *"AC"* | | | *Start next cycle on day 22* | |
|---|---|---|---|---|
| Doxorubicin | 60 mg/m²/day | i.v. | Day 1 | |
| Cisplatin | 40 mg/m²/day | i.v. | Day 1 | |

**Prg:**

| Tumor | Five-year survival (%) | Ten-year survival (%) |
|---|---|---|
| Papillary carcinoma | 85 | 80 |
| Follicular carcinoma | 70 | 60 |
| Medullary carcinoma | 70 | 55 |
| Undifferentiated carcinoma | < 10 | < 1 |

**F/U:**

- Monitoring of disease including medical history, physical examination, ultrasound (neck / abdomen), thyroglobulin / calcitonin / CEA, $^{131}$I whole body scan, chest x-ray; follow-up initially every 3–6 months, from 5th year every 12 months
- Life-long replacement therapy with l-thyroxine (150–250 µg/day) or triiodothyronine (80–120 µg/day); dosage according to basal TSH and T3 / FT3 (or T4 / FT4); aim: with differentiated carcinomas: suppressed TSH levels, with undifferentiated or medullary tumors: slightly subnormal TSH levels
- Monitoring of calcium metabolism (patients with treatment-induced hypoparathyroidism)
- With *medullary carcinomas*: exclusion of hereditary syndrome (MEN 2) → family screening for medullary carcinoma (pentagastrin test), pheochromocytoma (abdominal ultrasound, increased urinary levels of catecholamines / vanillylmandelic acid, metaiodobenzylguanidine scan, abdominal MRI), primary hyperparathyroidism ($Ca^{2+}$ ↑, phosphate ↓, parathormone ↑) possibly RET protooncogene assay

**Px:**
- *Medullary carcinoma:* possibly prophylactic thyroidectomy in patients with MEN 2 syndrome

**Ref:**

1. Baudin E, Schlumberger M. New therapeutic approaches for metastatic thyroid carcinoma. Lancet Oncol 2007;8:148–56
2. Fernandes JK, Day TA, Richardson MS et al. Overview of the management of differentiated thyroid cancer. Curr Treat Options Oncol 2005;6:47–57
3. Kebebew E, Greenspan FS, Clark OH et al. Anaplastic thyroid carcinoma. Cancer 2005;103:1330–5
4. Kondo T, Ezzat S, Asa SL. Pathogenetic mechanisms in thyroid follicular-cell neoplasia. Nat Rev Cancer 2006;6:292–306
5. Patel KN, Shaha AR. Poorly differentiated and anaplastic thyroid cancer. Cancer Control. 2006; 13:119–28
6. Sherman SI. Thyroid carcinoma. Lancet 2003;361:501–11
7. Traugott A, Moley JF. Medullary thyroid cancer: medical management and follow-up. Curr Treat Options Oncol 2005;6:339–46

**Web:**

| | | |
|---|---|---|
| 1. | http://www.endocrineweb.com/thyroidca.html | Endocrine Web |
| 2. | http://www.cancer.gov/cancertopics/types/thyroid | NCI Cancer Topics |
| 3. | http://www.nlm.nih.gov/medlineplus/thyroidcancer.html | MedlinePlus |
| 4. | http://www.emedicine.com/med/ONCOLOGY.htm | E-medicine |
| 5. | http://www.nccn.org/professionals/physician_gls/PDF/thyroid.pdf | NCCN Guideline |

## 8.7.2    Neuroendocrine Tumors (NET)

**F. Otto, R. Engelhardt, C.F. Waller**

**Def:**    Malignant tumors of neuroendocrine origin; characteristic secretion of serotonin and other hormones. Synonym: carcinoid

**ICD-10:**    C17, C34

**Ep:**    Rare disease; 0.5–2% of all gastrointestinal tumors; 0.4–1% of all neoplasias, incidence 1–2 cases/100,000 population; distribution male:female = 2:3; no age peak.

**Pg:**    The pathogenesis of sporadically occurring carcinoids is unknown. Increased risk in families with genetic syndromes (▶ Chap. 8.7.3):
- Multiple endocrine neoplasia type I (MEN 1)
- von Recklinghausen's disease (neurofibromatosis) type 1 (NF I)

**Path:**    *Histology*
Tumors originate from enterochromaffin, epithelial, or subepithelial neuroendocrine cells. Five histological subtypes: mixed, insular, trabecular, glandular, and undifferentiated forms.

*Location*
Carcinoids are most commonly located in the following organs:
- Appendix: 40% of all carcinoids
- Small intestine: 27%
- Rectum: 15%
- Bronchus: 12%
- Multiple locations: 30%

*Metastasis*
Depending on tumor size, extension into the muscle layer of the intestine, lymph node involvement, and tumor location (appendiceal carcinoids < 1 cm never metastasize, colon carcinoids metastasize frequently).

**Class:**    The classification of Williams and Sandler (1969) differentiates NET (carcinoids) depending on location and embryogenetic aspects:
- Origin in the foregut: thymus, lung, stomach, duodenum
- Origin in the midgut: ileum, appendix, proximal colon
- Origin in the hindgut: distal colon, rectum

The WHO classification of NET (2000) defines basic types of NET depending on their location:
1. Highly differentiated neuroendocrine tumor (carcinoid): benign or low malignant types, generally limited to the mucosa / submucosa
2. Highly differentiated neuroendocrine carcinoma (malignant carcinoid): low malignant course of disease, invasive
3. Poorly differentiated neuroendocrine carcinoma: always aggressive disease course, invasive growth and metastatic spread.

### WHO Classification of Gastrointestinal Neuroendocrine Tumors (NET) (2000)

*Stomach*
*Highly differentiated neuroendocrine tumors (carcinoid)*
- Enterochromaffin-like cell tumor (corpus / fundus): indolent; often multiple sites or carcinoid tumor associated with chronic atrophic gastritis (CAG) or MEN 1
- Tumor positive for serotonin or gastrin (rare)

*Highly differentiated neuroendocrine carcinoma (malignant carcinoid)*
- Functionally inactive: sporadic enterochromaffin-like cell carcinoma, in rare cases with chronic atrophic gastritis (CAG) or multiple endocrine neoplasia type I (MEN 1)
- Functionally active: carcinoma positive for serotonin (atypical carcinoid syndrome) or positive for gastrin (gastrinoma)

*Poorly differentiated neuroendocrine carcinoma*

### Duodenum / Proximal Jejunum
*Highly differentiated neuroendocrine tumors (carcinoid)*
- Tumor positive for gastrin (proximal duodenum)
- Functionally active gastrin-positive tumor (gastrinoma), sporadic or MEN 1
- Functionally active or inactive serotonin-positive tumor
- Gangliocytic paraganglioma (periampullary)
- Functionally inactive somatostatin-positive tumor (ampulla Vateri) with or without NF 1

*Highly differentiated neuroendocrine carcinoma (malignant carcinoid)*
- Functionally active gastrin-positive carcinoma (gastrinoma), sporadic or MEN 1
- Functionally inactive somatostatin-positive tumor (ampulla Vateri) with or without NF 1
- Functionally inactive or active carcinoma (with carcinoid syndrome)
- Malignant gangliocytic paraganglioma

*Poorly differentiated neuroendocrine carcinoma*

### Ileum, Cecum, Colon, and Rectum
*Highly differentiated neuroendocrine tumors (carcinoid)*
- Serotonin-positive tumor
- Enteroglucagon-positive tumor

*Highly differentiated neuroendocrine carcinoma (malignant carcinoid)*
- Functionally active or inactive serotonin-positive carcinoma
- Functionally inactive enteroglucagon-positive tumor

*Poorly differentiated neuroendocrine carcinoma*

### Appendix
*Highly differentiated neuroendocrine tumors (carcinoid)*
- Serotonin-positive tumor
- Enteroglucagon-positive tumor

*Highly differentiated neuroendocrine carcinoma (malignant carcinoid)*
- Functionally active or inactive serotonin-positive carcinoma

*Poorly differentiated neuroendocrine carcinoma*
- Goblet cell carcinoid

**Pathophysiology of carcinoid syndromes**

| Secreted polypeptide | Symptoms |
| --- | --- |
| Kallikrein (bradykinin) | Vasodilation (flushing), diarrhea, broncho-spasm |
| Serotonin | Flush, diarrhea, endocardial fibrosis, glucose intolerance, arthropathy, hypotension, edema, bronchoconstriction |
| Prostaglandin | Flushing, diarrhea, bronchospasm |
| Tachykinin (neurokinin A, neuropeptide K, substance P) | Vasodilation (flush) |
| Vasoactive intestinal polypeptide (VIP) | Diarrhea, telangiectasia |
| Hydroxytryptophan | Flush |

**Sy:**    *Nonspecific Symptoms*
- Abdominal symptoms, ileus of the small or large intestine, anemia

*Specific Symptoms Due to Hormonal Activity / Liver Metastases*
- Varying symptoms depending on hormonal release → acromegaly, Cushing's syndrome, recurrent ulcers of the stomach or duodenum (Zollinger-Ellison syndrome)

*Carcinoid Syndrome*
- Independent of the secretion of 5-hydroxyindoleacetic acid (5-HIAA), carcinoids may be accompanied by a carcinoid syndrome. Symptoms: flush attacks, intestinal hypermotility and hypersecretion with diarrhea, bronchospasm, endocardial fibrosis, hypotension, arthropathy, glucose intolerance
- Clinically symptomatic carcinoid syndrome often occurs only after metastatic invasion of the liver (reduced hepatic metabolization of polypeptides)

**Dg:**    *Medical History, Physical Examination*
- Medical history including symptoms of polypeptide secretion
- Physical examination including abdominal examination

*Laboratory Tests*
- Complete blood count, liver and renal function tests
- Tumor markers: chromogranin A, 5-HIES, serum levels of hormones (with functionally active tumors)

*Histology*
- Histology with histochemistry, immunoperoxidase stain (polypeptide hormones, ACTH, parathyroid hormone, gastrin, VIP, etc.), Ki-67 index
- Where applicable, electron microscopic analysis to detect potential membrane-bound neurosecretory granula

*Imaging*
- Abdominal ultrasound, chest x-ray, thoracic CT, abdominal CT
- Bone scan, octreotide scan; $^{187}$I-DOPA-PET
- Endoscopy (gastroscopy, rectosigmoidoscopy, colonoscopy, endosonography)
- Preoperatively: angiography, MRI, PET

**Co:**    Complications occur depending on location: ileus of the small or large intestine, hemorrhage, right heart failure with carcinoid syndrome.

Neuroendocrine tumors (NET)

| Location and subtype | Cell of origin and histology | Age (years) | Five-year survival | Clinical features |
|---|---|---|---|---|
| *Lungs and Bronchi* | | | | |
| Well-differentiated neuroendocrine tumor (typical carcinoid, mostly hilar region) | Epithelial endocrine cell, little atypia and mitoses | 40–50 | > 90% | Normally indolent; in some cases, secretion of corticotropin or serotonin |
| Well-differentiated neuroendocrine carcinoma (atypical carcinoid, peripheral) | Epithelial endocrine cell, cellular atypia, more mitoses, necrotic zone | 50–60 | 40–60% | Normally aggressive, high incidence of metastases (30–50%) |
| *Stomach* | | | | |
| Carcinoid tumor associated with chronic atrophic gastritis | Enterochromaffin-like cell Well differentiated Non-invasive | 60–70 | | Indolent; often multiple sites; no association with carcinoid syndrome; approximately 75% of gastric carcinoids, men > women, often < 1 cm |
| Carcinoid tumor and Zollinger-Ellison syndrome or MEN 1 | Enterochromaffin-like cell Well differentiated Non-invasive | | | Indolent; may occur in multiple sites, no carcinoid syndrome, 5–10% of gastric carcinoids, almost always patients with MEN 1 |
| Sporadic carcinoid | Enterochromaffin-like cell Well differentiated Often invasive | | | Aggressive growth with high incidence of metastasis, associated with atypical carcinoid syndrome (flush); 15–25% of gastric carcinoids, women > men |
| *Small Intestine* | | | | |
| Distal ileum, often multiple sites | Epithelial endocrine cell, well differentiated Presence of serotonin and substance P | 60–70 | 36% (metastasized) 65% (localized) | Often multiple sites, often occurring in ileum, 5–7% associated with carcinoid syndrome |

**Neuroendocrine tumors (NET)** (*continued*)

| Location and subtype | Cell of origin and histology | Age (years) | Five-year survival | Clinical features |
|---|---|---|---|---|
| *Appendix* | | | | |
| 75% distal third, 20% middle third, < 10% near base | Subepithelial endocrine cell, well differentiated<br>Presence of serotonin and substance P | 40–50 | 34% (metastasized)<br>94% (localized) | Normally indolent, men > women, > 95% less than 2 cm |
| *Colon* | | | | |
| Approximately 65% in right colon, particularly cecum | Epithelial endocrine cell, well differentiated<br>Presence of serotonin and substance P | 60–70 | 20% (metastasized)<br>70% (localized) | Often on right side, advanced stage at presentation, < 5% with carcinoid syndrome |
| *Rectum* | | | | |
| | Epithelial endocrine cell, well differentiated<br>Presence of serotonin and substance P | 50–60 | 18% (metastasized)<br>81% (localized) | Rarely associated with carcinoid syndrome, > 60% less than 1 cm, risk of metastasis is proportional to tumor size |

**Th:**

## Treatment Concept

The majority of carcinoids are malignant at presentation and cannot be cured by surgery alone, requiring a multimodal treatment approach.

## Types of Treatment

### Surgery

- Due to the slow growth of carcinoids, surgical resection is the key treatment option.
- Treatment with curative intent should involve radical resection of the primary tumor (even if multiple sites) including all accessible lymph nodes in the locoregional lymphatic drainage area of the tumor.
- In palliative situations, i.e., with locally incurable disease, the primary target is tumor debulking (particularly in cases of liver metastases, manifest carcinoid syndrome, and local obstruction).

### Radiotherapy / Nuclear Medicine

- Conventional radiotherapy only in patients with cerebral metastases or to control pain
- Treatment with radioactively marked agents ($^{90}$Y-DOTA-lanreotide, $^{177}$Lu-DOTA-octreotide) has demonstrated clinical benefit.

### Somatostatin Analogs

Symptomatic treatment; blocking somatostatin receptors.

- *Octreotide:* 50–200 µg 3 times daily by s.c. injection, for 6 weeks (minimum) → if good response: regularly; if no response or tachyphylaxis: dose increase to 1,000 µg twice daily; if given regularly, close monitoring of blood glucose and colon (colonoscopy → risk of colitis)
- *Lanreotide:* 750 µg 3 times daily by s.c. injection, days 1, 2, 3, 4 (repeat therapy after 2 weeks) or 30 mg by i.m. injection every 2 weeks; for 6 weeks (minimum)

### Interferon-α (IFNα)

- Anti-proliferative effect due to induction of nuclear enzymes; tumor regression (15%), stabilization (40%), and biochemical response (50%) have been described; median duration of response: 32 months; dosage: 3–9 million units by s.c. injection, 3–7 times weekly

### Chemotherapy

Carcinoids are moderately chemosensitive → chemotherapy only indicated after treatment failure with interferon / somatostatin analogs: response rate in NET of the pancreas with 5-FU + streptozocin or doxorubicin + streptozocin is 45% and 65%, respectively. Combination chemotherapy with etoposide and cisplatin (for protocol ▶ Chap. 8.2.1). Monotherapy with doxorubicin, melphalan or 5-FU achieves response in approximately 25% of patients.

**Prg:**

**Prognostic criteria for gastrointestinal NET**

| Biological behavior | Benign | Low malignancy | High malignancy |
| --- | --- | --- | --- |
| Metastases | – | + | + |
| Muscularis propria infiltration | – | +[b] | + |
| Grade differentiation | High | High | Low |
| Tumor size | ≤ 1 cm[a] | > 2 cm | Variable |
| Angioinvasion | – | + | + |
| Ki-67 index | < 2% | > 2% | > 30% |
| Hormonal syndrome | – | + | – |

[a] Except: malignant duodenal gastrinoma are generally smaller than 1 cm and limited to the submucosa
[b] Except: benign NET of appendix generally infiltrate lamina muscularis propria

**F/U:**          Clinical symptoms are the most important follow-up parameters. At the earliest 6 weeks after the start of treatment, follow-up by imaging and nuclear medical or biochemical procedures.

**Ref:**          1.    Durá I, Salazar R, Casanovas O et al. New drug development in digestive neuroendocrine tumors. Ann Oncol 2007;18:1307–13
                  2.    Kulke M. Advances in the treatment of neuroendocrine tumors. Curr Treat Options Oncol 2005;6:397–409
                  3.    Lal A, Chen H. Treatment of advanced carcinoid tumors. Curr Opin Oncol 2006;18:9–15
                  4.    Oberg K, Kvols L, Caplin M et al. Consensus report on the use of somatostatin analogs for the management of neuroendocrine tumors of the gastroenteropancreatic system. Ann Oncol 2004;15:966–73
                  5.    Ramage JK, Davies AH, Ardill J et al. Guidelines for the management of gastroenteropancreatic neuroendocrine (including carcinoid) tumours. Gut 2005;54(suppl 4):iv1–16
                  6.    Soga J. Early-stage carcinoids of the gastrointestinal tract. Cancer 2005;103:1587–95
                  7.    Zuetenhorst JM, Taal BG. Metastatic carcinoid tumors. Oncologist 2005;10:123–31

**Web:**          1.    http://www.carcinoid.org/                                            Carcinoid Foundation
                  2.    http://www.nlm.nih.gov/medlineplus/carcinoidtumors.html              Medline Plus
                  3.    http://www.cancer.gov/cancertopics/types/NCI
                        gastrointestinalcarcinoid/                                           Cancer Topics
                  4.    http://www.nccn.org/professionals/physician_gls/PDF/
                        neuroendocrine.pdf                                                   NCCN Guideline
                  5.    http://www.emedicine.com/med/topic271.htm                            E-medicine

### 8.7.3     Malignant Pheochromocytoma and MEN

**I. Brink, M. Engelhardt, H.P.H. Neumann**

**Def:**     Pheochromocytoma: malignant catecholamine-releasing tumor of the adrenal medulla or the paraganglia.

**ICD-10:**     C 74.1 (pheochromocytoma), C 85.8 (multiple endocrine neoplasia, MEN)

**Ep:**     Rare disease; no age peak; both sexes equally affected. Underlying cause of hypertension in 0.1% of cases

**Pg:**     There are no known exogenous causes of pheochromocytoma. Association with hereditary endocrine neoplastic syndromes in 35% of cases:
- von Hippel-Lindau (VHL) syndrome
- Multiple endocrine neoplasia type 2 (MEN 2)
- Neurofibromatosis type 1 (NF 1)
- Pheochromocytoma-paraganglioma syndrome (PGL 1, PGL 3, PGL 4)

Multiple endocrine neoplasias are hereditary (autosomal dominant) diseases with neoplastic changes of one or more of the following organs: pituitary gland, thyroid, parathyroid glands, exocrine pancreas, adrenal glands. Pathogenetic mutations of tumor suppressor genes, protooncogenes, or genes of the intracellular signal transduction are relevant (see table).

**Path:**     The majority of pheochromocytomas are benign, approximately 5% are malignant. In most pheochromocytoma-associated neoplastic syndromes (VHL syndrome, MEN 2, NF 1) malignant pheochromocytomas (1%) are rare. However, in patients with paraganglioma syndrome types (associated with SDHB mutations) the incidence is considerably high.

#### Malignancy Criteria
- Distant metastasis (liver, lung, bones)
- High mitotic index or vascular invasion, local invasion of retroperitoneal fat, or tumor in locoregional lymph nodes: suspicious, but no definite sign of malignancy

**Sy:**     Early symptoms are caused by endocrine activity (secretion of adrenaline / noradrenaline).
- Palpitations:                 > 80% of cases
- Headache:                    > 80%
- Excessive sweating:         > 80%
- Other symptoms caused by changes in the autonomic nervous system (paraganglia).

In advanced stages, symptoms due to tumor invasion and distant metastases.

**Dg:**     *Medical History, Physical Examination*
- Case history including family history (hereditary neoplastic syndromes?)
- Physical examination: hypertension (often intermittent), 24-h blood pressure assessment

#### Laboratory Tests
- Routine laboratory tests including liver and renal function tests
- Pathognomonic: detection of catecholamines in the urine → classical analyses include noradrenaline (NA), adrenaline (A), vanillylmandelic acid (VMS); determination of vanillylmandelic acid is less sensitive than noradrenaline. Currently the best marker is plasma metanephrine
- Molecular genetic examination to exclude hereditary tumor syndromes (see table)

### Imaging
- Abdominal CT / MRI
- Metaiodobenzylguanidine scan (MIBG) or DOPA-PET (using $^{18}$F-DOPA): DOPA-PET shows highest resolution
- MRI and MIBG scan and DOPA-PET have a higher sensitivity (95%) than CT scan; MIBG and DOPA-PET: key advantage is detection of whole body findings → exclusion of multilocular pheochromocytoma. MRI: esp. for imaging of retroperitoneum

**Recommended diagnostic approach with malignant pheochromocytoma: catecholamine levels in 24-h urine together with abdominal MRI.**

**Th:**

## Treatment Concept

1. Localized pheochromocytoma are primarily treated by surgery, if possible consider organ-preserving laparoscopic surgery.
2. Systemic treatment if resection not possible: therapeutic administration of MIBG, symptomatic blockade of catecholamine effects; with malignant pheochromocytoma: chemotherapy.
3. Symptoms, diagnosis, and treatment of malignant and benign pheochromocytomas are identical (apart from postoperative options).

## Treatment Modalities

### Receptor Blockade
Blockade of alpha- and beta-receptors. Indications:
- Preoperatively (to avoid intraoperative complications by catecholamine secretion)
- Palliative in inoperable cases

### Surgery
Localized malignant pheochromocytomas are resected by organ-preserving laparoscopic surgery if possible.

### MIBG Therapy
Therapeutic administration of $^{131}$Iodine metaiodobenzylguanidine ($^{131}$I-MIBG) in tumors with MIBG uptake (verified by diagnostic MIBG scan). Individual doses typically range from 3.7 to 7.4 GBq and will be repeatedly administered at intervals of several month.
"High dose" MIGB therapy (270-700 MBq/kg body weight, maximum 37 GBq) has been introduced by a San Francisco group achieving 13% CR and 50% PR in 30 patients. Side effects include severe thrombocytopenia and neutropenia, hypothyreodism, hypertension, ovarian failure, nausea, vomiting, secondary infections.

### Chemotherapy
- Conventional chemotherapy with cyclophosphamide, vincristine, and dacarbazine ("CVD", Averbuch protocol), 3–6 cycles depending on response
- Somatostatin analogs are not effective.
- Experimental therapies: sorafenib, sunitinib and VEGF antagonists are currently tested in clinical trials.

## Chemotherapy Protocol: Malignant Pheochromocytoma

| "CVD" Protocol 12.14.1 | | | Start next cycle on days 22–29 |
|---|---|---|---|
| Cyclophosphamide | 750 mg/m²/day | i.v. | Day 1 |
| Vincristine | 1.4 mg/m²/day | i.v. | Day 1, maximal 2 mg absolute |
| Dacarbazine | 600 mg/m²/day | i.v. | Days 1–2 |

**Prg:**    *Benign Pheochromocytoma*
Five-year overall survival: 95%

*Malignant Pheochromocytoma*
Available data limited due to low incidence of malignant pheochromocytomas; disease course can vary significantly; slow tumor growth or even stagnation are common; treatment with the Averbuch protocol achieves normalization of catecholamine levels in 79%, partial remission (PR) in 29%, complete remission (CR) in 14% of cases.

**Ref:**    1.    Kim WY, Kaelin WG. Role of VHL mutation in human cancer. J Clin Oncol 2004;24:4991–5004
2.    Lenders JWM, Eisenhofer G, Mannelli M et al. Phaeochromocytoma. Lancet 2005;366:665–75
3.    Lonser RR, Glenn GM, Walther M et al. Von Hippel-Lindau disease. Lancet 2003;361:2059–67
4.    Marx SJ. Molecular genetics of multiple endocrine neoplasia types 1 and 2. Nat Rev Cancer 2005;5:367–75
5.    Neumann HPH, Bausch B, McWhinney SR et al. Germline mutations in nonsyndromic pheochromocytoma. N Engl J Med 2002;346:1459–66
6.    Schiavi F, Boedecker cc, Bausch B et al. Predictors and prevalence of paraganglioma syndrome associated with mutations of the SDHC gene. JAMA 5005;294:2057–63
7.    Scholz T, Eisenhofer G, Pacak K et al. Current treatment of malignant pheochromocytoma. J Clin Endocrinol Metab 2007;92:121–25

**Web:**    1.    http://www.cancer.gov/cancertopics/types/pheochromocytoma/    NCI Cancer Topics
2.    http://www.nlm.nih.gov/medlineplus/pheochromocytoma.html    MedlinePlus
3.    http://www.emedicine.com/med/topic1816.htm    E-medicine

**Multiple endocrine neoplasia (MEN)**

| Hereditary syndrome | Gene | Manifestation | Basic diagnostics | Treatment concept |
|---|---|---|---|---|
| Multiple endocrine neoplasia 1 (MEN 1) | MEN 1 (11q13) | Primary hyperparathyroidism (90%), Endocrine pancreatic tumors (insulinoma) (60%), Pituitary tumors (5%) | Parathyroid hormone, gastrin, prolactin, molecular genetics | Subtotal parathyroid resection in HPT |
| Multiple endocrine neoplasia 2 (MEN 2) | c-RET (10q11,2) | Medullary thyroid cancer (95%), Pheochromocytoma (50%), Primary hyperparathyroidism (10%) | Calcitonin, pentagastrin test, molecular genetics | Thyroidectomy (even prophylactic), subtotal parathyroid resection in HPT |
| Von Hippel-Lindau (VHL) syndrome | VHL (3p25-26) | Angiomatosis retinae (50%), CNS hemangioblastoma (55%), Pheochromocytoma (30%), renal cysts (25%), renal cell cancer (25%), pancreatic cysts (15%), islet cell tumors (3%) | Fundoscopy, MRI CNS, abdomen, catecholamines in urine, ultrasound epididymis, molecular genetics | Retinal laser- / cryotherapy, adrenal resection, tumor resection of CNS tumors / pheochromocytoma / renal cell cancer |
| Neurofibromatosis type 1 (NF 1) | NF 1 (17q11,2) | Cutaneous café au lait spots (70–100%), axillary or inguinal speckling, neurofibromas (≥ 2 or 1 plexiform) (30%), Lisch nodules (≥ 2) (33–95%), optical glioma (15%), skeletal anomalies, Pheochromocytoma, abnormal vessels | Skin, eyes, MRI skull, abdomen, catecholamines in urine | Laser surgery of café au lait spots, resection of neurofibroma/ optical glioma |
| Pheochromocytoma- paraganglioma type 1 (PGL 1) | SDHD (11q23) | Pheochromocytoma Paraganglioma | MRI neck / thorax / abdomen, catecholamines in urine, molecular genetics | Tumor resection |
| Pheochromocytoma- paraganglioma type 2 (PGL 2) | 11q13 | Pheochromocytoma Paraganglioma | MRI neck / thorax / abdomen, catecholamines in urine, molecular genetics | Tumor resection |
| Pheochromocytoma- paraganglioma type 3 (PGL 3) | SDHC (1q21) | Pheochromocytoma Paraganglioma | MRI neck / thorax / abdomen, catecholamines in urine, molecular genetics | Tumor resection |
| Pheochromocytoma- paraganglioma type 4 (PGL 4) | SDHB (1p36) | Pheochromocytoma Paraganglioma | MRI neck / thorax / abdomen, catecholamines in urine, molecular genetics | Tumor resection |

*SDH* succinate dehydrogenase, *HPT* hyperparathyroidism, *MRI* magnetic resonance imaging

## 8.7.4 Tumors of the Adrenal Cortex

**M. Reincke, F. Flohr, J. Seufert**

**Def:** Predominantly benign tumors of the adrenal cortex (adenomas). Carcinomas of the adrenal cortex are rare.

**ICD-10:** D44.- (adrenal tumor)
C74.- (adreno cortical carcinoma)

**Ep:** Prevalence 1%, > 50 years: 3–7%. Incidence of adrenal cancer 2/100,000/year; distribution: male: female = 1:5. Two age peaks: before the age of 5, and between 40 and 70 years. Increasing frequency of "incidentaloma" (asymptomatic adrenal tumor) in the last 20 years due to improved imaging (CT /MRI/ultrasound).

**Pg:** *Adrenocortical Adenoma*
- Clonal expansion; underlying mutations unknown

*Adrenocortical Carcinoma*
- Clonal expansion after somatic oncogenic mutation (IGF II, p53), high genetic instability, loss of heterozygosity (e.g., ACTH receptor)
- Hereditary tumor syndromes: multistep carcinogenesis (Li–Fraumeni, Beckwith–Wiedemann syndrome, etc.)
- Risk factors: smoking, oral contraceptives

**Path:** *Histopathology (Adrenocortical Carcinomas)*
Adrenocortical cells with enlarged nuclei, multiple nucleoli and high rate of mitosis. Histological determination of malignant potential difficult in small tumors; search for additional macroscopic evidence: tumor weight > 500 g, typical lobulated surface, necroses, calcifications, hemorrhage, Ki67-lndex > 5%. Probability of malignancy is dependent on tumor size: < 4 cm: 3%; 4–6 cm: 6%; > 6 cm: 25%.

*Localisation*
No predominance for right or left adrenal, bilateral in 2–10% of cases.

**Staging of adrenal carcinoma**

| Stage | TNM |
|---|---|
| I | T1 N0 M0: tumor < 5 cm, limited to adrenal |
| II | T2 N0 M0: tumor > 5 cm, limited to adrenal |
| III | T1–2 N1 M0: tumor limited to adrenal and local lymph nodes, or T3 N0 M0 tumor outside adrenal, no organ invasion |
| IV | T3–T4 N1 M0 tumor outside adrenal, invading adjacent organs and local lymph node metastasis, or T1–4 N0–1 M1: tumor of any size with distant metastasis |

Carcinomas are characterized by dissemination: intracranial, cervical, lung, bone, liver.

**Sy:** *Adenoma (benign)*
- 80% of all cases are asymptomatic (incidentaloma)
- 20% hormonally active: subclinical Cushing's disease (11%), Conn's disease (2%), rarely androgen-producing tumor

*Adrenal Carcinoma*
- B symptoms: loss of weight, anorexia, fatigue
- Symptoms caused by size: abdominal pain, inferior vena cava syndrome
- Symptoms caused by metastasis (liver, lung, bone)

- Hormonal activity in 45–62% of cases (rapid onset):
  - Cushing's disease (hypercortisolism, 30–40%): striae, obesity, muscular atrophy, hypokalemia, hypertension, diabetes mellitus, depression
  - Virilization: (hyperandrogenism, 20–30%): acne, male hair growth pattern
  - Hyperaldosteronism (rare): hypertension, hypokalemia

**Dg:**    *Medical History, Physical Examination*
- Medical history including family history
- Physical examination including skin, abdomen, lymph nodes

*Laboratory Tests*
- Routine laboratory with blood count, liver and renal function tests; characteristic are anemia and hypokalemia
- With suspected Cushing's syndrome: 24 h urinary cortisol excretion ↑. No suppression of serum cortisol by dexamethasone (1 mg)
- With suspected Conn's syndrome: elevated aldosterone / renin ratio, metabolites of aldosterone in urine (aldosterone-18-glucuronide, tetrahydroaldosterone, THA)
- High secretion of androgens and/or estradiol, testosterone, DHEA-S or estradiol, pregnenolone

*Imaging (Staging)*
- Ultrasound of the abdomen, CT (native and contrast)
- If required MRI, FDG-PET
- Under development: $^{123}$I-Metomidate adrenal scintigraphy

*Histology*
- Surgical resection, histological processing. *NOTE:* no biopsy if adrenal carcinoma is suspected (risk of dissemination)

**Dd:**
- Metastases of extraadrenal primary tumors: 25–75%
- Infections: granuloma (tuberculosis, fungal), Echinococcus
- Tumor of adjacent organs: renal cell carcinoma, lipoma, etc.

**Co:**
- Adenoma and carcinoma: consequences of hormonal hypersecretion
- Carcinoma: local invasion (kidney, vena cava), tumor dissemination (lymphatic to retroperitoneal lymph nodes, hematogenous to lung, liver, bone)

**Th:**    *Tumor of Unknown Malignancy, Hormonally Active*
- Surgical resection
- Early consultation of endocrinologist. *NOTE:* watch for postoperative adrenal insufficiency even with asymptomatic patients (e.g., subclinical Cushing's syndrome)

*Tumors of Unknown Malignancy, Hormonally Inactive*
- Tumor < 4 cm: watch and wait, imaging every 6–12 months
- Tumor 4–6 cm: high resolution CT, if malignant tumor is suspected → surgical resection
- Tumor > 6 cm: open surgical resection
- Laparascopic surgical resection in specialized center, if tumor size < 4 cm

*Adrenocortical Carcinoma (ACC)*
- Stage I–II: surgical resection, "en bloc resection" with curative intent. Even with R0 resection often local relapse or spreading → consider adjuvant chemotherapy mitotane. *NOTE:* risk of adrenal insufficiency. Consider adjuvant radiotherapy within randomized prospective trials.
- Stage III–IV: standard therapy is primary surgical resection. In stage IV, the adrenolytic compound mitotane is part of first-line treatment, but often needs to be combined with cytotoxic chemotherapy. The benefit of adjuvant chemotherapy on overall survival has not been established. With tumor spreading: resection of primary tumor. Polychemotherapy with etoposide, doxorubicin and cisplatin or streptozotocin (response rate 30–54%).

**Prg:**

*Adrenal Adenoma*

100% cure by surgical resection.

*Adrenocortical Carcinoma: Poor prognosis*

- Stage I–II: mean overall survival 14 months to 3 years
- Stage III–IV: mean overall survival with chemotherapy 6–10 months

**F/U:**

- Hormonal hypersecretion: endocrinological function can be used as "tumor marker" (control of tumor progression)
- Postoperative adrenal insufficiency (Cushing's syndrome): cortisone substitution (diarrhea, surgery, etc.)
- Carcinoma: CT initially every 3 months

**Ref:**

1. Cobb WS, Kercher KW, Sing RF et al. Laparoscopic adrenalectomy for malignancy. Am J Surg 2005;189:405–11
2. Kirschner LS. Emerging treatment strategies for adrenocortical carcinoma. J Clin Endocrinol Metab 2006;91:14–21
3. Libe R, Bertherat J. Molecular genetics of adrenocortical tumours, from familial to sporadic diseases. Eur J Endocrinol 2005;153:477–87
4. Shen WT, Sturgeon C, Duh OY. From incidentaloma to adrenocortical carcinoma: the surgical management of adrenal tumors. J Surg Oncol 2005;89:186–92
5. Sidhu S, Sywak M, Robinson B et al. Adrenocortical cancer. Curr Opin Oncol 2004;16:13–18
6. Young WF. The incidentally discovered adrenal mass. N Engl J Med 2007;356:601–10

**Web:**

| | | |
|---|---|---|
| 1. | http://www.endotext.org/adrenal | Endotext |
| 2. | http://www.ensat.org/ | EU Network Adrenal Tumors |
| 3. | http://www.ganimed-net.de | GANIMED |
| 4. | http://www.firm-act.org | ACC Study |
| 5. | www.conn-register.de | Conn Register |
| 6. | http://www.cancer.gov/cancertopics/pdq/treatment/adrenocortical | Nci Cancer Topics |

## 8.7.5    Pituitary Gland Tumors

**F. Flohr, M. Reincke, J. Seufert**

**Def:**    Mainly benign pituitary adenoma, rarely pituitary carcinoma (< 0.5%)

**ICD-10:**    D44.3 (pituitary tumor); D35.2 (benign pituitary tumor)
C75.1 (pituitary carcinoma)

**Ep:**    Incidence of symptomatic pituitary tumors 0.4–7.4/100,000. No gender predominance. Asymptomatic microadenomas (≤ 10 mm) in 12–25% of all autopsies. Increase with age. "Incidentaloma" more frequently diagnosed by increasing use of imaging techniques (CT, MRI). 10–25% of all intracranial tumors.

**Pg:**    *Pituitary Adenoma/ Carcinoma*
- Clonal expansion; suspected role of "pituitary tumor transforming gene" (PTTG) oncogene in benign and malignant pituitary tumors.
- Familial: In Multiple Endocrine Neoplasia (MEN) tumor suppressor gene "Menin" mutated; however this explains only a small fraction (< 1%) of pituitary tumors

**Path:**    *Functional Histopathological Classification*

| *Pituitary Adenoma* | 99% |
|---|---|
| • Lactotroph adenoma (prolactinoma): | 35% |
| • Somatotroph adenoma (acromegaly): | 15–20% |
| • Corticotroph adenoma (Cushing's disease): | 5–10% |
| • Thyrotroph adenoma (hyperthyroidism): | < 1% |
| • Gonadotroph adenoma (amenorrhea): | rare |
| • Endocrine inactive tumors (null cell adenoma): | 30% |
| *Pituitary carcinomas* | |
| • No subtypes, metastases are indicative | 0.1–0.2% |

Carcinomas are defined by metastases: intracranial, cervical, lung, bones, liver (invasive growth per se is not a criterion for malignancy).

**Class:**    *Classification of Pituitary Tumors (Wilson)*

I:    normal/focally enlarged sella: tumor < 10 mm: microadenoma
II:    sella enlarged, tumor ≥ 10 mm: macroadenoma
III:    limited penetration into the basis of the sella
IV:    diffuse destruction of the basis of the sella
V:    extension within the sellar space or systemic dissemination

*Extension Beyond Sella*

0:    no
A:    infiltration in basal cisterna
B:    occlusion of recessus of 3rd ventricle
C:    displacement of 3rd ventricle
D:    parasellar extension
E:    extradural parasellar extension into or next to sinus cavernosus

**Sy:**    *Dependent on Sellar Mass*
- Headache of acute onset: pituitary apoplexy
- Diminished visual acuity (lead symptom in 40% of pituitary adenoma), hemianopia (bitemporal), oculomotory palsies (M. oculomotorius and M. abducens)
- Periorbital pain with sinus cavernosus infiltration
- Hydrocephalus
- "Obstructed nose," rhinoliquorrhea (large, invasive tumors)

### Failure of Anterior and Posterior Pituitary Gland
- Smaller tumor asymptomatic
- Secondary hypogonadism: amenorrhea, loss of libido, loss of secondary hair
- Secondary hypothyroidism: cold intolerance, puffy skin, attention deficit, slow pulse
- Secondary adrenal failure: wax-like skin color, reduced performance, fatigue, hypotension, hypoglycemia, nausea, adynamia, coma
- Growth hormone deficiency: weakness, increase of body fat, growth failure in children
- ADH deficiency: incomplete diabetes insipidus; polydipsia (nocturia)

### Endocrine Hypersecretion
- Acromegaly: acral growth, increased coarseness of figure, sweat, carpal tunnel syndrome, diabetes mellitus, joint pain, visceromegaly with heart failure
- Prolactinoma: galactorrhea, altered menstruation, loss of libido, amenorrhea, infertility, hypogonadism
- Cushing's syndrome: skin-related symptoms: acne, hirsutism, striae, ecchymoses; obesity, muscle atrophy, diabetes mellitus, hypertension, osteoporosis
- TSH- or gonadotropin-secreting tumors are rare: hyperthyroidism, amenorrhea

**Dg:**
### Medical History, Physical Examination
- Medical history, drug history
- Physical examination including neurological symptoms

### Laboratory Tests
- Routine laboratory evaluation
- Prolactin, TSH, fT3, fT4, FSH, LH
- Anterior lobe failure: hyponatremia, anemia; with hypersecretion: hypokalemia
- With suspected Cushing's syndrome: 24-h urine: cortisol excretion ↑. Missing suppression of serum cortisol following dexamethasone (1 mg). Abrogated circadian rhythm
- Growth hormone excess: IGF-I ↑, growth hormone secretion not suppressible by oral glucose load
- Suspected diabetes insipidus: water restriction test with osmolality in serum / urine

### Imaging (Staging)
- MRT skull (first choice): with dynamic sequences following gadolinium DTPA; CT only preoperative for evaluation of bone destruction

### Other Tests
- Ophthalmology: perimetry, fundoscopy, cranial nerves: III, IV, V1, VI
- Stereotactic biopsy: with suspected malignancy or craniopharyngioma
- Selective venous sampling (petrosal sinus catheter) with suspected central Cushing's syndrome

**Dd:**
- Inflammation: tuberculosis, sarcoidosis, lymphocytic hypophysitis
- Meningioma (15% of all intracranial tumors, 10% in sellar region)
- Craniopharyngioma, astrocytoma (hypothalamic tumor)
- Metastases: rarely clinically symptomatic; in post mortem series of patients with malignancy 27%
- Cystic tumors (Rathke's pouch)

**Co:**
- Continuing visual impairment (frequently normalization following surgery)
- Pituitary failure: most common anterior lobe, rarely posterior lobe (transiently following surgery)
- Hypothalamus affection with big tumors (disturbed appetite regulation, hypotonia)

**Th:**
### Surgery
- Indication: macroadenoma with extensive growth, failure of endocrine axis or endocrine hypersecretion. (Exception: in prolactinoma only drug treatment)

- Technique: transsphenoidal surgery possible in 90% (complications: CSF fistulae, meningitis < 1%), transcranial: necessary in rare cases with large tumors (complications: 3–5%)

### Radiation (< 45 Gy)
- Indication: invasive adenoma / recurrent tumors after surgical and medical treatment. Pituitary carcinoma, intractable endocrine hypersecretion
- Complications: hypopituitarism, optical nerve atrophy

### Medical Treatment
- Dopamine agonists are first-line treatment with prolactinoma
- Somatostatin analogs (octreotide, lanreotide) and GH-receptor antagonists (pegvisomant) in GH-secreting tumors (if not completely resectable)
- Hypopituitarism: substitution of cortisol, thyroxine, growth hormone, estrogens / gestagens, testosterone, desmopressin

### Pituitary Carcinoma
- Only case reports, surgery with radiation therapy
- Medical treatment: octreotide, dopamine agonists, and tamoxifen: may lower endocrine hypersecretion
- In palliative situation: chemotherapy with lomustine + 5-fluorouracil or platinum-based chemotherapy

**Prg:**
- Frequency of recurrent disease: 15% in the first 10 years following surgery
- Carcinoma: several years latency (7.7 years) between first diagnosis of pituitary tumor and appearance of metastases
- In metastatic disease: mean survival time 12 months

**F/U:**
- With endocrine hypersecretion: use normalization of endocrine function as marker
- Endocrinological follow-up 0, 3, and 12 months after surgery; from second year: at least once per year (valid for all pituitary tumors)

**Ref:**
1.    Bradshaw C, Kakar SS: Pituitary tumor transforming gene: an important gene in normal cellular functions and tumorigenesis. Histol Histopathol. 2007; 22:219–226.
2.    Melmed S, Acromegaly. N Engl J Med 2006; 355:2558–73.
3.    Minematsu T, Miyai S, Kajiya H, et al. Recent progress in studies of pituitary tumor pathogenesis. Endocrine 2005;28:37–41.
4.    Kaltsas GA, Grossmann AB: Malignant pituitary tumors. Pituitary 1998(1): 69–81.
5.    Simard MF: Pituitary tumor endocrinopathies and their endocrine evaluation. Neurosurg Clin N Am. 2003; 14:41–54.

**Web:**
1.    http://www.endotext.com/neuroendo
2.    http://www.ninds.nih.gov/disorders/pituitary_tumors/pituitary_tumors.htm
3.    http://www.cancer.gov/cancertopics/pdq/treatment/pituitary/healthprofessional

## 8.8 Malignant Tumors of the Skin

### 8.8.1 Melanoma

M. Schwabe, H. Veelken

**Def:** Malignant tumors of the melanocytic system.

**ICD-10:** C43

**Ep:** Incidence 6–14 cases/100,000/year in Europe, 30–50/100,000/year in Australia; 1.5–2% of all malignant tumors in Europe, 6–10% in Australia; incidence dependent on skin type / color of the skin and geographical factors; current incidence increase: 3–7% per year; distribution male:female = 2:3; age peak 40–60 years.

**Pg:** *Endogenous Genetic Risk Factors*
- Photosensitive bright skin and red or blond hair, blue or gray / green eyes, prone to sunburn (skin type I–III)
- Congenital nevus cell nevi: > 5 cm or large quantities (> 50)
- Dysplastic nevi or familial dysplastic nevus cell syndrome (familial atypical multiple mole and melanoma – FAMMM syndrome)
- Lentigo maligna
- Xeroderma pigmentosum
- Genetic abnormalities: mutations on chromosomes 9 (melanoma locus 9p21 with the tumor suppressor genes *INK4a* and *INK4b* → normal protein products p16$^{INK4a}$ and p15$^{INK4b}$ show tumor suppressor activity via Rb and p53); 1p; 6q22-27; 10q24-26 and 7

*Exogenous Risk Factors*
- High UV exposure (UV-A > UV-B)
- Repeated severe sunburn, especially during childhood

**Path:** *Histology*
Tumors originating from melanocytes (neural crest).

| Manifestation | Abbreviation | Frequency (%) |
|---|---|---|
| • Superficial spreading melanoma | SSM | 50–70 |
| • Nodular melanoma | NM | 10–30 |
| • Acrolentiginous melanoma | ALM | 5 |
| • Lentigo maligna melanoma | LMM | < 5 |
| • Unclassifiable cases, special types | | < 5 |

*Location*
- Skin (> 90%), eye (5%, most common intraocular tumor)
- Mucous membranes (GI tract, bronchial system), meninges

*Metastasis*
- At diagnosis, 80% primary tumors without metastasis
- "Satellite metastases": skin metastases ≤ 2 cm from primary tumor
- "In-transit metastases": skin metastases > 2 cm from primary tumor but not beyond the regional lymph nodes (skin metastases beyond the regional lymph nodes are considered distant metastases)
- Regional lymph node metastases
- Distant metastases, esp. skin, subcutaneous tissue, lymph nodes, CNS, visceral organs, bone, and bone marrow

**Class:**     Principles of the revised classification of the AJCC (2001):

- Depth of invasion according to Clark is only used for carcinoma in situ (Tis, equal to Clark level I) and T1 tumors.
- Key prognostic criteria of the primary tumor are vertical thickness (according to Breslow) and ulceration status.
- Lymph node metastases are subclassified according to size.
- Distant metastases are classified according to their location.

### Depth of invasion (Clark Level; 1969)

| Level | Depth of invasion |
|-------|-------------------|
| I     | Intraepidermal |
| II    | Extending beyond the basal membrane into the papillary dermis |
| III   | Tumor fills the entire papillary dermis |
| IV    | Invasion of the reticular dermis |
| V     | Invasion of the subcutaneous fat |

### TNM staging of melanoma (2002)

| *T* | *Primary Tumor: Thickness (Breslow)* |
|-----|--------------------------------------|
| Tx  | Primary tumor cannot be assessed |
| T0  | No primary tumor |
| Tis | Melanoma in situ, Clark level I |
| T1  | Tumor thickness (TT) ≤ 1.0 mm |
|     | A: not ulcerated and Clark level II–III |
|     | B: ulcerated or Clark level IV–V |
| T2  | TT 1.01–2.0 mm (A not ulcerated, B ulcerated) |
| T3  | TT 2.01–4.0 mm (A not ulcerated, B ulcerated) |
| T4  | TT > 4.0 mm (A not ulcerated, B ulcerated) |
| *N* | *Lymph Nodes (LN)* |
| Nx  | Lymph nodes cannot be assessed |
| N0  | No lymph node metastasis |
| N1  | 1 LN (A micrometastases[a], B macrometastases[b]) |
| N2  | 2–3 LN (A micrometastases, B macrometastases, C in-transit metastases or satellite(s) without lymph node metastasis) |
| N3  | ≥ 4 LN or matted LN or in-transit metastases or satellite tumors with lymph node metastatis |
| *M* | *Distant Metastasis* |
| Mx  | Distant metastasis cannot be assessed |
| M0  | No distant metastasis |
| M1  | Distant metastasis |
|     | A: cutaneous, subcutaneous, non-regional LN, LDH normal |
|     | B: lung, LDH normal |

*TT* tumor thickness (Breslow 1970), *LN* lymph node(s)
[a] Diagnosis of micrometastases via sentinel lymph node biopsy (SLNB) or elective lymphadenectomy
[b] Macrometastases: palpable lymph nodes with histologically confirmed tumor invasion or lymph nodes with extensive histological capsular invasion

**TNM staging of melanoma (2002)** *(continued)*

> C: all other visceral metastases with normal LDH or any distant metastases with increased LDH

*TT* tumor thickness (Breslow 1970), *LN* lymph node(s)
[a] Diagnosis of micrometastases via sentinel lymph node biopsy (SLNB) or elective lymphadenectomy
[b] Macrometastases: palpable lymph nodes with histologically confirmed tumor invasion or lymph nodes with extensive histological capsular invasion

**AJCC Staging (2002) and prognosis**

| Stage | TNM classification | | | Survival rates (%) | | |
|---|---|---|---|---|---|---|
| | T | N | M | 1 year | 5 years | 10 years |
| 0 | Tis | N0 | M0 | 99 | 97 | 95 |
| IA | T1a | N0 | M0 | 99 | 95 | 88 |
| IB | T1b, T2a | N0 | M0 | 99 | 90 | 81 |
| IIA | T2b, T3a | N0 | M0 | 98 | 93 | 64 |
| IIB | T3b, T4a | N0 | M0 | 95 | 65 | 53 |
| IIC | T4b | N0 | M0 | 90 | 45 | 32 |
| IIIA | Any T | N1 | M0 | 94 | 67 | 60 |
| IIIB | Any T | N2 | M0 | 85 | 52 | 42 |
| IIIC | Any T | N3 | M0 | 75 | 27 | 19 |
| IVA | Any T | Any N | M1A | 60 | 19 | 16 |
| IVB | Any T | Any N | M1B | 57 | 7 | 3 |
| IVC | Any T | Any N | M1C | 40 | 9 | 6 |

**Sy:**
- Asymmetric mark with irregular borders, light brown to black
- Sometimes ulcerating, bleeding, or itchy
- Also occurring in locations such as eye, sole of foot, subungual, oral mucosa, rectum, vulva, vagina, or penis
- Symptoms with metastatic disease dependent on involved area

**Dg:**

### Medical History, Physical Examination
- Medical history including family history, UV exposure, skin changes
- Physical examination including local symptoms, lymph node status

**ABCD rule: suspected melanoma**

| A | Asymmetry | Asymmetrical |
|---|---|---|
| B | Border | Irregular |
| C | Color | Inhomogeneous, light brown to black, sometimes speckled |
| D | Diameter | > 5 mm in diameter |

### Laboratory Tests
- Blood count, liver and renal function, LDH
- Alkaline phosphatase (evidence of bone metastases?)

### Imaging (Staging)
- Ultrasound (abdomen, lymph nodes), chest x-ray
- Thoracic / abdominal CT, cranial MRI
- Possibly PET (importance uncertain)
- Possibly bone scan, melanoma scan

### Histology
- *ATTENTION: suspect lesions must always be excised in total with a safety margin and histologically analyzed; no fine-needle biopsy to avoid risk of tumor cell spread*
- Immunohistochemistry (especially in cases with indistinct histology): detection of melanoma-specific antigens (e.g., HMB-45, MITF) and non-specific antigens (S-100)

### Sentinel Lymph Node (SLN) Biopsy
Intraoperative identification of the first lymph node into which the tumor drains ("sentinel node") via radiolymphoscintigraphy (labeled sulfur colloid) and/or peritumoral injection of vital dye. Frozen section → if sentinel lymph node positive for tumor cells: regional lymphadenectomy

**Dd:**
- Melanocytic nevi
- Epithelial tumors (e.g., pigmented basalioma)
- Vascular tumors (e.g., pyogenic granuloma)
- Hematoma

**Th:**

## Treatment Concept

1. *Initial therapy of melanoma is usually with curative intent.* Patients in early stages of the disease have a long-term cure rate > 50%. Only patients with multiple cerebral metastases or poor performance status (Karnofsky < 70%) are treated palliatively. Correct staging prior to treatment is essential.
2. *Surgery* is first-line treatment of the primary tumor, lymph nodes, and single metastases.
3. *Chemotherapy:* chemotherapy alone is indicated in selected cases only; response rates (mono- or combination chemotherapy) 10–40%. Effective drugs: dacarbazine (DTIC), temozolomide, fotemustine, platinum analogs, vinca alkaloids, taxanes, alkylating agents (ifosfamide, cyclophosphamide).
4. *Cytokines and biochemotherapy:* are standard treatments in advanced stages. Monotherapy with interferon alpha (IFNα) or interleukin-2 (IL-2) yields response rates of 15–20% in cases with stage IV disease. High-dose cytokines in combination with cytostatics ("biochemotherapy") lead to improved response rates.
5. *Radiotherapy:* patients with cerebral metastases, localized bone metastases, and adjuvant treatment after sphincter-preserving excision of perianal, rectal, or vaginal melanomas. The value of adjuvant radiotherapy of regional lymph nodes has not yet been established in randomized prospective phase III trials.

**Treatment of melanoma**

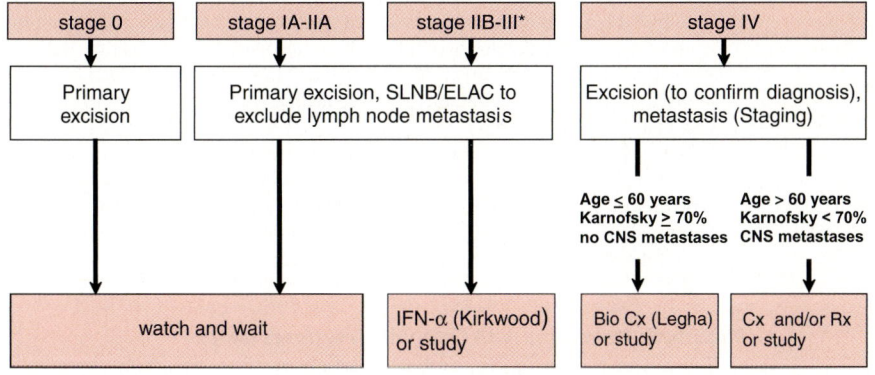

*SLNB* sentinel lymph node biopsy, *ELAC* elective lymphadenectomy, *Cx* chemotherapy, *Rx* radiotherapy, *BioCx* biochemotherapy

## Therapy Guidelines: Local Disease (Stages 0–III)

### Treatment according to metastatic potential
- With low risk of metastasis (e.g., carcinoma in situ, SLNB with no lymph node metastasis) → watch and wait
- High metastatic potential (e.g., micrometastases in the SLN, large tumors) → adjuvant chemotherapy is indicated.

### Localized Stages with Low Risk of Distant Metastasis (Stages IA–IIA)
- Wide surgical excision of the primary tumor, safety margin > 1 cm
- SLN biopsy (SLNB) or elective lymphadenectomy (ELAC)
- Adjuvant treatment not indicated

### Localized Stages with High Risk of Distant Metastasis (Stages IIB–III)
- Wide surgical excision of the primary tumor, safety margin ≥ 2 cm
- SLN biopsy or elective lymphadenectomy
- Adjuvant treatment is indicated
- Neoadjuvant treatment is currently tested in clinical studies (chemotherapy / biochemotherapy)
- In stage III disease and with N3 metastases (bulky lymph nodes; often invasion of nerve and vascular sheaths): R0 resection may not be feasible → treat like stage IV disease

### Adjuvant Treatment Options
- *High-dose IFN-$\alpha_{2b}$:* randomized studies have demonstrated a significant advantage with respect to relapse-free survival and overall survival; currently being tested in clinical trials: pegylated interferon α.
- *Adjuvant chemotherapy or radiotherapy:* no improvement in relapse-free or overall survival rate.
- *Experimental therapies:* current trials with autologous dendritic cells as well as other vaccination concepts (e.g., ganglioside vaccine, EORTC study 18961)

### Treatment Guidelines: Metastatic (Stage IV)

#### Metastatic Melanoma without Cerebral Metastases (M1a and M1b)
- Combined biochemotherapy is effective (cytokines + combination chemotherapy). Treatment according to the Legha protocol (cisplatin + vinblastine + dacarbazine + IFN$\alpha_{2b}$ + IL-2) yields response rates of > 50% and CR rates of 10–20%; improved relapse-free survival or overall survival has not yet been etablished. Replacement of dacarbazine by temozolomide leads to reduced CNS relapse rates.
- Patients with poor performance status (Karnofsky ≤ 70%) or > 60 years of age are not eligible for treatment according to the Legha protocol; alternative: palliative chemotherapy (dacarbazine or temozolomide).
- Combination chemotherapy (esp. Dartmouth regime: dacarbazine, cisplatin, CCNU, tamoxifen) is not superior to monotherapy with dacarbazine.
- Isolated organ metastases should be removed surgically.

#### Metastatic Melanoma with Cerebral Metastases (M1c)
- *Isolated cerebral metastases:* surgical resection, possibly stereotactic approach
- *Multiple cerebral metastases:* whole-brain radiotherapy, possibly concomitant chemotherapy with temozolomide
- *ATTENTION:* patients with symptomatic cerebral metastases should not be treated according to the Legha biochemotherapy protocol (risk of lethal side effects due to potentiation of perifocal cerebral edema by IFN$\alpha$ and IL-2)
- Alternative chemotherapies for patients with symptomatic cerebral metastases or poor performance status (Karnofsky ≤ 70%): temozolomide and fotemustine

#### Treatment of Relapse
- Often good response with second line chemotherapy (e.g., fotemustine) or biochemotherapy
- Inclusion in clinical trials (experimental treatment approaches)

#### Experimental Therapies
- *Active immunotherapy:* vaccination with melanoma-associated tumor antigens (MAGE-1, MAGE-3, Melan-A, gp100, tyrosinase, etc.), e.g., peptide vaccines or peptide-loaded autologous dendritic cells, genetically modified tumor cells.
- *Adoptive immunotherapy:* adoptive transfer of tumor-specific T-cells; if applicable, with non-myeloablative conditioning treatment.
- *High-dose chemotherapy:* allogeneic blood stem cell transplantation if HLA-identical related donor is available and ECOG performance status is 0–1, to induce graft-versus-tumor effects.
- *Regional therapies:* hyperthermic limb perfusion with melphalan and tumor necrosis factor (carried out in experienced centers in line with clinical studies). Liver metastases in trials choroidal melanoma: fotemustine 100 mg/m², infusion via hepatic arterial line.

### Melanoma Therapy Protocols

| "hd IFN-$\alpha_{2b}$ (Kirkwood)" | | | |
| --- | --- | --- | --- |
| IFN$\alpha_{2b}$ | 20 MIU/m² | i.v. | 5 times weekly for 4 weeks (induction) |
| | 10 MIU/m² | s.c. | 3 times weekly for 18 months (maintenance) |

| *"Biochemotherapy (Legha)"* ▶ Protocol 12.15.1 | | | *Start next cycle on day 43* |
|---|---|---|---|
| Dacarbazine | 800 mg/m²/day | i.v. | Days 1, 22 |
| Vinblastine | 1.5 mg/m²/day | i.v. | Days 1–4, 22–25 |
| Cisplatin | 20 mg/m²/day | i.v. | Days 1–4, 22–25 |
| IL-2 | 9 MIE/m²/day | i.v. | Days 5–8, 17–20, 26–29 |
| IFNα$_{2b}$ | 5 MIE/m²/day | s.c. | Days 5–9, 17–21, 26–30 |

| *"CVD"* ▶ Protocol 12.15.3 | | | *Start next cycle on day 22* |
|---|---|---|---|
| Dacarbazine | 800 mg/m²/day | i.v. | Days 1, 22 |
| Vinblastine | 2 mg/m²/day | i.v. | Days 1–4, 22–26 |
| Cisplatin | 20 mg/m²/day | i.v. | Days 1–4, 22–26 |

| *"DTIC mono"* ▶ Protocol 12.5.4 | | | *Start next cycle on day 22* |
|---|---|---|---|
| Dacarbazine | 1000 mg/m²/day | i.v. | Day 1 |

| *"Temozolomide mono"* ▶ Protocol 12.17.2 | | | *Start next cycle on day 29* |
|---|---|---|---|
| Temozolomide | 150 mg/m²/day | p.o. | Days 1–5 |

| *"Fotemustine mono"* | | | *Start next cycle on day 43* |
|---|---|---|---|
| Fotemustine | 100 mg/m²/day | i.v. | Days 1, 8, 15, for 1 h, protect from light |

| *"Temozolomide with Whole-brain Irradiation"* | | | |
|---|---|---|---|
| Temozolomide | 75 mg/m²/day | p.o. | Parallel to radiotherapy, then |
| | 200 mg/m²/day | p.o. | Days 1–5 (maintenance) |

**Prg:** Prognostic factors:
- Thickness and ulceration of the primary tumor
- Regional lymph node involvement (number of involved lymph nodes, micro- versus macro-metastases)
- Number and location of distant metastases: poor prognosis with visceral metastases (lung, GI tract, CNS)
- LDH, alkaline phosphatase, platelets: poor prognosis with increased LDH / ALP levels or pathological platelet count
- Performance status: ECOG ≥ 1 and Karnofsky < 70%: poor prognosis
- Gender: women have a more favorable prognosis

**Px:**
- Education on risk factors for melanoma
- Regular inspection of the skin (ABCD rule)
- Sun protection; sunburn must be avoided (particularly in children)

**F/U:**     Patients treated with curative intent should be monitored closely:
- First and 2nd year: physical examination every 3 months, chest x-ray and abdominal ultrasound every 6 months
- From 3rd year: physical examination every 6 months, chest x-ray and abdominal ultrasound every 12 months or whenever clinically indicated

With metastases or palliative situations: symptom-based approach

**Ref:**     1.   Curtin JA, Fridlyand J, Kageshita T et al. Distinct sets of genetic alterations in melanoma. N Engl J Med 2005;353:2135–47

**Ref:**     2.   ESMO Guidelines Working Group. Cutaneous malignant melanoma: ESMO Clinical Recommendations for diagnosis, treatment and follow-up. Ann Oncol 2007;18(suppl 2):ii71–3

3.   Fears TR, Guerry DP, Pfeiffer RM et al. Identifying individuals at high risk of melanoma: a practical predictor of absolute risk. J Clin Oncol 2006;24:3590–6

4.   Ives NJ, Stowe RL, Lorigan P et al. Chemotherapy compared with biochemotherapy for treatment of metastatic melanoma. J Clin Oncol 2007;25:5426–34

5.   Miller AJ, Mihm MC. Melanoma. N Engl J Med 2006;355:51–65

6.   Morton DL, Thompson JF, Chochran AJ et al. Sentinel-node biopsy or nodal observation in melanoma. N Engl j Med 2006;355:1307–17

7.   Scoggins CR, Chagpar AB, Martin RC et al. Should sentinel lymph-node biopsy be used routinely for staging melanoma and breast cancers? Nat Clin Pract Oncol 2005;2:448–55

8.   Thompson JF, Scolyer RA, Kefford RF. Cutaneous melanoma. Lancet 2005;365:687–701

9.   Verma S, Quirt I, McCready D et al. Systematic review of systemic adjuvant therapy for patients at high risk for recurrent melanoma. Cancer 2006;106:1431–42

**Web:**     1.   http://www.cancer.gov/cancertopics/types/melanoma            NCI Cancer Topics
2.   http://www.nlm.nih.gov/medlineplus/melanoma.html            MedlinePlus
3.   http://www.emedicine.com/DERM/topic257.html                  E-medicine
4.   http://www.nccn.org/professionals/physician_gls/PDF/melanoma.pdf   NCCN Guideline
5.   http://www.sign.ac.uk/pdf/sign72.pdf                          SIGN Guideline

**8.8.2**     **Basal Cell Carcinoma**

H. Veelken

**Def:**      Malignant epithelial neoplasia originating from epidermal basal cells and/or the outer root sheath of the hair follicle. Synonym: basalioma

**ICD-10:**   C44.-

**Ep:**       Most common malignant tumor of the skin. Incidence: 60–100 cases/100,000/year; distribution male:female = 1:1; median age: 60 years.

**Pg:**       *Risk Factors*
- Chronic UV exposure, radiation
- Carcinogenic chemicals (e.g., arsenic)
- Immunosuppression
- Genetic factors, e.g., hypopigmented skin

**Path:**     Basal cell carcinoma (BCC) is characterized by slow growth for months or years. They are regarded as semimalignant, due to their locally infiltrating and destructive growth (potential invasion of bones and cartilage) but usually non-metastatic nature.

*Histology (Often Mixed)*

| Type | Characteristics |
|------|-----------------|
| Nodular BCC | Nodular string-of-pearls margin (solid subtype, adenoid subtype, cystic subtype) |
| Superficial BCC | Superficial type, flat growth, string-of-pearls margin, mainly affecting area of the back |
| Sclerosing BCC | Sclerodermiform type ("morphea-like"), superficial encrusted skin lesion (resembling non-healing skin abrasion, red mark), string-of-pearls margin; aggressive growth, high relapse risk, more malignant than other types |

*Location*
Eighty percent on head / neck, mostly face → mainly in the eyelid region.

**Dg:**       *Medical History, Physical Examination*
- Case history with assessment of risk factors
- Skin inspection: initially, flesh-colored hardened patch of skin; later, hyaline yellow-red nodules with string-of-pearls margin (telangiectasis); in some cases, central ulceration or plate-like appearance; facial basal cell carcinomas are usually located above the line from angle of mouth to ear, often eyelid

*Histology*
- Excision with safety margin, histology

*Imaging*
Only with destructive basal cell carcinomas, tumors > 2 cm and/or clinically suspected invasion of deeper structures:
- Chest x-ray, abdominal ultrasound, lymph node ultrasound
- Where applicable, MRI scan of the affected region (head)

**Th:**  **Treatment Concept**

The type of treatment depends on the location and size of the tumor as well as the patient's performance status. Systemic chemotherapy does not play a role in the treatment of basal cell carcinoma.

### Surgical Treatment
- First-line therapy: excision
- Invasive basal cell carcinomas of the head / distal extremities, if located around nose, orbit or ear: > 5 mm, otherwise > 2 cm, relapsed tumor: Mohs' micrographic surgery (complete histological examination of excisional margins; lowest relapse risk)
- R1 and R2 resection of facial tumors and/or invasive tumor type: always secondary surgery aimed at R0 resection
- Where applicable, plastic surgery to compensate skin defects

### Radiotherapy
- In primarily inoperable situations as well as R1 and R2 resection → total dose 50–74 Gy
- Similar cure rate as surgery
- Better cosmetic and functional results

### Alternative Therapies
- Cryotherapy with liquid nitrogen or $CO_2$ laser therapy: with small superficial tumors in older patients (disadvantages: scarring, photosensitivity)
- Photodynamic therapy (PDT): superficial tumors only → application of photosensitizer cream (MAOP) followed by exposition to infrared light, very good cosmetic result, no scarring
- Topical therapy: superficial basal cell carcinoma and multiple basal cell carcinomas of the trunk: topical treatment with imiquimod 5% cream twice daily for 4–6 weeks; local (and experimental intralesional) chemotherapy with 5-fluorouracil

**Prg:**  Cure rate 90–99%; involvement of the eyelid may require removal of the eye.

**Px:**  **Protection**
- Intensive sun exposure should be avoided
- Use of sun blockers with high sun protection factor
- *Screening*: annual examination of the skin for potentially cancerous lesions: women from 20 years and men from 45 years of age

**F/U:**  First 3 years: annual follow-up; with local relapse or after R1/R2 resection more frequently.

**Ref:**
1. Bath FJ, Bong J, Perkins W et al. Interventions for basal cell carcinoma of the skin. Cochrane Database Syst Rev 2003;2:CD003412
2. Brooke RC. Basal cell carcinoma. Clin Med 2005;5:551–4
3. Rubin AI. Basal cell carcinoma. N Engl J Med 2005;353:2262–9

**Web:**
1. http://www.nlm.nih.gov/medlineplus/ency/article/000824.htm     MedlinePlus
2. http://www.emedicine.com/med/topic214.htm     E-medicine
3. http://www.skincancer.org/basal/index.php     Skin Cancer Foundation

**8.8.3 Squamous Cell Carcinoma**

H. Veelken

**Def:** Malignant tumor of the skin originating from cells of the epidermal stratum spinosum.

**ICD-10:** C44.-

**Ep:** Incidence approximately 9 cases/100,000/year; more common in fair-skinned people; men > women; median age 70 years.

**Pg:** *Risk Factors*
- Genetic factors
- Chronically stressed skin: chronic UV exposure, chronic inflammation, radiodermatitis, burn scars, lupus vulgaris, viral infections (e.g., condylomata acuminata due to oncogenic HPV), phimosis
- Pre-cancerous lesions: solar / actinic keratosis, leukoplakia
- Immunosuppression
- Ionizing radiation
- Chemical carcinogens (e.g., arsenic, asphalt, tar, paraffin)

**Path:** *Histology*

| Type | Characteristics |
|------|-----------------|
| Cutaneous spindle cell | Aggressive |
| Desmoplastic | – |
| Acantholytic / adenoid | – |
| Keratinizing | – |
| Lymphoepithelioma-like | Benign, no distant metastasis |
| Verrucous | – |

*Location*

Ninety percent are in the face (mainly bottom lip but also oral mucosa and tongue); 10%: other locations (e.g., hands, penis, vulva). Squamous cell carcinomas of the skin are characterized by locally destructive growth. Metastasis rate: approximately 5% (regional lymph nodes).

**TNM staging of squamous cell carcinoma of the skin**

| *T* | *Primary Tumor* |
|-----|-----------------|
| TX | Primary tumor cannot be assessed |
| T0 | No evidence of primary tumor |
| Tis | Carcinoma in situ (no metastasis) |
| T1 | Tumor ≤ 2 cm |
| T2 | Tumor > 2 cm, ≤ 5 cm |
| T3 | Tumor > 5 cm |
| T4 | Tumor invades deep extradermal structures (e.g., cartilage, skeletal muscle, or bone) |
| *N* | *Lymph Node Involvement* |
| NX | Regional lymph nodes cannot be assessed |
| N0 | No regional lymph node metastases |

**Class:**          **TNM staging of squamous cell carcinoma of the skin** *(continued)*

| | |
|---|---|
| N1 | Regional lymph node metastases |
| *M* | *Distant Metastasis* |
| MX | Distant metastasis cannot be assessed |
| M0 | No distant metastasis |
| M1 | Distant metastasis |

**AJCC Staging (2002)**

| Stage | TNM classification | | |
|---|---|---|---|
| 0 | Tis | N0 | M0 |
| I | T1 | N0 | M0 |
| II | T2 | N0 | M0 |
| | T3 | N0 | M0 |
| III | T4 | N0 | M0 |
| | Any T | N1 | M0 |
| IV | Any T | Any N | M1 |

**Histopathological classification according to tumor thickness**

| pT category | Definition of prognostic groups | Metastasis rate |
|---|---|---|
| pT1–3a | Limited to dermis, tumor thickness ≤ 2 mm | 0% |
| pT1–3b | Limited to dermis, tumor thickness > 2 mm, < 6 mm | 6% |
| pT1–3c | Invasion of subcutis and/or tumor thickness > 6 mm | 20% |
| pT4a | Invasion of deep extradermal structures (T4): tumor thickness ≤ 6 mm | 25% |
| pT4b | Invasion of deep extradermal structures (T4): tumor thickness > 6 mm | Up to 40% |

**Dg:**          *Medical History, Physical Examination*
- Medical history including risk factors
- Skin inspection: endophytically growing nodule with central crater and raised margin, mainly bottom lip but also forehead or cheek, usually on UV-damaged skin, sometimes bleeding Lymph nodes.

*Histology*
- Excision (biopsy). Typical: keratinization and formation of keratin pearls

*Imaging*
- Tumor > 2 mm: lymph node ultrasound scan
- Chest x-ray, abdominal ultrasound
- Where applicable, CT thorax / abdomen, MRI

**Dd:**          • Other skin tumors: basalioma, Merkel cell carcinoma, melanoma
- Tumors with skin affection: Paget's disease; lymphoma, metastasis, etc.

**Th:**   **Treatment Concept**

*Treatment must be initiated immediately after diagnosis.*

### Surgery
Standard treatment is immediate tumor excision; local cure rate 88–96%.
- With facial tumors or invasive desmoplastic tumors: micrographic surgery (3–5 mm safety margin, topographical marking, complete histological analysis), where required, secondary excision (always with desmoplastic tumors) aimed at R0 resection
- If necessary, conventional surgery with ≥ 1 cm safety margin, however: increased relapse risk
- Where applicable, sentinel lymph node biopsy
- Squamous cell carcinoma of the ear / tip of the nose: primary excision in combination with plastic surgery
- Involvement of regional lymph nodes: radical lymphadenectomy
- With extensive involvement of lips and concurrent lymph node spread: therapy analog to oral carcinoma of the floor of the mouth (▶ Chap. 8.1)

### Cryotherapy
- Indication: small superficial tumors in older patients, pre-cancerous lesions, carcinoma in situ

### Radiotherapy
- Indication: primarily inoperable tumors, carcinoma of skin appendages, following R1 and R2 resection, with regional lymph node metastases; total dose: 50–74 Gy
- Similar cure rate as surgical treatment
- Better cosmetic and functional results

### Palliative Chemotherapy
- Indication: stages III and IV, Karnofsky scale > 70%
- Standard treatment: methotrexate monotherapy (response rate 20–40%)
- Pain and other symptoms: combination chemotherapy, e.g., cisplatin / doxorubicin, cisplatin / 5-fluorouracil, cisplatin / 5-fluorouracil / bleomycin (response rate 50–90%)
- Compared to monotherapy, combination chemotherapy does not seem to confer a survival advantage

### Multimodal Therapies
- Patients with inoperable primary tumors may be treated with combined radiochemotherapy similar to the treatment of head / neck tumors (cisplatin / 5-fluorouracil / radiotherapy)

**Prg:**   Skin tumors < 2 cm: cure rate of approximately 97%; poor prognosis: cancer of the tongue, vulva, and penis.

**F/U:**   Risk-adapted follow-up:
- Tumor ≤ 2 mm in thickness: annual follow-up for up to 5 years
- Tumor 2.1–5 mm in thickness: 6-monthly follow-up for up to 5 years
- Tumor > 5 m in thickness and/or immunosuppression: 1st year: 3-monthly follow-up with clinical examination and ultrasound, 2nd to 3rd year: every 6 months, from 4th year: clinical examination every 12 months

**Ref:**
1. Albert MR, Weinstock MA. Keratinocyte carcinoma. CA Cancer J Clin 2003;53:292–302
2. Boukamp P. Non-melanoma skin cancer: what drives tumor development and progression? Carcinogenesis 2005;26:1657–65
3. Lane JE, Kent DE. Surgical margins in the treatment of nonmelanoma skin cancer and Mohs micrographic surgery. Curr Surg 2005;62:518–26
4. Rinker MH, Fenske NA, Scalf LA et al. Histologic variants of squamous cell carcinoma of the skin. Cancer Control 2001;8:354–63

**Web:**
1. http://www.cancer.gov/cancertopics/types/skin                   NCI Cancer Topics
2. http://www.nlm.nih.gov/medlineplus/ency/article/000829.htm       MedlinePlus
3. http://www.emedicine.com/DERM/topic401.htm                       E-medicine
4. http://www.skincancer.org/squamous/index.php                     Skin Cancer Foundation

## 8.8.4　Merkel Cell Carcinoma

H. Veelken

**Def:** Malignant neoplasia of Merkel cells (basal layer of the epidermis). Synonym: trabecular carcinoma, cutaneous neuroendocrine carcinoma

**ICD-10:** C44.-

**Ep:** Incidence: 0.23 cases/100,000 population/year (caucasian), 0.01 cases/100,000 population/year (noncaucasians); ratio male:female = 2.3:1; age peak approximately 70 years.

**Pg:** *Risk Factors*
- Immunosuppression (e.g., HIV, secondary neoplasia)
- High UV exposure (UV-A, UV-B), repeated sunburn
- Arsenic cytostatic drugs
- Genetic abnormalities: e.g., aberrations of chromosomes 1, 3, 13, del(1p36), p53 mutations, bcl-2 overexpression

**Path:** Merkel cells are part of the neuroendocrine system (APUD system); involved in mechanoreception. Characteristics of Merkel cell carcinoma are:
- *Macroscopic:* subepidermal tumor frequently extending to subcutaneous fat, rarely epidermis.
- *Histology:* small basophilic cells with hyperchromatic nuclei and minimal cytoplasm arranged in different size strands / solid cell complexes (trabecular pattern).
- *Immunohistochemistry:* immunophenotype of the malignant cells: positive for cytokeratin 20, cytokeratin 8, cytokeratin 18, neurofilament protein, NSE; negative for cytokeratin 7, S100.

*Histopathological Classification of Merkel Cell Carcinomas*

| Subtype | Frequency (%) | Prognosis |
|---|---|---|
| Trabecular | 8 | Good |
| Intermediate solid | 56 | Intermediate |
| Small cell diffuse | 32 | Poor |

*Location*
- Head / neck:　　　　50% of cases
- Extremities:　　　　40%
- Trunk and genitals:　10%

**Class:** Staging of Merkel cell carcinomas (according to Yiengpruksawan et al.)

| | |
|---|---|
| Stage I | Primary skin tumor without metastases |
| Stage Ia | Primary tumor ≤ 2 cm |
| Stage Ib | Primary tumor > 2 cm |
| Stage II | Primary skin tumor with regional lymph node metastases |
| Stage III | Distant metastases (cutaneous, liver, lung, bone, brain) |

Merkel cell carcinomas are characterized by aggressive growth, high relapse rates, and a strong tendency to metastasize. At presentation, approximately 20% of patients have stage II disease and 8% have stage III disease.

**Dg:**    *Medical History, Physical Examination*
- Medical history including risk factors
- Physical examination including local skin inspection: solid red-violet or flesh-colored painless nodule, sometimes plaque-shaped or ulcerated, average diameter < 2 cm, typical location: areas with high UV exposure (face, extremities). Examination of lymph node status

*Histology*
- Excision biopsy with safety margin, histology, immunohistochemistry

*Imaging*
- Lymph node ultrasound scan, possibly lymphscintigraphy
- Chest x-ray, abdominal ultrasound
- CT thorax / abdomen, cranial MRI (where applicable)
- Octreotide scan, $^{131}$iodine metaiodobenzylguanidine (MIBG) scan (where applicable)

## Treatment Concept

1. The primary treatment of Merkel cell carcinomas is surgical excision with adjuvant radiotherapy.
2. Merkel cell carcinomas are chemo- and radiosensitive. However, duration of remission is generally < 6 months. In adjuvant situations, chemotherapy is of no relevance. Chemotherapy is, however, recommended in the treatment of advanced metastatic disease (combination chemotherapy similar to small cell lung cancer) (▶ Chap. 8.2.1).
3. In inoperable situations, palliative treatment can significantly improve quality of life.

**Treatment of Merkel cell carcinoma**

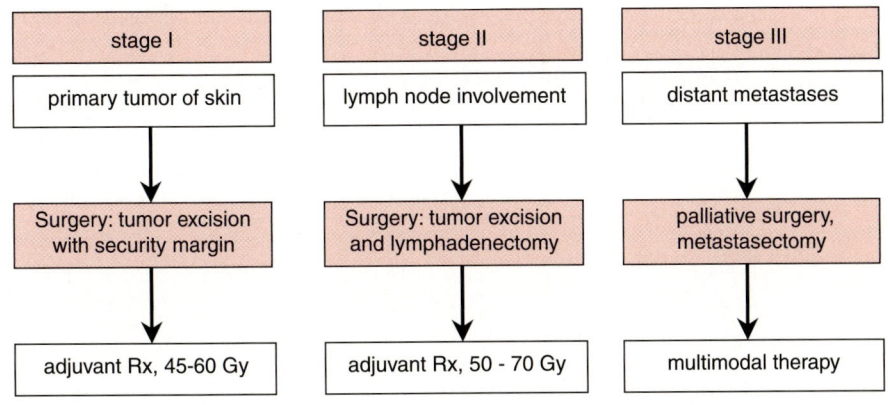

*Rx* radiotherapy

### Stage I:
- Complete tumor excision with 2–3 cm safety margin or Mohs' micrographic surgery (particularly facial area)
- Adjuvant radiotherapy of the primary tumor and the regional lymph nodes, total dose (TD) 45–60 Gy (elective lymphadenectomy if radiotherapy not possible)
- Nonresectable tumors: local radiotherapy including regional lymph nodes, TD 50 Gy with additional 20 Gy boost to the involved area (up to 70 Gy TD)

### Stage II:

- Tumor excision, radical lymphadenectomy, if required including contralateral lymph nodes
- Adjuvant radiotherapy including regional lymph nodes, RO resection: TD 50–55 Gy; R1 resection: 60–66 Gy, R2 resection: 70 Gy
- Cutaneous metastases limited to one extremity or locally advanced tumor which can only be resected by sacrificing the extremity: (hyperthermal) isolated limb perfusion with melphalan (± TNFα / IFNγ)
- Immunotherapy with interferon-α (experimental)

### Stage III:

- Where applicable, palliative surgery (excision, metastasectomy)
- Combined modality treatment: systemic chemotherapy ± radiotherapy TD 40–50 Gy ± excision or resection of metastasis

## Chemotherapy Protocols

| "CMF" | | | Start next cycle on day 29 |
|---|---|---|---|
| Cyclophosphamide | 600 mg/m²/day | i.v. | Days 1+8 |
| Methotrexate | 40 mg/m²/day | i.v. | Days 1+8 |
| 5-Fluorouracil | 600 mg/m²/day | i.v. | Days 1+8 |

| "ECAB" | | | Start next cycle on day 22 |
|---|---|---|---|
| Etoposide | 150 mg/m²/day | i.v. | Days 1+2 |
| Cisplatin | 80 mg/m² | i.v. | Day 1 |
| Doxorubicin | 50 mg/m² | i.v. | Day 1 |
| Bleomycin | 30 mg | i.v. | Day 1 |

**Prg:**

### Negative Prognostic Factors:

Advanced disease, men, age < 60 years, primary tumor located in head / neck region or extremities, small cell subtype.

| Stage | Two-year survival (%) | Median survival (months) |
|---|---|---|
| Stage I | 63 | 42 |
| Stage II | 58 | 32 |
| Stage III | 14 | 10 |

**F/U:**

Patients treated with curative intent should initially be checked every 6 weeks (medical history, physical examination). After 1 year: every 3 months, after 2 years: every 6 months (medical history, physical examination including lymph node palpation and ultrasound; once a year: ultrasound examination of the upper abdomen, chest x-ray). The follow-up period should be at least 5 years. In palliative situations: symptom-based approach.

**Ref:**

1. Goessling W, McKee PH, Mayer RJ. Merkel cell carcinoma. J Clin Oncol 2002;20:588–598
2. McAfee WJ, Morris GG, Mendenhall CM et al. Merkel cell carcinoma: treatment and outcomes. Cancer 2005;104:1761–4
3. Pectasides D, Pectasides M, Economopoulos T. Merkel cell cancer of the skin. Ann Oncol 2006;17:1489–95
4. Poulsen M. Merkel-cell carcinoma of the skin. Lancet Oncol 2004;5:593–9

**Web:**

1. http://www.cancer.gov/cancertopics/pdq/treatment/NCImerkelcell/HealthProfessional      Cancer Topics
2. http://www.emedicine.com/DERM/topic262.htm      E-medicine

# 8.9 Sarcomas

## 8.9.1 Soft Tissue Sarcoma

R. Marks, J. Finke, J. Heinz

**Def:**   Heterogeneous group of mesenchymal tumors located in and originating from soft tissue of the extremities, trunk, retroperitoneum, and head / neck region.

**ICD-10:**   C48, C49

**Ep:**   Incidence 2–3 cases/100,000 population/year; most common type of sarcoma; 10–15% of all malignancies in children (mostly rhabdomyosarcomas and undifferentiated sarcomas); 0.7% of all malignancies in adults; age peak: adolescence and 45–55 years.

**Pg:**   *Etiology*
- Possible influence of ionizing radiation (Thorotrast, radiotherapy) and chemicals (vinyl chloride, dioxin, arsenic, timber preservatives, herbicides)
- Genetic predisposition: neurofibromatosis, Li-Fraumeni syndrome, retinoblastoma, Gardner's syndrome
- Herpes virus (HHV-8) infection may be etiologically relevant in Kaposi's sarcoma

*Molecular Abnormalities*
Chromosomal / molecular genetic changes can be found in > 50% of cases (e.g., p53 mutations in patients with rhabdomyosarcoma, NF 1 mutations in Schwann cell tumors).

**Path:**   *Pathomorphology and Histogenesis of Soft Tissue Sarcomas*

| Normal tissue | Sarcoma type | Frequency (%) |
|---|---|---|
| Connective tissue | Malignant fibrous histiocytoma | 11 |
| | Fibrosarcoma | 18 |
| Fatty tissue | Liposarcoma | 19 |
| Smooth muscle | Leiomyosarcoma | 7 |
| Skeletal muscle | Rhabdomyosarcoma | |
| Vascular system | Angiosarcoma, hemangiopericytoma | |
| Synovial tissue | Synovial sarcoma, malignant synovialoma | |
| Peripheral nerve tissue | Malignant Schwann cell tumor, neurogenic sarcoma | |
| Sympathetic ganglia | Neuroblastoma | |
| Paraganglionic structures | Malignant chemodectoma | |
| Mixed tissue | Malignant mesenchymoma | |

*NOTE:* Therapy and prognosis of soft tissue sarcomas are influenced by tumor type, tumor grade (percentage of necrotic tissue, hemorrhage, mitotic index), tumor stage, and the size of the primary tumor (unfixed preparation, < or > 5 cm). Histopathological assessment has to be conducted by an experienced pathologist including determination of the grade of malignancy:
- Highly malignant tumors: early metastasis and rapid progression
- Practically all rhabdomyosarcomas and synovial sarcomas are highly malignant

*Location of Soft Tissue Sarcomas in Adults*
Extremities (46%), trunk (11%), visceral (16%), retroperitoneum (central abdominal) (15%), other (12%).

### Spread

Early metastasis, particularly to lung (85%), lymph nodes (25%, esp. rhabdomyosarcoma and synovial sarcoma), liver (25%), and bone (15%).

**TNM staging of soft tissue sarcoma**

| | |
|---|---|
| *T* | *Primary Tumor* |
| TX | Primary tumor cannot be assessed |
| T0 | No primary tumor |
| T1 | Primary tumor < 5 cm |
| | A: superficial tumor (above superficial fascia without invasion) |
| | B: deep[a] tumor (beneath the superficial fascia, or above the fascia with invasion) |
| T2 | Primary tumor > 5 cm |
| | A: superficial tumor (above superficial fascia without invasion) |
| | B: deep[a] tumor (beneath the superficial fascia, or above the fascia with invasion) |
| *N* | *Lymph Node Involvement[b]* |
| NX | Regional lymph nodes cannot be assessed |
| N0 | No regional lymph node metastasis |
| N1 | Regional lymph node metastasis |
| *M* | *Distant Metastasis* |
| MX | Distant metastasis cannot be assessed |
| M0 | No distant metastasis |
| M1 | Distant metastasis (including contralateral or distant lymph nodes) |

[a] Retroperitoneal, mediastinal, and pelvic soft tissue sarcomas
[b] Regional lymph nodes are those closest to the tumor

**Residual tumor after surgical resection**

| | |
|---|---|
| RX | Residual tumor cannot be assessed |
| R0 | No residual tumor |
| R1 | Microscopic residual tumor |
| R2 | Macroscopic residual tumor |

**Histopathological grade of differentiation (grading)**

| | |
|---|---|
| GX | Grade of differentiation cannot be assessed |
| G1 | Well differentiated → "low grade" |
| G2 | Moderately differentiated → "low grade" |
| G3 | Poorly differentiated → "high grade" |
| G4 | Undifferentiated → "high grade" |

**AJCC Staging (1997)**

| Stage | Grading | TNM stage | | |
|-------|---------|-----------|------|------|
| IA | G1, 2 | T1A–B | N0 | M0 |
| IB | G1, 2 | T2 A | N0 | M0 |
| IIA | G1, 2 | T2 B | N0 | M0 |
| IIB | G3, 4 | T1A–B | N0 | M0 |
| IIC | G3, 4 | T2 A | N0 | M0 |
| III | G3, 4 | T2 B | N0 | M0 |
| IV | Any G | Any T | N1 | M0 |
| | Any G | Any T | Any N | M1 |

**Sy:**
- Local mass (growth depending on grading), induration, usually painless
- Symptoms caused by tumor expansion, loss of function, weight loss

**Dg:**

### Medical History, Physical Examination
- Medical history including risk factors
- Physical examination including skeletal system

### Laboratory Tests
- Complete blood count with differential, liver and renal function tests, alkaline phosphatase

### Histology
- Surgical biopsy (incision biopsy) is recommended, fine-needle biopsy usually not adequate
- Samples for morphological, immunohistochemical (vimentin, cytokeratin, EMA, desmin, actin, proliferation antigen Ki-67), electron microscopic, and possibly molecular genetic analysis

### Imaging
- MRI of tumor (local spread)
- Chest x-ray, possibly CT
- Abdominal ultrasound, possibly CT abdomen and pelvis
- Selective arteriography; possibly phlebography, bone scan
- Possibly cranial CT / MRI, possibly PET

**Th:**

## Treatment Concept

1. Soft tissue sarcomas are treated according to stage, location, and grade of differentiation.
2. There is no standard treatment for soft tissue sarcomas. In certain situations, interdisciplinary multimodal treatment including surgery, radiotherapy, and/or chemotherapy (neoadjuvant, adjuvant, intra-arterial) is superior to surgical treatment alone. Postoperative adjuvant chemotherapy may be advantageous.
3. Patients should be treated in clinical studies (e.g., EORTC Soft Tissue and Bone Sarcoma Group Studies).
4. Once the diagnosis has been confirmed, patients should be immediately referred to centers experienced in treating soft tissue sarcomas.

## Treatment Options

### Localized Tumor < 5 cm, No Metastases
- Surgical excision (aimed at R0 resection), either limb-preserving techniques (compartment resection, wide excision) or amputation (last resort)
- Where applicable, postoperative radiotherapy, particularly with G2–3 tumors
- After R1 or R2 resection: consider additional surgery and adjuvant radiotherapy

- In selected cases: radiotherapy alone with curative intent, if patient objects to surgery or surgery is medically contraindicated

### Localized Tumor > 5 cm, No Metastases
- Neoadjuvant treatment options: chemotherapy (with/without hyperthermia or radiotherapy), limb perfusion with TNFα and melphalan (good results at experienced centers)
- Surgical treatment aimed at R0 resection
- Depending on surgical outcome, possibly adjuvant chemotherapy with/without radiotherapy

### Localized Tumor, No Metastases, Inoperable
- Neoadjuvant therapy aimed at reducing the tumor to resectable size; options: chemotherapy (with/without hyperthermia), limb perfusion with TNFα and melphalan (good results at experienced centers); alternatively: systemic chemotherapy with/without radiotherapy
- Surgical treatment aimed at R0 resection; retroperitoneal sarcomas: consider intraoperative radiotherapy (IORT)
- Depending on surgical outcome: adjuvant chemotherapy ± radiotherapy

### Metastatic Tumor
- Neoadjuvant chemotherapy in selected cases → if good response (partial or complete remission): resection of tumor and metastases, followed by radiotherapy and/or systemic chemotherapy (particularly with G3 tumors).
- Patients with diffuse metastasis (80–90% of cases): palliative chemotherapy and/or local treatment, particularly with symptomatic patients (surgery, radiotherapy, limb perfusion, intralesional interferon-β); chemotherapy should be adapted to the patient's age and performance status. With younger patients: more aggressive chemotherapy, older patients: monotherapy; with very slow growing tumors (G1) and in palliative situations: watch and wait, treatment as soon as symptoms occur.
- Most effective cytostatic drugs in the treatment of soft tissue sarcoma in adults: doxorubicin and ifosfamide, response rate (CR + PR) 20–30%; other effective compounds (response rate 10–20%): epirubicin, dactinomycin, dacarbazine, methotrexate (high-dose), cisplatin, gemcitabine, paclitaxel.
- Treatment alternatives: doxorubicin monotherapy, ifosfamide monotherapy, doxorubicin + ifosfamide, doxorubicin + dacarbazine, trofosfamide.

### Treatment of Relapse
- If possible, additional surgery (resection or amputation); possibly neoadjuvant therapy
- Patients who have not yet received radiotherapy: preoperative or postoperative radiotherapy, possibly adjuvant chemotherapy
- Pulmonary metastases: pulmonary metastasectomy (especially if ≤ 4–6 metastases); particularly with grade 3 tumors neoadjuvant / adjuvant chemotherapy; curative approach is possible in 20% of patients

## Chemotherapy Protocols

| "Adria / Ifo" ▶ Protocol 12.16.1 | | | | Start next cycle on day 29 |
|---|---|---|---|---|
| Doxorubicin | 50 mg/m²/day | i.v. | Day 1 | |
| Ifosfamide | 1,500 mg/m²/day | i.v. | Days 1–5 | |

| "Doxorubicin Monotherapy" | | | | Start next cycle on day 22 |
|---|---|---|---|---|
| Doxorubicin | 75 mg/m² | i.v. | Day 1 | |

| *"Gemcitabine Monotherapy"* ▶ *Protocol 12.8.1* | | | *Start next cycle on day 29* |
|---|---|---|---|
| Gemcitabine | 1,000 mg/m²/day | i.v. | Days 1, 8, 15 |

| *"Gemcitabine / Paclitaxel"* | | | *Start next cycle on day 29* |
|---|---|---|---|
| Gemcitabine | 675 mg/m²/day | i.v. | Days 1, 8 |
| Paclitaxel | 100 mg/m²/day | i.v. | Day 8 |

| *"DTIC Monotherapy"* ▶ *Protocol 12.15.4* | | | *Start next cycle on day 22* |
|---|---|---|---|
| Dacarbacine (DTIC) | 1,000 mg/m²/day | i.v. | Day 1 |

| *"Paclitaxel Monotherapy"* *(Angiosarcoma)* | | | *Start next cycle on day 22* |
|---|---|---|---|
| Paclitaxel | 175 mg/m² | i.v. | Day 1 |

### Experimental Treatments
- Radiotherapy with radiosensitizers or intralesional interferon β
- Regional hyperthermia and isolated limb perfusion
- Administration of ecteinascidin (ET 743) or temozolomide
- Tyrosine kinase inhibitor (imatinib) with dermatofibrosarcoma protuberans

**Prg:** Factors indicating favorable prognosis:
- Age < 60 years
- Tumor size < 5 cm, high grade of differentiation
- Local stage, tumor located on an extremity

Five-year survival depending on:
- Grade of differentiation: G1: 76%, G2: 56%, G3: 26%
- Tumor stage: stage I: > 90%, II: 70%: III: 20–50%, IV: < 20%

**F/U:** Patients treated with curative intent should be closely monitored (every 3 months) including imaging (depending on tumor location: ultrasound / x-ray / CT / MRI). If diagnosed early and treated adequately, local relapse does not constitute a survival disadvantage.
Palliative situations: symptom-based approach.

**Ref:**
1. Clark MA, Fisher C, Judson I et al. Soft-tissue sarcomas in adults. N Engl J Med 2005;353:701–11
2. Cormier JN, Pollock RE. Soft tissue sarcomas. CA Cancer J Clin 2004;54:94–109
3. ESMO Guidelines Working Group. Soft tissue sarcomas: ESMO Clinical Recommendations for diagnosis, treatment and follow-up. Ann Oncol 2007;18(Suppl.2):ii74–6
4. Kotilingam D, Lev DC, Lazar AJF et al. Staging soft tissue sarcoma: evolution and change. CA Cancer J Clin 2006;56:282–91
5. Mocellin S, Rossi CR, Brandes A et al. Adult soft tissue sarcomas: conventional therapies and molecularly targeted approaches. Cancer Treat Rev 2006;32:9–27

**Web:**
1. http://www.cancer.gov/cancertopics/types/soft-tissue-sarcoma/ — NCI Cancer Topics
2. http://www.nlm.nih.gov/medlineplus/softtissuesarcoma.html — MedlinePlus
3. http://www.nccn.org/professionals/physician_gls/PDF/sarcoma.pdf — NCCN Guideline

## 8.9.2    Gastrointestinal Stromal Tumor (GIST)

**J. Heinz**

| | |
|---|---|
| **Def:** | Mesenchymal tumor of the gastrointestinal tract. Characteristic expression of c-kit |
| **ICD-10:** | C26.9 |
| **Ep:** | Incidence: 10–20 cases/1,000,000 population/year, ratio male:female = 1:1; median age 55–65 years |

**Pg:** Tumors originate from interstitial cells of Cajal (gastrointestinal pacemaker of the myenteric plexus); GIST cells express CD117 (c-kit, stem cell factor SCF receptor). c-kit is involved in the regulation of cell growth, differentiation, and apoptosis; in 80% of cases, gain-of-function mutations in the c-kit gene (67% in exon 11, 17% in exon 9) detectable → gene activation leads to ligand-independent activation of the c-kit protein kinase → stimulation of proliferation, inhibition of apoptosis.

**Path:**
- *Histology:* spindle cell (70%), epitheloid (20%), mixed (10%)
- *Immunohistochemistry:* expression of CD117 (regularly), CD34 (60–80%), SMA (30–40%), desmin (< 2%), S100 (0–15%)
- *Location:* stomach (50–60%), small intestine (20–30%), colon / rectum (10%), omentum / mesentery (5%), esophagus (5%)

**Diagnostic criteria to assess the aggressiveness of GIST (WHO 2002)**

| Risk group | Tumor size (cm) | Number of mitoses per HPF |
|---|---|---|
| Very low risk | < 2 | < 0.1 |
| Low risk | 2–5 | < 0.1 |
| Intermediate risk | < 5 | 0.1-0.2 |
| | 5–10 | < 0.1 |
| High risk | > 5 | > 0.1 |
| | > 10 | Any number |
| | Any size | > 0.2 |

*HPF* high power field (microscopy)

**Sy:**
- Painless mass, in some cases incidental diagnosis during laparoscopy / laparotomy
- Palpable abdominal tumor, in advanced stages abdominal pain
- Gastrointestinal hemorrhage (in 10–25%), ulceration, anemia

**Dg:**    *Medical History, Physical Examination*
- Medical history, examination including rectal examination / fecal occult blood test

*Laboratory Tests*
- Full blood count, clinical chemistry

*Imaging / Histology*
- Endoscopy (gastro- / recto- / colonoscopy) with biopsy (CD117 expression)
- Ultrasound, abdominal CT / MRI (exclusion of liver and intra-abdominal metastasis), FDG-PET (best parameter for monitoring disease course)

**Dd:**    Other solid tumors (carcinomas / sarcomas / benign tumors) of the gastrointestinal tract

**Co:**    Hemorrhage, rupture of tumor, organ displacement

**Th:**  **Treatment Concept**

1. *Surgery:* only complete tumor resection is curative; lymphadenectomy is not required. At diagnosis, only 50% of GIST are localized; R0 resection is possible in 60–70% of patients. In the first 24 months after R0 resection, 50–80% of patients relapse.
2. *Systemic treatment:* indicated with advanced inoperable GIST (at diagnosis 15–50%). Current first-line treatment is imatinib (tyrosine kinase inhibitor):
   - Imatinib (400–800 mg/day) selectively inhibits the c-kit protein kinase → inhibition of cellular proliferation and apoptosis induction.
   - Median time to response 3–4 months; complete remission (CR) < 5%, partial remission (PR) 60–80%, progression-free survival (PFS) after 18 months 66%. In the course of treatment 20% of patients develop resistance.
   - Currently, adjuvant and neoadjuvant therapies with imatinib are being evaluated. Improved protein kinase inhibitors (e.g., dasatinib, sunitinib) are studied in clinical trials and are effective in imatinib-resistant GIST.
   - Chemotherapy achieves response rates of < 5–10%.
3. Radiotherapy: is of no relevance (radiation resistance).

**Prg:**  *Prognostic Factors*

- The most important prognostic factor is R0 resection (5-year survival after R0 resection: 50%). R1 or R2 resection constitute a poor prognosis.
- Tumor size > 5 cm and high mitosis rate: poor prognosis.
- Tumor location: poor prognosis: small intestine.
- Rupture of tumor and abdominal tumor cell metastasis during surgery: poor prognosis.
- c-kit mutation type: exon 11 mutation: good prognosis (response to imatinib 78%), exon 9 mutation: poor prognosis (response to imatinib 9%).

**F/U:**  Patients treated with curative intent should be closely monitored, initially every 3 months (including imaging: CT / MRI / abdominal ultrasound, chest x-ray, and FDG-PET).
Palliative situations: symptom-based approach.

**Ref:**
1. Blay JY, Bonvalot S, Casali P et al. Consensus meeting for the management of gastrointestinal stromal tumors (GISTs). Ann Oncol 2005;16:566–78
2. Chen LL, Sabripour M, Andtbacka RH et al. Imatinib resistance in gastrointestinal stromal tumors. Curr Oncol Rep 2005;7:293–9
3. Demetri G, Von Mehren M, Blanke CD et al. Efficacy and safety of imatinib mesylate in advanced gastro-intestinal stromal tumors. N Engl J Med 2002;347:472–80
4. ESMO Guidelines Working Group. Gastrointestinal stromal tumors: ESMO Clinical Recommendations for diagnosis, treatment and follow-up. Ann Oncol 2007;18(Suppl.2):ii27–9
5. Kosmadakis N, Visvardis EE, Kartsaklis P et al. The role of surgery in the management of GISTs in the era of imatinib mesylate effectiveness. Surg Oncol 2005;14:75–84
6. Rubin BP, Heinrich MC, Corless CL. Gastrointestinal stromal tumor. Lancet 2007;369:1731–41
7. Van der Zwan SM, De Matteo RP. Gastrointestinal stromal tumor. Cancer 2005;104:1781–8

**Web:**
1. http://www.emedicine.com/radio/topic388.htm                          E-medicine
2. http://www.cancer.org/docroot/CRI/CRI_2_3x.asp?dt=81                  Am Cancer Soc
3. http://www.nccn.org/professionals/physician_gls/PDF/sarcoma.pdf       NCCN Guideline

### 8.9.3    Primitive Neuroectodermal Tumors (PNET) and Ewing's Sarcoma

**R. Marks, M. Kleber, J. Finke, J. Heinz**

**Def:**    Primary bone tumor characterized by lack of fibroblastic proliferation as well as by small round anaplastic cells with intracytoplasmic accumulation of glycogen (PAS positive). PNET: primitive neuroectodermal tumors

**ICD-10:**    C40, C41

**Ep:**    Incidence 1–3 cases/1,000,000 population/year; ratio male:female = 1:2; age peak: 10–20 years.

**Pg:**    *Pathogenesis*
Ewing's sarcoma and primitive neuroectodermal tumors (PNET) are closely related and treated similarly. Ewing's sarcoma is pathogenetically characterized by translocations involving the EWS gene on chromosome 22:
- t(11;22)(q24;q12) → fusion gene EWS/FLI1 in 90–95% of cases
- t(21;22)(q22;q12) → fusion gene EWS/ERG in 5–10% of cases

*Differentiation*
Ewing's sarcoma and PNET both express the surface protein p30/32 mic2 but show differences in the expression of neuronal markers (e.g., NSE, Leu7, PGP9.5, S100):
- Ewing's sarcoma: expression of maximum 1 neuronal marker
- PNET: expression of > 2 neuronal markers
- Differentiation from leukemias and lymphomas: lack of CD53

**Path:**    *Histology*
- Hypercellular tissue with necroses, tumor tissue often located around small blood vessels ("pseudorosettes"); small lymphocyte-like tumor cells (differential diagnosis: osteomyelitis) with round nucleus, granular chromatin, and intracytoplasmic glycogen (PAS stain)
- Immunohistochemistry: positive for mesenchymal markers (vimentin) and occasionally neuronal markers (e.g., NSE, Leu7, PGP9.5, S100)
- Detection of surface protein p30/32 mic2

*Location and Spread*
- Primary location: all parts of the skeleton, most commonly pelvis, femur, ribs, tibia, and humerus
- Early hematogenous metastasis into lung, bone, and bone marrow; lymph node involvement is rare

**Class:**    At presentation:
- Localized Ewing's sarcoma: 70–80% of cases
- Metastasized Ewing's sarcoma: 20–30% of cases

**Sy:**    
- Local swelling, induration, hyperthermia, pain
- Symptoms due to tumor growth, impaired function

**Dg:**    *Medical History, Physical Examination*
- Physical examination including skeletal system

### Laboratory Tests
- Routine laboratory tests including complete blood count, LDH ↑, NSE (neuron-specific enolase, neuronal marker), ESR
- Prior to chemotherapy: liver and renal function tests, virology (CMV, EBV, VZV, HSV, HAV, HBV, HCV, HIV)

### Histology
- Surgical biopsy
- Bilateral bone marrow cytology and biopsy (to exclude invasion), including molecular diagnosis (PCR to detect rearrangements of chromosome 22)

### Imaging
- X-ray ("moth-eaten" pattern of necrosis) of affected area, CT / MRI (tumor mass assessment)
- Chest x-ray, thoracic CT, abdominal ultrasound
- Bone scan, MRI of suspected areas, angiography

### Other Tests
- Prior to chemotherapy: cardiac function (ECG, echocardiogram), pulmonary function tests

**Dd:**
- Osteomyelitis (difficult to differentiate clinically and histologically)
- Other bone tumors, skeletal metastases

**Th:**

## Treatment Concept

1. Ewing's sarcoma is to be regarded as a systemic disease at diagnosis. More than 90% of patients with clinically localized disease have occult micrometastases.
2. Treatment is always interdisciplinary, consisting of a combination of systemic chemotherapy and localized surgery and/or radiotherapy. The treatment approach is influenced by patient age, tumor location, response to chemotherapy, and tumor extent at presentation.
3. Most effective chemotherapeutic drugs: doxorubicin, cyclophosphamide, ifosfamide, vincristine, actinomycin D; always as combination chemotherapy. High-dose chemotherapy with autologous stem cell transplantation should only be performed in the setting of trials in patients with primary or secondary metastasis.
4. Surgical treatment: extremity-preserving techniques in combination with radiotherapy / chemotherapy. Amputation should be avoided.
5. Radiotherapy: preoperative, postoperative, or as local treatment in combination with chemotherapy. Radiation dose: > 55–60 Gy, in combination with chemotherapy: 45 Gy.
6. Patients should be treated in the setting of trials. Euro-E.W.I.N.G. 99 is the current trial of the "European Ewing tumor Working Initiative of National Groups" and represents the European standard treatment.

**Euro-E.W.I.N.G 99 Study**

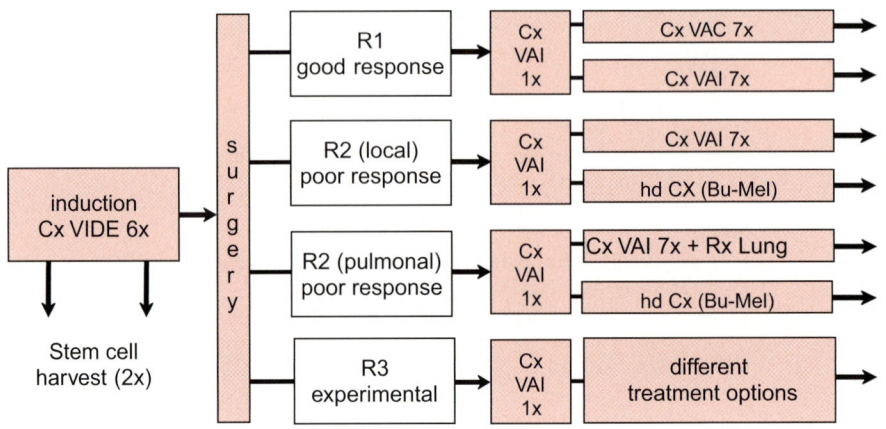

*Cx* chemotherapy, *hd Cx* high-dose chemotherapy, *Rx* radiotherapy, *VIDE* vincristine + ifosfamide + doxorubicin + etoposide, *VAI* vincristine + actinomycin D + ifosfamide, *VAC* vincristine + actinomycin D + cyclophosphamide, *Bu-Mel* busulfan + melphalan
Good response: < 10% vital cells in biopsy
Poor response: > 10% vital cells in biopsy

### Euro-E.W.I.N.G. 99

- *Basic concept:* sequence of neoadjuvant chemotherapy → surgery → adjuvant chemotherapy. Adjuvant chemotherapy according to risk factors and vital tumor cells in biopsy.
- *Objective:* comparison of different consolidation chemotherapy protocols according to response to induction chemotherapy: VAI versus VAC in patients with good histological response, role of high-dose chemotherapy in patients with poor response, value of radiotherapy in patients with pulmonary metastases.
- *Selection of patients (inclusion criteria):* all patients with histologically established primary or metastatic Ewing's sarcoma, atypical Ewing's sarcoma, or peripheral neuroectodermal tumors (PNET).
- *Treatment plan:* induction chemotherapy with VIDE (6 cycles), stem cell harvest between 2nd and 4th cycle; followed by surgery (if tumor is resectable) and one cycle of VAI protocol chemotherapy. Consolidation therapy: randomization into several groups on the basis of tumor response and tumor mass.

### Relapse

Any relapse should be treated with curative intent. Late relapse has the best prognosis. Myeloablative high-dose chemotherapy with autologous / allogeneic transplantation should be considered as salvage treatment.

### Chemotherapy Protocols

| "VIDE" ▶ Protocol 12.16.2. | | | Start next cycle according to study protocol |
|---|---|---|---|
| Vincristine | 1.5 mg/m²/day | i.v. | Day 1, max. single dose 2 mg |
| Ifosfamide | 3,000 mg/m²/day | i.v. | Days 1–3, for 1 h |
| Doxorubicin | 20 mg/m²/day | i.v. | Days 1–3, for 4 h |
| Etoposide | 150 mg/m²/day | i.v. | Days 1–3, for 1 h |

| *"VAI"* ► Protocol 12.16.3 | | | *Start next cycle according to study protocol* |
|---|---|---|---|
| Vincristine | 1.5 mg/m²/day | i.v. | Day 1, max. single dose 2 mg |
| Dactinomycin | 0.75 mg/m²/day | i.v. | Days 1–2, max. single dose 1.5 mg |
| Ifosfamide | 3,000 mg/m²/day | i.v. | Days 1–2 |

| *"VAC"* ► Protocol 12.16.4 | | | *Start next cycle according to study protocol* |
|---|---|---|---|
| Vincristine | 1.5 mg/m²/day | i.v. | Day 1, max. single dose 2 mg |
| Dactinomycin | 0.75 mg/m²/day | i.v. | Days 1–2, max. single dose 1.5 mg |
| Cyclophosphamide | 1,500 mg/m²/day | i.v. | Day 1 |

| *"Busulfan-Melphalan"* ► Protocol 14.7 | | | |
|---|---|---|---|
| Busulfan | 4mg/kg/day | p.o. | Days -6 to -3, 1 mg/kg every 6 h |
| Melphalan | 140 mg/m²/day | i.v. | Day -2 |

Stem cell re-infusion on day 0, at least $3 \times 10^6$ CD34-positive cells per kg body weight

**Prg:**

### Prognostic Factors

Prognosis depends on tumor stage at presentation (mass, dissemination), response to chemotherapy, and presence of the EWS/FLI1 translocation.

### Five-year Survival

- Localized Ewing's sarcoma, radiotherapy / surgery alone: < 10%
- Localized Ewing's sarcoma, multimodal therapy: 50–75%
- Ewing's sarcoma metastasized to the lung, multimodal therapy: 30–40%
- Ewing's sarcoma metastasized to bone, multimodal therapy: < 20%

**F/U:**

Patients treated with curative intent should be closely monitored including imaging.
Palliative situations: symptom-based approach.

**Ref:**

1. Bernstein M, Kovar H, Paulussen M et al. Ewing's sarcoma family of tumors: current management. Oncologist 2006;11:503–19
2. Ek ET, Choong PF. The role of high-dose therapy and autologous stem cell transplantation for pediatric bone and soft tissue sarcomas. Expert Rev Anticancer Ther 2006;6:225–37
3. ESMO Guidelines Working Group. Ewing's sarcoma of bone: ESMO Clinical Recommendations for diagnosis, treatment and follow-up. Ann Oncol 2007;18(Suppl.2):ii79–80
4. Janknecht R. EWS-ETS oncoproteins: the linchpins of Ewing tumors. Gene 2005;363:1–14
5. Kennedy JG, Frelinghuysen P, Hoang BH. Ewing sarcoma: current concepts in diagnosis and treatment. Curr Opin Pediatr 2003;15:53–7
6. Thacker MM, Temple HT, Scully SP. Current treatment for Ewing's sarcoma. Expert Rev Anticancer Ther 2005;5:319–31

**Web:**

1. http://euro-ewing.uni-muenster.de/     EURO-E.W.I.N.G. 99
2. http://www.cancer.gov/cancertopics/types/ewings     NCI Cancer Topics
3. http://www.nlm.nih.gov/medlineplus/ency/article/001302.htm     MedlinePlus
4. http://www.emedicine.com/RADIO/topic275.htm     E-medicine

### 8.9.4    Osteosarcoma

**R. Marks, M. Kleber, J. Heinz**

**Def:** Malignant tumors of the bone originating from malignant osteoblasts which may form osteoid, bone, or cartilage.

**ICD-10:** C40, C41

**Ep:** Frequency: 0.1% of all neoplasia; incidence 2 cases/1,000,000 population/year; ratio male:female = 3:2; age peaks: 10–20 years (90% of cases) and 50–70 years (10% of cases).

**Pg:** *Risk Factors*
- Genetic predisposition in patients with hereditary retinoblastoma, Li-Fraumeni syndrome
- Secondary osteosarcomas after radiotherapy, therapy with alkylating agents, fibrous dysplasia, bone cysts, or osteitis deformans (Paget's disease)

*Molecular Abnormalities*
- Inactivation of tumor suppressor genes such as pRB110 (Rb) and p53
- Expression of the c-sis protooncogene and subsequent secretion of platelet-derived growth factor (PDGF, stimulates proliferation of mesenchymal cells)
- Oncogene expression (ras, raf, mos, myc, fos) or oncornavirus

**Path:** *Classification*
- *Histology:* osteoblastic / chondroblastic / fibroblastic / telangiectatic / small cell osteosarcomas; low-grade forms are rare
- *Growth pattern:* central (classic intraosseous growth), periosteal, paraosteal (juxtacortical), craniofacial, and extraskeletal growth

*Location and Spread*
- In 80% of cases, located in the metaphysis of long bones, particularly around the knee joint (50%) and the humerus (15%), less common: skull and jaw bones
- At presentation, 10–20% of patients have clinically detectable metastases, 80–90% have occult metastases, esp. metastasis to the lung and skeletal system

**Class:** **TNM**

| *T* | *Primary Tumor* |
|-----|-----------------|
| TX | Primary tumor cannot be assessed |
| T0 | No evidence of primary tumor |
| T1 | Primary tumor ≤ 8 cm |
| T2 | Primary tumor > 8 cm |
| T3 | Discontinuous tumors in the primary bone site |
| *N* | *Lymph Node Involvement* |
| NX | Regional lymph nodes cannot be assessed |
| N0 | No regional lymph node metastasis |
| N1 | Regional lymph node metastasis |
| *M* | *Distant Metastases* |
| MX | Distant metastasis cannot be assessed |
| M0 | No distant metastasis |
| M1 | Distant metastasis (including nonregional lymph nodes) |
|  | A: Lung |
|  | B: Other |

**AJCC Staging staging of osteosarcoma**

| Stage | Grading | TNM stage | | |
|-------|---------|-----------|------|------|
| Ia | G1–2 | T1 | N0 | M0 |
| Ib | G1–2 | T2 | N0 | M0 |
| IIa | G3–4 | T1 | N0 | M0 |
| IIb | G3–4 | T2 | N0 | M0 |
| III | Any G | T3 | N0 | M0 |
| IVA | Any G | Any T | N1 | M0 |
| IVB | Any G | Any T | Any N | M1 |

**Sy:**
- Local mass, induration, pain
- Symptoms caused by tumor growth, impaired function

**Dg:**

### Medical History, Physical Examination
- Medical history including risk factors (previous radiation)
- Physical examination including skeletal system and lymph node status

### Laboratory Tests
- Routine laboratory tests including complete blood count, liver and renal function tests, coagulation status, alkaline phosphatase (in 60–80% ↑)

### Imaging
- Conventional x-ray and MRI of the affected area, possibly CT
- Chest x-ray, thoracic CT, abdominal ultrasound
- Bone scan with digital three-phase technique, in selected cases: angiography
- Possibly PET to assess vitality of residual tumor after treatment

### Histology
- Surgical biopsy

### Other Tests
- Prior to chemotherapy: cardiac function (ECG, echocardiography), audiometry

**Th:**

### Treatment Concept

1. Osteosarcoma is to be regarded a systemic disease at diagnosis (diffuse micrometastases in 80–90% of patients).
2. Interdisciplinary treatment with curative intent. Basic concept: *biopsy → preoperative chemotherapy → surgery → postoperative chemotherapy.*
   Exception: low-grade osteosarcomas: usually surgery only.
3. Most effective chemotherapeutic drugs: doxorubicin, cisplatin, ifosfamide, methotrexate (response rate with monotherapy: 20–40%); combination chemotherapy superior to monotherapy.
4. Surgical techniques: amputation, limb-sparing surgery; choice of treatment depends on patient's age, tumor location, and response to preoperative chemotherapy; resection of pulmonary metastases.
5. Due to the marked resistance of osteosarcomas to radiotherapy this treatment is only used in selected palliative cases or as part of multimodal therapies in trials.
6. All patients should be treated in trials, current trials: EURO-B.O.S.S. (EUROpean Bone Over 40 Sarcoma Study) for patients > 40 years, EURAMOS trial for patients < 40 years.

**EURO-B.O.S.S. Study ("EUROpean Bone Over 40 Sarcoma Study")**

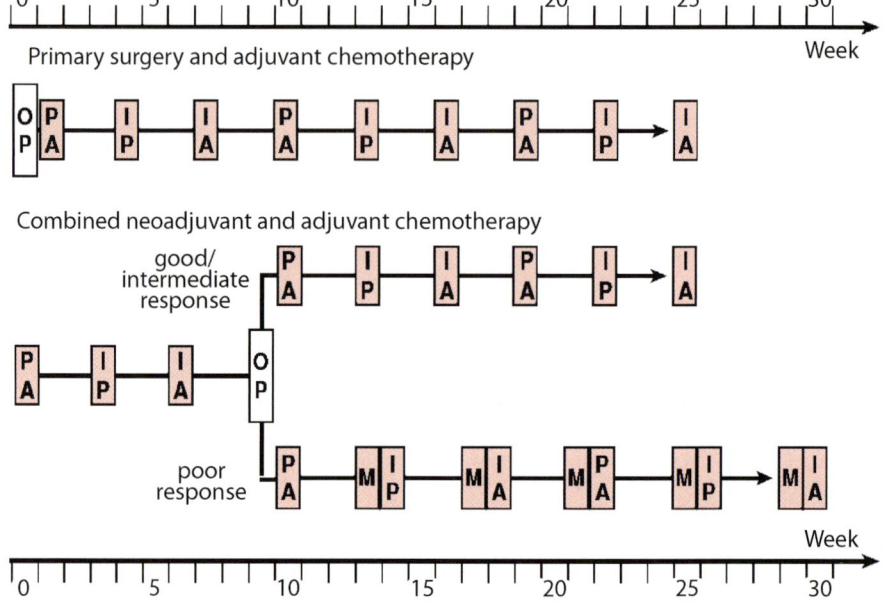

*OP* surgery, *A* doxorubicin, *I* ifosfamide, *M* methotrexate, *P* cisplatinum

## Treatment Plans

### EURO-B.O.S.S. Trial

- *Basic concept:* course of neoadjuvant chemotherapy → surgery → adjuvant chemotherapy
- *Objective:* evaluation of response and implementation of intensified chemotherapy in patients between 41 and 65 years with osteosarcoma
- *Selection of patients (inclusion criteria):* age 41–65 years, patients with established bone sarcoma (osteosarcoma, malignant fibrous histiocytoma, leiomyosarcoma, dedifferentiated chondrosarcoma, angiosarcoma)
- *Exclusion criteria:* bone marrow involvement, impaired organ function (hepatic / cardiac / renal), contraindications to chemotherapy
- *Treatment course:* first arm: adjuvant treatment of patients with primary surgery, second arm: combined therapy including neoadjuvant and adjuvant chemotherapy of patients with no primary surgery. The fraction of vital tumor cells in biopsy defines the classification of risk groups and intensity of adjuvant chemotherapy.
- All patients should be reported to the trial; cases with contraindications for chemotherapy or with exclusion criteria can be observed off study ("observation patients")

### EURAMOS Trial

- *Basic concept:* course of neoadjuvant chemotherapy → surgery → adjuvant chemotherapy
- *Objective:* after neoadjuvant chemotherapy: impact of postoperative maintenance chemotherapy (interferon-α treatment of patients with good response) or intensified chemotherapy (patients with poor response)
- See study details: http://www.euramos.org

### Treatment of Relapse

- Treatment depends on prior therapy, location and number of metastases
- If possible, R0 resection should be attempted.

- If surgical treatment is not possible: consider radiotherapy and/or secondary chemotherapy, high-dose chemotherapy, or isotope treatment with samarium[153] and autologous stem cell support
- Possibly recruitment to current trials

## Chemotherapy Protocols

| *"EURO-B.O.S.S: PA"* ► *Protocol 12.16.5* | | | *Start next cycle according to study protocol* |
|---|---|---|---|
| Cisplatin | 33,3 mg/m$^2$/day | c.i.v. | Days 1–3, continuous infusion |
| Doxorubicin | 60 mg/m$^2$/day | c.i.v. | Day 4, for 24 h |

| *"EURO-B.O.S.S: IP"* ► *Protocol 12.16.6* | | | *Start next cycle according to study protocol* |
|---|---|---|---|
| Ifosfamide | 3,000 mg/m$^2$/day | .i.v. | Days 1+2, for 1 h |
| Cisplatin | 33,3 mg/m$^2$/day | c.i.v. | Days 3–5, for 24 h |

| *"EURO-B.O.S.S: IPA"* ► *Protocol 12.16.7* | | | *Start next cycle according to study protocol* |
|---|---|---|---|
| Ifosfamide | 3,000 mg/m$^2$/day | i.v. | Days 1+2, for 1 h |
| Doxorubicin | 60 mg/m$^2$/day | c.i.v. | Day 3, for 24 h |

| *"EURO-B.O.S.S: MTX"* ► *Protocol 12.16.8* | | | *Start next cycle according to study protocol* |
|---|---|---|---|
| Methotrexate (MTX) | 8 g/m$^2$/day | i.v. | Day 1, for 4 h |
| Calcium folinate | Acc. to MTX level | p.o. | Days 2–4, starting 24 h after MTX |

*CAUTION: Folinic acid administration according to MTX levels is of vital importance. Non-compliance may cause life-threatening toxicity.*
- Usually: $4 \times 15$ mg/m$^2$/day p.o. (with vomiting / emesis: i.v.) starting 24 h after MTX treatment, every 6 h for 3 days
- MTX serum level: measured 4 h prior to MTX infusion, and 0, 4, 12, 24, 48 and 72 h after infusion. If necessary, measure serum levels daily until MTX < 0.4 µmol/l
- If MTX level is too high or signs of toxicity: intensified leucovorin rescue, see original protocol

**Prg:**

### *Prognostic Factors*
- Tumor stage (size, invasion) and location
- Histology (poor prognosis: poorly differentiated tumors, chondroblastic tumors, paraosteal or telangiectatic growth)
- Response to chemotherapy, initial tumor mass

### *Five-year Survival*
- With surgical treatment alone:          15%
- With combined treatment (surgery + chemotherapy): > 50–70%

**F/U:**

Patients treated with curative intent should be monitored closely including imaging. Follow-up: first 3 years: every 3 months, then every 6 months for 5 years.
Palliative situations: symptom-based approach.

**Ref:**

1. ESMO Guidelines Working Group. Osteosarcoma: ESMO Clinical Recommendations for diagnosis, treatment and follow-up. Ann Oncol 2007;18(Suppl.2):ii77–8
2. Ferguson WS, Goorin AM. Current treatment of osteosarcoma. Cancer Invest 2001;19:292–315
3. Grimer RJ. Surgical options for children with osteosarcoma. Lancet Oncol 2005;6:85–92
4. Heck RK, Peabody TD, Simon MA. Staging of primary malignancies of bone. CA Cancer J Clin 2006;56:366–75
5. Marina N, Gebhardt M, Teot L et al. Biology and therapeutic advances for pediatric osteosarcoma. Oncologist 2004;9:422–41
6. Miller SL, Hoffer FA. Malignant and benign bone tumors. Radiol Clin North Am 2001;39:673–99
7. Ngarajan R, Clohisy D, Weigel B. New paradigms for therapy of osteosarcoma. Curr Oncol Rep 2005;7:410–4
8. Wang LL. Biology of osteogenic sarcoma. Cancer J 2005;11:294–305
9. Wittig JC, Bickels J, Priebat D et al. Osteosarcoma: a multidisciplinary approach to diagnosis and treatment. Am Fam Physician 2002;65:1123–32

**Web:**

1. http://www.euramos.org/                                          Eur Am Osteosarc Grp
2. http://www.emedicine.com/orthoped/topic531.htm                   E-medicine
3. http://www.cancer.gov/cancertopics/pdq/treatment/
   osteosarcoma/HealthProfessional                                 NCI Cancer Topics
4. http://www.nlm.nih.gov/medlineplus/ency/article/001650.htm       MedlinePlus

# 8.10    CNS Tumors

### H. Henß

**Def:**    Malignant primary tumors of the brain, the spinal cord, the brainstem, or the cranial nerves.

**ICD-10:**    C70–C72

**Ep:**    Incidence approximately 6 cases/100,000 population/year; age peaks: 5–10 years (childhood tumors) and 50–55 years.

**Pg:**

### Etiology
- Genetic factors: rare (Li-Fraumeni syndrome, Turcot's syndrome, NF 1, NF 2, tuberous sclerosis)
- Toxic chemicals: exposure to vinyl chloride; possible associated with pesticides, herbicides, petrochemical products
- Ionizing radiation

### Molecular Genetic Aspects
- Frequently: amplification of genes encoding growth factors or receptors (TGFα, EGFR, PDGF, βFGF), deletions of negative-regulatory elements (p53, CDKN2, MTS2) particularly on chromosome 9p21, deletion 1p or 19q in oligodendrogliomas.

**Pathomorphology and histogenesis of CNS tumors**

| Normal tissue | Tumor (selection) |
| --- | --- |
| Astrocyte | Astrocytoma, anaplastic astrocytoma, glioblastoma multiforme |
| Ependymocyte | Ependymoma, anaplastic ependymoma |
| Oligodendrocyte | Oligodendroglioma, anaplastic oligodendroglioma; mixed gliomas (oligoastrocytoma) |
| Arachnoid fibroblast | Meningioma |
| Nerve cell, neuroblast | Ganglioneuroma, neuroblastoma, retinoblastoma |
| Neuroectoderm, neuroblast | Medulloblastoma |
| Schwann cell | Schwannoma (neurinoma) |
| Melanocyte | Malignant melanoma |
| Choroid epithelial cell | Papillomas / carcinomas of the choroid plexus |
| Pituitary | Adenoma (carcinoma) |
| Endothelial cell | Hemangioblastoma |
| Primitive germ cell | Germinoma, pinealoma, teratoma, cholesteatoma |
| Pineal parenchyma | Pineocytoma |
| Remnants of the notochord | Chordoma |

**Primary intracranial tumors in adults**

| Type | Frequency (%) |
|---|---|
| Glioblastoma multiforme | 30 |
| Astrocytomas (grade I–II) | 20 |
| Other gliomas | 7 |
| Meningiomas | 18 |
| Neurinomas, schwannomas | 9 |
| Pituitary tumors | 5 |
| Ependymomas | 5 |
| Plexus papillomas | 2 |
| Other (medulloblastomas[a], etc.) | 4 |
| Other (malignant lymphomas, germ cell tumors) | Rare |

[a] In children, 25% of intracranial tumors

## Malignant Gliomas: Classification

*Astrocytic Tumors (40–50% of all brain tumors)*
- Noninvasive: juvenile pilocytic astrocytoma, subependymal astrocytoma
- Grade I–II: well differentiated / moderately differentiated astrocytoma
- Grade III: anaplastic astrocytoma (semimalignant)
- Grade IV: glioblastoma multiforme (malignant, 50% of astrocytoma)

*Ependymal Tumors*
- Myxopapillary and highly differentiated ependymoma
- Anaplastic ependymoma
- Ependymoblastoma

*Oligodendroglial Tumors*
- Well differentiated / anaplastic oligodendroglioma

*Mixed Gliomas*
- Well differentiated / anaplastic oligoastrocytoma

*Medulloblastoma*

## Location of Malignant Gliomas
- Cerebral hemispheres:                          90%
- Brainstem and optic nerve:                     10%
- Multilocular:                                  < 5%
- Extracranial manifestations / metastases:      < 1%

**Sy:** Mainly uncharacteristic symptoms including headache, impaired vision, signs of intracranial pressure, focal symptoms, psychological disorders, progressive personality changes.
Clinical picture also depends on tumor location.

### Infratentorial Tumors
More common in children; differential diagnosis: medulloblastoma, astrocytoma grade I, ependymoma; classic triad: impaired vision + headache + vomiting

### Supratentorial Tumors
More common in adults; differential diagnosis: glioblastoma, astrocytoma, oligodendroglioma
- Focal symptoms (hemiparesis, aphasia, unilateral hearing impairment, homonymous hemianopia)
- Cerebral seizures (generalized or Jacksonian epilepsy), first symptom in 25% of cases
- Signs of intracranial pressure (papilledema, headache, vomiting, somnolence)

### Tumors of the Posterior Skull Base
- Ataxia (cerebellum)

### Tumors of the Pituitary Gland
- Hormonal disorders, bitemporal hemianopia

**Dg:** ### Medical History, Physical Examination
- Medical history including risk factors
- Physical examination, esp. neurological status (including EEG)

### Histology / Cytology
- Histological diagnosis and grading by (stereotactic) biopsy
- CSF analysis (ATTENTION: with infratentorial lesions, lumbar puncture may be contraindicated)

### Imaging
- CT, MRI
- Where applicable: angiographic procedures

**Dd:**
- Intracranial hemorrhage, particularly subdural hematoma
- Inflammation (cerebral abscess)
- Impaired CSF drainage (aqueduct stenosis, arachnopathy)

**Th:** ## Treatment of Malignant Gliomas

Treatment is conducted according to the histological type and the tumor grading.

### Supportive Treatment
- Therapy of cerebral edema: dexamethasone 40 mg bolus, then 4 mg 3 times daily (up to 8 mg 6 times daily)
- Antiepileptic treatment with generalized seizures

### Surgical Treatment
Where possible, surgery is the treatment of first choice: conventional operation or stereotactic techniques. Even partial tumor resection can prolong the patient's life. The objective is to remove as much of the tumor as possible. Relapsed patients should be considered for secondary surgery. The prevention of neurological deficits however has priority over the radicality of surgical treatment.

### Radiotherapy
- Always carried out; in addition to surgery (adjuvant situation)
- With palliative indication: possibly radiotherapy alone or in combination with chemotherapy
- Radiation field: focal radiotherapy (60 Gy); preferably use of more recent techniques (e.g., hyperfractionation, intensity-modulated radiotherapy IMRT)
- Where applicable, stereotactic radiotherapy (tumor ≤ 3 cm)

### Chemotherapy
- In adjuvant situations, combination of radiotherapy and chemotherapy (temozolomide + radiotherapy) is superior to radiotherapy alone
- In cases with inoperable glioblastoma, meta-analyses have shown combined radiochemotherapy to confer a better prognosis (than radiotherapy alone)
- The value of chemotherapy alone, especially with relapsed malignant gliomas, remains uncertain. Tumor remissions have been achieved, but significant survival improvement has so far only been demonstrated in large meta-analyses.

### Cytostatic Drugs
- Nitrosoureas (BCNU, ACNU): e.g., ACNU 100 mg/m²/day i.v., every 4–6 weeks
- Procarbazine: 150 mg/m²/day, days 1–28, orally
- Cytosine arabinoside (enters CSF only if continuously infused for > 2 h)
- Epipodophyllotoxins (etoposide): only effective if given in high doses
- Temozolomide: oral dacarbazine derivative

## Chemotherapy Protocols

| *"Nimustine Monotherapy"* ▶ *Protocol 12.17.1* | | | *Start next cycle after 4–6 weeks* |
|---|---|---|---|
| Nimustine | 100 mg/m²/day | i.v. | Day 1 |

| *"Temolozomide Monotherapy"* ▶ *Protocol 12.17.2* | | | *Start next cycle on day 29* |
|---|---|---|---|
| Temozolomide | 150 mg/m²/day | p.o. | Days 1–5 |

| *"PCV"* | | | *Start next cycle after 6–8 weeks* |
|---|---|---|---|
| Procarbazine | 60 mg/m²/day | p.o. | Days 8–21 |
| CCNU | 110 mg/m²/day | p.o. | Day 1 |
| Vincristine | 1.4 mg/m²/day | i.v. | Days 8, 29, max. single dose 2 mg |

### New Drugs / Experimental Therapies
- High-dose tamoxifen (100 mg daily)
- Gene therapy approaches
- Interstitial / focal radiotherapy ("gamma-knife")
- "Targeted therapies": angiogenesis inhibitors, EGFR inhibitors

## Treatment of Other CNS Tumors

### Malignant Ependymomas, Plexus Papillomas, Gangliogliomas
Treatment similar to therapy of malignant glioma

### Meningiomas
Small tumors: watch and wait strategy or, if necessary, surgical treatment

### Primary Cerebral Lymphomas
See malignant lymphoma (▶ Chap. 7.5.8)

### Medulloblastomas, Primitive Neuroectodermal Tumors (PNET)
Childhood tumors, rarely occurring in adults; often chemosensitive; recommended treatment: according to pediatric protocols, usually combination of surgery, radiotherapy, and chemotherapy.

**Prg:**     ### Prognosis of Malignant Gliomas According to Prognostic Criteria
- Histological type: oligodendrogliomas associated with favorable prognosis
- Grading: grade III significantly better than grade IV

- Age: patients < 40–50 years have better prognosis
- Performance status
- Resectability

### Prognosis of Other CNS Tumors
- Malignant ependymomas, plexus papillomas, gangliogliomas: see malignant gliomas
- Primary cerebral lymphomas (▶ Chap. 7.5.8)

**F/U:** Patients treated with curative intent should be monitored closely including physical examination and cranial CT / MRI.
Palliative situations: symptom-based approach.

**Ref:**
1. Behin A, Hoang-Xuan K, Carpentier AF et al. Primary brain tumors in adults. Lancet 2003;361:323–31
2. ESMO Guidelines Working Group. Malignant glioma: ESMO Clinical Recommendations for diagnosis, treatment and follow-up. Ann Oncol 2007;18(Suppl.2):ii69–70
3. Grier JT, Batchelor T. Low-grade gliomas in adults. Oncologist 2006;11:681–93
4. Jaeckle KA, Ballmann KV, Rao RD et al. Current strategies in treatment of oligodendroglioma: evolution of molecular signatures of response. J Clin Oncol 2006;24:1246–52
5. Lang FF, Gilbert MR. Diffusely infiltrative low-grade gliomas in adults. J Clin Oncol 2006;24:1236–45
6. Maris JM, Hogarty MD, Bagatell R et al. Neuroblastoma. Lancet 2007;369:2106–20
7. Reardon DA, Rich JN, Friedman HS et al. Recent advances in the treatment of malignant astrocytoma. J Clin Oncol 2006;24:1253–65
8. Stupp R, Hegi ME, Gilbert MR et al. Chemoradiotherapy in malignant glioma: standard of care and future directions. J Clin Oncol 2007;25:4127–36
9. Van den Bent MJ, Hegi ME, Stupp R. Recent developments in the use of chemotherapy in brain tumors. Eur J Cancer 2006;42:582–8

**Web:**
| | | |
|---|---|---|
| 1. | http://www.nlm.nih.gov/medlineplus/braincancer.html | MedlinePlus |
| 2. | http://www.cancer.gov/cancertopics/types/brain/ | NCI Cancer Topics |
| 3. | http://brain.mgh.harvard.edu | Harvard Univ |
| 4. | http://cbtrus.org | Brain Tumor Registry |
| 5. | http://www.tbts.org/ | Brain Tumor Society |
| 6. | http://www.abta.org/ | Brain Tumor Assoc |

## 8.11     Cancer of Unknown Primary (CUP)

H. Henß

**Def:**     Histologically confirmed malignancy which is not a primary tumor of the respective site of manifestation and the origin of which cannot be determined. Synonym: metastases from unknown primary tumor (MUP)

**ICD-10:**     C76, C80

**Ep:**     Incidence 7–9 cases/100,000 population/year, 3% of all solid tumors; ratio male:female = 2:1; age peak 50–70 years.

**Pg:**     *Possible Pathogenetic Concepts*
- Metastatic small primary tumor (< 1 cm), which is not detectable despite thorough investigation (CT, MRI, invasive diagnostic procedures)
- Resection of an unidentified malignant tumor before metastasis becomes evident (e.g., malignant skin tumors)
- Hemorrhagic infarction, necrosis, scarring, or involution of the primary tumor (e.g., testicular cancer, choriocarcinoma, malignant melanoma)
- Primary tumor unidentifiable due to extensive metastasis or rapid tumor progression (in 15–33% of cases, autopsy fails to identify primary tumor)

**Histological classification of CUP**

| Tumor type | Frequency (%) |
|---|---|
| Adenocarcinoma | 40–70 |
| Undifferentiated carcinoma | 30–40 |
| Squamous cell carcinoma | 10–15 |
| Malignant melanoma | 2–5 |
| Neuroblastoma | 1 |
| Other | < 1 |

Histopathological analysis plays a key role in the diagnosis and treatment of metastases from unknown primary tumors. Only an established histological diagnosis enables specific treatment according to tumor type. This requires the use of the entire spectrum of pathomorphological diagnosis (including immunohistology and molecular biology) as well as detailed clinical information.
- *Most common tumor types in CUP:* pancreatic carcinoma (up to 25% of cases), lung cancer (15–20%), gastric cancer (10%), colorectal tumors (10%), and hepatobiliary cancer (10%).
- *Squamous cell carcinomas:* most common primary location: head / neck, lung, or uterine cervix; other less common locations: esophagus, rectum, anus, penis, or skin.
- *Adenocarcinomas:* most common primary location: breast, ovaries, lung, gastrointestinal tract, thyroid, or prostate; 75% of adenocarcinomas originate from sites below the diaphragm.
- *Most common undifferentiated tumors:* melanoma, rhabdomyoblastoma, myeloma, small cell lung cancer, lymphomas, testicular cancer, Ewing's sarcoma, or neuroblastoma.
- Of all tumors of unknown primary origin, 3% are *prostate carcinomas* that can be identified by determination of the serum PSA level or immunohistochemistry.

**Metastatic pattern and possible primary locations**

| Location | Frequency (%) | Type | Possible primary location |
|---|---|---|---|
| Abdomen | 30 | Hepatic | Pancreas, stomach, colon, lung, breast |
| | | Ascites | Ovaries, pancreas, stomach, colon, lymphoma |
| Thorax | 22 | Pulmonary | Lung, breast, GIT, RCC, ovaries, testis, sarcoma |
| | | Pleural | Lung, breast, ovaries, lymphoma, GIT |
| | | Pericardial | Lung, breast, lymphoma, melanoma |
| Lymph nodes | 20 | Cervical | ENT, lung, breast, GIT, prostate, testis, thyroid |
| | | Axillary | Breast, melanoma, lung, upper extremities, stomach |
| | | Inguinal | Prostate, rectum, vulva, melanoma, bladder, testis |
| Skeletal system | 16 | Osteolytic | NSCLC, RCC, breast, thyroid, plasmacytoma |
| | | Osteoblastic | Prostate, breast, thyroid, GIT, carcinoid, Hodgkin's disease, sarcoma, NSCLC, urinary bladder |
| | | Mixed type | Breast, SCLC, prostate, thyroid |
| CNS | 6 | Cerebral | Lung, breast, melanoma, RCC, ENT, thyroid |
| | | Spinal | Breast, lung, lymphoma, prostate |
| Skin | 2 | Cutaneous | Lung, breast, kidney, ovaries, melanoma |

*ENT* ear / nose / throat, *GIT* gastrointestinal tract, *NSCLC* non-small cell lung cancer, *RCC* renal cell carcinoma, *SCLC* small cell lung cancer

**Sy:** In most cases, symptoms due to advanced malignancy
- Pain in the affected area:      75% of cases
- Fatigue, reduced performance:      60%
- Hepatomegaly, abdominal symptoms:      40%
- Lymphadenopathy:      20%
- Respiratory insufficiency:      15%
- Anorexia, weight loss:      15%
- Neurological symptoms (CNS metastasis):      5%

**Dg:** ### Diagnostic Guidelines

Most patients present with advanced and diffuse metastatic disease and require an individual diagnostic approach. Identification of the primary tumor is only relevant if it has therapeutic consequences. Diagnostic targets:
- Identification of patients who can potentially be treated with curative intent (10–15% of cases of CUP)
- Identification of patients who require palliative therapy
- Diagnostic procedures should be limited to avoid discomfort for the patient. Non-invasive tests should be conducted prior to invasive procedures.

## Diagnostic Procedures

### Medical History, Physical Examination
- Medical history including risk factors associated with common tumor types, dynamics of the disease, family history
- Physical examination, esp. lymph node status, skin, thyroid, breast, prostate, rectum, testis
- Where necessary, consultation of specialists (ENT, gynecology, urology)

### Laboratory Tests
- Routine laboratory tests including complete blood count, electrolytes, liver and renal function tests, LDH
- Fecal occult blood test, urinary status
- Tumor markers: PSA, βHCG, AFP, CEA, CA19-9, CA15-3, CK-7, CA125, calcitonin, SCC, thyroglobulin. Only PSA (prostate-specific antigen) is suitable for screening, other tumor markers are not diagnostic but may help monitor the disease course (▶ Chap. 2.4)

### Histology
- Biopsy: resection of a sufficient amount of tissue, possibly in combination with cytoreductive surgery
- Light microscopy and standard stains
- Additional tests: special stains, immunohistochemistry (PSA, estrogen receptors, cytokeratin, vimentin, leukocyte antigens, S100 protein, etc.), molecular biological tests, cytogenetics, electron microscopy
- Where applicable: chromosome analysis (isochromosome 12 with germ cell tumors; t(11;22) translocation with Ewing's sarcoma)

### Imaging
- Chest x-ray, abdominal ultrasound, CT / MRI
- CT / MRI of pelvis and abdomen lead to identification of the primary tumor in 35% of cases
- Endoscopy: esophago-gastro-duodenoscopy, rectoscopy, colonoscopy
- Other: mammography, barium x-ray
- PET, especially if no other detectable tumor manifestations

*NOTE:* anticancer treatment without an established histological diagnosis should be avoided. Exception: individual patients displaying definite clinical signs of malignancy and requiring immediate treatment (e.g., radiotherapy of painful localized tumors).

### Likelihood of a Diagnosis Being Established in CUP
- Repeated thorough investigation:              15%
- Autopsy:                             70–85%

*NOTE:* up to 25% of diagnoses are revised at autopsy

**Th:**      ## Treatment Concept

The treatment of cancer of unknown origin depends on the tumor histology, the suspected primary tumor, and the extent of metastasis.

### Curative Treatment
10 to 15% of patients can be treated with curative intent, especially in case of:
- Localized tumor stages → surgical treatment, radiotherapy, multimodal therapy concepts
- Tumor types which can be effectively treated even in advanced stages (testicular cancer / germ cell tumors, lymphomas, leukemias, small cell lung cancer) → chemotherapy, multimodal therapy concepts

### Indications for Treatment with Palliative Intent
- Improvement of the patient's quality of life
- Pain (▶ Chap. 4.5)
- Local complications, e.g., malignant effusions (▶ Chap. 4.8), superior vena cava syndrome (▶ Chap. 9.2), spinal cord compression (▶ Chap. 9.3), symptoms due to tumor expansion
- Metabolic complications, e.g., hypercalcemia (▶ Chap. 9.5), hyperuricemia (▶ Chap. 9.6)

If the differential diagnosis of a tumor of unknown origin includes potentially curable diseases, all curative treatment options should be used, e.g.:
- Cisplatin-containing therapy protocol and possibly high-dose chemotherapy with suspected testicular cancer or germ cell tumors (▶ Chaps. 8.5.1, 8.5.2)
- Intensified regimen with suspected small cell lung cancer ("limited disease") (▶ Chap. 8.2.1)
- Taxane- / anthracycline-containing therapies with suspected breast cancer (▶ Chap. 8.4.1)
- Multimodal therapy concepts with localized tumors of the head and neck (▶ Chap. 8.1)

### Chemotherapy Protocol

| "PCE" ▶ Protocol 12.18.1 | | | Start next cycle on day 22 |
|---|---|---|---|
| Paclitaxel | 200 mg/m²/day | i.v. | Day 1 |
| Carboplatin | AUC 6 | i.v. | Day 1 |
| Etoposide | 50 mg absolute | p.o. | Days 1, 3, 5, 7, 9 |
| | 100 mg absolute | p.o. | Days 2, 4, 6, 8, 10 |

**Prg:** Generally poor prognosis:
- Median survival: 3–4 months
- One-year survival: 25%
- Five-year survival: < 5%

**Ref:**
1. Chorost MI, Lee MC, Yeoh CB et al. Unknown primary. J Surg Oncol 2004;87:191–203
2. ESMO Guidelines Working Group. Cancer of unknown primary site: ESMO Clinical Recommendations for diagnosis, treatment and follow-up. Ann Oncol 2007;18(Suppl.2):ii81–2
3. Hillen HF. Unknown primary tumours. Postgrad Med J 2000;76:690–3
4. Pavlidis N, Fizazi K. Cancer of unknown primary (CUP). Crit Rev Oncol Hematol 2005;54:243–50
5. Van de Wouw AJ, Jansen RLH, Speel EJM et al. The unknown biology of the unknown primary tumour. Ann Oncol 2003;14:191–6
6. Varadhachary GR, Abbruzzese JL, Lenzi R. Diagnostic strategies for unknown primary cancer. Cancer 2004;100:1776–85

**Web:**
1. http://www.cancer.gov/cancertopics/types/unknownprimary — NCI Cancer Topics
2. http://www.emedicine.com/MED/topic1463.htm — E-medicine
3. http://www.unknownprimarycancer.com/ — Sarah Cannon Ctr

## 8.12     Metastasis

### R. Engelhardt, F. Otto

**Def:**     Migration of cells of a malignant primary tumor to different places within the same organ or to other organs.

### Terms
- *Micrometastases:* histological evidence only
- *Macrometastases:* detectable by imaging
- *Solitary metastasis:* a single metastasis in the entire organism
- *Singular metastasis:* a single metastasis in a particular organ
- *Anachronous metastasis:* detection prior to diagnosis of the primary tumor
- *Synchronous metastasis:* detection simultaneous to primary tumor
- *Metachronous metastasis:* detection after diagnosis of the primary tumor

**Ep:**     Organ metastasis and site of primary tumor:
- *Cerebral metastases:* lung cancer (48%), breast cancer (15%), malignant melanoma (9%), colon cancer (5%), cancer of unknown origin (11%)
- *Pulmonary metastases:* lung cancer (28%), breast cancer (14%), colorectal cancer (10%), renal cell carcinoma (10%), gastric cancer (8%), biliary tract carcinoma (7%), and others
- *Liver metastases:* mainly tumors drained by the portal venous system (48%).The most common extraportal tumors with liver metastases are lung cancer and breast cancer.
- *Bone metastases:* mainly prostate, breast, lung, thyroid, and renal cell carcinoma

**Pp:**     Organ metastases develop due to hematogenous or lymphatic migration of tumor cells as well as direct invasion.

### Hematogenous Spread
Initial spread usually following the blood flow to first capillary bed:
- Colorectal carcinomas: liver metastases (portal circulation)
- Lung cancer: brain (systemic circulation)
- Renal cell carcinomas, germ cell tumors: lungs (systemic circulation)

**Class:**     In the *TNM classification*, organ metastases are classified as tumor stage M1 (▶ Chap. 1.6). Further classification according to location via indices:
- ADR: adrenal gland
- BRA: brain
- HEP: liver
- LYM: lymph node
- MAR: bone marrow
- OSS: bone
- PER: peritoneum
- PUL: lung
- SKI: skin
- OTH: other

**Dg:**     *Diagnostic Procedure in Case of Metastases Without Known Primary Tumor*
- Biopsy for histological analysis
- Search for primary tumor (diagnostic procedures depending on histology)
- Staging
- Establishment of treatment concept according to tumor type, stage, and clinical picture

### Laboratory Tests

The following are indicators of the presence of organ metastases after removal of the primary tumor:

- Inflammation markers: ESR, fibrinogen, α2 globulin, ferritin
- Cell destruction: LDH
- Liver and bone metastases: alkaline phosphatase
- Tumor markers (depending on tumor type, ▶ Chap. 2.4)

*NOTE:* "Typical" medical history, clinical picture, or imaging are not sufficient for the diagnosis of metastases. Usually, cytological or histological analysis of at least one site is required.

**Dd:**
- Primary tumor
- Benign tumor (e.g., glioma)
- Deformities (e.g., hemangioma, cyst)
- Inflammatory processes (e.g., abscess)
- Result of trauma (e.g., hematoma, fracture)

**Th:**
The treatment of metastases is part of the overall treatment of the underlying disease. Treatment with curative intent is usually more aggressive → e.g., in case of:
- Primary tumor in remission
- Long disease-free interval (DFI)
- Solitary metastasis
- High chemo- and/or radiosensitivity (e.g., testicular cancer)

Palliative situations: symptom-based approach.

**Prg:**
Organ metastases usually constitute an unfavorable prognosis for the cancer patient. Disease-free interval (DFI, time between occurrence / resection of the primary tumor and occurrence of metastases) of > 12 months is regarded as a favorable prognostic factor.

**Ref:**
1. Bogenrieder T, Herlyn M. Axis of evil. Molecular mechanisms of cancer metastasis. Oncogene 2003;22:6524–36
2. Cao Y. Emerging mechanisms of tumor lymphangiogenesis and lymphatic metastasis. Nat Rev Cancer 2005;5:735–42
3. Eccles SA, Welch DR. Metastasis: recent discoveries and novel treatment strategies. Lancet 2007;369:1742–57
4. Entschladen F, Drell TL, Lang K et al. Tumor-cell migration, invasion and metastasis: navigation by neurotransmitters. Lancet Oncol 2004;5:254–8
5. Hunter K. Host genetics influence tumour metastasis. Nat Rev Cancer 2006;6:141–6
6. Liotta LA, Kohn EC. The microenvironment of the tumour-host interface. Nature 2001;411:375–9
7. Pantel K, Brakenhoff RH. Dissecting the metastatic cascade. Nat Rev Cancer 2004;4:448–56
8. Steeg PS. Tumor metastasis: mechanistics insights and clinical challanges. Nature Med 2006;12:895–904
9. Weigelt B, Peterse JL, Van't Veer LJ. Breast cancer metastasis: markers and models. Nat Rev Cancer 2005;5:591–602

**Web:**
1. http://www.nlm.nih.gov/medlineplus/ency/article/002260.htm    Metastasis, Medline Plus
2. http://www.path.sunysb.edu/courses/im/    Metastasis, New York University
3. http://www.cancer.gov/cancertopics/understandingcancer/angiogenesis    NCI Cancer Topics

## 8.12.1     Brain Metastases

### R. Engelhardt, F. Otto

**Def:**     Metastasis to the central nervous system.

**Ep:**     Of all cancer patients, 20–40% develop brain metastases. In most cases metachronous metastases (> 80%), singular metastasis in 25%. 60% of patients with brain metastases also have pulmonary lesions (primary tumor or pulmonary metastases).

**Pg:**     *Primary Tumors*
- Lung cancer                           48%
- Breast cancer                         15%
- Malignant melanoma                    9%
- Colon cancer                          5%
- Cancer of unknown primary origin      11%

*Location of Brain Metastases*
- Cerebral hemispheres                  80%
- Cerebellum                            15%
- Brainstem                             5%

**Sy:**
- Headaches                             42%
- Focal neurological weakness           31%
- Cognitive dysfunction                 27%
- Epileptic seizures                    20%
- Ataxia                                17%

**Dg:**     *Medical History, Physical Examination*
- Physical examination including neurological tests

*Imaging*
- MRI
- Search for primary tumor: chest x-ray, CT thorax / abdomen, abdominal ultrasound

*Histology*
- Particularly with solitary processes: stereotactic biopsy to confirm diagnosis

**Dd:**
- Primary brain tumor
- Infectious foci, cerebral abscesses
- Cerebral ischemia
- Brain hemorrhage
- Demyelinating disease

**Th:**     The treatment of brain metastases mainly focuses on the palliation of neurological defects. However, in certain cases of an isolated metastasis, surgery with curative intent is indicated (e.g., renal cell carcinoma).

*Treatment of Cerebral Edema*
- Dexamethasone p.o. or i.v., initially up to $6 \times 8$ mg/day
- Famotidine $1 \times 40$ mg/day (evenings, gastric mucosal protection)
- Trimethoprim-sulfamethoxazole (TMP-SMZ) p.o., mornings (prevention of *Pneumocystis carinii* pneumonia, especially in patients > 50 years and application of steroids > 2 weeks)

*ATTENTION: potential side effects: steroid diabetes (measure blood sugar levels regularly), steroid psychosis*
Alternatively: mannitol up to 3 times per day, intravenously via central venous line.

### Prophylaxis of Seizures

Use of anticonvulsive drugs (e.g., phenytoin) particularly to avoid relapse after primary seizures ("secondary prophylaxis"); primary prophylactic therapy (before first seizure) is indicated with:
- Cortical metastases
- EEG indicating seizure potential
- Patients with increased risk of fracture in case of a fall (osteoporosis, bone metastases)

*ATTENTION:* treatment with steroids can mask allergic reactions to phenytoin.

### Surgical Treatment

Treatment of brain metastases usually focuses on palliation of neurological symptoms; indication for surgery with curative intention only in selected cases:
- Singular/isolated metastasis
- Long disease-free interval (DFI > 1 year)
- No extracranial tumor growth
- Good performance status (Karnofsky scale > 70%)

### Radiotherapy

Conventional radiotherapy (whole brain radiotherapy) or high-dose local radiotherapy of individual metastases or areas of the brain ("radiosurgery," "gamma knife"). Indicated in cases of:
- Multiple metastases, short DFI (< 1 year) or inoperable lesions
- Postoperative

### Chemotherapy

The chemosensitivity of the primary tumor as well as the permeability of the blood-brain barrier for cytostatic drugs determine the efficacy of chemotherapy. Indicated in cases of:
- Small cell lung cancer (SCLC) with synchronous brain metastases
- Small cell tumors with synchronous brain metastases
- Breast cancer with inoperable brain metastases not previously treated with intensive cytostatic therapy or consolidation therapy after surgery

**Prg:**

| Stage | Median survival (months) |
|---|---|
| Solitary metastasis | 10–18 |
| Multiple metastases, with therapy | 6–9 |
| Multiple metastases, without therapy | 1–2 |

**Ref:**

1. Eichler AF, Loeffler JS. Multidisciplinary management of brain metastases. Oncologist 2007;12:884–98
2. Kaap EC, Niel CG, Vecht CJ. Therapeutic management of brain metastasis. Lancet Neurol 2005;4:289–98
3. Khuntia D, Brown P, Li J et al. Whole-brain radiotherapy in the management of brain metastasis. J Clin Oncol 2006;24:1295–304
4. Klimo P, Schmidt MH. Surgical management of spinal metastasis. Oncologist 2004;9:188–96
5. Langer CL, Mehta MP. Current management of brain metastases, with a focus on systemic options. J Clin Oncol 2005;23:6207–19
6. Van den Bent MJ. The role of chemotherapy in brain metastases. Eur J Cancer 2003;39:2114–20
7. Vogelbaum MA, Suh JH. Resectable brain metastases. J Clin Oncol 2006;24:1289–94

**Web:**

1. http://neuroscript.com/neuroscript.com/index.htm    Neuroscript
2. http://www.nlm.nih.gov/medlineplus/ency/
   article/000769.htm    Metastatic Brain Tumor, Medline Plus
3. http://www.emedicine.com/Radio/topic101.htm    E-medicine

### 8.12.2    Carcinomatous Meningitis (Leptomeningeal Metastases)

**M. Trepel**

**Def:**   Tumor spread to the leptomeninges (the soft membranes covering the brain and spinal cord)

**ICD-10:**   C79.3

**Ep:**   Up to 5% of patients with metastatic cancer suffer from symptomatic leptomeningeal metastases (LM), up to 20% have asymptomatic LM at the terminal stage of the disease. Most frequent tumors: breast cancer (12–34%), lung cancer (10–26%), melanoma (17–25%), gastrointestinal cancer (4–14%), and cancers of unknown primary (CUP) (1–7%).

**Pphys:**   Spread of malignant cells throughout the subarachnoid space. Tumor cells access the CSF in several ways:
- Hematogenous spread via the arachnoid vessels
- Extension from brain metastases
- Metastases to the choroid plexus which produces the CSF
- Extension from vertebral or cranial bone metastases
- Primary meningeal tumor (lymphoma, melanoma, sarcoma, e.g., arising from the nerve sheaths)

Tumor cells within the CSF are disseminated, invading the leptomeninges at multiple locations and sometimes obstructing CSF flow at any point along its pathway. Almost all patients with solid tumors suffering from LM also have other systemic metastases, while LM patients with hematological malignancies (leukemia, lymphoma) often have no evidence of additional systemic involvement.

**Sy:**   Multifocal involvement is a hallmark of diffuse LM, resulting in:
- Headache and meningeal signs (50% of patients) such as nuchal rigidity, nausea, vomiting, dizziness
- Hydrocephalus and elevated intracranial pressure (ICP)
- Dysfunction of cranial nerves (most common: diplopia) and spinal nerve roots (most common: radicular pain)
- Focal neurological signs and epileptic seizures

Clinical symptoms and signs vary, depending upon the site of leptomeningeal, nerve root, and brain parenchyma invasion.

**Dg:**
- History and neurological examination
- Gadolinium-enhanced cranial and/or spinal MRI (always prior to lumbar puncture) showing meningeal enhancement (more sensitive but less specific than CSF examination)
- Lumbar puncture or ventricular puncture. At least 15 ml CSF necessary for laboratory investigation. In > 80% cell count, protein and lactate ↑, and glucose ↓. Cytological and immunocytochemical detection of tumor cells is positive in 80–90%. Accompanying lymphocyte pleocytosis is common.
- Tumor markers in the CSF, if cytology is negative (CSF tumor marker concentrations > 3% of serum values are suggestive for LM, concentrations of CSF tumor markers > 80% of serum values are almost evidentiary)
- In exceptional cases with negative cytology and without evidence of disseminated cancer, open leptomeningeal biopsy should be considered

**Dd:**
- Brain parenchymal metastases causing focal neurological signs, increased ICP, or seizures
- Bacterial or viral meningitis
- Spine or skull metastases causing nerve root compression

**Th:**
- Treatment of meningeal involvement in lymphoma or leukemia can be curative.
- Treatment of LM in solid tumors is palliative, aiming at pain relief, improving neurological function, and prolongation of survival.
- Treatment decisions have to take into account the extent of meningeal involvement as well as systemic spread of the tumor to other sites.

### Treatment Strategy for Poor Risk Patients

Low Karnofsky performance status, multiple neurological deficits, and extensive systemic cancer spread predict poor prognosis even upon aggressive therapy. For these patients, treatment of LM should focus on symptom relief rather than tumor control, including:
- Radiation therapy involving certain segments of the neuraxis for symptoms caused by localized LM
- Analgesic medication
- Corticosteroids to improve analgesia and (particularly for LM in breast cancer, leukemia, lymphoma) to improve focal neurological symptoms
- Anticonvulsants only for patients with seizures

### Treatment Strategy for Good Risk Patients

Karnofsky performance scale > 60, few or no neurological deficits, low systemic tumor burden, or tumors sensitive to systemic therapy predict better prognosis. Therapy is directed at controlling tumor growth, including radiotherapy and intrathecal or systemic high-dose chemotherapy both directed at meningeal and extrameningeal cancer. Treatment options, which always have to involve the entire neuraxis, include:
- Systemic administration of dexamethasone 8 mg twice a day if signs of increased intracranial pressure (ICP) are present.
- Ventriculoperitoneal shunt for selected patients with elevated ICP resistant to dexamethasone (potential complications: infection, shunt obstruction by tumor cells, tumor spread to the abdominal cavity).
- Prior to radiotherapy (RT) or intrathecal chemotherapy (ITC), a radionuclide cisternogram is useful to study CSF flow and detect areas of obstruction preventing homogenous distribution of ITC (up to 60% of patients). RT to such areas can normalize CSF flow, improving the efficacy of ITC.

### Radiation Therapy (RT)
- More effective for symptom control (especially pain control) than intrathecal chemotherapy
- Should always be considered in bulky LM
- Total dose 30–36 Gy in daily 3-Gy fractions to sites of symptomatic disease and/or to sites of obstructed CSF flow prior to intrathecal chemotherapy
- Radiotherapy of the entire neuraxis can be applied but often results in substantial myelosuppression, especially if concomitant systemic or intrathecal chemotherapy is applied

### Intrathecal Chemotherapy (ITC): General Considerations
- ITC is the standard treatment for LM
- Application either directly into the lateral ventricle through a ventricular catheter via a subcutaneous reservoir (e.g., Ommaya reservoir) or into the spinal subarachnoid space by lumbar puncture (no data from randomized trials comparing both applications available)
- Four drugs are commonly used: methotrexate, (liposomal) cytarabine, thiotepa, and (in lymphoma and lymphoid leukemia) dexamethasone
- Superiority of ITC over systemic chemotherapy has not been proven in randomized trials
- Intrathecal chemotherapy is rarely effective for bulky meningeal disease > 1 mm, or LM along nerve root sleeves, or LM within the Virchow-Robin spaces due to limited drug diffusion
- Superiority of combinations of agents for ITC versus single-agent ITC for LM from solid tumors is unproven
- Complications of CSF drug administration: headache, nausea and vomiting, herniation, especially if the total CSF volume is increased due to impaired CSF flow and resorption. Therefore, equivalent volumes of CSF must be removed prior to injecting ITC

### Intrathecal Methotrexate (MTX)

- Most commonly used drug for ITC in LM. Active against breast cancer and hematological malignancies, less active against other solid tumors
- Applied in 10- to 15-mg doses twice a week
- Response rate approximately 20–60%
- Optimal duration of therapy in responding patients is uncertain (4–6 months)
- Concurrent oral leucovorin may be considered to minimize the risk of systemic MTX toxicity
- Neurological complications: chemical (aseptic) meningitis, delayed leukoencephalopathy, acute encephalopathy, transverse myelopathy

### Intrathecal Cytarabine (AraC)

- Available for ITC in conventional or liposomal formulations
- Liposomal cytarabine is preferred in solid tumor-derived LM in which conventional cytarabine is relatively ineffective. Conventional AraC is mainly used for leukemic or lymphomatous meningitis
- AraC is applied at 40 mg twice a week; liposomal AraC is applied in 50-mg doses every 2–4 weeks (intraventricular reservoir not needed)
- Response rate of liposomal AraC approximately 30–70%
- Liposomal AraC confers better progression-free and overall survival than MTX

### Intrathecal Thiotepa

- Very short CSF half-life (< 1 h)
- Usual ITC regimen is 10 mg twice a week
- Limited efficacy, particularly suited for patients failing MTX and AraC or receiving concomitant RT

### Systemic Chemotherapy

- Particularly suitable for hematological malignancies to treat both systemic and leptomeningeal disease simultaneously
- Systemic high-dose MTX (8,000 mg/m$^2$) with leucovorin rescue is the most commonly used systemic therapy for LM from solid tumors and lymphomas
- High-dose AraC (3,000 mg/m$^2$ twice a day) has not been proven to be useful in the treatment of LM from solid tumors but can be effective in hematological malignancies
- Oral capecitabine may be beneficial in some patients with LM from solid tumors such as breast cancer

### Investigational Intrathecal Therapies

- Cytostatics: mafosfamide, etoposide, dacarbazine, busulfan, topotecan
- Monoclonal antibodies such as trastuzumab or rituximab

### Response Evaluation

- CSF cell count, CSF cytology and flow cytometry / immunocytochemistry, CSF lactate (response is expected within 4–8 weeks after initiation of treatment)
- Cranial / spinal MRI is suitable only for monitoring bulky disease und unsuitable for diffuse LM because meningeal enhancement may persist long after cytological CSF clearance and may be sustained due to repeated lumbar puncture and/or ITC

## Intrathecal (IT) Chemotherapy Protocols

| *"MTX mono"* ▶ *Protocol 12.19.3* | | | *Repeat twice a week* |
|---|---|---|---|
| Methotrexate | 15 mg | i.t. | |

| *"Triple therapy"* ▶ *Protocol 12.19.2* | | | *Repeat twice a week* |
|---|---|---|---|
| Cytarabine | 40 mg | i.t. | |
| Dexamethasone | 4 mg | i.t. | |
| Methotrexate | 15 mg | i.t. | |

| *"Liposomal cytarabine"* ▶ *Protocol 12.19.4* | | | *Repeat day 15* |
|---|---|---|---|
| Liposomal cytarabine | 50 mg | i.t. | |

**Prg:**
- Leptomeningeal metastases from hematological malignancies are potentially curable
- Leptomeningeal metastases from solid tumors have a poor prognosis. Median survival for untreated patients is 6–8 weeks. If clinical improvement is achieved by ITC, progression-free survival is usually short and limited to 2–3 months. Median survival in aggressively treated patients is 3–4 months for most tumors (6–7 months for breast cancer, 2–3 months for high-grade glioma)

**Ref:**
1. Balm M, Hammack J. Leptomeningeal carcinomatosis: presenting features and prognostic factors. Arch Neurol 1996;53:626–32
2. Chamberlain MC. Combined-modality treatment of leptomeningeal gliomatosis. Neurosurgery 2003;52:324
3. Kesari S, Batchelor TT. Leptomeningeal metastases. Neurol Clin 2003;21:25–66
4. Omuro AM, Lallana EC, Bilsky MH, DeAngelis LM. Ventriculoperitoneal shunt in patients with leptomeningeal metastasis. Neurology 2005;64:1625–7

**Web:**
1. http://www.emedicine.com/neuro/topic188.htm
2. http://cancerweb.ncl.ac.uk/cancernet/103859.html

## 8.12.3    Lung Metastases

**R. Engelhardt, F. Otto**

**Def:**    Metastasis to the lung.

**Ep:**    Incidence 6 cases/100,000 population/year; 20–40% of all tumor patients develop lung metastases.

**Pg:**    *Primary Tumors*
- Lung cancer                           28%
- Breast cancer                         14%
- Colorectal cancer                     10%
- Renal cell carcinoma                  10%
- Gastric cancer                         8%
- Biliary tract carcinoma                7%

Pathological distinction between hematogenous and lymphatic metastasis (lymphangiosis carcinomatosa).

**Sy:**
- Cough, hemoptysis, dyspnea
- Chest pain (indicative of pleural invasion)
- Weakness, weight loss

**Dg:**    *Medical History, Physical Examination*
- Medical history including smoking, risk factors
- Physical examination (lung, signs of metastasis, neurology, etc.)

*Imaging*
- Chest x-ray, thoracic CT

*Histology*
- Fine-needle biopsy (*NOTE*: thoracic drainage required in 4% of patients)
- Video assisted thoracoscopy
- Open thoracotomy

**Dd:**    *Differential Diagnosis: Intrapulmonary Lesions*

| | |
|---|---|
| *Malignant tumors* | |
| • Lung cancer | 40–50% of cases (▶ Chap. 8.2.1) |
| • Metastases | 10% of cases |
| • Carcinoid | Originating from the APUD system (▶ Chap. 8.7.2) |
| • Cylindroma | Adenoid-cystic carcinoma, poor prognosis |
| *Benign tumors* | |
| • Bronchial adenoma | Malignant conversion possible |
| • Chondroma | Benign hamartoma |
| • Other | Neurinoma, lipoma, fibroma, osteoma, etc. |
| *Other* | |
| • Infection | Tuberculosis, actinomycosis, pneumonia |
| • Sarcoidosis | Stage II or III |

**Th:** *Surgical Treatment*

Indication for surgery in certain tumor types:
- Osteosarcoma, soft tissue sarcomas
- Colorectal carcinoma, renal cell carcinoma, breast cancer
- Germ cell tumors: after chemotherapy for further cytoreduction and histological evaluation (detection of vital tumor cells) → planning of further systemic treatment
- Melanoma: patients with solitary metastasis and long disease-free interval after primary treatment

Metastasectomy of multiple metastases is possible if:
- Local containment of the primary tumor
- No extrathoracic metastases
- Surgically accessible site / resectability

*Cytokine Therapy*

More effective with pulmonary metastases than with other types of metastases; e.g., with malignant melanoma (interferon-α), renal cell carcinoma (interleukin-2).

**Prg:** Prognosis is influenced by tumor histology.

Favorable prognostic factors: long disease-free interval (DFI), small number of metastases.

**Ref:**
1. Briccoli A, Rocca M, Salone M et al. Resection of recurrent pulmonary metastases in patients with osteosarcoma. Cancer 2005;104:1721–5
2. Kondo H, Okumura T, Ohde Y et al. Surgical treatment for metastatic malignancies. Pulmonary metastasis: indications and outcome. Int J Clin Oncol 2005;10:81–5
3. Schreiber G, Pitterle D, Kim YC et al. Molecular genetic analysis of primary lung cancer and cancer metastatic to the lung. Anticancer Res 1999;19:1109–15
4. Thao B, Schwartz LH, Moskowitz CS et al. Pulmonary metastases: effect of CT section thickness on measurement: initial experience. Radiology 2005;234:934–9
5. Van Putte BP, Hendriks JM, Romijn S et al. Isolated lung perfusion for the treatment of pulmonary metastases. Surg Oncol 2003;12:187–93
6. Yoneda KY, Louie S, Shelton DK. Approach to pulmonary metastases. Curr Opin Pulm Med 2000;6:356–63

**Web:**
1. http://www.nml.nih.gov/medlineplus/ency/article/000097.htm — Pulmonary Metastases, Medline Plus
2. http://www.emedicine.com/med/topic2987.htm — E-medicine
3. http://www.meddean.luc.edu/lumen/MedEd/medicine/pulmonar/cxr/met.htm — Loyola University
4. http://www.ctsnet.org/ — Cardiothoracic Surgery Network
5. http://cancernet.nci.nih.gov — CancerNet, National Cancer Institute

## 8.12.4     Liver Metastases

### R. Engelhardt, F. Otto

**Def:**     Metastasis to the liver.

**Ep:**     Of patients undergoing surgery for colorectal cancer, 10–25% have synchronous resectable liver metastases.

**Pg:**
- Mainly tumors drained by the portal venous system (48%)
- Most common extraportal primary tumors: lung cancer and breast cancer
- Isolated hepatic metastasis (no extrahepatic lesions): mainly with colorectal cancer → local treatment of liver metastases only relevant in this disease

**Sy:**     Fever, loss of appetite, fatigue, weight loss, abdominal fullness

**Dg:**     *Medical History, Physical Examination*
- Medical history including evidence of colorectal cancer (irregular bowel movement, constipation, diarrhea, perianal hemorrhage, etc.)
- Physical examination including liver palpation and rectal examination

*Laboratory Tests*
- Liver function parameters, clotting, tumor markers (depending on primary tumor)

*Imaging*
- Abdominal ultrasound, intraoperative ultrasound
- Abdominal CT / spiral CT / MRI

*Histology*
- Needle biopsy (Menghini) or fine-needle biopsy
- Laparoscopy (if uncertainty about indication for surgery)

**Dd:**     *Differential Diagnosis: Intrahepatic Lesions*

| *Malignant tumors* | |
| --- | --- |
| Metastases | Most common malignant process in the liver (90%) |
| Hepatocellular carcinoma | HCC |
| Cholangiocarcinoma | CCC, rare |
| Angiosarcoma | Vinyl chloride, arsenic, ionizing radiation |
| Hepatoblastoma | Embryonic tumor (in children) |
| *Benign tumors* | |
| Hemangioma | Most common benign liver tumor |
| Liver cell adenoma | Men > women, risk factor: contraceptives |
| Bile duct adenoma | Rare |
| Focal nodular hyperplasia | FNH, mainly women |
| *Cystic processes* | |
| Solitary hepatic cysts | Common |
| Dysontogenetic cysts | Rare, hereditary |
| Cystic echinococcosis | Caused by dog tapeworm (*Echinococcus granulosus*) |
| Alveolar echinococcosis | Caused by fox tapeworm (*Echinococcus multilocularis*) |
| Liver abscess | Pyogenic, amoebic |

**Th:**

### Surgical Treatment

Metastasectomy is the only potentially curative treatment of colorectal cancer with hepatic metastases. Surgical treatment is appropriate particularly in patients with solitary or unilobular metastases. The surgical mortality rate is < 5%.

### Systemic Chemotherapy

According to primary tumor, e.g., colorectal cancer (▶ Chap. 8.3.4)

### Local Chemotherapy

The rationale of local chemotherapy is a higher intratumoral concentration of the chemotherapeutic drug and lower systemic toxicity (particularly for drugs with high "first pass" effect). The chemotherapeutic drug is administered via portal line and transported to the liver via the hepatic artery. All published studies demonstrate significantly improved tumor response rates compared to systemic chemotherapy, i.e., better local tumor control, but without conferring a significant survival advantage.

Alternatively: chemoembolization or percutaneous tumor destruction (laser, alcohol injection, cryotherapy, etc.).

**Prg:**
Five-year survival of patients with liver metastases of colorectal carcinoma:
- After surgery: 30%
- Without surgical treatment: < 2%

**Ref:**

1. Khatri VP, Petrelli NJ, Belghiti J. Extending the frontiers of surgical therapy for hepatic colorectal metastases: is there a limit? J Clin Oncol 2005;23:8490–9
2. Malafosse R, Penna C, Sa Cunha A et al. Surgical management of hepatic metastases from colorectal malignancies. Ann Oncol 2001;12:887–94
3. Mocellin S, Pilati P, Lise M et al. Meta-analysis of hepatic arterial infusion for unresectable liver metastases from colorectal cancer: the end of an era? J Clin Oncol 2007;25:5649–54
4. Pawlik TM, Schulick RD, Choti MA. Expanding criteria for resectability of colorectal liver metastases. Oncologist 2008;13:51–64
5. Venook AP, Warren RS. Therapeutic approaches to metastasis confined to the liver. Curr Oncol Rep 2001;3:109–15

**Web:**

1. http://www.nlm.nih.gov/medlineplus/ency/article/000277.htm — Liver Metastases, Medline Plus
2. http://www.emedicine.com/RADIO/topic 394.htm — E-medicine
3. http://www.aasld.org/ — Liver Diseases
4. http://www.liverfoundation.org/ — American Liver Foundation
5. http://www.livercancer.com/ — Liver Cancer Network
6. http://www3.mdanderson.org/departments/liver/metastasis.htm — Liver Metastases, MD Anderson

**8.12.5    Bone Metastases**

R. Engelhardt, F. Otto

**Def:**  Metastasis to the skeletal system.

**Ep:**  Bone metastases (usually multiple metastases) from prostate, breast, lung, thyroid or renal cell cancer. Solitary bone metastases are rare (mainly with thyroid cancer, renal cell cancer, and myeloma).

**Pp:**  ***Type of Metastasis (Radiological Diagnosis)***
- *Osteolytic metastases:* osteoclast activation by tumor cells → secondary tumor cell invasion
- *Osteoblastic metastases:* osteoblast activation, osteosclerotic lesions
- *Mixed metastases:* activation of osteoblasts and osteoclasts → osteolytic-osteoblastic metastases

***Primary Tumors***
- Osteolytic metastases: lung cancer, renal cell carcinoma, hepatocellular carcinoma, ovarian cancer, pancreatic cancer, gastric cancer, breast cancer
- Osteoblastic metastases: prostate cancer, carcinoid, pancreatic cancer, gastric cancer, breast cancer
- Mixed metastases: colon cancer, breast cancer

**Sy:**
- Pain, impaired mobility
- Fatigue, reduced performance status, weight loss

**Dg:**  ***Medical History, Physical Examination***
- Medical history including pain, mobility
- Physical examination

***Laboratory Tests***
- Serum alkaline phosphatase (ALP), urinary hydroxyproline → markers of metastatic bone activity

***Imaging***
- Skeletal x-ray
- CT → particularly assessment of pelvis, shoulder, and spinal column
- MRI → particularly assessment of spine and spinal column
- $^{99}$Tc diphosphonate scan
*ATTENTION:* possibility of false-negative results with fast-growing purely osteolytic metastases (lung cancer, melanoma, plasmacytoma); limited suitability for monitoring of disease course ("flare effect" with treatment response)

***Histology***
- CT-guided fine-needle biopsy, particularly with osteolytic lesions
- Open biopsy, particularly with osteosclerotic metastases

**Dd:**
- Traumatic / osteoporotic fracture, osteomyelitis, cysts
- Primary benign or malignant bone tumors

**Co:**
- Bone instability → fracture
- Hypercalcemia

### Signs for Increased Risk of Fracture
- Pain with movement
- Painful cortical lesions > 2.5 cm in diameter
- Painful cortical osteolytic lesions longer than the diameter of the bone
- Painful medullary lesions measuring > 50% of the diameter of the bone

**Th:**

## Supportive Care

### Pain Control
- Particularly effective: nonsteroidal anti-inflammatory drugs, e.g., metamizole
- Bisphosphonates, e.g. zoledronate, 4 mg over 15 min i.v. every 3–4 weeks; also effective in preventing fractures (breast cancer, multiple myeloma)

### Treatment of Hypercalcemia
▶ Chap. 9.5

## Antineoplastic Treatment

### Surgical Metastasectomy: Indications
- Solitary metastases and long disease-free interval (DFI) since treatment of the primary tumor
- Spinal cord compression → laminectomy
- Fracture or imminent risk of fracture → internal fixator, bone cement

### Percutaneous Radiotherapy: Indications
- Postoperative radiotherapy (adjuvant radiotherapy)
- Prevention of fractures
- Pain control (almost always effective, independent of the histological type)

**ATTENTION:** except with chemosensitive tumors (lymphomas, germ cell tumors) or fully resectable tumors, percutaneous radiotherapy should initially be considered as a therapy option. Side effects of radiotherapy may include myelosuppression and may limit subsequent chemotherapy.

### Systemic Radionuclides
- $^{131}I$ (radioiodine): highly differentiated thyroid cancer
- $^{89}Sr$ (strontium): accumulates similar to calcium in areas of increased bone turnover

**Ref:**
1. Coleman RE. Management of bone metastases. Oncologist 2000;5:463–70
2. Mercadante S, Fulfaro F. Management of painful bone metastases. Curr Opin Oncol 2007;19:308–14
3. Roodman GD. Mechanisms of bone metastasis. N Engl J Med 2004;350:1655–64
4. Serafini AN. Therapy of metastatic bone pain. J Nucl Med 2001;42:895–906
5. Van Poznack C, Nadal C. Bone integrity and bone metastases in breast cancer. Curr Oncol Rep 2006;8:22–8

**Web:**
1. http://www.cancer.med.umich.edu/learn/bonemetsfacts.htm — Bone Metastases, Michigan University
2. http://www.emedicine.com/radio/topic88.htm — E-medicine
3. http://www.stat.washington.edu/TALARIA/LS2.3.1.html — Bone Metastases, Washington University
4. http://www.bonetumor.com/page67.html — Bone Metastases, Bonetumor.Org

## 8.13    Paraneoplastic Syndromes

### H. Henß

**Def:**   Non-malignant disorders caused by or associated with malignancies. Onset of symptoms is usually concurrent with diagnosis of the malignancy, but may occur before the disease or persist after remission.

**Ep:**   Up to 20% of all patients with malignant diseases develop paraneoplasia.

**Pg:**   Often unclear etiology. Possible factors are:
- Ectopic hormone production or hormonally active substances
- Synthesis of hematopoietic growth factors, cytokines, or inhibitors
- Synthesis of autoimmune antibodies or hemostasis inhibitors

**Class:**   *Paraneoplastic Syndromes*

- *Endocrine paraneoplastic syndromes:* ectopic production of hormones or hormone analogs with corresponding clinical symptoms.

- *Hematological paraneoplastic syndromes:* hematological disorders occurring with a number of malignant diseases. Differentiation between tumors directly affecting hematopoiesis and true paraneoplastic syndromes is often difficult.

- *Neurological paraneoplastic syndromes:* neurological complications occurring with malignant processes; often immunological mechanisms.

- *Cutaneous paraneoplastic syndromes:* skin changes occurring in malignant diseases.

**Sy:**   Variable; depending on the respective syndrome.

### Endocrine Paraneoplastic Syndromes

### Paraneoplastic Hypercalcemia (▶ also Chap. 9.5)

**Def:**   Increased serum calcium due to paraneoplastic osteoclast activation. In 10–20% of all cancer patients; severe hypercalcemia requiring treatment in 1–3% of cases

**Pg:**   Malignant cells secreting osteoclast-activating factors

**Sy:**   Often asymptomatic; with severe hypercalcemia:
- *Kidney:* polyuria, polydipsia
- *Gastrointestinal:* nausea, vomiting; ulcers or pancreatitis (rare)
- *Muscle:* myasthenia, constipation (ileus)
- *Cardiac:* bradycardia, atrial and ventricular fibrillation
- *CNS:* fatigue, lethargy, coma, impaired vision, psychosis

**Dg:**   
- *Laboratory:* routine laboratory tests including $Ca^{2+}$, electrolytes; where applicable: PTH or PTH-RP (parathyroid hormone-related protein)
- *ECG:* QT interval ↓, PQ interval ↓, broadened T-wave, bradycardia, arrhythmia

**Th:**   ▶ Chap. 9.5

### Hypertrophic Osteoarthropathy (Pierre-Marie-Bamberger)

**Def:** Clubbed fingers, periosteal proliferation of tubular bones

**Pg:** Pathogenesis not completely clear. Possibly ectopic production of vasoactive substances, GHRH (growth hormone releasing hormone) and other growth factors as well as inflammatory cytokines (PGDF, TNFα, and TGFβ). Hypoxia alone is not thought to be sufficient

**Sy:** Bone pain, joint pain, clubbed fingers

**Dg:** Bone scan, x-ray

**Dd:** Osteoarthropathy with chronic cardiac or pulmonary diseases

**Th:** Treatment of the underlying malignancy, symptomatic treatment with analgesics (nonsteroidal antiinflammatories), possibly vagotomy

### Paraneoplastic Cushing's Syndrome

**Pg:** Ectopic production of ACTH or functional ACTH prohormone or corticotropin-releasing factor (CRF)

**Sy:**
- Typical clinical signs: central obesity, moon face
- Edema, hypertension
- Hyperglycemia, hypokalemic alkalosis
- Hyperpigmentation of the skin

**Dg:** Physical examination, plasma cortisol level, possibly dexamethasone suppression test

**Dd:** Hypercortisolism of different origin (steroid medication, pituitary tumor, etc.)

**Th:** Treatment of underlying malignancy, possibly symptomatic treatment with aminoglutethimide or ketoconazole. In hypokalemic alkalosis: potassium and aldosterone antagonists

### Inadequate ADH Secretion (SIADH, Schwarz-Bartter Syndrome)

**Pg:** Ectopic production of ADH (antidiuretic hormone) or biologically similar substances by malignant tumor cells. Rare. Mainly with small cell lung cancer, pancreatic cancer, and malignant melanoma

**Sy:** Clinical picture of water intoxication: cough, dyspnea, "fluid lung," pulmonary edema, rapid weight gain, neurological disorders (headaches, agitation, amentia, cramps, apathy, stupor, coma)

**Dg:** Laboratory: inadequately increased ADH levels, serum sodium ↓, serum chloride ↓, serum hypo-osmolality, urinary hyperosmolarity

**Th:** Treatment of the underlying malignancy, restrict fluid intake (as far as possible)

### Paraneoplastic Hypoglycemia

**Def:** Hypoglycemia due to paraneoplastic secretion of hormone analogues. Common with insulinoma, otherwise rare

**Pg:** Paraneoplastic secretion of insulin or insulin analogs (e.g., insulin-like growth factor, IGF), in some cases preceding clinical diagnosis of the tumor. Occurring with insulinoma, mesenchymal tumors, gastrointestinal carcinomas, and tumors of adrenal cortex

**Sy:**    Symptoms of hypoglycemia in three phases:
- *Parasympathetic symptoms:* ravenous appetite, nausea / vomiting, reduced performance
- *Sympathetic symptoms:* restlessness, sweating, tremor, tachycardia, mydriasis, hypertension
- *Central nervous:* headache, lack of concentration, confusion, cramps, focal symptoms, somnolence, and coma

**Dg:**    Serum glucose < 40 mg/dl

**Dd:**
- Initial phase of diabetes mellitus
- Overdose of insulin or sulfonylurea (iatrogenic or self-inflicted as "hypoglycemia factitia")
- Drugs: sulfonamides, nonsteroidal antiinflammatories, beta-blockers, ACE inhibitors
- Severe hepatic disease (gluconeogenesis ↓), glycogenosis
- Renal dysfunction / uremia
- Postoperative, postgastrectomy syndrome following gastric resection
- Rare: anorexia (e.g., in case of vegetative syndrome, excessive alcohol consumption)

**Th:**    *Mild hypoglycemia:* conscious patient: glucose 5–20 g orally (soluble dextrose or saccharose), alternatively: fruit juice
*Severe hypoglycemia:* unconscious patient: 40% glucose 25–100 ml i.v.

### Further Measures
- Where applicable, glucagon 1 mg i.m. (confused / aggressive patients)
- Search for tumor and histological analysis with suspected malignancy
- Treatment of the underlying disease

## Paraneoplastic Gynecomastia, Galactorrhea, Precocious Puberty

**Def:**    Gynecomastia, galactorrhea, or precocious puberty occurring with malignant processes. Rare, occurring mainly with malignant germ cell tumors, small cell lung cancer (0.5–0.9%), and malignant liver tumors

**Pg:**    Ectopic secretion of chorionic gonadotropin or prolactin

**Sy:**    Breast changes, start of puberty

## Hematological Paraneoplastic Syndromes

## Paraneoplastic Erythroblastopenia (Pure Red Cell Aplasia)

**Def:**    Isolated erythropoietic abnormalities in patients with malignant tumors. Rare, mainly with malignant thymoma (50%), occasionally with adenocarcinomas (gastric cancer, breast cancer, adenocarcinomas of unknown primary origin)

**Pg:**    Pathogenetic mechanisms not finally established; possibly T-cell-mediated inhibition of erythropoiesis (in lymphoproliferative diseases)

**Dg:**    Full blood count with differential, bone marrow biopsy (smear, histology); exclusion of other causes of anemia (▶ Chap. 6.4)

**Th:**    Treatment of the underlying disease, therapy with cyclophosphamide or immunosuppressive drugs

### Microangiopathic Hemolytic Anemia (MAHA)

**Def:** Tumor-associated anemia with presence of fragmentocytes. Rare, mainly with mucin-producing adenocarcinomas

**Pg:** Unknown, possibly mechanical alteration of red bloods cells due to disseminated intravascular coagulation (DIC, ▶ Chap. 6.5.5), intima proliferation, pulmonary intraluminal tumor emboli

**Dg:** Hemolytic anemia with fragmentocytes, negative Coomb's test

**Th:** Treatment of the underlying disease, heparin is usually ineffective

### Paraneoplastic Polycythemia

**Def:** Increased red cell count associated with malignant tumors, e.g. renal cell cancer (35% of cases), hepatic carcinoma, cerebellar tumors

**Pg:** Aberrant secretion of erythropoietin or erythropoietic factors. In some cases increased erythrocytic differentiation due to tumor-associated prostaglandin secretion

**Dd:** Polycythemia vera rubra (▶ Chap. 7.3.2), other causes of polycythemia

**Dg:** Complete blood count with differential, erythropoietin level

**Th:** Treatment of the underlying disease; if necessary: venesection

### Paraneoplastic Granulocytopenia

**Def:** Low granulocyte count not caused by treatment. Very rare. Occurring with thymomas

**Pg:** Unknown, possibly T-cell mediated effect on granulopoiesis

**Dg:** Complete blood count and differential, bone marrow biopsy. Exclusion of other potential causes (▶ Chap. 6.2)

**Th:** Treatment of the underlying disease

### Paraneoplastic Granulocytosis, Eosinophilia

**Def:** Granulocytosis or eosinophilia associated with malignant diseases, mainly with gastrointestinal tumors (gastric / pancreatic cancer), lung cancer, melanoma, Hodgkin's disease

**Pg:** Aberrant production of hematopoietic factors or analogs by tumor tissue

**Dg:** Complete blood count with differential, exclusion of other potential causes

**Th:** Treatment of the underlying disease

### Paraneoplastic Thrombocytopenia

**Def:** Thrombocytopenia in patients with malignant tumors. Very rare. Occurring with malignant lymphomas (Hodgkin's disease, NHL), lung cancer, breast cancer

**Pg:** "ITP-like syndrome," mediated by autoantibodies against platelets or thrombopoietic factors

**Sy:**    Petechia, hematomas, hemorrhage

**Dg:**    Full blood count with differential, exclusion of other potential causes (chemotherapy-induced thrombocytopenia, bone marrow infiltration, ▶ Chap. 6.3)

**Th:**    Steroids (▶ Chap. 6.3.1), often ineffective. In severe cases: possibly splenectomy. Treatment of the underlying disease

### Paraneoplastic Thrombocytosis

**Def:**    Thrombocytosis associated with malignant tumors, mainly with lung cancer and gastrointestinal tumors.

**Pg:**    Aberrant cytokine production (thrombopoietin, IL-6)

**Dg:**    Full blood count with smear; exclusion of other potential causes (essential thrombocytosis, etc., ▶ Chap. 7.3.3)

**Th:**    In severe cases: low-dose acetylsalicylic acid (50–100 mg/day p.o.); treatment of the underlying disease

### Neurological Paraneoplastic Syndromes

### Paraneoplastic Polyneuropathy

**Def:**    Sensorimotor disorders occurring in the course of malignant disease, most commonly in lung cancer, but also occurring in other types of cancer

**Pg:**    Suspected autoimmune mechanism (autoantibodies detected in some cases)

**Sy:**    Pain, hypoesthesia, motor disturbances up to paresis

**Th:**    Treatment of the underlying disease; in certain cases: steroids (dexamethasone); neurotrophic vitamins usually ineffective

### Paraneoplastic Lambert-Eaton Syndrome

**Def:**    Presynaptic disorder of neuromuscular transmission associated with malignant tumors. Mainly lung cancer (3% of lung cancer patients)

**Pg:**    Cross-reacting antibodies causing functional impairment of specific voltage-operated calcium channels → release of acetylcholine ↓

**Sy:**
- Weakness of the pelvic and shoulder muscles, often difficulties in walking
- Dryness of the mouth, occasionally: paresthesia
- Impotence, in some cases: sphincter dysfunction → urination disturbances

**Dg:**
- Electrophysiological tests (differentiation from myasthenia gravis: pathologically low compound muscle action potentials)
- Tensilon test

**Th:**    Treatment of the underlying disease; where applicable calcium channel blockers (guanidine hydrochloride or 3-4-diaminopyridine or 4-aminopyridine, 4 × 40 up to 4 × 80 mg daily); also: pyridostigmine

### Paraneoplastic Myasthenia Gravis

**Def:** Impaired neuromuscular transmission associated with malignant diseases. 4–10 cases/100,000 population/year. Approximately 30% of patients with malignant thymoma (▶ Chap. 8.2.3)

**Pg:** Blockade of acetylcholine receptors by polyclonal antibodies

**Sy:**
- Skeletal muscle weakness, rapid exhaustion (in some cases, recovery after taking a break)
- Normal sensation

**Dg:**
- Electrophysiological examination
- Tensilon test
- Detection of antibodies to acetylcholine receptors

**Th:**
- Treatment of the underlying disease (thymectomy, ▶ Chap. 8.2.3)
- Cholinesterase inhibitors
- Corticosteroids (gradually increasing dose)
- In severe cases: plasma exchange to eliminate antibodies

### Cutaneous Paraneoplastic Syndromes

### Paraneoplastic Dermatomyositis

**Def:** Inflammation of muscle tissue and erythema associated with malignant diseases. Underlying malignancy in 20–25% of cases of newly diagnosed dermatomyositis (mainly lung cancer, breast cancer)

**Pg:** Unclear, possibly autoimmune mechanism

**Sy:**
- Muscle weakness, muscular atrophy particularly of the proximal extremities
- Dysphagia (if pharyngeal muscle affected)
- Heliotrope erythema around the eyelids, cheeks, front of the neck ("lilac disease")

**Dg:** Muscle biopsy: definite diagnosis (immunohistology)

**Th:** Treatment of the underlying disease; corticosteroids, in severe cases: immunosuppressives (azathioprine, methotrexate); where applicable, high-dose immunoglobulin therapy

### Acanthosis Nigricans

**Def:** Hyperpigmentation and hyperkeratosis in connection with malignant diseases. Underlying malignancy in 90% of cases; mainly abdominal adenocarcinomas

**Pg:** Unclear, possibly cytokine-mediated effect (insulin-like growth factor IGF, transforming growth factor α TGFα or homologous factors)

**Sy:**
- Erythema of the skin in the area of the hips, bottom, perineum, armpit, back of the neck
- Hyperkeratosis of the affected areas, roughening of the skin (tree bark-like scales, lichenification) with yellow-brown to gray-black discoloration

**Dg:** Skin biopsy: definite diagnosis

**Th:** Treatment of the underlying disease; local treatment usually ineffective

## Paraneoplastic acrokeratosis ("Bazex's Syndrome")

**Def:** Psoriasiform lesions of the fingers and toes associated with malignant diseases. Rare. Practically only affecting men with squamous cell carcinomas of the head and neck

**Sy:** Erythema and hyperkeratosis of the hands, nails, knees, elbows; other nail abnormalities

**Dg:** Morphology, biopsy: hyperkeratosis, acanthosis, perivascular lymphocytic infiltrates

**Th:** Treatment of the underlying disease; retinol derivatives (retinoids, e.g., acitretin); disease course can vary → complete regression is not guaranteed even if underlying disease has been treated successfully

## Erythema Gyratum Repens

**Def:** Migratory erythema affecting the trunk and extremities, wood grain appearance with concentric rings. Underlying malignancy in almost all cases, mainly lung cancer, but also breast cancer and esophageal cancer

**Pg:** Probably immune mechanisms (complement factors have been detected in the basal membrane of the skin)

**Sy:** Skin symptoms, severe pruritus

**Th:** Treatment of the underlying disease; local treatment usually ineffective

## Hypertrichosis Lanuginosa et Terminalis Acquisita

**Def:** Growth of lanugo-like hair in patients with malignant diseases. Rare, male:female = 1:3; occurring mainly in connection with advanced metastasized carcinomas (lung cancer)

**Pg:** Unclear; so far, no detection of hormonally active factors

**Sy:** Lanugo and in some cases terminal hair appearing around the face, back, ears, and legs

**Th:** Symptomatic (epilation), treatment of the underlying disease

**Ref:**
1.  Abu-Shakra M, Buskila D, Ehrenfeld M et al. Cancer and autoimmunity: autoimmune and rheumatic features in patients with malignancies. Ann Rheum Dis 2001;60:433–41
2.  Bollanti L, Riondino G, Strollo F. Endocrine paraneoplastic syndromes with special reference to the elderly. Endocrine 2001;14:151–7
3.  Darnell RB, Posner JB. Paraneoplastic syndromes involving the nervous system. N Engl J Med 2003;349:1543–54
4.  De Beukelaar JW, Smitt PAS. Managing paraneoplastic neurological disorders. Oncologist 2006;11:292–305
5.  Stone SP, Buescher LS. Life-threatening paraneoplastic neurological disorders. Oncologist 2006;23:301–6

**Web:**
1.  http://www.emedicine.com/MED/topic1747                                    E-medicine
2.  http://www.emedicine.com/derm/topic552                                    E-medicine
3.  http://www.neuro.wustl.edu/neuromuscular/nother/paraneo.htm               Washington University
4.  www.cancernetwork.com/handbook/emergencies.htm                           Cancer Network
5.  http://www.lungcanceronline.org/syndromes.htm                            Lung Cancer Online
6.  http://www.merck.com/pubs/mmanual/section14/chapter177/177e.htm          Merck Manual

## 9.1          Neutropenic Sepsis

### H. Bertz

**Def:**  Systemic reaction to an infection during neutropenia (particularly after chemotherapy or radio-therapy).
- *Severe sepsis:* temperature > 38.0°C or < 36°C, heart rate > 90/min, respiratory rate > 20/min or $PaCO_2$ < 32 mmHg
- *Septic shock:* hypotension with blood pressure (BP) < 90 mmHg (systolic) or BP decrease by 40 mmHg and signs of organ failure: lactate acidosis, oliguria, multiorgan failure (MOF)

**ICD-10:**  A41

**Ep:**  Fever during neutropenia (FN; ▶ Chap. 4.2) is a common side effect after myelosuppressive che-motherapy or radiotherapy; the incidence correlates directly with length and severity of the neu-tropenia. Up to 15% of patients with febrile neutropenia develop severe sepsis or septic shock.

**Path:**  *Risk factors → neutropenia → febrile neutropenia → sepsis*

### Risk of Sepsis in Case of Granulocytopenia
- *Low risk:* granulocytes $0.5–1 \times 10^9$/l for 2–7 days → in case of sepsis, mortality 14%
- *High risk:* granulocytes $< 0.1 \times 10^9$/l for > 7–10 days → in case of sepsis, mortality 47%

Both proinflammatory (TNFα, IL-6, IL-8) and antiinflammatory (IL-1 RA, IL-10) cytokines play an important role.

**Sy:**
- Fever, general symptoms, weakness, reduced performance
- Local signs of inflammation: catheter infection, skin infections, mucositis, gingivitis, acral fo-cal infections, abscesses
- Sinusitis, signs of pulmonary infection
- Gastrointestinal symptoms, pain, diarrhea
- Meningitis, headache, amentia
- Sepsis: decrease in blood pressure, tachycardia, hypothermia

**Dg:**  ### Medical History, Physical Examination
- Medical history (fever, diarrhea, dysuria, etc.)
- Physical examination: intravenous access sites, catheter ports, skin, oral mucous membranes, perianal region, pulmonary auscultation and percussion, abdominal pressure pain, pain on tapping / pressure pain of the paranasal air sinuses, lymphadenopathy, monitoring of blood pressure and pulse, meningism

### Laboratory Tests
- Routine laboratory tests, parameters of inflammation, plasmic coagulation, antithrombin III (ATIII), plasminogen activator inhibitor (PAI 1), liver and renal function tests

### Microbiology
- Peripheral blood cultures and cultures from intravenous access and catheters (▶ Chap. 10.8). Aerobic and anaerobic blood culture, isolator tube bottle. Where applicable, remove catheter, microbiological analysis of the catheter tip.
- Urine culture, sputum culture, swabs from suspicious lesions, lumbar / pleural / ascites punc-ture and culture
- *With pulmonary infiltrates:* bronchoalveolar lavage (BAL)
- *With diarrhea:* stool culture, detection of enterotoxins from *Clostridium difficile*, Gruber-Widal reaction

### Imaging
- Chest x-ray, possibly x-ray of paranasal air sinuses
- Abdominal ultrasound if indicated
- High-resolution CT scan if indicated

**Th:**

### Emergency Treatment
With fever during neutropenia, rapid initiation of treatment is essential:
1. Microbiological analysis
2. Immediate initiation of empirical antibiotic treatment: broad-spectrum antibiotic with effectiveness against pseudomonas spp., where applicable in combination with an aminoglycoside and a glycopeptide (particularly in case of catheter sepsis). Rapid escalation with antimycotics has proven benefit (amphotericin B, lipid formulation amphotericin B, azoles, echinocandins) (▶ Chap. 4.2)
3. Optimization of tissue oxygenation. Administration of oxygen via nasal tube or mask, 2 l/min up to 12 l/min. Where applicable, respiration support (non-invasive: CPAP; invasive: intubation)
4. Volume substitution; where applicable, administration of catecholamines
5. Initiate intensive medical care at an early stage

### Further Measures
- Further diagnosis (imaging, ultrasound, bronchoalveolar lavage (BAL), abscess aspiration / biopsy, etc.)
- In case of impaired renal function, initiate dialysis
- If persistence of neutropenia is expected, administer G-CSF to support bone marrow reconstitution. (▶ Chap. 4.3). Activated protein C demonstrated a positive effect on the overall survival of septic patients, but with marked side effects. Consider granulocyte transfusion (▶ Chap. 5.4).

**Px:**
- Basic hospital hygiene; conduct of invasive procedures under aseptic conditions
- Patient hygiene, especially skin care, dental care, mucositis prophylaxis; avoid foods with high germ counts
- If neutropenia persists for more than 7 days: regular monitoring, even if apyrexial → blood cultures, fecal cultures, throat swabs, sputum. Consequent treatment of fever in neutropenia (▶ Chap. 4.2)
- Administration of hematopoietic growth factors (G-CSF) according to current guidelines (ASCO / ESMO guideline; (▶ Chap. 4.3)

**Ref:**

1. Aapro MS, Cameron DA, Pettengell R et al. EORTC guidelines for the use of granulocyte-colony stimulating factor to reduce the incidence of chemotherapy-induced febrile neutropenia in adult patients with lymphomas and solid tumours. Eur J Cancer 2006;42:2433–53
2. Bertz H, Auner HW, Weissinger F et al. Antimicrobial therapy of febrile complications after high-dose chemo-/radiotherapy and autologous hematopoietic stem cell transplantation: guidelines of the AGIHO/ DGHO. Ann Hematol 2003;82(suppl 2):S167–74
3. Crawford J, Dale DC, Lyman GH. Chemotherapy-induced neutropenia: risks, consequences and new directions for its management. Cancer 2004;100:228–37
4. ESMO Guidelines Working Group. Hematopoietic growth factors: ESMO Recommendations for the application. Ann Oncol 2007;18(Suppl.2):ii89–91
5. Penack O, Beinert T, Buchheidt D et al. Management of sepsis in neutropenia: guidelines of the AGIHO/ DGHO. Ann Hematol 2006;85:424–33
6. Sipsas NV, Bodey GP, Kostoyiannis DP. Perspectives for the management of febrile neutropenic patients. Cancer 2005;103:1103–13
7. Smith TJ, Khatcheressian J, Lyman GJ et al. 2006 update of recommendations for the use of white blood cell growth factors: An evidence-based clinical practice guideline. J Clin Oncol 2006;24:3187–205

**Web:**

1. http://www.nccn.org/professionals/physician_gls/pdf/fever.pdf        NCCN

**9.2    Superior Vena Cava Syndrome (SVCS)**

H. Henß

**Def:**    Obstruction of the superior vena cava due to tumor compression, tumor-induced thrombosis, or other causes. Characteristic clinical picture of congestion of the superior vena cava. Underlying malignancy in 75–80% of cases.

**Ep:**    In approximately 5% of lung cancer patients (particularly small cell lung cancer, SCLC, ▶ Chap. 8.2.1) and approximately 2% of patients with aggressive non-Hodgkin's lymphoma (NHL, ▶ Chap. 7.5). Patients with indolent non-Hodgkin's lymphoma or Hodgkin's disease rarely develop SVCS.

**Pg:**    Obstruction of the superior vena cava by compression:
→ Secondary thrombosis due to venous stasis
→ Distal venous distension
→ Formation of collaterals if disease develops slowly

**Sy:**    Usually, rapid onset (within 6 weeks):
- Venous congestion with facial swelling, edema of the arm, visible veins on the chest wall: 80% of cases
- Headache, central nervous symptoms: 60%
- Dyspnea, tachypnea, cyanosis, cough (occasionally): 60%
- Dysphagia: 5%
- Horner's syndrome (miosis, ptosis, enophthalmus): 3%

**Dg:**    *Medical History, Physical Examination*
- Medical history (tumors, other risk factors)
- Physical examination including venous congestion, neurological signs, lymphadenopathy, spleen

*Histology*
- Sputum cytology, effusion cytology (pleural effusion), immunocytology (▶ Chap. 2.5)
- Bone marrow analysis (exclusion of tumor invasion, lymphoma)
- Bronchoscopy with biopsy or brush cytology
- Lymph node biopsy (in cases of peripheral lymphadenopathy)
- CT-guided fine-needle biopsy
- Mini-thoracotomy (low complication rate)
- Mediastinoscopy. *ATTENTION: high complication rate: hemorrhage, edema, impaired wound healing, infection; only if other procedures do not provide definitive diagnosis*

*Imaging*
- Chest x-ray (mediastinal or hilar expanding lesion in 80% of cases, pleural effusion, pulmonary infiltrates)
- Thoracic CT / MRI (where applicable)

**Dd:**    Differential diagnosis of SVCS

| Diagnosis | Frequency (%) |
|---|---|
| *Malignant tumors* | 85 |
| Lung cancer (esp. small cell lung cancer) | 65 |
| Lymphomas (esp. high-grade NHL) | 10 |
| Metastases (esp. from breast cancer, seminomas, sarcomas) | 10 |

**Dd:**      **Differential diagnosis of SVCS** *(continued)*

| Diagnosis | Frequency (%) |
|---|---|
| *Benign lesions* | 12 |
| Teratomas, thymomas, goiter, sarcoidosis | |
| *Mediastinal fibrosis* | 1 |
| Inflammatory disease (histoplasmosis, actinomycosis, tuberculosis) | |
| After mediastinal radiotherapy, thyroiditis, retroperitoneal fibrosis | |
| *Thrombosis of the Superior Vena Cava* | 2 |
| Behçet's disease, myeloproliferative syndromes (P. vera) | |
| Foreign body mediated (pacemaker, central venous line) | |

**Th:**      Indications for immediate therapy (emergency situations): cerebral symptoms, cardiac dysfunction (impairment of diastolic filling, LVEF ↓), respiratory obstruction

### Emergency Treatment

| | |
|---|---|
| 1. | Bed rest, upper body in elevated position, aspiration prophylaxis |
| 2. | Oxygen (nasal tube or mask), 2–12 l/min |
| 3. | Steroids (efficacy uncertain), e.g., prednisolone 100 mg i.v. |
| 4. | Anticoagulation, heparin 10,000–15,000 IU/day |

### Further Measures
- Histology (see above). ATTENTION: histological analysis is essential for effective antineoplastic treatment
- Treatment of the underlying disease:
  - Radiotherapy: only indicated in exceptional cases as emergency radiotherapy; total dose 30–50 Gy; response at the earliest after 3–7 days; response rate: 75% (lymphomas) to 25% (lung cancer)
  - Chemotherapy: indicated in patients with lung cancer and lymphomas
  - Surgery is not indicated (except for histology)
- In selected cases: stent insertion into the superior vena cava (decompression) possible

**Prg:**     According to the prognosis of the underlying disease; SVCS alone is not an independent prognostic factor.

**Ref:**
1. Aurora R, Milite F, Vander Els NJ. Respiratory emergencies. Semin Oncol 2000;27:256–69
2. Kanani RS, Drachmann DE. Malignant obstruction of the superior vena cava. N Engl J Med 2006;354:e7
3. Rowell NP, Gleeson FV. Steroids, radiotherapy, chemotherapy and stents for superior vena caval obstruction in carcinoma of the bronchus. Cochrane Database Syst Rev 2001;CD001316
4. Wilson LD, Detterbeck FC, Yahalom J. Superior vena cava syndrome with malignant causes. N Engl J Med 2007;356:1862–9

**Web:**
1. http://www.emedicine.com/emerg/topic561.htm                      E-medicine
2. http://www.cancer.gov/cancertopics/pdq/supportivecare/
   cardiopulmonary/patient                                          NCI Cancer Topics
3. http://www.fpnotebook.com/CV303.htm                              Family Practice

**9.3**   **Spinal Cord Compression / Cauda Equina Syndrome**

H. Henß

**Def:**   Malignancy-induced spinal cord compression with resulting neurological deficits.

**Ep:**   Cerebral metastases in 15% of all solid tumors, signs of spinal cord compression eventually occur in 5% of all tumor patients.

**Pg:**   *Etiology*
Occurrence with various solid tumors and hematological neoplasia → most common: lung cancer, breast cancer, prostate cancer, melanoma, lymphoma, multiple myeloma.

*Mechanisms of Tumor-Induced Spinal Cord Damage*
Usually extracordal compression of spinal cord or cauda equina:
- Tumor invasion from the vertebral body into the epidural space → spinal cord compression (common with lung cancer, breast cancer)
- Tumor invasion through the intervertebral foramina → spinal cord compression or nerve root compression (lymphoma)
- Direct metastasis into the spinal canal (rare)
- Tumor-induced vascular damage → malperfusion, spinal cord damage due to infarction
- Paraneoplastic syndromes (► Chap. 8.13)

**Path:**   Location of spinal cord compression:
- Cervical: 10%
- Thoracic: 70%
- Lumbosacral: 20%
- Multifocal: 25%

**Sy:**   Often protracted process over a longer period of time, however, neurological deficits may develop within a few hours (especially with rapidly proliferating neoplasia such as lung cancer, renal cell carcinoma, melanoma, or lymphoma).
- *Most common symptom:* pain (> 90% of patients) as "back ache," "lumbar syndrome," etc.
- *Radicular deficits:* dermatoma-specific sensory and motor deficits; band-like pain; in some cases unilateral
- *Segmental myelopathy:* motor deficits / paresis, segmental sensory deficits
- *Generalized myelopathy:* bilateral motor disorders / pareses, sensory deficits; compression around cauda equina: "saddle anesthesia," bladder / colon paralysis, anal sphincter tone ↓, tendon reflexes ↑, positive Babinski's sign

**Dg:**   *Medical History, Physical Examination*
- Medical history (tumors, risk factors)
- Physical examination including neurological status

*Imaging*
- Plain x-ray, spinal MRI
- CT or bone scan if diagnosis uncertain

*Histology*
- Lumbar puncture (spinal tap) if suspected meningeal involvement
- Needle biopsy (if surgery is contraindicated)

**Dd:**
- Benign tumors: meningioma
- Epidural expanding lesions: hematoma, abscess
- Slipped disk, spondylolisthesis, osteoporotic fracture of a vertebral body
- Guillain-Barré syndrome, plexus lesion (congenital / acquired)
- Infection (e.g., tuberculosis)

**Th:**    ***Emergency Treatment***

1.    Steroids, e.g., dexamethasone initially 10 mg i.v., then 4–8 mg every 6 h
2.    Neurosurgical options must be considered at an early stage. Surgery within 6 to maximum 24 h. If symptoms have persisted longer than 24 h, risk of irreversible damage

### Further Measures
- Histology
- Treatment of the underlying disease, taking into consideration the dynamics of progression and severity of neurological deficits:
    - Neurosurgery: laminectomy or resection of vertebral bodies
    - Radiotherapy: primary irradiation or adjuvant radiotherapy after surgical decompression, especially with radiosensitive tumors (breast cancer, lymphomas, plasmacytoma); target dose: 30–40 Gy over 2–4 weeks
    - Combined radiochemotherapy
    - Chemotherapy alone only with minor deficits, slow progression, or chemosensitive tumor

### Treatment Objectives
- Improvement or normalization of neurological deficits
- Mobility and stability preservation of the vertebral column / spine
- Analgesia

**Prg:**    ***Prognostic Factors***
- Time between diagnosis and initiation of therapy
- Extent of neurological deficits before start of treatment
- Nature of the primary tumor

**Ref:**    1.    Bagley CA, Gokaslan ZL. Cauda equina syndrome caused by primary and metastatic neoplasms. Neurosurg Focus 2004;16:e3
2.    Byrne T. Spinal cord compression from epidural metastases. N Engl J Med 1992;327:614–7
3.    Loblaw DA, Laperriere NJ. Emergency treatment of malignant extradural spinal cord compression: an evidence based guideline. J Clin Oncol 1998;16:1613–24
4.    Maranzano E, Bellavita R, Rossi R et al. Short-course versus split-course radiotherapy in metastatic spinal cord compression: results of a phase III, randomized, multicenter trial. J Clin Oncol 2005;23:3358–65
5.    Quinn JA, DeAngelis LM. Neurologic emergencies in the cancer patient. Semin Oncol 2000;27:311–21

**Web:**    1.    http://www.caudaequina.org/                Cauda Equina Portal
2.    http://www.emedicine.com/EMERG/topic85.htm        E-medicine
3.    http://www.merck.com/mmhe/sec06/ch093/ch093c.htm    Merck Manual

| | |
|---|---|
| **9.4** | **Malignant Cardiac Tamponade** |

H. Henß

**Def:** Severe hemodynamically significant pericardial effusion caused by tumor invasion of the pericardium or myocardium. Medical emergency.

**Ep:** Invasion of pericardium or myocardium in up to 15% of patients with solid tumors.

**Pg:** Direct invasion or lymphatic / hematogenous metastasis to the pericardium or myocardium in patients with solid tumors and hematological neoplasia.

**Pp:** *Cardiac Tamponade*
Metastasis to the pericardium / myocardium
→ Pericardial effusion, arrhythmia
→ Cardiac tamponade (critical effusion volume in cases of rapid onset: 300–400 ml)
→ Diastolic dysfunction (ventricular load)
→ Cardiac insufficiency, cardiogenic shock

**Sy:** Over 65% of pericardial and myocardial metastases are clinically asymptomatic. Symptoms develop with increasing severity and due to hemodynamic consequences of malignant pericardial effusion:
- Dyspnea, cough, weakness, reduced performance
- Retrosternal pain
- Arrhythmia, tachycardia
- Signs of cardiac insufficiency (jugular venous distension, hepatosplenomegaly, cyanosis)
- Syncope

**Dg:** *Medical History, Physical Examination*
Physical examination: rise in jugular venous pressure (increased on inspiration = Kussmaul's sign), pulsus paradoxus (end-inspiratory decrease in blood pressure by > 10 mmHg), muffled heart sounds, pulmonary rales, hepatosplenomegaly, ascites, edema

*Imaging*
- Chest x-ray: enlarged heart silhouette
- ECG changes are usually unspecific, sometimes electrical alternans and/or precordial low voltage; with concurrent pericarditis: sinus tachycardia, raised ST, changes in T-wave
- Echocardiography (most important diagnostic tool)
- In selected cases: right heart catheterization, angiocardiography

*Cytology*
Diagnostic pericardiocentesis with effusion analysis:
- Total protein, LDH, glucose, triglycerides, cholesterol
- Cell count, cytology, immunocytology
- Microbiological diagnosis: cultures (including tuberculosis), Gram stain, Ziehl-Neelsen stain

**Dd:** *In cases of underlying malignancy:*
- Superior vena cava syndrome (SVCS, ► Chap. 9.2)
- Radiogenic pericarditis (as a result of radiotherapy)

**Th:** Treatment of cardiac tamponade / malignant pericardial effusion depends on symptoms, patient's performance status, and prognosis:
- Asymptomatic effusion without hemodynamic significance: treatment not indicated
- Terminal disease: individual assessment in each case

Emergency pericardiocentesis may be indicated in case of:
- Dyspnea, cyanosis, shock, altered level of consciousness
- Blood pressure decrease by > 20 mmHg
- Increase of peripheral venous pressure to > 13 mmHg

### Emergency Treatment

1. Bed rest with upper body in an elevated position

2. Where required, analgesia (paracetamol, diclofenac), mild sedation

3. Oxygen (nasal tube or mask), 2–12 l/min

4. Anticoagulation, heparin 10,000–15,000 IU/day

   *ATTENTION: discontinue before pericardiocentesis or other invasive measures*

5. Emergency pericardiocentesis

   *ATTENTION: pericardiocentesis should only be performed by an experienced cardiologist and/or in an intensive care unit, ultrasound- or echocardiography-guided. Needle is pushed (while aspirating) from below the xiphoid process in the direction of the pericardial effusion*

### Further Measures
- *Aspiration* of hemodynamically significant effusions: pericardiocentesis and pericardial drainage; if necessary, subxiphoid emergency pericardiocentesis or emergency pericardiotomy.
- *Local treatment* of confirmed malignant pericardial effusion: instillation of cytostatics (e.g., methotrexate 25 mg, cisplatin 20–200 mg, or bleomycin 30–60 mg). Pericardial fenestration, e.g., by inferior pericardiotomy. Radiotherapy: total dose of 25–35 Gy in 3–4 weeks, response rates of up to 60%.
- *Systemic treatment* of the underlying disease: chemotherapy, particularly in previously untreated patients with chemosensitive malignancies (small cell lung cancer, lymphoma, leukemia).
- *Surgery:* pleuropericardial fenestration; pericardiectomy only in selected cases (e.g., chronic radiogenic pericarditis)

**Prg:**  Prognosis is determined by the underlying disease. Median survival: 6–24 months.

**Ref:**
1. Keefe DL. Cardiovascular emergencies in the cancer patient. Semin Oncol 2000;27:244–55
2. Little WC, Freeman GL. Pericardial disease. Circulation 2006;113:1622–32
3. Martinoni A, Cipolla CM, Civelli M et al. Intrapericardial treatment of neoplastic pericardial effusions. Herz 2000;25:787–93
4. Retter AS. Pericardial disease in the oncology patient. Heart Dis 2002;4:387–91
5. Soler-Soler J, Sagrista-Sauleda J, Permanyer-Miralda G. Management of pericardial effusion. Heart 2001;86:235–40
6. Spodick DH. Acute cardiac tamponade. N Engl J Med 2003;349:684–90

**Web:**
1. http://www.emedicine.com/med/topic1786.htm          E-medicine
2. http://www.emedicine.com/emerg/topic412.htm          E-medicine
3. http://www.nkm.nih.gov/medlineplus/ency/articl/000194.htm          MedlinePlus

## 9.5 Malignant Hypercalcemia

**H. Henß**

**Def:** Tumor-induced increase in serum calcium, usually paraneoplastic, with osteoclast activation.
Types:
- *Humoral hypercalcemia of malignancy* (HHM): hypercalcemia without detectable osteolysis, e.g., multiple myeloma, pancreatic cancer, lung cancer
- Hypercalcemia in case of advanced osteolytic metastasis (tumor-induced osteolysis, TIO): detectable osteolysis, e.g., breast cancer

**Ep:** Incidence: 10–20% of all cancer patients; severe hypercalcemia requiring treatment in 1–3% of cases.

**Pg:** *Tumor entities commonly associated with hypercalcemia:* breast cancer, lung cancer, renal cell cancer, multiple myeloma

**Pp:** Secretion of osteoclast-activating factors by malignant cells
- Parathyroid hormone-related protein (PTH-RP): detectable in 75–90% of patients with tumor-associated hypercalcemia (both humoral hypercalcemia and bone metastasis)
- Interleukin-1
- Interleukin-6 (particularly multiple myeloma)
- Transforming growth factor alpha (TGF-α)

### Consequences
- Osteoclast activation and proliferation → increased bone destruction, calcium release
- Inhibition of osteoblast activity → reduced bone regeneration
- Glomerular filtration rate ↓ , tubular calcium reabsorption ↑

**Sy:** The majority of patients with moderate hypercalcemia are asymptomatic.
Symptoms of advanced hypercalcemia (> 2.7 mmol/l) or hypercalcemic crisis (> 3.5 mmol/l):
- *Kidney:* polyuria, polydipsia, dehydration → later anuria, acute renal damage, nephrocalcinosis, nephrolithiasis
- *Gastrointestinal tract:* nausea, vomiting, weight loss, anorexia, gastroduodenal ulcers / pancreatitis (rare)
- *Muscle:* muscle weakness, constipation, ileus
- *Cardiac:* bradycardia, atrial and ventricular arrhythmias
- *CNS:* fatigue, lethargy, impaired vision, psychosis, somnolence, coma

**Dg:**
- Routine laboratory tests including $Ca^{2+}$, phosphate, $K^+$, $Na^+$, $Cl^-$, urea and electrolytes, serum creatinine, bilirubin, alkaline phosphatase, albumin
- Determination of serum PTH and, where applicable, PTH-RP
- ECG: QT interval ↓, PQ interval ↓, T-wave (widened), bradycardia, arrhythmia
- Imaging: exclusion of osteolysis (skull, vertebral column, pelvis, humerus, femur); with plasmacytomas: plain x-ray (skull, axial skeleton, pelvis, thorax, humerus, femur)

**Co:** Nephrolithiasis, gastric / duodenal ulcers, pancreatitis (rare)

**Dd:** **Differential diagnosis of hypercalcemia**

| Diagnosis | Frequency (%) |
| --- | --- |
| • Tumor-associated hypercalcemia | 60 |
| • Primary hyperparathyroidism | 20 |
| • Hyperthyroidism | Rare |
| • Adrenal failure | Rare |

**Dd:**        **Differential diagnosis of hypercalcemia** *(continued)*

| Diagnosis | Frequency (%) |
|---|---|
| • Drug-induced: vitamin D, vitamin A, tamoxifen, thiazide diuretics, lithium, theophyllines | 10 |
| • Sarcoidosis, tuberculosis | < 5 |
| • Immobilization | < 5 |

**Th:**        *Emergency Treatment*

1.    Hydration: NaCl 0.9%, minimum 2,000–3,000 ml/day; monitor urea, electrolytes, serum creatinine, and bilirubin; if necessary: $K^+$ / $Mg^{2+}$ replacement → improved renal function / calcium elimination ↑

2.    Furosemide (if diuresis is inadequate) → improved renal function, calcium elimination ↑

3.    Bisphosphonates, e.g., zoledronate i.v. (infusion, 1 mg/min) → inhibition of osteoclast activity

       *SE:* fever and/or flu-like symptoms, hypocalcemia

4.    Corticosteroids, e.g., prednisolone 1 mg/kg i.v., usually 40–100 mg, particularly with hematological diseases (multiple myeloma) → cytokine release (IL-1, IL-6) ↓, intestinal calcium absorption ↓

5.    If insufficient calcium level decrease: calcitonin 4–6 × 100 IU/day s.c. → osteoclast inhibition, calciuric effect

6.    Dialysis in case of chronic renal failure: → calcium elimination by calcium-free dialysate

*Further Measures*
• Histology (if malignancy uncertain)
• Treatment of the underlying disease

**Prg:**        Survival without treatment: < 4 weeks. After correction of electrolyte imbalance and successful antineoplastic treatment, hypercalcemia per se does not constitute an independent prognostic factor.

**Ref:**
1.    Bajorunas DR. Clinical manifestations of cancer-related hypercalcemia. Semin Oncol 1990;17:16–20
2.    Flombaum CD. Metabolic emergencies in the cancer patient. Semin Oncol 2000;27:322–34
3.    Perry CM, Figgitt DP. Zoledronic acid. Drugs 2004;64:1197–211
4.    Stewart AF. Hypercalcemia associated with cancer. N Engl J Med 2005;352:373–9

**Web:**
1.    http://www.cancer.gov/cancertopics/pdq/supportivecare/
       hypercalcemia/patient            NCI Cancer Topics
2.    http://www.emedicine.com/emerg/topic 260.htm        E-medicine

## 9.6 Tumor Lysis Syndrome

H. Henß

**Def:** Syndrome arising due to rapid destruction / decomposition of large amounts of tumor tissue with release of intracellular components, including $K^+$, phosphate, and uric acid.

**Ep:** Incidence 10% after effective treatment of acute leukemia, high-grade non-Hodgkin's lymphoma (particularly Burkitt's lymphoma), and myeloproliferative syndromes. Efficient prophylaxis (see below) can reduce the risk of tumor lysis syndrome to < 1%.

**Pg:** Effective antineoplastic treatment in patients with large tumor burden and/or rapidly proliferating malignancy:
- Leukemia, particularly acute lymphoblastic leukemia (ALL)
- High-grade non-Hodgkin's lymphomas (particularly Burkitt's lymphoma)
- Myeloproliferative syndromes (particularly chronic myeloid leukemia)
- Solid tumors (rare cases, e.g., germ cell tumors, small cell lung cancer)

### Risk Factors
- Renal failure, renal damage, dehydration
- Large retroperitoneal or mediastinal tumors, LDH ↑

**Pphys:**
- Hyperuricemia → acute urate nephropathy
- Hyperkalemia → cardiac disorders
- Hyperphosphatemia → hyperphosphaturia
- Formation / precipitation of calcium phosphate in glomeruli and tubules → additional renal damage, hypocalcemia

**Sy:** Acute disease usually occurring 12–24 h after start of chemotherapy.
- General symptoms: nausea, vomiting, malaise
- Hyperkalemia: arrhythmia, cardiac arrest, paresthesia, pareses
- Hyperphosphatemia: renal damage due to calcium phosphate precipitation
- Hyperuricemia: urate nephropathy, renal failure, lethargy, nausea / vomiting
- Hypocalcemia: muscle cramps, tetany, paresthesia, cardiac arrhythmia, diarrhea

**Dg:** ### Medical History, Physical Examination
- Medical history including chemotherapy, malignant diseases
- Physical examination including cardiovascular function, renal function, neurological status

### Laboratory Tests
- Blood count, liver and renal function parameters, including $K^+$, $Ca^{2+}$, phosphate, urea, serum creatinine, bilirubin, uric acid, LDH

### ECG
- Signs of hyperkalemia (prolonged PQ interval, P amplitude ↓, QRS complex widened, shortened QT, tall peaked symmetrical T-wave, ultimately "sinus wave") and signs of hypocalcemia (arrhythmia, impaired conduction, QT interval ↑)

**Dd:**
- *Acute tissue destruction:* rhabdomyolysis, burns, trauma, hemolytic crisis
- *Hyperuricemia:* metabolic syndrome
- *Electrolyte imbalance:* renal failure, hypoparathyroidism, pancreatitis, sepsis, acidosis, paraneoplastic syndromes, potassium-sparing diuretics

**Th:**     *Emergency Treatment*

1. Regular ECG monitoring; cardiac function monitoring if necessary
2. Hydration: NaCl 0.9%, minimum 2,000–3,000 ml/day
3. Hyperkalemia (> 5 mg/dl):
   - Cation exchange resin p.o. or enema every 6 h
   - Glucose plus insulin (1 U per 2 g of glucose). *ATTENTION: rebound effect when discontinued, as $K^+$ is not fully eliminated but bound intracellularly*
   - If necessary, dialysis to eliminate calcium
4. Hypocalcemia (< 2 mmol/l or < 8 mg/dl):
   - Calcium gluconate 10% i.v. 10–40 mg, repeat every 12 h if necessary
   - In mild cases: calcium 500–1,000 mg p.o.
5. Hyperuricemia:
   - Rasburicase (recombinant urate oxidase) 0.2 mg/kg/day, for 5–7 days. *ATTENTION: for measurement of uric acid during treatment with rasburicase use cooled serum; otherwise inaccurate (low) readings.*
6. Renal dysfunction / acute oliguria:
   - Dopamine 100–200 mg/24 h (infusion pump); benefit not fully established.
   - Dialysis (after exclusion of urinary tract obstruction)

### Further Measures
Close monitoring: ECG, central venous pressure (CVP, target: > 5), routine laboratory tests (urea + electrolytes, serum creatinine, bilirubin, uric acid)

**Px:**     *Most important: detection of risk factors and appropriate prophylaxis prior to initiation of treatment in high-risk patients:*
- Identification of high-risk patients (acute leukemias, Burkitt's lymphoma, high-grade non-Hodgkin's lymphomas, high tumor burden)
- Sufficient rehydration (target: > 2.5 l urine daily) while monitoring CVP
- Alkalization (target: urinary pH > 7) with $NaHCO_3$ p.o. or citrate p.o., intravenous bicarbonate (if required)
- Xanthine oxidase inhibitors (allopurinol 300 mg/day) → if not tolerated: benzbromarone (uricosuric agent)

**ATTENTION:** allopurinol inhibits the metabolization of 6-mercaptopurine, azathioprine, theophylline, and phenprocoumon → if given with allopurinol, the dose of 6-mercaptopurine must be lowered to 25%.

**Ref:**    1. Cairo MS, Bishop M. Tumor lysis syndrome: new therapeutic strategies and classification. Br J Hematol 2004;127:3–11
          2. Del Toro G, Morris E, Cairo MS. Tumor lysis syndrome: pathophysiology, definition and alternative treatment approaches. Clin Adv Hematol Oncol 2005;3:54–61
          3. Nicolin G. Emergencies and their management. Eur J Cancer 2002;38:1365–77

**Web:**    1. http://www.emedicine.com/MED/topic2327.htm          E-medicine
          2. http:www.answers.com/topic/tumor-lysis-syndrome          Infoportal

## 9.7 Hemorrhagic Complications / Malignant Vascular Erosion

### H. Henß

**Def:** Hemorrhagic complications associated with malignant diseases.

**Ep:** Of patients with solid tumors, 10% die due to hemorrhagic complications caused by vascular invasion / erosion or ischemic tumor lysis.

**Pg:** Often combination of several pathogenetic factors:
- Thrombocytopenia, thrombopathy
- Disseminated intravascular coagulopathy, hyperfibrinolysis, coagulation inhibitors
- Decrease in plasmatic coagulation factors / hepatic dysfunction
- Treatment-induced hemorrhage (hemorrhagic cystitis, mucositis, asparaginase therapy)
- Surgery-induced hemorrhage (biopsy, centesis, etc.)
- Tumor-induced hemorrhage: bleeding from tumor (gastrointestinal tumors, lung cancer) or malignant vascular erosion (head and neck tumors)

**Sy:**
- Hemorrhage (acute bleeding), e.g., hematemesis, hemoptysis, melena, hematuria
- Anemia (chronic bleeding)
- Signs of shock (tachycardia, hypotension)

**Th:** Treatment is determined by the severity of the hemorrhage.

#### Emergency Treatment

1. Bed rest
2. Rehydration
3. Oxygen (nasal tube or mask), 3–12 l/min
4. Blood typing, ordering of blood products

#### Further Measures
- Where applicable, red blood cell (RBC) transfusion; thrombocytopenic patients: platelet transfusion (▶ Chap. 6.3)
- Specification of the hemorrhage: local / punctate / diffuse / generalized
- Specific hemostatic measures: endoscopic obliteration; where applicable: surgical intervention (vascular ligation, tumor extirpation), transarterial embolization (angiography and subsequent embolization)

### Specific Types of Hemorrhage

### Hemorrhagic Cystitis

**Def:** Acute or subacute hemorrhagic inflammation of the mucous membrane of the urinary bladder, usually treatment-induced (cyclophosphamide, ifosfamide, radiotherapy)

**Sy:** Hematuria, pollakiuria, pain

**Th:** *Mild Hemorrhage*
Bladder irrigation; often spontaneous cessation.

*Severe Bleeding*
- Irrigation with large urinary catheter
- Removal of blood clots (if required, cystoscopically)
- Intravesicular treatment, e.g., 1% alum or prostaglandin E2 and F2
- With circumscribed hemorrhage: possibly cystoscopic obliteration of the source of bleeding

**Px:**          *Prophylactic treatment with mesna after cyclophosphamide / ifosfamide therapy. Severe hemorrhage may require surgery.*

### Severe Hemoptysis

**Def:**          Coughing up of large quantities of blood (bright red and foamy = arterial, dark = venous), usually vascular erosion by malignant tumor.

**Th:**          Emergency bronchoscopy, if possible: local coagulation, blockade / tamponade with balloon-tipped catheter

### Severe Hematemesis

**Def:**          Vomiting of large quantities of blood, due to a bleeding malignant tumor, hemorrhagic gastritis / mucositis, vascular erosion.

**Th:**          Endoscopy, local coagulation, if necessary: emergency surgery

### Melena (Tarry Stools) / Hematochezia (Perianal Hemorrhage)

**Def:**          Hemorrhage in the upper gastrointestinal tract (melena) or lower gastrointestinal tract (bright red blood in stools).

**Pg:**          • *Melena:* occurring in cases of hemorrhage > 100–200 ml from upper GI tract and slow passage (> 8 h) through the intestine. Bacterial fermentation of the blood in the intestine.
          • *Hematochezia:* usually colorectal hemorrhage; in rare cases: massive bleeding in the upper GI tract and rapid passage through the intestine.

**Sy:**          • Melena: black tarry stools
          • Hematochezia: symptoms depend on severity and location of the bleeding → rectal hemorrhage: blood covering the stools, bleeding from colon: bloody diarrhea or visible traces of blood in the stools

**Dg:**          • If necessary, fecal occult blood test to confirm presence of blood in stools
          • Investigation of the cause of hemorrhage: esophago-gastro-duodenoscopy, rectoscopy, colonoscopy, possibly radionuclide scintigraphy ($^{99m}$Tc-marked erythrocytes) or selective arteriography
          • Monitoring of blood quantity and cardiovascular parameters, renal function, coagulation

**Th:**          Specific hemostatic measures (endoscopic or surgical).

**Ref:**          1.   British Committee for Standards in Haematology. Guidelines on the management of massive blood loss. Br J Haematol 2006;135:634–41
          2.   Imbesi JJ, Kurtz RC. A multidisciplinary approach to gastrointestinal bleeding in cancer patients. J Support Oncol 2005;3:102–10
          3.   Mannucci PM, Levi M. Prevention and treatment of major blood loss. N Engl J Med 2007;356:2301–11
          4.   Pereira J, Phan T. Management of bleeding in patients with advanced cancer. Oncologist 2004;9:561–70
          5.   Reimann T, Butts CA. Upper gastrointestinal bleeding as a metastatic manifestation of breast cancer: a case report and review of the literature. Can J Gastroenterol 2001;15:67–71

**Web:**          1.   http://www.cancernetwork.com/textbook/morev42.htm#Cardiovascular%20Emergencies
          2.   http://www.ncbi.nlm.nih.gov/books/bv.fcgi?rid=cmed6.section.43920

## 9.8 Transfusion Reactions

### H. Bertz

**Def:** Complications occurring after transfusion of cellular blood products (packed red cells and platelet concentrates), fresh frozen plasma (FFP), coagulation factors, immunoglobulins, or human albumin. Transfusion reactions are classified according to pathogenesis, type of blood product, time of occurrence, and clinical picture.

### Acute Transfusion Reactions

**Ep:** Incidence: approximately 1–10% of all transfusions.

**Pg:** *Acute Hemolytic Transfusion Reaction (AHTR)*
- Most dangerous form of acute transfusion reactions, incidence 1:6,000 to 1:25,000 transfusions, 0.75 deaths per 100,000 transfusions
- Major ABO incompatibility → severe acute intravascular hemolysis with complement activation and cytokine release
- In rare cases, irregular preformed antierythrocytic allo- or autoantibodies in the recipient (Kell system, Kidd system, Duffy system, etc.)

*Febrile Non-hemolytic Transfusion Reaction (FNHTR)*
- Most common transfusion reaction, 5% of all transfusions
- Post-transfusion temperature increase by ≥ 1°C with no signs of hemolysis or other transfusion-induced reactions
- *Pathogenesis:* antibodies against platelets or leukocytes, active mediator release from viable leukocytes contained in the blood product (e.g., cytokines), bacterial contamination (very rare)

*Urticarial Reaction*
- Local or generalized allergic reaction to plasma proteins
- In case of *local urticarial reaction*: transfusion may be continued after antihistamine treatment (all other cases of transfusion reactions: stop the transfusion, return blood product to blood bank, see below)

*Anaphylactic Reaction to Plasma-containing Products (Platelet Concentrates, FFP)*
- Patients with congenital IgA deficiency (incidence 1:700) and presence of IgA antibodies. In the majority of cases, pathogenesis not clear.

*Transfusion-related Acute Lung Injury (TRALI)*
- Granulocyte- or monocyte-specific antibodies (HLA class I or II) in the donor plasma react with leukocyte antigens in the recipient (in rare cases, reverse antibody constellation) → agglutination and activation of granulocytes and monocytes, especially in the lungs
- Rare and potentially fulminant ARDS-like reaction occurring 1–6 h after transfusion; lethal in approximately 15%

*Non-immunological Side Effects (esp. with Massive Transfusions)*
- Citrate intoxication (platelet concentrates, FFP) and alkalosis
- Hypothermia, hypovolemia
- Hyperkalemia (neonates, anuric patients), hypocalcemia
- Embolism (rare), bacterial contamination (rare)

**Sy:** *Rapid onset after start of transfusion:*
- Shivers, fever, sweating, nausea, vomiting
- Skin reactions, urticaria, flush, pruritus (particularly with allergic transfusion reactions)

- Restlessness, drop in blood pressure, tachycardia, dyspnea, tachypnea
- Headache, back pain
- Hemolytic transfusion reactions: red-brown urine (hemoglobinuria), later: jaundice
- ATTENTION: in anesthetized patients, symptoms may be masked

**Dg:**    ### Medical History, Physical Examination
- Medical history including specifics of the transfusion, risk factors
- Physical examination including blood pressure, pulse, respiratory rate, cardiopulmonary auscultation; close monitoring

### Laboratory Tests
- Blood count, hemolysis parameters (haptoglobin, bilirubin, LDH, free plasma hemoglobin) → ideally compared to pretransfusion sample
- Urine sample (hemoglobinuria)
- Blood culture (exclusion of bacterial contamination)

### Notification of the Blood Bank (Side Effects of Medicinal Products)
- Retain blood bag (forensic reasons)
- Return blood bag and a recent blood sample of the patient to the blood bank
  - → Retesting of serological compatibility (before/after reaction), ABO compatibility between blood product and patient's blood, direct antiglobulin test, screening for irregular antibodies, bacteriological examination of the blood product

**Co:**
- AHTR: shock, disseminated intravascular coagulation (DIC), acute renal failure
- FNHTR, urticaria: usually self-limiting without serious complications
- TRALI: acute respiratory insufficiency, cardiopulmonary failure. Urgent indication for intensive medical care
- *Anaphylaxis:* shock

**Th:**    ### Emergency Treatment

| | |
|---|---|
| 1. | **Stop transfusion immediately** (most important measure) |
| 2. | Save the intravenous line or insert a new access |
| 3. | Diagnostic measures (see above), close monitoring (blood pressure, pulse, respiratory rate, urinary output, clinical examination) |
| 4. | Supportive treatment (depending on the severity / cause of the reaction): oxygen, blood pressure, stabilization, diuresis maintenance with fluids and/or osmodiuretics (mannitol); TRALI: early ventilation support may be required |
| 5. | Prednisolone 100 mg i.v., alternatively: dexamethasone 8 mg i.v. |
| 6. | Allergic reactions: antihistamines |

### Further Measures
- Volume substitution, alkalinization, monitoring of urinary output to prevent acute renal failure; with impending acute renal failure: hemodialysis; *ATTENTION:* hyperkalemia due to potassium release from erythrocytes
- Continued antiallergic treatment: steroids, antihistamines
- Close monitoring of coagulation parameters, exclusion of DIC (▶ Chap. 6.5.5)

**ATTENTION:** do not underestimate the dynamics of acute transfusion reactions. Patients may require intensive care from an early stage.

### Subacute Transfusion Reactions

**Pg:**
#### *Post-transfusion Purpura (Packed Red Cells or Platelet Concentrates)*
- Development of platelet-specific alloantibodies → severe thrombocytopenia approximately 5–9 days after transfusion involving the patient's own platelets ("innocent bystander"), usually occurring in women between 50 and 70 years of age
- *Treatment:* intravenous IgG (avoid platelet transfusion)

#### *Delayed Hemolytic Transfusion Reaction (DHTR)*
- Primary immunization or boosting of alloantibodies → delayed hemolysis, usually few clinical symptoms
- *Diagnosis:* immunohematological re-examination, hemolytic parameters

#### *Transfusion-associated Graft-versus-Host Reaction (tGvHR)*
Reaction of proliferating donor T-lymphocytes to the recipient; occurring with transfusion of immunosuppressed patients and transfusion of blood relatives ("one-way HLA match")
- Engraftment of transfused cells
- Later: transfusion-associated graft-versus-host disease (tGvHD)
- After latent period of 20–60 days, skin manifestations (dermatitis), intestinal symptoms (gastroenteritis), hepatitis; often not associated with transfusion due to latency period, mortality rate of up to 90%
- *Diagnosis:* detection of donor lymphocytes, DNA fingerprinting, skin biopsies
- *Prophylaxis:* irradiation of blood products (indications: ▶ Chap. 4.9.1)

### Hemosiderosis

**Pg:**
Iron deposition in the tissue due to iron overload by a factor of $\geq 5$ (normal iron level: men 3.5 g, women 2.2 g).
*Rule of thumb:* in chronically transfused patients risk of hemosiderosis after $\geq 100$ packed red cell transfusions (approximately 250 mg iron per transfusion).

**Sy:**
Symptoms depending on the affected organs:
- Hepatic dysfunction, diabetes mellitus, endocrine disturbances
- Dark pigmentation of the skin ("bronze diabetes")
- Cardiomyopathy, arrhythmia

**Dg:**
#### *Medical History, Physical Examination*
- Medical history
- Physical examination including skin pigmentation, cardiopulmonary status

#### *Laboratory Tests*
- Serum iron ↑, ferritin ↑, transferrin saturation ↑

#### *Histology*
- Detection of iron in the bone marrow (bone marrow biopsy / smear) or in the liver (ultrasound-guided liver biopsy)

**Dd:**
Primary iron storage disease: hemochromatosis

**Th:**
- Chelators, e.g., desferrioxamine: 2,000 U/day s.c. long-term therapy via pump or weekly bolus s.c.
- Oral therapy with deferasirox: 20–30 mg/kg body weight/day or deferiprone, 25 mg/kg body weight, × 3/day

### Infectious Complications

#### Human Immunodeficiency Virus (HIV)

Risk with cellular products: < 1: 1,000,000 → further minimized due to introduction of HIV genome testing of donors by nucleic acid amplification; significantly lower risk with cell-free products (FFP, immunoglobulins, and coagulation factor products) due to quarantine or virus inactivation.

#### Hepatitis B Virus (HBV)

Risk with cellular products: 1:50,000 to 1:200,000; significantly lower risk with cell-free products (due to quarantine or virus inactivation).

#### Hepatitis C Virus (HCV)

Risk with cellular products: < 1:500,000; risk minimization possible by statutory nucleic acid amplification testing (HCV-NAT) of cellular blood products; significantly lower risk with cell-free products (due to quarantine or virus inactivation).

#### Cytomegalovirus (CMV)

- Leukocyte-depleted cellular blood products are equally low risk as anti-CMV-negative blood products (according to guidelines). However, high-risk patients (e.g., anti-CMV-negative recipient of allogenic stem cell transplant, intrauterine transfusion) should strictly receive anti-CMV-negative blood products
- CMV reactivation / CMV coinfection in anti-CMV-positive immunosuppressed recipients by administration of blood products is unlikely (general leukocyte depletion)

#### Other Transfusion Relevant Viruses

- Parvovirus B19 (PV-B19): transfusions from PV-B19-IgG-positive donors recommended in patients needing regular transfusions
- HTLV I/II: risk identification and sequential testing of donors for HTLV I/II is recommended
- EBV (Epstein-Barr virus), HHV-6, HAV (hepatitis A virus)
- HGV (hepatitis G virus): relevance in relation to transfusions as yet uncertain
- TTV (transfusion-transmitted virus): isolated in 1998, significance as yet uncertain

#### Other Transfusion Relevant Infectious Agents

- *Bacteria:* bacterial contamination is rare with sterile preparation and use of single-use materials.
- *Parasitic diseases:* malaria, babesiosis, Chagas' disease etc; preventable by temporary abstinence from blood donation after travel to affected regions.
- *Creutzfeldt-Jakob disease (CJD) / new variant CJD (vCJD):* so far, no scientific data on transmission through blood products, however this possibility can not be definitively excluded. Individuals potentially at risk of CJD infection due to their medical history (e.g., treatment with human growth hormone derived from pituitary glands of corpses, > 6 month stay in Great Britain between 1980 and 1996) are excluded from donation.

Ref:
1. Davenport DD. Pathophysiology of hemolytic transfusion reactions. Semin Hematol 2005;42:165–9
2. Dzik WH. New technology for transfusion safety. Br J Haematol 2006;136:181–90
3. Pomper GJ, Wu Y, Snyder EL. Risks of transfusion-transmitted infections 2003. Curr Opin Hematol 2003;10:412–8
4. Popovsky MA (ed). Transfusion Reactions, 2nd edn. AABB Press, Bethesda, USA, 2001
5. Schroeder ML. Transfusion-associated graft-versus-host disease. Br J Haematol 2002;117:257–87
6. Sillmann CC, Ambrusi DR, Boshkov LK. Transfusion-related acute lung injury. Blood 2005;105:2266–73

Web:
1. http://www.emedicine.com/emerg/topic063.htm          E-medicine
2. http://www.nlm.nih.gov/medlineplus/ency/article/001303.htm    Medline Plus
3. http://www.psbc.org/medical/transfusion/bcrm/section_c/default.ht  Puget Sound Blood Ctr
4. http://www3.mdanderson.org/~citm/          MD Anderson, Transfusion Reactions

**9.9**  **Extravasation of Cytostatic Drugs**

B. Lubrich, H. Henß

**Def:** Extravasation / paravascular administration of cytostatic drugs.

**Ep:** Extravasation in 0.1–0.5% of all cases of intravenous administration of cytostatic drugs.

**Pp:** **Classification of cytostatic drugs according to local toxicity**

| | |
|---|---|
| ***Severely necrotizing compounds*** | |
| Amsacrine | Mitomycin |
| Cisplatin (> 0.4 mg/ml) | Mitoxantrone |
| Dactinomycin | Paclitaxel |
| Daunorubicin | Vinblastine |
| Docetaxel | Vincristine |
| Doxorubicin | Vindesine |
| Epirubicin | Vinorelbine |
| Idarubicin | |
| ***Moderately toxic compounds*** | |
| Bendamustine | Estramustine |
| Carmustine | Etoposide |
| Cisplatin | Fotemustine |
| Dacarbazine | Melphalan |
| Daunorubicin liposomal | Oxaliplatin |
| Epirubicin liposomal | Treosulfan |
| ***Compounds of low local toxicity*** | |
| Alemtuzumab | Irinotecan |
| Asparaginase | Methotrexate |
| Carboplatin | Nimustine |
| Cladribine | Pegaspargase |
| Cyclophosphamide | Pentostatin |
| Cytarabine | Raltitrexed |
| Etoposide phosphate | Rituximab |
| Fludarabine | Thiotepa |
| Fluorouracil | Topotecan |
| Gemcitabine | Trastuzumab |
| Ifosfamide | |

**Sy:** ***Acute Reaction***
- Edema, erythema, pain, hyperthermia
- Potential systemic reactions: vasovagal reaction, nausea, vomiting

***Delayed Symptoms***
- Compounds of severe local toxicity: tissue necrosis / ulceration from day 7
- Superinfection of skin lesions

**Dd:** Local allergic reactions (→ topical corticoid treatment is advisable)

**Th:**       ***Emergency Treatment***

*Check pulse, local symptoms, and vital signs every 30 min*

*Immediate therapy—even if no symptoms*

1.   *Basic measures:*

   • Stop infusion immediately, leave i.v. line, replace infusion set.

   • Place 5-ml syringe on i.v. access and extract extravasated fluid if possible, then remove needle.

   • In case of blistering or extensive extravasation: transcutaneous aspiration.

2.   *Substance-specific measures:*

   • Anthracyclines (doxorubicin, daunorubicin, epirubicin, idarubicin), anthracenediones (mitoxantrone), platinum compounds (cisplatin, carboplatin), and mitomycin C: DMS0 99% every 3–4 h for at least 3 days (up to 14 days) → apply with swab to the entire extravasation area and leave to dry.

   • Anthracyclines: dexrazoxane hydrochloride 1000 mg/m²/d i.v. 24 h and 48 h after extravasation, 500 mg/m² at 72 h.

3.   *Other measures:*

   • In the first 24–48 h: elevate legs.

   • *Cool* local areas as required (to alleviate pain).

   • *Exception:* etoposide, teniposide, vinblastine, vincristine, and vindesine: mild dry *warmth* (use blanket to keep extravasation site warm).

   • Avoid exposure to light (dacarbazine).

4.   *Surgical measures:*

   • Progressive necrosis / ulceration: surgical debridement / removal of necrotic tissue / plastic surgery (flap).

5.   *Documentation:*

   • All cases of extravasation as well as management and treatment must be accurately documented.

6.   *Observation of the patient for at least 6 weeks:*

   • Necrosis may occur weeks or months after the incident

### Further Measures (Optional)

A number of therapies have been reported to be effective in the treatment of extravasation of various cytostatic drugs. These reports are usually based on individual case studies or studies with small groups of patients rendering a comprehensive assessment impossible. The therapies described in the following lack proof of efficacy and may even cause additional toxicity:

• Local application of corticosteroids, topical or subcutaneously (highly controversial, potential increase in skin toxicity)

• Local infiltration of hyaluronidase

• Local infiltration of NaHCO₃ 8.4%, sodium thiosulfate, or heparin (particularly with vinca alkaloids)

• Local dilution by subcutaneous installation of NaCl 0.9% or glucose 5%

**F/U:**     Close monitoring for 6 months

**Px:**      *Prevention of extravasation by correct administration of cytostatic drugs:*

• For peripheral line: only use veins on the dorsum of the forearm, ensure good flow

• Only use intravenous catheters

• In patients with history of mastectomy, use contralateral arm for infusion (due to impaired lymph drainage and venous congestion after axillary dissection)

- Ensure correct position of the intravenous line (erythema, swelling, induration, local pain); if in doubt: resite the i.v. line
- Reliable fixation of the extremity, leave access visible
- If placement of intravenous line was unsuccessful at first attempt, avoid puncturing the same vein distal to the original access point
- Cytostatic drugs should only be added to a freely running infusion (NaCl 0.9% or glucose 5%); consider possible incompatibilities (▶ Chap. 3.2.6)
- Always administer cytostatic drugs with severe local toxicity as infusion via a central venous line
- Administration of cytostatic drugs of severe local toxicity via peripheral line: only as bolus by experienced physician / nurse

**Ref:**

1. Davies AG, Russell WC, Thompson JP. Extravasation and tissue necrosis due to central line infusions. Anaesthesia 2003;58:820–1
2. Ener RA, Meglathery SB, Styler M. Extravasation of systemic hemato-oncological therapies. Ann Oncol 2004;15:858–62
3. Goolsby TV, Lombardo FA. Extravasation of chemotherapeutic agents: prevention and treatment. Semin Oncol 2006;33:139–42
4. Kurul SP, Saip P, Aydin T. Totally implantable venous-access ports: local problems and extravasation injury. Lancet Oncol 2002;3:684–92
5. Napoli P, Corradino B, Badalamenti G et al. Surgical treatment of extravasation injuries. J Surg Oncol 2005;91:264–8
6. Schrijvers DL. Extravasation: a dreaded complication of chemotherapy. Ann Oncol 2003;14(suppl 3): iii26–30
7. Schulmeister L. Managing vesicant extravasations. Oncologist 2008;13:284–8

**Web:**

1. http://www.extravasation.org.uk/home.htm          Natl Extravasation Info

## 10.1    Thoracentesis

### R. Engelhardt

**Def:**    Insertion of a needle into the pleural cavity in order to remove excess pleural fluid.

**Ind:**
- *Diagnostic thoracentesis:* pleural effusion of unknown origin
- *Therapeutic thoracentesis:* symptomatic pleural effusion (dyspnea, pain, irritable cough), to relieve the patient before further treatment of the underlying disease

**Ci:**    *Relative contraindications:* hemorrhagic diathesis, anticoagulation

**Meth:**    **Thoracentesis set**

| Item | Type | Quantity |
| --- | --- | --- |
| Skin disinfectant | | 1 |
| Cotton swabs | Sterile | 3 packs |
| Compresses | Sterile, 7.5 × 7.5 cm | 3 packs |
| Drapes (fenestrated drapes) | Sterile | 1 |
| Gloves | Sterile, size as needed | 2 pairs |
| Bed pads | | 1 |
| Local anesthetic | Vials 1% | 2 |
| Cannulas | 22G, 0.7 mm | 2 |
| | 20G, 0.9 mm × 40 mm | 2 |
| | 20G, 0.9 mm × 70 mm | 2 |
| Intravenous catheter | 18G, 1.3 mm | 2 |
| | 16G, 1.7 mm | 2 |
| Disposable syringes | 2 ml, 5 ml, 50 ml | 2 of each |
| Three-way stopcocks | Sterile | 2 |
| Connecting tubes | Sterile, Luer-Lok system | 2 |
| Collection container | 1,000 ml | 1 |
| Sample tubes | Sterile | 5 |
| Dressing material | | 2 |

### Technique

#### Preparation
- *Position of the patient:* patient sitting comfortably, e.g., on edge of the bed
- *Puncture under sterile conditions:* skin disinfection, sterile cover

#### Puncture Site
- Posterior (e.g., posterior axillary line), upper border of a rib. ***ATTENTION:*** *subcostal neurovascular bundle on lower border of each rib.* Ultrasound location of effusion; alternatively: intercostal space below the fluid level
- ***ATTENTION:*** *puncture site should not be below the 6th or 7th intercostal space (danger of puncturing liver or spleen)*

#### Local Anesthesia of Skin and Parietal Pleura
- 22G or 20G needle. Thoracentesis needle is passed perpendicular to the chest wall on the upper border of the rib, if hitting bone, move skin and needle slightly upward

- Infiltration of the subcutaneous tissue and the upper border of the rib with local anesthetic
- Aspirate constantly. Infiltrate deeper tissues as far as the parietal pleura. If pleural fluid is aspirated, withdraw needle (*ATTENTION:* danger of pneumothorax)

### Puncture of the Pleural Cavity
- Same technique as with local anesthesia, but using a special thoracentesis needle or a large intravenous cannula (16G to 18G plastic cannula with metal trocar)
- If pleural fluid is aspirated: pull trocar back, move cannula forward a few more millimeters

### Aspiration of Pleural Fluid
- Diagnostic thoracentesis: 50–100 ml
- Therapeutic thoracentesis: up to 1,000 ml; monitor cardiovascular function
- Occurrence of cough/pain is due to contact of visceral and parietal pleura → drainage is complete, remove needle while having the patient perform a Valsalva maneuver (intrathoracic pressure increase)
- *ATTENTION:* aspiration of large quantities of pleural fluid may lead to decompression-induced pulmonary edema

### After Completion of Thoracentesis
- Check x-ray after 30–60 min


## Processing of Sample Material

*Clinical chemistry*
- 5 ml, serum tube (total protein, LDH, glucose, amylase, cholesterol, triglycerides, tumor markers)
- 5 ml, in blood gas tube (pH)
- 5 ml, EDTA tube (cell count, full blood count with differential, hematocrit)

*Pathology*
- 25–50 ml, heparinized (effusion cytology)
- Immunocytology (where applicable)

*Microbiology*
- 10 ml, sterile or blood bottle (aerobic and anaerobic cultures)
- 5 ml, sterile (tuberculosis and fungi)

**Co:**
- Pneumothorax (5–10% → compulsory chest x-ray after thoracentesis)
- Decompression-induced pulmonary edema (after aspiration of > 1,000–1,500 ml)
- Hemothorax, soft tissue injury, infection
- Vasovagal reaction
- Formation of effusion compartments after repeated thoracentesis

**Ref:**
1. Antunes G, Neville E. Management of malignant pleural effusions. Thorax 2000;55:981–3
2. Bass J, White DA. Thoracocentesis in patients with hematologic malignancy: yield and safely. Chest 2005;127:2101–5
3. Erasmus JJ, Goodman PC, Patz EF. Management of malignant pleural effusions and pneumothorax. Radiol Clin North Am 2000;38:375–83
4. Ferrer J, Roldan J. Clinical management of the patient with pleural effusion. Eur J Radiol 2000;34:76–86
5. Tassi GF, Cardillo G, Marchetti GP et al. Diagnostic and therapeutic management of malignant pleural effusion. Ann Oncol 2006;17(suppl 2):ii11–12

**Web:**
1. http://www.merck.com/pubs/mmanual/section6/chapter65/65c.htm — Thoracentesis, Merck Manual
2. http://www.nlm.nih.gov/medlineplus/ency/article/003420.htm — MedlinePlus
3. http://www.webmd.com/hw/lab_tests/hw233202.asp — WebMD
4. http://note3.blogspot.com/2004/02/thoracentesis-procedure-guide.html — Clinical Notes
5. http://www.emedicine.com/med/topic1843.htm — E-medicine

## 10.2    Pleurodesis

### R. Engelhardt

**Def:**    Palliative obliteration of the pleural space by adhesion of the pleural layers.

**Ind:**    First-line treatment of symptomatic recurrent malignant pleural effusion in palliative situations. Intrapleural application of substances with chemical, physical, or biological irritating effect → causing local inflammation (pleuritis) resulting in adhesion of the pleural layers.

### Prerequisites
1. Symptoms (dyspnea) are successfully relieved by aspiration of pleural fluid
2. Lungs fully expanded after thoracentesis (x-ray)

**Ci:**    *Relative contraindications:* hemorrhagic diathesis, therapeutic anticoagulation

**Meth:**    ### Technique

### Preparation
- Imaging (chest x-ray, ultrasound) to identify/exclude effusion compartments
- *Position of the patient:* patient sitting comfortably, e.g., on the edge of the bed
- *Sterile conditions:* skin disinfection, sterile cover

### Puncture Site
- Posterior (e.g., posterior axillary line), upper border of a rib. *ATTENTION: subcostal neurovascular bundle on lower border of each rib.* Ultrasound location of effusion; alternatively: intercostal space below the fluid level
- Local anesthesia of skin, periosteum, and parietal pleura
- Technique of puncture, see thoracentesis (▶ Chap. 10.1)

### Drainage of the Effusion
- Placement of a thoracic drainage tube in the dorsal costophrenic recess
- Attachment of a suction pump (15–20 cm $H_2O$ negative pressure)
- Drainage of the pleural fluid until lungs are fully expanded (x-ray), drainage with suction pump preferably down to < 200 ml/24 h
- In case of effusion compartments: repeated intrapleural instillation of fibrinolytics (e.g., 100,000 IU of urokinase in 50 ml NaCl 0.9% daily)

### Sclerosing
- Before sclerosing: systemic analgesia, intrapleural injection of a local anesthetic (e.g., 10 ml Xylocaine 2%)
- Injection of the sclerosing agent, flushed in with 20–50 ml NaCl
- Frequent turning of patient every 15 min for 2 h (drainage blocked off)
- Resume drainage of pleural fluid via pump for 1–3 days) until drainage volume is < 150 ml 24 h; gradual increase of the applied suction pressure reduces risk of decompression-induced pulmonary edema (e.g., suction without negative pressure for 3 h, followed by 2–5 cm $H_2O$ negative pressure for 3 h, then double negative pressure every 3 h until 20 cm $H_2O$)

### Sclerosing Agents
- *Talc:* usually administered by insufflation (2.5–6 g, requiring thoracoscopy), alternatively: suspension (e.g., 2 g in 50 ml NaCl 0.9%, via thoracic drainage tube). Most effective agent (efficacy: 90–95%). *Advantage:* inexpensive, highly effective, established method. *Adverse effects:* severe pain → administration requiring anesthesia (e.g., during thoracoscopy). *ATTENTION:* ARDS (acute respiratory distress syndrome), rare complication

- *Tetracyclines:* Supramycin 1 g absolute (or 20 mg/kg) in 30–50 ml NaCl 0.9%, efficacy: 70–75%. Alternatively: doxycycline 1 g absolute (or 10 mg/kg), often requiring second dose. *Adverse effects:* fever, pain (10% of cases). *Advantage:* inexpensive and effective, simple use
- *Bleomycin:* 60 mg absolute, efficacy: 70%. *Disadvantage:* expensive, compared to tetracyclines
- *Fibrin glue:* efficacy approximately 80%. *Disadvantage:* expensive

### Monitoring
- After removal of thoracic drainage tube: x-ray
- Over following weeks: regular ultrasound / chest x-rays

### Alternatives (in Case of Unsuccessful Pleurodesis)
- *Pleuroperitoneal shunt:* manually operated subcutaneous pump draining the pleural fluid into the peritoneal cavity via two catheters. *Indications:* non-expansion of the lungs after drainage; failure of pleurodesis. *Disadvantages:* requires general anesthesia; occasional shunt obstruction
- *Pleurectomy:* effective way of controlling malignant pleural effusion by removal of the parietal pleura; indicated only in selected cases
- *Long-term drainage:* via tunneled pleural catheter (e.g., Denver Pleurex kit)

**Co:**
- Pneumothorax (5–10% → chest x-ray after thoracocentesis)
- Decompression-induced pulmonary edema (aspiration of > 1,000–1,500 ml)
- ARDS: after talc pleurodesis (rare)
- Hemothorax, soft tissue injury, infection
- Vasovagal reaction (treatment: e.g., 1 mg atropine s.c.)

**Ref:**
1. Antony VB, Loddenkemper R, Astoul P et al. Management of malignant pleural effusions. Eur Respir J 2001;18:402–19
2. Antunes G, Neville E. Management of malignant pleural effusions. Thorax 2000;55:981–3
3. Dikensoy O, Light RW. Alternative widely available, inexpensive agents for pleurodesis. Curr Opin Pulm Med 2005;11:340–4
4. Janssen JP, Collier G, Astoul P et al. Safety of pleurodesis with talc poudrage in malignant pleural effusion: a prospective cohort study. Lancet 2007;369:1535–9
5. Pollak JS. Malignant pleural effusions: treatment with tunneled long-term drainage catheters. Curr Opin Pulm Med 2002;8:302–7
6. Shaw P, Agarwal R. Pleurodesis for malignant pleural effusions. Cochrane Database Syst Rev 2004;CD002916
7. West SD, Davies RJ, Lee YC. Pleurodesis for malignant pleural effusions. Curr Opin Pulm Med 2004;10:305–10

**Web:**
1. http://oncolink.upenn.edu/pdq_html/cites/09/09988.html — Pleurodesis, Oncolink
2. http://www.cochrane.org/reviews/en/ab002916 — Cochrane Library
3. http://www.vh.org/Providers/TeachingFiles/PulmonaryCoreCurric/PleuralEffusion/PleuralEffusion.html — Pleural Effusion and Pleurodesis, Virtual Hospital

## 10.3　Abdominal Paracentesis

### R. Engelhardt

**Def:**　Puncture of the peritoneal cavity to remove pathological intraperitoneal fluid (ascites).

**Ind:**
- *Diagnostic paracentesis:* obligatory to confirm the diagnosis and to exclude a primary or secondary infection.
- *Therapeutic paracentesis:* first-line treatment of symptomatic malignant ascites which cannot be treated conservatively.

**Ci:**　*Relative contraindications:* hemorrhagic diathesis, therapeutic anticoagulation

**Meth:**　**Paracentesis set**

| Item | Type | Quantity |
|---|---|---|
| Skin disinfectant | | 1 |
| Cotton swabs | Sterile | 3 packs |
| Compresses | Sterile, 7.5 × 7.5 cm | 3 packs |
| Drapes (fenestrated drapes) | Sterile | 1 |
| Gloves | Sterile, size as needed | 1 pair of each |
| Bed pads | | 1 |
| Local anesthetic | Vials 1% | 2 |
| Cannulas | 22G, 0.7 mm | 2 |
| | 20G, 0.9 mm × 40 mm | 2 |
| | 20G, 0.9 mm × 70 mm | 2 |
| Intravenous cannulas | 18G, 1.3 mm | 2 |
| | 16G, 1.7 mm | 2 |
| Disposable syringes | 2 ml, 5 ml, 50 ml | 2 of each |
| Three-way stopcock | Sterile | 2 |
| Connection tubes | Sterile, Luer-Lok system | 2 |
| Collection container | 1,000 ml | 3 |
| Sample tubes | Sterile | 5 |
| Dressing material | | 2 |

### Technique

#### Preparation
- Prerequisites: intravenous line, empty bladder
- Position of the patient: lying on back or side

#### Puncture Site
- Between the outer and middle third of the line connecting the anterior superior iliac spine and the navel
- Alternative: ultrasound-guided puncture

#### Puncture Under Sterile Conditions Using a Thin Needle
- Skin disinfection, sterile drapes
- If necessary *local anesthesia* of the skin (usually not required) → 22G or 20G needle, inject a subcutaneous depot, then advance needle carefully while constantly aspirating; infiltrate

deeper tissue as far as peritoneum; if ascites is aspirated, withdraw needle (*ATTENTION:* intestinal perforation)

- Insertion of paracentesis needle into the peritoneal cavity: same technique as with local anesthesia but using a special paracentesis needle or a large intravenous cannula (16G to 18G plastic cannula with metal trocar); once ascites is aspirated: pull trocar back and move cannula forward a few more millimeters

### *Aspiration of Ascites*

- Diagnostic paracentesis: 50–100 ml
- Therapeutic paracentesis: to relieve patient
- *ATTENTION:* aspiration of > 1,000 ml of ascites or repeated paracentesis: fluid replacement with NaCl 0.9%, protein replacement with human albumin 25%, 50 ml per 1,000 ml ascites

### Processing of Sample Material

*Clinical chemistry*
- 5 ml, serum tube (total protein, albumin, amylase, cholesterol, fibronectin, tumor markers)
- 5 ml, EDTA tube (cell count, full blood count with differential, hematocrit)

*Pathology*
- 25–50 ml, heparinized (effusion cytology)
- Immunocytology (where applicable)

*Microbiology*
- 10 ml, sterile or in blood culture bottles (aerobic and anaerobic culture)
- 5 ml, sterile (culture if suspected tuberculosis)

**Co:**  Complications are generally rare:
- Hematomas of the abdominal wall, intra-abdominal hemorrhage
- Intestinal perforation (particularly therapeutic paracentesis)
- Acute renal failure

**Ref:**
1. Adam RA, Adam YG. Malignant ascites. J Am Coll Surg 2004;198:999–1011
2. Becker G, Galandi D, Blum HE. Malignant ascites: systematic review and guideline for treatment. Eur J Cancer 2006;42:589–97
3. Covey AM. Management of malignant pleural effusions and ascites. J Support Oncol 2005;3:169–73
4. Parsons SL, Watson SA, Steele RJ. Malignant ascites. Br J Surg 1996;83:6–14
5. Runyon BA. Care of patients with ascites. N Engl J Med 1994;330:337–42

**Web:**
1. http://www.emedicine.com/med/topic173.htm — E-medicine
2. http://www.fpnotebook.com/GI33.htm — Family Practice Notebook
3. http://www.medstudents.com.br/medint/medint3.htm — Paracentesis, MedStudents
4. http://www.nlm.nih.gov/medlineplus/ency/article/0003896.htm — MedlinePlus

## 10.4    Bone Marrow Aspiration and Biopsy

### A. Engelhardt, R. Engelhardt

**Def:** Aspiration of bone marrow for cytology, histology, and further diagnosis. Differentiation between bone marrow aspiration and punch biopsy, with different diagnostic impact:
- *Aspirate:* for cytology, immunocytology, cytogenetics, FISH, molecular analysis, virology, bacteriology
- *Punch biopsy:* for histology, immunohistology

**Ind:**
- Diagnosis and monitoring of hematological diseases
- Diagnosis of bone marrow invasion by solid tumors, infections (e.g., miliary TB, CMV), storage diseases (e.g., Gaucher's disease)
- Evidence of bone marrow stroma disorders

**Ci:** *Relative contraindications:*
- Hemorrhagic diathesis, therapeutic anticoagulation (coumarins, heparin, acetylsalicylic acid / ASS)
- Local infection around the puncture site

**Meth:** **Bone marrow biopsy set**

| Item | Type | Quantity |
|------|------|----------|
| *Standard* | | |
| Skin disinfectant | | 1 |
| Cotton swabs or compresses 7.5 × 7.5 cm | Packages | 3–6 |
| Drapes (fenestrated drapes) | Sterile | 1 |
| Gloves | Sterile, size as needed | 1–2 |
| Bed pads | | 1 |
| Scalpel (or lancet) | No. 11 | 1 |
| BM biopsy needle (or sternal biopsy needle) | Jamshidi, G11×4 | 2 |
| Local anesthetic | Vials 1% / 2% | 4 of each |
| Cannulas (no. 1) | | 6 of each |
| Disposable syringes | 2 ml, 5 ml, 10 ml, 20 ml | 4 of each |
| Sodium EDTA solution | 0.25% | 2 |
| NaCl heparin | 25,000 IU, ampoules 5 ml | 2 |
| Fixation container | Containing descaler, e.g., formalin 1% + calcium acetate 0.16% + glutaraldehyde 0.5% in water for injection | 1 |
| Dressing material | | 2 |
| Petri dishes | | 1 |
| Microscope slides | | 8–12 |
| Midazolam | Ampoules 5 mg | 2 |
| Flumazenil | Ampoules 0.5 mg, 1.0 mg | 1 |
| *Extras as required:* | | |
| Sternal puncture needle | In isolated cases | 2 |
| Intravenous cannula | | 2 |

**Meth:**        **Bone marrow biopsy set (continued)**

| Item | Type | Quantity |
|------|------|----------|
| Swabs | | 2 |
| Sodium 0.9% | 250 ml | 1 |
| Midazolam | Vials 5 mg | 2 |
| Flumazenil | Vials 0.5 mg, 1.0 mg | 1 |

## Technique

### Pre-biopsy Check List
- Patient information and consent
- Medical history including bleeding / medication
- *Laboratory:* blood count (platelets); INR, PTT; platelet transfusion in case of thrombocytopenia (▶ Chaps. 4.9.1, 6.3)

### Premedication
- Analgesia: preferably peripheral analgesia, e.g., paracetamol p.o. or i.v., metamizole p.o.
- In case of severe pain / re-puncture: where applicable, analgesic such as morphine hemisulfate, 5–10 mg p.o. 15–30 min prior to bone marrow biopsy. *ATTENTION:* older patients, patients with pulmonary or cardiac diseases
- Where applicable, midazolam for sedation, slowly i.v., *ATTENTION: only if* standby resuscitation *and monitoring facilities available.* Caution with patients > 60 years, reduced general health, myasthenia, and chronic renal, hepatic or cardiac insufficiency. *Contraindications:* hypersensitivity, acute closed-angle glaucoma, alcohol or drug intoxication. *Antidote:* flumazenil
- In selected cases: short general anesthesia (in cooperation with anesthetist)

### Preparation
- *Positioning of the patient:* comfortable lateral position, bottom leg straight, upper leg bent (or: both legs bent). Alternatively: face-down position
- *Prepare syringes:* 20-ml syringes with 2 ml EDTA, for cytology (smears), immunocytology (cell marker) and molecular diagnosis, virology. Where applicable, 20-ml syringe with 5 ml Na-heparin (10,000 IU) for cytogenetics

### Puncture Site
- Posterior superior iliac spine. Puncturing of both sides recommended in case of high grade NHL, and in selected cases of solid tumors.
- Alternatively anterior superior iliac spine, experienced staff only (higher risk of puncturing other structures). Sternal biopsy (aspirate) only in selected cases (e.g., after pelvic radiotherapy) because of risk of puncturing the mediastinum (life-threatening complication).

### Skin Anesthesia and Biopsy
- Palpation of the posterior superior iliac spine, marking of puncture site if necessary
- Skin disinfection, sterile drapes, disinfect skin again, all further steps with sterile gloves
- Infiltration anesthesia: skin, subcutaneous tissue, puncture site, periosteum. Sufficient local anesthesia improves success of biopsy
- Skin incision. Insert needle (rotating movements) through the periosteum into spongy bone (less resistance)

### Bone Marrow Aspiration
- Remove trocar from biopsy needle, attach EDTA-containing syringe onto needle, aspirate bone marrow swiftly and firmly (4–6 ml)
- If cytogenetic analysis is planned: repeat with heparin-filled syringe
- *ATTENTION: aspiration is painful, warn and instruct patient to take deep breath*

- Agitate aspirate thoroughly; check successful biopsy by applying a sample of the aspirate to the petri dish; if bone marrow flecks: prepare smears
- Unsuccessful aspiration (dry tap): "roll" bone marrow core biopsy on the slide (touch preparation)

### Bone Marrow Biopsy (Punch Biopsy)
- After removing the stylus, push Jamshidi needle (rotating movements) at least 20 mm toward the anterior superior iliac spine
- Ensure that punch is long enough (by careful probing with the stylus), rotate needle several times (shearing movements) by 360° until the tip of the punch cylinder loosens in the pelvic bone (otherwise use recovery aid)
- Remove needle carefully (rotating movements)
- Apply pressure to puncture site, elastic dressing, 30 min bed rest, patient lying on his/her back, on a sand bag; if risk of hemorrhage: 1–2 h bed rest


### Processing of the Biopsy Material

*Aspirate*
- Hematology laboratory (approximately 5 ml bone marrow in 2 ml EDTA): smear; results within the same day
- Cell markers (5 ml bone marrow in EDTA): e.g., with AML, ALL, NHL; results after approximately 2–3 days (▶ Chap. 2.5)
- Cytogenetic analysis (5 ml bone marrow in EDTA; send off in heparin): e.g., with CML, ALL, AML, MDS, plasmacytoma; results after several days (▶ Chap. 2.1)
- Molecular genetic analysis (5 ml bone marrow in heparin); detection of bcr/abl translocation in CML or ALL, t(14;18) in NHL, translocation t(15;17) PML/RAR in AML type M3, t(8,21) in AML type M2, Inv(16) in AML type M4 Eo (▶ Chap. 2.2)
- Other: microbiological analysis (bone marrow sterile or in isolator bottle), Gram stain, anaerobic and aerobic cultures, Ziehl-Neelsen stain (tuberculosis), virological analysis (bone marrow in EDTA; e.g., CMV-PCR after bone marrow transplantation)

*Punch biopsy*
- Pathology: results after approximately 7 days


**Co:**
- Hemorrhage (particularly platelet function disorders, MPS, thrombocytopenia)
- Nerve lesions, infections
- Perforation of the iliac bone, psoas bleeding (puncture of other structures, particularly in the presence of osteolysis, pelvic deformities, osteoporosis, obesity)

**Ref:**
1. Bain BJ. Bone marrow biopsy morbidity and mortality. Br J Haematol 2003;121:949–51
2. Eikelboom JW. Bone marrow biopsy in cytopenic or anticoagulated patients. Br J Haematol 2005;129:562–3
3. Hodges A, Koury MJ. Needle aspiration and biopsy in the diagnosis and monitoring of bone marrow diseases. Clin Lab Sci 1996;9:349–53
4. Hyun BH, Stevenson AJ, Hanau CA. Fundamentals of bone marrow examination. Hematol Oncol Clin North Am 1994;8:651–63
5. Parapia LA. Trepanning or threphines: a history of bone marrow biopsy. Br J Haematol 2007;139:14–9
6. Wang J, Weiss LM, Chang KL et al. Diagnostic utility of bilateral bone marrow examination. Cancer 2002;94:1522


**Web:**
1. http://www.nlm.nih.gov/medlineplus/ency/article/003934.htm    MedlinePlus
2. http://www.emedicine.com/med/topic2971.htm    E-medicine
3. http://www.webmd.com/hw/lab_tests/hw200221.asp    WebMD
4. http://www.pathology.vcu.edu/education/lymph/How%20to%20marrow.pdf    Univ Virginia

**10.5**     **Basic Hematological Diagnostics**

F. Gärtner, R. Engelhardt

**Def:**     Quantitative, qualitative, and morphological characterization of the three components of hematopoiesis (erythrocytopoiesis, leukocytopoiesis, thrombocytopoiesis) in the peripheral blood (PB) and bone marrow (BM).

**Meth:**     *Sampling*
- Venous or capillary blood anticoagulated with EDTA (ethylenediaminetetraacetate) is suitable for most hematological tests
- For morphological analysis (e.g., differential blood count), blood should be processed within 3 h

*Peripheral Blood Smear: Technique*
- Place one drop of blood close to the end of a clean slide.
- Hold the end of a second slide against the surface of the first slide at an angle of 30–45°, so that blood clinches in the sharp angle of the slides.
- The upper slide spreads the blood swiftly and evenly on the back of the other slide → even, thin spreading on the bottom slide.
- Label and air dry the smear.

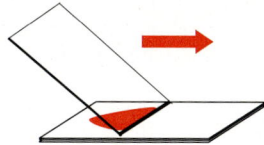

*Differential Blood Count: Staining Technique*
Panoptic Pappenheim's stain:
- May-Grünwald (eosin–methylene blue in methanol): 3–5 min, rinse with distilled water
- Giemsa solution (azure–eosin–methylene blue solution in distilled water): 15 min, rinse with distilled water
- Air dry, following fixation with methanol
  - → Eosin is an acidic dye and stains alkaline (= eosinophilic) cellular components
  - → Methylene blue is alkaline and stains acidic (= basophilic) cellular components

*Automated Hematology Analyzer (AHA)*
Automated analysis of hematological parameters. Principles of measurement:
- *Impedance method:* cells passing through an aperture cause a characteristic alteration of resistance within the electric circuit
- *Optical light scattering system:* cells passing a laser beam cause light to scatter characteristically
- *Automated cytochemical staining techniques:* optical detection
  - → Advantages: high precision, reproducibility, and analysis capacity
  - → Rapid performance of parallel analyses

**Erythrocytes**

*Red Blood Cell Count (RBC)*
**Def:**     Concentration of erythrocytes in full blood ($10^6/\mu l$ or $10^{12}/l$). Normal values: men 4.3–$5.7 \times 10^6/\mu l$, women 3.9–$5.3 \times 10^6/\mu l$

**Meth:**
- *Counting chamber:* blood is mixed with Hayem's solution in a red cell diluting pipette (1:100 to 1:200). Red cells contained in a defined volume (0.02 μl) are counted in a counting chamber under the microscope.
- *AHA:* counting of particles using impedance or light scattering methods (see above).

**Path:**
- ↓ E.g., anemia (▶ Chap. 6.4), hemodilution
- ↑ E.g., polyglobulia (▶ Chap. 7.3.2), exsiccosis

### Hematocrit (HCT, PCV = Packed Cell Volume)
**Def:**    Percentage of red blood cells in the blood. Normal values: men 40–52%, women 37–48%

**Meth:**
- *Microhematocrit method:* blood is centrifuged in a glass capillary, quotient of the pellet length to the length of blood column in the capillary (erythrocytes, plasma with platelets, leukocytes).
- *AHA:* RBC and MCV are directly measured by the AHA. Hematocrit is calculated with the formula PCV (%) = RBC ($10^6$/μl) × MCV (fl) / 10.

**Path:**
- ↓ E.g., anemia (▶ Chap. 6.4), hemodilution
- ↑ E.g., polyglobulia (▶ Chap. 7.3.2), exsiccosis

### Hemoglobin (Hb, HGB)
**Def:**    Hemoglobin concentration in the blood (g/dl). Normal values: men 14–18 g/dl, women 12–16 g/dl

**Meth:**
- *Hemiglobincyanide method:* blood hemoglobin derivatives (e.g., oxyhemoglobin, desoxyhemoglobin, carboxyhemoglobin, methemoglobin, hemiglobin) are stabilized with Drabkin's solution (oxidation of $Fe^{2+}$ to $Fe^{3+}$ by potassium ferricyanide, complexation of the resulting hemiglobin by cyanide ions) and photometric determination of the hemiglobincyanide concentration at 540 nm using a standard.
- *AHA:* automated analysis using the hemiglobincyanide method.

**Path:**
- ↓ E.g., anemia (▶ Chap. 6.4), hemodilution
- ↑ E.g., polyglobulia (▶ Chap. 7.3.2), exsiccosis

### Red Cell Indices (MCV, MCH, MCHC, RDW)
**Def:**
- *MCV:* mean corpuscular volume, normal value: 82–101 fl
- *MCH:* mean corpuscular hemoglobin, mean hemoglobin in one erythrocyte, normal value: 27–34 pg
- *MCHC:* mean cellular hemoglobin concentration, normal value: 31.5–36 g/dl
- *RDW:* red cell distribution width, variation coefficient of the erythrocyte distribution width, normal value: 11.5–14.5%

*ATTENTION:* the red cell indices are average values. Existence of different red cell populations can result in normal indices in spite of red cell disorders. In this case, consider the RDW.

**Meth:**    **Calculation Methods**
- MCV (fl) = PCV (%) × 10 / RBC ($10^6$/μl)
- MCH (pg) = Hb (g/dl) × 10 / RBC ($10^6$/μl)
- MCHC (g/dl) = Hb (g/dl) × 100 / PCV (%)
- RDW (%) = standard erythrocyte volume deviation / MCV × 100, AHA analysis

**Path:**
- MCV: normal → normocytic,          ↑ → macrocytic,      ↓ → microcytic
- MCH: normal → normochromic,     ↑ → hyperchromic,  ↓ → hypochromic
- RDW: normal → isocytic,               ↑ → anisocytic

### Red Cell Morphology
**Def:**    Analysis of size, shape, staining behavior, and cell inclusions of red cells

**Meth:**    Microscopic analysis of red cells in a peripheral blood smear.

**Path:**  *Size (normal diameter: approximately 6–8.5 μm)*
- *Macrocytosis:* diameter > 8.5 μm, e.g., pernicious anemia
- *Microcytosis:* diameter < 6 μm, e.g., iron deficiency anemia
- *Anisocytosis:* variable diameter, e.g., anemia of chronic disease

*Shape*
- *Poikilocytosis:* variable erythrocyte shape, e.g., with iron deficiency anemia
- *Elliptocytes:* oval erythrocytes, e.g., with hereditary elliptocytosis
- *Spherocytes:* spherical cells, e.g., with hereditary spherocytosis
- *Target cells:* target-like cell appearance with strong staining of central and peripheral areas of erythrocytes e.g., in thalassemia, following splenectomy
- *Acanthocytes:* spiculated shape, erythrocytes with spiked projections, e.g., in uremia
- *Schistocytes:* fragmentocytes, erythrocyte fragments, e.g., in microangiopathic disease (DIC, TTP), heart valve replacement, burns
- *Dacryocytes:* tear drop cells, drop-shaped erythrocytes, e.g., in myelofibrosis
- *Drepanocytes:* sickle cells, sickle-shaped erythrocytes, e.g., in sickle cell anemia

*Staining*
- *Hypochromia:* reduced staining of erythrocytes, ↓ e.g., with iron deficiency anemia
- *Hyperchromia:* increased staining of erythrocytes, ↑ e.g., in pernicious anemia
- *Polychromatophilia:* reddish grey-blue staining of erythrocytes, e.g., in reticulocytes

*Cell inclusions*
- *Howell-Jolly bodies:* basophilic inclusions (remnant of nucleus), e.g., following splenectomy
- *Basophilic stippling:* basophilic inclusions (ribosomes), e.g., in lead poisoning
- *Heinz bodies:* special stain necessary (denatured Hb), e.g., in hemoglobinopathies
- *Cabot rings:* basophilic ring (presumably nucleus remnants), e.g., following splenectomy
- *Normoblasts:* nucleated erythrocyte precursors, e.g., in extramedullary blood production
- *Plasmodia:* in malaria

### Reticulocytes
**Def:**
- Young erythrocytes in the peripheral blood which still produce hemoglobin in polyribosomes. Normal value: 0.8–2.2% of red cell population.
- In anemic patients, the corrected reticulocyte production index (RPI) is more suitable than the reticulocyte count for assessment of adequate regeneration of erythropoiesis.

**Meth:**
- Staining of full blood with supravital dye (e.g., brilliant cresyl blue) → intrareticulocytic precipitation of RNA as substantia reticulofilamentosa
- RPI = Reti (%) × (PCV (%) / 45) / C, with C being the correction factor for the reticulocyte maturation time (PCV 45% → C = 1, PCV 35% → C = 1.5, PCV 25% → C = 2, PCV 15% → C = 3)

**Path:**
- Reticulocytes (%): normal → normoregenerative, ↑ → hyperregenerative, ↓ → hyporegenerative
- RPI with anemia: > 2 → adequate regeneration, < 2 → inadequate regeneration

### Leukocytes

### White Blood Cell Count (WBC)
**Def:**  (Particle) concentration of leukocytes in the blood ($10^3$/μl or $10^9$/l), normal value $4$–$10 \times 10^3$/μl or $10^9$/l

**Meth:**
- *Counting chamber:* dilution of the blood and lysis of the red and white cells with Tuerk's solution using a white cell dilution pipette (1:10 to 1:20) and counting of the white cell nuclei contained in a defined volume (0.4 μl) in a counting chamber under the microscope

- *AHA:* counting of particles using impedance or light scattering methods (see above) after lysis of the erythrocytes

**Path:**
- ↓ Leukopenia (▶ Chap. 6.2)
- ↑ Leukocytosis, e.g., bacterial infections, leukemia (▶ Chaps. 7.1, 7.3, 7.5)

### Differential Cell Count

**Def:** Quantitative analysis of the types of leukocytes. Normal values:

| Cell type | | Occurrence |
|---|---|---|
| • Band forms (neutrophil granulocytes) | BAND | 3–5% |
| • Segmented (neutrophil granulocytes) | SEGM | 40–75% |
| • Eosinophils (granulocytes) | EOS | 2–4% |
| • Basophils (granulocytes) | BASO | 0–1% |
| • Lymphocytes | LYMP | 25–40% |
| • Monocytes | MONO | 2–8% |

**Meth:**
- *Manual:* counting and identification of 100 consecutive nucleated cells in Pappenheim's stained peripheral blood smears (see above)
- *AHA:* counting and identification of leukocytes using light scattering methods and cytochemistry after lysis of erythrocytes

### Special Stains / Cytochemistry
- *Myeloperoxidase (MPO):* staining of cells of granulocytopoiesis, differentiation between AML versus ALL
- *Leukocyte alkaline phosphatase (LAP score):* differentiation between CML (LAP ↓) versus other myeloproliferative syndromes (LAP ↑)
- *Iron stain:* identification of sideroblasts in myelodysplastic syndromes (▶ Chap. 7.2)

**Path:**
- Characteristic findings, e.g., with infections (leukocytosis with reactive left shift), with hemato-oncological diseases (e.g., blasts with acute leukemia, leukocytosis with pathological left shift with CML) or with allergic / parasitic diseases (eosinophilia)

## Thrombocytes

### Thrombocyte Count (PLT = Platelets)

**Def:** (Particle-) concentration of thrombocytes in whole blood per $10^3/\mu l$ or $10^9/l$. Normal value: $140–400 \times 10^3/\mu l$ or $10^9/l$

**Meth:**
- *Counting chamber:* dilution of blood and lysis of erythrocytes in an erythrocyte mixing pipette with Thrombo-Count reagent (1:100) and microscopic count of thrombocytes in a defined volume (0.02 µl) in a counting chamber.
- *AHA:* counting of particles using impedance or light scattering methods (see above).

**Path:**
- ↓ Thrombocytopenia (▶ Chap. 6.3)
- ↑ Thrombocytosis, e.g., with infections, iron deficiency, MPS (▶ Chap. 7.3)

## Bone Marrow Examination

**Def:** Quantitative, qualitative, and morphological evaluation of bone marrow preparations for:
- Hematopoietic cells (erythrocytopoiesis, leukocytopoiesis, thrombocytopoiesis)
- Bone marrow stroma

- Non-bone marrow cells

**Meth:** Aspiration of bone marrow (aspiration and biopsy) (▶ Chap. 10.4)

### Bone Marrow Smear
- Spreading of bone marrow particles on a glass slide and air drying
- Panoptic Pappenheim's stain
- If needed, special stains / cytochemistry (see above)

### Bone Marrow Biopsy
- Fixation, decalcifying, and paraffin embedding, alternatively methyl methacrylate embedding
- Different staining methods, analysis by pathologist

**Normal values of bone marrow cytology / myelography**

| Cell type | Mean value (%) | 95% Confidence interval (%) |
|---|---|---|
| *Neutrophil lineage* | 53.6 | 33.6–73.6 |
| • Myeloblasts | 0.9 | 0.1–1.7 |
| • Promyelocytes | 3.3 | 1.9–4.7 |
| • Myelocytes | 12.7 | 8.5–16.9 |
| • Metamyelocytes | 15.9 | 7.4–24.7 |
| • Band forms | 12.4 | 9.4–15.4 |
| • Segmented | 7.4 | 3.8–11.0 |
| *Eosinophil lineage* | 3.1 | 1.1–5.2 |
| *Basophils and mast cells* | 0.1 | |
| *Red Blood Cell lineage* | 25.6 | 15.0–36.2 |
| • Pronormoblasts | 0.6 | 0.1–1.1 |
| • Basophilic normoblasts | 1.4 | 0.4–2.4 |
| • Polychromatic normoblasts | 21.6 | 13.1–30.1 |
| • Orthochromatic normoblasts | 2.0 | 0.3–3.7 |
| *Lymphocytes* | 16.2 | 8.6–23.8 |
| *Plasma cells* | 1.3 | 0.0–3.5 |
| *Monocytes* | 0.3 | 0.0–0.6 |
| *Megakaryocytes* | 0.1 | |
| *Reticular cells* | 0.3 | 0.0–0.8 |
| *Ratio erythrocytopoiesis / granulocytopoiesis* | 2.3:1 | 1.1–3.5 |

**Path:** Evaluation of qualitative and quantitative defects of erythropoietic cells (e.g., MDS, aplastic anemia, polycythemia vera), of leukocytopoiesis (e.g., agranulocytosis, AML) or of thrombocytopoiesis (e.g., essential thrombocytosis). Diagnosis of pathological changes of bone marrow stroma (e.g., osteomyelofibrosis), detection of non-marrow cells (e.g., bone marrow infiltration by carcinoma).

**Ref:**
1. Bain BJ. Diagnosis from the blood smear. N Engl J Med 2005;353:498–507
2. Gulati GL, Hyun BH. Blood smear examination. Hematol Oncol Clin North Am 1994;8:631–50
3. Riley RS, Hogan TF, Pavot DR et al. Performing a bone marrow examination. J Clin Lab Anal 2004;18:70–90

**Web:**
1. http://www.hematologyatlas.com    Hematology Atlas
2. http://image.bloodline.net    Bloodline

## 10.6    Lumbar Puncture (Spinal Tap) and Intrathecal Instillation of Cytostatic Drugs

### R. Engelhardt

**Def:**    Puncture of the cerebrospinal fluid (CSF) space for diagnostic or therapeutic purposes. Instillation of antineoplastic drugs into the CSF space.

**Ind:**    Diagnosis or exclusion of:
- Cerebral / meningeal / spinal involvement in hematological diseases
- Carcinomatous or sarcomatous meningitis
- Inflammatory or demyelinating CNS diseases, meningitis
- Subarachnoid hemorrhage

**Ci:**
- Increased risk of hemorrhage: thrombocytopenia < 30,000/μl, anticoagulation (PT test < 60%), thrombopathy, thrombocyte aggregation inhibitors (e.g., ASS)
- Increased intracranial pressure

Always ensure normal intracranial pressure prior to lumbar puncture → ophthalmoscopy (papilledema?), CNS CT scan/MRI

**Meth:**    Usually lumbar puncture (intervertebral space L3/L4 or L4/L5). Suboccipital puncture: only in selected cases, carried out by an experienced physician (increased risk).

### Materials
- Standard spinal needle 22G × 3½ with stylet
- NaCl 0.9%, local anesthesia
- Sterile gloves, fenestrated drapes, sterile swabs, compresses
- Sample tube
- Dressing material

### Technique

#### Position of the Patient
- Lateral decubitus position (back and knees flexed, head down)
- Head should be level with puncture site
- Shoulders perpendicular to spinal column, avoid any torsion of the spine
- Alternatively: sitting position with flexed back and pulled-up legs (sitting on the edge of the bed, feet on a chair)

#### Puncture
- *Puncture site:* intervertebral space L3/L4 or below L4/L5. *Orientation:* the connecting line between the two iliac crests usually marks the dorsal process of L4.
- Skin disinfection and sterile drapes (*ATTENTION:* strictly aseptic technique)
- Local skin anesthesia only (not subcutaneous tissue nor needle track)
- Spinal tap using lumbar puncture needle with trocar (if applicable: with stylet), strictly medial and at a cranial angle of approximately 30°
- Firm resistance: interspinal ligament
- If hitting bone, withdraw needle and change direction
- Soft resistance: flaval ligament → advance needle only a little further
- Remove stylet → CSF will drip out

#### Diagnostic Collection of CSF
- Collection according to requirements (see below)
- If no instillation of cytostatic drugs: replace extracted CSF with equal amounts of sterile NaCl 0.9% (instill slowly)

### Intrathecal Instillation of Cytostatic Compounds

- Inject slowly in the following sequence: (1) cytosine arabinoside, (2) dexamethasone, (3) methotrexate
- Remove needle while injecting NaCl 0.9%
- Patient must lie flat immediately for 1 h, ideally in a face-down position; then bed rest for another 8 h (if possible)

## Processing of Collected CSF

*Routine laboratory tests*
- Color, cloudiness / blood
- Cell count (normal: < 4/μl)
- Cell differentiation (normal: 60–70% lymphocytes, 30% monocytes)
- Total protein (normal: 200–500 mg/l), albumin quotient (normal: < $7.5 \times 10^{-3}$)
- Intrathecal detection of IgG, IgM, IgA (normal: negative); oligoclonal IgG bands
- Glucose quotient (CSF glucose / serum glucose, normal: > 0.5)

*Screening for hematological diseases*
- Surface markers (FACS analysis)

*Pathology*
- CSF cytology

*Microbiology*
- Gram stain, anaerobic and aerobic cultures, Ziehl-Neelsen stain, mycobacteria, virological tests

**Co:**
- Headache after lumbar puncture (due to loss of CSF, "spontaneous low cerebrospinal fluid pressure syndrome")
- Nausea, vomiting, double vision, tinnitus, and loss of hearing
- Transtentorial or transforaminal herniation if increased intracranial pressure
- Clinical deterioration of paraplegic syndrome
- Subdural hematoma and hygroma
- Bleeding into the epidural or subarachnoid space (< 0.1% of cases)
- Infection (meningitis, empyema)
- *ATTENTION:* concentration of intrathecal methotrexate must be < 5 mg/ml

**Ref:**
1. Blaney SM, Poplack DG. New cytotoxic drugs for intrathecal administration. J Neurooncol 1998;38:219–23
2. Chamberlain MC. Neoplastic meningitis. J Clin Oncol 2005;23:3605–13
3. Mercadante S. Controversies over spinal treatment in advanced cancer patients. Support Care Cancer 1998;6:495–502
4. Roos KL. Lumbar puncture. Semin Neurol 2003;23:105–14

**Web:**
1. http://www.medstudents.com.br/proced/lumbpunc.htm     Lumbar Puncture, MedStudents
2. http://www.emedicine.com/neuro/topic557.htm     E-medicine

## 10.7    Central Venous Access (CVA), Central Venous Catheter (CVC)

**S. Mielke, R. Engelhardt**

**Def:**  Positioning of a venous indwelling catheter into a central venous vessel, e.g., internal jugular vein, subclavian vein, or femoral vein.

**Ind:**
- Intravenous administration of hyperosmolar parenteral nutrition, drugs, transfusions
- Measuring central venous pressure
- Poor peripheral venous access

**Ci:**  ***Relative Contraindications***
- Thrombocytopenia < 20,000/µl, anticoagulation, severe clotting disorders
- Carotid stenosis
- Contralateral pneumothorax
- Large struma, cervical space-occupying lesions, suspected cervical spine fracture
- Inflammation of the puncture site

**Meth:**  For central venous access, several sites for venous cannulation are possible. The internal jugular vein provides the easiest access and lowest rate of complications (easy sonographic imaging of the neck vessels, significantly reduced incidence of pneumothoraces in comparison with subclavian catheters). Alternatively: if cannulation of the internal jugular vein is not possible, the subclavian vein or femoral vein can be used.

**Materials**

| Item | Type | Quantity |
|------|------|----------|
| Skin disinfectant | | 1 |
| Round cotton swabs | Sterile | 2 packs |
| Bed pads | | 1 |
| Drapes (fenestrated drapes) | Sterile | 1–2 |
| Coat | Sterile | 1 |
| Gloves | Sterile, size as needed | 1 |
| Catheter set | Internal jugular vein catheter, 2- or 3-lumen | 1 |
| Cannulas | | 1 |
| Disposable syringes | 5 ml | 1 |
| | 10 ml | 3 |
| Local anesthesia | Vials 0.5–2.0% | 1 |
| NaCl 0.9% | Vials 10 ml | 3 |
| Dressing material | | 1 |
| Suture material | Sterile, non-resorbable | 1 |
| Needle holder | Sterile | 1 |
| If necessary, scalpel | Sterile, no. 11 | 1 |

### Technique of CVC Placement Via Internal Jugular Vein

#### Preparations
- Observe clotting parameters (platelets > 20,000/μl, Quick > 70%, pTT normal, stop heparin at least 1 h in advance).
- In hypovolemic patients, substitute 1–3 l parenteral fluid to fill veins → assists venous puncture. *ATTENTION: elderly subjects, cardiac disorders, volume load.*
- Information and informed consent.
- Make patient turn his/her head to the contralateral side, if possible, position head downward to dilate cervical veins and to prevent air embolism. *ATTENTION: not with increased intracranial pressure, with respiratory failure, thrombocytopenia, or right ventricular failure.*
- Ultrasound imaging of internal jugular vein. *ATTENTION: if cervical vein not compressible or hyperdense structures in vessel lumen consider cervical vein thrombosis and avoid puncture on this side.*
- Sterile gown, sterile gloves, skin disinfection, sterile drapes on the chosen side from mastoid to suprasternal fossa. Sterile handling of material. Fill two 10-ml syringes with NaCl 0.9% and one 5-ml syringe with local anesthesia 0.5–2%. Flush every catheter lumen with sterile saline. In doing so, check patency and impermeability of catheter. *ATTENTION: a damaged catheter can result in neck paravasation.*

#### Puncturing of Internal Jugular Vein with Seldinger Technique
- Palpation of A. carotis medial of vein, local anesthesia.
- Exploratory puncture of vein under continuous aspiration. Puncture direction: ipsilateral nipple at a 30 degree angle with the skin, insert needle with continuous aspiration slowly into neck. Usually, the vein position is rather superficial, therefore, a lateral and horizontal puncture direction should be preferred over a dorsal and medial direction. As soon as venous blood appears, the syringe is removed.
- Repeat puncture with puncture needle and attached 10-ml 0.9% NaCl syringe, under steady aspiration. As soon as venous blood appears, syringe is removed, while the needle stays in the vein (*ATTENTION: air aspiration with low central venous pressure*). Advance guide wire rapidly up to the second or third guidance mark (20–30 cm) and remove the guide cannula.
- Attach cleansed catheter on guide wire. Rule of thumb for extent of insertion: on the *right*: body height (cm) / 10 − 1 cm and on the *left*: body height (cm) / 10 + 1 cm.
- Remove guide wire. Aspirate all branches of the CVC, block with 0.9% NaCl solution and fix catheter to skin.

#### Confirmation of Correct Position
- Chest x-ray (in exhalation): confirmation of correct position and exclusion of pneumothorax. In optimal position the catheter tip lies almost distal to the right atrium, on the level of the carina tracheae.
- If necessary, correction of position, *in which the catheter may only be drawn back and not advanced.*

#### General Measures in Handling CVC
- Aspiration before every i.v. application, subsequent flushing with 0.9% NaCl to check patency, avoid backward flow of blood into the system.
- *Meticulous care of CVC:* daily change of dressing and control of CVC insertion site
- At interception / disconnection: flush with 0.9% NaCl, and block with 100 IU heparin in 2.5 ml NaCl 0.9% per branch, aspirate blood before reconnection. *ATTENTION: air embolism with low central venous pressure possible.*
- With immunocompromised patients: change of infusion system every 48 h.
- New infusion set after transfusions, lipid-containing solutions, cytostatic drugs.

**Co:** #### Acute Complications During Catheter Placing
- Malpuncture of A. carotis (1–2%): firm pressure for 5–10 min; if needed, platelet-substitution; if intravenous position is doubted, perform blood gas analysis
- Pneumothorax: after first unsuccessful attempt: contralateral repuncture only after exclusion of pneumothorax

- Bleeding and hematoma
- Air aspiration: always puncture with head positioned downward
- Injury of plexus brachialis, of neck sympathetic nerve with Horner syndrome, of trachea, or (rare) of A. vertebralis
- Arrhythmia: conduction disturbance due to catheter tip

### Complications with Catheter in Position
- Thrombosis, thrombophlebitis
- Infection of CVC, sepsis

**Ref:**

1. Boersma RS, Jie KSG Verbon A et al. Thrombotic and infectious complications of central venous catheters in patients with hematological malignancies. Ann Oncol 2008;19:433–42
2. Freytes CO. Indications and complications of intravenous devices for chemotherapy. Curr Opin Oncol 2000;12:303–7
3. Higgs ZJC, Macafee DAL, Braithwaite BD et al. The Seldinger technique: 50 years on. Lancet 2005;366:1407–9
4. Kuter DJ. Thrombolic complications of central venous catheters in patients. Oncologist 2004;9:207–16
5. Lee AY, Levine MN, Butler G et al. Incidence, risk factors and outcomes of catheter-related thrombosis in adult patients with cancer. J Clin Oncol 2006;24:1404–8
6. Lubelcheck RJ, Weinstein RA. Strategies for preventing catheter-related bloodstream infections: the role of new technologies. Crit Care Med 2006;34:905–7
7. Vescia S, Baumgärtner AK, Jacobs VR et al. Management of venous port systems in oncology: a review of current evidence. Ann Oncol 2008;19:9–15
8. Verso M, Agnelli G. Venous thromboembolism associated with long-term use of central venous catheters in cancer patients. J Clin Oncol 2003;21:3665–75

**Web:**

1. http://www.cdc.gov/ncidod/hip/iv/iv.htm          CDC Guidline Catheter Infections
2. http://www.nda.ox.ac.uk/wfsa/html/u12/u1213_01.html    Practical Procedures

## 10.8 Blood Cultures

### U. Frank, H. Bertz

**Def:**  Microbiological cultivation of blood samples in cases of suspected bacteremia, infection, or septicemia.

**Ind:**  Diagnosis or exclusion of bacteremia, infection, or septicemia, i.e., in case of:
- Clinical signs of infection
- Fever > 38°C (rectal or oral temperature)
- Increase in inflammatory parameters (ESR, CRP, acute phase reactions)
- Suspected septicemia (fever or hypothermia, decreased blood pressure, tachycardia, later: symptoms of shock)

Urgent indication for blood culture, microbiological diagnosis, and immediate treatment: fever in neutropenic patients (▶ Chap. 4.2).

**Meth:**  *Blood Sampling Technique*
Different techniques for qualitative (BacT/Alert-FAN blood culture bottles) and quantitative (isolator tubes) analysis. In general:
- Disinfect hands thoroughly, use gloves
- Venipuncture only after thorough skin disinfection; observe instructions for use of different disinfectants (usually skin disinfection for at least 1 min prior to venipuncture)
- Collect at least 35–42 ml of blood (8–12 ml per culture bottle, 3–6 bottles depending on disease, see below)
- Put sample into culture bottle (sterile conditions)
- Label bottles carefully (central or peripheral vessel, date, ward, with isolator tubes: time)
- Indicate puncture site (e.g., right or left cubital vein, central venous line, CVL)

*BacT/Alert-FAN Blood Culture Bottle*
- Collect blood as described above
- Disinfect rubber stopper of bottles (wipe with alcohol swab), insert blood (use same needle); no ventilation, place inside incubator immediately
- Temperature of blood culture bottle: at least room temperature, ideally body temperature

*Isolator Tube (Suspected Septic Line, Port Infection, etc.)*
- Thoroughly disinfect opening of the catheter, central line: handle with disinfected hands and gloves only
- Disinfect rubber stopper of bottles (wipe with alcohol swab)
- Collect at least 8–10 ml of blood from each arm of the catheter plus isolator tube with blood from peripheral vein
- Do not ventilate or incubate the isolator tube, store at room temperature
- Send samples immediately to microbiological laboratory; samples must be processed within 8 h to be suitable for quantitative analysis

### Number of Samples According to Disease

*Single Sampling Strategy*
I.e., collection of sufficient amounts of blood from a single venipuncture for all planned tests

*Suspected Systemic and/or Local Infection (Sepsis, Meningitis, Osteomyelitis, Arthritis, Pneumonia, Pyelonephritis) or Pyrexia of Unknown Origin*
Prior to antibiotic treatment, take blood from two different peripheral veins:
- First vein: 2 aerobic and 1 anaerobic blood culture samples
- Second vein: 2 aerobic blood culture samples

### Suspected Anaerobe Infection

Prior to antibiotic treatment, take blood from two different peripheral veins:
- First vein: 2 aerobic and 2 anaerobic blood culture samples
- Second vein: 1 aerobic blood culture sample

### Suspected Septic Intravenous Line

Prior to antibiotic treatment, take two separate samples from the intravenous line and one peripheral vein:
- 1 isolator tube from the intravenous line
- 1 isolator tube and 2 aerobic blood cultures from peripheral vein

### Suspected Infective Endocarditis

Prior to antibiotic treatment, take 6 samples from 3 different peripheral veins:
- First vein: 2 aerobic blood cultures
- Second vein: 1 aerobic and 1 anaerobic blood culture
- Third vein: 1 aerobic and 1 anaerobic blood culture

### Suspected Infection Despite Antibiotic Treatment

Take 6 samples from 3 different peripheral veins immediately before giving antibiotics:
- First vein: 2 aerobic blood cultures
- Second vein: 1 aerobic and 1 anaerobic blood culture
- Third vein: 1 aerobic and 1 anaerobic blood culture

**Ref:**

1. Chien JW. Making the most of blood cultures. Tips for optimal use of this time-honored test. Postgrad Med 1998;104:119–24,127
2. De Marie S. New developments in the diagnosis and management of invasive fungal infections. Haematologica 2000;85:88–93
3. Lamy B, Roy P, Carret G et al. What is the relevance of obtaining multiple blood samples for culture? A comprehensive model to optimize the strategy for diagnosing bacteremia. Clin Infect Dis 2002;35:842–50
4. Mylotte JM, Tayara A. Blood cultures: clinical aspects and controversies. Eur J Clin Microbiol Infect Dis 2000;19:157–63
5. Weinstein MP. Current blood culture methods and systems: clinical concepts, technology, and interpretation of results. Clin Infect Dis 1996;23:40–6

**Web:**

1. http://www.webmd.com/hw/lab_tests/hw3603.asp          WebMD

# 11    Standardized Treatment Protocols

D. Behringer, D.P. Berger, H. Bertz, W.D. Digel, M. Engelhardt, J. Finke, H. Henß,
M. Lübbert, R. Mertelsmann, C. Waller

## Selection of treatment protocols

In the following appendix current treatment protocols (chemotherapy, cytokine therapy) are summarized, which are used in Freiburg for the treatment of patients with malignant diseases. We have tried to reflect the state of the art in clinical practice and to establish standardized procedures for chemotherapy administration.

This resulted in a collection which deliberately does not intend to represent a complete account of all available treatment protocols, but rather describes selectively those protocols, which have proven to be of value in the setting of our department.

## Use of treatment protocols

The aim of the present protocol collection is to support standardized implementation and documentation of selected chemotherapeutic treatment procedures. However, in each single case, the indication, dose, selection and administration of therapy must be supervised by an experienced oncologist and treatment alternatives must be taken into consideration as applicable.

Information concerning epidemiology, pathogenesis, diagnosis, treatment and prognosis of individual disease entities is described in the previous chapters of this manual. In the following table and in each single treatment protocol reference is made to the corresponding chapter.

This selection is a basis for discussion. We welcome comments and suggestions.

**Standardized Treatment Protocols: Summary (1)**

| Protocol Nr. | Denomination, compounds | Indication |
|---|---|---|
| 11.1.1 | ALL Prephase | ALL |
| 11.1.2 | Induction I | ALL |
| 11.1.3 | Induction II | ALL |
| 11.1.4 | Consolidation I | ALL |
| 11.1.5 | Consolidation II, III,VI | ALL |
| 11.1.6 | Consolidation II HR/T-ALL | ALL (high risk, T-ALL) |
| 11.1.7 | Consolidation II HR/VHR | B-ALL, Burkitt Lymphoma |
| 11.1.8 | Consolidation IV | ALL |
| 11.1.9 | Consolidation V | ALL |
| 11.1.10 | Reinduction I | ALL |
| 11.1.11 | Reinduction II | ALL |
| 11.1.12 | Maintenance therapy | ALL |
| 11.1.13 | B-ALL, Prephase | B-ALL, Burkitt Lymphoma |
| 11.1.14 | B-ALL, block A | B-ALL, Burkitt Lymphoma |
| 11.1.15 | B-ALL, block B | B-ALL, Burkitt Lymphoma |
| 11.1.16 | B-ALL, block C | B-ALL, Burkitt Lymphoma |
| 11.1.17 | Consolidation I, B-ALL | B-ALL, Burkitt Lymphoma |
| 11.2.1 | Prephase (AML-SG 7-04) | AML |
| 11.2.2 | Induction (AML-SG 7-04) | AML |
| 11.2.3 | Consolidation (AML-SG 7-04) | AML |
| 11.2.4 | DNR/AraC (Intergroup) | AML |
| 11.2.5 | HD D-AraC (Intergroup) | AML |
| 11.2.6 | S-HAM | AML |
| 11.2.7 | MICE | AML |
| 11.2.8 | Mini ICE | AML |
| 11.2.9 | IDA 3 + 7 | AML |
| 11.3.1 | HD -13 | Hodgkin's disease |
| 11.3.2 | BEACOPP-II standard | Hodgkin's disease |
| 11.3.3 | BEACOPP-II escalated | Hodgkin's disease |
| 11.3.4 | Vinblastine | Hodgkin's disease |
| 11.3.5 | Stanford V | Hodgkin's disease |
| 11.4.1 | VACOP-B | aggressive NHL |
| 11.4.2 | CHOP | aggressive NHL |
| 11.4.3 | R-CHOP | aggressive NHL |
| 11.4.4 | R-CHOP 14 | aggressive NHL |
| 11.4.5 | COP | aggressive NHL |
| 11.4.6 | DHAP | aggressive NHL |
| 11.5.1 | Bendamustin | low malignant NHL |
| 11.5.2 | Fludarabine | low malignant NHL |
| 11.5.3 | Fludarabine / Cyclophosphamide | low malignant NHL |
| 11.5.4 | FCR | low malignant NHL |
| 11.5.5 | Chlorambucil/Prednisone | low malignant NHL |

**Standardized Treatment Protocols: Summary (1)** *(continued)*

| Protocol Nr. | Denomination, compounds | Indication |
|---|---|---|
| 11.5.6 | Alemtuzumab | low malignant NHL |
| 11.5.7 | Cladribine | low malignant NHL |
| 11.5.8 | Pentostatin | low malignant NHL |
| 11.5.9 | Rituximab | low malignant NHL |
| 11.5.10 | 90Y-Ibritumomab Tiuxetan+Rituximab | low malignant NHL |
| 11.6.1 | R-MCP | CNS- Lymphoma |
| 11.6.2 | "Freiburg protocol" | CNS- Lymphoma |
| 11.7.1 | Melphalan / Prednison | Multiple myeloma |
| 11.7.2 | HD Dexamethasone | Multiple myeloma |
| 11.7.3 | VAD | Multiple myeloma |
| 11.7.4 | Ind 1 Cyclo | Multiple myeloma |
| 11.7.5 | CTD | Multiple myeloma |
| 11.7.6 | LD Thalidomide+Dexamethasone | Multiple myeloma |
| 11.7.7 | Bortezomib | Multiple myeloma |
| 11.7.8 | DeCyBo | Multiple myeloma |
| 11.7.9 | HD-Dexa/IFN-alpha | Multiple myeloma |
| 11.7.10 | LD Thalidomide+ Prednisone | Multiple myeloma |

**Standardized Treatment Protocols: Summary (2)**

| Protocol Nr. | Denomination, compounds | Indication |
|---|---|---|
| 12.1.1 | 5-FU / Carboplatin | Head and neck tumors |
| 12.1.2 | EMB | Head and neck tumors |
| 12.2.1. | Cisplatin /Etoposide-Phosphate | Small Cell Lung Cancer |
| 12.2.2 | EPI-CO | Small Cell Lung Cancer |
| 12.2.3 | Paclitaxel weekly | Small Cell Lung Cancer |
| 12.2.4 | CE | Small Cell Lung Cancer |
| 12.2.5 | Topotecan | Small Cell Lung Cancer |
| 12.2.6 | TEC | Small Cell Lung Cancer |
| 12.2.7 | Vinorelbin / Carboplatin | Non Small Cell Lung Cancer |
| 12.2.8 | Paclitaxel / Carboplatin | Non Small Cell Lung Cancer |
| 12.2.9 | Gemcitabin / Cisplatin | Non Small Cell Lung Cancer |
| 12.2.10 | Docetaxel | Non Small Cell Lung Cancer |
| 12.2.11 | Cisplatin /Vinorelbine | Non Small Cell Lung Cancer |
| 12.2.12 | Pemetrexed 2. line | Non Small Cell Lung Cancer |

**Standardized Treatment Protocols: Summary (2)** *(continued)*

| Protocol Nr. | Denomination, compounds | Indication |
|---|---|---|
| 12.3.1 | Paclitaxel / Carboplatin RT | Pleural Mesothelioma |
| 12.3.2 | Pemetrexed /Cisplatin | Pleural Mesothelioma |
| 12.4.1 | PAC | Thymic Carcinoma |
| 12.5.1 | Rx / 5-FU / Cisplatin (Naunheim) | Esophageal Cancer |
| 12.6.1 | PELF | Gastric Cancer |
| 12.6.2 | ECF | Gastric Cancer |
| 12.6.3 | DCF (Docetaxel/Cisplatin/5FU) | Gastric Cancer |
| 12.7.1 | FOLFIRI | Colorectal Cancer |
| 12.7.2 | FOLFIRI + Bevacizumab | Colorectal Cancer |
| 12.7.3 | Irinotecan + Cetuximab | Colorectal Cancer |
| 12.7.4 | 5-FU / Leucovorin (Ardalan) | Colorectal Cancer |
| 12.7.5 | 5-FU / Leucovorin (Poon) | Colorectal Cancer |
| 12.7.6 | FOLFOX 4 | Colorectal Cancer |
| 12.7.7 | FOLFOX 6 | Colorectal Cancer |
| 12.7.8 | Oxaliplatin mono | Colorectal Cancer |
| 12.7.9 | Capecitabine mono | Colorectal Cancer |
| 12.7.10 | Rx / 5-FU / Mitomycin / Cisplatin | Anal Cancer |
| 12.8.1 | Gemcitabine | Pancreatic cancer |
| 12.9.1 | Gem Ox 3 | Cholangiocarcinoma |
| 12.10.1 | CMF (Bonadonna) | Breast cancer |
| 12.10.2 | FAC (FEC) | Breast cancer |
| 12.10.3 | AC (EC) | Breast cancer |
| 12.10.4 | Docetaxel | Breast cancer |
| 12.10.5 | Epirubicin | Breast cancer |
| 12.10.6 | EP | Breast cancer |
| 12.10.7 | Vinorelbine | Breast cancer |
| 12.10.8 | Liposomal Doxorubicine | Breast cancer |
| 12.10.9 | Trastuzumab / Paclitaxel | Breast cancer |
| 12.10.10 | EC + Paclitaxel | Breast cancer |
| 12.10.11 | EC + Paclitaxel (dose dense) | Breast cancer |

**Standardized Treatment Protocols: Summary (3)**

| Protocol Nr. | Denomination, compounds | Indication |
| --- | --- | --- |
| 12.11.1 | Taxol / Carboplatin | Ovarial cancer |
| 12.11.2 | Treosulfan | Ovarial cancer |
| 12.11.3 | PEB | Germ Cell Tumors |
| 12.11.4 | PEI | Germ Cell Tumors |
| 12.11.5 | PIV | Germ Cell Tumors |
| 12.12.1 | Doxorubicin | Prostate Cancer |
| 12.12.2 | Docetaxel /Prednisolone | Prostate Cancer |
| 12.13.1 | HD-IL-2 / IFN$\alpha$ | Renal Cell Cancer |
| 12.13.2 | M-VAC | Urothelial cancer |
| 12.14.1 | CycloVD | Pheochromocytoma |
| 12.15.1 | CVD / IL-2 / IFN$\alpha$ | Melanoma |
| 12.15.2 | Consolidation | Melanoma |
| 12.15.3 | CVD | Melanoma |
| 12.15.4 | Dacarbazine mono | Melanoma |
| 12.15.5 | Fotemustine | Melanoma |
| 12.16.1 | Adria / Ifo (Sarkom) | Soft tissue sarcoma |
| 12.16.2 | VIDE | Ewing -Sarcoma |
| 12.16.3 | VAI | Ewing Sarcoma |
| 12.16.4 | VAC | Ewing Sarcoma |
| 12.16.5 | PA EURO-BOSS | Osteosarcoma |
| 12.16.6 | IP EURO-BOSS | Osteosarcoma |
| 12.16.7 | IA EURO-BOSS | Osteosarcoma |
| 12.16.8 | HD-MTX EURO-BOSS | Osteosarcoma |
| 12.17.1 | Nimustine | CNS- Tumors |
| 12.17.2 | Temozolomide | CNS- Tumors |
| 12.18.1 | PCE | CUP |
| 12.19.1 | Bleomycin intrapericardial | pericardial effusion |
| 12.19.2 | AraC / Dexa / MTX intrathecal | CNS prophylaxis /treatment |
| 12.19.3 | MTX mono intrathecal | CNS prophylaxis /treatment |
| 12.19.4 | Liposomal Cytarabine | CNS treatment |
| 13.1.1 | VCP-E | PBSC Mobilisation |
| 13.1.2 | VIP-E | PBSC Mobilisation |
| 13.1.3 | Cyclo-Mob-1d | PBSC Mobilisation |
| 13.1.4 | Cyclo-Mob-2d | PBSC Mobilisation |
| 13.1.5 | Dexa-BEAM | PBSC Mobilisation |
| 13.1.6 | IEV < 60 years | PBSC Mobilisation |
| 13.1.7. | ECV< 60 years (instead IEV) | PBSC Mobilisation |

**Standardized Treatment Protocols: Summary (4)**

| Protocol Nr. | Denomination, compounds | Indication |
| --- | --- | --- |
| 14.1 | BEAM | High-Dose Chemotherapy |
| 14.2 | Melphalan 200 | High-Dose Chemotherapy |
| 14.3 | Melphalan 140 | High-Dose Chemotherapy |
| 14.4 | Bu / Cy | High-Dose Chemotherapy |
| 14.5 | Busulfan mono | High-Dose Chemotherapy |
| 14.6 | VIC | High-Dose Chemotherapy |
| 14.7 | BuMel | High-Dose Chemotherapy |
| 14.8 | CNS-NHL HD MTX | High-Dose Chemotherapy |
| 14.9 | CNS-NHL HD AraC Thiotepa | High-Dose Chemotherapy |
| 14.10 | CNS-NHL HD BCNU Thiotepa | High-Dose Chemotherapy |
| 14.11 | Prophylaxis delayed emesis | Emesis |
| 14.12 | Amphothericin B | FUO, Organ Mycoses |
| 14.13 | Leucovorin rescue | Methotrexate therapy |

**11.1.1**

| Prephase | GMALL 07/2003 | Indication: ALL |
|---|---|---|
| Study protocol: MTX (i.t.) /Dexa/Cyclo | all ALL patients: | week 1, days 1-5 |

## Chemotherapy

| Week | Day | Compounds (generic names) in chronological order | Dosage | Diluent | Route | Duration of Infusion | Comments |
|---|---|---|---|---|---|---|---|
| | 1 | **Methotrexate** | 15mg | in 3ml water | i.t. | bolus | before systemic therapy |
| | 1-5 | **Dexamethasone** | 10mg/m² | | oral | | in 3 divided doses |
| | 3-5 | **Cyclophosphamide** | 200mg/m² | 250ml Saline 0.9% | i.v. | 1h | |

**Please note: bone marrow biopsy on day 1; send sample for MRD evaluation! (See study protocol pages 34ff/141ff)**

**With an initial granulocytopenia < 500/µl, give Filgrastim 5 µg/kg from day 1**

**Cautions**

Cycle Diagram: d1 w1 | d8 w2 | d15 w3 | d22 w...
- Methotrexate i.t.
- Dexamethasone
- Cyclophos.

## Obligatory Pre- and Concurrent Medication

| Week | Day | Compounds (generic names) | Sequence and Timing | Amount Per Dose | Diluent | Route | Duration of Infusion | Comments |
|---|---|---|---|---|---|---|---|---|
| | 1-5 | Saline 0.9% + Sodium Bicarbonate | continuously | 40ml/1000ml | 2000ml | i.v. | 24h | in infusion fluid, urine target pH >7.4 |
| | 3-5 | Metoclopramide | 30' before Cyclophosphamide | 50mg | | oral | | may be given intravenously |
| | 1-5 | Allopurinol | 1-0-0 | 300mg | | oral | | dose according to uric acid level |
| | 1-5 | Amphotericin B | 1-1-1-1 | 500mg (5ml) | | oral | | as suspension |
| | 1-5 | Sucralfate | 1-0-0 | 1g | | oral | | |
| | from day 1 | Co-trimoxazole | 1-0-1 (2x/week) | 960mg | | oral | | for infection prophylaxis |
| | | Mesna | 0h, 4h, 8h, after Cycloph. | each dose 40mg/m² | | i.v. | | |

**Medicines As Required:** Allopurinol according to serum uric acid; alkalinization; Metoclopramide oral or i.v.

**Antibiotic Prophylaxis:** If neutrophils < 500/µl for >10 days: Colistin 95mg(1-1-1) every 6 hours

**Routine Tests:** FBC, U&Es, serum creatinine, creatinine clearance, uric acid, LDH, fluid balance, LFTs

**Dose Reduction:** See Dose Modification Table

**Max. Cum. Dose :** Not defined

**References:** Study protocol "Multicenter study for therapy optimization of acute lymphatic leukemia in adults and adolescents from 15 years, GMALL 07/2003"

| Induction I GMALL 07/2003 + Rituximab | | Indication: ALL (CD20+) | | | | ICD-10: C91.0 | 11.1.2 |

**Dexa/Vincristine/Daunorubicin/Asp/Ritux**

\* Rituximab application:  weeks 1-3, days 6-21

*This chemotherapy may cause life-threatening toxicity! It should only be administered under the supervision of an experienced medical oncologist! The protocol must first be reviewed and considered in relationship to the clinical situation of the patient.*

>20% CD 20 positive cells

## Chemotherapy

| Week | Day | Compounds (generic names) in chronological order | Dosage | Route | Diluent | Duration of Infusion | Comments |
|---|---|---|---|---|---|---|---|
| | 6 | **Rituximab\*** | 375mg/m² | i.v. | 500ml Saline 0.9% | initially 50mg/h | via separate access, monitor closely esp. with 1st infusion, resuscitation equipment! in 3 divided doses; do not tail off, continue in reduced dose with withdrawal symptoms |
| | 7-8/14-17 | **Dexamethasone** | 10mg/m² | oral | | | |
| | 7-8/³14-15 | **Daunorubicin** | 45mg/m² (30mg/m² >55 years) | i.v. | *100ml Saline 0.9% | 15min | via existing central line: 1h |
| | 7, ³14, 21 | **Vincristine** | 2mg (absolute) | i.v. | undiluted | bolus | Itraconazole NOT to be given in parallel! |
| | 21 | **PEG-Asparaginase** | 1000 units/m² (500 units/m² >55 years) | i.v. | 100ml Saline 0.9% | 2h | monitor, pharmacokinetics on days 21, 28, 34 |
| | from day 7 | **Filgrastim** (from day 1 if initial granulocytopenia) | 5µg/kg or 150µg/m² | s.c. | | | until granulocytes >1000 after nadir |

**Please note: Schedule radiotherapy! Bone marrow biopsy on day 12. Serum Asparaginase level on days 21, 28, 34.**

**Rituximab: first dose over 4 hours each time**

Day 1: 200mg, day 2: remainder up to 375mg/m², starting at 50mg/h and increasing by 50mg/h every 30min up to max. 300mg/h

³**Patients with an initial granulocyte count <500/µl (on presentation or on days 1-5):**
**With CR or PR on day 12: therapy may be delayed (Dauno/Dexa/Vincristine) until granulocytes >500/µl (1 week maximum)**
**With treatment failure /progressive disease: continue therapy**

| Cycle Diagram | d1 w1 | d8 w2 | d15 w3 | d22 w4 |
|---|---|---|---|---|
| Rituximab | | | | |
| Dexamethasone | | | | |
| Daunorubicin | | | | |
| Vincristine | | | | |
| Asparaginase | | | | |
| Filgrastim | | ------------------------> | | |

## Obligatory Pre- and Concurrent Medication

| Week | Day | Compounds (generic names) | Sequence and Timing | Amount Per Dose | Route | Diluent | Duration of Infusion | Comments |
|---|---|---|---|---|---|---|---|---|
| | 6 | Paracetamol | -1h | 1000mg | oral | | | |
| | 6 | Clemastine | -30min | 2mg | i.v. | | bolus | |
| | 6-8/14-15 | Allopurinol | 1 - 0 - 0 | 300mg | oral | | | dose according to uric acid level |
| | 7-8/14-15 | Saline 0.9% | 15' before chemotherapy | | i.v. | 1000ml | 4h | |
| | 21 | Saline 0.9% | 15' before chemotherapy | | i.v. | 500ml | 2h | |
| | 7-8/14-15 | Granisetron | 15' before chemotherapy | 3mg | i.v. | | bolus | |
| | 21 | Metoclopramide | 1 - 1 - 1 | 20mg | oral | | | |
| | 7, 14, 21 | Lactulose | 1 - 0 - 1 | 10g | oral | | | for constipation prophylaxis |
| | from day 1 | Co-trimoxazole | 1 - 0 - 1 | 960mg | oral | | | till granulocytes >500/µl, then 960mg on Mon. Wed. Fri. |
| | from day 1 | Amphotericin B (as suspension) | 1 - 1 - 1 - 1 | 500mg | oral | | | until granulocytes >500/µl + rinse with Dexpanthenol/Chlorhexidine |
| | from day 1 | Sucralfate | 1 - 0 - 0 | 1g | oral | | | |
| | from day 1 | Colistin | 1 - 1 - 1 - 1 | 150mg | oral | | | if granulocytes ≤ 500/µl (>10 days) |

| **Cautions** | | | | | | | | |

**Medicines As Required:** Metoclopramide oral i.v., Granisetron i.v., Heparin 2500-10,000 units i.v., Allopurinol

**Antibiotic Prophylaxis:** With neutropenia (< 500/µl) >10 days: Colistin 150mg every 6 hours

**Routine Tests:** FBC; Asparaginase: before therapy: LFTs, clotting studies; daily: fibrinogen, ATIII, TP, PTT (D-dimer test); 2-3x/ week: blood glucose profile, amylase, LFTs, transaminases, U&Es, serum creatinine, uric acid, urine testing; Daunorubicin: ECG/echocardiogram (before 1st dose + during therapy course), with pre-existing cardiac disease: consult Study Center; Rituximab: caution: cytokine release syndrome; Vincristine: neurotoxicity. 1/week: CXR

**Dose Reduction:** Asparaginase: fibrinogen < 80mg/dl or ATIII level drops to <70% -> give FFP; Contraindications: thrombotic tendency, severe coagulation disorders, severe hemorrhagic complications, hepatic impairment, past history of pancreatitis. Daunorubicin: reduce dose to 50% if bilirubin >2mg/dl. Contraindication: if bilirubin >5mg/dl. Vincristine: reduce dose with neurotoxicity and to 50% with pronounced paresthesias, discontinue with pareses or paralytic ileus; reduce dose with hepatic failure; stop with venous pain or spasm, inject remainder of solution into another large vein. Contraindication: if bilirubin >5mg/dl - unless due to hemolysis; see study protocol for details. Rituximab: see study protocol.

**Max. Cum. Dose:** Daunorubicin >550 mg/m²: Danger of cardiotoxicity; Vincristine 5-20mg: Danger of neurotoxicity

**References:** Study protocol "Multicenter study for therapy optimization of acute lymphatic leukemia in adults and adolescents from 15 years", with Rituximab to improve prognosis with CD20+ standard risk ALL"

# Induction II GMALL 07/2003 + Rituximab

**Indication: ALL (CD20+)**  ICD-10: C91.0  **11.1.3**

Study protocol: MTX (i.t.) /Cytarabine/Cyclo/Mercaptopurine/Rituximab

* Rituximab application:
>20% CD 20 positive cells

Rituximab application: weeks 4-7, days 27-48

*This chemotherapy may cause life-threatening toxicity! It should only be administered under the supervision of an experienced medical oncologist! The protocol must first be reviewed and considered in relationship to the clinical situation of the patient.*

## Chemotherapy

| Week | Day | Compounds (generic names) in chronological order | Dosage | Diluent | Route | Duration of Infusion | Comments |
|---|---|---|---|---|---|---|---|
| | 27 | **Rituximab*** | 375mg/m² | 500ml Saline 0.9% | i.v. | initially 50mg/h | monitor closely, resuscitation equipment! |
| | 30, 37, 44 | **Methotrexate** | 15mg | in 3ml water | i.t. | bolus | platelets >20,000/µl |
| | 28-48 | **Mercaptopurine** | 60mg/m² | | oral | | evenings before food, not to be taken with milk |
| | 28, 48 | **Cyclophosphamide** | 1000mg/m² | 500ml Saline 0.9% | i.v. | 1h | fluid balance, hydration + diuresis at least 2 liters of fluid /24 hours |
| | 30-33,37-40,44-47 | **Cytarabine** | 75mg/m² | 250ml Saline 0.9% | i.v. | 1h | |
| | from day 28 | **Filgrastim** | 5µg/kg | | s.c. | | until granulocytes >1000/µl |

Cycle Diagram columns: d1 w1, d8 w2, d15 w3, d22 w4, d29 w5, d36 w6, d43 w7, d50

Cycle Diagram rows: Rituximab., Methotrexate i.t., Mercaptopurine, Cyclophos., Cytarabine, Filgrastim

### Cautions

**Please note:** after days 27 and 48 protocol for prophylaxis of delayed emesis! (Please contact consultant in charge with queries regarding Dexamethasone)

**Please note:** days 27 & 48   bone marrow biopsy
days 27 & 48   send sample for MRD evaluation
days 27 to 48   CNS irradiation with 24 Gy!
days 30, 37, 44   lumbar puncture

With cytopenia: withhold all cytostatic agents but continue radiotherapy, see study protocol page 30

## Obligatory Pre- and Concurrent Medication

| Week | Day | Sequence and Timing | Compounds (generic names) | Amount Per Dose | Diluent | Route | Duration of Infusion | Comments |
|---|---|---|---|---|---|---|---|---|
| | 27 | -1h | Paracetamol | 1000mg | | oral | | |
| | 27 | -30min | Clemastine | 2mg | | i.v. | bolus | |
| | 28, 48 | 15' before chemotherapy | Saline 0.9% | | at least 2000ml | i.v. | | |
| | 28, 48 | 0h, 4h & 8h after start of Cycloph. | Mesna | each dose is 20% that of Cyclophos. | | i.v. | bolus | |
| | 28, 48 | 15' before Cyclophosphamide | Dexamethasone | 20mg | | i.v. | bolus | |
| | 28,30-33,37-40,44-48 | 15' before chemotherapy | Granisetron | 3mg | | i.v. | bolus | |
| | from day 1 | 1 - 1 - 1 | Co-trimoxazole | 960mg | | oral | | till granulocytes >500/µl, then 960mg on Mon. Wed. Fri. |

**Medicines As Required:** Dexamethasone, Metoclopramide, Allopurinol according to serum uric acid, Sucralfate, Lynestrenol (5mg every 12 hours) or Primosiston® (1 tablet every 12 hours)

**Antibiotic Prophylaxis:** If neutrophils < 500/µl: Colistin 200mg every 8 hours; Amphotericin B suspension 5ml every 6 hours, continue prophylaxis until granulocyte count stable at >500/µl

**Routine Tests:** 3x/ week: FBC, ATIII; daily: fibrinogen TP, PTT; serum Asparaginase level on days 28 and 34; at least 1/week: transaminases, amylase, blood glucose, U&Es; serum creatinine, uric acid, urine testing, ECG, CXR; Methotrexate overdose: cerebrospinal fluid exchange; Rituximab: caution: cytokine release syndrome

**Dose Reduction:** Mercaptopurine: if Allopurinol is necessary, then reduce dose to 1/3 (potentiation); TPMT deficiency: reduce dose to 10%; Cytarabine: reduce dose with renal failure

**Withhold Therapy:** With severe organotoxicity, severe infection or mucositis, granulocytes <200/µl, platelets <20,000/µl
Rituximab: immediately with occurrence of unwanted side effects; with abatement of symptoms, restart infusion at 50% normal rate

**References:** Study protocol "Multicenter study for therapy optimization of acute lymphatic leukemia in adults and adolescents from 15 years"; with Rituximab to improve prognosis with CD20+ standard risk ALL"

# Consolidation I GMALL 07/2003 + Rituximab

**Indication: ALL (CD20+)**　　**ICD-10: C91.0**　　**11.1.4**

Study protocol: Cytarabine/Dexa/Etopo/MTX/Vindesine /Ritux+ i.t.

**Rituximab application:** day 71, week 11

\* Rituximab application:
>20% CD 20 positive cells

This chemotherapy may cause life-threatening toxicity! It should only be administered under the supervision of an experienced medical oncologist! The protocol must first be reviewed and considered in relationship to the clinical situation of the patient.

## Chemotherapy

| Week | Day | Compounds (generic names) in chronological order | Dosage | Diluent | Route | Duration of infusion | Comments |
|---|---|---|---|---|---|---|---|
| | 0 | **Rituximab\*** | 375mg/m² | 500ml Saline 0.9% | i.v. | initially 50mg/h | monitor closely, resuscitation equipment! |
| | 1-5 | **Dexamethasone** | 10mg/m² | | oral | | in 3 divided doses |
| | 1 | **Vindesine (maximum single dose 5mg)** | 3mg/m² | in 5ml Saline 0.9% | i.v. | bolus | Itraconazole NOT to be given in parallel! |
| | 1 | **Methotrexate** | 1.5g/m² (1g/m² >55 years) | 500ml Saline 0.9% | i.v. | 24h | 10% in 30 minutes, 90% in 23.5 hours |
| | 4, 5 | **Etoposide (VP-16)** | 250mg/m² | 250ml Saline 0.9% | i.v. | 1h | dose at 12 noon, 6h after 1st Cytarabine dose |
| | 5 | **Cytarabine** | 2g/m² (1g/m² >55 years) twice a day | 250ml Saline 0.9% | i.v. | 3h | every 12 hours in each case; monitor |
| | from day 7 | **Filgrastim** | 5µg/kg | | s.c. | | continue until granulocytes >1000 |
| | 12 | **MTX/AraC/Dexa "triple prophylaxis"** | | | i.t. | | CSF exchange with overdose! |

Day 1 (71): bone marrow biopsy/ MRD evaluation
Note: Leucovorin Rescue according to MTX-ALL sheets in database (see appendix)

| Cycle Diagram | d0 | d1(71) w11 | d8(78)w12 |
|---|---|---|---|
| Rituximab | | | |
| Dexamethasone | | | |
| Vindesine | | | |
| Methotrexate | | | |

| Cycle Diagram continued | d0 | d1(71) w11 | d8(78)w12 |
|---|---|---|---|
| Etoposide | | | |
| Cytarabine | | | |
| Filgrastim | | | ----------> |
| MTX/AraC/Dexa i.t. | | | |

**Cautions**

## Obligatory Pre- and Concurrent Medication

| Week | Day | Sequence and Timing | Compounds (generic names) | Amount Per Dose | Diluent | Route | Duration of Infusion | Comments |
|---|---|---|---|---|---|---|---|---|
| | 0 | -1h | Paracetamol | 1000mg | | oral | bolus | |
| | 0 | -30min | Clemastine | 2mg | | i.v. | bolus | |
| | 1-3 | continuously | Saline 0.9% + Gluc.5% alternately | | 3000ml + 1000ml | i.v. | 24h | at least 3000ml/m² |
| | | | + Potassium Chloride | 20mmol/1000ml | in infusion fluid | | | check serum potassium |
| | | | + Sodium Bicarbonate | 40mmol/1000ml | in infusion fluid | | | urine pH >7.2 during MTX + for 48h after |
| | 1-4 | 1 - 1 - 1 - 1 | Sodium Bicarbonate | 2g | | oral | | |
| | 1 | 6h and 12h after start of Methotrexate | Furosemide | 40mg | | i.v. | bolus | |
| | 1 | 1 - 0 - 1 | Lactulose | 10g | | oral | | for constipation prophylaxis |
| | 1, 4, 5 | 15' before chemotherapy | Granisetron | 3mg | | i.v. | bolus | increase dose to 3mg with emesis |
| | 4 | 15' before chemotherapy | Saline 0.9% | | 1000ml | i.v. | 12h | |
| | 5-7 | continuously | Saline 0.9% | | 3000ml | i.v. | 24h | |
| | 5-7 | every 2 hours | Dexamethasone eye drops (1mg/ml) | 2-3 drops | | each eye | | in alternation |
| | | | Saline 0.9% eye drops | | | | | |
| | from day 1 | 1 - 1 - 1 | Co-trimoxazole | 960mg | | oral | | till granulocytes >500/µl, then 960mg on Mon. Wed. Fri. |
| | 1-5 | 1 - 0 - 0 - 0 | Sucralfate | 1g | | oral | | |

**Medicines As Required:** Metoclopramide, Sodium Bicarbonate orally, Furosemide 20mg i.v. with >1kg weight gain; conjunctivitis: Carbomer gel/Dexpanthenol eye ointment for 24 hours

**Antibiotic Prophylaxis:** If neutrophils < 500/µl: Colistin 200mg twice a day (1 - 0 - 1); Amphotericin B suspension 5ml every 6 hours, continue prophylaxis until granulocyte count stable at >500/µl

**Routine Tests:** Daily: serum creatinine, AST (SGOT), ALT (SGPT), bilirubin; 3x/ week: FBC; 1/week: ATIII, transaminases, amylase, U&Es, blood glucose, clotting studies, uric acid, urine testing, fluid balance, ECG, exclude third space fluid accumulation, neurotoxicity, conjunctivitis, conjunctivitis, serum Methotrexate level; Rituximab: caution: cytokine release syndrome; cytopenia: 1/week:CXR

**Dose Reduction:** With cytopenia, withhold therapy (no dose reduction); with cerebellar or cerebral symptoms, discontinue therapy; **Methotrexate, Etoposide Phosphate:** reduce dose with renal or hepatic failure; **Vindesine:** reduce dose with hepatotoxicity or neurotoxicity (by 50% with paresthesias, discontinue with pareses or paralytic ileus), with venous pain or spasm: stop and inject remainder into another large vein

**Withhold Therapy:** With **high-dose Cytarabine:** therapy-refractory conjunctivitis, severe allergic reactions, severe neurological symptoms, transaminases > 5 times upper limit of normal

**References:** Study protocol: GMALL 07/2003+Rituximab

# Consolidation II, III, VI GMALL 07/2003 + Rituximab

**Indication: ALL (CD20+)**  **ICD-10: C91.0**  **11.1.5**

**Study protocol: High-Dose Methotrexate/Asparaginase/Rituximab**

| * Rituximab application: | weeks 16, 30, 46 |
|---|---|
| >20% CD 20 positive cells | |

*This chemotherapy may cause life-threatening toxicity! It should only be administered under the supervision of an experienced medical oncologist! The protocol must first be reviewed and considered in relationship to the clinical situation of the patient.*

## Chemotherapy

| Week | Day | Compounds (generic names) in chronological order | Dosage | Diluent | Route | Duration of Infusion | Comments |
|---|---|---|---|---|---|---|---|
| 16 and 30 only | 0 | **Rituximab*** | 375mg/m² | 500ml Saline 0.9% | i.v. | initially 100mg/h | monitor closely, resuscitation equipment! |
| 16, 30, 46 | 1-7, 15-21 | **Mercaptopurine** | 60 mg/m² | | oral | | evenings before food, not to be taken with milk |
| 16, 30, 46 | 1, 15 | **Methotrexate** | 1.5g/m² (1g/m² >55 years) | 500ml Saline 0.9% | i.v. | 24h | 10% in 30 minutes, 90% in 23.5 hours |
| 16, 30, 46 | 2, 16 | **PEG-Asparaginase** | 500 IU/m² | 100ml Saline 0.9% | i.v. | 2h | monitor during infusion! |

| Cycle Diagram | d0 d1 | d8 | d15 | d22 |
|---|---|---|---|---|
| | w16, 30 | w17, 31 | w18, 32 | |
| Rituximab | | | | |
| Mercaptopurine | | | | |
| Methotrexate | | | | |
| Asparaginase | | | | |

| | d0 d1 | d8 | d15 | d22 |
|---|---|---|---|---|
| | w46 | w47 | w48 | w49 |

**Cautions**

Between Consolidation Blocks III-VI and after Consolidation VI, maintenance therapy until stratification according to MRD evaluation: (granulocytes >1500, platelets >100,000, hemoglobin >10)

| Mercaptopurine | once a day (1 - 0 - 0) | 60mg/m² | oral |
|---|---|---|---|
| Methotrexate | once a week | 20mg/m² | i.v. |

Bone marrow biopsy/MRD evaluation: day 1 of weeks 16, 30 and 52!
Week 46: bone marrow biopsy only! From week 52: triple prophylaxis
Rituximab only in weeks 16 and 30! Week 16: lumbar puncture
Serum Methotrexate level and Leucovorin rescue according to data sheets **Consider Leucovorin Rescue!**

## Obligatory Pre- and Concurrent Medication

| Week | Day | Compounds (generic names) | Amount Per Dose | Diluent | Route | Duration of Infusion | Comments |
|---|---|---|---|---|---|---|---|
| 16, 30, 46 | 0 | Paracetamol | 1000mg | | oral | | |
| 16, 30, 46 | 0 | Clemastine | 2mg | | i.v. | bolus | |
| 16, 30, 46 | 1-3,15-17 | Saline 0.9% + Gluc.5% alternately | 3000ml/m² | (3000ml) + 1000ml | i.v. | 24h | at least 3000ml/m² |
| | | + Potassium Chloride | 20mmol/1000ml | in infusion fluid | | | according to serum potassium |
| | | + Sodium Bicarbonate | 40mmol/1000ml | in infusion fluid | | | urine pH >7.2 during MTX + for 48h after |
| 16, 30, 46 | 1, 15 | Furosemide | 40mg | | i.v. | bolus | 6h and 12h after start of Methotrexate |
| 16, 30, 46 | 1, 15 | Dexamethasone | 20mg | | i.v. | bolus | 15' before chemotherapy |
| 16, 30, 46 | 1, 15 | Granisetron | 3mg | | i.v. | bolus | 15' before chemotherapy |
| 16, 30, 46 | from day 1 | Co-trimoxazole | 960mg | | oral | | till granulocytes >500/µl, then 960mg on Mon. Wed. Fri. |

| **Medicines As Required:** | Metoclopramide oral or i.v.; Granisetron i.v.; Sodium Bicarbonate orally |
|---|---|
| **Antibiotic Prophylaxis:** | If neutrophils < 500/µl: Amphotericin B suspension 5ml every 6 hours; in the case of neutropenia >10 days, add Colistin 150mg twice a day (1 - 0 - 1) |
| **Routine Tests:** | 3x/ week: FBC; Asparaginase: before therapy: LFTs, clotting studies; daily: fibrinogen, ATIII, TP, PTT (D-dimer test); 2-3x/ week: serum Asparaginase level, caution: hyperglycemia |
| **Contraindications:** | thrombotic tendency, coagulation disorders, severe hemorrhagic complications, hepatic impairment, past history of pancreatitis, caution: hypertension (danger of hemorrhage); Mercaptopurine: LFTs; Methotrexate: daily: serum creatinine, bilirubin, AST (SGOT), ALT (SGPT), neurotoxicity, fluid balance, serum Methotrexate level! |
| | Rituximab: caution: cytokine release syndrome; 1/week: blood glucose profile, amylase, transaminases, U&Es, serum creatinine, uric acid, urine testing, ECG |
| **Dose Reduction:** | L-Asparaginase: fibrinogen < 80mg/dl or ATIII level drops to <70% -> give FFP; stop infusion with complications that have previously occurred during administration |
| | Mercaptopurine: if Allopurinol is necessary, then reduce dose to 1/3, TPMT deficiency: reduce dose to 10% |
| | Methotrexate: reduce dose with 3rd space fluid accumulation, renal failure depending on serum creatinine (see study protocol), hepatic failure |
| | Rituximab: withhold with severe unwanted side effects; with abatement of symptoms, restart infusion at 50% normal rate |
| **References:** | Study protocol "Multicenter study for therapy optimization of acute lymphatic leukemia in adults and adolescents from 15 years", with Rituximab to improve prognosis with CD20+ standard risk ALL" |

| Consolidation II | GMALL 07/2003 | Indication: ALL | 11.1.6 |
|---|---|---|---|

high risk/T-ALL

Study protocol: Clad/VP16/Cytarabine + i.t.    **Week 16 Arm A**    high risk/T-ALL:    week 16

## Chemotherapy

| Week | Day | Compounds (generic names) in chronological order | Dosage | Diluent | Route | Duration of Infusion | Comments |
|---|---|---|---|---|---|---|---|
| | 1 | **Cytarabine** | 40mg | in 2ml water | i.t. | bolus | |
| | 1 | **Dexamethasone** | 4mg | undiluted | i.t. | bolus | |
| | 1 | **Methotrexate** | 15mg | in 3ml water | i.t. | bolus | |
| | 1-5 | **Cladribine (2-CdA)** | 0.2mg/m² | 500ml Saline 0.9% | i.v. | 2h | |
| | 1-5 | **Etoposide Phosphate** | 60mg/m² | 100ml Saline 0.9% | i.v. | bolus 15min | as Etoposide Phosphate |
| | 1-5 | **Cytarabine** | 1.5g/m² (1g/m² >55 years) | 250ml Saline 0.9% | i.v. | 1h30min | from +6 hours of therapy |
| | from day 6 | **Filgrastim** | 5μg/kg | | s.c. | | until granulocytes >1000/μl |

Please note: bone marrow biopsy on day 1; send sample for MRD evaluation! See study protocol pages 34ff/141ff

Cautions: **Cytarabine: pulmonary edema**

| Cycle Diagram | d1 w16 | d8 w17 | d15 w18 |
|---|---|---|---|
| Cytarabine i.t. | | | |
| Dexamethasone i.t. | | | |
| Methotrexate i.t. | | | |
| Cladribine | | | |
| Etoposide | | | |
| Cytarabine | | | |
| Filgrastim | | | |

## Obligatory Pre- and Concurrent Medication

| Week | Day | Sequence and Timing | Compounds (generic names) | Amount Per Dose | Diluent | Route | Duration of Infusion | Comments |
|---|---|---|---|---|---|---|---|---|
| | 1-5 | continuously | Saline 0.9% | | 2000ml | i.v. | 24h | |
| | 1-5 | 15' before chemotherapy | Dexamethasone | 8mg | | i.v. | bolus | |
| | 1-5 | 15' before chemotherapy | Granisetron | 1mg | | i.v. | bolus | increase dose to 3mg with emesis |
| | 1-5 | every 2-3 hours, in alternation | Dexamethasone eye drops (1mg/ml) | 2 drops | | each eye | | to be given throughout the night, |
| | 1-5 | every 2-3 hours, in alternation | Saline 0.9% eye drops | 2 drops | | each eye | | if possible |
| | from day 1 | 1 - 0 - 1 (2x/week) | Co-trimoxazole | 960mg | | oral | | for infection prophylaxis |

**Medicines As Required:** Metoclopramide oral or i.v., for conjunctivitis: Carbomer gel every 8 hours to each eye, alternating with Dexpanthenol eye ointment every 8 hours to each eye

**Antibiotic Prophylaxis:** If granulocytes < 500/μl: Amphotericin B suspension 5ml every 6 hour, in the case of granulocytopenia (<500/μl) >10 days, add Colistin 95mg every 6 hours (1-1-1-1)

**Routine Tests:** FBC (with **lymphocyte subpopulations**), U&Es, LFTs, clotting studies, serum creatinine, creatinine clearance, fluid balance, **caution:** pulmonary edema with Cytarabine

**Dose Reduction:** **Etoposide:** reduce dose with renal or hepatic failure; **Cytarabine:** reduce dose to 1g/m² with renal failure and in patients >55 years; discontinue treatment in patients with advanced therapy-refractive disease, conjunctivitis, severe allergic reactions, severe neurological symptoms, transaminases > 5x original level

**References:** Study protocol "Multicenter study for therapy optimization of acute lymphatic leukemia in adults and adolescents from 15 years, GMALL 07/2003"

*This chemotherapy may cause life-threatening toxicity! It should only be administered under the supervision of an experienced medical oncologist! The protocol must first be reviewed and considered in relationship to the clinical situation of the patient.*

| Consolidation II high/very high risk | GMALL 07/2003 | Indication: ALL | 11.1.7 |
|---|---|---|---|
| Study protocol: Idarubicin/FLAG | Week 16 Arm B | high/very high risk ALL:  precursor B-cell or T-cell ALL  week 16 | |

*This chemotherapy may cause life-threatening toxicity! It should only be administered under the supervision of an experienced medical oncologist! The protocol must first be reviewed and considered in relationship to the clinical situation of the patient.*

## Chemotherapy

| Week | Day | Compounds (generic names) in chronological order | Dosage | Diluent | Route | Duration of Infusion | Comments |
|---|---|---|---|---|---|---|---|
| | 1 | **Methotrexate** | 15mg | in 3ml water | i.t. | bolus | before systemic therapy |
| | 1 | **Dexamethasone** | 4mg | undiluted | i.t. | bolus | before systemic therapy |
| | 1 | **Cytarabine** | 40mg | in 2ml water | i.t. | bolus | before systemic therapy |
| | 1, 3 | **Idarubicin** | 10mg/m² (7mg/m² >55 years) | undiluted | i.v. | bolus 15min | 15min before Cytarabine |
| | 1-5 | **Fludarabine** | 30mg/m² | 250ml Saline 0.9% | i.v. | 1h | |
| | 1-5 | **Cytarabine** | 2g/m² (1g/m² >55 years) | 250ml Saline 0.9% | i.v. | 2h | 4h after end of Fludarabine infusion |
| | from day 7 | **Filgrastim** | 5µg/kg | | s.c. | | until granulocytes >1000/µl |

**Please note:** bone marrow biopsy on day 1; send sample for MRD evaluationl See study protocol pages 34ff/141ff

**Cautions**

Anthracycline dose reduction: with hepatic impairment, pre-existing cardiac impairment; see Dose Modification Table

| Cycle Diagram | | d1 w16 | d8 w17 | d15 w18 |
|---|---|---|---|---|
| Methotrexate i.t. | | | | |
| Dexamethasone i.t. | | | | |
| Cytarabine i.t. | | | | |
| Idarubicin | | | | |
| Fludarabine | | | | |
| Cytarabine | | | | |
| Filgrastim | | | | |

## Obligatory Pre- and Concurrent Medication

| Week | Day | Sequence and Timing | Compounds (generic names) | Amount Per Dose | Diluent | Route | Duration of Infusion | Comments |
|---|---|---|---|---|---|---|---|---|
| | 1-5 | continuously | Saline 0.9% | | 2000ml | i.v. | 24h | |
| | 1-5 | 15' before chemotherapy | Dexamethasone | 20mg | 100ml Saline 0.9% | i.v. | bolus 15min | |
| | 1-5 | 15' before chemotherapy | Granisetron | 1mg | | i.v. | bolus | increase dose to 3mg with emesis |
| | 1-7 | every 4 hours | Dexamethasone eye drops (1mg/ml) | 2 drops | | each eye | | alternating with Saline eye drops |
| | 1-14 | every 4 hours | Saline 0.9% eye drops | 2-3 drops | | each eye | | alternating with Dexamethasone eye drops |
| | from day 1 | 1 - 0 - 1 (2x/week) | Co-trimoxazole | 960mg | | oral | | for infection prophylaxis |

| Medicines As Required: | Metoclopramide; for conjunctivitis: Carbomer gel every 8 hours to each eye, alternating with Dexpanthenol eye ointment every 8 hours to each eye |
|---|---|
| Antibiotic Prophylaxis: | If neutrophils < 500/µl: Colistin 95mg twice a day (1 - 1 - 1 - 1) Amphotericin B suspension 5ml every 6 hours, continue prophylaxis until granulocyte count stable at >500/µl |
| Routine Tests: | FBC, U&Es, LDH, LFTs, clotting studies, serum creatinine, uric acid, blod gases, cardiac function, neurotoxicity, ECG before Idarubicin therapy |
| Dose Reduction: | With renal failure, cerebellar symptoms, exanthema, bilirubin >3.0 mg/dl, raised AST (SGOT) or ALP: Stop **Cytarabine**; with cytopenia, withhold therapy (no dose reduction); **Anthracycline:** see cautions above |
| References: | Study protocol "Multicenter study for therapy optimization of acutely phatic leukemia in adults and adolescents from 15 years, GMALL 07/2003" |

| Consolidation IV GMALL 07/2003 + Rituximab | Indication: ALL (CD20+) | ICD-10: C91.0    11.1.8 |
|---|---|---|

**Study protocol: Etoposide Phosphate/Cytarabine/Rituximab**

| * Rituximab application: | week 36 |
|---|---|
| >20% CD 20 positive cells | |

*This chemotherapy may cause life-threatening toxicity! It should only be administered under the supervision of an experienced medical oncologist! The protocol must first be reviewed and considered in relationship to the clinical situation of the patient.*

## Chemotherapy

| Week | Day | Compounds (generic names) in chronological order | Dosage | Diluent | Route | Duration of Infusion | Comments |
|---|---|---|---|---|---|---|---|
| | 0 | **Rituximab*** | 375mg/m² | 500ml Saline 0.9% | i.v. | initially 50mg/h | monitor closely, resuscitation equipment! |
| | 1-5 | **Cytarabine** | 150mg/m² | 250ml Saline 0.9% | i.v. | 1h | Cytarabine infusion before Etop.Phos.infusion |
| | 1-5 | **Etoposide Phosphate** | 100mg/m² | 100ml Saline 0.9% | i.v. | 1h | monitor |
| | 1 | **MTX/AraC/Dexa "triple prophylaxis"** | | | i.t. | | |

Between consolidation therapies IV and V: maintenance therapy with Mercaptopurine/Methotrexate
Note: lumbar puncture weekly on day 1
Rituximab: cytokine release syndrome

**Cautions**

| Cycle Diagram | dd d1 w1 | d8 w2 | d15 w3 | d |
|---|---|---|---|---|
| Rituximab | | | | |
| Cytarabine | | | | |
| Etoposide Phosph. | | | | |
| MTX/AraC/Dexa i.t. | | | | |

## Obligatory Pre- and Concurrent Medication

| Week | Day | Sequence and Timing | Compounds (generic names) | Dose | Diluent | Route | Duration of Infusion | Comments |
|---|---|---|---|---|---|---|---|---|
| | 0 | -1h | Paracetamol | 1000mg | | oral | | |
| | 0 | -30min | Clemastine | 2mg | | i.v. | bolus | |
| | 1-5 | 15' before chemotherapy | Granisetron | 3mg | | i.v. | bolus | |
| | 1-5 | 15' before chemotherapy | Dexamethasone | 8mg | | i.v. | 15min | |
| | 1-5 | 15' before chemotherapy | Saline 0.9% | | 250ml | i.v. | 2h30min | |
| | from day 1 | Mon. & Thurs. 1 - 0 - 1 | Co-trimoxazole | 960mg | | oral | | |
| | from day 1 | Mon. & Thurs. 1 - 0 - 1 | Folic Acid | 5mg | | oral | | |

| | |
|---|---|
| **Medicines As Required:** | Metoclopramide |
| **Routine Tests:** | 3x/ week: FBC; once a week: ATIII, transaminases, amylase, blood glucose, U&Es, serum creatinine, uric acid, urine testing, clotting studies, diuresis, neurotoxicity; |
| **Dose Reduction:** | **Methotrexate:** cerebrospinal fluid exchange with overdose; **Rituximab:** see **cautions** |
| | **Cytarabine:** reduce dose with renal failure, stop if transaminases > 5 times upper limit of normal, severe conjunctivitis, severe allergic reactions, severe neurological symptoms; with cytopenia, withhold therapy (no dose reduction); reduce dose with renal or hepatic failure (see Dose Modification Table); |
| | **Rituximab:** withhold therapy if severe side effects, with abatement of symptoms, restart infusion at 50% normal rate |
| **Max. Cum. Dose:** | Not defined |
| **References:** | Study protocol "Multicenter study for therapy optimization of acute lymphatic leukemia in adults and adolescents from 15 years", with Rituximab to improve prognosis with CD20+ standard risk ALL" |

# Consolidation V GMALL 07/2003 + Rituximab | Indication: ALL (CD20+) | ICD-10: C91.0 | 11.1.9

| Study protocol: Cyclophosphamide/Cytarabine/Rituximab | * Rituximab application: week 41 |
|---|---|
| | >20% CD 20 positive cells |

**This chemotherapy may cause life-threatening toxicity! It should only be administered under the supervision of an experienced medical oncologist! The protocol must first be reviewed and considered in relationship to the clinical situation of the patient.**

## Chemotherapy

| Week | Day | Compounds (generic names) in chronological order | Dosage | Diluent | Route | Duration of Infusion | Comments |
|---|---|---|---|---|---|---|---|
| | 0 | Rituximab* | 375mg/m² | 500ml Saline 0.9% | i.v. | initially 50mg/h | monitor closely, resuscitation equipment! |
| | 1 | Cyclophosphamide | 1000mg/m² | 500ml Saline 0.9% | i.v. | 1h | fluid balance |
| | 1 | Cytarabine | 500mg/m² | 250ml Saline 0.9% | i.v. | 24h | |
| | 1 | MTX/AraC/Dexa "triple prophylaxis" | | | i.t. | | |

Between consolidation therapies V and VI: maintenance therapy with Mercaptopurine/Methotrexate
Please note: day 1 - bone marrow biopsy
 - lumbar puncture
Please note: after day 1 protocol for prophylaxis of delayed emesis

**Cautions**

| Cycle Diagram | dd d1 w1 | d8 w2 | d15 w3 |
|---|---|---|---|
| Rituximab | | | |
| Cytarabine | | | |
| Etoposide Phosph. | | | |
| MTX/AraC/Dexa i.t. | | | |

## Obligatory Pre- and Concurrent Medication

| Week | Day | Sequence and Timing | Compounds (generic names) | Dose | Diluent | Route | Duration of Infusion | Comments |
|---|---|---|---|---|---|---|---|---|
| | 0 | -1h | Paracetamol | 1000mg | | oral | | |
| | 0 | -30min | Clemastine | 2mg | | i.v. | bolus | |
| | 1 | continuously | Saline 0.9% | | 2000ml | i.v. | 24h | hydration + diuresis at least 2000ml of fluid/24 hours |
| | 1 | 0h, 4h & 8h after start of Cycloph. | Mesna | each dose is 20% that of Cyclophos. | | i.v. | bolus | |
| | 1 | 15' before chemotherapy | Granisetron | 3mg | | i.v. | bolus | |
| | 1 | 15' before chemotherapy | Dexamethasone | 20mg | | i.v. | 15min | |
| | from day 1 | 960mg on Mon. Wed. and Fri. | Co-trimoxazole | 960mg | | oral | | |

**Medicines As Required:** Metoclopramide

**Routine Tests:** 3x/ week: FBC; once a week: ATIII, transaminases,amylase, blood glucose, U&Es, serum creatinine, uric acid, urine testing, clotting studies, ECG, neurotoxicity, conjunctivitis, fluid balance, diueresis + give at least 2 liters fluid per 24h; Methotrexate: cerebrospinal fluid exchange with overdose; cytopenia: 1/ week: CXR; Rituximab: cytokine release syndrome

**Dose Reduction:** With cerebellar symptoms, exanthema, bilirubin >3.0 mg/dl; with cytopenia, withhold therapy (no dose reduction); for patients with hepatic or renal failure, see Dose Modification Table
Cytarabine: reduce dose with renal failure, stop if severe conjunctivitis, severe allergic reactions, severe neurological symptoms, transaminases >5 times upper limit of normal;
Rituximab: withhold therapy if severe side effects; with abatement of symptoms, restart infusion at 50% normal rate

**Max. Cum. Dose:** Not defined

**References:** Study protocol "Multicenter study for therapy optimization of acute lymphatic leukemia in adults and adolescents from 15 years", with Rituximab to improve prognosis with CD20+ standard risk ALL"

| Reinduction I GMALL 07/2003 + Rituximab | Indication: ALL (CD20+) | ICD-10: C91.0 | 11.1.10 |
|---|---|---|---|

Study protocol: Vindesine/Doxorubicin/Rituximab

**\* Rituximab application:**
**>20% CD 20 positive cells**

**This chemotherapy may cause life-threatening toxicity! It should only be administered under the supervision of an experienced medical oncologist! The protocol must first be reviewed and considered in relationship to the clinical situation of the patient.**

**week 22**

## Chemotherapy

| Week | Day | Compounds (generic names) in chronological order | Dosage | Diluent | Route | Duration of Infusion | Comments |
|---|---|---|---|---|---|---|---|
| | 0 | **Rituximab\*** | 375mg/m² | 500ml Saline 0.9% | i.v. | Initially 50mg/h | monitor closely, resuscitation equipment! gradually withdraw in 3 stages every 3 |
| | 1-14 | **Prednisolone** | 20mg/m² every 8 hours | | oral | | days (giving 1/2, 1/4 and 1/8 of the dose) |
| | 1, 7 | **Vindesine (maximum single dose 5mg)** | 3mg/m² | in 5ml Saline 0.9% | i.v. | bolus | |
| | 1, 7 | **Doxorubicin** | 50mg/m² | undiluted | i.v. | 15min | via central line: 1h |
| | 1 | **MTX/AraC/Dexa "triple prophylaxis"** | | | i.t. | | |

Please note: day 1 - bone marrow biopsy
- lumbar puncture
Rituximab: cytokine release syndrome

| Cycle Diagram | d0 | d1 | w1 | d8 | w2 | d15 | w3 | d |
|---|---|---|---|---|---|---|---|---|
| Rituximab | | | | | | | | |
| Prednisolone | | | | | | | | |
| Vindesine | | | | | | | | |
| Doxorubicin | | | | | | | | |
| MTX/AraC/Dexa i.t. | | | | | | | | |

## Obligatory Pre- and Concurrent Medication

| Week | Day | Compounds (generic names) | Dose | Diluent | Route | Duration of Infusion | Comments |
|---|---|---|---|---|---|---|---|
| | 0 | Paracetamol | 1000mg | | oral | | |
| | 0 | Clemastine | 2mg | | i.v. | bolus | |
| | 1 | Zoledronic Acid | 4mg | | i.v. | | |
| | 1, 7 | Saline 0.9% | | 1000ml | i.v. | 4h | |
| | 1, 7 | Granisetron | 3mg | | i.v. | 15min | |
| | 1, 7 | Lactulose | 10g | | oral | | for constipation prophylaxis |
| | from day 1 | Sucralfate | 1g | | oral | | until Prednisolone withdrawn |
| | from day 1 | Co-trimoxazole | 960mg | | oral | | for infection prophylaxis |

**Medicines As Required:** Metoclopramide, Allopurinol

**Antibiotic Prophylaxis:** If neutrophils < 500/µl: Amphotericin B suspension 5ml every 6 hours; if neutrophils < 500/µl >10 days: Colistin 200mg twice a day (1 - 0 - 1)

**Routine Tests:** 3x/ week: FBC; once a week: ATIII, transaminases, amylase, blood glucose, U&Es, clotting studies, serum creatinine, uric acid, urine testing; cytopenia: 1/week: CXR;

**Doxorubicin:** ECG/echocardiogram before 1st dose + during therapy course, neurotoxicity; **Methotrexate:** CSF exchange with overdose; **Rituximab:** see **cautions**

**Dose Reduction:** With cytopenia, withhold therapy (no dose reduction); **Doxorubicin:** reduce dose with hepatic failure, reduce dose to 50% if bilirubin >2g/dl, contraindicated if bilirubin >5g/dl

**Vindesine:** reduce dose by 50% with pronounced paresthesia, hepatic failure, contraindicated with pareses, paralytic ileus;

**Rituximab:** withhold therapy if severe side effects; with abatement of symptoms, restart infusion at 50% normal rate

**Max. Cum. Dose:** **Doxorubicin** >550 mg/m²: Danger of cardiotoxicity; **Vindesine** 5-20mg: Danger of neurotoxicity

**References:** Study protocol "Multicenter study for therapy optimization of acute lymphatic leukemia in adults and adolescents from 15 years"; with Rituximab to improve prognosis with CD20+ standard risk ALL"

| Reinduction II | GMALL 07/2003 | Indication: ALL | 11.1.11 |
|---|---|---|---|

Study protocol: Cytarabine/Cyclo/Thioguanine

low risk ALL: weeks 24-25
high/very high risk ALL: weeks 24-25 (only patients without PBSCT)

*This chemotherapy may cause life-threatening toxicity! It should only be administered under the supervision of an experienced medical oncologist! The protocol must first be reviewed and considered in relationship to the clinical situation of the patient.*

## Chemotherapy

| Week | Day | Compounds (generic names) in chronological order | Dosage | Diluent | Route | Duration of Infusion | Comments |
|---|---|---|---|---|---|---|---|
| | 15 | Cytarabine | 40mg | in 2ml water | i.t. | bolus | |
| | 15 | Dexamethasone | 4mg | undiluted | i.t. | bolus | |
| | 15 | Methotrexate | 15mg | in 3ml water | i.t. | bolus | |
| | 15 | Cyclophosphamide | 1000mg/m² | 500ml Saline 0.9% | i.v. | 1h | |
| | 15-28 | Thioguanine | 60mg/m² | | oral | | with plenty of fluid, preferably on an empty stomach |
| | 17-20, 24-27 | Cytarabine | 75mg/m² | 250ml Saline 0.9% | i.v. | 1h | |

Cycle Diagram

| | d1 w22 | d8 w23 | d15 w24 | d22 w25 | d29 w26 | d36 |
|---|---|---|---|---|---|---|
| Cytarabine i.t. | | | | | | |
| Dexamethasone i.t. | | | | | | |
| Methotrexate i.t. | | | | | | |
| Cyclophosphamide | | | | | | |
| Thioguanine | | | | | | |
| Cytarabine | | | | | | |

**Cautions**

## Obligatory Pre- and Concurrent Medication

| Week | Day | Sequence and Timing | Compounds (generic names) | Amount Per Dose | Diluent | Route | Duration of Infusion | Comments |
|---|---|---|---|---|---|---|---|---|
| | regularly | 1-0-0 | Sucralfate | 1g | | oral | | until Prednisolone withdrawn |
| | 15 | 15' before chemotherapy | Saline 0.9% | | 1000ml | i.v. | 4h | |
| | 15 | 15' before, 4h, 8h after Cycloph. | Mesna | each dose is 20% that of Cyclophos. | | i.v. | bolus | |
| | 15 | 15' before chemotherapy | Granisetron | 1mg | | i.v. | bolus | |
| | 15, 17-20, 24-27 | 15' before chemotherapy | Dexamethasone | 8mg | | i.v. | bolus | |
| | 17-20, 24-27 | 15' before & 8h after chemo. | Metoclopramide | 50mg | | oral/i.v. | bolus | |
| | 16 | 1 - 1 - 1 - 1 | Metoclopramide | 30mg | | oral | bolus | = prophylaxis for delayed emesis |
| | 16 | 1 - 0 - 0 - 1 | Dexamethasone | 8mg | | oral | bolus | = prophylaxis for delayed emesis |
| | from day 1 | 1 - 0 - 1 (2x/week) | Co-trimoxazole | 960mg | | oral | | for infection prophylaxis |

Medicines As Required: Granisetron

Antibiotic Prophylaxis: If neutrophils < 500/µl: Amphotericin B suspension 5ml every 6 hours  If neutrophils < 500/µl >10 days: Colistin 95mg twice a day (1 - 1- 1 - 1)

Routine Tests: FBC, U&Es, LFTs, clotting studies, serum creatinine, creatinine clearance, uric acid

Dose Reduction: Thioguanine, Cyclophosphamide: impaired liver or renal function (Cyclophosphamide: see Dose Modification Table), w cytopenia, withhold therapy (no dose reduction)
Methotrexate: see Dose Modification Table

Max. Cum. Dose: Not defined

References: Study protocol "Multicenter study for therapy optimization of acute lymphatic leukemia in adults and adolescents from 15 years, GMALL 07/2003"

# Maintenance Therapy    GMALL 07/2003    Indication: ALL    11.1.12

low risk ALL patients: **weeks 26-29; 33-35; 37-40; 42-45**

high/very high risk ALL (only patients without PBSCT): **weeks 26-29; 33-35; 37-40; 42-45**

*This chemotherapy may cause life-threatening toxicity! It should only be administered under the supervision of an experienced medical oncologist! The protocol must first be reviewed and considered in relationship to the clinical situation of the patient.*

## Chemotherapy

| Week | Day | Compounds (generic names) in chronological order | Dosage | Diluent | Route | Duration of Infusion | Comments |
|---|---|---|---|---|---|---|---|
| | 1, 8, 15 (22) | **Methotrexate** | 20mg/m² | undiluted | i.v. | bolus | |
| | 1-21 (-28) | **Mercaptopurine** | 60mg/m² | | oral | | mornings, on an empty stomach |

**Cautions**

Cycle Diagram — Weeks: 1-25 | 26 | 27 | 28 | 29 | 30 | 31 | 32 | 33 | 34 | 35 | 36 | 37 | 38 | 39 | 40 | 41 | 42 | 43 | 44 | 45

| Cycle Diagram | d1 w1 | d8 w2 | d15 w3 | d22 w4 | d29 w5 |
|---|---|---|---|---|---|
| Methotrexate | | | | | |
| Mercaptopurine | | | | | |

## Obligatory Pre- and Concurrent Medication

| Week | Day | Sequence and Timing | Compounds (generic names) | Amount Per Dose | Diluent | Route | Duration of Infusion | Comments |
|---|---|---|---|---|---|---|---|---|
| | 1, 8, 15 (22) | -15 min | Saline 0.9% | | 500ml | i.v. | 1h | |
| | 1, 8, 15 (22) | -15 min | Dexamethasone | 4mg | | i.v. | bolus | |
| | from day 1 | 1 - 0 - 1 (2x/week) | Co-trimoxazole | 960mg | | oral | | for infection prophylaxis |

| | |
|---|---|
| Medicines As Required | Metoclopramide |
| Antibiotic Prophylaxis: | If neutrophils < 500/µl: Colistin 95mg(1-1-1) (granulocytopenia >10 days), Amphotericin B suspension 5ml every 6 hours |
| Routine Tests: | FBC, U&Es, LFTs, clotting studies, serum creatinine, creatinine clearance, uric acid |
| Dose Reduction: | If Allopurinol is necessary, reduce **Mercaptopurine** dose to 1/3 (potentiation); with cytopenia, reduce dose as follows: leukocytes 3000-2000 or platelets 100,000-150,000: reduce **Mercaptopurine+Methotrexate** to 66%; leukocytes 2000-1500 or platelets 50,000-100,000: reduce **Mercaptopurine+Methotrexate** to 50%; leukocytes <1500 or platelets < 50,000: withhold therapy |
| References: | Study protocol "Multicenter study for therapy optimization of acute lymphatic leukemia in adults and adolescents from 15 years, GMALL 07/2003" |

# Prephase: GMALL B-ALL/NHL 2002

## Indication: B-ALL/Burkitt's Lymphoma

**11.1.13**

*This chemotherapy may cause life-threatening toxicity! It should only be administered under the supervision of an experienced medical oncologist! The protocol must first be reviewed and considered in relationship to the clinical situation of the patient.*

## Chemotherapy

| Block Day | Protocol Day | Compounds (generic names) in chronological order | Dosage | Diluent | Route | Duration of Infusion | Comments |
|---|---|---|---|---|---|---|---|
| | 1-5 | **Prednisone** | 60mg/m² | | oral | | 3 doses |
| | 1-5 | **Cyclophosphamide** | 200mg/m² | 250ml Saline 0.9% | i.v. | 1h | |

**Please note: bone marrow biopsy before start of therapy: send bone marrow and peripheral blood samples for MRD evaluation**

**Cautions**

| Cycle Diagram | d1 w1 | d8 w2 | d15 w3 | d22 w4 |
|---|---|---|---|---|
| Prednisone | | | | |
| Cyclophos. | | | | |

## Obligatory Pre- and Concurrent Medication

| Block Day | Protocol Day | Compounds (generic names) | Sequence and Timing | Dose | Diluent | Route | Duration of Infusion | Comments |
|---|---|---|---|---|---|---|---|---|
| | 1-5 | Saline 0.9%+Sodium Bicarbonate | 12h before Cyclophosphamide | 40ml/1000ml | 2000ml | i.v. | 24h | in prehydration infusion, urine target pH >7.5 |
| | 1-5 | Mesna | 15' before, 4h & 8h after chemo. | 400mg/m² | | i.v. | | increase dose to 3mg with emesis |
| | 1-5 | Granisetron | 15' before chemotherapy | 1mg | | i.v. | bolus | may be given intravenously |
| | 1-5 | Metoclopramide | 30' before Cyclophosphamide | 50mg | | oral | | dose according to uric acid level |
| | 1-5 | Allopurinol | 1 - 0 - 0 | 300mg | | oral | | for infection prophylaxis |
| | from day 1 | Amphotericin B (as suspension) | 1 - 1 - 1 - 1 | 500mg | | oral | | for infection prophylaxis |
| | from day 1 | Co-trimoxazole | 1 - 0 - 1 (2x/week) | 960mg | | oral | | |

| | |
|---|---|
| Medicines As Required | Metoclopramide oral or i.v.; if not tolerated replace with 5-HT3 antagonists; Rasburicase |
| Antibiotic Prophylaxis: | If neutrophils < 500/µl: Colistin 95mg(1-1-1-1) three times a day |
| Routine Tests: | FBC, U&Es, serum creatinine, serum bilirubin, clotting studies, uric acid, weight, fluid balance |
| Dose Reduction: | Not defined |
| Max. Cum. Dose : | Unknown |
| References: | See multicenter study for therapy optimization in B-ALL and hg B-NHL in adults (GMALL-B-ALL/NHL 2002). |

## Block A: GMALL B-ALL/NHL 2002 | Indication: B-ALL/Burkitt's Lymphoma | 11.1.14

*This chemotherapy may cause life-threatening toxicity! It should only be administered under the supervision of an experienced medical oncologist! The protocol must first be reviewed and considered in relationship to the clinical situation of the patient.*

### Chemotherapy

Block: A1: days 7-12
A2: days 77-82

| Block Day | Protocol Day | Compounds (generic names) in chronological order | Dosage | Diluent | Route | Duration of Infusion | Comments |
|---|---|---|---|---|---|---|---|
| 1 | 7, 77 | Rituximab | 375mg/m² | 500ml Saline 0.9% | i.v. | initially 50mg/h | |
| 2-6 | 8-12, 78-82 | Dexamethasone | 10mg/m² | | oral | in 3 doses | |
| 2 | 8, 78 | Vincristine | 2mg absolute | undiluted | i.v. | bolus | |
| 2 | 8, 78 | Methotrexate | 1500mg/m² | 500ml Saline 0.9% | i.v. | 24h | 10% in 30min, 90% in 23 1/2 hours |
| 2-6 | 8-12, 78-82 | Ifosfamide | 800mg/m² | 500ml Saline 0.9% | i.v. | 1h | |
| 5-6 | 11-12, 81-82 | Cytarabine | 150mg/m² twice a day | 250ml Saline 0.9% | i.v. | 1h | every 12 hours |
| 5-6 | 11-12, 81-82 | Teniposide | 100mg/m² | 500ml Saline 0.9% | i.v. | 1h | ECG monitor |
| from day 8 | from days 14, 84 | Filgrastim | 5µg/kg (or 150µg/m²) | | s.c. | | until granulocytes >1000/µl for 2 days |
| 2+6 | 8+12, 78+82 | Cytarabine | 40mg | in 2ml water | i.t. | bolus | |
| 2+6 | 8+12, 78+82 | Dexamethasone | 4mg | undiluted | i.t. | bolus | |
| 2+6 | 8+12, 78+82 | Methotrexate | 15mg | in 2ml water | i.t. | bolus | |

**Cautions:** The combination of Vincristine and Itraconazole is neurotoxic!
For Methotrexate serum level determination and Leucovorin rescue: see attachment High-Dose Methotrexate

| Cycle Diagram (i.t.) | d1 w1 | d8 w2 | d71 w11 | d78 w12 | d85 w13 |
|---|---|---|---|---|---|
| Cytarabine i.t. | | | | | |
| Dexameth. i.t. | | | | | |
| Methotrexate i.t. | | | | | |

| Cycle Diagram | d1 w1 | d8 w2 | d71 w11 | d78 w12 | d |
|---|---|---|---|---|---|
| Rituximab | | | | | |
| Dexameth. | | | | | |
| Vincristine | | | | | |
| Methotrexate | | | | | |
| Ifosfamide | | | | | |
| Cytarabine | | | | | |
| Teniposide | | | | | |
| Filgrastim | | | | | |

### Obligatory Pre- and Concurrent Medication

| Block Day | Protocol Day | Compounds (generic names) | Sequence and Timing | Dose | Diluent | Route | Duration of Infusion | Comments |
|---|---|---|---|---|---|---|---|---|
| 1 | 7, 77 | Paracetamol | 1h before Rituximab | 1000mg | | oral | | |
| 1 | 7, 77 | Clemastine | 30' before Rituximab | 2mg | | i.v. | bolus | |
| 2-4 | 8-10, 78-80 | Saline 0.9% + Gluc.5% alternately + Potassium Chloride + Sodium Bicarbonate | continuously | | 3000ml + 1000ml in infusion fluid / 20ml/1000ml in infusion fluid / 40ml/1000ml in infusion fluid | i.v. | 24h | up to 3000ml/m² if possible, check serum potassium, urine target pH >7.5 |
| 5-6 | 11-12, 81-82 | Saline 0.9% | continuously | 2000ml | | i.v. | 24h | |
| 2 | 8, 78 | Furosemide | 6h and 12h after Methotrexate | 40mg | | i.v. | bolus | increase dose to 3mg with emesis |
| 2-6 | 8-12, 78-82 | Granisetron | 15' before chemotherapy | 1mg | | i.v. | bolus | |
| 2-6 | 8-12, 78-82 | Mesna | 15' before, 4h & 8h after chemo. | 160mg/m² | | i.v. | bolus | |
| 5-6 | 11-12, 81-82 | Metoclopramide | 15' before 2nd Cytarabine dose | 50mg | | i.v. | bolus | |
| 2-4 | 8-10, 78-80 | Sodium Bicarbonate | 1-1-1-1 | 2g | | oral | | |
| from day 1 | | Amphotericin B (as suspension) | 1-1-1-1 | 500mg | | oral | | for infection prophylaxis |
| from day 1 | | Folic Acid | 1-0-0 | 5mg | | oral | | |
| from day 1 | | Co-trimoxazole | 1-0-0-1 (2x/week) | 960mg | | oral | | for infection prophylaxis |

**Medicines As Required:** Metoclopramide oral or i.v.; if not tolerated replace with 5-HT3 antagonists; Rasburicase; Sodium Bicarbonate
**Antibiotic Prophylaxis:** If neutrophils < 500/µl: Colistin 200mg three times a day
**Routine Tests:** FBC, U&Es, LFTs, clotting studies, serum creatinine, creatinine clearan e, fluid balance, exclude third space fluid accumulation, serum Methotrexate level
**Dose Reduction:** Withhold therapy with cytopenia (no dose reduction): see study protocol
**References:** See multicenter study for therapy optimization in B-ALL and hg B-NHL in adults (GMALL-B-ALL/NHL 2002).

| Block A*: GMALL B-ALL/NHL 2002 | Indication: B-ALL/Burkitt's Lymphoma >55 years | 11.1.14 |

**Chemotherapy**

Block: A1*: days 7-12
A2*: days 49-54
A3*: days 98-103

*This chemotherapy may cause life-threatening toxicity! It should only be administered under the supervision of an experienced medical oncologist! The protocol must first be reviewed and considered in relationship to the clinical situation of the patient.*

| Block Day | Protocol Day | Compounds (generic names) in chronological order | Dosage | Diluent | Route | Duration of Infusion | Comments |
|---|---|---|---|---|---|---|---|
| 1 | 7, 49, 98 | Rituximab | 375mg/m² | 500ml Saline 0.9% | i.v. | initially 50mg/h | |
| 2-6 | 8-12,50-54,99-103 | Dexamethasone | 10mg/m² | | oral | | 3 doses |
| 2 | 8, 50, 99 | Methotrexate | 500mg/m² | 500ml Saline 0.9% | i.v. | 24h | 10% in 30min, 90% in 23 1/2 hours |
| 2-6 | 8-12,50-54,99-103 | Ifosfamide | 400mg/m² | 500ml Saline 0.9% | i.v. | 1h | *9+11, 51+53, 100+102 optional* |
| 5-6 | 11-12,53-54,102-103 | Cytarabine | 60mg/m² twice a day | 250ml Saline 0.9% | i.v. | 1h | every 12 hours |
| 5-6 | 11-12,53-54,102-103 | Teniposide | 60mg/m² | 500ml Saline 0.9% | i.v. | 1h | ECG monitor |
| from day 8 | daily from days 14,56,105 | Filgrastim | 5µg/kg (or 150µg/m²) | | s.c. | | until granulocytes >1000/µl for 2 days |
| 2 | 8, 50, 99 | Methotrexate | 12mg | in 2ml water | i.t. | bolus | |

**Cycle Diagram**

| | d1 w1 | d8 w2 | d43 w7 | d50 w8 | d92 w14 | d99 w15 | d |
|---|---|---|---|---|---|---|---|
| Rituximab | | | | | | | |
| Dexameth. | | | | | | | |
| Methotrexate | | | | | | | |
| Ifosfamide | | | | | | | |
| Cytarabine | | | | | | | |
| Teniposide | | | | | | | |
| Filgrastim | | | | | | | |
| Methotrexate i.t. | | | | | | | |

**Cautions**

For Methotrexate serum level determination and Leucovorin rescue: see attachment High-Dose Methotrexate!
The combination of Vincristine and Itraconazole is neurotoxic!

## Obligatory Pre- and Concurrent Medication

| Day | Sequence and Timing | Compounds (generic names) | Dose | Diluent | Route | Duration of Infusion | Comments |
|---|---|---|---|---|---|---|---|
| 7, 49, 98 | 1h before Rituximab | Paracetamol | 1000mg | | oral | | |
| 7, 49, 98 | 30' before Rituximab | Clemastine | 2mg | | i.v. | bolus | |
| 8-10,50-52,99-101 | continuously | Saline 0.9% + Gluc.5% alternately + Potassium Chloride + Sodium Bicarbonate | 20ml/1000ml 40ml/1000ml | 3000ml + 1000ml in infusion fluid in infusion fluid | i.v. | 24h | up to 3000ml/m² if possible check serum potassium urine target pH >7.5 |
| 11-12,53-54,102-103 | continuously | Saline 0.9% | 2000ml | | i.v. | 24h | |
| 8, 50, 99 | 6h and 12h after Methotrexate | Furosemide | 40mg | | i.v. | bolus | |
| 8-12,50-54,99-103 | 15' before chemotherapy | Granisetron | 1mg | | i.v. | bolus | increase dose to 3mg with emesis |
| 8-12,50-54,99-103 | 15' before, 4h & 8h after chemo. | Mesna | 80mg/m² | | i.v. | bolus | |
| 11-12,53-54,102-103 | 15' before 2nd Cytarabine dose | Metoclopramide | 50mg | | i.v. | bolus | |
| 8-10,50-52,99-101 | 1 - 1 - 1 | Sodium Bicarbonate | 2g | | oral | | |
| from day 1 | 1 - 1 - 1 - 1 | Amphotericin B (as suspension) | 500mg | | oral | | for infection prophylaxis |
| from day 1 | 1 - 0 - 1 | Folic Acid | 5mg | | oral | | |
| from day 1 | 1 - 0 - 1 (2x/week) | Co-trimoxazole | 960mg | | oral | | for infection prophylaxis |

**Medicines As Required:** Metoclopramide oral or i.v.; if not tolerated replace with 5-HT3 antagonists; Rasburicase; Sodium Bicarbonate

**Antibiotic Prophylaxis:** If neutrophils < 500/µl: Colistin 200mg three times a day

**Routine Tests:** FBC, U&Es, LFTs, clotting studies, serum creatinine, clearance, fluid balance, exclude third space fluid accumulation, serum Methotrexate level

**Dose Reduction:** Withhold therapy with cytopenia (no dose reduction); see study protocol

**References:** See multicenter study for therapy optimization in B-ALL and hg B-NHL in adults (GMALL-B-ALL/NHL 2002).

## Block B: GMALL B-ALL/NHL 2002

**Indication: B-ALL/Burkitt's Lymphoma**    11.1.15

*This chemotherapy may cause life-threatening toxicity! It should only be administered under the supervision of an experienced medical oncologist! The protocol must first be reviewed and considered in relationship to the clinical situation of the patient.*

### Chemotherapy

Block: B1: days 7-12
B2: days 77-82

| Block Day | Protocol Day | Compounds (generic names) in chronological order | Dosage | Diluent | Route | Duration of Infusion | Comments |
|---|---|---|---|---|---|---|---|
| 1 | 28, 98 | **Rituximab** | 375mg/m² | 500ml Saline 0.9% | i.v. | initially 50mg/h | |
| 2-6 | 29-33, 99-103 | **Dexamethasone** | 10mg/m² | undiluted | oral | | 3 doses |
| 2 | 29, 99 | **Vincristine** | 2mg absolute | | i.v. | bolus | |
| 2 | 29, 99 | **Methotrexate** | 1500mg/m² | 500ml Saline 0.9% | i.v. | 24h | 10% in 30min, 90% in 23 1/2 hours |
| 2-6 | 29-33, 99-103 | **Cyclophosphamide** | 200mg/m² | 250ml Saline 0.9% | i.v. | 1h | |
| 5-6 | 32-33, 102-103 | **Doxorubicin** | 25mg/m² | undiluted | i.v. | bolus 15min | |
| from day 8 | from days 35, 105 | **Filgrastim** | 5µg/kg (or 150µg/m²) | | s.c. | | until granulocytes >1000/µl for 2 days |
| 2+6 | 29+33, 99+103 | **Cytarabine** | 40mg | in 2ml water | i.t. | bolus | |
| 2+6 | 29+33, 99+103 | **Dexamethasone** | 4mg | undiluted | i.t. | bolus | |
| 2+6 | 29+33, 99+103 | **Methotrexate** | 15mg | in 3ml water | i.t. | bolus | |

*Cautions*

For Methotrexate serum level determination and Leucovorin rescue: see attachment High-Dose Methotrexate
Anthracycline: Danger of cardiotoxicity - echocardiogram

Cycle Diagram (i.t.): columns d22 w4 | d29 w5 | d92 w14 | d99 w15 | d106 w16
- Cytarabine i.t.
- Dexameth. i.t.
- Methotrexate i.t.

Cycle Diagram: columns d22 w4 | d29 w5 | d92 w14 | d99 w15 | d1
- Rituximab
- Dexameth.
- Vincristine
- Methotrexate
- Cyclophos.
- Doxorubicin
- Filgrastim

### Obligatory Pre- and Concurrent Medication

| Block Day | Protocol Day | Sequence and Timing | Compounds (generic names) | Dose | Diluent | Route | Duration of Infusion | Comments |
|---|---|---|---|---|---|---|---|---|
| 1 | 28, 98 | 1h before Rituximab | Paracetamol | 1000mg | | oral | | |
| 1 | 28, 98 | 30' before Rituximab | Clemastine | 2mg | | i.v. | bolus | |
| 2-4 | 29-31, 98-100 | continuously | Saline 0.9% + Gluc.5% alternately + Potassium Chloride + Sodium Bicarbonate | | 3000ml + 1000ml / 20ml/1000ml in infusion fluid / 40ml/1000ml in infusion fluid | i.v. | 24h | up to 3000ml/m² if possible check serum potassium urine target pH >7.5 |
| 5-6 | 23-33, 101-103 | continuously | Saline 0.9% | | 2000ml | i.v. | 24h | |
| 2 | 29, 99 | 6h and 12h after Methotrexate | Furosemide | 40mg | | i.v. | bolus | |
| 2-6 | 29-33, 99-103 | 15' before chemotherapy | Granisetron | 1mg | | i.v. | bolus | increase dose to 3mg with emesis |
| 2-6 | 29-33, 99-103 | 15' before, 4h & 8h after chemo. | Mesna | 40mg/m² | | i.v. | bolus | |
| 2-4 | 29-31, 98-100 | 2 - 2 - 2 - 2 | Sodium Bicarbonate | 1g | | oral | | |
| from day 1 | | 1 - 1 - 1 - 1 | Amphotericin B (as suspension) | 500mg | | oral | | for infection prophylaxis |
| from day 1 | | 1 - 0 - 1 (2x/week) | Co-trimoxazole | 960mg | | oral | | for infection prophylaxis |

**Medicines As Required:** Metoclopramide oral or i.v.; if not tolerated replace with 5-HT3 antagonists; Rasburicase
**Antibiotic Prophylaxis:** If neutrophils <500/µl: Colistin 95mg(1-1-1-1) three times a day
**Routine Tests:** see **cautions** above; FBC, U&Es, LFTs, clotting studies, serum creatinine, creatinine clearance, fluid balance, exclude third space fluid accumulati on, neurotoxicity
serum Methotrexate level
**Dose Reduction:** Withhold therapy with cytopenia (no dose reduction); see study protocol
**Max. Cum. Dose.:** **Anthracycline:** see **cautions** above; max. cum. dose is 550mg/m². **Vincristine** 5-20mg/m². **Vincristine** 5-20mg absolute: Danger of neurotoxicity
**Doxorubicin:** Danger of cardiotoxicity; max. cum. dose is 550mg/m² in B-ALL and hg B-NHL in adults (GMALL-B-ALL/NHL 2002).
**References:** See multicenter study for therapy optimization in B-ALL and hg B-NHL in adults (GMALL-B-ALL/NHL 2002).

# Block B*: GMALL B-ALL/NHL 2002 — Indication: B-ALL/Burkitt's Lymphoma >55 years — 11.1.15

**Block:** B1*: days 28-33
B2*: days 77-82
B3*: days 119-124

*This chemotherapy may cause life-threatening toxicity! It should only be administered under the supervision of an experienced medical oncologist! The protocol must first be reviewed and considered in relationship to the clinical situation of the patient.*

## Chemotherapy

| Block Day | Protocol Day | Compounds (generic names) in chronological order | Dosage | Diluent | Route | Duration of Infusion | Comments |
|---|---|---|---|---|---|---|---|
| 1 | 28, 77, 119 | Rituximab | 375mg/m² | 500ml Saline 0.9% | i.v. | initially 50mg/h | |
| 2-6 | 29-33,78-82,120-124 | Dexamethasone | 10mg/m² | | oral | | 3 doses |
| 2 | 29, 78, 120 | Vincristine | 1mg absolute | undiluted | i.v. | bolus | |
| 2 | 29, 78, 120 | Methotrexate | 500mg/m² | 500ml Saline 0.9% | i.v. | 24h | 10% in 30min, 90% in 23 1/2 hours |
| 2-6 | 29-33,78-82,120-124 | Cyclophosphamide | 200mg/m² | 250ml Saline 0.9% | i.v. | 1h | 30+32, 79+81, 121+123 *optional* |
| 5-6 | 32-33,81-82,123-124 | Doxorubicin | 25mg/m² | undiluted | i.v. | bolus 15min | |
| from day 8 | daily from days 35, 84, 126 | Filgrastim | 5µg/kg (or 150µg/m³) | | s.c. | | until granulocytes >1000/µl for 2 days |
| 2 | 29, 78, 120 | Methotrexate | 12mg | in 3ml water | i.t. | | |

**Cautions**

For Methotrexate serum level determination and Leucovorin rescue:
see attachment High-Dose Methotrexate
Anthracycline: Danger of cardiotoxicity - echocardiogram

| Cycle Diagram (i.t.) | d22 w4 | d29 w5 | d71 w11 | d78 w12 | d113 w17 | d120 w18 |
|---|---|---|---|---|---|---|
| Methotrexate i.t. | | | | | | |

| Cycle Diagram | d22 w4 | d29 w5 | d71 w11 | d78 w12 | d113 w17 | d120 w18 | d |
|---|---|---|---|---|---|---|---|
| Rituximab | | | | | | | |
| Dexameth. | | | | | | | |
| Vincristine | | | | | | | |
| Methotrexate | | | | | | | |
| Cyclophos. | | | | | | | |
| Doxorubicin | | | | | | | |
| Filgrastim | | | | | | | |

## Obligatory Pre- and Concurrent Medication

| Block Day | Protocol Day | Sequence and Timing | Compounds (generic names) | Dose | Diluent | Route | Duration of Infusion | Comments |
|---|---|---|---|---|---|---|---|---|
| 1 | 28, 77, 119 | 1h before Rituximab | Paracetamol | 1000mg | | oral | | |
| 1 | 28, 77, 119 | 30' before Rituximab | Clemastine | 2mg | | i.v. | bolus | |
| 2-4 | 29-31,78-80,120-12 | continuously | Saline 0.9% + Gluc.5% alternately + Potassium Chloride + Sodium Bicarbonate | 20ml/1000ml 40ml/1000ml | 3000ml + 1000ml in infusion fluid in infusion fluid | i.v. | 24h | up to 3000ml/m² if possible check serum potassium urine target pH >7.5 |
| 5-6 | 32-33,81-82,123-124 | continuously | Saline 0.9% | | 2000ml | i.v. | 24h | |
| 2 | 29, 78, 120 | 6h and 12h after Methotrexate | Furosemide | 1mg | | i.v. | bolus | increase dose to 3mg with emesis |
| 2-6 | 29-33,78-82,120-124 | 15' before chemotherapy | Granisetron | 1mg | | i.v. | bolus | |
| 2-6 | 29-33,78-82,120-124 | 15' before, 4h & 8h after chemo. | Mesna | 40mg/m² | | i.v. | bolus | |
| 2-4 | 29-31,78-80,120-122 | 2 - 2 - 2 - 2 | Sodium Bicarbonate | 1g | | oral | | for infection prophylaxis |
| | from day 1 | 1 - 1 - 1 - 1 | Amphotericin B (as suspension) | 500mg | | oral | | for infection prophylaxis |
| | from day 1 | 1 - 0 - 1 (2x/week) | Co-trimoxazole | 960mg | | oral | | |

**Medicines As Required:** Metoclopramide oral or i.v.; if not tolerated replace with 5-HT3 antagonists; Rasburicase; Sodium Bicarbonate

**Antibiotic Prophylaxis:** If neutrophils <500/µl: Colistin 95mg(1-1-1-1) three times a day

**Routine Tests:** **cautions** above; FBC, U&Es, LFTs, clotting studies, serum creatinine, creatinine clearance, fluid balance, exclude third space fluid accumulati on, neurotoxicity serum Methotrexate level

**Dose Reduction:** Withhold therapy with cytopenia (no dose reduction); see study protocol

**Max. Cum. Dose :** **Doxorubicin:** Danger of cardiotoxicity; max. cum. dose is 550mg/m². **Vincristine** 5-20mg absolute: Danger of neurotoxicity

**References:** See multicenter study for therapy optimization in B-ALL and hg B-NHL in adults (GMALL-B-ALL/NHL 2002).

845

**Block C: GMALL B-ALL/NHL 2002** | **Indication: B-ALL/Burkitt's Lymphoma** | **11.1.16**

*This chemotherapy may cause life-threatening toxicity! It should only be administered under the supervision of an experienced medical oncologist! The protocol must first be reviewed and considered in relationship to the clinical situation of the patient.*

## Chemotherapy

Block: C1: days 49-54
C2: days 119-124

| Block Day | Protocol Day | Compounds (generic names) in chronological order | Dosage | Diluent | Route | Duration of Infusion | Comments |
|---|---|---|---|---|---|---|---|
| 1 | 49, 119 | **Rituximab** | 375mg/m² | 500ml Saline 0.9% | i.v. | initially 50mg/h | |
| 2-6 | 50-54, 120-124 | **Dexamethasone** | 10mg/m² | | oral | | 3 doses |
| 2 | 50, 120 | **Vindesine** | 3mg/m²(5mgmax.) | | i.v. | bolus | |
| 2 | 50, 120 | **Methotrexate** | 1500mg/m² (>55 years: 500mg/m²) | in 5ml Saline 0.9% | i.v. | 24h | 10% in 30min, 90% in 23 1/2 hours |
| 5-6 | 53-54, 123-124 | **Etoposide Phosphate** | 250mg/m² (>55 years: 500mg/m²) | 100ml Saline 0.9% (from 200mg in 250ml) | i.v. | 1h | dose expressed in terms of Etoposide base |
| 6 | 54, 124 | **Cytarabine** | 2g/m² (>55 years: 1g/m²) twice a day | 250ml Saline 0.9% | i.v. | 1h | every 12 hours in each case |
| from day 8 | from days 56, 126 | **Filgrastim** | 5µg/kg (or 150µg/m²) | | s.c. | | until granulocytes >1000/µl for 2 days |

**Cautions**

Etoposide Phosphate and Sodium Bicarbonate must not be administered concomitantly through the same infusion site!
For Methotrexate serum level determination and Leucovorin rescue: see attachment High-Dose Methotrexate
Stem cell apheresis: following block C1 for all high-risk patients without a related donor

Cycle Diagram (d43 w7, d50 w8, d113 w17, d120 w18, d1...): Rituximab, Dexameth., Vindesine, Methotrexate, Etop. Phos., Cytarabine, Filgrastim

## Obligatory Pre- and Concurrent Medication

| Block Day | Protocol Day | Sequence and Timing | Compounds (generic names) | Dose | Diluent | Route | Duration of Infusion | Comments |
|---|---|---|---|---|---|---|---|---|
| 1 | 49, 119 | 1h before Rituximab | Paracetamol | 1000mg | | oral | | |
| 1 | 49, 119 | 30' before Rituximab | Clemastine | 2mg | | i.v. | bolus | |
| 2-4 | 50-52, 120-122 | continuously | Saline 0.9% + Gluc.5% alternately + Potassium Chloride + Sodium Bicarbonate | 3000ml + 1000ml, 20ml/1000ml, 40ml/1000ml | in infusion fluid, in infusion fluid | i.v. | 24h | up to 3000ml/m² if possible, check serum potassium, urine target pH >7.5 |
| 2-6 | 50-54, 120-124 | 2 - 2 - 2 - 2 | Sodium Bicarbonate | 1g | | oral | | |
| 2 | 50, 120 | 6h and 12h after start of chemo. | Furosemide | 40mg | | i.v. | bolus | |
| 2.5 | 50, 53, 120, 123 | 15' before chemotherapy | Granisetron | 1-3mg | | i.v. | bolus | |
| 5 | 53, 123 | 15' before chemotherapy | Saline 0.9% | | 1000ml | i.v. | 12h | |
| 6 | 54, 124 | 15' before Cytarabine dose | Granisetron | 3mg | | i.v. | bolus | |
| 6-8 | 54-56, 124-126 | continuously | Saline 0.9% | | 2000ml | i.v. | 24h | |
| 6-7 | 54-55, 124-125 | every 6 hours | Dexamethasone eye drops (1mg/ml) | 2 drops | | each eye | | |
| 8-10 | 56-58, 126-128 | every 6 hours | Dexpanthenol eye drops (50mg/ml) | 1 drop | | each eye | | |
| from day 1 | | 1 - 1 - 1 - 1 | Amphotericin B (as suspension) | 500mg | | oral | | for infection prophylaxis |
| from day 1 | | 1 - 0 - 1 (2x/ week) | Co-trimoxazole | 960mg | | oral | | for infection prophylaxis |

**Medicines As Required:** Metoclopramide oral or i.v.; if not tolerated replace with 5-HT3 antagonists; Rasburicase; Sodium Bicarbonate
**Antibiotic Prophylaxis:** If neutrophils <500/µl: Colistin 95mg(1-1-1-1) three times a day
**Routine Tests:** FBC, U&Es, LFTs, clotting studies, serum creatinine, creatinine clearance, fluid balance, exclude third space fluid accumulation, serum Methotrexate level
**Dose Reduction:** Withhold therapy with cytopenia (no dose reduction); see study protocol
**References:** See multicenter study for therapy optimization in B-ALL and hg B-NHL in adults (GMALL-B-ALL/NHL 2002).

| Consolidation: GMALL B-ALL/NHL 2002 | | Indication: B-ALL/Burkitt's Lymphoma | | | | | 11.1.17 |

**Chemotherapy**

*This chemotherapy may cause life-threatening toxicity! It should only be administered under the supervision of an experienced medical oncologist! The protocol must first be reviewed and considered in relationship to the clinical situation of the patient.*

| Block Day | Protocol Day | Compounds (generic names) in chronological order | Dosage | Diluent | Route | Duration of Infusion | Comments |
|---|---|---|---|---|---|---|---|
| 1 | 140, 161 | **Rituximab** | 375mg/m² | 500ml Saline 0.9% | i.v. | Initially 50mg/h | |
| | | | | | | | |

**Cautions**

Rituximab Infusion Rate:

**First Dose:** start at 50mg/h for 1hour; then if well tolerated increase every 30min by 50mg/h up to max. 400mg/h

**Subsequent Doses (excluding high-risk patients):** give 1/10 of the total dose in first 30min, then 9/10 of the total dose over the next 3.5 hours up to max. 400mg/h

**High-risk Patients** (high tumor burden, cardiovascular/respiratory disease, antibody incompatibility): start at 25mg/h for 1hour, then increase every 30min by 25mg/h up to max. 200mg/h

**Monitoring: every 15 min in the first hour, then hourly: blood pressure, heart rate, respiratory rate, temperature;**

**FULL RESUSCITATION FACILITIES SHOULD BE AT HAND!**

If an allergic/anaphylactic reaction occurs (chills, fever et ), stop infusion IMMEDIATELY, Corticosteroids, intensive care treatment may be necessary.

With improvement of symptoms: therapy may be resumed slowly with a 50% reduction in infusion rate

| Cycle Diagram | d134 | w20 | d141 | w21 | 148 | w22 | 155 | w23 | d162 | w |
|---|---|---|---|---|---|---|---|---|---|---|
| Rituximab | | | | | | | | | | |

**Obligatory Pre- and Concurrent Medication**

| Block Day | Protocol Day | Compounds (generic names) | Sequence and Timing | Dose | Diluent | Route | Duration of Infusion | Comments |
|---|---|---|---|---|---|---|---|---|
| 1 | 140, 161 | Paracetamol | 1h before Rituximab | 1000mg | | oral | | |
| 1 | 140, 161 | Clemastine | 30' before Rituximab | 2mg | | i.v. | bolus | |
| 1 | 140, 161 | Saline 0.9% | with Rituximab | | 500ml | i.v. | | |
| | from day 1 | Co-trimoxazole | 1 - 0 - 1 (2x/ week) | 960mg | | oral | | for infection prophylaxis |
| | | | | | | | | |

| Medicines As Required | Prednisolone 50mg i.v. before and during Rituximab infusion |
|---|---|
| Antibiotic Prophylaxis: | If neutrophils < 500/µl: Colistin 95mg/µl (1-1-1) three times a day |
| Routine Tests: | Uric acid, blood urea, serum creatinine, serum bilirubin; during infusion signs of intolerance/anaphylaxis, especially if leukocytes >50,000/µl |
| Dose Reduction: | Withhold therapy with cytopenia (no dose reduction); see study protocol |
| References: | See multicenter study for therapy optimization in B-ALL and hg B-NHL in adults (GMALL–B-ALL/NHL 2002). Updated: 12th August 200 2 |

# AMLSG 7-04 study: Prephase

**Indication: AML**

**11.2.1**

## Chemotherapy

*This chemotherapy may cause life-threatening toxicity! It should only be administered under the supervision of an experienced medical oncologist! The protocol must first be reviewed and considered in relationship to the clinical situation of the patient.*

| Week | Day | Compounds (generic names) in chronological order | Dosage | Diluent | Route | Duration of Infusion | Comments |
|------|-----|-----|--------|---------|-------|----------------------|----------|
| | 1 | **Cytarabine** | 100mg/m² | 250ml Saline 0.9% | i.v. | 24h | |
| | | | | | | | |
| | | | | | | | |
| | | | | | | | |
| | | | | | | | |

**Commence first induction cycle as soon as leukocyte count is under 50,000.**

**Cytarabine therapy may be shortened in Induction I due to its administration in the Prephase**

**Incompatibility: Cytarabine<>Heparin**

| Cycle Diagram | d1 w1 | d8 w2 | d15 w3 | d22 w4 | d29 w5 |
|---------------|-------|-------|--------|--------|--------|
| Cytarabine | | | | | |
| | | | | | |
| | | | | | |
| | | | | | |

**Cautions**

## Obligatory Pre- and Concurrent Medication

| Week | Day | Compounds (generic names) | Dose | Diluent | Route | Duration of Infusion | Comments |
|------|-----|---------------------------|------|---------|-------|----------------------|----------|
| | 1 | Saline 0.9% | | 2000ml | i.v. | 24h | leukapheresis if necessary |
| | | +....mmol KCl +....mmol Magnesium | | | | | correspondig to electroytes control |
| | 1 | Granisetron | 3mg | | i.v. | bolus | |
| | | | | | | | |
| | | | | | | | |
| | | | | | | | |
| | | | | | | | |
| | | | | | | | |
| | | | | | | | |
| | | | | | | | |
| | | | | | | | |
| | | | | | | | |
| | | | | | | | |
| | | | | | | | |
| | | | | | | | |

| | |
|---|---|
| **Medicines As Required** | Allopurinol according to serum uric acid; alkalinization; Metoclopramide oral or i.v. |
| **Antibiotic Prophylaxis:** | |
| **Routine Tests:** | FBC, clotting studies, U&Es, serum creatinine, creatinine clearance, uric acid, LDH, fluid balance, LFTs |
| **Dose Reduction:** | See Dose Modifier |
| **Max. Cum. Dose :** | Not defined |
| **References:** | Study protocol  AMLSG 7-04 |

# AMLSG 7-04 study Arm A: Induction ICE | Indication: AML | 11.2.2 A

*This chemotherapy may cause life-threatening toxicity! It should only be administered under the supervision of an experienced medical oncologist! The protocol must first be reviewed and considered in relationship to the clinical situation of the patient.*

## Chemotherapy

| Week | Day | Compounds (generic names) in chronological order | Dosage | Diluent | Route | Duration of Infusion | Comments |
|---|---|---|---|---|---|---|---|
| | 1,3,5 | **Idarubicin** | 12mg/m² | 100ml Saline 0.9% | i.v. | 2h | 2nd Induction: only on days 1 and 3 |
| | 1-3 | **Etoposide Phosphate** | 100mg/m² | 100ml Saline 0.9% | i.v. | 1h | |
| | 1-7 | **Cytarabine** | 100mg/m² | 250ml Saline 0.9% | i.v. | 22h | |

| Cycle Diagram | d1 w1 | d8 w2 | d15 w3 | d22 w4 | d29 w5 | d3 |
|---|---|---|---|---|---|---|
| Idarubicin | | | | | <—N.C.—> | |
| Etop. Phos. | | | | | | |
| Cytarabine | | | | | | |

**Cautions**

Etoposide Phosphate and Sodium Bicarbonate must not be administered concomitantly through the same infusion site!

Incompatibilities: Idarubicin<>Heparin, Cytarabine<>Heparin

**Note:** On day 21 and/orday 28, evaluation of the first and/or second induction cycles with FBC and differential and bone marrow cytology and/or bone marrow punch biopsy and with the existence of extramedullary involvement before therapy, biopsy of the relevant tissue.

## Obligatory Pre- and Concurrent Medication

| Week | Day | Compounds (generic names) | Sequence and Timing | Dose | Diluent | Route | Duration of Infusion | Comments |
|---|---|---|---|---|---|---|---|---|
| | 1-7 | Saline 0.9% | continuously | | 2000ml | i.v. | 24h | |
| | | +....mmol KCl +....mmol Magnesium | | | | | | correspondig to electroytes control |
| | 1-7 | Heparin | continuously | 5000-15000 units | | i.v. | 24h | via central line |
| | 1-7 | Granisetron | 15' before chemotherapy | 3mg | | i.v. | bolus | |
| | from day 1 | Co-trimoxazole | 1 - 0 - 1 (2x/ week) | 960mg | | oral | | for infection prophylaxis |

| | |
|---|---|
| Routine Tests: | FBC, U&Es, LFTs, diuresis, cardiac function (echocardiogram before 1st therapy), neurotoxicity. |
| Dose Reduction: | **Anthracycline** with hepatic impairment, **caution**: previous cardiac impairment, see Dose Modification Table |
| Next Cycle (N.C): | Between days 22 and 29; **day 15**: aplasia assessment including FBC and differential and bone marrow cytology |
| Max. Cum. Dose : | **Idarubicin** >120mg/m² i.v.: Danger of cardiotoxicity |
| References: | Study protocol (Int.Nr. 0478) with Valproate, ATRA and their combination with both  induction and consolidation therapies as well as Pegfilgrastim in the consolidation therapy for younger patients with newly diagnosed AML |

| AMLSG 7-04 study Arm A: Consolidation | | Indication: AML | | | | | 11.2.3 A |
|---|---|---|---|---|---|---|---|

*This chemotherapy may cause life-threatening toxicity! It should only be administered under the supervision of an experienced medical oncologist! The protocol must first be reviewed and considered in relationship to the clinical situation of the patient.*

## Chemotherapy

| Week | Day | Compounds (generic names) in chronological order | Dosage | Diluent | Route | Duration of Infusion | Comments |
|---|---|---|---|---|---|---|---|
| | 1,3,5 | **Cytarabine** | 3g/m² twice a day | 250ml Saline 0.9% | i.v. | 3h | every 12 hours |
| | | | | | | | |
| | | | | | | | |

**Cautions:** Evaluation, including FBC and differential and bone marrow cytology, between days 36 and 43 of the previous consolidation cycle

| Cycle Diagram | d1 w1 | d8 w2 | d15 w3 | d22 w4 | d29 w5 | d36 w6 | d43 w7 | d5 |
|---|---|---|---|---|---|---|---|---|
| Cytarabine | | | | | | | <--N.C.--> | |

## Obligatory Pre- and Concurrent Medication

| Week | Day | Compounds (generic names) | Dose | Diluent | Route | Duration of Infusion | Comments |
|---|---|---|---|---|---|---|---|
| | 1,3,5 | Saline 0.9% +....mmol KCl +....mmol Magnesium | 2000ml | | i.v. | 24h | corresponding to electroytes control |
| | 1,3,5 | Heparin | 5000-15000 units | | i.v. | 24h | via central line |
| | 1,3,5 | Granisetron | 3mg | | i.v. | bolus | |
| | 1 | Allopurinol | 300mg | | oral | | further doses according to serum uric acid level |
| | from day 1 | Folic Acid | 5mg | | oral | | |
| | from day 1 | Co-trimoxazole | 960mg | | oral | | for infection prophylaxis |
| | 10 | Pegfilgrastim | 6mg | | s.c. | | |
| | | Dexamethasone eye drops (1mg/ml) | 1-2 drops | | each eye | | until end of Cytarabine therapy |
| | | | | | | | |

**Sequence and Timing:** continuously (1,3,5); continuously (1,3,5); 15' before chemotherapy (1,3,5); one dose only (1); 1 - 0 - 0 (from day 1); 1 - 0 - 1 (2x/week) (from day 1); one dose only (10); every 6 hours

**Medicines As Required:** Metoclopramide oral or i.v., Sodium Bicarbonate 2g every 6 hours orally or NaHCO₃ i.v.

**Routine Tests:** FBC, U&Es, LFTs, diuresis, blood gases, cardiac function (echocardiogram before 1st course of chemotherapy), neurotoxicity

**Dose Reduction:**

**Next Cycle (N.C.):** Between days 36 and 43

**References:** Study protocol (Int.Nr. 0478) with Valproate, ATRA and their combination with both  induction and consolidation therapies as well as Pegfilgrastim in the consolidation therapy for younger patients with newly diagnosed AML

| AMLSG 7-04 study Arm B: Consolidation | | Indication: AML | | | | | 11.2.3 B |

## Chemotherapy

*This chemotherapy may cause life-threatening toxicity! It should only be administered under the supervision of an experienced medical oncologist! The protocol must first be reviewed and considered in relationship to the clinical situation of the patient.*

| Week | Day | Compounds (generic names) in chronological order | Dosage | Diluent | Route | Duration of Infusion | Comments |
|------|-----|--------------------------------------------------|--------|---------|-------|----------------------|----------|
| | 1,3,5 | **Cytarabine** | 3g/m² twice a day | 250ml Saline 0.9% | i.v. | 3h | every 12 hours |
| | 6–21 | **Tretinoin (ATRA)** | 15mg/m² | | oral | | in 3 divided daily doses; |
| | | | | | | | to be taken with or shortly after food |

**Cautions**

Evaluation, including FBC and differential and bone marrow cytology, between days 35 and 42 of a particular cycle
Discontinue ATRA and give high-dose Dexamethasone (10 mg/12h i.v.) with leukocyte increase >10,000/µl before or during ATRA therapy or with signs of ATRA syndrome (deterioration of pulmonary function, unexplained renal failure)

| Cycle Diagram | d1 w1 | d8 w2 | d15 w3 | d22 w4 | d29 w5 | d36 w6 | d43 w7 | d5 |
|---------------|-------|-------|--------|--------|--------|--------|--------|-----|
| Cytarabine | | | | | | | <---N.C.---> | |
| Tretinoin | | | | | | | | |

## Obligatory Pre- and Concurrent Medication

| Week | Day | Compounds (generic names) | Dose | Diluent | Route | Duration of Infusion | Comments |
|------|-----|---------------------------|------|---------|-------|----------------------|----------|
| | 1,3,5 | Saline 0.9% | | 2000ml | i.v. | 24h | |
| | | +....mmol KCl +....mmol Magnesium | | | | | after electroytes control |
| | 1,3,5 | Heparin | 5000–15000 units | | i.v. | 24h | via central line |
| | 1,3,5 | Granisetron | 3mg | | i.v. | bolus | |
| | 1 | Allopurinol | 300mg | | oral | | further doses according to serum uric acid level |
| | from day 1 | Folic Acid | 5mg | | oral | | |
| | from day 1 | Co-trimoxazole | 960mg | | oral | | for infection prophylaxis |
| | 10 | Pegfilgrastim | 6mg | | s.c. | | until end of Cytarabine therapy |
| | | Dexamethasone eye drops (1mg/ml) | 1–2 drops | | each eye | | every 6 hours |

| | |
|--|--|
| Medicines As Required | Metoclopramide oral or i.v., Sodium Bicarbonate 2g every 6 hours orally or NaHCO₃ i.v. |
| Routine Tests: | FBC, U&Es, LFTs, diuresis, blood gases, cardiac function (echocardiogram before 1st course of chemotherapy), neurotoxicity |
| Dose Reduction: | |
| Next Cycle (N.C.): | Between days 36 and 43 |
| References: | Study protocol (Int.Nr. 0478) with Valproate, ATRA and their combination with both  induction and consolidation therapies as well as Pegfilgrastim in the consolidation therapy for younger patients with newly diagnosed AML. |

| Daunorubicin/Cytarabine | AML 1/99 Intergroup: Induction | | Indication: AML, RAEB-t until 60 years | | | | 11.2.4 |

*This chemotherapy may cause life-threatening toxicity! It should only be administered under the supervision of an experienced medical oncologist! The protocol must first be reviewed and considered in relationship to the clinical situation of the patient.*

## Chemotherapy

| Week | Day | Compounds (generic names) in chronological order | Dosage | Diluent | Route | Duration of Infusion | Comments |
|---|---|---|---|---|---|---|---|
| | 1-7 | **Cytarabine** | 100mg/m² | 250ml Saline 0.9% | i.v. | 22h | |
| | 3-5 | **Daunorubicin** | 60mg/m² | 100ml Saline 0.9% | i.v. | 2h | |
| | | | | | | | |
| | | | | | | | |
| | | | | | | | |

**Cautions**

Previous cardiac impairment, s ee Dose Modification Table and study protocol

Incompatibilities: Daunorubicin<>Dexamethasone, Cytarabine<>Heparin

| Cycle Diagram | d1 w1 | d8 w2 | d15 w3 | d22 w4 | d29 w5 |
|---|---|---|---|---|---|
| Cytarabine | | | | N.C. | |
| Daunorubicin | | | | | |
| | | | | | |

## Obligatory Pre- and Concurrent Medication

| Week | Day | Compounds (generic names) | Dose | Diluent | Route | Duration of Infusion | Comments |
|---|---|---|---|---|---|---|---|
| | 1-7 | Saline 0.9% | | 2000ml | i.v. | 24h | |
| | 1-7 | Heparin | 5000-15000 units | | i.v. | 24h | via Hickman catheter or central line |
| | 1-7 | Dexamethasone | 8mg | | oral | | |
| | 1-7 | Granisetron | 1mg | | i.v. | | increase dose to 3mg with emesis |
| | 1-7 | Famotidin | 20mg | | oral | | |
| | from day 1 | Co-trimoxazole | 960mg | | oral | | for infection prophylaxis |
| | | | | | | | |
| | | | | | | | |
| | | | | | | | |

| | |
|---|---|
| **Medicines As Required** | Metoclopramide oral or i.v., Sodium Bicarbonate 2g every 6 hours orally or NaHCO₃ i.v. |
| **Routine Tests:** | FBC, intestinal toxicity, U&Es, LFTs, clotting studies, serum creatinin , creatinine clearance, fluid balance, cardiac function (echocardiogram before 1st course of chemotherapy). neurotoxicity |
| **Dose Reduction:** | **Anthracycline** with hepatic impairment, **caution**: previous cardiac impairment, see Dose Modification Table |
| **Max. Cum. Dose :** | **Daunorubicin** 550mg/m² |
| **Efficacy Assess.** | Bone marrow biopsy on day 15 for aplasia assessment |
| **Next Cycle (N.C.):** | Day 22 repeat induction course: may be earlier if blasts persist (see study protocol page 4) |
| **References:** | Mayer RJ et al, N Engl J Med 1994; 331:896-903; "multicenter study for the treatment of patients with acute myeloid leukemia (AML) or RAEB-t ≤ 60 years" (AML 1/99 SHG protocol) |

852

| High-Dose Cytarabine | AML 1/99 Intergroup:<br>Post-Remission | Indication: AML, RAEB-t until 60 years | 11.2.5 |
|---|---|---|---|

*This chemotherapy may cause life-threatening toxicity! It should only be administered under the supervision of an experienced medical oncologist! The protocol must first be reviewed and considered in relationship to the clinical situation of the patient.*

## Chemotherapy

| Week | Day | Compounds (generic names) in chronological order | Dosage | Diluent | Route | Duration of Infusion | Comments |
|---|---|---|---|---|---|---|---|
| | 1,3,5 | **Cytarabine** | 3g/m² twice a day | 250ml Saline 0.9% | i.v. | 3h | every 12 hours |
| | | | | | | | |
| | | | | | | | |
| | | | | | | | |

**Cautions**

| Cycle Diagram | d1 w1 | d8 w2 | d15 w3 | d22 w4 | d29 w5 |
|---|---|---|---|---|---|
| Cytarabine | | | | | |
| | | | | | |
| | | | | | |

## Obligatory Pre- and Concurrent Medication

| Week | Day | Compounds (generic names) | Dose | Diluent | Route | Duration of Infusion | Comments |
|---|---|---|---|---|---|---|---|
| | 1-6 | Saline 0.9% | | 2000ml | i.v. | 24h | |
| | 1,3,5 | Dexamethasone | 8mg | | i.v. | bolus | |
| | 1,3,5 | Granisetron | 1mg | | i.v. | bolus | increase dose to 3mg with emesis |
| | 1-6 | Dexamethasone eye drops (1mg/ml) | 2 drops | | each eye | | |
| | 7-11 | Dexpanthenol eye drops (50mg/ml) | 1 drop | | each eye | | |
| | from day 1 | Co-trimoxazole | 960mg | | oral | | for infection prophylaxis |
| | | | | | | | |
| | | | | | | | |
| | | | | | | | |
| | | | | | | | |
| | | | | | | | |
| | | | | | | | |
| | | | | | | | |

| | |
|---|---|
| **Medicines As Required** | Metoclopramide |
| **Routine Tests:** | FBC, intestinal toxicity, U&Es, LFTs, clotting studies, serum creatinine, creatinine clearance, fluid balance, cardiac function, neurotoxicity |
| **Dose Reduction:** | With cerebellar symptoms, exanthema, bilirubin > 3.0mg/dl, raised AST (SGOT) or ALP: Stop **Cytarabine**; with cytopenia, withhold therapy (no dose reduction) |
| **Max. Cum. Dose :** | None |
| **Efficacy Assess.** | Bone marrow biopsy and blood count after complete hematopoietic regeneration |
| **Next Cycle (N.C.):** | 1 week after hematological normalization of peripheral blood (day +28 at the earliest) |
| **References:** | See "multicenter study for the treatment of patients with acute myeloid leukemia (AML) or RAEB-t ≤60 years" (AML 1/99 SHG protocol); Mayer RJ et al, N Engl J Med 1994; 331:896-903 |

853

# S-HAM

## Indication: Relapsed AML

11.2.6

*This chemotherapy may cause life-threatening toxicity! It should only be administered under the supervision of an experienced medical oncologist! The protocol must first be reviewed and considered in relationship to the clinical situation of the patient.*

## Chemotherapy

| Week | Day | Compounds (generic names) in chronological order | Dosage | Diluent | Route | Duration of Infusion | Comments |
|---|---|---|---|---|---|---|---|
| | 1,2,8,9 | **Cytarabine** | 1g/m² twice a day | 250ml Saline 0.9% | i.v. | 3h | every 12 hours |
| | 3,4,10,11 | **Mitoxantrone** | 10mg/m² | 250ml Saline 0.9% | i.v. | 30min | |
| | | | | | | | |
| | | | | | | | |

**Cautions**

| Cycle Diagram | d1 w1 | d8 w2 | d15 w3 | d22 w4 |
|---|---|---|---|---|
| Cytarabine | | | | |
| Mitoxantrone | | | | |
| | | | | |

## Obligatory Pre- and Concurrent Medication

| Week | Day | Sequence and Timing | Compounds (generic names) | Dose | Diluent | Route | Duration of Infusion | Comments |
|---|---|---|---|---|---|---|---|---|
| | 1-4,8-11 | continuously | Saline 0.9% | | 2000ml | i.v. | 24h | |
| | 1,2,8,9 | 15' before Cytarabine | Dexamethasone | 8mg | | i.v. | bolus | |
| | 1,2,8,9 | 15' before Cytarabine | Granisetron | 1mg | | i.v. | bolus | |
| | 3,4,10,11 | 15' before chemotherapy | Dexamethasone | 8mg | | i.v. | bolus | |
| | 1,2,3,8,9,10 | 1 - 1 - 1 - 1 | Dexamethasone eye drops (1mg/ml) | 2 drops | | each eye | | |
| | 4,11 | 1 - 1 - 1 - 1 | Povidone eye drops (50mg/ml) | 2 drops | | each eye | | |
| | from day 1 | 1 - 0 - 1 (2x/week) | Co-trimoxazole | 960mg | | oral | | for infection prophylaxis |
| | from day 1 | every 2 days | Amphotericin B | 0.5mg/kg | | i.v. | 6-12h | for infection prophylaxis; min.dose: 50mg |
| | from day 18* | once a day | Filgrastim | 5µg/kg | | s.c. | | *after aplasia assessment:<br>give Filgrastim only if aplasia is achieved<br>and till WBC>1000/µl;<br>withhold Filgrastim if blasts persist |
| | | | | | | | | |
| | | | | | | | | |
| | | | | | | | | |
| | | | | | | | | |
| | | | | | | | | |

| | |
|---|---|
| **Medicines As Required** | Metoclopramide oral or i.v., Sodium Bicarbonate 2g every 6 hours orally or 200 ml i.v. |
| **Routine Tests:** | FBC, U&Es, LFTs, serum creatinine, diuresis, cardiac function (echocardiogram before 1st therapy), neurotoxicity |
| **Dose Reduction:** | With cerebral symptoms, exanthema, bilirubin >3.0 mg/dl, raised AST (SGOT) or ALP: Stop **Cytarabine** |
| **Max. Cum. Dose :** | **Mitoxantrone** >100mg/m²: Danger of cardiotoxicity |
| **References:** | Kern W. et al., Cancer, 1997, 59-68; Kern W. et al., Ann Hematol., 1998, 115-122 |

| MICE | induction therapy analogous to EORTC-LCG AML 17 (61-80years) | | Indication: AML (induction therapy) | | | | 11.2.7 |

*This chemotherapy may cause life-threatening toxicity! It should only be administered under the supervision of an experienced medical oncologist! The protocol must first be reviewed and considered in relationship to the clinical situation of the patient.*

## Chemotherapy

| Week | Day | Compounds (generic names) in chronological order | Dosage | Route | Diluent | Duration of Infusion | Comments |
|------|-----|---------------------------------------------------|--------|-------|---------|----------------------|----------|
| | 1,3,5 | **Mitoxantrone** | 7mg/m² | i.v. | 250ml Saline 0.9% | 30min | |
| | 1-3 | **Etoposide Phosphate** | 100mg/m² | i.v. | 100ml Saline 0.9% | 30min | |
| | 1-7 | **Cytarabine** | 100mg/m² | i.v. | 250ml Saline 0.9% | 22h | |

| Cycle Diagram | d1 w1 | d8 w2 | d15 w3 | d22 w4 | d29 w5 |
|---------------|-------|-------|--------|--------|--------|
| Mitoxantrone | | | | | N.C. |
| Etop. Phos. | | | | | |
| Cytarabine | | | | | |

**Cautions:** Etoposide Phosphate and Sodium Bicarbonate must not be administered concomitantly through the same infusion site!
Incompatibilities: Cytarabine<>Heparin, Mitoxantrone<>Heparin

## Obligatory Pre- and Concurrent Medication

| Week | Day | Compounds (generic names) | Dose | Route | Diluent | Duration of Infusion | Comments |
|------|-----|---------------------------|------|-------|---------|----------------------|----------|
| | 1-7 | Saline 0.9% | | i.v. | 2000ml | 24h | |
| | | +....ml KCl | | | | | according to serum potassium |
| | | +....ml Magnesium | | | | | according to serum magnesium |
| | 1-7 | Granisetron | 1mg | i.v. | | bolus | |
| | from day 15* | Filgrastim | <70kg: 300µg, >=70kg: 480µg | s.c. | | | *after aplasia assessment: give Filgrastim only if aplasia is achieved and till WBC>1000/µl; withhold Filgrastim if blasts persist |
| | from day 1 | Sodium Bicarbonate | 2g every 6 hours | oral | | | or mmol NaHCO₃ i.v. |
| | from day 1 | Co-trimoxazole | 960mg | oral | | | for infection prophylaxis |

| | |
|---|---|
| Medicines As Required | Metoclopramide oral or i.v., Allopurinol, Dexamethasone oral or i.v. (avoid if possible on account of Aspergillosis) |
| Routine Tests: | FBC, U&Es, LFTs, diuresis, neurotoxicity, serum creatinine, cardiac function (echocardiogram before 1st therapy), creatinine clearance |
| Dose Reduction: | No dose modification during induction therapy |
| Next Cycle (N.C.): | Day 29 (after hematopoietic regeneration, bone marrow biopsy and FBC on days 8 and 29); aplasia assessment 1 week after therapy ends |
| Max. Cum. Dose : | Mitoxantrone >100mg/m²: Danger of cardiotoxicity |
| References: | Jehn et al., Blood, 2002: 100 (suppl. 1): 859a |

# Mini ICE (i.v.)

consolidation therapy analogous to EORTC-LCG AML 17 (61-80years)

## Indication: AML (consolidation therapy)

**11.2.8**

*This chemotherapy may cause life-threatening toxicity! It should only be administered under the supervision of an experienced medical oncologist! The protocol must first be reviewed and considered in relationship to the clinical situation of the patient.*

## Chemotherapy

| Week | Day | Compounds (generic names) in chronological order | Dosage | Diluent | Route | Duration of Infusion | Comments |
|---|---|---|---|---|---|---|---|
| | 1,3,5 | **Idarubicin** | 8mg/m² | undiluted | i.v. | bolus 15min | |
| | 1-3 | **Etoposide Phosphate** | 100mg/m² | 100ml Saline 0.9% | i.v. | 30min | |
| | 1-5 | **Cytarabine** | 100mg/m² | 250ml Saline 0.9% | i.v. | 22h | |
| | | | | | | | |
| | | | | | | | |

| Cycle Diagram | d1 w1 | d8 w2 | d15 w3 | d22 w4 | d29 w5 |
|---|---|---|---|---|---|
| Idarubicin | | | | | N.C. |
| Etop. Phos. | | | | | |
| Cytarabine | | | | | |

**Cautions:** Etoposide Phosphate and Sodium Bicarbonate must not be administered concomitantly through the same infusion site!

Incompatibilities: Idarubicin<>Heparin, Cytarabine<>Heparin

## Obligatory Pre- and Concurrent Medication

| Week | Day | Compounds (generic names) | Dose | Diluent | Route | Duration of Infusion | Comments |
|---|---|---|---|---|---|---|---|
| | 1-5 | Saline 0.9% | | 2000ml | i.v. | 24h | |
| | | +....mmol KCl | | | | | according to serum potassium |
| | | +....mmol Magnesium | | | | | according to serum magnesium |
| | 1-5 | Granisetron | 1mg | | i.v. | bolus | |
| | from day 15* | Filgrastim | <70kg: 300µg, >=70kg: 480µg | | s.c. | | *after aplasia assessment: give Filgrastim only if aplasia is achieved and till WBC>1000/µl; withhold Filgrastim if blasts persist |
| | from day 1 | Co-trimoxazole | 960mg | | oral | | for infection prophylaxis |

**Medicines As Required** Metoclopramide oral or i.v., Allopurinol, Dexamethasone oral or i.v. (avoid if possible on account of Aspergillosis)

**Routine Tests:** FBC, U&Es, LFTs, diuresis, cardiac function (echocardiogram before 1st therapy), neurotoxicity.

**Dose Reduction:** **Anthracycline** with hepatic impairment; **caution:** previous cardiac impairment, see Dose Modification Table

**Next Cycle (N.C.):** Day 29 (after hematopoietic regeneration, bone marrow biopsy and full blood count); aplasia assessment 1 week after therapy ends

**Max. Cum. Dose :** **Idarubicin** >120mg/m² i.v.: Danger of cardiotoxicity

**References:** Jehn et al., Blood, 2002; 100 (suppl. 1): 859a

# Ida/Cytarabine 3+7 — Induction Therapy — Indication: AML — 11.2.9

*This chemotherapy may cause life-threatening toxicity! It should only be administered under the supervision of an experienced medical oncologist! The protocol must first be reviewed and considered in relationship to the clinical situation of the patient.*

## Chemotherapy

| Week | Day | Compounds (generic names) in chronological order | Dosage | Diluent | Route | Duration of Infusion | Comments |
|---|---|---|---|---|---|---|---|
| | 1-7 | **Cytarabine** | 100mg/m² | 250ml Saline 0.9% | i.v. | 22h | |
| | 3-5 | **Idarubicin** | 12mg/m² | 100ml Saline 0.9% | i.v. | bolus 15min | |
| | | | | | | | |
| | | | | | | | |
| | | | | | | | |

| Cycle Diagram | d1 w1 | d8 w2 | d15 w3 | d22 w4 | d29 w5 |
|---|---|---|---|---|---|
| Cytarabine | | | | <--N.C.--> | |
| Idarubicin | | | | | |

### Cautions

Previous cardiac impairment, s ee Dose Modification Table and study protocol

Incompatibilities: Idarubicin<>Heparin, Cytarabine<>Heparin

## Obligatory Pre- and Concurrent Medication

| Week | Day | Compounds (generic names) | Dose | Diluent | Route | Duration of Infusion | Comments |
|---|---|---|---|---|---|---|---|
| | 1-7 | Saline 0.9% | | 2000ml | i.v. | 24h | |
| | 1-7 | Heparin | 5000-15000 units | | i.v. | 24h | via central line |
| | 1-7 | Dexamethasone | 8mg | | oral | | |
| | 1-2, 6-7 | Metoclopramide | 30mg | | oral | | |
| | 3-5 | Granisetron | 1mg | | i.v. | | increase dose to 3mg with emesis |
| | from day 1 | Co-trimoxazole | 960mg | | oral | | for infection prophylaxis |
| | from day 14* | Filgrastim | 5µg/kg | | s.c. | | *after aplasia assessment: give Filgrastim only if aplasia is achieved and till WBC>1000/µl; withhold Filgrastim if blasts persist |
| | | | | | | | |
| | | | | | | | |
| | | | | | | | |
| | | | | | | | |

| | |
|---|---|
| Medicines As Required | Metoclopramide oral or i.v., Sodium Bicarbonate 2g every 6 hours orally or NaHCO₃ i.v. |
| Routine Tests: | FBC, U&Es, LFTs, diuresis, blood gases, cardiac function (echocardiogram before 1st course of chemotherapy), neurotoxicity |
| Dose Reduction: | **Anthracycline** with hepatic impairment, **caution:** previous cardiac impairment, see Dose Modification Table |
| Max. Cum. Dose : | **Idarubicin** >120mg/m² i.v.: Danger of cardiotoxicity |
| Next Cycle (N.C.): | In 3-4 weeks (after hematopoietic regeneration, bone marrow biopsy and full blood count); aplasia assessment 1 week after therapy ends |
| References: | Berman et al., Blood, 1991; 77(8): 1666-1674 |

| HD 13-protocol | Arm A, B, C, D | Indication: Hodgkin's Disease | 11.3.1 |
|---|---|---|---|

*This chemotherapy may cause life-threatening toxicity! It should only be administered under the supervision of an experienced medical oncologist! The protocol must first be reviewed and considered in relationship to the clinical situation of the patient.*

## Chemotherapy

| Week | Day | Compounds (generic names) in chronological order | Dosage | Diluent | Route | Duration of Infusion | Comments |
|---|---|---|---|---|---|---|---|
| | 1,15 | **Doxorubicin** | 25mg/m² | | i.v. | bolus 15min | |
| | 1,15 | **Bleomycin** | 10mg/m² | | i.v. | bolus 15min | |
| | 1,15 | **Vinblastine** | 6mg/m² | | i.v. | bolus 10min | |
| | 1,15 | **Dacarbazine (DTIC)** | 375mg/m² | 500ml Saline 0.9% | i.v. | 2h | protect from light |

**Cautions**

Cycle Diagram:

| Cycle Diagram | d1 w1 | d8 w2 | d15 w3 | d22 w4 | d29 w5 |
|---|---|---|---|---|---|
| Doxorubicin | | | | | N.C. |
| Bleomycin | | | | | |
| Vinblastine | | | | | |
| Dacarbazine | | | | | |

| | A | B | C | D |
|---|---|---|---|---|

## Obligatory Pre- and Concurrent Medication

| Week | Day | Compounds (generic names) | Sequence and Timing | Dose | Diluent | Route | Duration of Infusion | Comments |
|---|---|---|---|---|---|---|---|---|
| | 1,15 | Saline 0.9% | 15' before chemotherapy | | 1000ml | i.v. | 2h | |
| | 1,15 | Dexamethasone | 15' before, 4h & 8h after chemo. | 8mg | 100ml Saline 0.9% | i.v. | 15 min | |
| | 1,15 | Granisetron | 15' before chemotherapy | 1mg | | i.v. | bolus | |
| | 1,15 | Clemastine | before Bleomycin | 2mg | | i.v. | bolus | |

| | A | B | C | D |
|---|---|---|---|---|

| | |
|---|---|
| Medicines As Required | With chemical phlebitis, Heparin 5000 units in hydration infusion, Granisetron i.v. |
| Routine Tests: | FBC, U&Es, LFTs, serum creatinine, cardiac function, pulmonary function tests, neurotoxicity, high resolution CT scan with suspected Bleomycin induced pneumonitis |
| Dose Reduction: | GFR < 60ml/min: **Bleomycin** 75%, **Dacarbazine** 75%; s see Dose Modification Table and study protocol |
| Max. Cum. Dose : | **Doxorubicin** >550mg/m²: Danger of cardiotoxocity; **Bleomycin** >400mg absolute: Danger of pulmonary toxicity **Doxorubicin** >400mg absolute: Danger of Bleomycin induced pneumonitis |
| Next Cycle (N.C.): | Day 29 |
| Efficacy Assess. | After 2 cycles (HD13) |
| References: | Study protocol |

# BEACOPP-II-Standard Dose

## Indication: Hodgkin's Disease

11.3.2

### Chemotherapy

German Hodgkin's Lymphoma
Study Group; study protocol

*This chemotherapy may cause life-threatening toxicity! It should only be administered under the supervision of an experienced medical oncologist! The protocol must first be reviewed and considered in relationship to the clinical situation of the patient.*

| Week | Day | Compounds (generic names) in chronological order | Dosage | Diluent | Route | Duration of Infusion | Comments |
|---|---|---|---|---|---|---|---|
| | 1-7 | **Procarbazine** | 100mg/m² | | oral | | |
| | 1-14 | **Prednisone** | 40mg/m² | | oral | | |
| | 1 | **Cyclophosphamide** | 650mg/m² | 500ml Saline 0.9% | i.v. | 1h | |
| | 1 | **Doxorubicin** | 25mg/m² | undiluted | i.v. | bolus 15min | |
| | 1-3 | **Etoposide Phosphate** | 100mg/m² | 100ml Saline 0.9% | i.v. | bolus 15min | dose expressed in terms of Etoposide base |
| | 8 | **Vincristine** | 1.4mg/m² | undiluted | i.v. | bolus 15min | maximum dose 2mg absolute |
| | 8 | **Bleomycin** | 10mg/m² | undiluted | i.v. | bolus 15min | |

**Cautions**

Etoposide Phosphate and Sodium Bicarbonate must not be administered concomitantly through the same infusion site!

Pegfilgrastim is for patients outside the study. Study patients are to have Filgrastim only.

**Anthracycline:** Danger of cardiotoxicity - echocardiogram

**Bleomycin:** Pulmonary function tests before start of therapy and after every second cycle

| Cycle Diagram | d1 w1 | d8 w2 | d15 w3 | d22 w4 |
|---|---|---|---|---|
| Procarazine | | | | N.C. |
| Prednisone | | | | |
| Cyclophos. | | | | |
| Doxorubicin | | | | |
| Etop. Phos. | | | | |
| Vincristine | | | | |
| Bleomycin | | | | |

### Obligatory Pre- and Concurrent Medication

| Week | Day | Sequence and Timing | Compounds (generic names) | Dose | Diluent | Route | Duration of Infusion | Comments |
|---|---|---|---|---|---|---|---|---|
| | 0 | 12h before chemotherapy | oral fluids | | 1000-2000ml | oral | | or Saline 0.9% i.v. |
| | 1 | with chemotherapy | Saline 0.9% | | 2000ml | i.v. | 3h | |
| | 2,3 | 15' before chemotherapy | Saline 0.9% | | 500ml | i.v. | 1h30min | |
| | 8 | 15' before chemotherapy | Saline 0.9% | | 250ml | i.v. | 30min | |
| | 1 | 15' before & 4h after chemo. | Dexamethasone | 8mg | 100ml Saline 0.9% | i.v. | 15min | or orally at home |
| | 2,3 | 15' before chemotherapy | Dexamethasone | 8mg | 100ml Saline 0.9% | i.v. | 15min | or orally at home |
| | 1 | 15' before chemotherapy | Granisetron | 1mg | | i.v. | bolus | increase dose to 3mg with emesis |
| | 1 | 0h, 4h & 8h after Cyclophos. | Mesna | 130/260mg/m² | | i.v. | bolus | or orally at home |
| | 8 | before Bleomycin | Clemastine | 2mg | | i.v. | bolus | |
| | 8-15 | 1 - 0 - 1 (2x week) | Co-trimoxazole | 960mg | | oral | | |
| | 1-15 | 0 - 0 - 0 - 1 | Sucralfate | 1g | | oral | | |
| 1st neutropenic cycle* | | once a day | Filgrastim | 5µg/kg | | s.c. | | *when WBC<1000/µl; give until >2000/µl |
| from cycle 2** | 9** | prophyl. admin. 24h after i.v. chemo. | Pegfilgrastim | 6mg | | s.c. | | **only for pts. outside the study if decreased WBC in previous cycle; give instead of Filgrastim |

**Medicines As Required** Granisetron 1mg i.v., Famotidine

**Routine Tests:** **Anthracycline** and **Bleomycin:** see cautions above; FBC, U&Es, serum creatinine, clotting studies, LFTs, creatinine clearance, neurotoxicity

**Dose Reduction:** See Dose Modification Table and study protocol HD14/HD15 (on day 8. **Bleomycin & Vincristine** can be given even if neutropenia present)

**Max. Cum. Dose :** **Doxorubicin:** Danger of cardiotoxicity; max. cum. dose is 550mg/m². **Bleomycin:** Danger of pulmonary fibrosis esp. if cum. dose exceeds 400mg absolute

**Next Cycle (N.C.):** Day 22

**Efficacy Assess.** After cycles 4 and 8

**References:** German Hodgkin's Lymphoma Study Group study protocol; Diehl V et al., N Engl J Med, 2003; 348(24): 2386-95

# BEACOPP-II-Escalated Dose

## Indication: Hodgkin's Disease

**11.3.3**

### Chemotherapy

German Hodgkin's Lymphoma
Study Group; study protocol

*This chemotherapy may cause life-threatening toxicity! It should only be administered under the supervision of an experienced medical oncologist! The protocol must first be reviewed and considered in relationship to the clinical situation of the patient.*

| Week | Day | Compounds (generic names) in chronological order | Dosage | Diluent | Route | Duration of Infusion | Comments |
|---|---|---|---|---|---|---|---|
| | 1-7 | **Procarbazine** | 100mg/m² | | oral | | |
| | 1-14 | **Prednisone** | 40mg/m² | | oral | | |
| | 1 | **Cyclophosphamide** | 1250mg/m² | 500ml Saline 0.9% | i.v. | 1h | |
| | 1 | **Doxorubicin** | 35mg/m² | undiluted | i.v. | bolus 15min | |
| | 1-3 | **Etoposide Phosphate** | 200mg/m² | 250ml Saline 0.9% | i.v. | 30min | dose expressed in terms of Etoposide base |
| | 8 | **Vincristine** | 1.4mg/m² | undiluted | i.v. | bolus | maximum dose 2mg absolute |
| | 8 | **Bleomycin** | 10mg/m² | undiluted | i.v. | bolus | |

| Cycle Diagram | d1 w1 | d8 w2 | d15 w3 | d22 w4 |
|---|---|---|---|---|
| Procarbazine | | | | N.C. |
| Prednisone | | | | |
| Cyclophos. | | | | |
| Doxorubicin | | | | |
| Etop. Phos. | | | | |
| Vincristine | | | | |
| Bleomycin | | | | |

**Etoposide Phosphate and Sodium Bicarbonate must not be administered concomitantly through the same infusion site!**

**Cautions:**

**Anthracycline:** Danger of cardiotoxicity - echocardiogram

**Bleomycin:** Pulmonary function tests before start of therapy and after every second cycle

### Obligatory Pre- and Concurrent Medication

| Week | Day | Sequence and Timing | Compounds (generic names) | Dose | Diluent | Route | Duration of Infusion | Comments |
|---|---|---|---|---|---|---|---|---|
| | once only | at start of therapy | Zoledronic Acid | 4mg | 500ml Saline 0.9% | i.v. | 4h | |
| | every 3 months | | Zoledronic Acid | 4mg | 250ml Saline 0.9% | i.v. | 1h | |
| | regularly | 0 - 0 - 1 | Calcium Carbonate | 1000mg | | oral | | |
| | 0 | 12h before chemotherapy | oral fluids | | 1000ml-2000ml | oral | | or Saline 0.9% i.v. |
| | 1 | with chemotherapy | Saline 0.9% | | 1000ml | i.v. | 6-12h | or orally at home |
| | 1 | 15' before & 4h after chemo. | Dexamethasone | 8mg | 100ml Saline 0.9% | i.v. | 15min | or orally at home |
| | 1 | 15' before chemotherapy | Granisetron | 1mg | | i.v. | bolus | increase dose to 3mg with emesis |
| | 2,3,8 | 0h, 4h & 8h after Cyclophos. | Mesna | 250/500mg/m² | | i.v. | bolus | or orally at home |
| | 2,3 | with chemotherapy | Saline 0.9% | | 500ml | i.v. | 1h | |
| | 8 | 15' before chemotherapy | Dexamethasone | 8mg | | i.v. | bolus 15min | |
| | 8-15 | before Bleomycin | Clemastine | 2mg | | i.v. | bolus | |
| | 8-15 | 1 - 0 - 1 (2x week) | Co-trimoxazole | 960mg | | oral | | |
| | 1-15 | 0 - 0 - 0 - 1 | Sucralfate | 1g | | oral | | |
| | 8-12* | once a day | Filgrastim | <70kg: 300µg; >70kg: 480µg | | s.c. | | *till WBC>1000/µl for 3 days (after passing nadir) |
| from cycle 2** | 9** | prophyl. admin. 24h after i.v. chemo. | Pegfilgrastim | 6mg | | s.c. | | **only for pts. outside the study if decreased WBC in previous cycle: give instead of Filgrastim |

| | |
|---|---|
| **Medicines As Required** | Metoclopramide oral or i.v., Granisetron i.v., Famotidine |
| **Routine Tests:** | **Anthracycline and Bleomycin:** see **cautions** above; FBC, U&Es, serum creatinine, clotting studies, LFTs, creatinine clearance, neurotoxicity |
| **Dose Reduction:** | See Dose Modification Table. Toxicity Grade 4, see study protocol HD14/HD15 (on day 8. **Bleomycin & Vincristine** can be given even if neutropenia present) |
| **Max. Cum. Dose :** | **Doxorubicin:** Danger of cardiotoxicity; max. cum. dose is 550mg/m²; **Bleomycin:** Danger of pulmonary fibrosis esp. if cum. dose exceeds 400mg absolute |
| **Next Cycle (N.C.):** | Day 22 |
| **Efficacy Assess.** | After cycles 4 and 8 |
| **References:** | German Hodgkin's Lymphoma Study Group study protocol; Diehl V et al., N Engl J Med, 2003; 348(24); 2386-95 |

# Vinblastine

## Indication: Hodgkin's Disease

**11.3.4**

*This chemotherapy may cause life-threatening toxicity! It should only be administered under the supervision of an experienced medical oncologist! The protocol must first be reviewed and considered in relationship to the clinical situation of the patient.*

## Chemotherapy

| Week | Day | Compounds (generic names) in chronological order | Dosage | Diluent | Route | Duration of Infusion | Comments |
|------|-----|-------------------------------------------------|--------|---------|-------|---------------------|----------|
| | 1,8,15,22,29,36 | **Vinblastine** | 6mg/m² | undiluted | i.v. | bolus 1min | only inject into running infusion |
| | | | | | | | |
| | | | | | | | |
| | | | | | | | |

### Cautions

| Cycle Diagram | d1 w1 | d8 w2 | d15 w3 | d22 w4 | d29 w5 | d36 w6 | d43 w7 | d50 w8 | d57 w9 |
|---------------|-------|-------|--------|--------|--------|--------|--------|--------|--------|
| Vinblastine | | | | | | | | N.C. | |

## Obligatory Pre- and Concurrent Medication

| Week | Day | Sequence and Timing | Compounds (generic names) | Dose | Diluent | Route | Duration of Infusion | Comments |
|------|-----|---------------------|---------------------------|------|---------|-------|---------------------|----------|
| | 1,8,15,22,29,36 | 15' before chemotherapy | Saline 0.9% | | 500ml | i.v. | 1h | |

| | |
|---|---|
| Medicines As Required | Metoclopramide oral or i.v., Dexamethasone |
| Routine Tests: | FBC, LFTs, neurotoxicity |
| Dose Reduction: | Bilirubin >3mg/dl: **Vinblastine** 25%, bilirubin>5mg/dl: withhold **Vinblastine** |
| Max. Cum. Dose : | Unknown |
| Next Cycle (N.C.): | Week 8 or according to myelosuppression |
| Efficacy Assess. | After 6 weeks |
| References: | Warren RD et al., Am J Hematol, 1978;4(1):47-55 |

| Stanford V | Indication: Hodgkin's Disease | 11.3.5 |

*This chemotherapy may cause life-threatening toxicity! It should only be administered under the supervision of an experienced medical oncologist! The protocol must first be reviewed and considered in relationship to the clinical situation of the patient.*

## Chemotherapy

| Week | Day | Compounds (generic names) in chronological order | Dosage | Diluent | Route | Duration of Infusion | Comments |
|---|---|---|---|---|---|---|---|
| | 1, 15 | **Doxorubicin** | 25mg/m² | undiluted | i.v. | bolus 15min | |
| | 1, 15 | **Vinblastine** | 6mg/m² | undiluted | i.v. | bolus 10min | |
| | 1 | **Mechlorethamine** | 6mg/m² | undiluted | i.v. | bolus 15min | during Saline infusion |
| | 15, 16 | **Etoposide Phosphate** | 60mg/m² | 250ml Saline 0.9% | i.v. | 1h | if Etop. dose is >200mg, 500ml Saline 0.9% |
| | 8, 22 | **Vincristine** | 1,4mg/m² | undiluted | i.v. | bolus | max. 2mg absolute |
| | 8, 22 | **Bleomycin** | 5units/m² | undiluted | i.v. | bolus 15min | |
| | continuous | **Prednisone** | 40/10mg/m² | | oral | | |

**Cautions**

Etoposide Phosphate and Sodium Bicarbonate must not be administered concomitantly through the same infusion site.

Anthracycline: Danger of cardiotoxicity - echocardiogram

Bleomycin: Pulmonary function tests before start of therapy and after every second cycle

If the patient is >50 years old: Vincristine week 10 and 12 (cycle 3) max. 1mg; Vinblastine week 9 and 11 (cycle 3) max. 4mg/m²

| Cycle Diagram | week 1-10/week 11 and 12 | | | |
|---|---|---|---|---|
| | d1 w1 | d8 w2 | d15 w3 | d22 w4 |
| Doxorubicin | | | | |
| Vinblastine | | | | |
| Mechloreth. | | | | |
| Etop. Phos. | | | | |
| Vincristine | | | | |
| Bleomycin | | | | |
| Prednisone | | | | |

## Obligatory Pre- and Concurrent Medication

| Week | Day | Compounds (generic names) | Sequence and Timing | Dose | Diluent | Route | Duration of Infusion | Comments |
|---|---|---|---|---|---|---|---|---|
| 1-12 | regularly | Ranitidin | 1-0-1 | | | oral | | |
| 1-12 | regularly | Co-trimoxazole | 1-0-1 (2x/week) | 960mg | | oral | | during the meal |
| 1-12 | regularly | Ketoconazol | once daily | 200mg/day | | oral | | |
| 1-12 | regularly | Acyclovir | 1-0-1 | 200mg | | oral | | |
| d17(cycle1-3) d2(cycle2+3) | 1, 2, 3 | Filgrastim | -1h before chemotherapy | 5µg/kg | | s.c. | | |
| | 1-4 | Aprepitant | d1-15min, d2-4 in the morning | * | | oral | | * d1: 125mg, d2+3: 80mg |
| | 1-4 | Dexamethasone | 1-4 | * | | i.v./oral | | * d1: 12mg/d2-4: 8mg |
| | 1, 15, 16 | Saline 0.9% | -15min before chemotherapy | | 1000ml | i.v. | 2h | |
| | 1, 15 | Granisetron | -15min before chemotherapy | 1mg | | i.v. | bolus | |
| | 15/16 | Dexamethasone | -15 min, +4 and 8h/-15min | 8mg | | i.v./oral/oral | | |
| | 8, 22 | Saline 0.9% | 0h | | 500ml | i.v. | 1h | |
| | 8, 22 | Clemastine | -15min bevore Bleomycin | 2mg | | i.v. | bolus | |

**Medicines As Required:** Metoclopramide oral or i.v., Granisetron i.v., Heparin

**Anthracycline and Bleomycin:** see **cautions** above.

**Routine Tests:** FBC, U&Es, serum creatinine, clotting studies, LFTs, creatinine clearance, neurotoxicity

**Dose Reduction:** Mechlorethamine, Doxorubicin, Vinblastine and Etoposide Phosphate reduc.d to 65% of the dose if ANC 500-1000/µl, delay about 1 week if ANC<500/µl

**Max. Cum. Dose:** Doxo.: Danger of cardiotoxocity; max. cum. dose is 550mg/m²; **Bleo.**: Danger of pulmonary fibrosis esp. if cum. dose exceeds 400mg abs.; **Vincristine**: 5-20mg abs.; Danger of neurotox.

**Next Cycle (N.C.):** Day 29

**Efficacy Assess.:** After cycle 3

# VACOP-B  weeks 1, 5, 9   Page 1   Indication: NHL   11.4.1

*This chemotherapy may cause life-threatening toxicity! It should only be administered under the supervision of an experienced medical oncologist! The protocol must first be reviewed and considered in relationship to the clinical situation of the patient.*

## Chemotherapy

| Week | Day | Compounds (generic names) in chronological order | Dosage | Diluent | Route | Duration of Infusion | Comments | 1 | 2 | 3 | 4 | 5 | 6 | 7 | 8 | 9 | 10 | 11 | 12 |
|---|---|---|---|---|---|---|---|---|---|---|---|---|---|---|---|---|---|---|---|
| 1 | 1-7 | **Prednisone** | BSA<1.6m²: 75mg / BSA>1.6m²:100mg | | oral | | mornings | x | | | | | | | | | | | |
| 5,9 | 1,3,5,7 | **Prednisone** | | | | | | x | | | | x | | | | x | | | |
| 1,5,9 | 1 | **Doxorubicin** | 50mg/m² | undiluted | i.v. | bolus 15min | | x | | | | x | | | | x | | | |
| 1,5,9 | 1 | **Cyclophosphamide** | 350mg/m² | 250ml Saline 0.9% | i.v. | 1h | | x | | | | x | | | | x | | | |

### Cautions

Etoposide Phosphate and Sodium Bicarbonate must not be administered concomitantly through the same infusion site!

Because of possible CNS side effects (esp. in young patients) Metoclopramide may be replaced by Granisetron

**Anthracycline:** Danger of cardiotoxicity - echocardiogram

**Bleomycin:** Pulmonary function tests before start of therapy and after every second cycle

#### Weeks:

| | Dosage | Route | Duration |
|---|---|---|---|
| Doxorubicin | 50mg/m² | | |
| Cyclophosphamide | 350mg/m² | | |
| Vincristine | 1.2mg/m² | | |
| Bleomycin | 10mg/m² | | |
| Etoposide Phosphate | 50mg/m² | i.v. | day 1 |
| Etoposide | 100mg/m² | oral | days 2-3 |
| CNS Prophylaxis: | | | |

| Cycle Diagram | d1 w1 | d8 w2 | d15 w3 | d22 w4 | d29 w5 | d36 w6 | d43 w7 | d50 w8 | d57 w9 |
|---|---|---|---|---|---|---|---|---|---|
| Prednisone | | | | | | | | | |
| Doxorubicin | | | | | | | | | |
| Cyclophos. | | | | | | | | | |

## Obligatory Pre- and Concurrent Medication

| Week | Day | Compounds (generic names) | Sequence and Timing | Dose | Diluent | Route | Duration of Infusion | Comments |
|---|---|---|---|---|---|---|---|---|
| | 1 | Saline 0.9% | 15' before chemotherapy | 1000ml | | i.v. | 3h | |
| | 1 | Dexamethasone | 15' before Doxorubicin | 8mg | 100ml Saline 0.9% | i.v. | 15min | |
| | 1 | Metoclopramide | 15' before, 2h & 6h after Doxo. | 50mg | | i.v. | bolus | or 10-20mg orally (outpatients) |
| | 1 | Mesna | with start of Cyclophosphamide | 70mg/m² | | i.v. | bolus | |
| | 1 | Mesna | 2h and 6h after Cyclophosp. | 70mg/140mg/m² | | oral | 15min | or orally |
| | regularly | Co-trimoxazole | 1-0-1 (2x/week) | 960mg | | oral | | |
| | regularly | Amphotericin B | 1-1-1-1 | 100mg (1ml) | | oral | | assuspension |
| | regularly | Famotidine | evenings | 20mg | | oral | | |

| | |
|---|---|
| **Medicines As Required** | Metoclopramide, Famotidine 20mg evenings, Sucralfate |
| **Routine Tests:** | **Anthracycline** and **Bleomycin:** see cautions above; FBC, U&Es, serum creatinine, clotting studies, LFTs, creatinine clearance, neurotoxicity |
| **Dose Reduction:** | See Dose Modification Table |
| **Max. Cum. Dose :** | **Doxorubicin:** Danger of cardiotoxicity; max. cum. dose is 550 mg/m² |
| **Next Cycle (N.C.):** | Every 12 weeks |
| **Efficacy Assess.** | Interim evaluation after 6 weeks |
| **References:** | Connors JM et al., Ann Oncol 1991; 2 Suppl 1:17-23; Raanani P, Leuk Res 1998;22:997-1002 und 1999; 23:1 |

**11.4.1**

| VACOP-B   weeks 2, 4, 6, 8, 10, 12   Page 2 | Indication: NHL |
|---|---|

*This chemotherapy may cause life-threatening toxicity! It should only be administered under the supervision of an experienced medical oncologist! The protocol must first be reviewed and considered in relationship to the clinical situation of the patient.*

## Chemotherapy

| Week | Day | Compounds (generic names) in chronological order | Dosage | Diluent | Route | Duration of Infusion | Comments |
|---|---|---|---|---|---|---|---|
| 2,4,6,8,10,12 | 1,3,5,7 | **Prednisone** | BSA<1.6m²: 75mg / BSA>1.6m²: 100mg | | oral | | mornings |
| 2,4,6,8,10,12 | 1 | **Vincristine** | 1.2mg/m² | undiluted | i.v. | bolus 5min | |
| 2,4,6,8,10,12 | 1 | **Bleomycin** | 10mg/m² | undiluted | i.v. | bolus 5min | |
| 2,6,10 | 1 | **Cytarabine**[a] | 40mg | | i.t. | | |
| 2,6,10 | 1 | **Dexamethasone** | 4mg | undiluted | i.t. | | |
| 2,6,10 | 1 | **Methotrexate** | 15mg | | i.t. | | |

a: Accompanying CNS Prophylaxis: with orbital, testicular, parana al sinus, bone and bone marrow involvement as well as peripheral spread in weeks 2, 6 and 10 of the 3x/week systemic therapy, then triple intrathecal therapy: Cytarabine 40mg absolute, Dexamethasone 4mg absolute, Methotrexate 15mg absolute. Lit.: Liang et al., Hem Oncol, 1990;8(3):141-145

Bleomycin: Pulmonary function tests before start of therapy and after every second cycle

Because of possible CNS side effects (esp. in young patients) Metoclopramide may be replaced by Granisetron

### Cycle Diagram

| | d1 w1 | d8 w2 | d22 w4 | d36 w6 | d50 w8 | d64 w10 | d78 w12 |
|---|---|---|---|---|---|---|---|
| Prednisone | | | | | | | |
| Vincristine | | | | | | | |
| Bleomycin | | | | | | | |
| Cytarabine | | | | | | | |
| Dexameth. | | | | | | | |
| Methotrexate | | | | | | | |

### Weeks:

| Compound | Dosage | Diluent | Route | Duration of Infusion | 1 | 2 | 3 | 4 | 5 | 6 | 7 | 8 | 9 | 10 | 11 | 12 |
|---|---|---|---|---|---|---|---|---|---|---|---|---|---|---|---|---|
| Doxorubicin | 50mg/m² | | | | x | | x | | x | | x | | x | | x | |
| Cyclophosphamide | 350mg/m² | | | | x | | | | x | | | | x | | | |
| Vincristine | 1.2mg/m² | | | | | x | | x | | x | | x | | x | | x |
| Bleomycin | 10mg/m² | | | | | x | | x | | x | | x | | x | | x |
| Etoposide Phosphate | 50mg/m² | i.v. | day 1 | | x | | | | x | | | | x | | | |
| Etoposide | 100mg/m² oral | | days 2-3 | | x | | | | x | | | | x | | | |
| CNS Prophylaxis: | | | | | | x | | | | x | | | | x | | |

*(left margin: Cautions)*

## Obligatory Pre- and Concurrent Medication

| Week | Day | Compounds (generic names) | Sequence and Timing | Dose | Diluent | Route | Duration of Infusion | Comments |
|---|---|---|---|---|---|---|---|---|
| | 1 | Saline 0.9% | 15' before chemotherapy | | 250ml | i.v. | 30min | |
| | 1 | Prednisolone | before Bleomycin | 50mg | | i.v. | bolus | |
| | regularly | Co-trimoxazole | 1-0-1 (2x/week) | 960mg | | oral | | |
| | regularly | Amphotericin B | 1-1-1-1 | 100mg (1ml) | | oral | | as suspension |
| | regularly | Famotidine | evenings | 20mg | | oral | | |

| | |
|---|---|
| Medicines As Required | Metoclopramide oral or i.v., Sucralfate |
| Routine Tests: | **Bleomycin:** see **cautions** above; FBC, U&Es, blood glucose, LFTs, serum creatinine |
| Dose Reduction: | See Dose Modification Table; if due to neurological or pulmonary side effects **Vincristine** or **Bleomycin** cannot be given, **Methotrexate** 50mg absolute should be substituted instead |
| Max. Cum. Dose: | **Doxorubicin:** Danger of cardiotoxicity; max. cum. dose is 550 mg/m² |
| Next Cycle (N.C.): | Every 12 weeks |
| Efficacy Assess. | Interim evaluation after 6 weeks |
| References: | Connors JM et al., Ann Oncol 1991; 2 Suppl 1:17-23; Raanani P, Leuk Res 1998;22:997-1002 und 1999; 23:I |

| VACOP-B weeks 3, 7, 11 | Page 3 | Indication: NHL | 11.4.1 |
|---|---|---|---|

*This chemotherapy may cause life-threatening toxicity! It should only be administered under the supervision of an experienced medical oncologist! The protocol must first be reviewed and considered in relationship to the clinical situation of the patient.*

## Chemotherapy

| Week | Day | Compounds (generic names) in chronological order | Dosage | Diluent | Route | Duration of Infusion | Comments |
|---|---|---|---|---|---|---|---|
| 3,7,11 | 1,3,5,7 | **Prednisone** | BSA<1.6m²: 75mg / BSA>1.6m²:100mg | | oral | | |
| 3,7,11 | 1 | **Doxorubicin** | 50mg/m² | undiluted | i.v. | bolus 15min | |
| 3,7,11 | 1 | **Etoposide Phosphate** | 50mg/m² | 100ml Saline 0.9% | i.v. | 30min | dose expressed in terms of Etoposide base |
| 3,7,11 | 2,3 | **Etoposide Phosphate** | 100mg/m² | | oral | | |

Because of possible CNS side effects (esp. in young patients) Metoclopramide may be replaced by Granisetron

Anthracycline: Danger of cardiotoxicity - echocardiogram

**Cautions**

| Cycle Diagram | d1 w1 | d8 w2 | d15 w3 | d43 w7 | d71 w11 | d78 w12 |
|---|---|---|---|---|---|---|
| Prednisone | | | | | | |
| Doxorubicin | | | | | | |
| Etop.Phos. | | | | | | |
| Etoposide | | | | | | |

| | Weeks: | 1 | 2 | 3 | 4 | 5 | 6 | 7 | 8 | 9 | 10 | 11 | 12 |
|---|---|---|---|---|---|---|---|---|---|---|---|---|---|
| Doxorubicin | 50mg/m² | × | | × | | × | | × | | × | | × | |
| Cyclophosphamide | 350mg/m² | × | | × | | × | | × | | × | | × | |
| Vincristine | 1.2mg/m² | | × | | × | | × | | × | | × | | × |
| Bleomycin | 10mg/m² | | × | | × | | × | | × | | × | | × |
| Etoposide Phosphate | 50mg/m² i.v. day 1 | | × | | × | | × | | × | | × | | |
| Etoposide | 100mg/m² oral days 2-3 | | × | | × | | × | | × | | × | | |
| CNS Prophylaxis: | | × | | | | | | | | | | | |

## Obligatory Pre- and Concurrent Medication

| Week | Day | Compounds (generic names) | Dose | Diluent | Route | Duration of Infusion | Comments |
|---|---|---|---|---|---|---|---|
| | 1 | Saline 0.9% | 500ml | | i.v. | 3h | |
| | 1 | Dexamethasone | 8mg | 100ml Saline 0.9% | i.v. | 15min | |
| | 1 | Metoclopramide | 50mg | | i.v. | bolus | or 10mg orally |
| | regularly | Co-trimoxazole | 960mg | | oral | | |
| | regularly | Amphotericin B | 100mg (1ml) | | oral | | as suspension |
| | regularly | Famotidine | 20mg | | oral | | |

| | |
|---|---|
| Medicines As Required | Metoclopramide 50mg 2-3x/day, Sucralfate |
| Routine Tests: | **Anthracycline:** see **cautions** above; FBC, U&Es, serum creatinine, clotting studies, LFTs, creatinine clearance, neurotoxicity |
| Dose Reduction: | See Dose Modification Table |
| Max. Cum. Dose : | **Doxorubicin:** Danger of cardiotoxicity; max. cum. dose is 550 mg/m² |
| Next Cycle (N.C.): | Every 12 weeks |
| Efficacy Assess. | Interim evaluation after 6 weeks |
| References: | Connors JM et al., Ann Oncol 1991; 2 Suppl 1:17-23; Raanani P, Leuk Res 1998;22:997-1002 und 1999; 23:l |

| CHOP | | Indication: NHL (Follicular, Mantle Cell, Lymphoplasmacytic) | | | | | 11.4.2 |
|---|---|---|---|---|---|---|---|

*This chemotherapy may cause life-threatening toxicity! It should only be administered under the supervision of an experienced medical oncologist! The protocol must first be reviewed and considered in relationship to the clinical situation of the patient.*

## Chemotherapy

| Week | Day | Compounds (generic names) in chronological order | Dosage | Diluent | Route | Duration of Infusion | Comments |
|---|---|---|---|---|---|---|---|
| | 1 | **Cyclophosphamide** | 750mg/m² | 500ml Saline 0.9% | i.v. | 1h | |
| | 1 | **Doxorubicin** | 50mg/m² | undiluted | i.v. | bolus 15min | |
| | 1 | **Vincristine** | 1.4mg/m² | undiluted | i.v. | bolus | maximum dose 2mg absolute |
| | 1-5 | **Prednisone** | 100mg | | oral | | |

**Cautions**

Incompatibility: Doxorubicin<>Vincristine
Anthracycline: Danger of cardiotoxicity - echocardiogram

| Cycle Diagram | d1 w1 | d8 w2 | d15 w3 | d22 w4 |
|---|---|---|---|---|
| Cyclophos. | | | | N.C. |
| Doxorubicin | | | | |
| Vincristine | | | | |
| Prednisone | | | | |

## Obligatory Pre- and Concurrent Medication

| Week | Day | Compounds (generic names) | Sequence and Timing | Dose | Diluent | Route | Duration of Infusion | Comments |
|---|---|---|---|---|---|---|---|---|
| | 1 | Saline 0.9% | continuously | | 1000ml | i.v. | 2h | |
| | 1 | Dexamethasone | 15' before, 4h after chemo. | 8mg | 100ml Saline 0.9% | i.v. | 15min | or orally at home |
| | 1 | Metoclopramide | 15' before, 4h & 8h after chemo. | 50mg | | i.v. | bolus | or 10-20mg orally at home |
| | 1 | Mesna | 15' before, 4h, 8h after Cycloph. | 150/300mg/m² | | i.v. | bolus | or orally at home |
| | regularly | Amphotericin B | 1 - 1 - 1 - 1 | 100mg (1ml) | | oral | | as suspension |
| 1st neutropenic cycle* | 1 | Filgrastim | once a day | 5µg/kg | | s.c. | | *when WBC<1000/µl; give until >1000/µl |
| subsequent cycles | 2** | Pegfilgrastim | one dose only | 6mg | | s.c. | | **prophyl. admin. 24h after i.v. chemo. if decreased WBC in previous cycle |

| | |
|---|---|
| Medicines As Required | Metoclopramide oral or i.v., if not tolerated replace with 5-HT3 antagonists; Famotidine 20mg evenings. Sucra fate |
| Routine Tests: | **Anthracycline:** see **cautions** above; FBC, U&Es, blood glucose, serum creatinine, LFTs, creatinine clearance, diuresis, neurotoxicity |
| Dose Reduction: | If leukocytes < 1000/µl and / or platelets < 75,000/µl on 2 days, reduce doses in next cycle as follows: **1. Doxorubicin** to 40mg/m². **Cyclophosphamide** to 600mg/m². With additional fall in leukocyte and/or platelet count, reduce doses further: **2. Doxorubicin** to 30mg/m². **Cyclophosphamide** to 450mg/m². **3. Doxorubicin** to 20mg/m². **Cyclophosphamide** to 300mg/m² |
| Max. Cum. Dose : | **Doxorubicin:** Danger of cardiotoxicity; max. cum. dose is 550mg/m². **Vincristine** 5-20mg absolute: Danger of neurotoxicity |
| Next Cycle (N.C.): | Day 22 |
| Efficacy Assess. | After cycle 2 |
| References: | McKelvey EM et al., Cancer, 1976; 38: 1484-1493; Balducci L et al., Oncology (Huntingt), 2000; 14: 221-227 |

# R-CHOP

## Indication: Aggressive NHL

**11.4.3**

*This chemotherapy may cause life-threatening toxicity! It should only be administered under the supervision of an experienced medical oncologist! The protocol must first be reviewed and considered in relationship to the clinical situation of the patient.*

## Chemotherapy

| Week | Day | Compounds (generic names) in chronological order | Dosage | Diluent | Route | Duration of Infusion | Comments |
|---|---|---|---|---|---|---|---|
| | 0 | **Rituximab** | 375mg/m² | 500ml Saline 0.9% | i.v. | initially 25ml/h | -24h to -4 h before CHOP |
| | 1 | **Cyclophosphamide** | 750mg/m² | 500ml Saline 0.9% | i.v. | 1h | |
| | 1 | **Doxorubicin** | 50mg/m² | undiluted | i.v. | bolus 15min | |
| | 1 | **Vincristine** | 1.4mg/m² | undiluted | i.v. | bolus | maximum dose 2mg absolute |
| | 1-5 | **Prednisone** | 100mg | | oral | bolus | withdraw gradually in older patients |

| Cycle Diagram | d1 w1 | d8 w2 | d15 w3 | d22 w4 |
|---|---|---|---|---|
| Rituximab | | | | N.C. |
| Cycloph. | | | | |
| Doxorubicin | | | | |
| Vincristine | | | | |
| Prednisone | | | | |

### Cautions

**Rituximab Infusion Rate:**
**First Dose:** start at 50mg/h for 1hour; then if well tolerated increase every 30min by 50mg/h up to max. 400mg/h

**Subsequent Doses (excluding high-risk patients):** give 1/10 of the total dose in first 30min, then 9/10 of the total dose over the next 3.5 hours up to max. 400mg/h

**High-risk Patients** (high tumor burden, cardiovascular/respiratory disease, antibody incompatibility): start at 25mg/h for 1hour, then increase every 30min by 25mg/h up to max.200mg/h

**Anthracycline: Danger of cardiotoxicity - echocardiogram**

## Obligatory Pre- and Concurrent Medication

| Week | Day | Compounds (generic names) | Sequence and Timing | Dose | Diluent | Route | Duration of Infusion | Comments |
|---|---|---|---|---|---|---|---|---|
| | 0 | Omeprazole | mornings | 20mg | | oral | | |
| | 0 | Allopurinol | mornings | 300mg | | oral | | |
| | 0 | Saline 0.9% | -2h | | 1000ml | i.v. | 6h | |
| | 0 | Paracetamol | -1h | 1000mg | | oral | | |
| | 0 | Clemastine | -30min | 2mg | | i.v. | bolus | |
| | 1 | Saline 0.9% | -15min | | 1000ml | i.v. | 2h | |
| | 1 | Dexamethasone | 15' before, 4h after chemo. | 8mg | 100ml Saline 0.9% | i.v. | 15min | or orally at home |
| | 1 | Granisetron | 15' before chemotherapy | 1mg | | i.v. | bolus | or orally at home |
| | 1 | Mesna | 15' before, 4h, 8h after Cycloph. | 150/300mg/m² | | i.v. | bolus | assuspension |
| 1st neutropenic cycle* | regularly | Amphotericin B | 1 - 1 - 1 - 1 | 100mg (1ml) | | oral | | |
| | | Filgrastim | once a day | 5µg/kg | | s.c. | | *when WBC<1000/µl; give until >1000/µl |
| subsequent cycles | 2** | Pegfilgrastim | one dose only | 6mg | | s.c. | | **prophyl. admin. 24h after i.v. chemo. if decreased WBC in previous cycle |

| | |
|---|---|
| Medicines As Required | Metoclopramide oral or i.v., if not tolerated replace with 5-HT3 antagon sts; Pantoprazole 40mg, Sucralfate, Ciprofloxacin 500mg if WBC<1000/µl |
| Routine Tests | **Anthracycline**: see **cautions** above; FBC, U&Es, blood glucose, LFTs, serum creatinine, creatinine clearance, diuresis, **Rituximab** neurotoxicity: signs of intolerance/anaphylaxis |
| Max. Cum. Dose : | **Doxorubicin**: Danger of cardiotoxicity; max. cum. dose is 55 mg/m², **Vincristine** 5-20mg/m² absolute: Danger of neurotoxicity |
| Dose Reduction: | With delay > 7 days, see protocol |
| Next Cycle (N.C.): | Day 21 |
| Efficacy Assess. | Staging after 4 cycles |
| References: | Study protocol for Aggressive Non-Hodgkin's Lymphoma, Prof. Pfreundschuh, German Study Group, Homburg April 2001 |

| R-CHOP-14 | Indication: NHL | 11.4.4 |
|---|---|---|

*This chemotherapy may cause life-threatening toxicity! It should only be administered under the supervision of an experienced medical oncologist! The protocol must first be reviewed and considered in relationship to the clinical situation of the patient.*

## Chemotherapy

| Week | Day | Compounds (generic names) in chronological order | Dosage | Diluent | Route | Duration of Infusion | Comments |
|---|---|---|---|---|---|---|---|
| | 0 | **Rituximab** | 375mg/m² | 500ml Saline 0.9% | i.v. | initially 25mg/h | -24h to -4 h before CHOP-14 |
| | 1 | **Cyclophosphamide** | 750mg/m² | 500ml Saline 0.9% | i.v. | 1h | |
| | 1 | **Doxorubicin** | 50mg/m² | undiluted | i.v. | bolus 15min | |
| | 1 | **Vincristine** | 1.4mg/m² | | i.v. | bolus | maximum dose 2mg absolute |
| | 1-5 | **Prednisone** | 100mg | | oral | | withdraw gradually in older patients |

| Cycle Diagram | d1 w1 | d8 w2 | d15 w3 | d22 |
|---|---|---|---|---|
| Rituximab | | | | |
| Cyclophos. | | | | |
| Doxorubicin | | | | |
| Vincristine | | | | |
| Prednisone | | | | N.C. |

**Cautions**

**Rituximab Infusion Rate:**

**First Dose:** start at **50mg/h** for 1hour; then if well tolerated increase every 30min by 50mg/h up to max. 400mg/h

**Subsequent Doses (excluding high-risk patients):** give 1/10 of the total dose in the first 30min, then 9/10 of the total dose over the next 3.5 hours up to max. 400mg/h

**High-risk Patients** (high tumor burden, cardiovascular/respiratory disease, antibody incompatibility): start at 25mg/h for 1hour, then increase every 30min by 25mg/h up to max. 200mg/h

## Obligatory Pre- and Concurrent Medication

| Week | Day | Compounds (generic names) | Sequence and Timing | Dose | Diluent | Route | Duration of Infusion | Comments |
|---|---|---|---|---|---|---|---|---|
| | 0 | Omeprazole | mornings | 20mg | | oral | | |
| | 0 | Allopurinol | mornings | 300mg | | oral | | |
| | 0 | Saline 0.9% | -2h | | 1000ml | i.v. | 6h | |
| | 0 | Paracetamol | -1h | 1000mg | | oral | | |
| | 0 | Clemastine | -30min | 2mg | | i.v. | bolus | |
| | 1 | Saline 0.9% | -15min | | 1000ml | i.v. | 2h | |
| | 1 | Dexamethasone | 15' before, 4h after chemo. | 8mg | 100ml Saline 0.9% | i.v. | 15min | or orally at home |
| | 1 | Granisetron | 15' before chemotherapy | 1mg | | i.v. | bolus | |
| | 1 | Mesna | 15' before, 4h, 8h after Cycloph. | each dose is 20% that of Cyclophos. | | i.v. | bolus | or orally at home |
| | each cycle | Pegfilgrastim | once a day | 6mg | | s.c. | | |
| | regularly | Amphotericin B | 1 - 1 - 1 | 100mg (1ml) | | oral | | as suspension |
| | regularly | Co-trimoxazole | 1 - 0 - 1 (2x/week) | 960mg | | oral | | weeks 1-6 |

| | |
|---|---|
| Medicines As Required | Metoclopramide oral or i.v., if not tolerated replace with 5-HT3 antagonists; Pantoprazole 40mg, Sucralfate |
| Routine Tests: | CBC, U&Es, blood glucose, uric acid, serum creatinine, creatinine clearance, cardiac function, neurotoxicity; during **Rituximab** therapy: signs of intolerance/anaphylaxis |
| Dose Reduction: | With delay >7 days see protocol |
| Max. Cum. Dose : | **Daunorubicin** >550 mg/m²: Danger of cardiotoxicity; **Vincristine** 5-20mg absolute: Danger of neurotoxicity |
| Next Cycle (N.C.): | Day 15 |
| Efficacy Assess. | Staging after 4 cycles |
| References: | Tirelli et al. J Clin Oncol 16:27-34 (1998) |

# COP

## Indication: B-CLL, NHL, Relapsed NHL

**11.4.5**

*This chemotherapy may cause life-threatening toxicity! It should only be administered under the supervision of an experienced medical oncologist! The protocol must first be reviewed and considered in relationship to the clinical situation of the patient.*

### Chemotherapy

| Week | Day | Compounds (generic names) in chronological order | Dosage | Diluent | Route | Duration of Infusion | Comments |
|---|---|---|---|---|---|---|---|
| | 1–5 | **Cyclophosphamide** | 400mg/m² | 250ml Saline 0.9% | i.v. | 1h | the same dose may be given orally |
| | 1 | **Vincristine** | 1.4mg/m² | undiluted | i.v. | bolus | maximum dose 2mg absolute |
| | 1–5 | **Prednisone** | 100mg | | oral | | absolute |
| | | | | | | | |
| | | | | | | | |

| Cautions | Cycle Diagram | d1 w1 | d8 w2 | d15 w3 | d22 w4 |
|---|---|---|---|---|---|
| | Cyclophos. | | | | N.C. |
| | Vincristine | | | | |
| | Prednisone | | | | |

### Obligatory Pre- and Concurrent Medication

| Week | Day | Compounds (generic names) | Sequence and Timing | Dose | Diluent | Route | Duration of Infusion | Comments |
|---|---|---|---|---|---|---|---|---|
| | 1 | Saline 0.9% | 15' before chemotherapy | | 1000ml | i.v. | 3h | |
| | 1–5 | Granisetron | 15' before chemotherapy | 1mg | | i.v. | bolus | |
| | 1–5 | Dexamethasone | 15' before chemotherapy | 4mg | | i.v. | bolus 15min | |
| | 1–5 | Mesna | 0h, 4h, 8h after Cyclophosp. | 80/160mg/m² | | i.v. | bolus | may be given orally |
| 1st neutropenic cycle* | | Filgrastim | once a day | 5µg/kg | | s.c. | | *when WBC<1000/µl; give until >1000/µl |
| subsequent cycles | 6** | Pegfilgrastim | one dose only | 6mg | | s.c. | | **prophyl. admin. 24h after i.v. chemo. if decreased WBC in previous cycle |
| | | | mucositis prophylaxis | | | | | |

| | |
|---|---|
| **Medicines As Required** | Metoclopramide oral or i.v., if not tolerated replace with 5-HT3 antagonists; Famotidine 20mg evenings, Sucralfate |
| **Routine Tests:** | FBC, U&Es, blood glucose, serum creatinine, blood pressure, diuresis, neurotoxicity |
| **Dose Reduction:** | See Dose Modification Table |
| **Max. Cum. Dose :** | Vincristine 5-20mg absolute: Danger of neurotoxicity |
| **Next Cycle (N.C.):** | Day 22 |
| **Efficacy Assess.** | After 2-3 cycles |
| **References:** | Bagley CM et al., Ann Int Med, 1972;76:227-34; McKelvey EM et al., Cancer, 1976;38:1484-93 |

| DHAP | | | Indication: Relapsed NHL | | | | 11.4.6 |
|---|---|---|---|---|---|---|---|

*This chemotherapy may cause life-threatening toxicity! It should only be administered under the supervision of an experienced medical oncologist! The protocol must first be reviewed and considered in relationship to the clinical situation of the patient.*

## Chemotherapy

| Week | Day | Compounds (generic names) in chronological order | Dosage | Diluent | Route | Duration of Infusion | Comments |
|---|---|---|---|---|---|---|---|
| | 1 | **Cisplatin** | 100mg/m² | undiluted | i.v. | 22h | |
| | 2 | **Cytarabine** | 2g/m² twice a day | 250ml Saline 0.9% | i.v. | 3h | at 12 hourly intervals |
| | 1-4 | **Dexamethasone** | 40mg | | i.v. | 15min | may also be given orally |

| Cycle Diagram | d1 w1 | d8 w2 | d15 w3 | d22 w4 | d29 w5 |
|---|---|---|---|---|---|
| Cisplatin | | | | N.C. or | N.C. |
| Cytarabine | | | | | |
| Dexameth. | | | | | |

**Cautions**

**Please note: crystallization may occur with high concentration Mannitol solutions**

## Obligatory Pre- and Concurrent Medication

| Week | Day | Compounds (generic names) | Dose | Diluent | Route | Duration of Infusion | Comments |
|---|---|---|---|---|---|---|---|
| | 1 | Saline 0.9% | | 1000ml | i.v. | 12h | |
| | 1 | Saline 0.9% | | 2500ml | i.v. | 24h | |
| | 2-4 | Saline 0.9% | | 2000ml | i.v. | 24h | |
| | 1 | Mannitol 10% | | 1000ml | i.v. | 24h | |
| | 1-2 | Granisetron | 1mg | | i.v. | bolus | |
| | 1-4 | Sodium Bicarbonate | 1g | | oral | | |
| | 2-3 | Dexamethasone eye drops (1mg/ml) | 2 drops | | each eye | | |
| | 4-6 | Dexpanthenol eye drops (50mg/ml) | 1 drop | | each eye | | |
| | regularly | Co-trimoxazole | 240mg | | oral | | except on Cisplatin days |
| | regularly | Amphotericin B | 100mg (1ml) | | oral | | as suspension |
| 1st neutropenic cycle* | once a day | Filgrastim | 5μg/kg | | s.c. | | *when WBC<1000/μl; give until >1000/μl |
| subsequent cycles | 3** | Pegfilgrastim | 6mg | | s.c. | | **prophyl. admin. 24h after i.v. chemo. if decreased WBC in previous cycle |
| | 1, 2, 3 | Aprepitant | * | | oral | | * d1: 125mg, d2+3: 80mg |

| **Medicines As Required** | Granisetron i.v., Famotidine 20mg evenings, Sucralfate |
|---|---|
| **Routine Tests:** | FBC, U&Es, esp. Mg²⁺, blood glucose, serum creatinine, creatinine clearance, fluid balance, ototoxicity, neurotoxicity |
| **Dose Reduction:** | Withhold **Cisplatin** if creatinine clearance < 60ml/min; see Dose Modification Table |
| **Next Cycle (N.C.):** | Day 22 or 29 |
| **References:** | Velasquez WS et al., Blood, 1988;71:117-22 |

# Bendamustine

**Indication: NHL (e.g. CLL, Multiple Myeloma)** relapsed / therapy refractory in Binet Stages B+C / Rai stages II–IV

**11.5.1**

*This chemotherapy may cause life-threatening toxicity! It should only be administered under the supervision of an experienced medical oncologist! The protocol must first be reviewed and considered in relationship to the clinical situation of the patient.*

## Chemotherapy

| Week | Day | Compounds (generic names) in chronological order | Dosage | Diluent | Route | Duration of Infusion | Comments |
|---|---|---|---|---|---|---|---|
|  | 1–2 | **Bendamustine** | 100mg/m² | 500ml Saline 0.9% | i.v. | 1h | incompatible with other solutions |

### Cautions

| Cycle Diagram | d1 w1 | d8 w2 | d15 w3 | d22 w4 | d29 w5 d |
|---|---|---|---|---|---|
| Bendamustine |  |  |  |  | N.C. |

## Obligatory Pre- and Concurrent Medication

| Week | Day | Sequence and Timing | Compounds (generic names) | Dose | Diluent | Route | Duration of Infusion | Comments |
|---|---|---|---|---|---|---|---|---|
|  | 1–2 | 15' before chemotherapy | Metoclopramide | 50mg |  | i.v. | bolus |  |
|  | 1–2 | with chemotherapy | Saline 0.9% |  | 1000ml | i.v. | 2h |  |
|  |  | 1 - 0 - 1 (2x/week) | Co-trimoxazole | 960mg |  | oral |  | with CD4 cell counts<250/µl PCP prophylaxis |
|  |  | 1 - 0 - 0 | Folic Acid | 5mg |  | oral |  | with CD4 cell counts<250/µl PCP prophylaxis |

**Medicines As Required:** Metoclopramide oral or i.v., if not tolerated replace with 5-HT3 antagonists

**Routine Tests:** FBC, LFTs, renal function, U&Es, total protein, immune status

**Dose Reduction:** With occurrence of a hematological toxic reaction WHO Grade 4 (Gran. <0 5/nl for 2 days and/or platelets < 25/nl for 2 days): reduce dose by 25% to 75mg/m² i.v. on days 1 and 2 of the following cycle. This dose reduction does not apply to the cytopenia due to bone marrow infiltration

**Requirements:** Granulocytes at least 1500/µl; CD4 lymphocytes at least 100,000/µl as well as GFR > 30 ml/min and exclusion of severe liver parenchymal damage

**Max. Cum. Dose :** Unknown

**Next Cycle (N.C.):** Day 29 till CR achieved, 4 to 6 cycles maximum. With progression, discontinue therapy after 2 cycles at the earliest!

**Efficacy Assess.** After 2 cycles at the earliest; bone marrow biopsy 4 weeks after completing the last cycle

**References:** Aivado M et al, Sem Oncol, 2002; 29 (Suppl 13):19–22; Preiss R et al., Hematol. Journal, 2003, 4 (Suppl 1): Abstract 394

# Fludarabine

## Indication: NHL, CLL

**11.5.2**

*This chemotherapy may cause life-threatening toxicity! It should only be administered under the supervision of an experienced medical oncologist! The protocol must first be reviewed and considered in relationship to the clinical situation of the patient.*

## Chemotherapy

| Week | Day | Compounds (generic names) in chronological order | Dosage | Diluent | Route | Duration of Infusion | Comments |
|------|-----|-----|--------|---------|-------|----------------------|----------|
|      | 1–5 | **Fludarabine** | 25mg/m² | 250ml Saline 0.9% | i.v. | 1h | |
|      |     |     |        |         |       |                      |          |
|      |     |     |        |         |       |                      |          |
|      |     |     |        |         |       |                      |          |
|      |     |     |        |         |       |                      |          |
|      |     |     |        |         |       |                      |          |

| Cycle Diagram | d1 w1 | d8 w2 | d15 w3 | d22 w4 | d29 w5 | d36 |
|---------------|-------|-------|--------|--------|--------|-----|
| Fludarabine   |       |       |        |        | N.C.   |     |

**Cautions**

## Obligatory Pre- and Concurrent Medication

| Week | Day | Compounds (generic names) | Dose | Diluent | Route | Duration of Infusion | Comments |
|------|-----|---------------------------|------|---------|-------|----------------------|----------|
|      | 1–5 | Saline 0.9% | | 500ml | i.v. | 1h | |
|      | regularly | Co-trimoxazole | 960mg | | oral | | |
|      | regularly | Amphotericin B | 100mg (1ml) | | oral | | |

**Medicines As Required** With HSV or VZV seropositive patients: prophylaxis with Acyclovir 200mg every 12 hours, Metoclopramide oral or i.v.

**Routine Tests** FBC, U&Es, serum creatinine, LFTs, inflammation parameters

**Dose Reduction:** Undefined

**Max. Cum. Dose :** Unknown

**Next Cycle (N.C.):** Day 28

**Efficacy Assess.** After 3 cycles

**References:** Cheson BD et al., Semin Oncol, 1990;17(5):1-71

# Fludarabine/Cyclophosphamide — Indication: CLL/PLL/NHL — 11.5.3

*This chemotherapy may cause life-threatening toxicity! It should only be administered under the supervision of an experienced medical oncologist! The protocol must first be reviewed and considered in relationship to the clinical situation of the patient.*

## Chemotherapy

| Week | Day | Compounds (generic names) in chronological order | Dosage | Diluent | Route | Duration of Infusion | Comments |
|---|---|---|---|---|---|---|---|
| | 1-3 | **Fludarabine** | 30mg/m² | 250ml Saline 0.9% | i.v. | 30min | |
| | 1-3 | **Cyclophosphamide** | 300mg/m² | 250ml Saline 0.9% | i.v. | 1h | |

**Cautions**

Full blood count
Option: Filgrastim from day 4

| Cycle Diagram | d1 w1 | d8 w2 | d15 w3 | d22 w4 | d29 w5 | D36 |
|---|---|---|---|---|---|---|
| Fludarabine | | | | | | |
| Cyclophos. | | | | | N.C. | |

## Obligatory Pre- and Concurrent Medication

| Week | Day | Sequence and Timing | Compounds (generic names) | Dose | Diluent | Route | Duration of Infusion | Comments |
|---|---|---|---|---|---|---|---|---|
| | from day 1 | 1 - 0 - 0 | Allopurinol | 300mg | | oral | bolus | plus hydration if tumor lysis syndrome suspected |
| | 1-3 | with chemotherapy | Saline 0.9% | | 1500ml | i.v. | 4h | |
| | 1-3 | 15' before chemotherapy | Dexamethasone | 4mg | | i.v. | bolus | |
| | 1-3 | 0h, 4h & 8h after Cyclophos. | Mesna | 60mgm² | | i.v. | bolus | |
| | regularly | 1 - 0 -1 (2x/week) | Co-trimoxazole | 960mg | | oral | | |
| | regularly | 1 - 1 - 1 - 1 | Amphotericin B | 100mg (1ml) | | oral | | as suspension |

**Medicines As Required** Filgrastim, Metoclopramide oral or i.v., Granisetron 1mg i.v., with HSV or VZV seropositive patients: prophylaxis with Acyclovir 200mg every 12 hours

**Routine Tests** FBC, U&Es, serum creatinine, LFTs, inflammation parameters

**Dose Reduction:** If creatinine 1.6-2mg/dl, reduce **Fludarabine** to 20mg/m²; if creatinine > 2mg/m²; with cystitis Grade 2-4 reduce **Cyclophosphamide** to 200mg/m²

**Max. Cum. Dose :** Unknown

**Next Cycle (N.C.):** Day 28 as long as neutrophils > 1500/µl and platelets > 75,000/µl, maximum 6 cycles

**Efficacy Assess.** After 3 cycles

**References:** O'Brien et al., Ann of Oncol, 1996, 7 (Supl.6) S. 27-33

**Fludarabine/Cyclophosphamide/Rituximab**                    **Indication: CLL/PLL/NHL**                    **11.5.4**

*This chemotherapy may cause life-threatening toxicity! It should only be administered under the supervision of an experienced medical oncologist! The protocol must first be reviewed and considered in relationship to the clinical situation of the patient.*

## Chemotherapy

| Week | Day | Compounds (generic names) in chronological order | Dosage | Diluent | Route | Duration of Infusion | Comments |
|---|---|---|---|---|---|---|---|
| | 1 | **Rituximab** | 375mg/m² | 500ml Saline 0.9% | i.v. | initially 25mg/h | |
| | 2-4 | **Fludarabine** | 30mg/m² | 250ml Saline 0.9% | i.v. | 30min | |
| | 2-4 | **Cyclophosphamide** | 300mg/m² | 250ml Saline 0.9% | i.v. | 1h | |
| | | | | | | | |
| | | | | | | | |

| | | Cycle Diagram | d1 w1 | d8 w2 | d15 w3 | d22 w4 | d29 w5 |
|---|---|---|---|---|---|---|---|
| **Full blood count** | | Rituximab | | | | | N.C. |
| | | Fludarabine | | | | | |
| **Cautions** | | Cyclophos. | | | | | |

## Obligatory Pre- and Concurrent Medication

| Week | Day | Compounds (generic names) | Dose | Diluent | Route | Duration of Infusion | Comments |
|---|---|---|---|---|---|---|---|
| | 1 | Omeprazole | 20mg | | oral | | |
| | 1 | Allopurinol | 300mg | | oral | | |
| | 1 | Saline 0.9% | | 1000ml | i.v. | 6h | |
| | 1 | Paracetamol | 1000mg | | oral | | |
| | 1 | Clemastine | 2mg | | i.v. | bolus | |
| | 2-4 | Saline 0.9% | | 1500ml | i.v. | 4h | |
| | 2-4 | Dexamethasone | 4mg | | i.v. | bolus | |
| | 2-4 | Mesna | 60mg/m² | | i.v. | bolus | as suspension |
| | Mon. & Thurs. | Co-trimoxazole | 960mg | | oral | | |
| | regularly | Amphotericin B | 100mg (1ml) | | oral | | |
| 1st neutropenic cycle* | once a day | Filgrastim | 5µg/kg | | s.c. | | *when WBC<1000/µl: give until >1000/µl |
| subsequent cycles | 5** | one dose only | Pegfilgrastim | 6mg | | s.c. | | **prophyl. admin. 24h after i.v. chemo. if decreased WBC in previous cycle |

| | |
|---|---|
| Medicines As Required | Metoclopramide oral/i.v., Granisetron 1mg orally; with HZV or VZV seropositive patients: prophylaxis with Aciclovir 200mg twice a day |
| Routine Tests: | FBC, U&Es, LFTs, serum creatinine, inflammation parameters |
| Dose Reduction: | If creatinine 1.6-2mg/dl, reduce **Fludarabine** to 20mg/m²; if creatinine > 2mg/dl reduce **Fludarabine** to15mg/m²; with cystitis Grade 2-4 reduce **Cyclophosphamide** to 200mg/m² |
| Max. Cum. Dose : | Unknown |
| Next Cycle (N.C.): | Day 28 provided neutrophils >1500/µl and platelets >75,000/µl; 6 cycles |
| Efficacy Assess. | After 3 cycles |
| References: | Analogous to Flinn et al., Blood, 2000: 96: 71-75 and Byrd et al., Blood, 2003: 101: 6-14 |

# Chlorambucil/Prednisone ("Knospe")

## Indication: CLL, Low Grade NHL

**11.5.5**

*This chemotherapy may cause life-threatening toxicity! It should only be administered under the supervision of an experienced medical oncologist! The protocol must first be reviewed and considered in relationship to the clinical situation of the patient.*

## Chemotherapy

| Week | Day | Compounds (generic names) in chronological order | Dosage | Diluent | Route | Duration of Infusion | Comments |
|---|---|---|---|---|---|---|---|
| | 1 | **Chlorambucil** | 18mg/m² | | oral | | dose may be increased by 5mg/m² per cycle depending on compatibility |
| | 1 | **Prednisone** | 75mg | | oral | | |
| | 2 | **Prednisone** | 50mg | | oral | | |
| | 3 | **Prednisone** | 25mg | | oral | | |

**Cautions**

| Cycle Diagram | d1 w1 | d8 w2 | d15 w3 | d22 w4 |
|---|---|---|---|---|
| Chlorambucil | | | | |
| Prednisone 75 | | | N.C. | |
| Prednisone 50 | | | | |
| Prednisone 25 | | | | |

## Obligatory Pre- and Concurrent Medication

| Week | Day | Compounds (generic names) | Dose | Diluent | Route | Duration of Infusion | Comments |
|---|---|---|---|---|---|---|---|
| | | | | | | | |

| | |
|---|---|
| Medicines As Required | Metoclopramide oral or i.v., Sucralfate, Famotidine 20mg evenings |
| Routine Tests | FBC, U&Es, blood glucose, serum creatinine, diuresis, cardiac function |
| Dose Reduction: | Undefined |
| Max. Cum. Dose : | Unknown |
| Next Cycle (N.C.): | Day 15 |
| Efficacy Assess. | After 2-3 months |
| References: | Knospe WH et al., Cancer 1974;33:555-62 |

| Alemtuzumab | analogous to MabCampath Study (0372) Arm A | Indication: CLL | 11.5.6 |

*This chemotherapy may cause life-threatening toxicity! It should only be administered under the supervision of an experienced medical oncologist! The protocol must first be reviewed and considered in relationship to the clinical situation of the patient.*

## Chemotherapy

| Week | Day | Compounds (generic names) in chronological order | Dosage | Diluent | Route | Duration of Infusion | Comments |
|---|---|---|---|---|---|---|---|
| 1 | 1 | **Alemtuzumab** | 3mg | | s.c. | | **Check Dose Escalation Table.** With severe dose-related side effects ≥CTC Grade 3: repeat same dose at daily intervals. |
| 1 | 2 | **Alemtuzumab** | 10mg | | s.c. | | With serious skin reactions from s.c. admin.: dose escalation may be effected by i.v. admin. (as a 2-hourly infusion) |
| 1 | 3 | **Alemtuzumab** | *30mg | 2x1.5ml | s.c. | | |
| 2-13 | 1,3,5 | **Alemtuzumab** | *30mg | 2x1.5ml | **s.c. | | **3x per week (Mon, Wed, Fri) for 4-12 weeks.** The first day of the 30mg administration marks the start of a 4-12 week course of treatment |

*For the 30mg s.c. dose: give 1 injection of 1.5ml into each thigh

**In patients, who have serious skin reactions after one s.c. dose escalation despite maximum premedication, changing Alemtuzumab from s.c. to i.v. administration may be considered

### Cautions

Week 1:

**Alemtuzumab Dose Escalation Table**

Day 1: 3mg Alemtuzumab s.c. → well tolerated toxicity < CTC Grade 3 / poorly tolerated toxicity ≥ CTC Grade 3

Day 2: 10mg Alemtuzumab s.c. → well tolerated toxicity < CTC Grade 3 / poorly tolerated toxicity ≥ CTC Grade 3

Day 3: 30mg Alemtuzumab s.c.

4-12 weeks in total: 30mg Alemtuzumab s.c.; 3x per week (Mon, Wed, Fri)

**Cycle Diagram**

| | d1 w1 | d8 w2 | d15 w3 | d22 w4 | weeks 5-11 | d78 w12 | d85 w13 |
|---|---|---|---|---|---|---|---|
| Alemtuzumab 3mg | | | | | | | |
| Alemtuzumab 10 mg | | | | | | | |
| Alemtuzumab 30mg | | | | | | | |
| Alemtuzumab 30mg | | | | | etc | | |

## Obligatory Pre- and Concurrent Medication

| Week | Day | Compounds (generic names) | Sequence and Timing | Dose | Diluent | Route | Duration of Infusion | Comments |
|---|---|---|---|---|---|---|---|---|
| 1-13 | from day 1 | Pegfilgrastim | every 2 weeks | 6mg | | s.c. | | for neutropenia prophylaxis; not if WBC>20,000/µl |
| 1-13 | from day 1 | Allopurinol | 1-0-0 | 300mg | | oral | | |
| 1 (-13) | 1-3 (1,3,5) | Paracetamol | 30' before Alemtuzumab | 500mg | | oral | | during dose escalation; gradually withdraw afterwards if well tolerated |
| 1 (-13) | 1-3 (1,3,5) | Clemastine | 30' before Alemtuzumab | 2mg | | i.v. | 15min | |
| 1 | 1-3 | Prednisolone | 30' before Alemtuzumab | 100mg | 100ml Saline 0.9% | i.v. | 15min | for severe dose-related side effects |
| 1 | 1-3 | Pethidine | 30' before Alemtuzumab | 25-50mg | | i.v. | | during dose escalation; no long-term use |
| | from day 8 | Folic Acid | 1-0-1 | 5mg | | oral | | |
| | from day 8 | Co-trimoxazole | 1-0-1 (2x/week) | 960mg | | oral | | until at least 4 months after Alemtuzumab therapy or till CD4 > 200/µl |
| | from day 8 | Aciclovir | 1-1-1 daily | 400mg | | oral | | |

**Medicines As Required:** For bone pain during Pegfilgrastim therapy: Paracetamol 500mg orally; for patients with a susceptibility to infection, antifungals (e.g. Amphotericin suspension) and antibacterials (e.g. Ciprofloxacin) may be given; with CMV reactivation: Ganciclovir 5mg/kg/day i.v.; if a transfusion is required, irradiated blood products must be given

**Routine Tests:** Weekly: FBC, WBC differential; in addition, after 4, 8 and 12 weeks of Alemtuzumab 30mg: Quick's test, U&Es, renal function, LFTs, upper abdominal ultrasound, CXR; bone marrow cytology and histology when appropriate e.g. with cytopenia/remission

**Dose Reduction:** With hematologic toxicity Grade 4 (platelets <25,000/µl, neutrophils <250/µl, Hb <56.5g/dl): **1st occurrence:** restart Alemtuzumab at 30mg after recovery; **2nd occurrence:** 10mg; with therapy interruptions >7days, gradual dose escalation must be restarted each time; **3rd occurrence, severe infection or symptomatic CMV infection:** discontinue treatment. After complete recovery and repeatedly negative CMV testing, therapy may be resumed

**Efficacy Assess.:** After 4, 8 and 12 weeks of Alemtuzumab 30mg

**Repeat Therapy:** Therapy duration with Alemtuzumab 30mg is between 4 weeks (minimum) and 12 weeks (maximum)

**References:** Study protocol (0372); Keating MJ et al, BLOOD;2002;99(10);3554-61; Rai KR et al,J Clin Onc;2002;20(18);3891-97

# 2-CdA

**Indication: Hairy Cell Leukemia, CLL, PLL, Cutaneous T-NHL**

11.5.7

*This chemotherapy may cause life-threatening toxicity! It should only be administered under the supervision of an experienced medical oncologist! The protocol must first be reviewed and considered in relationship to the clinical situation of the patient.*

## Chemotherapy

| Week | Day | Compounds (generic names) in chronological order | Dosage | Diluent | Route | Duration of Infusion | Comments |
|---|---|---|---|---|---|---|---|
| 1 | 1-5 | **Cladribine (2-CdA)** | 0.14mg/kg | 500ml Saline 0.9% | i.v. | 2h | |
| | | **alternative for Hairy Cell Leukemia:** | | | | | |
| 1 | 1-5 | **Cladribine (2-CdA)** | 0.14mg/kg | undiluted | s.c. | bolus | |

**Cautions**

| Cycle Diagram | d1 w1 | d8 w2 | d15 w3 | d22 w4 | d29 w5 | d36 |
|---|---|---|---|---|---|---|
| Cladribine | | | | therapy cycle is not normally repeated | | |

## Obligatory Pre- and Concurrent Medication

| Week | Day | Compounds (generic names) | Sequence and Timing | Dose | Diluent | Route | Duration of Infusion | Comments |
|---|---|---|---|---|---|---|---|---|
| | regularly | Co-trimoxazole | 1 - 0 - 1 (2x/week) | 960mg | | oral | | |

**Medicines As Required:** For HSV or VZV seropositive patients: prophylaxis with Aciclovir 200mg every 12 hours orally; Metoclopramide oral or i.v.; Allopurinol orally

**Routine Tests** In particular, regular FBC for the first 4-8 weeks after the start of therapy, inflammation parameters, neurotoxicity, serum creatinine, LFTs

**Dose Reduction:** Subcutaneous preparation of **Cladribine** contraindicated in patients with a creatinine clearance ≤ 50ml/min and/or with moderate to severe liver insuffiency

**Max. Cum. Dose :** Unspecified

**Next Cycle (N.C.):** Normally only one cycle with hairy cell leukemia; therapy may be repeated after remission control

**References:** von Rohr A et al., Ann Oncol. 2002;13(10):1641-9; Guchelaar HJ et al., Ann Hematol 1994, 69(5): 223- 230; Beutler E et al., Blo od Cells 1993, 19(3): 559- 568;

# Pentostatin

## Indication: Hairy Cell Leukemia

**11.5.8**

*This chemotherapy may cause life-threatening toxicity! It should only be administered under the supervision of an experienced medical oncologist! The protocol must first be reviewed and considered in relationship to the clinical situation of the patient.*

## Chemotherapy

| Week | Day | Compounds (generic names) in chronological order | Dosage | Diluent | Route | Duration of Infusion | Comments |
|------|-----|--------------------------------------------------|--------|---------|-------|---------------------|----------|
| | 1 | **Pentostatin** | 4mg/m² | 500ml Saline 0.9% | i.v. | 30min | |
| | | | | | | | |
| | | | | | | | |
| | | | | | | | |

**Cautions**

| Cycle Diagram | d1 w1 | d8 w2 | d15 w3 | d22 w4 | d29 w5 | d36 |
|---------------|-------|-------|--------|--------|--------|-----|
| Pentostatin | | | N.C. | | | |

## Obligatory Pre- and Concurrent Medication

| Week | Day | Sequence and Timing | Compounds (generic names) | Dose | Diluent | Route | Duration of Infusion | Comments |
|------|-----|---------------------|---------------------------|------|---------|-------|---------------------|----------|
| | 1 | 30' before chemotherapy | Glucose 5% | | 1500ml | i.v. | 1h30min | |
| | 1 | 15' before chemotherapy | Dexamethasone | 4mg | | i.v. | bolus | |

**Medicines As Required:** Paracetamol 500-1000mg orally, Metoclopramide oral or i.v.

**Routine Tests:** FBC, serum creatinine, creatinine clearance, urea, uric acid, LFTs

**Dose Reduction:** With creatinine clearance <60ml/min--> discontinue; with impaired liver function: bilirubin 1.5-3mg/d or AST 60-180U/l --> reduce dose to 75%, bilirubin 3-5mg/dl or AST >180U/l --> reduce dose to 50%, bilirubin>5mg/dl--> discontinue

**Therapy Deferral:** Interrupt therapy if neutrophils <200/µl (in patients with neutrophils >500/µl before therapy)

**Interactions:** In combination with **Fludarabine**, severe pulmonary toxicity is possible! Avoid combination with **Cyclophosphamide**

**Next Cycle (N.C.):** Day 15; 3-5 cycles

**References:** Flinn IW et al. Blood (2000) 96: 2981-2986;Goodman GR et al Curr Opin Hematol (2003) 10: 258-266; Maloisel F et al. Leukemia (2003) 17: 45-51

# Rituximab

## Indication: Follicular B-cell NHL

**11.5.9**

## Chemotherapy

| Week | Day | Compounds (generic names) in chronological order | Dosage | Diluent | Route | Duration of Infusion | Comments |
|---|---|---|---|---|---|---|---|
| | 1, 8, 15, 22 | **Rituximab** | 375mg/m² | 500ml Saline 0.9% | i.v. | initially 50mg/h | |

| Cycle Diagram | d1 w1 | d8 w2 | d15 w3 | d22 w4 | d29 w5 | d36 w6 | d43 w7 | d50 w8 | d57 w9 |
|---|---|---|---|---|---|---|---|---|---|
| Rituximab | | | | | | | | | N.C. |

**Cautions**

**Rituximab Infusion Rate:**

**First Dose:** start at 50mg/h for 1hour; then if well tolerated increase every 30min by 50mg/h up to max. 400mg/h

**Subsequent Doses (excluding high-risk patients):** give 1/10 of the total dose in first 30min, then 9/10 of the total dose over the next 3.5 hours up to max. 400mg/h

**High-risk Patients** (high tumor burden, cardiovascular/respiratory disease, antibody incompatibility): start at 25mg/h for 1hour, then increase every 30min by 25mg/h up to max.200mg/h

**Monitoring:** every 15 min in the first hour, then hourly: blood pressure, heart rate, respiratory rate, temperature;

**FULL RESUSCITATION FACILITIES SHOULD BE AT HAND!**

If an allergic/anaphylactic reaction occurs (chills, fever et ), stop infusion IMMEDIATELY, Corticosteroids, intensive care treatment may be necessary.

With improvement of symptoms: therapy may be resumed slowly with a 50% reduction in infusion rate

## Obligatory Pre- and Concurrent Medication

| Week | Day | Sequence and Timing | Compounds (generic names) | Dose | Diluent | Route | Duration of Infusion | Comments |
|---|---|---|---|---|---|---|---|---|
| | 1, 8, 15, 12 | 0h | Saline 0.9% | | 500ml | i.v. | | with the chemotherapy |
| | 1, 8, 15, 22 | -1h | Paracetamol | 1000mg | | oral | | |
| | 1, 8, 15, 22 | -1h | Saline 0.9% | | 1000ml | i.v. | 5h | |
| | 1, 8, 15, 22 | -30min | Clemastine | 2mg | | i.v. | bolus | |

| | | |
|---|---|---|
| Medicines As Required | Prednisolone 50mg i.v. before and during Rituximab therapy | |
| Routine Tests: | Uric acid, urea, bilirubin, serum creatinine; during infusion: signs of incompatibility/anaphylaxis especially if leukocytes > 50,000/µl | |
| Next Cycle (N.C.): | Depending on clinical course | |
| Efficacy Assess. | 5 weeks after the end of the first cycle (4 doses), i.e. in week 9 | |
| References: | Maloney DG et al., Blood 1994, 84:2457-2466, Maloney DG et al., Blood 1997, 90:2188-2195 | |

# 90Y-Ibritumomab Tiuxetan + Rituximab

**Indication:** FL +
Mantle Cell Lymphoma

**11.5.10**

*This chemotherapy may cause life-threatening toxicity! It should only be administered under the supervision of an experienced medical oncologist! The protocol must first be reviewed and considered in relationship to the clinical situation of the patient.*

## Immunotherapy

| Week | Day | Compounds (generic names) in chronological order | Dosage | Diluent | Route | Duration of Infusion | Comments |
|---|---|---|---|---|---|---|---|
| | 1, 8 | **Rituximab** | 250mg/m² | | i.v. | Initially 50mg/h | |
| | 8 | **90Y-Ibritumomab Tiuxetan** | 14.8MBq/kg (0.4mCi/kg) | | i.v. | 10min | immediately following Rituximab |

**Cycle Diagram**

| | d1 w1 | d8 w2 | d15 w3 | d22 w4 |
|---|---|---|---|---|
| Rituximab | | | | |
| 90Y-Ibritumomab Tiuxetan | | | | |

### Cautions

**Please note: therapy contraindicated if bone marrow infiltration >25%**

**Rituximab Infusion Rate:**

**First Dose:** start at 50mg/h for 1hour; then if well tolerated increase every 30min by 50mg/h up to max. 400mg/h

**Subsequent Doses (excluding high-risk patients):** give 1/10 of the total dose over the next 3.5 hours up to max. 400mg/h

**High-risk Patients** (high tumor burden, cardiovascular/respiratory disease, antibody incompatibility): start at 25mg/h for 1hour, then increase every 30min by 25mg/h up to max.200mg/h

**Monitoring: every 15 min in the first hour, then hourly: blood pressure, heart rate, respiratory rate, temperature;**

**FULL RESUSCITATION FACILITIES SHOULD BE AT HAND!**

If an allergic/anaphylactic reaction occurs (chills, fever et ), stop infusion IMMEDIATELY, Corticosteroids, intensive care treatment may be necessary.

With improvement of symptoms: therapy may be resumed slowly with a 50% reduction in infusion rate

## Obligatory Pre- and Concurrent Medication

| Week | Day | Compounds (generic names) | Dose | Diluent | Route | Duration of Infusion | Comments |
|---|---|---|---|---|---|---|---|
| | 1, 8 | Paracetamol | 1000mg | | oral | | before Rituximab dose |
| | 1, 8 | Clemastine | 2mg | | i.v. | bolus | before Rituximab dose |

| | |
|---|---|
| **Medicines As Required** | Prednisolone 50mg i.v. before and during Rituximab infusion |
| **Routine Tests:** | FBC, clinical chemistry, signs of intolerance/anaphylaxis during Rituximab or 90Y-Ibritumomab Tiuxetan therapy |
| **Dose Reduction:** | Reduce dose of 90Y-Ibritumomab Tiuxetan to 11.1MBq/kg (0.3mCi/kg) if platelets <150,000 or past history of autologous PBSCT |
| **Max. Cum. Dose :** | Maximum allowable dose of 90Y-Ibritumomab Tiuxetan is 1184 MBq, but 888MBq if platelets 100,000-150,000 |
| **Next Cycle (N.C):** | None |
| **Efficacy Assess.** | After 6 weeks and 3, 6, 9, 12 months |
| **References:** | Hagenbeek A. Leuk.Lymphoma 2003, vol44,S37-S47, |

# R-MCP

## Indication: CNS - NHL >65 years  —  11.6.1

*This chemotherapy may cause life-threatening toxicity! It should only be administered under the supervision of an experienced medical oncologist! The protocol must first be reviewed and considered in relationship to the clinical situation of the patient.*

## Chemotherapy

| Week | Day | Compounds (generic names) in chronological order | Dosage | Diluent | Route | Duration of Infusion | Comments |
|---|---|---|---|---|---|---|---|
| | -6, 1, 15, 29 | **Rituximab** | 375mg/m² | 500ml Saline 0.9% | i.v. | initially 50mg/h | |
| | 2 to 11 | **Procarbazine** | 60 mg/m² | | oral | | |
| | 2 | **Lomustine** | 110mg/m² | | oral | | |
| | 2, 16, 30 | **Methotrexate** | 3000mg/m² | | i.v. | 4h | |
| | 3-6, 17-20, 31-34 | **Calcium Folinate (Leucovorin)** | 15 mg/m² | | i.v./oral | | every 6 hours, **1st dose i.v.**; commence 24h after start of Methotrexate |

### Cautions

| Cycle Diagram | d 1 w1 | d8 w2 | d15 w3 | d22 w4 | d29 w5 | d36 w6 | d |
|---|---|---|---|---|---|---|---|
| Procarbazine | | | | | | | |
| Lomustine | | | | | | | N.C. |
| Methotrexate * | * | | * | | * | | |
| Leucovorin | | | | | | | |

**1st Staging:** after 2 cycles Methotrexate; PD/NC: whole brain irradiation >/= 50Gy with response: 3 further cycles until best response or side effects

**2nd Staging:** after 3 cycles; if residual tumor, radiotherapy may be given

**Rituximab:** **First Dose: start at 50mg/h for 1h; if well tolerated increase every 30min by 50mg/h up to max. 400mg/h. High-risk Pat.: start at 25mg/h for 1h, increase e ery 30min by 25mg/h up to max 200mg/h. Subsequent Dose: 1/10 of the total dose in 30min, then 9/10 over next 3.5h**

With delayed Methotrexate elimination: extension and dose increase of Leucovorin rescue in accordance with the Methotrexate Document in the COSS Database (chapter 3.5)

## Obligatory Pre- and Concurrent Medication

| Week | Day | Compounds (generic names) | Sequence and Timing | Dose | Diluent | Route | Duration of Infusion | Comments |
|---|---|---|---|---|---|---|---|---|
| | -6, 1, 15, 29 | Paracetamol | -1h | 1000mg | | oral | | before Rituximab |
| | -6, 1, 15, 29 | Clemastine | -30min | 2mg | | i.v. | bolus | before Rituximab |
| | 2, 16, 30 | Saline 0.9% | 3h before chemotherapy | | 1000ml | i.v. | 3h | urine pH must remain >7.4! |
| | | Sodium Bicarbonate | | 60ml/m² | in infusion fluid | | | |
| | 2-3, 16-17, 30-31 | Saline 0.9% + Gluc. 5% alternately | 15min before chemotherapy | | 2000ml + 1000ml | i.v. | 24h | urine target pH = 8 |
| | 2-3, 16-17, 30-31 | Sodium Bicarbonate | continuously | 200ml | | i.v. | 24h | |
| | 2, 16, 30 | Dexamethasone | 15min before chemotherapy | 8mg | | i.v. | bolus | **\* Rituximab:** |
| | 2, 16, 30 | Granisetron | 15min before chemotherapy | 1mg | | i.v. | bolus | First cycle day -6, 1, 15, 29 |
| | 2, 16, 30 | Furosemide | 6h after Methotrexate | 40mg | | i.v. | bolus | Following cycles: day 1, 15, 29 |

| | |
|---|---|
| Medicines As Required | Potassium orally, NaHCO₃ infusion 50ml/2 hours, Metoclopramide, Famotidine, Prednisolone 50mg i.v. before and during Rituximab infusion |
| Routine Tests: | FBC, U&Es, LFTs, serum creatinine, creatinine clearance, fluid balance, exclude third space fluid accumulation, urine pH >7.4, serum Methotrexate level; normal values according to Rescue Sheets |
| Dose Reduction: | Contraindication: if GFR <50ml/min or serum creatinine > 1.5 mg/min or serum creatinine > 1.5 mg% as well as serum bilirubin >2mg/dl |
| Max. Cum. Dose : | Unknown |
| Next Cycle (N.C.): | Day 43 |
| Efficacy Assess. | After 1 course (6weeks) |
| References: | adapted according to Provencio M et al., Ann Oncol 2006;17(6):1027-8  nd cerebral NHL protocol University of Freiburg |

881

| CNS - NHL High-Dose Methotrexate    Freiburg Protocol    Page 1 | Indication: CNS - NHL | ICD-10: C85.9 | 11.6.2 |
|---|---|---|---|

*This chemotherapy may cause life-threatening toxicity! It should only be administered under the supervision of an experienced medical oncologist! The protocol must first be reviewed and considered in relationship to the clinical situation of the patient.*

## Chemotherapy

| Week | Day | Compounds (generic names) in chronological order | Dosage | Diluent | Route | Duration of Infusion | Comments |
|---|---|---|---|---|---|---|---|
| | **Prephase:** | **Dexamethasone** | 4mg every 6 hours | | oral/i.v. | | withdraw gradually over 6 days beginning with start of Methotrexate |
| | | diagnostic L.P. if intracranial pressure normal; with CSF involvement: assessment on day 20 after i.v. Methotrexate dose | | | | | |
| | -6, 0, 10, 20, 30 | **Rituximab** | 375 mg/m² | | i.v. | 4h | |
| | 1, 11, 21, 31 | **Methotrexate** | 8000 mg/m² | | i.v. | | |
| | 2-6, 12-16, 22-26 | **Calcium Folinate (Leucovorin)** | 15 mg/m² | | i.v./oral | | every 6 hours, **1st dose i.v.;** commence 24h after start of Methotrexate |
| | 32-36 | | | | | | see Rescue Protocol |

**Note:** with delayed Methotrexate elimination: extension and dose increase of Leucovorin rescue in accordance with the Methotrexate Document

**cave:** no aminoglycosides or NSAR during MTX application

Days 16-20  1st staging: if **PR/CR**, repeat therapy (cycle 2)
if PD/SD, start AraC/Thiotepa therapy

Days 38-40  2nd staging before AraC/Thiotepa therapy

**continue therapy with AraC/Thiotepa, starting on day 41**

Cycle Diagram

| | d-7 w0 | d1 w1 | d8 w2 | d15 w3 | d22 w4 | d29 w5 | d36 w6 | d43 w7 | d50 w8 | d57 w9 | d64 w10 |
|---|---|---|---|---|---|---|---|---|---|---|---|
| Dexameth. | | | | | | | | | | | |
| Rituximab | | | | | | | | | | | |
| Methotrexate | | | | | | | | | | | |
| | | | | PR/CR staging | | | staging | | | | |
| | | | | PD/SD =>CNS-NHL HD, continue therapy with AraC/TT | | | | | | | |
| Leucovorin | | | | | | | | | | | |

## Obligatory Pre- and Concurrent Medication

| Week | Day | Sequence and Timing | Compounds (generic names) | Dose | Diluent | Route | Duration of Infusion | Comments |
|---|---|---|---|---|---|---|---|---|
| | -5 till end of Dex. | 1 - 1 - 1 - 1 | Sucralfate | 1g | | oral | | during Dexamethasone therapy |
| | 0, 10, 20, 30 | 2 - 2 - 2 - 2 | Sodium Bicarbonate | 2g | | oral | | |
| | 1, 11, 21, 31 | 3h before chemotherapy | Saline 0.9% | | 1000ml | i.v. | 3h | urine pH must remain >7.4! |
| | 1, 11, 21, 31 | | Sodium Bicarbonate | 60mmol/m² | in infusion fluid | | | urine target pH = 8 |
| | 1-2, 11-12, 21-22, 31-32 | 15min before chemotherapy | Saline 0.9% + Gluc.5% alternately | | 2000ml + 1000ml | i.v. | 24h | |
| | 1-2, 11-12, 21-22, 31-32 | continuously | Sodium Bicarbonate | 200mmol | | i.v. | 24h | |
| | 1, 11, 21, 31 | 15min before chemotherapy | Dexamethasone | 8mg | | i.v. | 15min | |
| | 1, 11, 21, 31 | 15min before chemotherapy | Granisetron | 1mg | | i.v. | bolus | |
| | 1, 11, 21, 31 | 6h after Methotrexate | Furosemide | 40mg | | i.v. | bolus | |

| | |
|---|---|
| **Medicines As Required:** | Potassium orally, NaHCO₃ infusion 50mmol/2 hours, Famotidine, Furosemide 40mg |
| **Routine Tests:** | FBC, U&Es, LFTs, serum creatinine, creatinine clearance, fluid balance, exclude third space fluid accumulation, urine pH >7.4, serum Methotrexate level; normal values according to Rescue Sheets |
| **Dose Reduction:** | Contraindication: if GFR < 50ml/min or serum creatinine > 1.5 mg% or serum bilirubin >2mg/dl |
| **Max. Cum. Dose:** | Unknown |
| **Next Cycle (N.C.):** | With **PR/CR**, continue therapy with next cycle starting on day 21 (cycle2) |
| **Efficacy Assess.** | Days 18-20, days 38-40 |
| **References:** | Freiburg protocol: therapy for primary cerebral NHL. |

Cautions

882

| CNS - NHL AraC/Thiotepa   Freiburg Protocol   Page 2 | Indication: CNS - NHL | ICD-10: C85.9 | 11.6.2 |
|---|---|---|---|

*This chemotherapy may cause life-threatening toxicity! It should only be administered under the supervision of an experienced medical oncologist! The protocol must first be reviewed and considered in relationship to the clinical situation of the patient.*

## Chemotherapy

| Week | Day | Compounds (generic names) in chronological order | Dosage | Diluent | Route | Duration of Infusion | Comments |
|---|---|---|---|---|---|---|---|
| | 0, 21 | **Rituximab** | 375 mg/m² | | i.v. | | |
| | 1, 2, 22, 23 | **Cytarabine (AraC)** | 3000 mg/m² | | i.v. | 3h | |
| | 2, 23 | **Thiotepa** | 40mg/m² | | i.v. | 1h | |
| | 10 | **Harvest** | | | | | |

Cycle Diagram: d-7 w0 | d1 w1 | d8 w2 | d15 w3 | d22 w4 | d29 w5 | d36 w6 | d43 w7 | d50 w8

Rituximab, Cytarabine, Thiotepa, Filgrastim, Harvest, Staging, BCNU, PBSCT

**Cautions**

PBSCT to be carried out not less than 3 days after the last dose of Thiotepa

Thiotepa is secreted in sweat! In order to avoid a toxic induced erythroderma especially in the axillary and inguinal regions, frequent washing with a wet flannel is recommended

MRT before 2nd cycle AraC/Thiotepa

- PR,CR or SD and reduction of neurologic symptoms: continue with 2nd cycle AraC/Thiotepa
- PD or SD without reduction of neurologic symptoms: continue with HD-BCNU/Thiotepa

## Obligatory Pre- and Concurrent Medication

| Week | Day | Sequence and Timing | Compounds (generic names) | Dose | Diluent | Route | Duration of Infusion | Comments |
|---|---|---|---|---|---|---|---|---|
| | 1, 2, 22, 23 | 30min before chemotherapy | Saline 0.9% | | 2000ml | i.v. | 24h | |
| | 1, 2, 22, 23 | 30min before chemotherapy | Dexamethasone | 8mg | | i.v. | 15min | |
| | 1, 2, 22, 23 | 30min before chemotherapy | Granisetron | 1mg | | i.v. | bolus | |
| | 1-3, 21, 22, 23 | every 6 hours | Dexamethasone eye drops (1mg/ml) | 2 drops | | each eye | | |
| | 4-8, 25-29 | every 6 hours | Dexpanthenol eye drops (50mg/ml) | 1 drop | | each eye | | |
| | 6-10, 27-31 | mornings | Filgrastim | 300µg absolute | | s.c. | | |

| Medicines As Required | Famotidine |
|---|---|
| Routine Tests: | FBC, U&Es, LFTs, serum creatinine |
| Dose Reduction: | GFR < 10ml/min is a relative contraindication |
| Max. Cum. Dose: | Unknown |
| Next Cycle (N.C.): | None |
| Efficacy Assess. | 3rd staging between days 18 and 20, 4th staging between days 38 and 40 |
| References:- | Freiburg protocol: therapy for primary cerebral NHL; Illerhaus et al. J Clin Onc 2006. |

## CNS - NHL High-Dose BCNU/Thiotepa  Freiburg Protocol   Page 3   Indication: CNS - NHL   ICD-10: C 85.9   11.6.2

*This chemotherapy may cause life-threatening toxicity! It should only be administered under the supervision of an experienced medical oncologist! The protocol must first be reviewed and considered in relationship to the clinical situation of the patient.*

### Chemotherapy

| Week | Day | Compounds (generic names) in chronological order | Dosage | Diluent | Route | Duration of Infusion | Comments |
|---|---|---|---|---|---|---|---|
| | 42 (-7) | **Rituximab** | 375 mg/m² | | i.v. | 1h | |
| | 43 (-6) | **Carmustine (BCNU)** | 400 mg/m² | | i.v. | 2h | |
| | 44 & 45 (-5 & -4) | **Thiotepa** | 5mg/kg twice a day | | i.v. | | at 12 hourly intervals |
| | 49 (0) | **Peripheral Blood Stem Cell Transplantation** | | | | | |

**Cycle Diagram**

| | d-7 w0 | d1 w1 | d8 w2 | d15 w3 | d22 w4 | d29 w5 | d36 w6 | d43 w7 | d50 w8 |
|---|---|---|---|---|---|---|---|---|---|
| Rituximab | | | | | | | | | |
| Cytarabine | | | | | | | | | |
| Thiotepa | | | | | | | | | |
| Filgrastim | | | | | | | | | |
| Harvest | | | <--> | | | | | | |
| Staging | | | | | | <--> | | | ---> |
| BCNU | | | | | | | | | |
| PBSCT | | | | | | | | | |

**Cautions**

PBSCT to be carried out not less than 3 days after the last dose of Thiotepa

Thiotepa is secreted in sweat! In order to avoid a toxic induced erythroderma especially in the axillary and inguinal regions, frequent washing with a wet flannel is recommended.

### Obligatory Pre- and Concurrent Medication

| Week | Day | Compounds (generic names) | Sequence and Timing | Dose | Diluent | Route | Duration of Infusion | Comments |
|---|---|---|---|---|---|---|---|---|
| | 43 | Saline 0.9% | 30min before chemotherapy | | 2000ml | i.v. | 24h | |
| | 44, 45 | Saline 0.9% | 30min before chemotherapy | | 3000ml | i.v. | 24h | |
| | 43, 44, 45 | Heparin | 30min before chemotherapy | 15000 units | | i.v. | 24h | |
| | 43, 44, 45 | Granisetron | 30min before chemotherapy | 1mg | | i.v. | bolus | |
| | 43, 44, 45 | Dexamethasone | 30min before chemotherapy | 8mg | | i.v. | 15min | |
| | 43, 44, 45 | Dexamethasone | +4h, +8h | 8mg | | i.v. | 15min | |
| | 53 (+5) | Pegfilgrastim | mornings | 6 mg | | s.c. | | |
| | regularly | Amphotericin B | 1 - 1 - 1 - 1 | 100mg (1ml) | | oral | | as suspension |
| | regularly | Co-trimoxazole | 1 - 0 - 0 | 960mg | | oral | | |

**Medicines As Required:** Metoclopramide, Famotidine

**Routine Tests:** FBC, U&Es, LFTs, serum creatinine., pulmonary function tests including carbon monoxide diffusion capacity, echocardiogram

**Dose Reduction:** GFR < 10ml/min, bilirubin >2mg/dl are relative contraindications

**Max. Cum. Dose:** Carmustine: increased risk of pulmonary toxicity when total cumulative dose >1000 mg/m²

**Next Cycle (N.C.):** None

**Efficacy Assess.:** Day 30 after PBSCT

**References:** Freiburg protocol: therapy for primary cerebral NHL. Illerhaus et al. J Clin Onc 2006

# Melphalan/Prednisone ("Alexanian")   Indication: Multiple Myeloma   11.7.1

*This chemotherapy may cause life-threatening toxicity! It should only be administered under the supervision of an experienced medical oncologist! The protocol must first be reviewed and considered in relationship to the clinical situation of the patient.*

## Chemotherapy

| Week | Day | Compounds (Generic names) in chronological order | Dosage | Diluent | Route | Duration of infusion | Comments |
|---|---|---|---|---|---|---|---|
| | 1–4 | **Melphalan** | 8mg/m² | | oral | | should be taken on an empty stomach |
| | 1–4 | **Prednisone** | 60mg/m² | | oral | | should be taken after food |
| | | | | | | | |
| | | | | | | | |
| | | | | | | | |
| | | | | | | | |

**Cautions**

| Cycle diagram | d1 w1 | d8 w2 | d15 w3 | d22 w4 | d29 w5 | d36 w6 | d |
|---|---|---|---|---|---|---|---|
| Melphalan | ▓ | | | | ▓ | | |
| Prednisone | | | | | | | |

## Obligatory Pre- and Concurrent Medication

| Week | Day | Sequence and Timing | Compound (Generic name) | Dose | Diluent | Route | Duration of infusion | Comments |
|---|---|---|---|---|---|---|---|---|
| every 4 weeks | 1–4 | 2 - 0 - 2 | Calcium–Sodium–Citrate (Acetolyt®) | 5g | | oral | | |
| | | | Zoledronic Acid | 4mg | | i.v. | 15min | |
| | | mucositis prophylaxis, hydration > 200ml orally per day | | | | | | |

| | |
|---|---|
| **Medicines As Required** | Metoclopramide oral or i.v.; Allopurinol according to uric acid, Sucralfate |
| **Routine Tests:** | FBC, U&Es esp. Ca²⁺, blood glucose, bilirubin, serum creatinine, creatinine clearance |
| **Dose Reduction:** | See Dose Modification Table |
| **Max. Cum. Dose :** | Unknown |
| **Repeat Therapy:** | Every 4 weeks; **Melphalan** dose may be increased by 20% depending on effectiveness and side effects; may be given intravenously |
| **Efficacy Assess.** | After 3 cycles |
| **References:** | Alexanian R et al., JAMA, 1969;208:1680–1685 |

# High-Dose Dexamethasone

## Indication: Multiple Myeloma

**11.7.2**

consider high dose therapy esp. with hyperkalemia or pancytopenia as well as concurrent radiotherapy

*This chemotherapy may cause life-threatening toxicity! It should only be administered under the supervision of an experienced medical oncologist! The protocol must first be reviewed and considered in relationship to the clinical situation of the patient.*

## Chemotherapy

| Week | Day | Compounds (Generic names) in chronological order | Dosage | Diluent | Route | Duration of infusion | Comments |
|---|---|---|---|---|---|---|---|
| | 1-4, 9-12, 17-20 | **Dexamethasone** | 40mg/m² | | oral | | mornings |
| | | | | | | | |

Cycle diagram: d1 w1 | d8 w2 | d15 w3 | d22 w4 | d29 w5 | d36 w6 | d43 w7 | d50 w8 | d57 w9
Dexameth.

**Cautions**

## Obligatory Pre- and Concurrent Medication

| Week | Day | Sequence and Timing | Compound (Generic name) | Dose | Diluent | Route | Duration of infusion | Comments |
|---|---|---|---|---|---|---|---|---|
| | | 1-0-1 (2x/week) | Co-trimoxazole | 960mg | | oral | | till end of therapy |
| | | 1-0-0 | Folic Acid | 5mg | | oral | 15min | till end of therapy |
| | regularly | 1-0-0 | Omeprazole | 20mg | | oral | | |
| | 1-7 | after food | Allopurinol | 100mg | | oral | | |
| | 1-4 | 1-1-1 | Sodium Bicarbonate | 2g | | oral | | |
| | regularly | 1-1-1-1 | Amphotericin B | 100mg (1ml) | | oral | | as suspension |
| | every 4 weeks | | Zoledronic Acid | 4mg | | i.v. | 15min | |

| | |
|---|---|
| **Medicines As Required** | Famotidine |
| **Routine Tests:** | FBC, U&Es, blood glucose, blood pressure monitoring, diuresis, psychological status |
| **Dose Reduction:** | Adjust dose with side effects: diabetes, hypertension, psychological changes; interval may be extended if necessary |
| **Repeat Therapy:** | After treatment-free interval of 14 days (day 35), then dose may be reduced by 20-40% according to side effects |
| **Efficacy Assess.** | After 6 weeks |
| **References:** | Alexanian R et al., Blood, 1992;80:887-890 |

| VAD | | | **Indication:** | **Multiple Myeloma** Stages II, III | | with primary chemo. resistance, consider high dose therapy | **11.7.3** |

*This chemotherapy may cause life-threatening toxicity! It should only be administered under the supervision of an experienced medical oncologist! The protocol must first be reviewed and considered in relationship to the clinical situation of the patient.*

## Chemotherapy

| Week | Day | Compounds (generic names) in chronological order | Dosage | Diluent | Route | Duration of Infusion | Comments |
|---|---|---|---|---|---|---|---|
| | 1-4 | **Vincristine** | 0.4mg | in 50ml Saline 0.9% | i.v. | 24h | infusion pump via central line |
| | 1-4 | **Doxorubicin** | 9mg/m² | in 50ml Saline 0.9% | i.v. | 24h | infusion pump via central line |
| | 1-4,17-20 | **Dexamethasone** | 40mg | | oral | | 1 - 0 - 0 |
| | | **(in cycle 1 Dexamethasone also on days 9-12)** | | | | | |

Anthracycline: Danger of cardiotoxicity - monitor cardiac function (echocardiogram)

**Cautions**

| Cycle Diagram | d1 w1 | d8 w2 | d15 w3 | d22 w4 | d29 w5 | d36 w6 | d43 w7 | d5 |
|---|---|---|---|---|---|---|---|---|
| Vincristine | | | | | | | N.C. | |
| Doxorubicin | | | | | | | | |
| Dexameth. | | cycle1 | | | | | | |

## Obligatory Pre- and Concurrent Medication

| Week | Day | Compounds (generic names) | Sequence and Timing | Dose | Diluent | Route | Duration of Infusion | Comments |
|---|---|---|---|---|---|---|---|---|
| every 4 weeks | 1-4 | Saline 0.9% | with chemotherapy | 1000ml | | i.v. | 24h | |
| | | Zoledronic Acid | 1 - 0 - 1 - 0 | 4mg | | i.v. | 15min | |
| | 1-4 | Calcium-Sodium-Citrate (Acetolyt®) | 1 - 0 - 1 (2x/week) | 10g | | oral | | |
| | regularly | Co-trimoxazole | 1 - 1 - 1 - 1 | 960mg | | oral | | |
| | regularly | Sucralfate | 1 - 1 - 1 - 1 | 1g | | oral | | |
| | regularly | Amphotericin B | 1 - 1 - 1 - 1 | 100mg (1ml) | | oral | | assuspension |
| | | | mucositis prophylaxis | | | | | |

| | |
|---|---|
| Medicines As Required | Arrhythmias, Allopurinol for large tumor mass, Metoclopramide oral or i.v., Famotidine 20mg |
| Routine Tests: | **Anthracycline:** see **cautions** above; FBC, blood glucose, neurotoxicity, signs of paralytic ileus (Vincristine), blood pressure |
| Dose Reduction: | See Dose Modification Table |
| Max. Cum. Dose : | **Doxorubicin:** Danger of cardiotoxicity; max. cum. dose is 550mg/m²; **Vincristine** 5-20mg/m² absolute: Danger of neurotoxicity |
| Next Cycle (N.C.): | Day 43 |
| Efficacy Assess. | After 3 cycles |
| References: | Barlogie B et al., N Engl J Med, 1984;310:1353-1356 |

| Ind1Cyclo | | Indication: Induction Therapy (MM) | 11.7.4 |
|---|---|---|---|

## Chemotherapy

*This chemotherapy may cause life-threatening toxicity! It should only be administered under the supervision of an experienced medical oncologist! The protocol must first be reviewed and considered in relationship to the clinical situation of the patient.*

| Week | Day | Compounds (generic names) in chronological order | Dosage | Diluent | Route | Duration of Infusion | Comments |
|---|---|---|---|---|---|---|---|
| | 1 | **Cyclophosphamide** | 1000mg/m² | 500ml Saline 0.9% | i.v. | 1h | |
| | | | | | | | |
| | | | | | | | |

**Cautions**

After day 1 protocol for prophylaxis of delayed emesis

| Cycle Diagram | d1 w1 | d8 w2 | d15 w3 | d22 w4 |
|---|---|---|---|---|
| Cyclophos. | | | | |
| | | | | |
| | | | | |

## Obligatory Pre- and Concurrent Medication

| Week | Day | Compounds (generic names) | Sequence and Timing | Dose | Diluent | Route | Duration of Infusion | Comments |
|---|---|---|---|---|---|---|---|---|
| | 1 | Saline 0.9% | 15' before chemotherapy | 1000ml | | i.v. | 2h | |
| | 1 | Dexamethasone | 15' before chemotherapy | 8mg | 100ml Saline 0.9% | i.v. | 15min | |
| | 1 | Granisetron | 15' before chemotherapy | 1mg | | i.v. | bolus | |
| | 1 | Mesna | 0h, 4h & 8h after chemotherapy | each dose is 20% that of Cyclophos. | | i.v. | bolus | or orally (outpatients) |
| | | | mucositis prophylaxis | | | | | |

| | |
|---|---|
| **Medicines As Required** | Metoclopramide, Ondansetron, Dexamethasone |
| **Routine Tests** | FBC, U&Es, serum creatinine, creatinine clearance, diuresis |
| **Dose Reduction:** | Reduce **Cyclophosphamide** with liver and renal impairment, see Dose Modification Table |
| **Repeat Therapy:** | Every 2 weeks, staging after 4 cycles |
| **References:** | Medical Research Council. Br. J. Cancer 1980;42:823. |

| CTD | Indication: | Multiple Myeloma | 11.7.5 |

## Chemotherapy

*This chemotherapy may cause life-threatening toxicity! It should only be administered under the supervision of an experienced medical oncologist! The protocol must first be reviewed and considered in relationship to the clinical situation of the patient.*

| Week | Day | Compounds (generic names) in chronological order | Dosage | Diluent | Route | Duration of Infusion | Comments |
|---|---|---|---|---|---|---|---|
| | 1-5; 15-19 | **Thalidomide** | 50mg* | | oral | | 0 - 0 - 0 - 1 |
| | 1-5 | **Cyclophosphamide** | 150mg/m²*** | | oral | | 1 - 0 - 0 - 0 |
| | 1-5; 15-19 | **Dexamethasone** | 20mg/m² | | oral | | 1 - 0 - 0 - 0 |

| Cycle Diagram | d1 w1 | d8 w2 | d15 w3 | d22 w4 | d29 w5 | d |
|---|---|---|---|---|---|---|
| Thalidomide | | | | | N.C. | |
| Cyclophos. | | | | | | |
| Dexameth. | | | | | | |

**Dose Increases:**

*Thalidomide: increase by 50mg every 2 weeks up to a maximum of 200mg/day

**Cyclophosphamide: increase to 150mg/m² twice a day if response inadequate

Cyclophosphamide should be taken before food and Dexamethasone after food

*(left margin: Cautions)*

## Obligatory Pre- and Concurrent Medication

| Week | Day | Compounds (generic names) | Sequence and Timing | Dose | Diluent | Route | Duration of Infusion | Comments |
|---|---|---|---|---|---|---|---|---|
| | | Co-trimoxazole | 1 - 0 - 1 - 0 | 960mg | | oral | | |
| | | Folic Acid | 1 - 0 - 0 - 0 | 5mg | | oral | | |
| | regularly | Amphotericin B | 1 - 1 - 1 - 1 | 100mg (1ml) | | oral | | as suspension |

| | |
|---|---|
| Medicines As Required: | Metoclopramide orally, Pantoprazole orally, constipation prophylaxis, p.ssibly prophylactic anticoagulation to patients at risk of deep vein thrombosis; possibly prophylactic antifungals |
| Routine Tests: | FBC, U&Es, blood glucose, uric acid, serum creatinine, bilirubin; with multiple myeloma: tumor lysis syndrome, thrombosis risk |
| Dose Reduction: | According to **Thalidomide** side effect profile e.g. deep vein thrombosis, polyneuropathy |
| Max. Cum. Dose : | None |
| Next Cycle (N.C.): | Every 28 days, 3 cycles in total; repeat course monthly in responsive patients, giving therapy on days 1-5 only |
| References: | Analogous to Dimopoulos A. et al., Hematol J. 2004;5(2):112-7 |

# Low-Dose Thalidomide +Dexamethasone    Indication:    Multiple Myeloma    11.7.6

*This chemotherapy may cause life-threatening toxicity! It should only be administered under the supervision of an experienced medical oncologist! The protocol must first be reviewed and considered in relationship to the clinical situation of the patient.*

## Chemotherapy

| Week | Day | Compounds (generic names) in chronological order | Dosage | Diluent | Route | Duration of Infusion | Comments |
|------|-----|-----|-----|-----|-----|-----|-----|
| | regularly | **Thalidomide** | 50mg* | | oral | | 0 - 0 - 0 - 1 |
| | see Cycle Diagram | **Dexamethasone** | 20mg absolute | | oral | | 1 - 0 - 0 - 0 |
| | | | | | | | |
| | | | | | | | |
| | | | | | | | |

**Cautions**

***Thalidomide Dose Increase:**
increase by 50mg every 2 weeks up to a maximum of 400mg/day
(on average, the best toleranced dose is 200mg/day)

| Cycle Diagram Dexameth. | d1 w1 | d8 w2 | d15 w3 | d22 w4 | d29 w5 |
|------|------|------|------|------|------|
| Cycle 1 | | | | | N.C. |
| Cycle 2 | | | | | |
| Cycle 3 | | | | | |

## Obligatory Pre- and Concurrent Medication

| Week | Day | Compounds (generic names) | Sequence and Timing | Dose | Diluent | Route | Duration of Infusion | Comments |
|------|-----|-----|-----|-----|-----|-----|-----|-----|
| | | Co-trimoxazole | 1 - 0 - 1 - 0 (2x/week) | 960mg | | oral | | |
| | | Folic Acid | 1 - 0 - 0 - 0 | 5mg | | oral | | |
| | regularly | Amphotericin B | 1 - 1 - 1 - 1 | 100mg (1ml) | | oral | | as suspension |
| | regularly | Enoxaparin Sodium | 1 - 0 - 0 | 20mg | | s.c. | | |
| | | | | | | | | |
| | | | | | | | | |
| | | | | | | | | |
| | | | | | | | | |
| | | | | | | | | |
| | | | | | | | | |
| | | | | | | | | |
| | | | | | | | | |

**Medicines As Required:** Metoclopramide orally, Pantoprazole orally, constipation prophylaxis, prophylactic anticoagulation to patients at risk of deep vein thrombosis; possibly prophylactic antifungals

**Routine Tests:** FBC, U&Es, blood glucose, uric acid, serum creatinine, bilirubin; with multiple myeloma: tumor lysis syndrome, thrombosis risk

**Dose Reduction:** According to **Thalidomide** side effect profile e.g. deep vein thrombosis, polyneuropathy

**Max. Cum. Dose :** None

**Next Cycle (N.C.):** Regular administration of **Thalidomide** throughout, **Dexamethasone** according to **Cycle Diagram** above, with next cycle starting on day 30

**Efficacy Assess.** After 3 cycles

**References:** analogous to: Weber et al. J Clin Oncol. 2003 Jan 1;21(1):16-9; Rajku ar et al. J Clin Oncol. 2002 Nov 1;20(21):4319-23; Singhal et al. N Engl J Med;341(21):1565-71

# Bortezomib

**Indication: Multiple Myeloma**    **11.7.7**

*This chemotherapy may cause life-threatening toxicity! It should only be administered under the supervision of an experienced medical oncologist! The protocol must first be reviewed and considered in relationship to the clinical situation of the patient.*

## Chemotherapy

| Cycle | Day | Compounds (generic names) in chronological order | Dosage | Diluent | Route | Duration of Infusion | Comments |
|---|---|---|---|---|---|---|---|
| 1–8 | 1,4,8,11 | **Bortezomib** | 1.3mg/m² | undiluted | i.v. | bolus | induction therapy |
| 9–11 | 1,8,15,22 | **Bortezomib** | 1.3mg/m² | undiluted | i.v. | bolus | maintenance therapy |

**Cycle Diagram**

| | d1 w1 | d8 w2 | d15 w3 | d22 w4 | d29 w5 | d36 w6 |
|---|---|---|---|---|---|---|
| Bortezomib (cycles 1–8) | ▨ | ▨ | ▨ | N.C. | | |
| Bortezomib (cycles 9–11) | ▨ | ▨ | ▨ | ▨ | | N.C. |

A time interval of at least 72 hours between Bortezomib doses is recommended

### Bortezomib Dose Reduction

| | Hematologic Toxicity (esp. thrombocytopenia) | Neuropathy |
|---|---|---|
| | Grades 1 or 2 : no dose reduction | **Grade 1:** no dose reduction |
| | | **Grade 1+ pain or Grade 2:** reduce dose to 1mg/m² |
| | **Grade 3:** no dose reduction, transfuse if necessary, evaluate therapy risks | **Grade 2+ pain or Grade 3:** withhold therapy, then give 0.7mg/m² once a week |
| | **Grade 4:** withhold therapy; restart after recovery, but reduce dose by 25% | **Grade 4:** discontinue therapy |

*Cautions*

## Obligatory Pre- and Concurrent Medication

| Cycle | Day | Compounds (generic names) | Sequence and Timing | Dose | Diluent | Route | Duration of Infusion | Comments |
|---|---|---|---|---|---|---|---|---|
| 1–11 | every 4 weeks | Zoledronic Acid | | 4mg | | i.v. | 15min | |

**Medicines As Required:** Loperamide, Famotidine, Sucralfate

**Routine Tests:** FBC, clinical chemistry, TTP analysis, radiographic skeletal survey (weeks 12 & 30), Karnofsky Index, paraprotein measurements (serum and urine), HbA1c/CRP (weeks 9,18,27), neurotoxicity, bone marrow biopsy if >Grade 3 infection

**Dose Reduction:** See **Cautions** above and Summary of Product Characteristics - SmPC)

**Next Cycle (N.C.):** Day 22 for cycles 1–8; day 36 for cycles 9–11

**References:** Richardson PG et al., N Engl J Med. 2005 Jun 16; 352(24): 2487–98; Lonial et al., Blood. 2005 Dec 1;106(12):3777–84

# DeCyBo

**Indication:    Multiple Myeloma**    **11.7.8**

*This chemotherapy may cause life-threatening toxicity! It should only be administered under the supervision of an experienced medical oncologist! The protocol must first be reviewed and considered in relationship to the clinical situation of the patient.*

## Chemotherapy

| Cycle | Day | Compounds (generic names) in chronological order | Dosage | Diluent | Route | Duration of Infusion | Comments |
|---|---|---|---|---|---|---|---|
| 1-8 | 1,4,8,11 | **Bortezomib** | 1.3mg/m² | undiluted | i.v. | bolus | |
| 1-8 | 1,2,4,5,8,9,11,12 | **Dexamethasone** | 20mg absolute | | oral | | |
| 1-8 | 1-21 | **Cyclophosphamide** | 50mg absolute | | oral | | |
| 9-11 | 1,8,15,22 | **Bortezomib** | 1.3mg/m² | undiluted | i.v. | bolus | |
| 9-11 | 1,2,8,9,15,16,22,23 | **Dexamethasone** | 20mg absolute | | oral | | |
| 9-11 | 1-35 | **Cyclophosphamide** | 50mg absolute | | oral | | |

**Cycle Diagram**

| | | d1 w1 | d8 w2 | d15 w3 | d22 w4 | d29 w5 | d36 w6 |
|---|---|---|---|---|---|---|---|
| Bortezomib | (cycles 1-8) | | | | | | |
| Dexameth. | (cycles 1-8) | | | | N.C. | | |
| Cyclophos. | (cycles 1-8) | | | | | | |
| Bortezomib | (cycles 9-11) | | | | | | |
| Dexameth. | (cycles 9-11) | | | | | | N.C. |
| Cyclophos. | (cycles 9-11) | | | | | | |

A time interval of at least 72 hours between Bortezomib doses is recommended

### Cautions

**Bortezomib Dose Reduction**

| Hematologic Toxicity (esp. thrombocytopenia) | Neuropathy |
|---|---|
| **Grades 1 or 2:** no dose reduction | **Grade 1: no dose reduction** |
| | **Grade 1+ pain or Grade 2:** reduce dose to 1mg/m² |
| **Grade 3:** no dose reduction, transfuse if necessary, evaluate therapy risks | **Grade 2+ pain or Grade 3:** withhold therapy, then give 0.7mg/m² once a week |
| **Grade 4:** withhold therapy; restart after recovery, but reduce dose by 25% | **Grade 4: discontinue therapy** |

## Obligatory Pre- and Concurrent Medication

| Cycle | Day | Sequence and Timing | Compounds (generic names) | Dose | Diluent | Route | Duration of Infusion | Comments |
|---|---|---|---|---|---|---|---|---|
| 1-11 | regularly | 1 - 0 - 0 - 0 | Pantoprazole | 40mg | | oral | | |
| 1-11 | regularly | 1 - 1 - 1 - 1 | Amphotericin B | 100mg (1ml) | | oral | | as suspension |
| 1-11 | | 1 - 0 - 1 - 0 | Co-trimoxazole | 960mg | | oral | | to be started on week 3 |
| 1-11 | | 1 - 0 - 0 - 0 | Folic Acid | 5mg | | oral | | |
| 1-11 | every 4 weeks | | Zoledronic Acid | 4mg | | i.v. | 15min | |
| 1-11 | regularly | 1 - 1 - 1 - 1 | Aciclovir | 200mg | | oral | | |

**Medicines As Required:** Loperamide, Granisetron, Sucralfate, if necessary Filgrastim 5µg/kg/day with febrile neutropenia

**Routine Tests:** FBC, U&Es, serum creatinine, uric acid, LFTs, total protein, albumin, paraprotein measurements (serum and urine), TTP analysis, Karnofsky Index, physical examination

**Dose Reduction:** For **Bortezomib** dose reduction, see **Cautions** above and Summary of Product Characteristics - SmPC); with repeated toxicity, reduce **Cyclophosphamide** to 50%

**Next Cycle (N.C.):** Day 22 for cycles 1-8; day 36 for cycles 9-11

**References:** Bauchmüller et al. # 512 Onkologie 2005;28(suppl 3):1-275; Kropff t al. # 513 Onkologie 2005;28(suppl 3):1-275; Lonial et al., Blood. 2005 Dec 1;106(12):3777-84

# High-Dose Dexa/ IFN-alpha (analogous to SWOG study S9628)

## Indication: Systemic Amyloidosis

**11.7.9**

*This chemotherapy may cause life-threatening toxicity! It should only be administered under the supervision of an experienced medical oncologist! The protocol must first be reviewed and considered in relationship to the clinical situation of the patient.*

## Chemotherapy

| Week | Day | Compounds (generic names) in chronological order | Dosage | Diluent | Route | Duration of Infusion | Comments |
|------|-----|--------------------------------------------------|--------|---------|-------|---------------------|----------|
| **Induction Therapy (for 3 cycles)** | | | | | | | |
| | 1–4; 9–12; 17–20 | **Dexamethasone** | 40mg absolute | | oral | | mornings |
| **Maintenance Therapy I (for 2 years)** | | | | | | | |
| 1 | 1–4 | **Dexamethasone** | 40mg absolute | | oral | | mornings |
| 1–4 | 3 x /week | **Interferon-alpha-2b** | 5million IU absolute | | s.c. | | |
| **Maintenance Therapy II (for 3 years)** | | | | | | | |
| | 3 x /week | **Interferon-alpha-2b** | 5million IU absolute | | s.c. | | |

**INDUCTION THERAPY (for 3 cycles)**

| Cycle Diagram | d1 w1 | d8 w2 | d15 w3 | d22 w4 | d29 w5 | d36 w6 |
|---------------|-------|-------|--------|--------|--------|--------|
| Dexameth. | | | | | | N.C. |

**MAINTENANCE THERAPY I (for 2 years)**

| Cycle Diagram | d1 w1 | d8 w2 | d15 w3 | d22 w4 | d29 w5 | d36 w6 |
|---------------|-------|-------|--------|--------|--------|--------|
| Dexameth. | | | | | | |
| Interferon | | | | | N.C. | |

**MAINTENANCE THERAPY II (for 3 years)**

| Cycle Diagram | d1 w1 | d8 w2 | d15 w3 | d22 w4 | d29 w5 | dn wn |
|---------------|-------|-------|--------|--------|--------|-------|
| Interferon | | | | | | |

**Cautions**

See Summary of Product Charactistics (SmPC) with regard to Routine Tests and Dose Reduction

## Obligatory Pre- and Concurrent Medication

| Week | Day | Sequence and Timing | Compounds (generic names) | Dose | Diluent | Route | Duration of Infusion | Comments |
|------|-----|---------------------|---------------------------|------|---------|-------|---------------------|----------|
| | | 1 – 0 – 1 (2x/week) | Co-trimoxazole | 960mg | | oral | | until the end of Maintenance Therapy I |
| | | 1 – 0 – 0 | Folic Acid | 5mg | | oral | | until the end of Maintenance Therapy I |
| | regularly | 0 – 0 – 1 | Pantoprazole | 20mg | | oral | | until the end of Maintenance Therapy I |
| | regularly | 1 – 1 – 1 – 1 | Amphotericin B (as suspension) | 100mg (1ml) | | oral | | until the end of Maintenance Therapy I |
| | every 3 months | | Zoledronic Acid | 4mg | | i.v. | 15min | long-term therapy* |
| from w1 Maint.I | daily | every 8 hours | Paracetamol | 1000mg | | oral | | if possible, discontinue after 2 weeks |

**Medicines As Required** Possibly Allopurinol, Zoledronic Acid as long-term medication may even be given 1x/month especially if there is osteolysis

**Routine Tests:** (See SmPC) **Lab.:** FBC, LFTs, renal function, blood glucose, lipids levels, serum proteins; **CNS side effects:** depression, suicide; **eyes:** examination before starting therapy, regular checkups, discontinue therapy with worsening ophth. side effects; **cardiac:** echocardiogram, regular ECG; **lungs:** CXR with cough or dyspnea; reduce dose with **edema** + overhydration

**Dose Reduction:** (See SmPC) Initial dose of **20mg Dexamethasone** for patients >70 years, to be increased on cycle 2 if possible; reduce dose with hematologic side effects: leukocytes <1500/μl, granulocytes <1000/μl, platelets <100,000/μl, discontinue thera py if leukocytes <1200/μl, neutropenia <750/μl, thrombocytopenia <70,000/μl.

**Next Cycle (N.C.):** **Induction Therapy:** next cycle: day 35, duration: 3 cycles; **Maintenance Therapy I:** repeat therapy every 4 weeks, duration: 2 years; **Maintenance Therapy II:** duration: 3 years

**Efficacy Assess.** Analogous to plasmacytoma/amyloidosis course parameters

**References:** Dhodapkar et al., Blood, 104(12);3520–6, 2004

| Low-Dose Thalidomide + Prednisone | Indication: | Myelofibrosis | 11.7.10 |
|---|---|---|---|

*This chemotherapy may cause life-threatening toxicity! It should only be administered under the supervision of an experienced medical oncologist! The protocol must first be reviewed and considered in relationship to the clinical situation of the patient.*

## Chemotherapy

| Week | Day | Compounds (generic names) in chronological order | Dosage | Diluent | Route | Duration of Infusion | Comments |
|---|---|---|---|---|---|---|---|
| | 1-28 | **Thalidomide** | 50mg | | oral | | 0 - 0 - 0 - 1 |
| | 1-28 | **Prednisone** | 0.5mg/kg* | | oral | | 1 - 0 - 0 |

**Cautions**

| Cycle Diagram | d1 w1 | d8 w2 | d15 w3 | d22 w4 | d29 w5 |
|---|---|---|---|---|---|
| Thalidomide | | | | | |
| Prednisone* | | | | | N.C. |

*Prednisone Dosage:
Cycle 1: 0.5mg/kg/day
Cycle 2: 0.25mg/kg/day
Cycle 3: 0.125mg/kg/day

With multiple myeloma, there is a risk of thrombosis

## Obligatory Pre- and Concurrent Medication

| Week | Day | Sequence and Timing | Compounds (generic names) | Dose | Diluent | Route | Duration of Infusion | Comments |
|---|---|---|---|---|---|---|---|---|
| | | 1 - 0 - 1 (2x/week) | Co-trimoxazole | 960mg | | oral | | |
| | | 1 - 0 - 0 | Folic Acid | 5mg | | oral | | |
| | regularly | 1 - 1 - 1 - 1 | Amphotericin B | 100mg (1ml) | | oral | | as suspension |

| | |
|---|---|
| Medicines As Required | Metoclopramide orally, Pantoprazole orally, constipation prophylaxis, prophylactic anticoagulation for patients at risk of deep vein thrombosis; possibly prophylactic antifungals |
| Routine Tests: | FBC, U&Es, blood glucose, uric acid, serum creatinine, bilirubin; with multiple myeloma: thrombosis risk |
| Dose Reduction: | According to **Thalidomide** side effect profile e.g. deep vein thrombosis, polyneuropathy |
| Max. Cum. Dose : | None |
| Next Cycle (N.C.): | Day 29: if response after 3 cycles, then continue for a further 3 cycles (but without Prednisone) |
| Efficacy Assess. | Blood count: increasing Hb, platelets, spleen size (ultrasound) |
| References: | Mesa RA et al. Blood. 2003;101(7):2534-41 |

# 5FU / Carboplatin

**Indication:** **Head and Neck Tumors, Esophageal Cancer**
(Squamous cell carcinoma, mainly T4M1)

**12.1.1**

*This chemotherapy may cause life-threatening toxicity! It should only be administered under the supervision of an experienced medical oncologist! The protocol must first be reviewed and considered in relationship to the clinical situation of the patient.*

## Chemotherapy

| Week | Day | Compounds (generic names) in chronological order | Dosage | Diluent | Route | Duration of Infusion | Comments |
|---|---|---|---|---|---|---|---|
| 1 | 1 | **Carboplatin** | #AUC 6mg/m²xmin | 500ml Glucose 5% | i.v. | 1h | #dose (mg) = AUC (mg/ml x min) x [GFR (ml/min)+25] |
| 1 | 1-5 | **Fluorouracil (5FU)** | 1000mg/m² | 250ml Saline 0.9% | i.v. | 4h | (or by Baxter pump over 24h as outpatient) |

**Cycle Diagram**

| | d1 w1 | d8 w2 | d15 w3 | d22 w4 |
|---|---|---|---|---|
| Carboplatin | | | | <--N.C.--> |
| Fluorouracil | | | | |

**Recommended dosage for Carboplatin from AUC** — target AUC (mg/ml x min)

| | |
|---|---|
| Carboplatin monotherapy, patients untreated | 5-7 |
| Carboplatin monotherapy, myelosuppressive pretreatment | 4-6 |
| Combination therapy with Carboplatin in standard dosage, patients untreated | 4-6 |

### Cautions

Reduce 5-FU to 50% with preceding radiotherapy

Incompatibility: 5FU<>Carboplatin, 5FU<>Metoclopramide

Oral fluids: at least 2 liters/day

Brivudine must <u>not</u> be given together with 5FU. This also includes topical applications (Fluorouracil, Capecitabine, Floxuridine, Tegafur).

Lethal consequences are possible for up to 4 weeks, due to inhibition of DPD enzyme activity.

## Obligatory Pre- and Concurrent Medication

| Week | Day | Compounds (generic names) | Sequence and Timing | Dose | Diluent | Route | Duration of Infusion | Comments |
|---|---|---|---|---|---|---|---|---|
| 1 | 1 | Saline 0.9% | 15' before chemotherapy | | 2000ml | i.v. | 5h30min | |
| 1 | 1 | Dexamethasone | 15' before chemotherapy | 8mg | 100ml Saline 0.9% | i.v | 15min | |
| 1 | 1 | Granisetron | 15' before chemotherapy | 1mg | | i.v | bolus | |
| 1 | 2-5 | Metoclopramide | 8.00 and 20.00 hours | 50mg | | oral | | |
| 1 | 2-5 | Saline 0.9% | with chemotherapy | | 500ml | i.v | 4h | |

| | |
|---|---|
| **Medicines As Required** | Metoclopramide oral or i.v., if not tolerated replace with 5-HT3 antagonists or on days 2-5 with Dexamethasone 8mg |
| **Routine Tests:** | FBC, U&Es esp. Mg²⁺, LFTs, serum creatinine, creatinine clearance, creatinine, ototoxicity, neurotoxicity |
| **Dose Reduction:** | Reduce **5FU** to 50% with preceding radiotherapy; if bilirubin increased, see Dose Modification Table; if platelet count < 50,000/µl, reduce **Carboplatin** to 80% |
| **Max. Cum. Dose :** | Unknown |
| **Next Cycle (N.C.):** | Day 22 - 29 |
| **Efficacy Assess.** | After cycles 2 and 4; 2 additional cycles if in complete remission |
| **References:** | Kaasa S et al., Eur J Cancer, 1991; 27:576-579; Jassem J et al., Cancer Chemother Pharmacol, 1993; 31:489-494 |

| EMB | | **Indication:** | **Head and Neck Tumors**<br>(Squamous Cell Carcinoma) | | | | | 12.1.2 |

*This chemotherapy may cause life-threatening toxicity! It should only be administered under the supervision of an experienced medical oncologist! The protocol must first be reviewed and considered in relationship to the clinical situation of the patient.*

## Chemotherapy

| Week | Day | Compounds (generic names) in chronological order | Dosage | Diluent | Route | Duration of Infusion | Comments |
|---|---|---|---|---|---|---|---|
| | 1 | **Epirubicin** | 50mg/m² | undiluted | i.v. | bolus 15min | |
| | 4,11,18 | **Bleomycin** | 10mg/m² | undiluted | i.v. | bolus 5min | |
| | 11,18 | **Methotrexate** | 40mg/m² | undiluted | i.v. | bolus 5min | |
| | | | | | | | |
| | | | | | | | |

**Cautions**

**Incompatibility: Bleomycin<>Methotrexate**

**Anthracycline: Danger of cardiotoxicity - monitor cardiac function**

| | Cycle Diagram | d1 w1 | d8 w2 | d15 w3 | d22 w4 |
|---|---|---|---|---|---|
| | Epirubicin | | | | N.C. |
| | Bleomycin | | | | |
| | Methotrexate | | | | |

## Obligatory Pre- and Concurrent Medication

| Week | Day | Compounds (generic names) | Sequence and Timing | Dose | Diluent | Route | Duration of Infusion | Comments |
|---|---|---|---|---|---|---|---|---|
| | 1,4,11,18 | Saline 0.9% | 15' before chemotherapy | | 500ml | i.v. | 1h | |
| | 1 | Dexamethasone | 15' before Epirubicin | 8mg | | i.v. | bolus | |
| | 1 | Metoclopramide | 15' before & 4h after Epirubicin | 50mg | | i.v. | bolus | |
| | 4,11,18 | Prednisone | 15' before Bleomycin | 50mg | | i.v. | bolus | |
| | 4,11,18 | Clemastine | 15' before Bleomycin | 2mg | | i.v. | bolus | |
| | | | | | | | | |

| Medicines As Required | Metoclopramide oral or i.v., Granisetron i.v. |
|---|---|
| Routine Tests: | **Anthracycline**: see **cautions** above; pulmonary function tests before start of therapy and after every 2 cycles, FBC 2x/week, U&Es, serum creatinine, LFTs |
| Dose Reduction: | See Dose Modification Table |
| Max. Cum. Dose : | **Epirubicin**: Danger of cardiotoxicity; max. cum. dose is 1000mg/m²; **Bleomycin**: Danger of pulmonary fibrosis esp. if cum. dose is over 400mg absolute, this would be exceeded from cycle 6 |
| Next Cycle (N.C.) : | Day 22 |
| Efficacy Assess. | After cycles 2 and 4; 2 additional cycles if in complete remission |
| References: | Paccaguella A et al., Eur J Cancer, 1993; 29A :704 |

# Cisplatin/Etoposide Phosphate

## Indication: SCLC Limited Disease

**12.2.1**

*This chemotherapy may cause life-threatening toxicity! It should only be administered under the supervision of an experienced medical oncologist! The protocol must first be reviewed and considered in relationship to the clinical situation of the patient.*

## Chemotherapy

| Week | Day | Compounds (generic names) in chronological order | Dosage | Diluent | Route | Duration of Infusion | Comments |
|------|-----|--------------------------------------------------|--------|---------|-------|---------------------|----------|
| | 1 | **Cisplatin** | 75mg/m² | 250ml Saline 0.9% | i.v. | 1h | |
| | 1-3 | **Etoposide Phosphate** | 100mg/m² | x*ml Saline 0.9% | i.v. | 30min | *conc. of 0.4mg/ml due to its shelf life |
| | | | | | | | |
| | | | | | | | |
| | | | | | | | |

**Cautions:**

After day 1 protocol for prophylaxis of delayed emesis
Granisetron: increase dose to 3mg with emesis

| Cycle Diagram | d1 w1 | d8 w2 | d15 w3 | d22 w4 |
|---------------|-------|-------|--------|--------|
| Cisplatin | | | | N.C. |
| Etoposide | | | | |

## Obligatory Pre- and Concurrent Medication

| Week | Day | Compounds (generic names) | Sequence and Timing | Dose | Diluent | Route | Duration of Infusion | Comments |
|------|-----|---------------------------|---------------------|------|---------|-------|---------------------|----------|
| | 1 | Saline 0.9% | 30' before chemotherapy | | 3000ml | i.v. | 6-8h | |
| | 1 | Granisetron | 30' before chemotherapy | 1mg | | i.v. | bolus | |
| | 2-3 | Granisetron | 30' before chemotherapy | 1mg | | i.v. | bolus | |
| | 1 | Mannitol 10% | 30' before and after Cisplatin | | 250ml | i.v. | 15 min | |
| | 2-3 | Saline 0.9% | 30' before chemotherapy | | 1000ml | i.v. | 2h | |
| | 1 | Dexamethasone | 30' before chemotherapy | 12mg | | i.v. | | |
| | 1, 2, 3 | Aprepitant | -1h before chemotherapy | * | | oral | | * d1: 125mg, d2+3: 80mg |
| | 2-4 | Dexamethasone | d2-4 in the morning | 8mg | | oral | | |
| | | | | | | | | |
| | | | | | | | | |
| | | | | | | | | |
| | | | | | | | | |

| | |
|---|---|
| **Medicines As Required** | Metoclopramide, Dexamethasone, Granisetron, Famotidine |
| **Routine Tests:** | FBC, U&Es, serum creatinine, serum bilirubin, creatinine clearance, fluid balance, neurotoxicity |
| **Dose Reduction:** | **Cisplatin:** if creatinine clearance < 60ml/min, dose reduction guidelines should be considered; if creatinine clearance =40-60ml/min, reduce dose in accordance with protocol; if creatinine clearance <40 ml/min, change to Carboplatin (AUC 5) \ see Dose Modification Table (study protocol page 10/14 of the ABC Study |
| **Next Cycle (N.C.):** | Every 21 days, 6 cycles |
| **Efficacy Assess.** | Before cycles 3 and 5; implement next chemotherapy cycle only if there  re no signs of tumor progression. For patients with PD , Epi-CO is recommended |
| **References:** | Sundstrom et al. J Clin. Onco. 2002: pp 4665-4672 |

| Epi-CO | | Indication: SCLC | | | | | 12.2.2 |
|---|---|---|---|---|---|---|---|

*This chemotherapy may cause life-threatening toxicity! It should only be administered under the supervision of an experienced medical oncologist! The protocol must first be reviewed and considered in relationship to the clinical situation of the patient.*

## Chemotherapy

| Week | Day | Compounds (generic names) in chronological order | Dosage | Diluent | Route | Duration of Infusion | Comments |
|---|---|---|---|---|---|---|---|
| | 1 | **Vincristine** | 2mg | undiluted | i.v. | bolus | |
| | 1 | **Epirubicin** | 70mg/m² | undiluted | i.v. | bolus 15min | |
| | 1 | **Cyclophosphamide** | 1000mg/m² | 500ml Saline 0.9% | i.v. | 1h | |
| | | | | | | | |
| | | | | | | | |

**Cautions**: Anthracycline: Danger of cardiotoxicity - monitor cardiac function (echocardiogram)

| Cycle Diagram | d1 w1 | d8 w2 | d15 w3 | d22 w4 |
|---|---|---|---|---|
| Vincristine | | | | N.C. |
| Epirubicin | | | | |
| Cyclophos. | | | | |

## Obligatory Pre- and Concurrent Medication

| Week | Day | Compounds (generic names) | Dose | Diluent | Route | Duration of Infusion | Comments |
|---|---|---|---|---|---|---|---|
| | 1 | Saline 0.9% | | 1000ml | i.v. | 2h | |
| | 1 | Dexamethasone | 20mg | 100ml Saline 0.9% | i.v. | 15min | |
| | 1 | Granisetron | 1mg | | i.v. | bolus | |
| | 1 | Mesna | each dose is 20% that of Cyclophos. | | i.v. | bolus | or orally at home |
| 1st neutropenic cycle* | | Filgrastim | 5µg/kg | | s.c. | | *when WBC<1000/µl; give until >1000/µl |
| subsequent cycles | 2** | Pegfilgrastim | 6mg | | s.c. | | **prophyl. admin. 24h after i.v. chemo. if decreased WBC in previous cycle |

| | |
|---|---|
| Medicines As Required | Metoclopramide oral or i.v., if not tolerated replace with 5-HT3 antagonists |
| Routine Tests: | **Anthracycline:** see **cautions** above; FBC, U&Es, LFTs, diuresis, neurotoxicity |
| Dose Reduction: | See Dose Modification Table |
| Max. Cum. Dose : | **Epirubicin:** Danger of cardiotoxicity; max. cum. dose is 1000 mg/m²; **Vincristine** 5-20mg absolute: Danger of neurotoxicity |
| Next Cycle (N.C.): | Day 22 |
| Efficacy Assess. | After every cycle |
| References: | Drings P et al., Onkol, 1986;9(1):14-20 |

# Paclitaxel weekly

## Indication: Head, Neck, Ovarian and Breast Cancer; NSCLC

**12.2.3**

*This chemotherapy may cause life-threatening toxicity! It should only be administered under the supervision of an experienced medical oncologist! The protocol must first be reviewed and considered in relationship to the clinical situation of the patient.*

## Chemotherapy

| Week | Day | Compounds (generic names) in chronological order | Dosage | Diluent | Route | Duration of Infusion | Comments |
|------|-----|--------------------------------------------------|--------|---------|-------|---------------------|----------|
| 1-6 | 1 | **Paclitaxel** | 80mg/m² | 500ml Saline 0.9% | i.v. | 3h | PVC-free infusion set |
| | | | | | | | |
| | | | | | | | |
| | | | | | | | |

**Cautions**

| Cycle Diagram | d1 w1 | d8 w2 | d15 w3 | d22 w4 | d29 w5 | d36 w6 | d43 w7 | d |
|---------------|-------|-------|--------|--------|--------|--------|--------|---|
| Paclitaxel | | | | | | | | N.C. |
| | | | | | | | | |
| | | | | | | | | |

## Obligatory Pre- and Concurrent Medication

| Week | Day | Compounds (generic names) | Sequence and Timing | Dose | Diluent | Route | Duration of Infusion | Comments |
|------|-----|---------------------------|---------------------|------|---------|-------|---------------------|----------|
| 1-6 | 1 | Dexamethasone | 30' before Paclitaxel | 8mg | 100ml | i.v. | 15min | |
| 1-6 | 1 | Clemastine | 30' before Paclitaxel | 2mg | | i.v. | bolus | |
| 1-6 | 1 | Ranitidine | 30' before Paclitaxel | 50mg | | i.v. | bolus | |
| 1-6 | 1 | Saline 0.9% | parallel to Paclitaxel | | 500ml | i.v. | 4h | |

| | |
|---|---|
| Medicines As Required | Dexamethasone i.v. or Metoclopramide oral or i.v. |
| Routine Tests: | FBC, WBC differential (twice weekly), U&Es esp. Mg²⁺, serum creatinine, ALP, AST (SGOT), ALT (SGPT), clinically: in particular polyneuropathy |
| Dose Reduction: | By 25% with leukopenia Grade 4 (<1000µl) or febrile neutropenia, by 25% with thrombocytopenia Grade 4 (<10,000/µl), by 25% with polyneuropathy 4-6 |
| Therapy Delay: | If leukocytes < 1500/µl or platelets < 75,000/µl (check twice weekly) |
| Max. Cum. Dose : | None |
| Next Cycle (N.C.): | Week 7 (1 cycle = 6 weeks treatment) |
| Efficacy Assess. | After every cycle |
| References: | Perez EA et al., J Clin Oncol, 2001; 19:4216-23; Vaughn DJ et al., J Clin Oncol, 2002; 20:937-40; Sikov WM et al., ASCO 2002, Abstract 134 |

# CE

## Indication: SCLC

### 12.2.4

*This chemotherapy may cause life-threatening toxicity! It should only be administered under the supervision of an experienced medical oncologist! The protocol must first be reviewed and considered in relationship to the clinical situation of the patient.*

## Chemotherapy

| Week | Day | Compounds (generic names) in chronological order | Dosage | Diluent | Route | Duration of Infusion | Comments |
|---|---|---|---|---|---|---|---|
| | 1 | **Carboplatin** | #AUC 6mg/ml×min | 500ml Glucose 5% | i.v. | 30min | #dose (mg) = AUC (mg/ml x min) x [GFR (ml/min)+25] |
| | 1-3 | **Etoposide Phosphate** | 120mg/m² | 100ml Saline 0,9% (from 200mg in 250ml) | i.v. | 1h | dose expressed in terms of Etoposide base |

| Recommended dosage for Carboplatin from AUC | target AUC (mg/ml×min) | Cycle Diagram | d1 w1 | d8 w2 | d15 w3 | d22 w4 | d29 w5 |
|---|---|---|---|---|---|---|---|
| Carboplatin monotherapy, patients untreated | 5-7 | Carboplatin | | | | | N.C. |
| Carboplatin monotherapy, myelosuppressive pretreatment | 4-6 | Etop. Phos. | | | | | |
| Combination therapy with Carboplatin in standard dosage, patients untreated | 4-6 | | | | | | |

**Cautions:** Etoposide Phosphate and Sodium Bicarbonate must not be administered concomitantly through the same infusion site!

## Obligatory Pre- and Concurrent Medication

| Week | Day | Compounds (generic names) | Sequence and Timing | Dose | Diluent | Route | Duration of Infusion | Comments |
|---|---|---|---|---|---|---|---|---|
| | 1-3 | Saline 0.9% | 15' before chemotherapy | | 1000ml | i.v. | 2h | |
| | 1 | Dexamethasone | 15' before & 4h after chemo. | 8mg | 100ml Saline 0.9% | i.v. | 15min | or orally at home |
| | 1 | Granisetron | 15' before chemotherapy | 1mg | | i.v. | bolus | |
| | 2-3 | Dexamethasone | 30' before chemotherapy | 8mg | | oral | | |
| 1st neutropenic cycle* | | Filgrastim | once a day | 5µg/kg | | s.c. | | *when WBC<1000/µl: give until >1000/µl |
| subsequent cycles | 4** | Pegfilgrastim | one dose only | 6mg | | s.c. | | **prophyl. admin. 24h after i.v. chemo. if decreased WBC in previous cycle |

| | |
|---|---|
| **Medicines As Required:** | Metoclopramide oral or i.v., if not tolerated may be replaced with 5-HT3 antagonists |
| **Routine Tests:** | FBC, U&Es, esp. Mg²⁺, serum creatinine, creatinine clearance before giving therapy, ototoxicity, neurotoxicity |
| **Dose Reduction:** | See Dose Modification Table |
| **Next Cycle (N.C.):** | Day 29 |
| **Efficacy Assess.** | After every cycle |
| **References:** | Heckmayr M et al., Pneumologie, 1990;44(1):256-257; Gatzemeier U et al., Pneumologie, 1990;44(1):584-585 |

# Topotecan — Indication: SCLC, Ovarian Carcinoma — 12.2.5

*This chemotherapy may cause life-threatening toxicity! It should only be administered under the supervision of an experienced medical oncologist! The protocol must first be reviewed and considered in relation to the clinical situation of the patient.*

## Chemotherapy

| Week | Day | Compounds (generic names) in chronological order | Dosage | Diluent | Route | Duration of Infusion | Comments |
|---|---|---|---|---|---|---|---|
| | 1–5 | **Topotecan** | 1.5 mg/m² | 100ml Saline 0.9% | i.v. | 30min | see below: Dose Increase & Dose Reduction |
| | | | | | | | |
| | | | | | | | |
| | | | | | | | |
| | | | | | | | |

**Cautions**

| Cycle Diagram | d1 w1 | d8 w2 | d15 w3 | d22 w4 |
|---|---|---|---|---|
| Topotecan | | | | N.C. |
| | | | | |
| | | | | |

## Obligatory Pre- and Concurrent Medication

| Week | Day | Compounds (generic names) | Sequence and Timing | Dose | Diluent | Route | Duration of Infusion | Comments |
|---|---|---|---|---|---|---|---|---|
| | 1–5 | Saline 0.9% | -15' before chemotherapy | | 500ml | i.v. | 1h | |
| | 1–5 | Dexamethasone | -15' before chemotherapy | 8mg | | i.v. | bolus | given as outpatient |
| | 6 | Pegfilgrastim | 24 h after chemotherapy | 6mg | | s.c. | | *when WBC<1000/µl; give until >1000/µl |
| 1st neutropenic cycle* | | Filgrastim | once a day | 5µg/kg | | s.c. | | **prophyl. admin. 24h after i.v. chemo. if |
| subsequent cycles | 6** | Pegfilgrastim | one dose only | 6mg | | s.c. | | decreased WBC in previous cycle |
| | | | | | | | | |
| | | | | | | | | |
| | | | | | | | | |

**Medicines As Required** Granisetron

**Routine Tests:** FBC (before start of therapy neutrophils>1500/µl, platelets>100,000/µl), U&Es; renal function tests and creatinine clearance (if <40ml/min reduce **Topotecan** to 50%).

LFTs (no dose reduction necessary till bilirubin ≥10 mg%)

**Dose Reduction:** * with significant thrombocytopenia, neutropenia or anemia (Grade 4 ) reduce dose in the next cycle to 1.25mg/m² per day, or even to 1.0 mg/m² if necessary

**Dose Increase:** * possible increase depending on effectiveness and side effects after 1st cycle: 2mg/m² to maximum 3mg/m²

**Next Cycle (N.C.):** Day 22

**Efficacy Assess.** After 4-5 cycles (= ca. 12 weeks; sometimes, response only after 24 weeks)

**References:** Kudelka et al., J. Clin. Oncol. 14, 1552–7, 1996

# TEC

## Indication: SCLC (Limited Disease)

**12.2.6**

*This chemotherapy may cause life-threatening toxicity! It should only be administered under the supervision of an experienced medical oncologist! The protocol must first be reviewed and considered in relationship to the clinical situation of the patient.*

## Chemotherapy

| Week | Day | Compounds (generic names) in chronological order | Dosage | Diluent | Route | Duration of Infusion | Comments |
|---|---|---|---|---|---|---|---|
|  | 1-3 | **Etoposide Phosphate** | 125mg/m² | 100ml Saline 0.9% (from 200mg in 250ml) | i.v. | 30min |  |
|  | 4 | **Paclitaxel** | 175mg/m² | 500ml Saline 0.9% | i.v. | 3h | PVC-free infusion set |
|  | 4 | **Carboplatin** | AUC 5 | 500ml Glucose 5% | i.v. | 1h |  |

**Cautions:** Etoposide Phosphate and Sodium Bicarbonate must not be administered concomitantly through the same infusion site!

| Cycle Diagram | d1 w1 | d8 w2 | d15 w3 | d22 w4 | d29 w5 |
|---|---|---|---|---|---|
| Etop. Phos. |  |  |  | N.C. |  |
| Paclitaxel |  |  |  |  |  |
| Carboplatin |  |  |  |  |  |

## Obligatory Pre- and Concurrent Medication

| Week | Day | Sequence and Timing | Compounds (generic names) | Dose | Diluent | Route | Duration of Infusion | Comments |
|---|---|---|---|---|---|---|---|---|
|  | 1-3 | 15' before chemotherapy | Saline 0.9% |  | 1000ml | i.v. | 2h |  |
|  | 1-3 | 30' before chemotherapy | Dexamethasone | 8mg | 100ml Saline 0.9% | i.v. | 15min | or orally at home |
|  | 4 | 30' before Paclitaxel | Saline 0.9% |  | 2000ml | i.v. | 5h | IVAC infusion pump must be used |
|  | 4 | 30' before Paclitaxel | Dexamethasone | 20mg | 100ml Saline 0.9% | i.v. | 15min |  |
|  | 4 | 30' before Paclitaxel | Clemastine | 2mg |  | i.v. | bolus |  |
|  | 4 | 30' before Paclitaxel | Ranitidine | 50mg |  | i.v. | bolus |  |
|  | 4 | 30' before chemotherapy | Granisetron | 1mg |  | i.v. | bolus |  |

| | |
|---|---|
| **Medicines As Required:** | Metoclopramide oral or i.v.. Granisetron i.v. |
| **Routine Tests:** | FBC, LFTs, U&Es esp. Mg²⁺, serum creatinine, creatinine clearance, ototoxicity, neurotoxicity |
| **Dose Reduction:** | Hematology: leukocytes <1000/µl (Grade 4) and/or platelets <10,000/µl (Grade 4) >7days: reduce dosages by 1level; with neutropenic fever and/or infection >7days, or with hemorrhage Grade 3: reduce dosages by 2 levels; if platelets <10000/µl (Grade 4): **Carboplatin** AUC 4: non-hematologic toxicity (mucositis, neurotoxicity, nephrotoxicity, etc.) |
| **Max. Cum. Dose:** | Unknown |
| **Next Cycle (N.C.):** | Every 21 days (with corresponding FBC: neutrophils ≥1500/µl and platelets ≥100,000/µl, growth factor from day 28 if necessary, therapy delay till day 35 maximum), 6 cycles maximum |
| **Efficacy Assess.** | After 2 cycles |

# Vinorelbine / Carboplatin  Indication: NSCLC  12.2.7

*This chemotherapy may cause life-threatening toxicity! It should only be administered under the supervision of an experienced medical oncologist! The protocol must first be reviewed and considered in relationship to the clinical situation of the patient.*

## Chemotherapy

| Week | Day | Compounds (generic names) in chronological order | Dosage | Diluent | Route | Duration of Infusion | Comments |
|---|---|---|---|---|---|---|---|
| | 1 | **Carboplatin** | #AUC 6mg/ml×min | 500ml Glucose 5% | i.v. | 1h | #dose (mg) = AUC (mg/ml x min) x [GFR (ml/min)+25] |
| | 1,8,15 | **Vinorelbine** | 25mg/m² | 100ml Saline 0.9% | i.v. | 10min | max. single dose 60mg absolute |

**Recommended dosage for Carboplatin from AUC**  target AUC (mg/ml×min)

| | |
|---|---|
| Carboplatin monotherapy, patients untreated | 5-7 |
| Carboplatin monotherapy, myelosuppressive pretreatment | 4-6 |
| Combination therapy with Carboplatin in standard dosage, patients untreated | 4-6 |

Cycle Diagram: Carboplatin d1 w1 | Vinorelbine d1 w1, d8 w2, d15 w3 | d22 w4 | d29 w5 N.C.

**Cautions**

Patients >70 years and Karnofsky Index <70%:
- Monotherapy regimen!
- Combination therapy not to be given!

## Obligatory Pre- and Concurrent Medication

| Week | Day | Sequence and Timing | Compounds (generic names) | Dose | Diluent | Route | Duration of Infusion | Comments |
|---|---|---|---|---|---|---|---|---|
| | 1 | 15' before chemotherapy | Saline 0.9% | | 1000ml | i.v. | 2h | |
| | 8,15 | 15' before chemotherapy | Saline 0.9% | | 500ml | i.v | 1h | |
| | 1 | 15' before and 4h after chemo. | Dexamethasone | 8mg | 100ml Saline 0.9% | i.v | 15min | |
| | 8,15 | 30' before chemotherapy | Dexamethasone | 8mg | | oral | | 2nd dose orally at home |
| | 1 | 15' before chemotherapy | Granisetron | 1mg | | i.v | bolus | |

| | |
|---|---|
| Medicines As Required | Metoclopramide oral or i.v. |
| Routine Tests: | FBC, U&Es, esp. Mg²⁺, LFTs, serum creatinine, creatinine clearance, ototoxicity, neurotoxicity, intestinal motility |
| Dose Reduction: | Bilirubin=2.5-5mg/dl: 50%, bilirubin=5-10mg/dl: 25%, bilirubin>10mg/dl: contraindicated; discontinue if leukocytes<1500/µl; see Dose Modification Table |
| | If leukocytes<1500/µl, platelets<50,000/µl after 1st cycle: **Vinorelbine** 20mg/m² |
| Next Cycle (N.C.): | Day 29 |
| Efficacy Assess. | After 2 cycles |
| References: | According to Jacoulet P et al., Lung Cancer, 1994;11(Suppl2),Abst438:115 |

# Paclitaxel /Carboplatin | Indication: NSCLC | 12.2.8

*This chemotherapy may cause life-threatening toxicity! It should only be administered under the supervision of an experienced medical oncologist! The protocol must first be reviewed and considered in relationship to the clinical situation of the patient.*

## Chemotherapy

| Week | Day | Compounds (generic names) in chronological order | Dosage | Diluent | Route | Duration of Infusion | Comments |
|---|---|---|---|---|---|---|---|
| | 1,8,15 | **Paclitaxel** | 100mg/m² | 500ml Saline 0.9% | i.v. | 3h | PVC-free infusion set |
| | 1 | **Carboplatin** | #AUC 6mg/mlxmin | 500ml Glucose 5% | i.v. | 1h | #dose (mg) = AUC (mg/ml x min) x [GFR (ml/min)+25] |

**Cautions**

| target AUC (mg/mlxmin) | |
|---|---|
| **Recommended dosage for Carboplatin from AUC** | |
| Carboplatin monotherapy, patients untreated | 5-7 |
| Carboplatin monotherapy, myelosuppressive pretreatment | 4-6 |
| Combination therapy with Carboplatin in standard dosage, patients untreated | 4-6 |

| Cycle Diagram | d1 w1 | d8 w2 | d15 w3 | d22 w4 | d29 w5 |
|---|---|---|---|---|---|
| Paclitaxel | | | | | |
| Carboplatin | | | | | N.C. |

## Obligatory Pre- and Concurrent Medication

| Week | Day | Sequence and Timing | Compounds (generic names) | Dose | Diluent | Route | Duration of Infusion | Comments |
|---|---|---|---|---|---|---|---|---|
| | 1,8,15 | 30' before Paclitaxel | Saline 0.9% | | 2000ml | i.v. | 5h | IVAC infusion pump must be used |
| | 1,8,15 | 30' before Paclitaxel | Dexamethasone | 8mg | | i.v. | bolus | |
| | 1,8,15 | 30' before Paclitaxel | Clemastine | 2mg | | i.v. | bolus | |
| | 1,8,15 | 30' before Paclitaxel | Ranitidine | 50mg | | i.v. | bolus | |
| | 8,15 | 30' before Paclitaxel | Saline 0.9% | | 500ml | i.v. | 5h | IVAC infusion pump must be used |
| | 1 | 30' before chemotherapy | Granisetron | 1mg | | i.v. | bolus | increase dose to 3mg with emesis |
| | 8,15 | 30' before Paclitaxel | Granisetron | 1mg | | i.v. | bolus | |
| | *daily except on days 8 & 15 | once a day | Filgrastim | 5µg/kg | | s.c. | | *when WBC<1000/µl; give until >1000/µl not on chemotherapy days |

**Medicines As Required:** Metoclopramide oral or i.v., Granisetron i.v.

**Routine Tests:** FBC, U&Es esp. $Mg^{2+}$, serum creatinine, creatinine clearance, ALP, AST (SGOT), ALT (SGPT), clinically: in particular polyneuropathy, ototoxicity, neurotoxicity

**Dose Reduction:** Paclitaxel: by 25% with leucopenia Grade 4 (<1000µl) or febrile neutropenia, by 25% with thrombocytopenia Grade 4 (<10,000/µl), by 25% with polyneuropathy 4-6

**Therapy Delay:** Paclitaxel: if leukocytes < 1500/µl or platelets < 75,000/µl (check twice weekly). Discontinue therapy if allergic to polyoxyethylene-3,5 castor oil

**Next Cycle (N.C.):** Day 29

**Efficacy Assess.:** After cycle 2

**References:** Belani CP et al., J Clin Oncol. 2003 Aug 1;21(15):2933-9; Schiller JH et al., N Engl J Med. 2002;346(2):92-98

# Gemcitabine / Cisplatin

**Indication:** NSCLC, Pleural Mesothelioma, Pancreatic Cancer, Urothelial Carcinoma

**12.2.9**

*This chemotherapy may cause life-threatening toxicity! It should only be administered under the supervision of an experienced medical oncologist! The protocol must first be reviewed and considered in relationship to the clinical situation of the patient.*

## Chemotherapy

| Week | Day | Compounds (generic names) in chronological order | Dosage | Diluent | Route | Duration of Infusion | Comments |
|------|-----|--------------------------------------------------|--------|---------|-------|---------------------|----------|
| | 1,8 | **Gemcitabine** | 1000mg/m² | 250ml Saline 0.9% | i.v. | 30min | |
| | 1 | **Cisplatin** | 70mg/m² | 250ml Saline 0.9% | i.v. | 1h | |
| | | | | | | | |
| | | | | | | | |

**After day 1 protocol for prophylaxis of delayed emesis**

| Cycle Diagram | d1 w1 | d8 w2 | d15 w3 | d22 w4 |
|---------------|-------|-------|--------|--------|
| Gemcitabine | | | | N.C. |
| Cisplatin | | | | |

(vertical label: **Cautions**)

## Obligatory Pre- and Concurrent Medication

| Week | Day | Sequence and Timing | Compounds (generic names) | Dose | Diluent | Route | Duration of Infusion | Comments |
|------|-----|--------------------|---------------------------|------|---------|-------|---------------------|----------|
| | 1 | 15' before chemotherapy | Saline 0.9% | | 3000ml | i.v. | 6-8h | |
| | 8 | 15' before chemotherapy | Saline 0.9% | | 500ml | i.v. | 1h | |
| | 8 | 15' before chemotherapy | Dexamethasone | 8mg | | i.v. | bolus | |
| | 1 | 15' before chemotherapy | Granisetron | 1mg | | i.v. | bolus | |
| | 1 | 30' before and after Cisplatin | Mannitol 10% | | 250ml | i.v. | 15min | |
| | *daily, except on days 1 & 8 | once a day | Filgrastim | 5µg/kg | | s.c. | | *when WBC<1000/µl: give until >1000/µl. |
| | 1, 2, 3 | -1h before chemo./d2+3 in the morning | Aprepitant | * | | oral | | * d1: 125mg, d2+3: 80mg |
| | 1-4 | d1 -15min, d2-4 in the morning | Dexamethasone | * | | i.v./oral | | * d1: 12mg/d2-4: 8mg |
| | | | | | | | | |
| | | | | | | | | |
| | | | | | | | | |

| | |
|---|---|
| **Medicines As Required** | Ondansetron i.v. or oral, Dexamethasone 8mg, |
| **Routine Tests:** | FBC, U&Es esp Mg²⁺, serum creatinine, creatinine clearance, diuresis |
| **Dose Reduction:** | Withhold **Cisplatin** if creatinine clearance < 60ml/min; see Dose Modification Table |
| | WBC<2000/µl or platelets<75,000/µl: withhold therapy; other side effects: WHO 3° (but not vomiting or hair loss): 50% or withhold therapy. |
| **Next Cycle (N.C.):** | Day 22 |
| **Efficacy Assess.** | After 2 cycles |
| **References:** | Sandler AB et al., J Clin Oncol. 2000;18:122-30, Schiller JH et al., N ngl J Med. 2002;346:92-8 (NSCLC); Nowak AK et al., Br J Cancer. 2002,87:491-6 (Pleura); |
| | Philip PA et al., Cancer. 2001;92:569-77 (Pankreas); von der Maase H et al, J Clin Oncol 2000;18:3068-77(Urothel): |

| Docetaxel | | Indication: NSCLC (2nd line therapy) | | | | | 12.2.10 |

*This chemotherapy may cause life-threatening toxicity! It should only be administered under the supervision of an experienced medical oncologist! The protocol must first be reviewed and considered in relationship to the clinical situation of the patient.*

## Chemotherapy

| Week | Day | Compounds (generic names) in chronological order | Dosage | Diluent | Route | Duration of Infusion | Comments |
|---|---|---|---|---|---|---|---|
| | 1 | **Docetaxel** | 75mg/m² | *250ml Saline 0.9% | i.v. | 1h | * if dose >200mg, increase volume (max. conc. 0.74mg/ml); PVC-free infusion set |
| | | | | | | | |
| | | | | | | | |

| Cautions | Extravasation | | | | | | |

| | Cycle Diagram | d1 w1 | d8 w2 | d15 w3 | d22 w4 |
|---|---|---|---|---|---|
| | Docetaxel | | | | N.C. |
| | | | | | |
| | | | | | |

## Obligatory Pre- and Concurrent Medication

| Week | Day | Sequence and Timing | Compounds (generic names) | Dose | Diluent | Route | Duration of Infusion | Comments |
|---|---|---|---|---|---|---|---|---|
| | 1 | 30' before chemotherapy | Saline 0.9% | | 500ml | i.v. | 1h30min | |
| | 1 | 30' before chemotherapy | Dexamethasone | 20mg | 100ml Saline 0.9% | i.v. | 15min | |
| | 1 | 30' before chemotherapy | Ranitidine | 50mg | | i.v. | bolus | |
| | 1 | 30' before chemotherapy | Clemastine | 2mg | | i.v. | bolus | |
| | 2-3 | twice a day | Dexamethasone | 8mg | | oral | | |
| 1st neutropenic cycle* | | once a day | Filgrastim | 5µg/kg | | s.c. | | *when WBC<1000/µl; give until >1000/µl |
| subsequent cycles | 2** | one dose only | Pegfilgrastim | 6mg | | s.c. | | **prophyl. admin. 24h after i.v. chemo. if decreased WBC in previous cycle |
| | | | | | | | | |
| | | | | | | | | |
| | | | | | | | | |

**Medicines As Required** Metoclopramide oral or i.v., Dexamethasone 8mg i.v./oral

**Side Effects:** Myelotoxicity, neuropathy, skin toxicity, fluid retention, allergic reactions, nausea/vomiting, **caution:** Extravasation

**Routine Tests:** FBC, clinical chemistry, U&Es, bilirubin, serum creatinine, LFTs

**Dose Reduction:** With Grade 4 neutropenia >7 days, febrile neutropenia, severe skin reactions or Grade 3–4 non-hematological toxic reaction: after 1st toxic reaction withhold therapy for 2 weeks then reduce to 55mg/m². If persisent > Grade 3 peripheral neuropathy, Grade 4 hypertension, raised bilirubin, 2.5-fold increase in ALP and 1.5-fold increase above no rmal in AST (SGOT) or ALT (SGPT) or previous dose reduction: discontinue therapy

**Next Cycle (N.C.):** Day 22

**Efficacy Assess.** After every cycle

**References:** Fossella FV et al : J Clin Oncol. 2000 Jun;18(12):2354-62; Quoix E et al : Ann Oncol. 2004 Jan;15(1):38-44

906

# Cisplatin/Vinorelbine

## Indication: NSCLC, adjuvant therapy IIA-IIIA

**12.2.11**

*This chemotherapy may cause life-threatening toxicity! It should only be administered under the supervision of an experienced medical oncologist! The protocol must first be reviewed and considered in relationship to the clinical situation of the patient.*

## Chemotherapy

| Cycle | Day | Compounds (generic names) in chronological order | Dosage | Diluent | Route | Duration of Infusion | Comments |
|---|---|---|---|---|---|---|---|
| 1-4 | 1 | **Cisplatin** | 80mg/m² | 1000ml Saline 0.9% | i.v. | 1h | |
| 1-4 | 1, 8 | **Vinorelbine** | 30mg/m² | 100ml Saline 0.9% | i.v. | 10min | |

After day 1 protocol for prophylaxis of delayed emesis

**Cautions**

| Cycle Diagram | d1 w1 | d8 w2 | d15 w3 | d22 w4 |
|---|---|---|---|---|
| Cisplatin | | | | N.C. |
| Vinorelbine | | | | |

## Obligatory Pre- and Concurrent Medication

| Cycle | Day | Sequence and Timing | Compounds (generic names) | Dose | Diluent | Route | Duration of Infusion | Comments |
|---|---|---|---|---|---|---|---|---|
| | 1 | 15' before chemotherapy | Saline 0.9% | | 3000ml | i.v. | 6-8h | |
| | 8 | 15' before chemotherapy | Saline 0.9% | | 500ml | i.v. | 2h | |
| | 8 | 15' before chemotherapy | Dexamethasone | 8mg | | i.v. | 10min | |
| | 1 | 15' before & 8h after Cisplatin | Granisetron | 1mg | | i.v. | bolus | increase dose to 3mg with emesis |
| | 1 | 30' before and after Cisplatin | Mannitol 10% | | 250ml | i.v. | 15min | |
| | 1, 2, 3 | -1h before chemo. d2+3 in the morning | Aprepitant | * | | oral | | * d1: 125mg, d2+3: 80mg |
| | 1-4 | d1 -15min, d2-4 in the morning | Dexamethasone | * | | i.v./oral | | * d1: 12mg/d2-4: 8mg |

**Medicines As Required:** Granisetron i.v. or oral, Dexamethasone 8mg, Metoclopramide oral or i.v.

**Routine Tests:** FBC, U&Es, esp. Mg²⁺, serum creatinine, serum bilirubin, creatinine clearance, diuresis

**Dose Reduction:** **Cisplatin** and **Vinorelbine:** see Dose Modification Table

**Next Cycle (N.C.):** Day 22. Chemotherapy will finish either after 4 cycles, with unacceptable toxicity or with the withdrawal of informed consent

**Efficacy Assess.:** After the end of the adjuvant therapy

**References:** Douillard, J. Y. et al. ASCO 2005 Abstract # 7031

# Pemetrexed - 2nd line therapy

## Indication: NSCLC/2nd line therapy

**12.2.12**

*This chemotherapy may cause life-threatening toxicity! It should only be administered under the supervision of an experienced medical oncologist! The protocol must first be reviewed and considered in relationship to the clinical situation of the patient.*

## Chemotherapy

| Week | Day | Compounds (generic names) in chronological order | Dosage | Diluent | Route | Duration of Infusion | Comments |
|---|---|---|---|---|---|---|---|
| | 1 | **Pemetrexed** | 500mg/m² | 100ml Saline 0.9% | i.v. | 15min | has shelf life of 24 hours after dilution in 100ml Saline 0.9% |
| | | | | | | | |
| | | | | | | | |

**Cautions**

| Cycle Diagram | d1 w1 | d8 w2 | d15 w3 | d22 w4 |
|---|---|---|---|---|
| Pemetrexed | | | | N.C. |
| | | | | |
| | | | | |

## Obligatory Pre- and Concurrent Medication

| Week | Day | Sequence and Timing | Compounds (generic names) | Dose | Diluent | Route | Duration of Infusion | Comments |
|---|---|---|---|---|---|---|---|---|
| | 1 | 30 min before chemotherapy | Saline 0.9% | 500ml | | i.v. | 1h | |
| | 0-2 | 1 - 0 - 1 | Dexamethasone | 4mg | | oral | | |
| | regularly | 1 - 0 - 0 | Folic Acid | 500µg | | oral | | start 5-7 days before 1st dose of Pemetrexed |
| one week before 1st dose of Pemetrexed, then every 9 weeks | | | Vitamin B12 | 1000µg | | i.m. | | |
| | | | | | | | | |

| | |
|---|---|
| Medicines As Required: | For diarrhea: intravenous infusion, Loperamide; with leukopenia/thrombocytopenia Grade 4: Leucovorin (see protocol for dose); with neutrophils less than 0.5 x10⁹/l, fever or infection: Filgrastim may be given; **NSAIDs/Salicylates must not be given from 2 days before and until 2 days after Pemetrexed therapy!** |
| Routine Tests: | Hemoglobin, hematocrit, leucocytes, lymphocytes, platelets, neutrophils, sodium, potassium, total bilirubin, ALP, ALT (SGPT), AST (SGOT), serum creatinine, LDH |
| Dose Reduction: | If platelet nadir ≥ 50x10⁹/l and leukocyte nadir < 0.5 x10⁹/l: reduce dose to 75%; if platelet nadir < 50x10⁹/l: reduce dose to 50% |
| Next Cycle (N.C.): | Every 21 days, leukocytes must be ≥ 1.5 x10⁹, platelets ≥ 100x10⁹/l |
| Efficacy Assess. | Every two or three cycles |
| References: | De Marinis et al., Oncol (Huntington). 18(13 Suppl 8):38-42. 2004 Nov; Ardizzoni et al., J of Chem. 16(4):104-7. 2004 Nov. |

# Paclitaxel/Carboplatin/RT — Page 1

## Indication: Epithelial Pleural Mesothelioma  12.3.1

(adjuvant therapy) Karnofsky Index <70%

*This chemotherapy may cause life-threatening toxicity! It should only be administered under the supervision of an experienced medical oncologist! The protocol must first be reviewed and considered in relationship to the clinical situation of the patient.*

## Chemotherapy

| Week | Day | Compounds (generic names) in chronological order | Dosage | Diluent | Route | Duration of Infusion | Comments |
|---|---|---|---|---|---|---|---|
| 1,4 | 1 | **Paclitaxel** | 200mg/m² | 500ml Saline 0.9% | i.v. | 3h | PVC-free infusion set |
| 1,4 | 1 | **Carboplatin** | #AUC 6mg/ml×min | 500ml Glucose 5% | i.v. | 1h | #dose (mg) = AUC (mg/ml × min) × [GFR (ml/min)+25] |
| 7,8,etc. | | **Fractionated Radiotherapy (Frctd. RT)** | 30 - 54 Gy | | | | |

### Cautions

Recommended dosage for Carboplatin from AUC — target AUC (mg/ml×min)

| | target AUC |
|---|---|
| Carboplatin monotherapy, patients untreated | 5-7 |
| Carboplatin monotherapy, myelosuppressive pretreatment | 4-6 |
| Combination therapy with Carboplatin in standard dosage, patients untreated | 4-6 |

Cycle Diagram

| | |
|---|---|
| Surg.: Extrapleur. pneumonectomy | |
| Paclitaxel 200mg/m² | |
| Carboplatin AUC 6 mg/ml × min | |
| Paclitaxel 50 mg/m² (1×/week under RT) | |

Frctd. RT: Hemithorax (total dose=30Gy), mediastinum (total dose= 40Gy), poss. boost up to 54Gy total dose

Cycle Diagram columns: d1 w1 | d8 w2 | d15 w3 | d22 w4 | d29 w5 | d36 w6 | d43 w7 ... 4-6 week interval

## Obligatory Pre- and Concurrent Medication

| Week | Day | Compounds (generic names) | Sequence and Timing | Dose | Diluent | Route | Duration of Infusion | Comments |
|---|---|---|---|---|---|---|---|---|
| 1,4 | 1 | Saline 0.9% | 30' before Paclitaxel | | 2000ml | i.v. | 5h | IVAC infusion pump must be used |
| 1,4 | 1 | Dexamethasone | 30' before Paclitaxel | 8mg | | i.v. | 15min | |
| 1,4 | 1 | Clemastine | 30' before Paclitaxel | 2mg | | i.v. | bolus | |
| 1,4 | 1 | Famotidine | 30' before Paclitaxel | 40mg | | oral | bolus | |
| 1,4 | 1 | Granisetron | 30' before chemotherapy | 1mg | | i.v. | bolus | |

| | |
|---|---|
| Medicines As Required: | Metoclopramide oral or i.v., Granisetron i.v. |
| Routine Tests: | FBC, U&Es esp. Mg²⁺, serum creatinine, creatinine clearance, ototoxicity, neurotoxicity |
| Dose Reduction: | Discontinue if leukocytes < 1500/μl or if allergic to polyoxyethylene-3,5 castor oil |
| Max. Cum. Dose : | None |
| Next Cycle (N.C.): | See Cycle diagram |
| References: | Sugarbaker-DJ et al. Journal of Thoracic and Cardiovascular Surgery 1999; 117:54-65 |

| Paclitaxel/Carboplatin/RT | Page 2 | Indication: | Epithelial Pleural Mesothelioma | 12.3.1 |

(adjuvant therapy) Karnofsky Index <70%

*This chemotherapy may cause life-threatening toxicity! It should only be administered under the supervision of an experienced medical oncologist! The protocol must first be reviewed and considered in relationship to the clinical situation of the patient.*

## Chemotherapy

| Week | Day | Compounds (generic names) in chronological order | Dosage | Diluent | Route | Duration of Infusion | Comments | d1 w1 | d8 w2 | d15 w3 | d22 w4 | d29 w5 | d36 w6 | d43 w7 |
|---|---|---|---|---|---|---|---|---|---|---|---|---|---|---|
| 7,8,etc. | 1 | **Paclitaxel** | 50mg/m² | 500ml Saline 0.9% | i.v. | 3h | PVC-free infusion set | | | | | | | |
| 7,8,etc. | | **Fractionated Radiotherapy (Frctd. RT)** | 30 - 54 Gy | | | | | | | | | | | |

**Cycle Diagram**

Surg.: Extrapleur. pneumonectomy

Paclitaxel 200mg/m²   | 4-6week interval

Carboplatin AUC 6 mg/ml x min

Paclitaxel 50 mg/m² (1x/week under RT)

Frctd. RT: Hemithorax (total dose=30Gy), mediastinum (total dose= 40Gy), poss. boost up to 54 Gy total dose

*Cautions*

## Obligatory Pre- and Concurrent Medication

| Week | Day | Sequence and Timing | Compounds (generic names) | Dose | Diluent | Route | Duration of Infusion | Comments |
|---|---|---|---|---|---|---|---|---|
| 7,8,etc. | 1 | 30' before Paclitaxel | Dexamethasone | 4mg | | i.v. | 15min | |
| 7,8,etc. | 1 | 30' before Paclitaxel | Clemastine | 2mg | | i.v. | bolus | |
| 7,8,etc. | 1 | 30' before Paclitaxel | Famotidine | 40mg | | oral | bolus | |
| 7,8,etc. | 1 | parallel to Paclitaxel | Saline 0.9% | | 500ml | i.v. | 4h | |

| | |
|---|---|
| Medicines As Required | Metoclopramide oral or i.v., Granisetron i.v. |
| Routine Tests: | FBC, U&Es esp. Mg²⁺, serum creatinine, creatinine clearance, ototoxicity, neurotoxicity |
| Dose Reduction: | Discontinue if leukocytes < 1500/µl or if allergic to polyoxyethylene-3,5 castor oil |
| Max. Cum. Dose : | None |
| Next Cycle (N.C.): | See Cycle diagram |
| References: | Sugarbaker-DJ et al. Journal of Thoracic and Cardiovascular Surgery 1999; 117:54-65 |

| Pemetrexed/Cisplatin | Indication: Pleural Mesothelioma | 12.3.2 |

**Cautions**

*This chemotherapy may cause life-threatening toxicity! It should only be administered under the supervision of an experienced medical oncologist! The protocol must first be reviewed and considered in relationship to the clinical situation of the patient.*

## Chemotherapy

| Week | Day | Compounds (generic names) in chronological order | Dosage | Diluent | Route | Duration of Infusion | Comments |
|---|---|---|---|---|---|---|---|
| 1 | 1 | **Pemetrexed** | 500mg/m² | 100ml Saline 0.9% | i.v. | 15min | stable for 24h after dilution in 100ml saline; maximum single dose is 1000mg absolute |
| 1 | 1 | **Cisplatin** | 75mg/m² | 250ml Saline 0.9% | i.v. | 1h | maximum single dose is 150mg absolute |

*Please note: on days 2-4, protocol for prophylaxis of delayed emesis

| Cycle Diagram | d1 w1 | d8 w2 | d15 w3 | d22 w4 |
|---|---|---|---|---|
| Pemetrexed | | | | N.C. |
| Cisplatin | | | | |

## Obligatory Pre- and Concurrent Medication

| Week | Day | Compounds (generic names) | Sequence and Timing | Dose | Diluent | Route | Duration of Infusion | Comments |
|---|---|---|---|---|---|---|---|---|
| from 1-2 weeks before chemo. | daily | Folic Acid | 1 - 0 - 0 | 500µg | | oral | | until 3 weeks after end of therapy |
| once every 9 weeks | | Vitamin B12 | | 1000µg | | i.m. | | until 3 weeks after end of therapy |
| 1 | 1 | Saline 0.9% | 15' before chemotherapy | | 3000ml | i.v. | 8h | |
| 1 | 1 | Granisetron | 15' before chemotherapy | 1mg | | i.v. | bolus | |
| 1 | 1 | Mannitol 10% | 30' before and after Cisplatin | | each 250ml | i.v. | 15min | |
| 1 | 1, 2, 3 | Aprepitant | -1h before chemo., d2+3 in the morning | * | | oral | | * d1 : 125mg, d2+3: 80mg |
| 1 | 1-4 | Dexamethasone | d1 -15min, d2-4 in the morning | * | | i.v./oral | | * d1 : 12mg/d2-4: 8mg |

| | |
|---|---|
| **Medicines As Required** | Granisetron oral or i.v., Filgrastim may be given if WBC <500/µl (>2 days) or with fever or infection in the neutropenic phase; **NSAIDs/Salicylates must not be given from 2 days before and until 2 days after Pemetrexed therapy.** Leucovorin rescue (see protocol for dose) with: leukopenia CTC Grade 4, thrombocytopenia Grade 4 or Grade 3 with hemorrhage and with mucositis Grade 3/4 |
| **Routine Tests:** | No later than 3 days before cycle and on day 7 or 8: Hb, FBC and differential, serum bilirubin, ALP, AST (SGOT), ALT (SGPT), serum creatinine; creatinine clearance no later than 3 days before cycle; radiology: CT or MRI scan after every 2nd cycle |
| **Dose Reduction:** | **With toxicity in previous cycles, reduce dose until end of therapy: hematologic: reduce dose by 25%** if: 1.Neutrophil nadir <1000/µl with fever ≥38.5°C; 2.Neutrophil nadir < 500/µl + platelet nadir ≥50,000/µl; 3.Platelet nadir < 50,000/µl without recovery; **reduce dose by 50%** if platelet nadir < 50,000/µl with hemorrhage; **mucositis: reduce Pemetrexed dose by 50%** with CTC Grade 3-4; **neurotoxicity: reduce Cisplatin dose by 50%** with CTC Grade 2; **other non-hematologic toxic reactions: reduce Pemetrexed dose by 25%** with other CTC Grade 3-4; **discontinue therapy:** creatinine clearance<45ml/min, neurotoxicity CTC Grade 3-4; other CTC toxicity Grade 3-4 after second dose reduction (except for raised serum transaminases) |
| **Next Cycle (N.C.):** | Day 22; 6 cycles maximum; start cycle only if WBC >1500/µl and platelets >100,000/µl |
| **Efficacy Assess.:** | After every 2nd cycle using the same procedures as used with initial ex mination (CT or MRI scan); with response, a confirmatory examination must be carried out within 4-6 weeks |
| **References:** | Munoz et al, N Engl J Med. 2006 Jan 19;354(3):305-7 |

# PAC

## Indication: Thymic Carcinoma

**12.4.1**

*This chemotherapy may cause life-threatening toxicity! It should only be administered under the supervision of an experienced medical oncologist! The protocol must first be reviewed and considered in relationship to the clinical situation of the patient.*

## Chemotherapy

| Week | Day | Compounds (generic names) in chronological order | Dosage | Diluent | Route | Duration of Infusion | Comments |
|---|---|---|---|---|---|---|---|
| | 1 | **Doxorubicin** | 50mg/m² | undiluted | i.v. | bolus 15min | |
| | 1 | **Cisplatin** | 50mg/m² | 250ml Saline 0.9% | i.v. | 1h | |
| | 1 | **Cyclophosphamide** | 500mg/m² | 250ml Saline 0.9% | i.v. | 1h | |
| | | | | | | | |
| | | | | | | | |

| Cycle Diagram | d1 w1 | d8 w2 | d15 w3 | d22 w4 |
|---|---|---|---|---|
| Doxorubicin | | | | N.C. |
| Cisplatin | | | | |
| Cyclophos. | | | | |

**Cautions**

After day 1 protocol for prophylaxis of delayed emesis

Incompatibilities: Cisplatin<>Mesna, Cisplatin<>NaHCO₃ Mg²⁺<>NaHCO₃

Anthracycline: Danger of cardiotoxicity - monitor cardiac function (echocardiogram)

## Obligatory Pre- and Concurrent Medication

| Week | Day | Compounds (generic names) | Sequence and Timing | Dose | Diluent | Route | Duration of Infusion | Comments |
|---|---|---|---|---|---|---|---|---|
| | -1 to +1 | Sodium Bicarbonate | regularly | 2g every 6 hours | | oral | | |
| | 1 | Saline 0.9% + 6.3mmol Mg²⁺ in hydration infusion | 15' before chemotherapy | | 3000ml | i.v. | 24h | |
| | 1 | Granisetron | 15' before chemotherapy | 1mg | | i.v. | bolus | |
| | 1 | Mannitol 10% | 30' before and after Cisplatin | | 250ml | i.v. | bolus | |
| | 1 | Mesna | 0h, 4h & 8h after Cyclophos. | 100/200mg/m² | | i.v. | bolus | or orally at home |
| | 1, 2, 3 | Aprepitant | -1h before chemo., d2+3 in the morning | * | | oral | | * d1: 125mg, d2+3: 80mg |
| | 1-4 | Dexamethasone | d1-15min,d2-4 in the morning | * | | i.v./oral | | * d1: 12mg/d2-4: 8mg |

**Medicines As Required** Metoclopramide oral or i.v., if not tolerated replace with 5–HT3 antagonists, fluid intake at least 2 liters/day

**Routine Tests:** **Anthracycline:** see **cautions** above; FBC, U&Es esp. Mg²⁺, serum creatinine, LFTs, diuresis

**Dose Reduction:** Withhold **Cisplatin** if creatinine clearance < 60ml/min; see Dose Modification Table

**Max. Cum. Dose :** **Doxorubicin:** Danger of cardiotoxicity; max. cum. dose is 550mg/m²

**Next Cycle (N.C.):** Day 22

**References:** Loehrer PJ Sr. et al, J Clin Oncol. 1997; 15(9);3093-9

# RX/5FU/Cisplatin ("Naunheim")

**Indication: Esophageal Cancer**
Preop. Radiochemotherapy $T_{2-4} N_{0-1} M_0$

**12.5.1**

*This chemotherapy may cause life-threatening toxicity! It should only be administered under the supervision of an experienced medical oncologist! The protocol must first be reviewed and considered in relationship to the clinical situation of the patient.*

## Chemotherapy

| Week | Day | Compounds (generic names) in chronological order | Dosage | Diluent | Route | Duration of Infusion | Comments |
|------|-----|------|------|------|------|------|------|
| 1+4 | 1-5 | **Cisplatin** | $20mg/m^2$ | 250ml Saline 0.9% | i.v. | 1h | |
| 1+4 | 1-5 | **Fluorouracil (5FU)** | $500mg/m^2$ | 250ml Saline 0.9% | i.v. | 20h | central line recommended |

| | | | $T_1$ $N_1$ $M_0$ | primary operation | pT>1 pN>0 | postoperative RCT1 | |
| | | | T1 N1 M0 or | pre-op. RCT I | Pre-op restaging (surgical dept.) as initial staging | PR,CR | operability + | Op | R 0 | monitor |
| 1-5 | | **+ Radiotherapy (RX) 1.8 Gy/day (total dose: 36Gy)** | T2-4 N0-1 M0 | | | | operability + | Op | R 1, 2 | RCT II |
| | | | | | | NC,MR,PD | operability + | Op | R 0, 1, 2 | RCT II |
| | | | | | | | operability - | RCT II | | |

MLYN &/or M1 5FU/Carbo/Plt. or Paclitaxel± 5FU

| | Week: | 1 | 2 | 3 | 4 | 5 | 6 | 7 | | 1 | 2 | 3 | |
|---|---|---|---|---|---|---|---|---|---|---|---|---|---|
| | | Radiochemotherapy (RCT) I | | | | Restaging I + surg. consult. | | RCT II | | Radiochemotherapy (RCT) II | | | |
| Fluorouracil **days 1-5** | | Z | Z | Z | Z | | | Further therapy see diagram | 5FU 500mg/m² days1-5 | Z | Z | Z | |
| Cisplatin **days 1-5** | | Z | Z | Z | Z | | | surgery or RCT II | Cisplatin 20mg/m²days1-5 | Z | | | |
| RT **d1-5**(1.8Gy5x/week) | | Z | Z | Z | Z | | | | RT 23Gy(1.8Gy/day;13days) | Z | Z | | |

| Cycle Diagram | d1 w1 | d8 w2 | d15 w3 | d22 w4 | w5 | w6 | w7 | d50 w8 | d57 w9 | d64 w10 | d7 |
|---|---|---|---|---|---|---|---|---|---|---|---|
| Cisplatin | | | | | | | | | | | |
| Fluorouracil | | | | | | | | | | | |
| RT 1.8Gy/day | | | | | | | | | | | |

*SmPC = Summary of Product Characteristics

**Cautions**

Apreptiant is a moderate inhibitor and inducer of CYP3A4 (see SmPC*) #
- additional caution with Etoposide, Vinorelbine, Docetaxel, Paclitaxel, Irinotecan and Ketoconazole
- not to be given concomitantly with Pimozide, Terfenadine, Astemizole or Cisapride
- avoid concomitant use with Rifampicin, Phenytoin, Carbamazepine or other CYP3A4 inducers
- reduce the normal dose of oral Dexamethasone to 50%
- the effectiveness of oral contraceptives may be decreased until 2 months after the last dose of Aprepitant
After day 5 in weeks 1+4 protocol for prophylaxis of delayed emesis

## Obligatory Pre- and Concurrent Medication

| Week | Day | Sequence and Timing | Compounds (generic names) | Dose | Diluent | Route | Duration of Infusion | Comments |
|------|-----|------|------|------|------|------|------|------|
| 1+4 | 0-5 | with chemotherapy | Saline 0.9% | | 2000ml | i.v. | 24h | |
| 2-3 | 1-5 | with chemotherapy | Saline 0.9% | | 1000ml | i.v. | 24h | |
| 2-3 | 1-5 | 30' before radiotherapy | Metoclopramide | 50mg | | oral | | except d8, w2 see above (delayed emesis) |
| 1+4 | 1-5 | 15' before Cisplatin | Heparin | 15000 units | | i.v. | 24h | |
| 1+4 | 1-7 | d1-5 1h before chemo./ d6+7 mornings | Aprepitant | day1: 125mg/ days 2-7: 80mg | | oral | | see **Cautions** above |
| 1+4 | 1-5 | 30' before Cisplatin | Granisetron | 1mg | | i.v. | bolus | |
| 1+4 | 1-8 | d1-5 30' before chemo./ d6-8 mornings | Dexamethasone | day1: 12mg/ days 2-8: 8mg | | oral | | |
| 1+4 | 1-5 | 30' before and 30' after Cisplatin | Mannitol 10% | | 250ml | i.v. | 15min | |

**Medicines As Required** Dexamethasone 8mg + Granisetron 1mg i.v.; with 5FU weeks 2 and 3: Alizapride or Metoclopramide

**Routine Tests:** FBC, U&Es, esp. Mg²⁺, serum creatinine, creatinine clearance, diuresis, ototoxicity, neurotoxicity

**Dose Reduction:** Withhold **Fluorouracil** if bilirubin > 5mg/dl; withhold **Cisplatin** if creatinine clearance < 60ml/min; also see Dose Modification Table

**Next Cycle (N.C.):** 4 weeks chemotherapy in combination with radiotherapy 1.8Gy/day on days 1-5 (weeks1-4, planned total dose: 36Gy), treatment-free interval, restaging, then surgery if appropriate

**Efficacy Assess.** After complete cycle (= after 4 weeks)

**References:** Naunheim KS et al., JThorac Cardiovasc Surg, 1992;103:887-895.

**Aprepitant:** SmPC, Bokemeyer C. Arzneimitteltherapie 2004;22:129-35, MASCC Antiemetic guidelines 2004 www.mascc.orgNavari RM. Cancer Invest. 2004;22(4);569-76.

# PELF (modified)*

## Indication: Gastric Cancer

**12.6.1**

*This chemotherapy may cause life-threatening toxicity! It should only be administered under the supervision of an experienced medical oncologist! The protocol must first be reviewed and considered in relationship to the clinical situation of the patient.*

## Chemotherapy

| Week | Day | Compounds (generic names) in chronological order | Dosage | | Diluent | Route | Duration of Infusion | Comments |
|---|---|---|---|---|---|---|---|---|
| 1-6 | 1 | **Cisplatin** | 40mg/m² | | 250ml Saline 0.9% | i.v. | 30min | |
| 1-6 | 1 | **Epirubicin** | 35mg/m² | | undiluted | i.v. | bolus 15min | |
| 1-6 | 1 | **Calcium Folinate (Leucovorin)** | 500mg/m² | | 100ml Saline 0.9% | i.v. | 30min | |
| 1-6 | 1 | **Fluorouracil (5FU)** | 500mg/m² | | 100ml Saline 0.9% | i.v. | 15min | |

| Cycle Diagram | d1 w1 | d8 w2 | d15 w3 | d22 w4 | d29 w5 | d36 w6 | d43 w7 | d50 w8 |
|---|---|---|---|---|---|---|---|---|
| Cisplatin | | | | | | | | N.C. |
| Epirubicin | | | | | | | | |
| Leucovorin | | | | | | | | |
| Fluorouracil | | | | | | | | |

**Cautions**

After day 1 protocol for prophylaxis of delayed emesis

Granisetron: increase dose to 3mg with emesis

**Anthracycline: Danger of cardiotoxicity - monitor cardiac function**

Brivudine must **not** be given together with 5FU. This also includes topical applications (Fluorouracil, Capecitabine, Floxuridine, Tegafur). Lethal consequences are possible for up to 4 weeks, due to inhibition of DPD enzyme activity.

## Obligatory Pre- and Concurrent Medication

| Week | Day | Compounds (generic names) | Sequence and Timing | Dose | Diluent | Route | Duration of Infusion | Comments |
|---|---|---|---|---|---|---|---|---|
| 1-6 | 1 | Saline 0.9% | start 2h before chemotherapy | | 3000ml | i.v. | 6-8h | |
| 1-6 | 1 | Granisetron | 15' before Cisplatin | 1mg | | i.v. | bolus | |
| 1-6 | 1 | Mannitol 10% | 30' before & 1h after Cisplatin | | 250ml | i.v. | 15min | |
| 1-6 | 1, 2, 3 | Aprepitant | -1h before chemotherapy | * | | oral | | * d1: 125mg, d2+3: 80mg |
| 1-6 | 1-4 | Dexamethasone | d1-15min, d2-4 in the morning | * | | i.v./oral | | * d1: 12mg/d2-4: 8mg |

**Medicines As Required** Granisetron; Filgrastim

| | |
|---|---|
| **Routine Tests:** | **Anthracycline: see cautions** above; FBC, U&Es, liver and renal function parameters, audiometry, cardiac status |
| **Therapy Delay:** | If leukocytes <4000/μl, platelets <100,000/μl, with Grade 2 or 3 ucositis, diarrhea, delay therapy for about a week; with occurrence of Grade 4 toxic reaction: discontinue therapy |
| **Dose Reduction:** | With polyneuropathy and ototoxcity from Grade 2 onwards, reduce **Cisplatin** dose |
| **Max. Cum. Dose :** | **Epirubicin:** Danger of cardiotoxicity; max. cum. dose of 1000mg/m² would be exceeded from cycle 29 |
| **Next Cycle (N.C):** | Week 8 (1 cycle = 6 weeks treatment) |
| **Efficacy Assess.** | After every cycle |
| **References:** | Cascinu et al., J Clin Oncol 15, 3313-3319 (1997)    *original protocol is with Glutathione; but the effect is uncertain and its very difficult to procare |

# ECF　　　Indication: Gastric Cancer　　　12.6.2

*This chemotherapy may cause life-threatening toxicity! It should only be administered under the supervision of an experienced medical oncologist! The protocol must first be reviewed and considered in relationship to the clinical situation of the patient.*

## Chemotherapy

| Week | Day | Compounds (generic names) in chronological order | Dosage | Diluent | Route | Duration of Infusion | Comments |
|---|---|---|---|---|---|---|---|
|  | 1 | **Epirubicin** | 50mg/m² | undiluted | i.v. | bolus |  |
|  | 1 | **Cisplatin** | 60mg/m² | 250ml Saline 0.9% | i.v. | 1h |  |
|  | 1-21 | **Fluorouracil (5FU)** | 200mg/m²/day | Saline 0.9% | i.v. | 24h | in a 7 day infusion pump |

| Cycle Diagram | d1 w1 | d8 w2 | d15 w3 | d22 w4 | d29 w5 | d36 w |
|---|---|---|---|---|---|---|
| Epirubicin |  |  |  | N.C. |  |  |
| Cisplatin |  |  |  |  |  |  |
| Fluorouracil |  |  |  |  |  |  |

**Cautions:**

Incompatibility: Cisplatin<>5FU

Add Heparin 2500 units/day (17,500 units / 7 days) to Fluorouracil in pump in order to avoid thrombotic complications.
Change pump every 7 days

Brivudine must **not** be given together with 5FU. This also includes topical applications (Fluorouracil, Capecitabine, Floxuridine, Tegafur). Lethal consequences are possible for up to 4 weeks, due to inhibition of DPD enzyme activity.

## Obligatory Pre- and Concurrent Medication

| Week | Day | Compounds (generic names) | Sequence and Timing | Dose | Diluent | Route | Duration of Infusion | Comments |
|---|---|---|---|---|---|---|---|---|
|  | 1 | Saline 0.9% | 2h before chemotherapy |  | 1500ml | i.v. | 3h |  |
|  | 1 | Mannitol 10% | 30' before & 1h15min after Cisplatin |  | each 250ml | i.v. | 15min |  |
|  | 1 | Granisetron | 30' before chemotherapy | 1mg |  | i.v. | bolus |  |
|  | 1 | Heparin | 30' before chemotherapy | 15000 units |  | i.v. | 24h |  |
|  | 1 | Saline 0.9% | with Cisplatin administration |  | 3000ml | i.v. | 24h |  |
|  | 1, 2, 3 | Aprepitant | -1h before chemo., d2+3 in the morning | * |  | oral |  | * d1: 125mg, d2+3: 80mg |
|  | 1-4 | Dexamethasone | d1 -30min, d2-4 in the morning | * |  | i.v./oral |  | * d1: 12mg/d2-4: 8mg |

| | |
|---|---|
| **Routine Tests** | FBC, U&Es esp. Ca²⁺, serum creatinine, creatinine clearance, total protein, albumin, bilirubin, LFTs, ototoxicity, neurotoxicity, weight |
| **Dose Reduction:** | With neutropenia<1500/µl and/or thrombocytopenia<100,000/µl on day 21: postpone cycle by max. of 2 weeks. With diarrhea>=Grade 3 or stomatitis Grade 3: reduce **5FU** dose by 20%. With serum creatinine>=Grade 2 (>1.5x normal value): creatinine clearance (=CCL) before every cycle, with CCL <60ml/min and >=40ml/min: reduce **Cisplatin** dose to 50%. With absence of recovery and with CCL <40ml/min: withhold **Cisplatin** in the following cycle. |
| **Next Cycle (N.C.):** | Day 22 |
| **Efficacy Assess.** | Neurological examination and radiological measurement of tumor after cycles 2, 4 and 6; with neoadjuvant intention, surgery after 3 cycles |
| **References:** | Cunningham D., ASCO 2005, Abstract # 4001; Webb A. et al., J. Clin. Oncol. 15; 261-267;1997 |

# DCF (Docetaxel/Cisplatin/5FU)

## Indication: Gastric Cancer

**12.6.3**

## Chemotherapy

*This chemotherapy may cause life-threatening toxicity! It should only be administered under the supervision of an experienced medical oncologist! The protocol must first be reviewed and considered in relationship to the clinical situation of the patient.*

| Week | Day | Compounds (generic names) in chronological order | Dosage | Diluent | Route | Duration of Infusion | Comments |
|---|---|---|---|---|---|---|---|
| | 1 | **Docetaxel** | 75mg/m² | 250ml Saline 0.9% | i.v. | 1h | |
| | 1 | **Cisplatin** | 75mg/m² | undiluted | i.v. | 1h | <100mg in 250ml Saline 0.9% |
| | 1 | **Fluorouracil (5FU)** | 2400mg/m² | 500ml Saline 0.9% | i.v. | 48h | |

Cycle Diagram: d1 w1 | d8 w2 | d15 w3 | d22 w4

Docetaxel / Cisplatin / Fluorouracil — N.C.

**Cautions**

- **Aprepitant** is a moderate inhibitor and inducer of CYP3A4 (see Summary of Product Characteristics - SmPC)
- additional caution with Etoposide, Vinorelbine, *Docetaxel*, Paclitaxel, Irinotecan and Ketoconazole
- not to be given concomitantly with Pimozide, Terfenadine, Astemizole or Cisapride
- avoid concomitant use with Rifampicin, Phenytoin, Carbamazepine or other CYP3A4 inducers
- reduce the normal dose of oral Dexamethasone to 50%
- the effectiveness of oral contraceptives may be decreased until 2 months after the last dose of Aprepitant
**Docetaxel:** Run in very slowly for the first 5 minutes
During 1st & 2nd infusions monitor blood pressure and pulse very closely (danger of anaphylaxis)
Incompatibilities: Cisplatin<>Mesna, Cisplatin<>NaHCO₃, Cisplatin<>5FU
**Brivudine** must not be given together with 5FU. Lethal consequences are possible for up to 4 weeks, due to inhibition of DPD enzyme activity.
Floxuridine, Tegafur). Lethal consequences are possible for up to 4 weeks, due to inhibition of DPD enzyme activity.

## Obligatory Pre- and Concurrent Medication

| Week | Day | Sequence and Timing | Compounds (generic names) | Dose | Diluent | Route | Duration of Infusion | Comments |
|---|---|---|---|---|---|---|---|---|
| | 1 | 30' before chemotherapy | Saline 0.9% | | 3000ml | i.v. | 6-8h | |
| | 1 | 1h before chemotherapy | Aprepitant | 125mg | | oral | | see **Cautions** |
| | 2 and 3 | mornings | Aprepitant | 80mg | | oral | | |
| | 1 | 30' before chemotherapy | Dexamethasone | 12mg | | oral | | |
| | 2-4 | mornings | Dexamethasone | 8mg | | oral | | |
| | 1 | 30' before chemotherapy | Granisetron | 1mg | | i.v. | bolus | |
| | 1 | 15' before chemotherapy | Clemastine | 2mg | | i.v. | bolus | |
| | 1 | 15' before chemotherapy | Ranitidine | 50mg | | i.v. | bolus | |
| | 1 | 30' before & after Cisplatin admin. | Mannitol 10% | | each 250ml | i.v. | 15min | |
| | 4 | 24h after end of chemotherapy | Pegfilgrastim | 6mg | | s.c. | | given as outpatient |

| | |
|---|---|
| **Medicines As Require** | Granisetron 1mg i.v., Loperamide |
| **Routine Tests** | FBC, U&Es esp. Ca²⁺, serum creatinine, creatinine clearance, total protein, albumin, serum bilirubin, LFTs, ototoxicity, neurotoxicity, weight |
| **Dose Reduction:** | With neutropenia<500/µl longer than 7 days and/or with febrile neutropenia or if platelets <25,000/µl: reduce **Docetaxel** dose by 20%. With neutropenia<1500/µl and/or platelets <100,000/µl: postpone cycle by max. of 2 weeks. With raised LFTs: **Docetaxel** dose may be reduced by 20%. With diarrhea or stomatitis Grade 3: reduce **Docetaxel** dose by 20%. With serum creatinine>=Grade 2 (>1.5x normal value): creatinine clearance (=CCL) before each cycle, with CCL<60ml/min and >=40ml/min: reduce **Cisplatin** dose to 50% - with absence of recovery and with CCL<40ml/min: withhold **Cisplatin** in the following cycle. With Grade 2 neuropathy: reduce **Cisplatin** dose by 20%. |
| **Next Cycle (N.C.):** | Day 22 |
| **Efficacy Assess.** | After cycles 2, 4 and 6: neurological examination, radiological measurement of tumor |
| **References:** | **DCF:** Roth AD et al. Ann Oncol 2004 15: 759-64; Janinis J et al. Am J Clin Oncol 2001 24:227-31; Ajani J et al. ASCO Proc 2003; **Aprepitant:** SmPC, Bokemeyer C. Arzneimitteltherapie 2004;22:129-35; MASCC Antiemetic guidelines 2004 www.mascc.org |

**FOLFIRI**                    **Indication: Colorectal Cancer**                    **12.7.1**

*This chemotherapy may cause life-threatening toxicity! It should only be administered under the supervision of an experienced medical oncologist! The protocol must first be reviewed and considered in relationship to the clinical situation of the patient.*

## Chemotherapy

| Week | Day | Compounds (Generic names) in chronological order | Dosage | Diluent | Route | Duration of infusion | Comments |
|---|---|---|---|---|---|---|---|
| | 1,15 | Irinotecan (CPT11) | 180mg/m² | 250ml Saline 0.9% | i.v. | 1h 30min | |
| | 1,15 | **Calcium Folinate (Leucovorin)** | 400mg/m² | 100ml Saline 0.9% | i.v. | 30min | |
| | 1,15 | Fluorouracil (5FU) | 400mg/m² | undiluted | i.v. | bolus | |
| | 1,15 | Fluorouracil (5FU) | *2400-3000mg/m² | 500ml Saline 0.9% | i.v. | 48h | |

**Cautions**: Brivudine must **not** be given together with 5FU. This also includes topical applications  (Fluorouracil, Capecitabine, Floxuridine, Tegafur). Lethal consequences are possible for up to 4 weeks, due to inhibition of DPD enzyme activity.

| Cycle diagram | d1 w1 | d8 w2 | d15 w3 | d22 w4 | d29 w5 | d |
|---|---|---|---|---|---|---|
| Irinotecan | | | | | N.C. | |
| Leucovorin | | | | | | |
| 5FU bolus | | | | | | |
| 5FU 48h | | | | | | |

## Obligatory Pre- and Concurrent Medication

| Week | Day | Compound (Generic name) | Dose | Diluent | Route | Duration of infusion | Comments |
|---|---|---|---|---|---|---|---|
| | 1,15 | Saline 0.9% | | 1000ml | i.v. | 2h45min | |
| | 1,15 | Dexamethasone | 8mg | 50ml | i.v. | 10min | |
| | 1,15 | Granisetron | 1mg | | i.v. | bolus | |

| | |
|---|---|
| Medicines As Required | Give patient Loperamide to take home! With acute cholinergic syndrome: Atropine 0.25 mg s.c. one dose |
| Routine Tests: | Bilirubin, LFTs, creatinine clearance, FBC and differential, clotting studies |
| Therapy Delay: | If neutrophils<500/μl or neutrophils<1000/μl+fever, then reduce by 20% |
| Dose Reduction: | If neutrophils<500/μl or neutrophils<1000/μl+fever, then reduce by 20%. |
| Dose Increase: | *If **Fluorouracil is** well tolerated in cycles 1 and 2, then the dose may be increased to 3g/m² from cycle 3. |
| Max. Cum. Dose : | Unknown |
| Next Cycle (N.C.): | Day 29 |
| Efficacy Assess. | Every 8 weeks |
| References: | Tournigand C et al. J Clin Oncol 2004; 22: 229- 237; André T et al., Europ J Cancer, 1999;35:1333-47 |

# FOLFIRI + Bevacizumab

## Indication: Colorectal Cancer

**12.7.2**

*This chemotherapy may cause life-threatening toxicity! It should only be administered under the supervision of an experienced medical oncologist! The protocol must first be reviewed and considered in relationship to the clinical situation of the patient.*

## Chemotherapy

| Week | Day | Compounds (Generic names) in chronological order | Dosage | Diluent | Route | Duration of infusion | Comments |
|------|-----|------|------|------|------|------|------|
| | 1,15 | **Bevacizumab** | 5mg/kg | 100ml Saline 0.9% | i.v. | 30min | 1st dose 90min, 2nd dose 60min |
| | 1,15 | **Irinotecan (CPT11)** | 180mg/m² | 250ml Saline 0.9% | i.v. | 1h 30min | |
| | 1,15 | **Folinic acid** | 400mg/m² | 100ml Saline 0.9% | i.v. | 30min | |
| | 1,15 | **Fluorouracil (5FU)** | 400mg/m² | undiluted | i.v. | bolus | |
| | 1,15 | **Fluorouracil (5FU)** | *2400-3000mg/m² | 500ml Saline 0.9% | i.v. | 48h | |

| Cycle diagram | d1 w1 | Duration of infusion | d8 w2 | d15 w3 | d22 w4 | d29 w5 | d3 |
|------|------|------|------|------|------|------|------|
| Bevacizumab | | 2h45min | | | | N.C. | |
| Irinotecan | | | | | | | |
| Leucovorin | | 10min | | | | | |
| 5FU bolus | | bolus | | | | | |
| 5FU 48h | | | | | | | |

**Cautions**

**Bevacizumab: (see Summary of Product Characteristics - SmPC)**

<u>1st dose:</u> Bevacizumab to be given over 90 min after chemotherapy, 2nd dose to be given over 60 min before chemotherapy, but may be given over 30 min if well tolerated.

**Cautions:** hemorrhage (GI), gastrointestinal perforation, thromboemboli, hypertensive crisis, allergic/anaphylactic reactions, proteinuria, impaired wound healing, congestive cardiac failure, cardiomyopathy.

- Treatment should only be started 28 days after major surgery at the earliest or with full wound healing

**Contraindications:** Pregnancy/lactation (contraception), untreated CNS metastases

**Brivudine must not be given together with 5FU. This also includes topical applications (Fluorouracil, Capecitabine, Floxuridine, Tegafur).**

**Lethal consequences are possible for up to 4 weeks, due to inhibition of DPD enzyme activity.**

## Obligatory Pre- and Concurrent Medication

| Week | Day | Sequence and Timing | Compound (Generic name) | Dose | Diluent | Route | Duration of infusion | Comments |
|------|-----|------|------|------|------|------|------|------|
| | 1,15 | 15' before chemotherapy | Saline 0.9% | | 1000ml | i.v. | 2h45min | |
| | 1,15 | 15' before chemotherapy | Dexamethasone | 8mg | 50ml | i.v. | 10min | |
| | 1,15 | 15' before chemotherapy | Graniseton | 1mg | | i.v. | bolus | |
| | | | | | | | | |
| | | | | | | | | |

| | |
|------|------|
| **Medicines As Required** | Give patient Loperamide to take home! With acute cholinergic syndrome: Atropine 0.25 mg s.c. one dose |
| **Routine Tests:** | Blood pressure, bilirubin, LFTs, creatinine clearance, FBC and differential, clotting studies, potassium, phosphorus, blood glucose, urinary protein, alkaline phosphatase |
| **Therapy Delay:** | If neutrophils<500/μl or neutrophils<1000/μl+fever, then reduce by 20% |
| **Dose Reduction:** | If neutrophils<500/μl or neutrophils<1000/μl+fever, then reduce by 20%.     *If **Fluorouracil** is well tolerated in cycles 1 and 2, then the dose may be increased to 3g/m² from cycle 3. With the occurrence of side effects from **Bevacizumab**, this drug should be withheld (see Summary of Product Characteristics - SmPC) |
| **Max. Cum. Dose :** | Unknown |
| **Next Cycle (N.C.):** | Day 29 |
| **Efficacy Assess.** | Every 8 weeks |
| **References:** | FOLFIRI: Tournigand C et al. J Clin Oncol 2004; 22: 229- 237; FOLFIRI-Bevacizumab: Hurwitz H et al, N Engl J Med. 2004 Jun 3;350(23):2335-42. |

# Irinotecan/Cetuximab

## Indication: Metastatic Colorectal Cancer

**12.7.3**

*This chemotherapy may cause life-threatening toxicity! It should only be administered under the supervision of an experienced medical oncologist! The protocol must first be reviewed and considered in relationship to the clinical situation of the patient.*

### Chemotherapy

| Week | Day | Compounds (Generic names) in chronological order | Dosage | Diluent | Route | Duration of infusion | Comments |
|---|---|---|---|---|---|---|---|
| | 1, 8 | **Cetuximab** | *250mg/m² | undiluted | i.v. | *1h | *use separate infusion set |
| | 1 | **Irinotecan (CPT11)** | 180mg/m² | 250ml Saline 0.9% | i.v. | 1h | Irinotecan infusion 1 hour after the end of |
| | | | | | | | Cetuximab at the earliest |

**Cautions**

***CETUXIMAB:***
- **First dose:** 400mg/m² i.v. over 2 hours
- Subsequent doses: 250mg/m² i.v. over 1 hour
- maximum infusion rate 5 ml/min = 10mg/min
- when infusion has finished, flush infusion line with Saline 0.9%

**Allergic /anaphylactic reactions**

| Cycle diagram | d1 w1 | d8 w2 | d15 w3 | d22 w4 | d29 w5 |
|---|---|---|---|---|---|
| Cetuximab | | | N.C. | | |
| Irinotecan | | | | | |

### Obligatory Pre- and Concurrent Medication

| Week | Day | Sequence and Timing | Compound (Generic name) | Dose | Diluent | Route | Duration of infusion | Comments |
|---|---|---|---|---|---|---|---|---|
| | 1, 8 | 30' before Cetuximab | Clemastine | 2mg | | i.v. | bolus | premed. obligatory with first Cetuximab |
| | 1, 8 | 30' before Cetuximab | Ranitidine | 50mg | | i.v. | bolus | dose and recommended with subsequent |
| | 1 | 30' before Irinotecan | Saline 0.9% | | 1500ml | i.v. | 4h | |
| | 1 | 30' before Irinotecan | Dexamethasone | 8mg | | i.v. | 10min | |
| | 1 | 30' before Irinotecan | Granisetron | 1mg | | i.v. | bolus | |

| | |
|---|---|
| **Medicines As Required** | With start of diarrhea, Loperamide 4mg orally, then 2mg every 2 hours, then 2mg every 2 hours until 12 hours after cessation of diarrhea; if no improvement after 48 hours/diarrhea+ neutropenic fever/ |
| | CTC Grade 4 diarrhea: start broad-spectrum antibiotic therapy (Quinolone); with acute cholinergic syndrome: Atropine 0.25 mg s.c. one dose |
| **Routine Tests:** | FBC and differential, renal function tests, LFTs |
| **Dose Reduction:** | **Cetuximab: allergic reactions:** CTC Grade: decrease infusion rate by 50%; duration of infusion not >4h in total; CTC Grade 2: stop infusion until improvement t o at least CTC Grade 1 ; |
| | then proceed as before; CTC Grade 3/4: discontinue therapy; **skin toxicity:** CTC Grade 3: withhold therapy for up to 14 days, with improvement after 1st occurrence: restart at |
| | 250mg/m², after 2nd occurrence: 200mg/m², after 3rd occurrence: 150mg/m²; if no improvement or 4th occurrence of CTC Grade 3 : discontinue therapy ; **Irinotecan:** reduce by 20% |
| | with CTC Grade 4 neutropenia, CTC Grade 4 emesis, other CTC Grade 3/4 (except for nausea, alopecia); with CTC Grades 2-4 cardiotoxicity: discontinue therapy |
| **Therapy Delay:** | Up to 28 days, if longer then discontinue therapy; start only if neutrophils ≥1500/µl+platelets ≥75,000/µl; serum bilirubin >1.5x upper limit of normal; CTC from Grade 2 (except for emesis; |
| | from Grade 3, nausea, alopecia) |
| **Next Cycle (N.C.):** | Day 15 |
| **Efficacy Assess.** | Every 8 weeks |
| **References:** | Cunningham D et al. NEJM 2004, 351:337–45 |

# Ardalan

**Indication:** Colon Cancer, Pancreatic Cancer, Cholangiocarcinoma    **12.7.4**

*This chemotherapy may cause life-threatening toxicity! It should only be administered under the supervision of an experienced medical oncologist! The protocol must first be reviewed and considered in relationship to the clinical situation of the patient.*

## Chemotherapy

| Week | Day | Compounds (generic names) in chronological order | Dosage | Diluent | Route | Duration of Infusion | Comments |
|---|---|---|---|---|---|---|---|
| 1-6 | 1 | **Calcium Folinate (Leucovorin)** | 100mg/m² | 100ml Saline 0.9% | i.v. | 30min | |
| 1-6 | 1 | **Fluorouracil (5FU)** | 2.6g/m² | 500ml Glucose 5% | i.v. | 24h | |
| | | | | | | | |
| | | | | | | | |
| | | | | | | | |

| Cycle Diagram | d1 w1 | d8 w2 | d15 w3 | d22 w4 | d29 w5 | d36 w6 | d43 w7 | d50 w8 |
|---|---|---|---|---|---|---|---|---|
| Fluorouracil | | | | | | | | N.C. |
| Leucovorin | | | | | | | | |
| | | | | | | | | |

**Cautions**

Brivudine must **not** be given together with 5FU. This also includes topical applications (Fluorouracil, Capecitabine, Floxuridine, Tegafur). Lethal consequences are possible for up to 4 weeks, due to inhibition of DPD enzyme activity.

## Obligatory Pre- and Concurrent Medication

| Week | Day | Compounds (generic names) | Sequence and Timing | Dose | Diluent | Route | Duration of Infusion | Comments |
|---|---|---|---|---|---|---|---|---|
| 1-6 | 1 | Saline 0.9% | with chemotherapy | | 250ml | i.v. | 30min | |
| 1-6 | 1 | Dexamethasone | 30' before chemotherapy | 8mg | | oral | | may be given intravenously |
| 1-6 | 1 | Metoclopramide | 30' before chemotherapy | 30mg | | oral | | may be given intravenously |

| | |
|---|---|
| **Medicines As Required** | Metoclopramide 10-50mg oral or i.v. |
| **Routine Tests:** | FBC, U&Es, LFTs, serum creatinine, bilirubin |
| **Dose Reduction:** | Reduce dose by 25% with mucositis > Grade 2; withhold **Fluorouracil** if bilirubin > 5mg/dl, see Dose Modification Table |
| **Max. Cum. Dose :** | None |
| **Therapy Delay:** | As long as neutrophils < 1500/µl or platelets < 70,000/µl; max. 2 weeks |
| **Next Cycle (N.C.):** | Day 50, 4 cycles maximum |
| **Efficacy Assess.** | Every 7 weeks |
| **References:** | According to Ardalan et al., JCO, 1991;9:625-30 |

920

# 5FU/Leucovorin "Poon" adjuvant & metastatic stages     Indication: Colorectal Cancer     12.7.5

*This chemotherapy may cause life-threatening toxicity! It should only be administered under the supervision of an experienced medical oncologist! The protocol must first be reviewed and considered in relationship to the clinical situation of the patient.*

## Chemotherapy

| Week | Day | Compounds (generic names) in chronological order | Dosage | Diluent | Route | Duration of Infusion | Comments |
|---|---|---|---|---|---|---|---|
| | 1-5 | **Calcium Folinate (Leucovorin)** | 20mg/m² | | i.v. | bolus | |
| | 1-5 | **Fluorouracil (5FU)** | 425mg/m² | undiluted | i.v. | bolus | |
| | | | | | | | |
| | | | | | | | |
| | | | | | | | |

| | Cycle Diagram | d1 w1 | d8 w2 | d15 w3 | d22 w4 | d29 w5 | d |
|---|---|---|---|---|---|---|---|
| | Leucovorin | | | | | N.C. | |
| | Fluorouracil | | | | | | |
| | | | | | | | |

**Cautions:** Increase dose of 5FU by 10% if well tolerated in previous cycle

Brivudine must not be given together with 5FU. This also includes topical applications (Fluorouracil, Capecitabine, Floxuridine, Tegafur). Lethal consequences are possible for up to 4 weeks, due to inhibition of DPD enzyme activity.

## Obligatory Pre- and Concurrent Medication

| Week | Day | Compounds (generic names) | Dose | Diluent | Route | Duration of Infusion | Comments |
|---|---|---|---|---|---|---|---|
| | 1-5 | Saline 0.9% | | 250ml | i.v. | 30min | |
| | 1-5 | Dexamethasone | 8mg | | oral | | may be given intravenously |
| | | mucositis prophylaxis | | | | | |
| | | | | | | | |
| | | | | | | | |
| | | | | | | | |
| | | | | | | | |
| | | | | | | | |
| | | | | | | | |

| | |
|---|---|
| Medicines As Required: | Metoclopramide 10-50mg oral or i.v. |
| Routine Tests: | FBC, U&Es, LFTs, diuresis |
| Dose Reduction: | Withhold **Fluorouracil** if bilirubin > 5mg/dl, see Dose Modification Table |
| Max. Cum. Dose : | None |
| Next Cycle (N.C.): | Day 29 |
| Efficacy Assess. | After 2-3 cycles (1 cycle = 5FU days 1-5) |
| References: | Poon MA et al., J Clin Oncol, 1991;9:1967-1972 |

# FOLFOX 4

## Indication: Colorectal Cancer, adjuvant therapy    12.7.6

*This chemotherapy may cause life-threatening toxicity! It should only be administered under the supervision of an experienced medical oncologist! The protocol must first be reviewed and considered in relationship to the clinical situation of the patient.*

## Chemotherapy

| Week | Day | Compounds (Generic names) in chronological order | Dosage | Diluent | Route | Duration of infusion | Comments |
|---|---|---|---|---|---|---|---|
| | 1 | **Oxaliplatin** | 85mg/m² | 250ml Glucose 5% | i.v. | 2h | **incompatible with saline** |
| | 1,2 | **Folinic acid** | 200mg/m² | 250ml Saline 0.9% | i.v. | 2h | |
| | 1,2 | **Fluorouracil (5FU)** | 400mg/m² | undiluted | i.v. | bolus | |
| | 1,2 | **Fluorouracil (5FU)** | 600mg/m² | 500ml Saline 0.9% | i.v. | 22h | |

| Cycle diagram | d1 w1 | d8 w2 | d15 w3 | d22 w4 | d29 |
|---|---|---|---|---|---|
| Oxaliplatin | | | N.C. | | |
| Leucovorin | | | | | |
| 5FU bolus | | | | | |
| 5FU 22h | | | | | |

**Cautions**

Incompatibility: Oxaliplatin<>Saline 0.9%
Do not give Magnesium or Calcium with cardiac glycosides, thiazide diuretics or if patient is hypercalcemic or hypermagnesemic. Brivudine must <u>not</u> be given together with 5FU. This also includes topical applications (Fluorouracil, Capecitabine, Floxuridine, Tegafur). Lethal consequences are possible for up to 4 weeks, due to inhibition of DPD enzyme activity.

## Obligatory Pre- and Concurrent Medication

| Week | Day | Compound (Generic name) | Sequence and Timing | Dose | Diluent | Route | Duration of infusion | Comments |
|---|---|---|---|---|---|---|---|---|
| | 1 | Dexamethasone | 30' before chemotherapy | 8mg | | i.v. | 10min | |
| | 1 | Granisetron | 30' before chemotherapy | 1mg | | i.v. | bolus | |
| | 1 | Magnesium 10% | 20' before Oxaliplatin, after Oxaliplatin | 3.15mmol | 125ml Glucose 5% | i.v. | 20min | |
| | 1 | Calcium 10% | | 2.3mmol | | | | |
| | 1 | Glucose 5% | with Oxaliplatin | | 500ml | i.v. | 2h | |
| | 1 | Glucose 5% | 2h20min after Oxaliplatin | | 250ml | i.v. | 1h | |
| | 2 | Saline 0.9% | 30' before chemotherapy | | 1000ml | i.v. | 3h | |
| | 2 | Dexamethasone | 30' before chemotherapy | 8mg | | i.v. | 10min | |

| | |
|---|---|
| Routine Tests: | FBC, U&Es, LFTs, serum creatinine, haptoglobin |
| Dose Increase: | *If **Fluorouracil** is well tolerated in cycles 1 and 2, increase dose to 3g/m² from cycle 3 |
| Dose Reduction: | Reduce dose of **Fluorouracil** by 25% with mucositis >Grade 2; withhold **Fluorouracil** if bilirubin >5mg/dl, see Dose Reduction Table |
| Next Cycle (N.C.): | Day 15 |
| Efficacy Assess. | Every 8 weeks |
| References: | Andre T et al., NEJM 2004, 350: 2343–51 |

# FOLFOX 6

**Indication:** Colorectal Cancer, palliative therapy
**Pancreatic Cancer**

**12.7.7**

*This chemotherapy may cause life-threatening toxicity! It should only be administered under the supervision of an experienced medical oncologist! The protocol must first be reviewed and considered in relationship to the clinical situation of the patient.*

## Chemotherapy

| Week | Day | Compounds (Generic names) in chronological order | Dosage | Diluent | Route | Duration of infusion | Comments |
|---|---|---|---|---|---|---|---|
| | 1,15 | **Oxaliplatin** | 100mg/m² | 500ml Glucose 5% | i.v. | 2h | **incompatible with saline** |
| | 1,15 | **Folinic acid** | 400mg/m² | 100ml Saline 0.9% | i.v. | 30min | |
| | 1,15 | **Fluorouracil (5FU)** | 400mg/m² | undiluted | i.v. | bolus | |
| | 1,15 | **Fluorouracil (5FU)** | *2400–3000mg/m² | 500ml Saline 0.9% | i.v. | 48h | |

| Cycle diagram | d1 w1 | d8 w2 | d15 w3 | d22 w4 | d29 |
|---|---|---|---|---|---|
| Oxaliplatin | | | | | N.C. |
| Leucovorin | | | | | |
| 5FU bolus | | | | | |
| 5FU 48h | | | | | |

**Cautions**

**Incompatibility: Oxaliplatin <> Saline 0.9%**
Do not give Magnesium or Calcium with cardiac glycosides, thiazide diuretics or if patient is hypercalcemic or hypermagnesemic.
Brivudine must not be given together with 5FU. This also includes topical applications (Fluorouracil, Capecitabine, Floxuridine, Tegafur). Lethal consequences are possible for up to 4 weeks, due to inhibition of DPD enzyme activity.

## Obligatory Pre- and Concurrent Medication

| Week | Day | Sequence and Timing | Compound (Generic name) | Dose | Diluent | Route | Duration of infusion | Comments |
|---|---|---|---|---|---|---|---|---|
| | 1,15 | 30' before chemotherapy | Dexamethasone | 8mg | | i.v. | 10min | |
| | 1,15 | 30' before chemotherapy | Granisetron | 1mg | | i.v. | bolus | |
| | 1,15 | 20' before Oxaliplatin, after Oxaliplatin | Magnesium 10% | 3.15mmol | 125ml Glucose 5% | i.v. | 20min | see **Cautions** |
| | | | Calcium 10% | 2.3mmol | | | | |
| | 1,15 | with Oxaliplatin | Glucose 5% | | 500ml | i.v. | 2h | |
| | 1,15 | 2h20' after Oxaliplatin | Glucose 5% | | 250ml | i.v. | 1h | |

| | |
|---|---|
| **Routine Tests:** | FBC, U&Es, LFTs, serum creatinine, haptoglobin |
| **Dose Increase:** | *If **Fluorouracil** is well tolerated in cycles 1 and 2, increase dose to 3g/m² from cycle 3 |
| **Dose Reduction:** | Reduce dose of **Fluorouracil** by 25% with mucositis >Grade 2; withhold **Fluorouracil** if bilirubin >5mg/dl, see Dose Reduction Table |
| **Next Cycle (N.C.):** | Day 29 |
| **Efficacy Assess.** | Every 8 weeks |
| **References:** | Tournigand C et al. J Clin Oncol 2004; 22: 229-237; Maindrault-Goebel F et al. European Journal of Cancer 1999; 35(9):1338-42; Gamelin et al. Clin Cancer Res 2004; 10: 4055-4061 |

# Oxaliplatin monotherapy | Indication: Colorectal Cancer | 12.7.8

*This chemotherapy may cause life-threatening toxicity! It should only be administered under the supervision of an experienced medical oncologist! The protocol must first be reviewed and considered in relationship to the clinical situation of the patient.*

## Chemotherapy

| Week | Day | Compounds (Generic names) in chronological order | Dosage | Diluent | Route | Duration of infusion | Comments |
|---|---|---|---|---|---|---|---|
| | 1 | **Oxaliplatin** | 130mg/m² | 250ml Glucose 5% | i.v. | 3h | incompatible with saline |

Incompatibility: Oxaliplatin <> Saline 0.9%
Do not give Magnesium or Calcium with cardiac glycosides, thiazide diuretics or if patient is hypercalcemic or hypermagnesemic

**Cautions**

| Cycle diagram | d1 w1 | d8 w2 | d15 w3 | d22 w4 |
|---|---|---|---|---|
| Oxaliplatin | | | | N.C. |

## Obligatory Pre- and Concurrent Medication

| Week | Day | Compound (Generic name) | Sequence and Timing | Dose | Diluent | Route | Duration of infusion | Comments |
|---|---|---|---|---|---|---|---|---|
| | 1 | Dexamethasone | 30' before and 4h after chemo. | 8mg | | i.v. | bolus | dose at 4h may be given orally |
| | 1 | Magnesium 10% | 20' before Oxaliplatin, after Oxaliplatin | 3.15mmol | 125ml Glucose 5% | i.v. | 20min | see **Cautions** |
| | | Calcium 10% | | 2.3mmol | | | | |
| | 1 | Glucose 5% | with Oxaliplatin | | 750ml | i.v. | 3h | |

| | |
|---|---|
| Medicines As Required | Metoclopramide 10-50mg oral or i.v. |
| Routine Tests: | FBC, LFTs, LDH, haptoglobin (hemolysis possible) |
| Dose Reduction: | If platelet nadir in previous cycle < 50,000/mm³, reduce dose to 80% |
| Next Cycle (N.C.): | Day 22 |
| Efficacy Assess. | After 2 cycles (6 weeks) |
| References: | Oxaliplatin Product Information, Sanofi-Synthelabo (manufacturer) 1999; Gamelin et al. Clin Cancer Res 2004; 10: 4055-4061 |

# Capecitabine monotherapy

## Indication: Colorectal Cancer

**12.7.9**

*This chemotherapy may cause life-threatening toxicity! It should only be administered under the supervision of an experienced medical oncologist! The protocol must first be reviewed and considered in relationship to the clinical situation of the patient.*

## Chemotherapy

| Week | Day | Compounds (generic names) in chronological order | Dosage | Diluent | Route | Duration of Infusion | Comments |
|------|-----|--------------------------------------------------|--------|---------|-------|---------------------|----------|
| | 1-14 | **Capecitabine** | 1250mg/m² twice a day | | oral | | To be taken 30' after a meal<br>150mg and 500 mg film-coated tablets available |
| | | | | | | | |
| | | | | | | | |
| | | | | | | | |

| Cycle Diagram | d1 w1 | d8 w2 | d15 w3 | d22 w4 | d29 w5 | d36 w6 |
|---------------|-------|-------|--------|--------|--------|--------|
| Capecitabine | | | | N.C. | | |
| | | | | | | |
| | | | | | | |

### Dose modification according to therapy course:

| Toxicity according to NCI | During therapy | Next cycle |
|---------------------------|----------------|------------|
| Grade 1 | Maintain dose | Maintain dose |
| Grade 2 | Withhold therapy till decrease in intensity to Grade 1 | 1st Event Dose => 100%<br>2nd Event Dose => 75%<br>3rd Event Dose => 50%<br>4th Event Dose => 0% |
| Grade 3 | Withhold therapy till decrease in intensity to Grade 1 | 1st Event Dose => 75%<br>2nd Event Dose => 50%<br>3rd Event Dose => 0% |
| Grade 4 | Discontinue therapy | 1st Event Dose => 50% |

**Cautions**

Increased incidence of side effects in patients with impaired renal function

## Obligatory Pre- and Concurrent Medication

| Week | Day | Compounds (generic names) | Dose | Diluent | Route | Duration of Infusion | Comments |
|------|-----|---------------------------|------|---------|-------|---------------------|----------|
| | | | | | | | |
| | | | | | | | |
| | | | | | | | |
| | | | | | | | |
| | | | | | | | |
| | | | | | | | |
| | | | | | | | |

| | |
|---|---|
| **Medicines As Required** | Metoclopramide oral or i.v., if not tolerated replace with 5-HT3 antagonists ; Loperamide after discussion with Consultant |
| **Routine Tests:** | FBC, U&Es (Calcium), serum creatinine, LFTs, hand and foot checks, neurotoxicity, cardiac function |
| **Therapy Deferral:** | Hand-and-Foot Syndrome: interrupt therapy or possibly reduce dose, diarrhea Grade 2-4, bilirubin > 3 fold increase above normal; see "Summary of Product Characteristics (SmPC)" |
| **Interactions:** | Folic Acid: maximum tolerated dose of **Capecitabine** is decreased; plasma Phenytoin concentration is increased |
| **Next Cycle (N.C.):** | Day 22 |
| **Efficacy Assess.** | After 3 cycles |
| **References:** | Cutsem VE et al., J Clin Oncol, 2001; 19 : 4097-106 |

# RX/5FU/Mitomycin/Cisplatin ("Nigro")

**Indication:** Anal Cancer

Preop. Radiochemotherapy $T_{1-4}$ $N_{0-3}$ $M_0$

**12.7.10**

*This chemotherapy may cause life-threatening toxicity! It should only be administered under the supervision of an experienced medical oncologist! The protocol must first be reviewed and considered in relationship to the clinical situation of the patient.*

## Chemotherapy

| Week | Day | Compounds (generic names) in chronological order | Dosage | Diluent | Route | Duration of Infusion | Comments |
|---|---|---|---|---|---|---|---|
| 1 | 1 | **Mitomycin** | 15mg/m² | undiluted | i.v. | bolus | |
| 1,5,10,14,18 | 1-4 | **Fluorouracil (5FU)** | 1000mg/m² | 250ml Saline 0.9% | i.v. | 22h | |
| 10,14,18 | 1 | **Cisplatin** | 100mg/m² | 250ml Saline 0.9% | i.v. | 1h | |
| 1-3 and 10,11 | 1-5 | **RX 2Gy/day (50Gy in total)** | | | | | |

**Cautions**

On days 2-4 of weeks 1, 10, 14, 18, protocol for prophylaxis of delayed emesis

Incompatibility: 5FU<>Cisplatin

Brivudine must not be given together with 5FU. This also includes topical applications (Fluorouracil, Capecitabine, Tegafur). Lethal consequences are possible for up to 4 weeks, due to inhibition of DPD enzyme activity.

| Week: | 1 | 2 | 3 | 4 | 5 | 6 | 7 | 8 | 9 | 10 | 11 | 12 | 13 | 14 | 15 | 16 | 17 | 18 | 19 | 20 | 21 | 22 |
|---|---|---|---|---|---|---|---|---|---|---|---|---|---|---|---|---|---|---|---|---|---|---|
| | Radiochemotherapy I | | | | | | | | Restaging | Radiochemotherapy II | | | | | | | | | | | | Restaging II + surg. cons. |
| Mitomycin  day 1 | z | | | | | | | | | z | | | | | | | | | | | | |
| Fluorouracil days 1-4 | z | | | | z | | | | | z | | | z | | z | | | z | | | | |
| Cisplatin  day 1 | | | | | | | | | | z | | | z | | z | | | z | | | | |
| RT d1-5 (2Gy 5x/week) | z | z | z | | | | | | | z | z | | | | | | | | | | | |

| Cycle Diagram | d1 w1 | d8 w2 | d15 w3 | d22 w4 | d29 w5 | w6 | w7 | w8 | w9 | d64 w10 | d71 w11 | w12 | w13 | d92 w14 | w15 | w16 | w17 | d120 w18 | w19 | w20 | w21 w22 | w23 |
|---|---|---|---|---|---|---|---|---|---|---|---|---|---|---|---|---|---|---|---|---|---|---|
| Mitomycin | | | | | | | | | | | | | | | | | | | | | | |
| Fluorouracil | | | | | | | | | | | | | | | | | | | | | | |
| Cisplatin | | | | | | | | | | | | | | | | | | | | | | |
| RT 2Gy/day | | | | | | | | | | | | | | | | | | | | | | |

## Obligatory Pre- and Concurrent Medication

| Week | Day | Compounds (generic names) | Sequence and Timing | Dose | Diluent | Route | Duration of Infusion | Comments |
|---|---|---|---|---|---|---|---|---|
| 1,10,14,18 | 1 | Saline 0.9% | 15' before chemotherapy | | 2000ml | i.v. | 24h | |
| 1,10,14,18 | 2-4 | Saline 0.9% | continuously | | 500ml | i.v. | 24h | |
| 5 | 1-4 | Saline 0.9% | continuously | | 500ml | i.v. | 24h | |
| 5 | 1-4 | Metoclopramide | 8.00 and 20.00 | 50mg | | oral | | may be given intravenously |
| 1,10,14,18 | 1 | Granisetron | 15' before chemotherapy | 1mg | | i.v. | bolus | or orally |
| 10,14,18 | 1 | Mannitol 10% | 30' before and after Cisplatin | | 250ml | i.v. | 15min | |
| 10,14,18 | 1, 2, 3 | Aprepitant | -1h before chemotherapy | * | | oral | | * d1: 125mg, d2+3: 80mg |
| 10,14,18 | 1-4 | Dexamethasone | d1-15min, d2-4 in the morning | * | | i.v./oral | | * d1: 12mg/d2-4: 8mg |

**Medicines As Required:** Dexamethasone 8mg, Granisetron or Metoclopramide

**Routine Tests:** FBC, U&Es esp .Mg²⁺, LFTs, serum creatinine, creatinine clearance, diuresis, ototoxicity, neurotoxicity

**Dose Reduction:** Withhold **Cisplatin** if GFR < 60ml/min; withhold **Fluorouracil** if bilirubin > 5mg/dl; also see Dose Modification Table

**Max. Cum. Dose :** **Mitomycin** >50mg/m²: Danger of nephrotoxicity

**Repeat Therapy:** Continue for a total of 22 weeks chemotherapy in combination with radio therapy (2Gy/day); treatment-free interval possibly followed by surgery

**References:** Analogous to Nigro ND, World J Surg, 1987;11:446-451

# Gemcitabine

## Indication: Pancreatic Cancer, NSCLC

**12.8.1**

*This chemotherapy may cause life-threatening toxicity! It should only be administered under the supervision of an experienced medical oncologist! The protocol must first be reviewed and considered in relationship to the clinical situation of the patient.*

### Chemotherapy

| Week | Day | Compounds (generic names) in chronological order | Dosage | Route | Diluent | Duration of Infusion | Comments |
|---|---|---|---|---|---|---|---|
| | 1, 8, 15 | **Gemcitabine** | 1000mg/m² | i.v. | 250ml Saline 0.9% | 30min | |
| | | | | | | | |
| | | | | | | | |
| | | | | | | | |
| | | | | | | | |

| Cycle Diagram | d1 w1 | d8 w2 | d15 w3 | d22 w4 | d29 w5 | d |
|---|---|---|---|---|---|---|
| Gemcitabine | | | | | N.C. | |

**Cautions**

### Obligatory Pre- and Concurrent Medication

| Week | Day | Compounds (generic names) | Dose | Route | Diluent | Duration of Infusion | Comments |
|---|---|---|---|---|---|---|---|
| | 1,8,15 | Saline 0.9% | 500ml | i.v. | | 1h | |
| | 1,8,15 | Dexamethasone | 8mg | i.v. | | bolus | |
| | | | | | | | |
| | | | | | | | |
| | | | | | | | |
| | | | | | | | |
| | | | | | | | |

| | |
|---|---|
| **Medicines As Required** | Metoclopramide oral or i.v., Paracetamol orally |
| **Routine Tests:** | FBC, LFTs, renal function tests |
| **Dose Reduction:** | Leukocytes 500-1000/µl or platelets 50,000-100,000/µl: 75%; leukocytes < 500/µl or platelets < 50,000/µl: delay therapy; primary hyperbilirubinemia >2mg/dl: 80% |
| **Side Effects:** | Myelosuppression, reversible hepatotoxiciy, rarely renal disturbances, nausea/vomiting, flu-like symptoms, edema |
| **Next Cycle (N.C.):** | Day 29 (3 weeks of therapy, 1 week without therapy); discontinue with tumor progression |
| **References:** | Carmichael J et al., Brit J Cancer, 1996;73(1):101-105; Casper ES et al., Invest New Drugs, 1994;12(1):29-34, Venook AP et al., JCO, 2000; 18: 2780-2787; Gillenwater et al; Clin Lung Cancer. 2000 Nov;2(2):133-8; Louvert et al. J-Clin Oncol 2005;23:3509-16 |

| GemOx3 | Indication: Cholangiocarcinoma | 12.9.1 |

*This chemotherapy may cause life-threatening toxicity! It should only be administered under the supervision of an experienced medical oncologist! The protocol must first be reviewed and considered in relationship to the clinical situation of the patient.*

## Chemotherapy

| Week | Day | Compounds (Generic names) in chronological order | Dosage | Diluent | Route | Duration of infusion | Comments |
|---|---|---|---|---|---|---|---|
| | 1, 8, 15 | **Gemcitabine** | 1000mg/m² | 250ml Saline 0.9% | i.v. | 30min | |
| | 1, 15 | **Oxaliplatin** | 100mg/m² | 500ml Glucose 5% | i.v. | 2h | |

| Cycle diagram | d1 w1 | d8 w2 | d15 w3 | d22 w4 | d29 N.C. |
|---|---|---|---|---|---|
| Gemcitabine | | | | | |
| Oxaliplatin | | | | | |

**Cautions**

Do not give Magnesium or Calcium with cardiac glycosides, thiazide diuretics or if patient is hypercalcemic or hypermagnesemic

Incompatibilities: Oxaliplatin<>Saline 0.9%
Gemcitabine<>Glucose 5%

Oxaliplatin is analogous to Carboplatin but is less renal toxic and less emetogenic

Side effects: post-infusion sensitivity to cold (central cause, harmless, resolves spontaneously)
peripheral neuropathy, mild myelosuppression, moderately emetogenic
because of the possibility of hemolysis, serum haptoglobin levels should be done

## Obligatory Pre- and Concurrent Medication

| Week | Day | Sequence and Timing | Compound (Generic name) | Dose | Diluent | Route | Duration of infusion | Comments |
|---|---|---|---|---|---|---|---|---|
| | 1, 8, 15 | 15' before chemotherapy | Saline 0.9% | | 500ml | i.v. | 1h | |
| | 1, 15 | 15' before chemotherapy | Granisetron | 1mg | | i.v. | bolus | increase dose to 3mg with emesis |
| | 1, 15 | 15' before and 4h after chemo. | Dexamethasone | 8mg | | i.v. | bolus | may also be given orally |
| | 1, 15 | 20' before Oxaliplatin, after Oxaliplatin | Magnesium 10% / Calcium 10% | 3.15mmol / 2.3mmol | 125ml Glucose 5% | i.v. | 20min | see **Cautions** |
| | 1, 15 | with Oxaliplatin | Glucose 5% | | 500ml | i.v. | 2h | |
| | 1, 15 | 2h20min after Oxaliplatin | Glucose 5% | | 250ml | i.v. | 1h | |
| | 8 | 15' before chemotherapy | Dexamethasone | 8mg | | i.v. | | |

| | |
|---|---|
| Medicines As Required | Metoclopramide 10–50mg oral or i.v.; Filgrastim for febrile neutropenia Grade 3-4. Filgrastim may also be given prophylactically (see study protocol, page 15) |
| Routine Tests: | FBC, LFTs, LDH (see study protocol, page 16) |
| Dose Reduction: | See Dose Modification Table (study protocol, page 13) |
| Next Cycle (N.C.): | Day 28 |
| Efficacy Assess. | After 2 cycles |
| References: | Gamelin et al., Clin Cancer Res 2004; 10: 4055–4061 |

# CMF "Bonadonna"

## Indication: Breast Cancer, adjuvant therapy

**12.10.1**

*This chemotherapy may cause life-threatening toxicity! It should only be administered under the supervision of an experienced medical oncologist! The protocol must first be reviewed and considered in relationship to the clinical situation of the patient.*

## Chemotherapy

| Week | Day | Compounds (generic names) in chronological order | Dosage | Diluent | Route | Duration of Infusion | Comments |
|---|---|---|---|---|---|---|---|
| | 1 | **Cyclophosphamide** | 600mg/m² | 500ml Saline 0.9% | i.v. | 1h | |
| | 1 | **Methotrexate** | 40mg/m² | undiluted | i.v. | bolus | dose reduction in patients > 60 years |
| | 1 | **Fluorouracil (5FU)** | 600mg/m² | 250ml Saline 0.9% | i.v. | 1h | |
| | | | | | | | |
| | | | | | | | |
| | | | | | | | |

**Cautions**

Incompatibility: Methotrexate<>5FU

Brivudine must not be given together with 5FU. This also includes topical applications (Fluorouracil, Capecitabine, Floxuridine, Tegafur). Lethal consequences are possible for up to 4 weeks, due to inhibition of DPD enzyme activity.

| Cycle Diagram | d1 w1 | d8 w2 | d15 w3 | d22 w4 |
|---|---|---|---|---|
| Cyclophos. | | | | N.C. |
| Methotrexate | | | | |
| Fluorouracil | | | | |

## Obligatory Pre- and Concurrent Medication

| Week | Day | Sequence and Timing | Compounds (generic names) | Dose | Diluent | Route | Duration of Infusion | Comments |
|---|---|---|---|---|---|---|---|---|
| | 1 | 15' before chemotherapy | Saline 0.9% | | 1000ml | i.v. | 3h | |
| | 1 | 15' before chemotherapy | Dexamethasone | 8mg | 100ml saline 0.9% | i.v. | 15min | |
| | 1 | 0h, 4h & 8h after Cyclophos. | Mesna | 120/240mg/m² | | i.v. | bolus | orally if necessary |
| | 1 | 15' before chemotherapy | Granisetron | 1mg | | i.v. | bolus | |
| 1st neutropenic cycle* | | once a day | Filgrastim | 5µg/kg | | s.c. | | *when WBC<1000/µl; give until >1000/µl |
| subsequent cycles | 2** | one dose only | Pegfilgrastim | 6mg | | s.c. | | **prophyl. admin. 24h after i.v. chemo. |
| | | | | | | | | if decreased WBC in previous cycle |
| | | mucositis prophylaxis | | | | | | |
| | | | | | | | | |
| | | | | | | | | |
| | | | | | | | | |
| | | | | | | | | |
| | | | | | | | | |
| | | | | | | | | |

| | |
|---|---|
| **Medicines As Required:** | Metoclopramide oral or i.v. |
| **Routine Tests:** | FBC, U&Es, LFTs, serum creatinine, creatinine clearance, exclude third space fluid accumulation |
| **Dose Reduction:** | Dose reduction in patients > 60 years: **Methotrexate** 40mg absolute, withhold **Fluorouracil** if bilirubin > 5mg/dl, see Dose Modification Table |
| **Max. Cum. Dose :** | None |
| **Next Cycle (N.C.):** | Day 22 |
| **Efficacy Assess.** | Before cycle 3 |
| **References:** | Buzzoni R et al., J Clin Oncol, 1991;9(12):2134-2140; Bonadonna G et al., Semin Oncol, 1987;14(1):8-22 |

# FAC (FEC)                    Indication: Breast Cancer                    12.10.2

*This chemotherapy may cause life-threatening toxicity! It should only be administered under the supervision of an experienced medical oncologist! The protocol must first be reviewed and considered in relationship to the clinical situation of the patient.*

## Chemotherapy

| Week | Day | Compounds (generic names) in chronological order | Dosage | Diluent | Route | Duration of Infusion | Comments |
|---|---|---|---|---|---|---|---|
| | 1 | **Cyclophosphamide** | 500mg/m² | 250ml Saline 0.9% | i.v. | 1h | |
| | 1 | **Doxorubicin (Epirubicin)** | 50 (100)mg/m² | undiluted | i.v. | bolus 15min | |
| | 1 | **Fluorouracil (5FU)** | 500mg/m | 250ml Saline 0.9% | i.v. | 1h | |

| | | | | |
|---|---|---|---|---|
| Cycle Diagram | d1 w1 | d8 w2 | d 15 w3 | d22 w4 |
| Cyclophos. | | | | N.C. |
| Doxo (Epi) | | | | |
| Fluorouracil | | | | |

**Cautions:** Brivudine must not be given together with 5FU. This also includes topical applications (Fluorouracil, Capecitabine, Floxuridine, Tegafur). Lethal consequences are possible for up to 4 weeks, due to inhibition of DPD enzyme activity.
Anthracycline: Danger of cardiotoxicity -monitor cardiac function (echocardigram)
Incompatibility: Doxorubicin<>5FU

## Obligatory Pre- and Concurrent Medication

| Week | Day | Compounds (generic names) | Sequence and Timing | Dose | Diluent | Route | Duration of Infusion | Comments |
|---|---|---|---|---|---|---|---|---|
| | 1 | Saline 0.9% | 15' before chemotherapy | | 1000ml | i.v. | 4h | |
| | 1 | Dexamethasone | 15' before chemotherapy | 20mg | 100ml Saline 0.9% | i.v. | 15min | |
| | 1 | Granisetron | 15' before chemotherapy | 1mg | | i.v. | bolus | increase dose to 3mg with emesis |
| | 1 | Mesna | 0h, 4h & 8h after Cyclophos. | 100/200mg/m² | | i.v. | bolus | or orally at home |
| | * | Filgrastim | once a day | 5µg/kg | | s.c. | | *when WBC<1000/µl; give until >1000/µl |

| | |
|---|---|
| **Medicines As Required** | Metoclopramide oral or i.v., if not tolerated replace with 5-HT3 antagonists. Oral fluids: at least 2 liters/day |
| **Routine Tests:** | Antracycline: see cautions above; FBC, U&Es, serum creatinine, LFTs, cardiac function |
| **Dose Reduction:** | Withhold **Fluorouracil** if bilirubin > 5mg/dl. See Dose Modification Table |
| **Max. Cum. Dose :** | **Doxorubicin: Danger of cardiotoxicity; max. cum. dose is 550mg/m²/Epirubicin:** Danger of cardiotoxicity; max. cum. dose is 1000 mg/m² |
| **Next Cycle (N.C.):** | Day 22 |
| **References:** | Smally RV et al., Cancer, 1977;40:625-632/French Adjuvant Study Group, J Clin Oncol. 2001 Feb 1;19(3):602-11 |

# AC (EC)

**Indication: Breast Cancer**

## Chemotherapy

*This chemotherapy may cause life-threatening toxicity! It should only be administered under the supervision of an experienced medical oncologist! The protocol must first be reviewed and considered in relationship to the clinical situation of the patient.*

| Week | Day | Compounds (generic names) in chronological order | Dosage | Diluent | Route | Duration of Infusion | Comments |
|------|-----|------|------|------|------|------|------|
| | 1 | **Doxorubicin (Epirubicin)** | 60 (90)mg/m² | undiluted | i.v. | bolus | |
| | 1 | **Cyclophosphamide** | 600mg/m² | 500ml Saline 0.9% | i.v. | 1h | |
| | | | | | | | |
| | | | | | | | |
| | | | | | | | |

**Cautions** — **Anthracycline: Danger of cardiotoxicity - monitor cardiac function (echocardiogram)**

| Cycle Diagram | d1 w1 | d8 w2 | d15 w3 | d22 w4 |
|------|------|------|------|------|
| Dox (Epi) | | | | N.C. |
| Cyclophos. | | | | |

## Obligatory Pre- and Concurrent Medication

| Week | Day | Sequence and Timing | Compounds (generic names) | Dose | Diluent | Route | Duration of Infusion | Comments |
|------|-----|------|------|------|------|------|------|------|
| | 1 | 15' before chemotherapy | Saline 0.9% | | 1000ml | i.v. | 2h | |
| | 1 | 15' before chemotherapy | Dexamethasone | 8mg | 100ml Saline 0.9% | i.v. | 15min | |
| | 1 | 15' before, 2h & 6h after chemo. | Metoclopramide | 50mg | | i.v. | bolus | |
| | 1 | 0h, 4h & 8h after Cyclophos. | Mesna | 120/240mg/m² | | i.v. | bolus | or orally at home |
| 1st neutropenic cycle* | | once a day | Filgrastim | 5µg/kg | | s.c. | | *when WBC<1000/µl; give until >1000/µl |
| subsequent cycles | 2** | one dose only | Pegfilgrastim | 6mg | | s.c. | | **prophyl. admin. 24h after i.v. chemo. if decreased WBC in previous cycle |
| | | | | | | | | |
| | | | | | | | | |

| | |
|------|------|
| **Medicines As Required** | Metoclopramide oral or i.v., Dexamethasone i.v. |
| **Routine Tests:** | **Anthracycline:** see **cautions** above; FBC, U&Es, serum creatinine, LFTs |
| **Dose Reduction:** | See Dose Modification Table |
| **Max. Cum. Dose :** | **Doxorubicin (Epirubicin):** Danger of cardiotoxicity; max. cum. dose is 550 (1000)mg/m² |
| **Next Cycle (N.C.):** | Day 22 |
| **Efficacy Assess.** | Before cycle 3 |
| **References:** | Fischer B et al, J Clin Oncol 1990; 8,1483-96; Wood WC et al, N Engl J ed 1994; 330:1253; adapted from Henderson IC et al, J Clin Oncol. 2003 Mar 15; 21(6): 976-83 |

| Docetaxel | Indication: Breast Cancer (2nd line therapy) | 12.10.4 |
|---|---|---|

*This chemotherapy may cause life-threatening toxicity! It should only be administered under the supervision of an experienced medical oncologist! The protocol must first be reviewed and considered in relationship to the clinical situation of the patient.*

## Chemotherapy

| Week | Day | Compounds (generic names) in chronological order | Dosage | Diluent | Route | Duration of Infusion | Comments |
|---|---|---|---|---|---|---|---|
| | 1 | **Docetaxel** | 100mg/m² | *Saline 0.9% | i.v. | 1h | * concentration: 0.3–0.74mg/ml |
| | | | | | | | |
| | | | | | | | |
| | | | | | | | |
| | | | | | | | |

| | Cycle Diagram | d1 w1 | d8 w2 | d15 w3 | d22 w4 |
|---|---|---|---|---|---|
| | Docetaxel | | | | N.C. |

**Extravasation**

Cautions

## Obligatory Pre- and Concurrent Medication

| Week | Day | Sequence and Timing | Compounds (generic names) | Dose | Diluent | Route | Duration of Infusion | Comments |
|---|---|---|---|---|---|---|---|---|
| | 1 | 30' before chemotherapy | Saline 0.9% | 500ml | | i.v. | 1h30min | |
| | 1 | 30' before chemotherapy | Dexamethasone | 20mg | 100ml Saline 0.9% | i.v. | 15min | |
| | 1 | 30' before chemotherapy | Ranitidine | 50mg | | i.v. | bolus | |
| | 1 | 30' before chemotherapy | Clemastine | 2mg | | i.v. | bolus | |
| | 2–3 | twice a day | Dexamethasone | 8mg | | oral | | |
| | | | | | | | | |
| | | | | | | | | |
| | | | | | | | | |
| | | | | | | | | |
| | | | | | | | | |

| | |
|---|---|
| **Medicines As Required** | Metoclopramide oral or i.v., Dexamethasone 8mg i.v./oral |
| **Routine Tests:** | FBC, U&Es, serum creatinine, LFTs, weight |
| **Side Effects:** | Myelotoxicity, neuropathy, skin toxicity, fluid retention, allergic reactions, nausea/vomiting; **Caution:** Extravasation |
| **Dose Reduction:** | No dose reduction; if granulocytes < 1500/µl delay therapy |
| **Next Cycle (N.C.):** | Day 22 (if granulocytes > 1500/µl) |
| **Therapy Duration:** | Dependent on the tolerance of the individual patient |
| **Efficacy Assess.** | After 6 weeks |
| **References:** | Aapro MS, Seminars in Oncology, 1995;22 (Suppl 4):1-33 |

# Epirubicin

Therapy may be given as outpatient

## Indication: Breast Cancer and other Solid Tumors  12.10.5

*This chemotherapy may cause life-threatening toxicity! It should only be administered under the supervision of an experienced medical oncologist! The protocol must first be reviewed and considered in relationship to the clinical situation of the patient.*

## Chemotherapy

| Week | Day | Compounds (generic names) in chronological order | Dosage | Diluent | Route | Duration of Infusion | Comments |
|------|-----|--------------------------------------------------|--------|---------|-------|---------------------|----------|
|  | 1 | **Epirubicin** | 20 mg/m² | undiluted | i.v. | bolus |  |
|  |  |  |  |  |  |  |  |
|  |  |  |  |  |  |  |  |
|  |  |  |  |  |  |  |  |
|  |  |  |  |  |  |  |  |

| Cycle Diagram | d1 w1 | d8 w2 | d15 w3 | d22 w4 |
|---------------|-------|-------|--------|--------|
| Epirubicin |  |  |  |  |

**Cautions**

Extravasation

Anthracycline: Danger of cardiotoxicity - monitor cardiac function

## Obligatory Pre- and Concurrent Medication

| Week | Day | Sequence and Timing | Compounds (generic names) | Dose | Diluent | Route | Duration of Infusion | Comments |
|------|-----|---------------------|---------------------------|------|---------|-------|---------------------|----------|
|  | 1 | 15' before chemotherapy | Saline 0.9% | 250ml |  | i.v. | 1h |  |
|  | 1 | 15' before chemotherapy | Dexamethasone | 8mg |  | i.v. | bolus |  |
|  | 1 | 15' before chemotherapy | Metoclopramide | 30mg |  | i.v. | bolus |  |

| | |
|---|---|
| **Medicines As Required** | Metoclopramide oral or i.v. |
| **Side Effects:** | Cardiotoxicity, rarely allergic reactions/nausea/vomiting, **caution**: extravasation |
| **Routine Tests:** | **Anthracycline**: see **cautions** above; FBC, U&Es, serum creatinine, LFTs |
| **Dose Reduction:** | See Dose Modification Table |
| **Max. Cum. Dose :** | **Epirubicin**: Danger of cardiotoxicity; max. cum. dose is 1000 mg/m² |
| **Repeat Therapy:** | Weekly administration (if granulocytes < 1500/μl delay therapy) |
| **Efficacy Assess.** | After 6 weeks |
| **References:** | Ebbs et al., Acta Oncologica, 1989; 28:887-92 |

933

# EP

## Indication: Breast Cancer

**12.10.6**

## Chemotherapy

| Week | Day | Compounds (generic names) in chronological order | Dosage | Diluent | Route | Duration of Infusion | Comments |
|---|---|---|---|---|---|---|---|
| | 1 | **Epirubicin** | 60 mg/m² | undiluted | i.v. | bolus 15min | |
| | 1 | **Paclitaxel** | 175 mg/m² | 500ml Saline 0.9% | i.v. | 3 h | PVC-free infusion set |
| | | | | | | | |
| | | | | | | | |
| | | | | | | | |

**Cautions**

Beware of cardiotoxicity! Epirubicin must therefore be given prior to Paclitaxel!
Anthracycline: Danger of cardiotoxicity - monitor cardiac function

| Cycle Diagram | d1 w1 | d8 w2 | d15 w3 | d22 w4 |
|---|---|---|---|---|
| Epirubicin | | | | N.C. |
| Paclitaxel | | | | |
| | | | | |

## Obligatory Pre- and Concurrent Medication

| Week | Day | Sequence and Timing | Compounds (generic names) | Dose | Diluent | Route | Duration of Infusion | Comments |
|---|---|---|---|---|---|---|---|---|
| | 1 | 30' before Paclitaxel | Dexamethasone | 20mg | 100ml Saline 0.9% | i.v. | 15min | |
| | 1 | 30' before Paclitaxel | Clemastine | 2mg | | i.v. | bolus | |
| | 1 | 30' before Paclitaxel | Ranitidine | 50mg | | i.v. | bolus | |
| | 1 | 15' before and 4h after Epirubicin | Metoclopramide | 50mg | | i.v. | | 2nd dose may be taken orally at home |
| | 1 | with chemotherapy | Saline 0.9% | | 1000ml | i.v. | 5h | saline infusion with Paclitaxel by IVAC |
| 1st neutropenic cycle* | | once a day | Filgrastim | 5µg/kg | | s.c. | | *when WBC<1000/µl; give until >1000/µl |
| subsequent cycles | 2** | one dose only | Pegfilgrastim | 6mg | | s.c. | | **prophyl. admin. 24h after i.v. chemo. if decreased WBC in previous cycle |
| | | | | | | | | |
| | | | | | | | | |
| | | | | | | | | |

| | |
|---|---|
| **Medicines As Required** | Metoclopramide, possibly increase with 5HT antagonists i.v. or oral |
| **Routine Tests:** | **Anthracycline :** see **cautions** above; FBC, U&Es, esp. Mg²⁺, LFTs, neurotoxicity |
| **Dose Reduction:** | Discontinue if leukocytes < 1500/µl or if allergic to polyoxyethylene-3,5 castor oil, see Dose Modification Table |
| **Max. Cum. Dose :** | **Epirubicin:** Danger of cardiotoxicity; max. cum. dose is 1000mg/m² |
| **Next Cycle (N.C.):** | Day 22 |
| **Efficacy Assess.** | After 2 cycles |
| **References:** | Luck HJ et al. Oncology 1998; 12(Sup):36-39; Fountzilas G et al. J Clin Oncol 2001; 19:2232-39; Luck H et al. Abstract 280, ASCO 2000:7; Konecny G et al., Abstract 88, ASCO 2001:31 |

# Vinorelbine

Therapy may be given as outpatient

**Indication: Breast Cancer, Esophageal Cancer; NSCLC**

**12.10.7**

*This chemotherapy may cause life-threatening toxicity! It should only be administered under the supervision of an experienced medical oncologist! The protocol must first be reviewed and considered in relationship to the clinical situation of the patient.*

## Chemotherapy

| Week | Day | Compounds (Generic names) in chronological order | Dosage | Diluent | Route | Duration of infusion | Comments |
|---|---|---|---|---|---|---|---|
| | 1,8,15,22,29,36 | **Vinorelbine** | 30mg/m² | 100ml Saline 0.9% | i.v. | 10min | max. single dose 60mg absolute |
| | | | | | | | |
| | | | | | | | |
| | | | | | | | |

**Cautions**

| Cycle diagram | | d1 w1 | d8 w2 | d15 w3 | d22 w4 | d29 w5 | d36 w6 | d4 |
|---|---|---|---|---|---|---|---|---|
| Vinorelbine | | | | | | | | |

**Extravasation**

## Obligatory Pre- and Concurrent Medication

| Week | Day | Sequence and Timing | Compound (Generic name) | Dose | Diluent | Route | Duration of infusion | Comments |
|---|---|---|---|---|---|---|---|---|
| | 1,8,15,22,29,36 | 15' before chemotherapy | Saline 0.9% | | 500ml | i.v. | 1h | |
| | 1,8,15,22,29,36 | 15' before chemotherapy | Dexamethasone | 8mg | 100ml Saline 0.9% | i.v. | 15min | |

**Medicines As Required** Metoclopramide oral or i.v., if not tolerated replace with 5-HT3 antagonists

| | |
|---|---|
| **Side Effects:** | Myelotoxicity, peripheral and autonomic neurotoxicity, rarely allergic reactions/nausea/vomiting, constipation, **Caution:** Extravasation |
| **Routine Tests:** | FBC, U&Es, serum creatinine, LFTs |
| **Dose Reduction:** | Bilirubin 2.5-5mg/dl: 50%, Bilirubin 5-10mg/dl: 25%, Bilirubin > 10mg/dl: contraindicated, see Dose Modification Table |
| **Repeat Therapy:** | Weekly (if granulocytes <1500/µl delay therapy) |
| **Therapy Duration:** | With tumor response, continue therapy for a further 3 months |
| **Efficacy Assess.** | 2 weeks after the end of a cycle (comprises 6 doses) |
| **References:** | Furmoleau P et al, J Clin Oncol, 1993;11:1245-52; Rossi A et al, Anticancer Res, 2003;23:1657-64; Gridelli C, Hainsworth J, Lung Cancer, 2002;38:37-41 |

# Liposomal Doxorubicin

## Indication: Breast Cancer

**12.10.8**

*This chemotherapy may cause life-threatening toxicity! It should only be administered under the supervision of an experienced medical oncologist! The protocol must first be reviewed and considered in relationship to the clinical situation of the patient.*

### Chemotherapy

| Week | Day | Compounds (generic names) in chronological order | Dosage | Diluent | Route | Duration of Infusion | Comments |
|---|---|---|---|---|---|---|---|
| | 1 | **Liposomal Doxorubicin** | 50mg/m² | Glucose 5% | i.v. | 1h | |
| | | | | | | | |
| | | | | | | | |
| | | | | | | | |

**Cautions**

| Cycle Diagram | d1 w1 | d8 w2 | d15 w3 | d22 w4 | d29 w5 | d3 |
|---|---|---|---|---|---|---|
| Liposomal Doxorubicin | | | | | N.C. | |

### Obligatory Pre- and Concurrent Medication

| Week | Day | Sequence and Timing | Compounds (generic names) | Dose | Diluent | Route | Duration of Infusion | Comments |
|---|---|---|---|---|---|---|---|---|
| | 1 | 30min before chemotherapy | Granisetron | 1mg | 100ml Saline 0.9% | i.v. | 15min | |
| | | | Dexamethasone | 20mg | | i.v. | bolus | |
| | 1 | 30min before chemotherapy | Clemastine | 2mg | | i.v. | bolus | |
| | 1 | 30min before chemotherapy | Cimetidine | 400mg | | i.v. | bolus | |
| | 1 | 1h after chemotherapy | Glucose 5% | 250ml | | i.v. | 30min | |
| | 1 | 0 - 0 - 1 | Dexamethasone | 4mg | | oral | | |
| | 2, 3 | 1 - 0 - 0 | Granisetron | 2mg | | oral | | |
| | 2, 3 | 1 - 0 - 1 | Dexamethasone | 4mg | | oral | | |
| | | | | | | | | |

**Medicines As Required**: Metoclopramide oral or i.v., Dexamethasone i.v., Pyridoxine (Vitamin B6) 100mg every 8 hours

**Routine Tests**: FBC once a week, differential WBC, differential WBC, LFTs, U&Es, serum creatinine, urine testing, ECG 2 days prior to each chemotherapy, echocardiogram before start of therapy and after every 3rd dose of Liposomal Doxorubicin

**Dose Reduction**: See Dose Modification Table

**Max. Cum. Dose :** Not defined

**Next Cycle (N.C.):** Day 28

**Efficacy Assess.** Before the 3rd cycle

**References:** Keller et al. J Clin Oncol, Vol 22, No 19 (October 1), 2004

# Trastuzumab/Paclitaxel

## Indication: Metastatic Breast Cancer

**12.10.9**

*This chemotherapy may cause life-threatening toxicity! It should only be administered under the supervision of an experienced medical oncologist! The protocol must first be reviewed and considered in relationship to the clinical situation of the patient.*

## Chemotherapy

| Cycle | Day | Compounds (Generic names) in chronological order | Dosage | Diluent | Route | Duration of infusion | Comments |
|---|---|---|---|---|---|---|---|
| 1 | 1 | **Trastuzumab** | 4mg/kg | 250ml Saline 0.9% | i.v. | 90min | Please note: 4mg/kg for first dose only |
| | 2 | **Paclitaxel** | 175mg/m² | 500ml Saline 0.9% | i.v. | 3h | |
| | 8,15 | **Trastuzumab** | 2mg/kg | 250ml Saline 0.9% | i.v. | 30min | 30min only if well tolerated |
| 2 etc. | 1,8,15 | **Trastuzumab** | 2mg/kg | 250ml Saline 0.9% | i.v. | 30min | |
| | 1 | **Paclitaxel** | 175mg/m² | 500ml Saline 0.9% | i.v. | 3h | |

Cycle diagram

| | d1 w1 | d8 w2 | d15 w3 | d22 w4 | d2 |
|---|---|---|---|---|---|
| Trastuzumab | | | | | N.C. |
| Paclitaxel (cycle1 only) | | | | | |
| Paclitaxel (cycle2 etc.) | | | | | |

**Cautions**

**Indication: HER2/neu protein overexpression (immunohistochemically: DAKO-Score 3+ or FISH +)**

**Side Effects: anaphylaxis, cardiotoxicity, polyneuropathy, bone marrow toxicity**

**Due to the danger of anaphylaxis in the first cycle, Paclitaxel and Trastuzumab should be given on 2 successive days**

## Obligatory Pre- and Concurrent Medication

| Cycle | Day | Sequence and Timing | Compound (Generic name) | Dose | Diluent | Route | Duration of infusion | Comments |
|---|---|---|---|---|---|---|---|---|
| 1etc. | 1,2 | 30' before Paclitaxel | Dexamethasone | 20mg | 100ml Saline 0.9% | i.v. | 15min | |
| | 1,2 | 30' before Paclitaxel | Clemastine | 2mg | | i.v. | bolus | |
| | 1,2 | 30' before Paclitaxel | Ranitidine | 50mg | | i.v. | bolus | |
| | 1,2 | parallel to Paclitaxel | Saline 0.9% | | 1000ml | i.v. | 4,5h | |
| | 1, 8, 15 | with Trastuzumab | Saline 0.9% | | 500ml | i.v. | 1h | |

| | |
|---|---|
| **Medicines As Required** | Dexamethasone i.v. or Metoclopramide oral or i.v. |
| **Routine Tests:** | FBC, differential blood count (twice weekly), U&Es esp. Mg²⁺, serum creatinine, LFTs; clinically: check for polyneuropathy; echocardiogram and ECG (cardiotoxicity) 3 monthly |
| **Dose Reduction:** | **Paclitaxel** by 25% if leukopenia Grade 4 (<1000/μl), febrile neutropenia, thrombocytopenia Grade 4 (<10,000/μl) or polyneuropathy Score 3 |
| **Next Cycle (N.C.):** | Day 22 |
| **Efficacy Assess.** | After 2 cycles |
| **References:** | Slamon D.J. et al., N Engl J Med 2001; 344:783–92; Burstein HJ et al., J Clin Oncol 2003; 21(1):46–53; Summary of Product Characteristics (SmPC) Hoffmann/ La Roche March 2002 |

| EC+Paclitaxel | Indication: Breast Cancer | 12.10.10 |

*This chemotherapy may cause life-threatening toxicity! It should only be administered under the supervision of an experienced medical oncologist! The protocol must first be reviewed and considered in relationship to the clinical situation of the patient.*

## Chemotherapy

| Week | Day | Compounds (generic names) in chronological order | Dosage | Diluent | Route | Duration of Infusion | Comments |
|---|---|---|---|---|---|---|---|
| 1,4,7,10 | 1 | **Epirubicin** | 90mg/m² | undiluted | i.v. | bolus 15min | |
| 1,4,7,10 | 1 | **Cyclophosphamide** | 600mg/m² | 500ml Saline 0.9% | i.v. | 1h | |
| 13,16,19,22 | 1 | **Paclitaxel** | 175mg/m² | 500ml Saline 0.9% | i.v. | 3h | PVC-free infusion set |

Cycle Diagram — Weeks: 1 2 3 4 5 6 7 8 9 10 11 12 13 14 15 16 17 18 19 20 21 22 Weeks
- Epirubicin
- Cyclophos.
- Paclitaxel

**Cautions:** Anthracycline: Danger of cardiotoxicity - monitor cardiac function

## Obligatory Pre- and Concurrent Medication

| Week | Day | Compounds (generic names) | Sequence and Timing | Dose | Diluent | Route | Duration of Infusion | Comments |
|---|---|---|---|---|---|---|---|---|
| 1,4,7,10 | 1 | Saline 0.9% | 15' before chemotherapy | | 1000ml | i.v. | 2h | |
| 1,4,7,10 | 1 | Dexamethasone | 15' before chemotherapy | 8mg | 100ml Saline 0.9% | i.v. | 15min | |
| 1,4,7,10 | 1 | Metoclopramide | 15' before, 2h & 6h after chemo. | 50mg | | i.v. | bolus | |
| 1,4,7,10 | 1 | Mesna | 0h, 4h & 8h after Cyclophos. | 120mg/m² | | i.v. | bolus | |
| 13,16,19,22 | 1 | Dexamethasone | 30' before Paclitaxel | 8mg | 100ml | i.v. | 15min | |
| 13,16,19,22 | 1 | Clemastine | 30' before Paclitaxel | 2mg | | i.v. | bolus | |
| 13,16,19,22 | 1 | Ranitidine | 30' before Paclitaxel | 50mg | | i.v. | bolus | |
| 13,16,19,22 | 1 | Saline 0.9% | parallel to Paclitaxel | | 500ml | i.v. | 4h | |
| 1st neutropenic cycle* | 1 | Filgrastim | once a day | 5µg/kg | | s.c. | | *when WBC<1000/µl; give until >1000/µl |
| subsequent cycles | 2** | Peg-filgrastim | one dose only | 6mg | | s.c. | | **prophyl. admin. 24h after i.v. chemo. if decreased WBC in previous cycle |

**Medicines As Required:** Dexamethasone i.v. or Metoclopramide oral or i.v.

**Routine Tests:** Anthracycline: see cautions above; FBC & differential (twice weekly), U&Es esp. $Mg^{2+}$, serum creatinine, ALP, AST (SGOT), ALT (SGPT), clinically: In particular polyneuropathy

**Therapy Delay:** Paclitaxel if leukocytes < 1500/µl or platelets < 75,00C/µl (check twice weekly).

**Dose Reduction:** Paclitaxel by 25% with leukopenia Grade 4 (<1000µl) or febrile neutropenia, by 25% with thrombocytopenia Grade 4 (<10,000/µl), by 25% with polyneuropathy 4-6

**Max. Cum. Dose:** Epirubicin: Danger of cardiotoxicity; max. cum. dose is 1000 mg/m²

**Next Cycle (N.C.):** EC every three weeks (four cycles in total), thereafter **Paclitaxel** every three weeks (four cycles in total)

**References:** Möbus V et al., analogous to Untch et al., ASCO 2003, Vol.22, 35, pp9, abstract; analogous to Henderson et al., J Clin Oncol 2003; 21; 976-83

| AC+Paclitaxel (Dose-dense) | Indication: Breast Cancer | 12.10.11 |
|---|---|---|

**This chemotherapy may cause life-threatening toxicity! It should only be administered under the supervision of an experienced medical oncologist! The protocol must first be reviewed and considered in relationship to the clinical situation of the patient.**

## Chemotherapy

| Week | Day | Compounds (generic names) in chronological order | Dosage | Diluent | Route | Duration of Infusion | Comments |
|---|---|---|---|---|---|---|---|
| 1,3,5,7 | 1 | **Doxorubicin** | 60mg/m² | undiluted | i.v. | bolus 15min | |
| 1,3,5,7 | 1 | **Cyclophosphamide** | 600mg/m² | 500ml Saline 0.9% | i.v. | 1h | |
| 9,11,13,15 | 1 | **Paclitaxel** | 175mg/m² | 500ml Saline 0.9% | i.v. | 3h | PVC-free infusion set |

| Cycle Diagram | 1 | 2 | 3 | 4 | 5 | 6 | 7 | 8 | 9 | 10 | 11 | 12 | 13 | 14 | 15 | 16 | 17 | 18 | 19 | 20 | 21 | 22 | Weeks |
|---|---|---|---|---|---|---|---|---|---|---|---|---|---|---|---|---|---|---|---|---|---|---|---|
| Doxorubicin | ■ | ■ | ■ | ■ | | | | | | | | | | | | | | | | | | | |
| Cyclophos. | ■ | ■ | ■ | ■ | | | | | | | | | | | | | | | | | | | |
| Paclitaxel | | | | | | | | | ■ | ■ | ■ | ■ | | | | | | | | | | | |

**Cautions**

## Obligatory Pre- and Concurrent Medication

| Week | Day | Compounds (generic names) | Dose | Diluent | Route | Duration of Infusion | Comments |
|---|---|---|---|---|---|---|---|
| 1,3,5,7 | 1 | Saline 0.9% | | 1000ml | i.v. | 2h | |
| 1,3,5,7 | 1 | Dexamethasone | 8mg | 100ml Saline 0.9% | i.v. | 15min | |
| 1,3,5,7 | 1 | Metoclopramide | 50mg | | i.v. | bolus | |
| 1,3,5,7 | 1 | Mesna | 120/240mg/m² | | i.v. | bolus | |
| 9,11,13,15 | 1 | Dexamethasone | 8mg | 100ml | i.v. | 15min | |
| 9,11,13,15 | 1 | Clemastine | 2mg | | i.v. | bolus | |
| 9,11,13,15 | 1 | Ranitidine | 50mg | | i.v. | bolus | |
| 9,11,13,15 | 1 | Saline 0.9% | | 500ml | i.v. | 4h | |
| 1st neutropenic cycle* | 1 | Filgrastim | 5µg/kg | | s.c. | | *when WBC<1000/µl; give until >1000/µl |
| subsequent cycles | 2** | Pegfilgrastim | 6mg | | s.c. | | **prophyl. admin. 24h after i.v. chemo. if decreased WBC in previous cycle |

| | |
|---|---|
| Medicines As Required | Dexamethasone i.v. or Metoclopramide oral or i.v. |
| Routine Tests: | FBC & differential (twice weekly), U&Es esp. Mg²⁺, serum creatinine, ALP, AST (SGOT), ALT (SGPT), clinically: In particular polyneuropathy |
| Dose Reduction: | **Paclitaxel** by 25% with leukopenia Grade 4 (<1000µl) or febrile neutropenia, by 25% with thrombocytopenia Grade 4 (<10,000/µl), by 25% w with polyneuropathy 4–6 |
| Therapy Delay: | **Paclitaxel** if leukocytes <1500/µl or platelets <75,000/µl (check twice weekly). |
| Max. Cum. Dose : | **Doxorubicin**: Danger of cardiotoxicity; max. cum. dose is 550 mg/m² |
| Next Cycle (N.C.): | **AC** every two weeks (four cycles in total), thereafter **Paclitaxel** every two weeks (four cycles in total) |
| References: | Analogous to Citron ML et al., J Clin Oncol. 2003 Apr 15; 21(8): 1431–9 |

| Paclitaxel/Carboplatin | Indication: Ovarian Cancer | 12.11.1 |
|---|---|---|

## Chemotherapy

This chemotherapy may cause life-threatening toxicity! It should only be administered under the supervision of an experienced medical oncologist! The protocol must first be reviewed and considered in relationship to the clinical situation of the patient.

| Week | Day | Compounds (generic names) in chronological order | Dosage | Diluent | Route | Duration of Infusion | Comments |
|---|---|---|---|---|---|---|---|
| 1 | 1 | **Paclitaxel** | 175mg/m² | 500ml Saline 0.9% | i.v. | 3h | PVC-free infusion set |
| | 1 | **Carboplatin** | #AUC 6mg/ml×min | 500ml Glucose 5% | i.v. | 1h | #dose (mg) = AUC (mg/ml x min) x [GFR (ml/min)+25] |

Cycle Diagram: d1 w1 | d8 w2 | d15 w3 | d22 w4 — Paclitaxel, Carboplatin; N.C.

### Cautions

| Recommended dosage for Carboplatin from AUC | target AUC (mg/ml×min) |
|---|---|
| Carboplatin monotherapy, patients untreated | 5-7 |
| Carboplatin monotherapy, myelosuppressive pretreatment | 4-6 |
| Combination therapy with Carboplatin in standard dosage, patients untreated | 4-6 |

## Obligatory Pre- and Concurrent Medication

| Week | Day | Compounds (generic names) | Sequence and Timing | Dose | Diluent | Route | Duration of Infusion | Comments |
|---|---|---|---|---|---|---|---|---|
| | 1 | Saline 0.9% | 30' before Paclitaxel | | 2000ml | i.v. | 5h | IVAC infusion pump must be used |
| | 1 | Dexamethasone | 30' before Paclitaxel | 20mg | | i.v. | 15min | |
| | 1 | Clemastine | 30' before Paclitaxel | 2mg | | i.v. | bolus | |
| | 1 | Ranitidine | 30' before Paclitaxel | 50mg | | i.v. | bolus | |
| | 1 | Granisetron | 30' before chemotherapy | 1mg | | i.v. | bolus | increase dose to 3mg with emesis |
| 1st neutropenic cycle* | | Filgrastim | once a day | 5µg/kg | | s.c. | | *when WBC<1000/µl; give until >1000/µl |
| subsequent cycles | 2** | Pegfilgrastim | one dose only | 6mg | | s.c. | | **prophyl. admin. 24h after i.v. chemo. if decreased WBC in previous cycle |

**Medicines As Required:** Metoclopramide oral or i.v., Granisetron i.v.

**Routine Tests:** FBC, U&Es esp. Mg²⁺: serum creatinine, serum bilirubin, creatinine clearance, ototoxicity, neurotoxicity

**Dose Reduction:** Discontinue if leukocytes <1500/µl or if allergic to polyoxyethylene-3,5 castor oil; in patients with previous bone marrow toxicity Paclitaxel may be started at 135mg/m² if necessary

**Max. Cum. Dose:** None

**Next Cycle (N.C.):** Day 22

**Efficacy Assess.:** After 2 cycles

**References:** Parmar et al., Lancet. 2003 Jun 21;361(9375):2099-106 ; Du Bois et al., J Natl Cancer Inst. 2003 Sep 3;95(17):1320-9.

# Treosulfan

## Indication: Ovarian Cancer

**12.11.2**

*This chemotherapy may cause life-threatening toxicity! It should only be administered under the supervision of an experienced medical oncologist! The protocol must first be reviewed and considered in relationship to the clinical situation of the patient.*

## Chemotherapy

| Week | Day | Compounds (generic names) in chronological order | Dosage | Diluent | Route | Duration of Infusion | Comments |
|------|-----|--------------------------------------------------|--------|---------|-------|----------------------|----------|
| | 1–28 | **Treosulfan** | 5g/m² | undiluted | i.v. | 1h | **Caution**: Extravasation |
| | | | | | | | |
| | | | | | | | |
| | | | | | | | |
| | | | | | | | |

### Cautions

**Extravasation**

| Cycle Diagram | d1 w1 | d8 w2 | d15 w3 | d22 w4 | d29 w5 |
|---------------|-------|-------|--------|--------|--------|
| Treosulfan | | | | | N.C. |
| | | | | | |
| | | | | | |

## Obligatory Pre- and Concurrent Medication

| Week | Day | Sequence and Timing | Compounds (generic names) | Dose | Diluent | Route | Duration of Infusion | Comments |
|------|-----|---------------------|---------------------------|------|---------|-------|----------------------|----------|
| | 1 | 15' before chemotherapy | Saline 0.9% | | 1000ml | i.v. | 1h15min | |
| | 1 | 15' before chemotherapy | Metoclopramide | 30mg | | i.v. | bolus | |
| | 1 | 15' before chemotherapy | Dexamethasone | 8mg | | i.v. | bolus 15min | |
| | | | | | | | | |

| | |
|---|---|
| **Medicines As Required** | Metoclopramide oral or i.v. |
| **Routine Tests:** | FBC, U&Es, liver and renal function parameters, pulmonary function |
| **Dose Increase:** | If well tolerated, dose may be increased to 7g/m² |
| **Max. Cum. Dose :** | Unknown |
| **Next Cycle (N.C.):** | Day 29 |
| **Efficacy Assess.** | After 2 cycles |
| **References:** | Meier et al., Proc ASCO, 1995;14:266 abstract, Gropp M et al, Gyn Onc 1998; 71(1):94-8; du Ba et al, Ann Onc 2002;13(2):251-7; Breitbach GP et al, Anticancer Res 2002; 22(5):2923-32 |

| PEB | Indication: Testicular Cancer | 12.11.3 |
|---|---|---|

*This chemotherapy may cause life-threatening toxicity! It should only be administered under the supervision of an experienced medical oncologist! The protocol must first be reviewed and considered in relationship to the clinical situation of the patient.*

## Chemotherapy

| Week | Day | Compounds (generic names) in chronological order | Dosage | Diluent | Route | Duration of Infusion | Comments |
|---|---|---|---|---|---|---|---|
| | 1-5 | **Cisplatin** | 20mg/m² | 250ml Saline 0.9% | i.v. | 15-30min | |
| | 1-5 | **Etoposide Phosphate** | 100mg/m² | 100ml Saline 0.9% | i.v. | 30min | dose expressed in terms of Etoposide base |
| | 1,8,15 | **Bleomycin** | 30mg absolute | undiluted | i.v. | bolus 15min | |

**Cautions:** Etoposide Phosphate and Sodium Bicarbonate must not be administered concomitantly through the same infusion site! After day 5 protocol for prophylaxis of delayed emesis

| Cycle Diagram | d1 w1 | d8 w2 | d15 w3 | d22 w4 |
|---|---|---|---|---|
| Cisplatin | | | | N.C. |
| Etop. Phos. | | | | |
| Bleomycin | | | | |

## Obligatory Pre- and Concurrent Medication

| Week | Day | Compounds (generic names) | Sequence and Timing | Dose | Diluent | Route | Duration of Infusion | Comments |
|---|---|---|---|---|---|---|---|---|
| | 1-5 | Saline 0.9% | continuously | 3000ml | | i.v. | 24h | |
| | 1-5 | Granisetron | 30' before chemotherapy | 1mg | | i.v. | bolus | increase dose to 3mg with emesis |
| | 1-5 | Mannitol 10% | 30' before and 6h after Cisplatin | | 250ml | i.v. | 30min | |
| | 1-5 | Heparin | continuously | 15000 units | | i.v. | 24h | |
| | 15 | Dexamethasone | before Bleomycin | 8mg | 100ml Saline 0.9% | i.v. | 15min | |
| | 1,8,15 | Clemastine | before Bleomycin | 2mg | | i.v. | bolus | |
| | 1-5 | Sucralfate | 0 - 0 - 0 - 1 | 1g | | oral | | |
| | *daily, except on days 1-5, 8, 15 | Filgrastim | once a day | 5µg/kg | | s.c. | | *when WBC<1000/µl; give until >1000/µl; but not on chemotherapy days |
| | 1-5/6+7 | Aprepitant | -1h before Cispl/d6+7 in the morning | * | | oral | | * d1: 125mg, d2-7: 80mg |
| | 1-5/6-8 | Dexamethasone | d1-5-15min before Cispl, d6-8 in the morning | * | | i.v./oral | | * d1: 12mg/d2-8: 8mg |
| | | mucositis prophylaxis | | | | | | |

| | |
|---|---|
| Medicines As Required | Metoclopramide, Dexamethasone, Granisetron, Famotidine |
| Routine Tests: | FBC, U&Es esp. Mg²⁺: serum creatinine, fluid balance, ototoxicity, neurotoxicity, pulmonary function before therapy and every 3 weeks |
| Dose Reduction: | Withhold **Cisplatin** if creatinine clearance < 60ml/min; see Dose Modification Table |
| Max. Cum. Dose : | **Bleomycin**: 400 mg absolute: Danger of pulmonary toxicity, discontinue if lung function deteriorates. |
| Next Cycle (N.C.): | Day 22, independent of leukopenia, delay only with fever and clinical symptoms |
| Efficacy Assess. | After 2 cycles, MRI scan/tumor markers; "low risk": with CR, no more th n 3 cycles; with PR: surgical resection of the remaining tumor after the 3rd cycle |
| References: | Williams SD et al., N Engl J Med, 1987;316:1435-1440 |

# PEI

## Indication: Metastatic Testicular Cancer

**12.11.4**

*This chemotherapy may cause life-threatening toxicity! It should only be administered under the supervision of an experienced medical oncologist! The protocol must first be reviewed and considered in relationship to the clinical situation of the patient.*

### Chemotherapy

| Week | Day | Compounds (generic names) in chronological order | Dosage | Diluent | Route | Duration of Infusion | Comments |
|---|---|---|---|---|---|---|---|
| | 1-5 | **Cisplatin** | 20mg/m² | 250ml Saline 0.9% | i.v. | 1h | |
| | 1-5 | **Ifosfamide** | 1200mg/m² | 500ml Saline 0.9% | i.v. | 4h | |
| | 1-5 | **Etoposide Phosphate** | 100mg/m² | 100ml Saline 0.9% | i.v. | bolus 15min | dose expressed in terms of Etoposide base |

**Cautions**

Etoposide Phosphate and Sodium Bicarbonate must not be administered concomitantly through the same infusion site!

After day 5 protocol for prophylaxis of delayed emesis

| Cycle Diagram | d1 w1 | d8 w2 | d15 w3 | d22 w4 |
|---|---|---|---|---|
| Cisplatin | | | | N.C. |
| Ifosfamide | | | | |
| Etop. Phos. | | | | |

### Obligatory Pre- and Concurrent Medication

| Week | Day | Compounds (generic names) | Sequence and Timing | Dose | Diluent | Route | Duration of Infusion | Comments |
|---|---|---|---|---|---|---|---|---|
| | 0 | Saline 0.9% + Gluc.5% alternately | prehydration fluid | | 1000ml + 1000ml | i.v. | 12h | |
| | 1-6 | Saline 0.9% + Gluc.5% alternately | continuously | | 2000ml + 1000ml | i.v. | 24h | |
| | | +Magnesium | | 3.15mmol/1000ml Saline 0.9% | | i.v. | 24h | in saline infusion |
| | 1-6 | Potassium Chloride | continuously | 40ml | | i.v. | 24h | check serum potassium |
| | 1-6 | Mesna | start before Ifosfamide | 240/1200/600mg/m² | | i.v. | 4h | |
| | 1-5 | Mannitol 10% | before and 1h after Cisplatin | | 250ml | i.v. | 15min | |
| | 1-5 | Dopamine | continuously | 200mg | | i.v. | 24h | |
| | 1-5 | Granisetron | 30' before chemotherapy | 1mg | | i.v. | bolus | |
| | 1-5 | Heparin | continuously | 15000 units | | i.v. | 24h | reduce if platelets <30,000/µl |
| | 1-5 | Sucralfate | 0 - 0 - 0 - 1 | 1g | | oral | | |
| 1st neutropenic cycle* | | Filgrastim | once a day | 5µg/kg | | s.c. | | *when WBC<1000/µl; give until >1000/µl |
| subsequent cycles | 6** | Pegfilgrastim | one dose only | 6mg | | s.c. | | **prophyl. admin. 24h after i.v. chemo. if decreased WBC on previous cycle |
| | | Aprepitant | -1h before chemo/d6+7 in the morning | * | | oral | | * d1: 125mg, d2-7: 80mg |
| | 1-5/6-8 | Dexamethasone | d1-5 -30min, d6-8 in the morning | * | | i.v./oral | | * d1: 12mg/d2-8: 8mg |

| | |
|---|---|
| Medicines As Required: | Metoclopramide, Dexamethasone, Granisetron i.v., Famotidine orally |
| Routine Tests: | FBC, U&Es esp. Mg²⁺, serum creatinine, fluid balance, diuresis, ototoxicity, neurotoxicity; check weight every 6-12h: if +1kg: 20mg Furosemide i.v. |
| Dose Reduction: | Withhold **Cisplatin** if creatinine clearance < 60ml/min; see Dose Modification Table |
| Next Cycle (N.C.): | Day 22 |
| Efficacy Assess. | After 2 cycles |
| References: | Harstrick et al., J Clin Oncol, 1991; 9 (9): 1549-55 |

| PIV with Pegfilgrastim | Indication: Testicular Cancer | 12.11.5 |
|---|---|---|

*This chemotherapy may cause life-threatening toxicity! It should only be administered under the supervision of an experienced medical oncologist! The protocol must first be reviewed and considered in relationship to the clinical situation of the patient.*

## Chemotherapy

| Week | Day | Compounds (generic names) in chronological order | Dosage | Diluent | Route | Duration of Infusion | Comments |
|---|---|---|---|---|---|---|---|
| | 1-5 | **Cisplatin** | 25mg/m² | 250ml Saline 0.9% | i.v. | 1h | |
| | 1-5 | **Ifosfamide** | 1200mg/m² | 500ml Saline 0.9% | i.v. | 4h | |
| | 1-5 | **Etoposide Phosphate** | 150mg/m² | 100ml Saline 0.9% (from 200mg in 250ml) | i.v. | 1h | |

| Cycle Diagram | d1 w1 | d8 w2 | d15 w3 | d22 w4 | d29 w5 |
|---|---|---|---|---|---|
| Cisplatin | | | | | N.C. |
| Ifosfamide | | | | | |
| Etop. Phos. | | | | | |

**Etoposide Phosphate and Sodium Bicarbonate must not be administered concomitantly through the same infusion site!**

When stem cell harvesting planned after cycle 2 Filgrastim 5µg/kg day+6 until end of leukapheresis

Mucositis prophylaxis

## Obligatory Pre- and Concurrent Medication

| Week | Day | Compounds (generic names) | Sequence and Timing | Dose | Diluent | Route | Duration of Infusion | Comments |
|---|---|---|---|---|---|---|---|---|
| | 0 | Saline 0.9% + Gluc.5% alternately | prehydration fluid | | 1000ml + 1000ml | i.v. | 12h | |
| | | +Magnesium | | 3.15mmol/1000ml Saline 0.9% | | i.v. | 12h | in prehydration infusion |
| | 0 | Potassium Chloride | prehydration fluid | 40ml | | i.v. | 12-24h | check serum potassium |
| | 1-5 | Saline 0.9% + Gluc.5% alternately | continuously | | 2000ml + 1000ml | i.v. | 24h | |
| | 1-5 | Dopamine | continuously | 200mg | | i.v. | 24h | |
| | 1-5 | Heparin | continuously | 15000 units | | i.v. | 24h | |
| | 1-5 | Mannitol 10% | 30' before and after Cisplatin | | 250ml | i.v. | 15min | |
| | 1-5 | Granisetron | 15' before chemotherapy | 1mg | | i.v. | bolus | increase dose to 3mg with emesis |
| | 1-6 | Mesna | 15' before Ifosfamide | 1200mg/m² | | i.v. | 22h | not in the same infusion line as Cisplatin |
| | 1-5 | Sucralfate | 0 - 0 - 0 - 1 | 1g | | oral | | |
| | 1-5/6+7 | Aprepitant | -1h before chemo/d6+7 in the morning | * | | oral | | * d1: 125mg, d2-7: 80mg |
| | 1-5/6-8 | Dexamethasone | d1-5 -15min ,d6-8 in the morning | * | | i.v./oral | | * d1: 12mg/d2-8: 8mg |
| | 6 | Pegfilgrastim | 24 h after chemotherapy ends | 6mg | | s.c. | | given as outpatient |
| | from day 6 | Ciprofloxacin | 1 - 0 - 1 | 500mg | | oral | | until WBC > 1000/µl |

| | |
|---|---|
| **Medicines As Required** | Granisetron i.v., Famotidine orally |
| **Routine Tests:** | FBC, U&Es esp. Mg²⁺, serum creatinine, fluid balance, diuresis, ototoxicity, neurotoxicity; every 6-12h check weight: if +1kg: 20mg Furosemide i.v. |
| **Dose Reduction:** | Withhold **Cisplatin** if creatinine clearance < 60ml/m n; see Dose Modification Table |
| **Filgrastim Dosage:** | Before planned leukapheresis 5µg/kg body weight (>75kg: 480µg, <75kg: 300µg) |
| **Next Cycle (N.C.):** | Day 29 |
| **Efficacy Assess.** | After 2 cycles |
| **References:** | Harstrick A et al., J Cancer Res Clin Oncol, 1991;117:198-202 |

| Doxorubicin | Therapy may be given as outpatient | Indication: Prostate Cancer | 12.12.1 |
|---|---|---|---|

*This chemotherapy may cause life-threatening toxicity! It should only be administered under the supervision of an experienced medical oncologist! The protocol must first be reviewed and considered in relationship to the clinical situation of the patient.*

## Chemotherapy

| Week | Day | Compounds (Generic names) in chronological order | Dosage | Route | Diluent | Duration of infusion | Comments |
|---|---|---|---|---|---|---|---|
| 1, 2, 3, 4 | 1 | **Doxorubicin** | 20mg/m² | i.v. | undiluted | bolus 15min | **Caution:** Extravasation; accompanying infusion must be freely running |
| | | | | | | | |
| | | | | | | | |
| | | | | | | | |
| | | | | | | | |

| Cycle diagram | d1 w1 | d8 w2 | d15 w3 | d22 w4 | d29 w5 | d36 w6 |
|---|---|---|---|---|---|---|
| Doxorubicin | | | | | | N.C. |
| | | | | | | |
| | | | | | | |

**Cautions**

**Anthracycline:** Danger of cardiotoxicity - monitor cardiac function (echocardiogram)
Extravasation; infusion must be freely running while i.v. chemotherapy is being injected

## Obligatory Pre- and Concurrent Medication

| Week | Day | Compound (Generic name) | Dose | Route | Diluent | Duration of infusion | Comments |
|---|---|---|---|---|---|---|---|
| 1, 2, 3, 4 | 1 | Saline 0.9% | | i.v. | 250ml | 1h | |
| 1, 2, 3, 4 | 1 | Dexamethasone | 8mg | i.v. | 100ml Saline 0.9% | 15min | |
| 1, 2, 3, 4 | 1 | Metoclopramide | 50mg | i.v. | | bolus | or 10-20mg orally at home |
| | | | | | | | |

| | |
|---|---|
| Medicines As Required | Dexamethasone, Metoclopramide, if not tolerated replace with 5-HT3 antagonists |
| Routine Tests: | **Anthracycline:** see **cautions** above; FBC, LFTs |
| Dose Reduction: | See Dose Modification Table |
| Max. Cum. Dose : | **Doxorubicin:** Danger of cardiotoxicity; max. cum. dose is 550 mg/m² |
| Next Cycle (N.C.): | Day 36 |
| Efficacy Assess. | After 4 injections |
| References: | Torti F et al., J Clin Oncol, 1983;1(8):477–482 |

# Docetaxel/Prednisolone

# Indication: Prostate Ca

**12.12.2**

*This chemotherapy may cause life-threatening toxicity! It should only be administered under the supervision of an experienced medical oncologist! The protocol must first be reviewed and considered in relationship to the clinical situation of the patient.*

## Chemotherapy

| Week | Day | Compounds (generic names) in chronological order | Dosage | Diluent | Route | Duration of Infusion | Comments |
|---|---|---|---|---|---|---|---|
| 1 | 1 | **Docetaxel** | 75mg/m² | *250ml Saline 0.9% | i.v. | 1h | *maximum concentration: 0.74mg/ml |
| 1-3 | 1-21 | **Prednisolone** | 5mg absolute twice a day | | oral | | |

**Extravasation**

| Cycle Diagram | d1 w1 | d8 w2 | d15 w3 | d22 w4 |
|---|---|---|---|---|
| Docetaxel | | | | |
| Prednisolone | | | | N.C. |

**Cautions**

## Obligatory Pre- and Concurrent Medication

| Week | Day | Sequence and Timing | Compounds (generic names) | Dose | Diluent | Route | Duration of Infusion | Comments |
|---|---|---|---|---|---|---|---|---|
| 1 | 1 | 30' before chemotherapy | Saline 0.9% | | 500ml | i.v. | 1h30min | |
| 1 | 1 | 30' before chemotherapy | Dexamethasone | 20mg | 100ml Saline 0.9% | i.v. | bolus 15min | |
| 1 | 1 | 30' before chemotherapy | Ranitidine | 50mg | | i.v. | bolus | |
| 1 | 1 | 30' before chemotherapy | Clemastine | 2mg | | i.v. | bolus | |

**Medicines As Required:** Metoclopramide, Pantoprazole, Granisetron

**Routine Tests:** FBC (start therapy only if neutrophils ≥1500/µl), U&Es, serum creatinine, LFTs, weight

**Side Effects:** Particularly bone marrow toxicity, neuropathy, skin toxicity, fluid retention, allergic reactions, **Caution**: Extravasation

**Dose Reduction:** With febrile neutropenia, neutropenia <500/µl > 7days, severe skin reactions or else Grade 3 to 4 non-hematological toxic reaction: after 1st occurrence, reduce dose in subsequent cycles to 60mg/m², with further occurrences despite dose reduction: discontinue therapy : if persistent ≥ Grade 3 peripheral neuropathy, Grade 4 hypertension, raised serum bilirubin and/or transaminases >1.5x above normal, or if ALP > 2.5x above normal: discontinue therapy

**Next Cycle (N.C.):** Day 22, 10 cycles maximum

**Efficacy Assess.** After 2 cycles

**References:** Tannock IF et al: N Engl J Med. 2004 Oct 7;351(15):1502-12; Picus J et al: Semin Oncol. 1999 Oct;26(5 Suppl 17):14-8

# High-Dose IL-2/IFN-alpha

## Indication: Renal Cell Carcinoma

**12.13.1**

*This chemotherapy may cause life-threatening toxicity! It should only be administered under the supervision of an experienced medical oncologist! The protocol must first be reviewed and considered in relationship to the clinical situation of the patient.*

## Immunotherapy

| Week | Day | Compounds (generic names) in chronological order | Dosage | Route | Duration of Infusion | Diluent | Comments |
|---|---|---|---|---|---|---|---|
| | 1, 2 | **Interleukin-2 (IL-2)** | 24 million IU/m² | i.v. | 24 h | 500 ml Glucose 5% | 0.1% Human Albumin |
| | 2, 4, 6 | **Interferon-alpha-2a (IFN-alpha)** | 6 million IU absolute | s.c. | | | |

| Cycle Diagram | d1 w1 | d8 w2 | d15 w3 | d22 w4 | d29 w5 | d36 w6 | d43 w7 | d50 w8 | d57 w9 | d64 w |
|---|---|---|---|---|---|---|---|---|---|---|
| IL-2 | | | | | | | | | | |
| IFN-alpha | | | | | | | | | | |

**Cautions**

ECG monitor, fluid balance, respiratory rate/pulse every 4 hours,

CVP measurement 2x /day in weeks 1 & 2

Start therapy in the mornings.

Put high-dose IL-2 intervention sheet with patient's charts.

Do not give steroids!

Incompatibility: IL-2 <> Saline 0.9%

## Obligatory Pre- and Concurrent Medication

| Week | Day | Sequence and Timing | Compounds (generic names) | Dose | Route | Duration of Infusion | Diluent | Comments |
|---|---|---|---|---|---|---|---|---|
| | 1, 2 | with cytokine therapy | Saline 0.9% | 3000 ml | i.v. | 24 h | | |
| | 1, 2 | continuously | Heparin | 15000 units | i.v. | 24 h | | |
| | 1, 2, 3 | continuously | Dopamine | 200 mg | i.v. | 24 h | | continue for 12h after end of IL-2 infusion |
| | 1, 2 | 0h, 6h, 12h & 18h after cytokines | Metoclopramide | 50 mg | i.v. | bolus | | 18h dose if awake |
| | 1, 2 | evenings | Famotidine | 40 mg | oral | | | with emesis, may be given intravenously |
| | 1, 2 | every 6 hours | Sucralfate | 1 g | oral | | | may be taken orally |
| | 1, 2 | every 6 hours | Paracetamol | 1000 mg | p.r. | | | with emesis, may be given i.v. instead |

| | |
|---|---|
| **Medicines As Required** | Metoclopramide, Granisetron, Loperamide oral or i.v. |
| **Routine Tests:** | Document vital signs every 4 hours, ECG monitor, blood pressure, twice daily CVP, fluid balance, twice daily weight, U&Es, serum creatinine, bilirubin, psychological state, T₃/T₄/TSH before start of therapy, after one cycle and at 3, 6 and 12 months respectively |
| **Dose Reduction:** | With treatment incompatibility (after consultation) |
| **Repeat Therapy:** | Every 7 days. Preferably start on a Monday or a Tuesday because of routine laboratory tests. 3 weeks therapy, 3 weeks treatment-free interval, 3 more weeks therapy. Repeat if responsive |
| **Efficacy Assess.** | 4 weeks after the end of two 3x/week therapy cycles (see Cycle Diagram) |
| **References:** | Engelhardt M et al, Eur J Cancer, 1997;33(7):1050–54; Negrier S et al, N Engl J Med, 1998;338(18):1272–8. |

# M-VAC

## Indication: Urothelial Carcinoma

**12.13.2**

*This chemotherapy may cause life-threatening toxicity! It should only be administered under the supervision of an experienced medical oncologist! The protocol must first be reviewed and considered in relationship to the clinical situation of the patient.*

## Chemotherapy

| Week | Day | Compounds (generic names) in chronological order | Dosage | Diluent | Route | Duration of Infusion | Comments |
|------|-----|------|--------|---------|-------|---------|----------|
| | 1,15,22 | **Methotrexate** | 30mg/m² | undiluted | i.v. | bolus | |
| | 2,15,22 | **Vinblastine** | 3mg/m² | undiluted | i.v. | bolus | |
| | 2 | **Doxorubicin** | 30mg/m² | undiluted | i.v. | bolus 15min | |
| | 2 | **Cisplatin** | 70mg/m² | 250ml Saline 0.9% | i.v. | 1h | |

| Cycle Diagram | d1 w1 | d8 w2 | d15 w3 | d22 w4 | d29 w5 |
|------|------|------|------|------|------|
| Methotrexate | | | | | N.C. |
| Vinblastine | | | | | |
| Doxorubicin | | | | | |
| Cisplatin | | | | | |

**Cautions**

After day 2 protocol for prophylaxis of delayed emesis
Anthracycline: Danger of cardiotoxicity - monitor cardiac function (echocardiogram)

## Obligatory Pre- and Concurrent Medication

| Week | Day | Compounds (generic names) | Dose | Diluent | Route | Duration of Infusion | Comments |
|------|-----|------|------|---------|-------|---------|----------|
| | 1,15,22 | Saline 0.9% | | 500ml | i.v. | 1h | |
| | 2 | Saline 0.9% | | 2000ml | i.v. | 6h | |
| | 2 | Granisetron | 1mg | | i.v. | bolus | |
| | 2 | Mannitol 10% | | 250ml | i.v. | 15min | |
| | 2-4 | Aprepitant | * | | oral | | * d2: 125mg, d3+4: 80mg |
| | 2-5 | Dexamethasone | * | | i.v/oral | | * d2: 12mg/d3-5: 8mg |
| | *daily, except on days 1, 2, 15, 22 | Filgrastim | 5µg/kg | | s.c. | | *when WBC<1000/µl; give until >1000/µl. |

| | |
|---|---|
| Medicines As Required | Metoclopramide 50mg i.v. 2-3x/day |
| Routine Tests: | **Anthracycline**: see **cautions** above; FBC, U&Es esp Mg²⁺ serum creatinine, creatinine clearance, diuresis, exclude third space fluid accumulation, ototoxicity, neurotoxicity |
| Dose Reduction: | Preceding radiotherapy: **Doxorubicin** 15mg/m² with > 20 Gy (pelvis), therapy contraindicated if creatinine clearance < 40ml/min; see Dose Modification Table |
| Max. Cum. Dose : | **Doxorubicin**: Danger of cardiotoxicity; max. cum. dose is 550mg/m² |
| Next Cycle (N.C.): | Day 29 |
| Efficacy Assess. | After 2 cycles |
| References: | Shipley WU et al., Semin Oncol, 1988;15:390-395; Sternberg CN et al., Cancer, 1989;64:2448-2458; Sternberg CN et al., J Clin Oncol, 2001;19(10):2638-2646 |

# CycloVD     Indication: Malignant Phaeochromocytoma     12.14.1

*This chemotherapy may cause life-threatening toxicity! It should only be administered under the supervision of an experienced medical oncologist! The protocol must first be reviewed and considered in relationship to the clinical situation of the patient.*

## Chemotherapy

| Week | Day | Compounds (generic names) in chronological order | Dosage | Diluent | Route | Duration of Infusion | Comments |
|---|---|---|---|---|---|---|---|
| | 1 | **Cyclophosphamide** | 750mg/m² | 250ml Saline 0.9% | i.v. | 1h | |
| | 1 | **Vincristine** (maximum dose 2mg absolute) | 1.4mg/m² | undiluted | i.v. | bolus | |
| | 1-2 | **Dacarbazine (DTIC)** | 600mg/m² | 500ml Saline 0.9% | i.v. | 2h | protect from light |

**Cautions:** Please note: after day 4 protocol for prophylaxis of delayed emesis

| Cycle Diagram | d1 w1 | d8 w2 | d15 w3 | d22 w4 | d29 w5 | d |
|---|---|---|---|---|---|---|
| Cyclophos. | | | | N.C. | | |
| Vincristine | | | | | | |
| Dacarbazine | | | | | | |

## Obligatory Pre- and Concurrent Medication

| Week | Day | Compounds (generic names) | Sequence and Timing | Dose | Diluent | Route | Duration of Infusion | Comments |
|---|---|---|---|---|---|---|---|---|
| | 1 | Saline 0.9% + 20ml KCl 7.45% | 15' before chemotherapy | 1000ml | | i.v. | 3h30min | |
| | 1 | Mesna | 0h, 4h & 8h after Cyclophos. | 150mg/m² | | i.v. | bolus | |
| | 1-2 | Dexamethasone | 30' before chemotherapy | 20mg | 100ml Saline 0.9% | i.v. | 15min | |
| | 1-2 | Granisetron | 15' before chemotherapy | 1mg | | i.v. | bolus | |
| | 2 | Saline 0.9% | 15' before chemotherapy | 250ml | | i.v. | 2h30min | |

| | |
|---|---|
| Medicines As Required | Metoclopramide, Filgrastim |
| Routine Tests: | FBC, U&Es, LFTs, creatinine clearance, serum creatinine, diuresis. Seru and urinary catecholamines and degradation products (e.g. metanephrine, VMA) every 3-4 weeks |
| Dose Reduction: | See Dose Modification Table |
| Next Cycle (N.C.): | Day 22. Increase doses of **Cyclophosphamide** and **Dacarbazine** by 10% per cycle until myelosuppression occurs |
| Efficacy Assess. | After 2 cycles |
| References: | Averbuch et al. Ann Int Med 1988;109:267-73 |

## CVD/IL-2/IFN-alpha ("Legha")

### Indication: Melanoma

**12.15.1**

### Chemoimmunotherapy

| Week | Day | Compounds (generic names) in chronological order | Dosage | Diluent | Route | Duration of Infusion | Comments |
|---|---|---|---|---|---|---|---|
| CVD: | 1/22 | **Dacarbazine (DTIC)** | 800mg/m² | 500ml Saline 0.9% | i.v. | 1h | |
| | 1-4/22-25 | **Vinblastine** | 1.5mg/m² | in 5ml Saline 0.9% | i.v. | bolus (1min) | |
| | 1-4/22-25 | **Cisplatin** | 20mg/m² | 250ml Saline 0.9% | i.v. | 30min | |
| IL2/IFN-alpha : | 5-8/17-20/26-29 | **Interleukin-2 (IL-2)** | 9million IU/m² | 500ml Glucose 5% | i.v. | 24h | 0.1% Human Albumin |
| | 5-9/17-21/26-30 | **Interferon-alpha-2a (IFN-alpha)** | 5million IU/m² | | s.c. | | |

**After day 4 and day 25 protocol for prophylaxis of delayed emesis without Dexamethasone**
**Do not give steroids!**

| Cycle Diagram | d1 w1 | d8 w2 | d15 w3 | d22 w4 | d29 w5 | d36 w6 | d43 w7 | d |
|---|---|---|---|---|---|---|---|---|
| Dacarbazine | | | | | | | | |
| Vinblastine | | | | | | | | N.C. |
| Cisplatin | | | | | | | | |
| IL-2 | | | | | | | | |
| IFN-alpha | | | | | | | | |

### Obligatory Pre- and Concurrent Medication

| Week | Day | Sequence and Timing | Compounds (generic names) | Dose | Diluent | Route | Duration of Infusion | Comments |
|---|---|---|---|---|---|---|---|---|
| CVD : | 1-4 | 2h before chemotherapy | Saline 0.9%+20ml KCl 7,45%/1000ml | | 3000ml | i.v. | 8h | |
| | 22-25 | 2h before chemotherapy | Saline 0.9%+20ml KCl 7,45%/1000ml | | 1000ml | i.v. | 4h | |
| | 22-25 | after chemotherapy | Saline 0.9%+20ml KCl 7,45%/1000ml | | 2000ml | i.v. | 20h | |
| | 22,23-25 | 30' , 2h before chemotherapy | Heparin | 15000 units | | i.v. | 24h | |
| | 1-4/22-25 | 30' before & 30' after Cisplatin | Mannitol 10% | | 250ml | i.v. | 15min | |
| | 1-4/22-25 | 30' before chemotherapy | Granisetron | 1mg | | i.v. | bolus | increase dose to 3mg with emesis |
| | 1-4/22-25 | 30' before & 4h, 8h after chemo | Metoclopramide | 50mg | | i.v. | bolus | |
| | 1-4/22-25 | 0-0-0-1 | Famotidine | 20mg | | oral | | |
| | 1-6/22-27 | d1-4/22-25 -1h before chemo/5+6,26+27 | Aprepitant | * | | oral | | * d1/22: 125mg, d2-6/23-27: 80mg |
| IL2/IFN-alpha : | 5-9/17-21/26-30 | parallel to therapy | Gluc. 5%+20ml KCl 7,45%/1000ml | | 2000ml | i.v. | 24h | |
| | 5-9/17-21/26-30 | parallel to therapy | Dopamine | 200mg | | i.v. | 24h | |
| | 5-9/17-21/26-30 | parallel to therapy | Heparin | 15000 units | | i.v. | 24h | |
| | 5-9/17-21/26-30 | every 8 hours | Paracetamol | 1000mg | | oral | | |
| | 5-9/17-21/26-30 | 0-0-0-1 | Famotidine | 20mg | | oral | | |

| | |
|---|---|
| Medicines As Required: | Paracetamol, Metoclopramide, Loperamide, Filgrastim, Lorazepam 1mg |
| Routine Tests: | FBC, U&Es, serum creatinine, creatinine clearance, diuresis, ototoxicity, neurotoxicity; with addition of IL-2/IFN-alpha until end of therapy (=24h after IL-2): ECG monitor, fluid balance, 4 hourly blood pressure, twice daily weight, neurological status; $T_3/T_4$/TSH before start of therapy, after the end of a cycle and at 3, 6 and 12 months respectively |
| Dose Reduction: | See Dose Modification Table |
| Next Cycle (N.C.): | Day 43 |
| Efficacy Assess. | Day 41 |
| References: | Eton O et al., J Clin Oncol, 2002;20(8):2045-52 |

| CVD/IL-2/IFN Consolidation | Indication: Metastatic Melanoma | 12.15.2 |
|---|---|---|

*This chemotherapy may cause life-threatening toxicity! It should only be administered under the supervision of an experienced medical oncologist! The protocol must first be reviewed and considered in relationship to the clinical situation of the patient.*

## Chemotherapy

| Week | Day | Compounds (generic names) in chronological order | Dosage | Diluent | Route | Duration of Infusion | Comments |
|---|---|---|---|---|---|---|---|
| | 1 | **Dacarbazine (DTIC)** | 800mg/m² | 500ml Saline 0.9% | i.v. | 1h | **protect from light** |
| | 1-4 | **Vinblastine** | 1.5mg/m² | in 5ml Saline 0.9% | i.v. | bolus 1min | |
| | 1-4 | **Cisplatin** | 20mg/m² | 250ml Saline 0.9% | i.v. | 30min | |
| | 1-4 | **Interleukin-2 (IL-2)** | 9million IU/m² | 500ml Glucose 5% | i.v. | 22h | 0.1% Human Albumin |
| | 1-5 | **Interferon-alpha-2a (IFN-alpha)** | 5million IU/m² | | s.c. | | |

| Cycle Diagram | d1 w1 | d8 w2 | d15 w3 | d22 w4 | d29 w5 | d36 w6 | d43 w7 |
|---|---|---|---|---|---|---|---|
| Dacarbazine | | | | | | | N.C. |
| Vinblastine | | | | | | | |
| Cisplatin | | | | | | | |
| IL2 | | | | | | | |
| IFN-alpha | | | | | | | |

**Cautions**

Incompatibilities: Vinblastine<>Heparin, IL-2<>Saline 0.9%
After day 4 protocol for prophylaxis of delayed emesis without Dexamethasone
**Do not give steroids!**

## Obligatory Pre- and Concurrent Medication

| Week | Day | Sequence and Timing | Compounds (generic names) | Dose | Diluent | Route | Duration of Infusion | Comments |
|---|---|---|---|---|---|---|---|---|
| | 1-4 | 2h before chemotherapy | Saline 0.9%+20ml KCl/1000ml | | 1000ml | i.v. | 4h | |
| | 5 | 2h before chemotherapy | Saline 0.9%+20ml KCl/1000ml | | 2000ml | i.v. | 24h | |
| | 1-4 | after chemotherapy | Gluc. 5%+20ml KCl/1000ml | | 2000ml | i.v. | 20h | |
| | 1-5 | parallel to chemotherapy | Dopamine | 200mg | | i.v. | 24h | |
| | 1-5 | 2h before chemotherapy | Heparin | 15000 units | | i.v. | 24h | |
| | 1-4 | 30' before & 30' after Cisplatin | Mannitol 10% | | 250ml | i.v. | 15min | |
| | 1-4 | 30' before chemotherapy | Granisetron | 1mg | | i.v. | bolus | increase dose to 3mg with emesis |
| | 1-4 | 30' before & 4h, 8h after chemo | Metoclopramide | 50mg | | i.v. | bolus | |
| | 1-5 | 0 - 0 - 1 | Famotidine | 20mg | | oral | | |
| | 1-5 | every 8 hours | Paracetamol | 1000mg | | oral | | |
| | 1-4/5+6 | -1h before chemo/d5+6 in the morning | Aprepitant | * | | oral | | * d1: 125mg, d2-6: 80mg |

| Medicines As Required | Paracetamol, Metoclopramide, Loperamide, Filgrastim, Lorazepam 1mg |
|---|---|
| Routine Tests: | FBC, U&Es, serum creatinine, creatinine clearance, diuresis, ototoxicity, neurotoxicity; with addition of IL-2/IFN-alpha until end of therapy (=24h after IL-2): ECG monitor, fluid balance, 4 hourly blood pressure, twice daily weight, neurological status; $T_3/T_4$/TSH before start of therapy, after the end of a cycle and at 3, 6 and 12 months respectively |
| Dose Reduction: | See Dose Modification Table |
| Next Cycle (N.C.): | Day 43: 4 cycles in total |
| Efficacy Assess.: | Day 41 |
| References: | Eton O et al., J Clin Oncol, 2002;20(8):2045-52; Legha SS et al., Ann Oncol, 1996;7(8):827-35 |

**CVD**  |  **Indication: Melanoma**  |  **12.15.3**

*This chemotherapy may cause life-threatening toxicity! It should only be administered under the supervision of an experienced medical oncologist! The protocol must first be reviewed and considered in relationship to the clinical situation of the patient.*

## Chemotherapy

| Week | Day | Compounds (generic names) in chronological order | Dosage | Diluent | Route | Duration of Infusi- | Comments |
|---|---|---|---|---|---|---|---|
| | 1 | **Dacarbazine (DTIC)** | 800mg/m² | 500ml Saline 0.9% | i.v. | 1h | protect from light |
| | 1-4 | **Vinblastine** | 2mg/m² | in 5ml Saline 0.9% | i.v. | bolus | |
| | 1-4 | **Cisplatin** | 20mg/m² | 250ml Saline 0.9% | i.v. | 30min | |
| | | | | | | | |
| | | | | | | | |

| Cycle Diagram | d1 w1 | d8 w2 | d15 w3 | d22 w4 |
|---|---|---|---|---|
| Dacarbazine | | | | N.C. |
| Vinblastine | | | | |
| Cisplatin | | | | |

**Cautions** — After day 4 protocol for prophylaxis of delayed emesis

## Obligatory Pre- and Concurrent Medication

| Week | Day | Compounds (generic names) | Sequence and Timing | Dose | Diluent | Route | Duration of Infu- | Comments |
|---|---|---|---|---|---|---|---|---|
| | 1-4 | Saline 0.9%+20mmol KCl/1000ml | 2h before chemotherapy | | 3000ml | i.v. | 8h | |
| | 1-4 | Mannitol 10% | 30' before & 30' after Cisplatin | | 250ml | i.v. | 15min | |
| | 1-4 | Granisetron | 30' before chemotherapy | 1mg | | i.v. | bolus | |
| | 1-4/5+6 | Aprepitant | -1h before chemo/d5+6 in the morning | * | | oral | | * d1: 125mg, d2-6: 80mg |
| | 1-4/5-7 | Dexamethasone | d1-4 -15min, d5-7 in the morning | * | | i.v./oral | | * d1: 12mg/d2-7: 8mg |

| | |
|---|---|
| Medicines As Required | Metoclopramide, Loperamide, Filgrastim, Lorazepam 1mg |
| Routine Tests: | FBC, U&Es, serum creatinine, LFTs, creatinine clearance, diuresis, ototoxicity, neurotoxicity; |
| Dose Reduction: | See Dose Modification Table |
| Next Cycle (N.C.): | Day 22: 8 cycles maximum |
| Efficacy Assess. | Day 41 |
| References: | Analogous to Legha et al., Proc Am Soc Clin Oncol. 1994;13:394 (abstr.1343); Legha SS et al., Ann Oncol. 1996;7(8):827-35 |

# Dacarbazine monotherapy

**Indication: Melanoma**

**12.15.4**

*This chemotherapy may cause life-threatening toxicity! It should only be administered under the supervision of an experienced medical oncologist! The protocol must first be reviewed and considered in relationship to the clinical situation of the patient.*

## Chemotherapy

| Week | Day | Compounds (generic names) in chronological order | Dosage | Diluent | Route | Duration of Infusion | Comments |
|------|-----|--------------------------------------------------|--------|---------|-------|----------------------|----------|
|      | 1   | **Dacarbazine (DTIC)**                           | 1000mg/m² | 500ml Saline 0.9% | i.v. | 2h | protect from light |
|      |     |                                                  |        |         |       |                      |          |
|      |     |                                                  |        |         |       |                      |          |
|      |     |                                                  |        |         |       |                      |          |
|      |     |                                                  |        |         |       |                      |          |

**Cautions**

After day1 protocol for prophylaxis of delayed emesis
Veno-occlusive disease

| Cycle Diagram | d1 w1 | d8 w2 | d15 w3 | d22 w4 |
|---------------|-------|-------|--------|--------|
| Dacarbazine   |       |       |        | N.C.   |
|               |       |       |        |        |

## Obligatory Pre- and Concurrent Medication

| Week | Day | Compounds (generic names) | Dose | Diluent | Route | Duration of Infusion | Comments |
|------|-----|---------------------------|------|---------|-------|----------------------|----------|
|      | 1   | Saline 0.9%               |      | 250ml   | i.v.  | 2h30min              |          |
|      | 1   | Dexamethasone             | 20mg | 100ml Saline 0.9% | i.v. | 15min         |          |
|      | 1   | Granisetron               | 1mg  |         | i.v.  | bolus                |          |

| | |
|---|---|
| **Medicines As Required** | Dexamethasone, Metoclopramide, Granisetron |
| **Routine Tests:** | FBC (nadir after 14-28 days), eosinophils, diuresis, LFTs |
| **Dose Reduction:** | See Dose Modification Table |
| **Next Cycle (N.C.):** | Day 22 |
| **References:** | Chapman PB et al., J Clin Oncol, 1999;17(9):2745-51 |

# Fotemustine

## Indication: Melanoma

**12.15.5**

## Chemotherapy

| Cycle | Day | Compounds (generic names) in chronological order | Dosage | Diluent | Route | Duration of Infusion | Comments |
|---|---|---|---|---|---|---|---|
| 1 | 1, 8, 15 | **Fotemustine** | 100mg/m² | 500ml Glucose 5% | i.v. | 1h | protect from light |
| 2-n | 1 | **Fotemustine** | 100mg/m² | 500ml Glucose 5% | i.v. | 1h | protect from light |

| Cycle Diagram | d1 w1 | d8 w2 | d15 w3 | d22 w4 | d29 w5 | d36 w6 | d43 w7 | d50 |
|---|---|---|---|---|---|---|---|---|
| Fotemustine (cycle 1 only) | | | | | | | | |
| Fotemustine (cycles 2-n) | | | | | | | | |

**Cautions**

## Obligatory Pre- and Concurrent Medication

| Cycle | Day | Sequence and Timing | Compounds (generic names) | Dose | Diluent | Route | Duration of Infusion | Comments |
|---|---|---|---|---|---|---|---|---|
| 1 | 1, 8, 15 | 15' before chemotherapy | Gluc. 5% | 500ml | | i.v. | 1h30min | |
| 1 | 1, 8, 15 | 15' before chemotherapy | Dexamethasone | 8mg | | i.v. | bolus 15min | |
| 1 | 1, 8, 15 | 15' before chemotherapy | Granisetron | 1mg | | i.v. | bolus | |
| 2-n | 1 | 15' before chemotherapy | Gluc. 5% | 500ml | | i.v. | 1h30min | |
| 2-n | 1 | 15' before chemotherapy | Dexamethasone | 8mg | | i.v. | bolus 15min | |
| 2-n | 1 | 15' before chemotherapy | Granisetron | 1mg | | i.v. | bolus | |

| | |
|---|---|
| Medicines As Required | Metoclopramide or Alizapride |
| Routine Tests: | FBC (delayed neutropenia and thrombocytopenia: **nadir days 35-44**), U&Es, serum creatinine, LFTs, diuresis |
| Dose Reduction: | Unknown |
| Max. Cum. Dose : | None |
| Repeat Therapy: | 1 x per week for 3 consecutive weeks; 4 week therapy-free interval: with response, 100mg/m² every 3 weeks |
| Efficacy Assess. | 8 weeks after start of therapy |
| References: | Jacquillat C et al., Cancer, 1990;66:1873-1878; Kleeberg UR et al., Melanoma Res., 1995;5(3):195-200 |

# Doxorubicin/Ifosfamide

## Indication: Soft Tissue Sarcoma  12.16.1

*This chemotherapy may cause life-threatening toxicity! It should only be administered under the supervision of an experienced medical oncologist! The protocol must first be reviewed and considered in relationship to the clinical situation of the patient.*

## Chemotherapy

| Week | Day | Compounds (generic names) in chronological order | Dosage | Diluent | Route | Duration of Infusion | Comments |
|---|---|---|---|---|---|---|---|
| | 1 | **Doxorubicin** | 50mg/m² | undiluted | i.v. | bolus | |
| | 1–5 | **Ifosfamide** | 1500mg/m² | 250ml Saline 0.9% | i.v. | 4h | |
| | | | | | | | |
| | | | | | | | |
| | | | | | | | |

| Cycle Diagram | d1 w1 | d8 w2 | d15 w3 | d22 w4 | d29 w5 |
|---|---|---|---|---|---|
| Doxorubicin | | | | | N.C. |
| Ifosfamide | | | | | |

**Cautions:** Anthracycline: Danger of cardiotoxicity - monitor cardiac function

## Obligatory Pre- and Concurrent Medication

| Week | Day | Compounds (generic names) | Sequence and Timing | Dose | Diluent | Route | Duration of Infusion | Comments |
|---|---|---|---|---|---|---|---|---|
| | 1–5 | Saline 0.9% + Gluc.5% alternately | continuously | | 2000ml + 1000ml | i.v. | 24h | |
| | 1–5 | Dexamethasone | 15' before chemotherapy | 4mg | | i.v. | bolus | |
| | 1–5 | Granisetron | 15' before chemotherapy | 1mg | | i.v. | bolus | |
| | 1–6 | Mesna | 15' before, 0h, +4h | 300/1500750mg/m² | | i.v. | 15min/4h/6h | |

| | |
|---|---|
| **Medicines As Required** | Granisetron, Dexamethasone |
| **Routine Tests:** | **Anthracycline:** see **cautions** above ; FBC, LFTs |
| **Dose Reduction:** | See Dose Modification Table |
| **Max. Cum. Dose :** | **Doxorubicin:** Danger of cardiotoxicity; max. cum. dose is 550 mg/m² |
| **Next Cycle (N.C.):** | Day 29; 6 cycles in total |
| **References:** | According to CWS 91 original protocol |

955

| VIDE | EURO - E.W.I.N.G. 99 | Indication: Ewing's Sarcoma | 12.16.2 |
|------|---------------------|----------------------------|---------|

**Cautions:** This chemotherapy may cause life-threatening toxicity! It should only be administered under the supervision of an experienced medical oncologist! The protocol must first be reviewed and considered in relationship to the clinical situation of the patient.

## Chemotherapy

| Week | Day | Compounds (generic names) in chronological order | Dosage | Diluent | Route | Duration of Infusion | Comments |
|------|-----|--------------------------------------------------|--------|---------|-------|---------------------|----------|
| | 1 | **Vincristine** | $1.5mg/m^2$ | undiluted | i.v. | bolus | maximum dose 2mg absolute |
| | 1,2,3 | **Ifosfamide** | $3000mg/m^2$ | 500ml Saline 0.9% | i.v. | 1h | |
| | 1,2,3 | **Doxorubicin** | $20mg/m^2$ | 250ml Saline 0.9% | i.v. | 4h | only give via central line |
| | 1,2,3 | **Etoposide Phosphate** | $150mg/m^2$ | 250ml Saline 0.9% | i.v. | 1h | dose expressed in terms of Etoposide base |

Etoposide Phosphate and Sodium Bicarbonate must not be administered concomitantly through the same infusion site!

All patients to have 6 cycles of VIDE as Induction Therapy

Two stem cell harvests

| Cycle Diagram | d1 w1 | d8 w2 | d15 w3 | d22 w4 |
|---------------|-------|-------|--------|--------|
| Vincristine | | | | N.C. |
| Ifosfamide | | | | |
| Doxorubicin | | | | |
| Etop. Phos. | | | | |

## Obligatory Pre- and Concurrent Medication

| Week | Day | Compounds (generic names) | Dose | Diluent | Route | Duration of Infusion | Comments |
|------|-----|---------------------------|------|---------|-------|---------------------|----------|
| | 1-4 | Saline 0.9% + Gluc.5% alternately + Potassium Chloride | 10ml/500ml in hydration infusion | 3000ml + 2000ml | i.v. | 24h | check serum potassium |
| | 1 | Mesna | $600mg/m^2$ | | i.v. | bolus | |
| | 1,2,3 | Sodium Bicarbonate | 200ml | | i.v. | 24h | venous gases, pH measurement |
| | 1,2,3 | Dexamethasone | 4mg | | i.v. | bolus | |
| | 1,2,3 | Granisetron | 1mg | | i.v. | bolus | |

| | |
|---|---|
| Medicines As Required | Granisetron, Dexamethasone, Furosemide |
| Routine Tests: | FBC, U&Es, LFTs, serum creatinine, creatinine clearance, clotting studies, cardiac function (echocardiogram), neurotoxicity (see study protocol) |
| Dose Reduction: | Leukocytes < 2000/µl or granulocytes < 1000/µl, platelets < 80,000/µl see study protocol |
| Max. Cum. Dose : | **Doxorubicin:** Danger of cardiotoxicity; max. cum. dose is 550 mg/m²; **Vincristine** 5-20mg absolute: Danger of neurotoxicity |
| Next Cycle (N.C): | Day 22 (see study protocol) |
| References: | Study protocol (0202) |

| VAI | | | EURO - E.W.I.N.G. 99 | | Indication: Ewing's Sarcoma | | | 12.16.3 |

*This chemotherapy may cause life-threatening toxicity! It should only be administered under the supervision of an experienced medical oncologist! The protocol must first be reviewed and considered in relationship to the clinical situation of the patient.*

## Chemotherapy

| Week | Day | Compounds (generic names) in chronological order | Dosage | Diluent | Route | Duration of Infusion | Comments |
|---|---|---|---|---|---|---|---|
| | 1 | **Vincristine** | 1.5mg/m² | undiluted | i.v. | bolus | maximum dose 2mg absolute |
| | 1,2 | **Dactinomycin** | 0.75mg/m² | 250ml Saline 0.9% | i.v. | bolus 10min | max. 1.5mg absolute, protect from light |
| | 1,2 | **Ifosfamide** | 3000mg/m² | 500ml Saline 0.9% | i.v. | 1h | |
| | | | | | | | |
| | | | | | | | |

**Cautions**

Incompatibility: Doxorubicin<->Vincristine
Patients to have cycle 7 as VAI

| Cycle Diagram | d1 w1 | d8 w2 | d15 w3 | d22 w4 |
|---|---|---|---|---|
| Vincristine | | | | N.C. |
| Dactinomycin | | | | |
| Ifosfamide | | | | |

## Obligatory Pre- and Concurrent Medication

| Week | Day | Compounds (generic names) | Sequence and Timing | Dose | Diluent | Route | Duration of Infusion | Comments |
|---|---|---|---|---|---|---|---|---|
| | 1-3 | Saline 0.9% + Gluc.5% alternately + Potassium Chloride | continuously | 3000ml + 2000ml | | i.v. | 24h | check serum potassium |
| | 1 | Mesna | 15' before, 4h and 8h after Ifo | 600mg/m² | 10ml/500ml in hydration infusion | i.v. | bolus | |
| | 1-3 | Mesna | during and after Ifosfamide | 3000mg/m² | | i.v. | 24h | |
| | 1,2 | Sodium Bicarbonate | 15' before chemotherapy | 200ml | | i.v. | 24h | venous gases, pH measurement |
| | 1,2 | Dexamethasone | 15' before chemotherapy | 4mg | | i.v. | bolus | |
| | 1,2 | Granisetron | 15' before chemotherapy | 1mg | | i.v. | bolus | |

| | |
|---|---|
| Medicines As Required | Granisetron, Dexamethasone, Furosemide |
| Routine Tests: | FBC, U&Es, LFTs, serum creatinine, creatinine clearance, clotting studies, cardiac function (echocardiogram), neurotoxicity |
| Dose Reduction: | Leukocytes < 2000/µl or granulocytes < 1000/µl, platelets < 80,000/µl or if delay >6 days see study protocol |
| Max. Cum. Dose : | Vincristine 5-20mg absolute: Danger of neurotoxicity |
| Next Cycle (N.C.): | Day 22 (see study protocol) |
| References: | Study protocol (0202) |

| VAC | | EURO - E.W.I.N.G. 99 | | Indication: Ewing's Sarcoma | | | 12.16.4 |

*This chemotherapy may cause life-threatening toxicity! It should only be administered under the supervision of an experienced medical oncologist! The protocol must first be reviewed and considered in relationship to the clinical situation of the patient.*

## Chemotherapy

| Week | Day | Compounds (generic names) in chronological order | Dosage | Diluent | Route | Duration of Infusion | Comments |
|---|---|---|---|---|---|---|---|
| | 1 | **Vincristine** | 1.5mg/m² | undiluted | i.v. | bolus | maximum dose 2mg absolute |
| | 1,2 | **Dactinomycin** | 0.75mg/m² | in 10ml Saline 0.9% | i.v. | bolus 10min | maximum dose 1.5mg absolute |
| | 1 | **Cyclophosphamide** | 1500mg/m² | 500ml Saline 0.9% | i.v. | 1h | |

**Cautions** — Incompatibility: Doxorubicin<>Vincristine

Cycle Diagram: d1 w1, d8 w2, d15 w3, d22 w4 — Vincristine, Dactinomycin, Cyclophos. N.C.

## Obligatory Pre- and Concurrent Medication

| Week | Day | Compounds (generic names) | Dose | Diluent | Route | Duration of Infusion | Comments |
|---|---|---|---|---|---|---|---|
| | 1-3 | Saline 0.9% + Gluc.5% alternately +.....mmol KCl/500ml (if required) | | 3000ml + 2000ml | i.v. | 24h | |
| | 1 | Mesna | 300mg/m² | | i.v. | bolus | |
| | 1 | Mesna | 300mg/m² | | i.v. | 24h | |
| | 1,2 | Granisetron | 1mg | | i.v. | bolus | |
| | 1,2 | Dexamethasone | 4mg | | i.v. | bolus | |

Medicines As Required: Granisetron, Dexamethasone, Furosemide
Routine Tests: FBC, U&Es,LFTs, serum creatinine, creatinine clearance, clotting studies, cardiac function (echocardiogram), neurotoxicity
Dose Reduction: Leukocytes < 2000/μl or granulocytes < 1000/μl, plate ets < 80,000/μl or if delay >6 days see study protocol
Max. Cum. Dose: **Doxorubicin** > 550mg/m²: Danger of cardiotoxicity; **Vincristine** 5–20mg absolute: Danger of neurotoxicity
Next Cycle (N.C.): Day 22 (see study protocol)
References: Study protocol (0202)

# Euro- B.O.S.S: Cisplatin/Doxorubicin Block  Indication: Osteosarcoma  12.16.5

## Chemotherapy

*This chemotherapy may cause life-threatening toxicity! It should only be administered under the supervision of an experienced medical oncologist! The protocol must first be reviewed and considered in relationship to the clinical situation of the patient.*

*only adjuvant: weeks 0, 9, 18
neoadjuvant+post-op GR: weeks 0, 9, 10, 19
neoadjuvant+post-op PR: weeks 0, 9, 10, 22

| Week | Day | Compounds (generic names) in chronological order | Dosage | Diluent | Route | Duration of Infusi- | Comments |
|---|---|---|---|---|---|---|---|
| * | 1, 2, 3 | **Cisplatin** | 33.3mg/m² | 250ml Saline 0.9% | i.v. | 24h | protect from light |
| * | 4 | **Doxorubicin** | 60mg/m² | in 100ml Saline 0.9% | i.v. | 24h | if peripherally administered, not>1mg/40ml; start after end of Cisplatin infusion |

| Cycle Diagram | d1 w1 | d8 w2 | d15 w3 | d22 w4 | d29 |
|---|---|---|---|---|---|
| Cisplatin | ▨ | | | | |
| Doxorubicin | ▨ | | | | |

### Cautions

After day 4 protocol for prophylaxis of delayed emesis
Incompatibilities: Cisplatin<>Metoclopramide, Doxorubicin/Cisplatin<>aluminium in infusion set, Doxorubicin<>Heparin, Doxorubicin<>Diazepam, Doxorubicin<>Furosemide, Doxorubicin<>Hydrocortisone Sodium Succinate
Anthracycline: Danger of cardiotoxicity - monitor cardiac function (echocardiogram)

## Obligatory Pre- and Concurrent Medication

| Week | Day | Compounds (generic names) | Sequence and Timing | Dose | Diluent | Route | Duration of Infu- | Comments |
|---|---|---|---|---|---|---|---|---|
| | 1 | Saline 0.9% | 4h before Cisplatin | | 750ml | i.v. | 4h | |
| | 1,2,3,4 | Granisetron | 30' before, 8h after start of chemo. | 1mg | | i.v. | bolus | |
| | 1,2,3 | Mannitol 10% | 15' before, 8h,16h,24h after start of Cisplatin | | 80ml,50ml,50ml,150ml | i.v. | 15min | |
| | 1,2,3 | Saline 0.9% + Gluc.5% alternately | with Cisplatin | | 1500ml + 1500ml | i.v. | 24h | |
| | 4 | Saline 0.9% + Gluc.5% alternately | with Doxorubicin | | 1000ml + 1000ml | i.v. | 24h | |
| | 1-4 | + Potassium Chloride 7.45% | | 30ml | in every 1000ml of infusion | | | check serum potassium regularly |
| | 1-4 | + Magnesium 10% | | 3.15mmol | | | | |
| | 1-4 | + Calcium 10% | | 2.3mmol | | | | |
| | from day 1 | Magnesium | once a day | 180mg/m² | | oral | | recommended for 3 months after chemo. |
| | days 7-14** | Filgrastim | once a day | 5µg/kg | | s.c. | | **with cycle delay due to neutropenia or neutropenic fever (>35.8°C, WBC<1000/µl) until WBC>5000/µl max. |
| | 1-3/4+5 | Aprepitant | -1h before chemo/d4+5 in the morning | * | | oral | | * d1: 125mg, d2-5: 80mg |
| | 1-4/5+6 | Dexamethasone | d1-4 -30min,d4-6 in the morning | * | | i.v./oral | | * d1: 12mg/d2-6: 8mg |

**Medicines As Required:** Metoclopramide, Granisetron, with insufficient diuresis Mannitol 20% 40ml/m² every 6 hours, Furosemide, Pantoprazole

**Routine Tests:** Anthracycline: see cautions above; start cycle only if: WBC≥3000/µl and/or neutrophils≥1000/µl, platelets≥10⁵/µl, echocardiogram or radionuclide ventriculography: FS>28% or LVEF >55%, LVEF decrease not >10% from baseline, normal serum creatinine, creatinine clearance ≥70ml/min x1.73³: serum bilirubin≤1.5 x upper limit of normal, audiogram (hearing loss<30dB at <2kHz); **other tests:** U&Es, fluid balance, transaminases, ALP, LDH, urinalysis; **after each cycle:** days 9-16: FBC every 2 days (longer time interval possible)

**Cisplatin Dose Reduction:** Neutropenic (<500/µl) fever: reduce dose by 25% (with recurrence, by 50%), serum creatinine >1.5mg/dl: reduce dose by 25% (with recurrence, withhold **Cisplatin**). peripheral neuropathy ≥CTC Grade 3, withhold **Cisplatin**

**Doxorubicin Dose Reduction:** Bilirubin: 1.25-2.09mg/dl --> reduce dose by 25%, 2.1-3.05mg/dl --> reduce dose by 50%, 3.06-5mg/dl --> reduce dose by 75%, >5mg/dl --> withhold **Doxorubicin,** with suspected cardiac dysfunction withhold **Doxorubicin** and see above-mentioned tests

**Max. Cum. Dose:** **Doxorubicin:** Danger of cardiotoxicity; max. cum. dose is 550mg/m²

**Next Cycle (N.C.):** Refer to ᵃ above

**References:** Study protocol EURO-B.O.S.S.: "A European treatment protocol for bone sarcoma in patients older than 40 years"

## Euro- B.O.S.S: Ifosfamide/Cisplatin

**Indication: Osteosarcoma**    **12.16.6**

### Chemotherapy

*only adjuvant:  weeks 3, 12, 21
neoadjuvant+post-op GR: weeks 3, 13, 22
neoadjuvant+post-op PR: weeks 3, 14, 26

*This chemotherapy may cause life-threatening toxicity! It should only be administered under the supervision of an experienced medical oncologist! The protocol must first be reviewed and considered in relationship to the clinical situation of the patient.*

| Week | Day | Compounds (generic names) in chronological order | Dosage | Diluent | Route | Duration of Infusion | Comments |
|---|---|---|---|---|---|---|---|
| * | 1, 2 | **Ifosfamide** | 3000mg/m² | 500ml Saline 0.9% | i.v. | 1h | |
| * | 3, 4, 5 | **Cisplatin** | 33.3mg/m² | 250ml Saline 0.9% | i.v. | 24h | protect from light, do not mix with Mesna |

**After day 5 protocol for prophylaxis of delayed emesis**
**Incompatibilities: Cisplatin<>Mesna (in vitro), Cisplatin<>Metoclopramide, Cisplatin<>aluminium in infusion set**

Cycle Diagram: d1 w1 | d8 w2 | d15 w3 | d22 w4 | d29
Ifosfamide
Cisplatin

### Obligatory Pre- and Concurrent Medication

| Week | Day | Sequence and Timing | Compounds (generic names) | Dose | Diluent | Route | Duration of Infusion | Comments |
|---|---|---|---|---|---|---|---|---|
| | 1-5 | 30' before, 8h after start of chemo.# | Granisetron | 3mg | | i.v. | bolus | #no 8h dose on days 1 and 2 |
| | 1-2 | 30' before, 4h & 8h after start of chemo. | Dexamethasone | 8mg | | i.v. | bolus | |
| | 1,2 | after Ifosfamide | Saline 0.9% + Gluc.5% alternately | | 1500ml + 1500ml in infusion | i.v. | 23h | |
| | 1,2 | 0h, 4h, 8h, after ifosfamide | +Mesna | 600mg/m² | | i.v. | | |
| | 1,2 | | + Potassium Chloride 7.45% | 30ml | in every 1000ml of infusion | | | check serum potassium regularly |
| | 1,2 | | + Magnesium 10% | 3.15mmol | | | | |
| | 1,2 | | + Calcium 10% | 2.3mmol | | | | |
| | 3-5 | 8,16,24h after start of Cisplatin | Mannitol 10% | | 50,50,150ml | i.v. | 15min | |
| | 3-6 | with Cisplatin & after end of Ifos. | Saline 0.9% + Gluc.5% alternately | | 1500ml + 1500ml in every 1000ml of infusion | i.v. | 24h | |
| | 3-6 | | + Potassium Chloride 7.45% | 30ml | | | | check serum potassium regularly |
| | 3-6 | | + Magnesium 10% | 3.15mmol | | | | |
| | 3-6 | | + Calcium 10% | 2.3mmol | | | | |
| | from day 1 | once a day | Megnesium | 180mg/m² | | oral | | recommended for 3 months after chemo. |
| | days 8-15** | once a day | Filgrastim | 5µg/kg | | s.c. | | **with cycle delay due to neutropenia or neutropenic fever (>35.8°C, WBC<1000/µl) until WBC>5000/µl max. |
| | 3-5/6+7 | -1h before chemo/d6+7 in the morning | Aprepitant | * | | oral | | * d3: 125mg, d4-7: 80mg |
| | 3-5/6-8 | d3-5 -15min, d6-8 in the morning | Dexamethasone | * | | i.v./oral | | * d3: 12mg/d4-8: 8mg |

**Medicines As Required:** Metoclopramide, Granisetron, with insufficient diuresis Mannitol 20% 40ml/m² every 6 hours, Furosemide, Pantoprazole

**Routine Tests:** **Start cycle only if:** WBC>3000/µl and/or neutrophils ≥1030/µl, platelets ≥10⁵/µl, echocardiogram or radionuclide ventriculography: FS>28% or LVEF>55%, LVEF decrease not >10% from baseline, normal serum creatinine, creatinine clearance ≥70ml/min x1.73², audiogram (hearing loss <30dB at <2kHz);

**other tests:** U&Es, fluid balance, serum bilirubin, transaminases, ALP, LDH, urinalysis; **after each cycle :** days 9-16: FBC every 2 days (longer time interval possible)

**Ifosfamide Dose Reduction:** Neutropenic (<500/µl) fever: reduce dose by 25% (with recurrence, by 50%); AST (SGOT)>300IU/l or bilirubin >3mg/dl: reduce dose by 75% with hematuria: double Mesna dose and increase hydration

**Cisplatin Dose Reduction:** Serum creatinine >1.5mg/dl: reduce dose by 25% (with recurrence, withhold Cisplatin), peripheral neuropathy ≥ CTC Grade 3, withhold Cisplatin

**Max. Cum. Dose :** Not specified
**Next Cycle (N.C):** Refer to * above
**References:** Study protocol EURO-B.O.S.S.: "A European treatment protocol for bone sarcoma in patients older than 40 years"

# Euro- B.O.S.S.: Ifosfamide/Doxorubicin Block — Indication: Osteosarcoma — 12.16.7

## Chemotherapy

*only adjuvant:* **weeks 6, 15, 24**
neoadjuvant+post-op GR: **weeks 6, 16, 25**
neoadjuvant+post-op PR: **weeks 6, 18, 30**

*This chemotherapy may cause life-threatening toxicity! It should only be administered under the supervision of an experienced medical oncologist! The protocol must first be reviewed and considered in relationship to the clinical situation of the patient.*

| Week | Day | Compounds (generic names) in chronological order | Dosage | Diluent | Route | Duration of Infusion | Comments |
|---|---|---|---|---|---|---|---|
| * | 1, 2 | **Ifosfamide** | 3000mg/m² | 500ml Saline 0.9% | i.v. | 1h | |
| * | 3 | **Doxorubicin** | 60mg/m² in 100ml Saline 0.9% | | i.v. | 24h | if peripherally administered, not>1mg/40ml |

### Cautions

**Incompatibilities: Doxorubicin<>aluminium in infusion set, Doxorubicin<>Heparin, Doxorubicin<>Diazepam,**
**Doxorubicin<>Furosemide, Doxorubicin<>Hydrocortisone Sodium Succinate**
**Anthracycline: Danger of cardiotoxicity - monitor cardiac function (echocardiogram)**

**Cycle Diagram**

| | d1 w1 | d8 w2 | d15 w3 | d22 w4 | d29 |
|---|---|---|---|---|---|
| Ifosfamide | | | | | |
| Doxorubicin | | | | | |

## Obligatory Pre- and Concurrent Medication

| Week | Day | Sequence and Timing | Compounds (generic names) | Dose | Diluent | Route | Duration of Infusion | Comments |
|---|---|---|---|---|---|---|---|---|
| | 1-3 | 30' before, 8h after start of chemo.# | Granisetron | 3mg | | i.v. | bolus | #no 8h dose on days 1 and 2 |
| | 1-3 | 30' before, 4h & 8h after start of chemo. | Dexamethasone | 8mg | | i.v. | bolus | |
| | 1,2 | after Ifosfamide | Saline 0.9% + Gluc.5% alternately | | 1500ml + 1500ml | i.v. | 23h | |
| | 1,2 | 0h, 4h, 8h after Ifosfamide | +Mesna | 600mg/m² | in infusion | i.v. | | check serum potassium regularly |
| | 1,2 | | + Potassium Chloride 7.45% | 30ml | in every 1000ml of infusion | | | |
| | 1,2 | | + Magnesium 10% | 3.15mmol | | | | |
| | 1,2 | | + Calcium 10% | 2.3mmol | | | | |
| | 3 | with Doxorubicin | Saline 0.9% + Gluc.5% alternately | | 1000ml + 1000ml | i.v. | 24h | check serum potassium regularly |
| | 3 | | + Potassium Chloride 7.45% | 30ml | in every 1000ml of infusion | | | |
| | 3 | | + Magnesium 10% | 3.15mmol | | | | |
| | 3 | | + Calcium 10% | 2.3mmol | | | | |
| | from day 1 | once a day | Magnesium | 180mg/m² | | oral | | recommended for 3 months after chemo. |
| | days 6-13** | once a day | Filgrastim | 5µg/kg | | s.c. | | **with cycle delay due to neutropenia or neutropenic fever (>35.8°C, WBC<1000/µl) until WBC<5000/µl max. |

| | |
|---|---|
| Medicines As Required | Metoclopramide, Granisetron, Furosemide, Pantoprazole |
| Routine Tests: | **Anthracycline:** see **cautions** above; **start cycle only if:** WBC≥3000/µl and/or neutrophils≥1000/µl, platelets≥10⁵/µl, echocardiogram or radionuclide ventriculography: FS>28% or LVEF>55%, LVEF decrease not ≥10% from baseline, no urinary dysfunction, normal serum creatinine, creatinine clearance ≥70ml/min x1.73², serum bilirubin ≤1.5 x upper limit of normal; **other tests:** U&Es, fluid balance, transaminases, ALP, LDH, urinalysis; **after each cycle:** days 9-16: FBC every 2 days (longer time interval possible) |
| Ifosfamide Dose Reduction: | Neutropenic (<500/µl) fever: reduce dose by 25% (with recurrence, by 50%); AST(SGOT)>300IU/l or bilirubin>3mg/dl: reduce dose b y 75%; with hematuria: double **Mesna** dose and increase hydration |
| Doxorubicin Dose Reduction: | **Bilirubin:** 1.25-2.09mg/dl --> reduce dose by 25%, 2.1-3.05mg/dl --> reduce dose by 50%, 3.06-5mg/dl --> reduce dose by 75%, >5mg/dl --> withhold **Doxorubicin,** **with suspected cardiac dysfunction** withhold **Doxorubicin** and see above-mentioned tests |
| Max. Cum. Dose : | **Doxorubicin:** Danger of cardiotoxicity; max. cum. dose is 550mg/m² |
| Next Cycle (N.C): | Refer to * above |
| References: | Study protocol EURO-B.O.S.S.: "A European treatment protocol for bone sarcoma in patients older than 40 years" |

| Euro-B.O.S.S: High-Dose Methotrexate | Indication: Osteosarcoma | 12.16.8 |

**Chemotherapy**   *neoadjuvant + post-op PR: weeks 13, 17, 21, 25, 29

*This chemotherapy may cause life-threatening toxicity! It should only be administered under the supervision of an experienced medical oncologist! The protocol must first be reviewed and considered in relationship to the clinical situation of the patient.*

| Week | Day | Compounds (generic names) in chronological order | Dosage | Diluent | Route | Duration of Infusion | Comments |
|---|---|---|---|---|---|---|---|
| * | 1 | **Methotrexate** | 8000mg/m² | 10g in 500ml Gluc.5% | i.v. | 4h | add sodium bicarbonate 1molar soln. (40ml/500ml) |
| * | 2, 3, 4 | **Calcium Folinate (Leucovorin)** | **15mg/m² 4 times a day | | i.v./oral | | start 24h after end of Methotrexate, give every 6hours, 1st dose i.v., thereafter oral administration |

| Cycle Diagram | d1 w1 | d8 w2 | d15 w3 | d22 w4 |
|---|---|---|---|---|
| Methotrexate | 4h | | | |
| Leucovorin | | | | |

**Cautions**

* Indications for high-dose Methotrexate in patients with the following histological findings at operation:
- Huvos Stage I and/or
- Salzer-Kuntschik Stage 5-6 and/or
- <50% tumor cell necrosis

** Leucovorin administration: stated dose is for patients with a serum Methotrexate level falling within the normal range (see Leucovorin Rescue sheet); administer every 6 hours; first dose i.v.; start 24 hours after end of Methotrexate infusion; if delayed Methotrexate excretion: dosage is according to Leucovorin Rescue sheet

| Week | Day | Sequence and Timing | Compounds (generic names) | Dose | Diluent | Route | Duration of Infusion | Comments |
|---|---|---|---|---|---|---|---|---|
| | 1 | 4h before chemotherapy | Saline 0.9% | | 1000ml | i.v. | 4h | |
| | | | + Sodium Bicarbonate 1 molar soln. | 60ml/m² | in infusion | | | or until urine pH > 7.4 |
| | 1 | 30' before chemotherapy | Granisetron | 3mg | | i.v. | bolus | |
| | 1 | 30' before, 4h & 8h after start of chemo. | Dexamethasone | 8mg | | i.v. | bolus | |
| | 1, 2 | continuously, starting after Metho. | Saline 0.9% + Gluc.5% alternately | | 1500ml + 1500ml | i.v. | 24h | |
| | | | + Sodium Bicarbonate 1 molar soln. | 60ml | in every 1000ml | | | check serum potassium regularly |
| | | | + Potassium Chloride 7.45% | 30ml | of infusion | | | |
| | 1 | 6h after start of Methotrexate | Furosemide | 20mg | | i.v. | bolus | |

**Medicines As Required:** If urine pH < 7.4: give an additional dose of Sodium Bicarbonate 1 molar solution 30ml/m² as a short infusion over 5–10min, Metoclopramide, Granisetron, Furosemide, Pantoprazole

**Routine Tests:** **Start cycle only if:** >3 fever-free days after an infection, at least 2 days after last Filgrastim dose, WBC >2000/µl and/or neutrophils >500/µl, platelets >80,000/µl, no urinary outflow dysfunction, serum creatinine, BUN, urinalysis, normal serum creatinine, creatinine clearance ≥ 70ml/min x1.73², urine pH >7.4 before start of Methotrexate, normal serum bilirubin; **other tests:** urine pH with each voiding; serum Methotrexate level at 4, 28, 44, 52, 76 hours after start of Methotrexate, further levels if necessary until serum Methotrexate<0.2µmol/l, U&Es, LFTs, weight

**Dose Reduction:** No dose reduction due to previous toxicity provided, if delayed Methotrexate excretion from nephrotoxicity: no further **Methotrexate** to be given; with body weight 75% – 84% of initial weight: every second Methotrexate block may be withheld

**Max. Cum. Dose:** Not specified

**Next Cycle (N.C.):** Refer to * above

**References:** Study protocol EURO-B.O.S.S.: "A European treatment protocol for bone sarcoma in patients older than 40 years". Salzer-Kuntschik et al, J Cancer Clin Oncol 1983; 106: 21–24

# Nimustine

## Indication: CNS Tumors

**12.17.1**

### Chemotherapy

*This chemotherapy may cause life-threatening toxicity! It should only be administered under the supervision of an experienced medical oncologist! The protocol must first be reviewed and considered in relationship to the clinical situation of the patient.*

| Week | Day | Compounds (generic names) in chronological order | Dosage | Diluent | Route | Duration of Infusion | Comments |
|---|---|---|---|---|---|---|---|
| | 1 | **Nimustine** | 100mg/m² | 250ml Saline 0.9% | i.v. | 30min | with prolonged cytopenia: see "Dose Reduction" below |

**Cautions**

| Cycle Diagram | d1 w1 | d8 w2 | d15 w3 | d22 w4 | d29 w5 | d36 |
|---|---|---|---|---|---|---|
| Nimustine | | | | | N.C. | |

### Obligatory Pre- and Concurrent Medication

| Week | Day | Sequence and Timing | Compounds (generic names) | Dose | Diluent | Route | Duration of Infusion | Comments |
|---|---|---|---|---|---|---|---|---|
| | 1 | 15' before chemotherapy | Saline 0.9% | | 500ml | i.v. | 1h | |
| | 1 | 15' before chemotherapy | Dexamethasone | 20mg | 100ml | i.v. | 15min | |
| | 1 | 15' before chemotherapy | Granisetron | 1mg | | i.v. | bolus | |
| | | mucositis prophylaxis | | | | | | |

| | |
|---|---|
| Medicines As Required | Metoclopramide, Granisetron, Dexamethasone |
| Routine Tests: | FBC, U&Es, LFTs, renal function |
| Dose Reduction: | Leukocytes 1500-2000/µl or platelets 40,000-60,000/µl: reduce dose to 75%; leukocytes 1000-1500/µl or platelets 20,000-40,000/µl: reduce dose to 50%; |
| Max. Cum. Dose : | Unknown |
| Next Cycle (N.C.): | Day 29; with prolonged cytopenia, day 43 |
| Efficacy Assess. | After 2 cycles |
| References : | Fiebig HH et al., Onkologie, 1984;7:370-377 |

| Temozolomide | Indication: Malignant Glioma | 12.17.2 |

*This chemotherapy may cause life-threatening toxicity! It should only be administered under the supervision of an experienced medical oncologist! The protocol must first be reviewed and considered in relationship to the clinical situation of the patient.*

## Chemotherapy

| Week | Day | Compounds (generic names) in chronological order | Dosage | Diluent | Route | Duration of Infusion | Comments |
|---|---|---|---|---|---|---|---|
| | 1-5 | **Temozolomide** | 150mg/m² | | oral | | should be taken on an empty stomach |

**Cautions**

For patients with previous chemotherapy treatment:
initial dose: 150mg/m²
from cycle 2: 200mg/m² if neutrophils >1500/µl and platelets >100,000/µl

| Cycle Diagram | Duration of Infusion | d 1 w1 | d8 w2 | d15 w3 | d22 w4 | d29 w5 | d36 |
|---|---|---|---|---|---|---|---|
| Temozolomide | | | | | | N.C. | |

## Obligatory Pre- and Concurrent Medication

| Week | Day | Compounds (generic names) | Sequence and Timing | Dose | Diluent | Route | Duration of Infusion | Comments |
|---|---|---|---|---|---|---|---|---|
| | | | | | | | | |

| | |
|---|---|
| Medicines As Required | Metoclopramide oral or i.v. |
| Routine Tests: | FBC |
| Dose Reduction: | If leukocytes <1000/µl or platelets <50,000/µl: reduce dose level*     *Dose levels: 100mg/m²; 150mg/m² and 200mg/m². Lowest dose: 100mg/m² |
| Max. Cum. Dose : | Unknown |
| Next Cycle (N.C.): | Day 29 |
| Efficacy Assess. | After 2 cycles |
| References: | Yung WKA et al., Br J Cancer, 2000,83:588-93: Summary of Product Characteristics (SmPC) March 2003 |

# PCE

## Indication: Primary Tumor Unknown

**12.18.1**

### Chemotherapy

| Week | Day | Compounds (generic names) in chronological order | Dosage | Diluent | Route | Duration of Infusion | Comments |
|---|---|---|---|---|---|---|---|
| | 1 | **Paclitaxel** | 200mg/m² | 250ml Saline 0.9% | i.v. | 1h | |
| | 1 | **Carboplatin** | #AUC 6 mg/ml×min | 500ml Glucose 5% | i.v. | 1h | #dose (mg) = AUC (mg/ml x min) x [GFR (ml/min)+25] |
| | 1, 3, 5, 7, 9 | **Etoposide Phosphate** | 50mg | | oral | | |
| | 2, 4, 6, 8, 10 | **Etoposide Phosphate** | 100mg | | oral | | |

*This chemotherapy may cause life-threatening toxicity! It should only be administered under the supervision of an experienced medical oncologist! The protocol must first be reviewed and considered in relationship to the clinical situation of the patient.*

**Cautions**

| | target AUC (mg/ml×min) | Cycle Diagram | d1 w1 | d8 w2 | d15 w3 | d22 w4 |
|---|---|---|---|---|---|---|
| Recommended dosage for Carboplatin from AUC | | Paclitaxel | | | | |
| Carboplatin monotherapy, patients untreated | 5-7 | Carboplatin | | | | N.C. |
| Carboplatin monotherapy, myelosuppressive pretreatment | 4-6 | Etoposide 50 | | | | |
| Combination therapy with Carboplatin in standard dosage, patients untreated | 4-6 | Etoposide 100 | | | | |

### Obligatory Pre- and Concurrent Medication

| Week | Day | Compounds (generic names) | Sequence and Timing | Dose | Diluent | Route | Duration of Infusion | Comments |
|---|---|---|---|---|---|---|---|---|
| | 1 | Saline 0.9% | 15' before chemotherapy | | 2000ml | i.v. | 6h | |
| | 1 | Dexamethasone | 15' before chemotherapy | 20mg | | i.v. | bolus | |
| | 1 | Granisetron | 15' before chemotherapy | 1mg | | i.v. | bolus | |
| | 1 | Clemastine | 15' before chemotherapy | 2mg | | i.v. | bolus | |
| | 1 | Ranitidine | 15' before chemotherapy | 50mg | | i.v. | bolus | |

| | |
|---|---|
| **Medicines As Required** | Metoclopramide, Dexamethasone |
| **Routine Tests:** | FBC, WBC differential, U&Es esp. Mg²⁺, serum creatinine, bilirubin, LFTs |
| **Dose Reduction:** | **Paclitaxel:** by 25% with leukopenia or febrile neutropenia, by 25% with thrombocytopenia Grade 4, by 25% with polyneuropathy Score 3 |
| **Therapy Delay:** | If leukocytes <1500/µl or platelets <75,000/µl |
| **Next Cycle (N.C.):** | 1 cycle = 21 days |
| **Efficacy Assess.** | After 1 cycle |
| **References:** | Hainsworth J D et al., J Clin Oncol 1997; 15: 2385-93. |

# Intrapericardial Bleomycin

## Indication: Malignant Pericardial Effusion

**12.19.1**

*This chemotherapy may cause life-threatening toxicity! It should only be administered under the supervision of an experienced medical oncologist! The protocol must first be reviewed and considered in relationship to the clinical situation of the patient.*

## Chemotherapy

| Week | Day | Compounds (generic names) in chronclogical order | Dosage | Diluent | Route | Duration of Infusion | Comments |
|------|-----|--------------------------------------------------|--------|---------|-------|----------------------|----------|
|      | 1   | **Bleomycin**                                    | 30mg absolute | 20ml Saline 0.9% | i.p. | bolus 5min |          |
|      |     |                                                  |        |         |       |                      |          |
|      |     |                                                  |        |         |       |                      |          |
|      |     |                                                  |        |         |       |                      |          |
|      |     |                                                  |        |         |       |                      |          |
|      |     |                                                  |        |         |       |                      |          |

| Cycle Diagram | d1 w1 | d8 w2 | d15 w3 | d22 w4 |
|---------------|-------|-------|--------|--------|
| Bleomycin     |       |       |        |        |

**Cautions**

**"Pericardiocentesis - Bleomycin"**
- drain effusion fully before intrapericardiac chemotherapy administration
- after administration, rinse catheter with a little Saline 0.9% and then clamp it for 2-4 hours
- attention: with intracavity administration, approx. 45% of the Bleomycin will be absorbed systemically!
- note: there may be gastrointestinal, hematological and renal side effects of any concomitant therapy!
- for alternative compounds: contact GCP (Tel. +49 761 270 3248)

| Week | Day | Compounds (generic names) | Sequence and Timing | Dose | Diluent | Route | Duration of Infusion | Comments |
|------|-----|---------------------------|---------------------|------|---------|-------|----------------------|----------|
|      | 1   | Indomethacin              | with Bleomycin administration | 50mg |         | oral  |                      |          |
|      |     |                           |                     |      |         |       |                      |          |
|      |     |                           |                     |      |         |       |                      |          |
|      |     |                           |                     |      |         |       |                      |          |
|      |     |                           |                     |      |         |       |                      |          |
|      |     |                           |                     |      |         |       |                      |          |
|      |     |                           |                     |      |         |       |                      |          |
|      |     |                           |                     |      |         |       |                      |          |

| | |
|---|---|
| **Medicines As Required** | Indomethacin 50mg or Paracetamol 500mg orally |
| **Routine Tests:** | FBC, U&Es, possibly pulmonary function tests with cumulative intrapericardial dose of >300mg absolute |
| **Dose Reduction:** | Initial dose 30mg, reduce dose to 15mg if therapy repeated within 48h |
| **Next Cycle (N.C.):** | If rate of fluid accumulation >25ml/12 hours, treat with initial dose at 48hour intervals till cessation |
| **Efficacy Assess.** | Daily by means of transthoracic echocardiography and quantity of fluid draining |
| **References:** | Liu G et al., J Clin Oncol, 1996, 14:3141-47; v.der Gaast et al., Eur J Cancer Clin Oncol 1989,10 (10):1505-6 |

# Triple Intrathecal Chemotherapy

**Indication:** Therapy/Prophylaxis of Hematological Neoplasia with CNS Involvement **12.19.2**

*This chemotherapy may cause life-threatening toxicity! It should only be administered under the supervision of an experienced medical oncologist! The protocol must first be reviewed and considered in relationship to the clinical situation of the patient.*

## Chemotherapy

| Week | Day | Compounds (generic names) in chronological order | Dosage | Diluent | Route | Duration of Infusion | Comments |
|------|-----|--------------------------------------------------|--------|---------|-------|---------------------|----------|
|      | 1   | **Cytarabine**                                   | 40mg   | in 2ml water | i.t. | bolus |  |
|      | 1   | **Dexamethasone**                                | 4.0mg  | undiluted | i.t. | bolus |  |
|      | 1   | **Methotrexate**                                 | 15.0mg | in 3ml water | i.t. | bolus |  |
|      |     |                                                  |        |         |       |       |  |
|      |     |                                                  |        |         |       |       |  |
|      |     |                                                  |        |         |       |       |  |

**Cycle Diagram:** d1 w1 | d8 w2 | d15 w3 | d22 w4
- Cytarabine
- Dexameth.
- Methotrexate

**Cautions**

Incompatibility: Cytarabine<>Methotrexate; draw up separately, administer in order listed

Methotrexate concentration should not exceed 5mg/ml - arachnoid irritation

Cumulative Methotrexate dose of more than 160mg increases risk of leukoencephalopathy

Occasionally, a potentially myelosuppressive Methotrexate blood level can be reached 24-48h post injection

Leucovorin rescue: not routinely recommended; only with strongly limited bone marrow reserve

Transient paralysis may occur with both Methotrexate and Cytarabine

With lymphomatous brain involvement after 1st cycle CHOP-14, radiotherapy to the whole cranium (36Gy) with boost (up to 50.4Gy)

## Obligatory Pre- and Concurrent Medication

| Week | Day | Sequence and Timing | Compounds (generic names) | Dose | Diluent | Route | Duration of Infusion | Comments |
|------|-----|--------------------|---------------------------|------|---------|-------|---------------------|----------|
|      |     |                    |                           |      |         |       |                     |          |
|      |     |                    |                           |      |         |       |                     |          |
|      |     |                    |                           |      |         |       |                     |          |
|      |     |                    |                           |      |         |       |                     |          |

| | |
|---|---|
| Medicines As Required | Leucovorin rescue only in high risk patients (see **Cautions**) in low dose (5mg/m² every 6 hours) for 72h, but only from 24h post injection as active Leucovorin metabolites can enter CSF |
| Routine Tests: | FBC, neurological status with signs of meningism; serum Methotrexate level only in exceptional cases ( see **Cautions**) |
| Dose Reduction: | **Cytarabine** to 20mg and **Methotrexate** to 5-10mg but only with marked primary meningeal symptoms; otherwise extend therapy intervals |
| Next Cycle (N.C.): | See therapy protocol corresponding to entity and/or prophylaxis versus therapy |
| Efficacy Assess. | According to symptoms; diagnostic lumbar puncture according to the appropriate therapy protocol |
| References: | Therapy protocol for adult ALL 06/99; SmPC MTX, AraC; Crom and Evans, 1993 Ch.29 in "Principles of therapeutic monitoring" |

| Intrathecal "Methotrexate monotherapy" | Indication: Carcinomatous Meningitis | 12.19.3 |

*This chemotherapy may cause life-threatening toxicity! It should only be administered under the supervision of an experienced medical oncologist! The protocol must first be reviewed and considered in relationship to the clinical situation of the patient.*

## Chemotherapy

| Week | Day | Compounds (generic names) in chronological order | Dosage | Diluent | Route | Duration of Infusion | Comments |
|---|---|---|---|---|---|---|---|
| 1 | 1 | **Methotrexate** | 15.0mg | in 3ml water | i.t. | bolus | |

| Cycle Diagram | d1 w1 | d8 w2 | d15 w3 | d22 w4 | d29 w5 | d... |
|---|---|---|---|---|---|---|
| Methotrexate | | | | | | |

**Cautions**

- **Methotrexate concentration should not exceed 5mg/ml** - arachnoid irritation
- **Cumulative Methotrexate dose of more than 160mg increases risk of leukoencephalopathy**
- Occasionally, a potentially myelosuppressive **Methotrexate blood level can be reached 24-48h post injection**
- **Leucovorin rescue: not routinely recommended; only with strongly limited bone marrow reserve**
- Renal insufficiency or known previous systemic toxicity after intrathecal (i.t.) administration
- **Transient paralysis may occur**

## Obligatory Pre- and Concurrent Medication

| Week | Day | Compounds (generic names) | Sequence and Timing | Dose | Diluent | Route | Duration of Infusion | Comments |
|---|---|---|---|---|---|---|---|---|
| | | | | | | | | |

**Medicines As Required:** **Leucovorin rescue** only in high-risk patients in low dose (5mg/m² every 6 hours) for 72h, but only from 24h post injection as active Leucovorin metabolites can enter CSF with marked arachnoid irritation (primary or secondary to drug administration): **Dexamethasone 4mg**

**Routine Tests:** FBC, neurological status with signs of meningism; serum Methotrexate level only in exceptional cases (see **Cautions**)

**Dose Reduction:** **Methotrexate** to 5-10mg but only with marked primary meningeal symptoms; otherwise extend therapy intervals

**Repeat Therapy:** Initially 2-3x/week till clinical/cytological response, then weekly till negative CSF cytology, then 3x every 2-3 weeks, extending to monthly later

**Efficacy Assess.** According to symptoms; CNS imaging (MRI scan) and CSF examination

**References:** Grossmann and Krabak, Cancer Treat Rev 1999, 25:103-19; Fachinfo. MTX; Crom and Evans, 1993 Ch.29 in "Principles of therapeutic monitoring"

# Liposomal Cytarabine — Indication: Lymphomatous Meningitis — 12.19.4

*This chemotherapy may cause life-threatening toxicity! It should only be administered under the supervision of an experienced medical oncologist! The protocol must first be reviewed and considered in relationship to the clinical situation of the patient.*

## Chemotherapy

| Week | Day | Compounds (generic names) in chronological order | Dosage | Diluent | Route | Duration of Infusion | Comments |
|---|---|---|---|---|---|---|---|
| **Induction Therapy** | | | | | | | |
| 1-4 | 1, 15 | Cytarabine Liposome | 50mg | | i.t. | 1-5min | |
| **Consolidation Therapy** | | | | | | | |
| 5-16 | 29, 43, 57, 85 | Cytarabine Liposome | 50mg | | i.t. | 1-5min | |
| **Maintenance Therapy** | | | | | | | |
| 17-30 | 113, 141, 169, 190 | Cytarabine Liposome | 50mg | | i.t. | 1-5min | |

**Cautions**

**INDUCTION THERAPY**
Cycle Diagram Phase 1 — Cytarabine Liposome
d1 w1 | d8 w2 | d15 w3 | d22 w4

**CONSOLIDATION THERAPY**
Cycle Diagram Phase 1 — Cytarabine Liposome
d29 w5 | d36 w6 | d43 w7 | d50 w8 | d57 w9 | d64 w10 | d78 w12 | d85 w13 | d92 w14 | d99 w15 | d106 w16

**MAINTENANCE THERAPY**
Cycle Diagram Phase 2 — Cytarabine Liposome
d113 w17 | d120 w18 | d127 w19 | d134 w20 | d141 w21 | d148 w22 | d155 w23 | d162 w24 | d169 w25 | d176 w26 | d183 w27 | d190 w28 | d197 w29 | d204 w30

**Please note: patient must lie flat for 1 hour after therapy!**

## Obligatory Pre- and Concurrent Medication

| Week | Day | Compounds (generic names) | Sequence and Timing | Dose | Route | Diluent | Duration of Infusion | Comments |
|---|---|---|---|---|---|---|---|---|
| | 1-5 | Dexamethasone | to be commenced with every Cytarbine Liposome dose | 4mg every 12 hours | oral/i.v. | | | |

| | |
|---|---|
| Dose Reduction: | Reduce dose to 25mg with symptoms of neurotoxicity |
| Next Cycle (N.C.): | See Cycle Diagram and Summary of Product Characteristics (SmPC) |
| Efficacy Assess. | After Induction Therapy and after Consolidation Therapy |
| References: | Summary of Product Characteristics (SmPC), Glantz M et al., J Clin Onc (1999); 17: 3110-3116 |

| VCP-E | Indication: | PBSC Mobilization (NHL, Lung Cancer, Breast Cancer, etc.) | 13.1.1 |
|---|---|---|---|

*This chemotherapy may cause life-threatening toxicity! It should only be administered under the supervision of an experienced medical oncologist! The protocol must first be reviewed and considered in relationship to the clinical situation of the patient.*

## Chemotherapy

| Week | Day | Compounds (generic names) in chronological order | Dosage | Diluent | Route | Duration of Infusion | Comments |
|---|---|---|---|---|---|---|---|
| | 1 | Epirubicin | 50mg/m² | undiluted | i.v. | bolus 15min | |
| | 1 | Etoposide Phosphate | 500mg/m² | 500ml Saline 0.9% | i.v. | 1h | dose expressed in terms of Etoposide base |
| | 1 | Cisplatin | 50mg/m² | 250ml Saline 0.9% | i.v. | 1h | |
| | 1 | Cyclophosphamide | 1350mg/m² | 500ml Saline 0.9% | i.v. | 1h | |

**Cautions:** Etoposide Phosphate and Sodium Bicarbonate must not be administered concomitantly through the same infusion site!
After day 1 protocol for prophylaxis of delayed emesis
Anthracycline: Danger of cardiotoxicity - monitor cardiac function

| Cycle Diagram | d1 w1 | d8 w2 | d15 w3 | d22 w4 |
|---|---|---|---|---|
| Epirubicin | | | | |
| Etop. Phos. | | | | |
| Cisplatin | | | | |
| Cyclophos. | | | | |

## Obligatory Pre- and Concurrent Medication

| Week | Day | Compounds (generic names) | Sequence and Timing | Dose | Diluent | Route | Duration of Infusion | Comments |
|---|---|---|---|---|---|---|---|---|
| | 0 | Saline 0.9% | prehydration | | 1000ml | i.v. | 12h | |
| | 0,1 | Magnesium | before & with chemotherapy | 6.3 mmol/day | in Saline 0.9% | i.v. | | in saline infusion |
| | 0-2 | Sodium Bicarbonate | before & with chemotherapy | 2g every 6 hours | | oral | | |
| | 1 | Saline 0.9% | continuously | | 3000ml | i.v. | 24h | |
| | 1 | Granisetron | 15' before chemotherapy | 1mg | | i.v. | bolus | |
| | 1 | Mannitol 10% | 30' before and after Cisplatin | | 250ml | i.v. | 15min | |
| | 1 | Mesna | 15' before, 4 and 8h after Cycloph. | 270mg/m² | | i.v. | 15min | |
| | from day 7 | Filgrastim | mornings | 5µg/kg *(see below) | | s.c. | | till end of leukapheresis |
| | 1, 2, 3 | Aprepitant | -1h before chemo/d2+3 in the morning | * | | oral | | * d1 : 125mg, d2+3: 80mg |
| | 1-4 | Dexamethasone | d1-15min,d2-4 in the morning | * | | i.v./oral | | * d1 : 12mg/d2-4: 8mg |

| | |
|---|---|
| **Medicines As Required** | Metoclopramide, Dexamethasone, Granisetron, Heparin 15000 units on days 1 and 2, Sodium Bicarbonate oral or i.v. |
| **Routine Tests:** | **Anthracycline**: see **cautions** above; FBC, U&Es esp. Ca²⁺ and Mg²⁺, LFTs, serum creatinine, creatinine clearance, diuresis, ototoxicity, neurotoxicity |
| **Dose Reduction:** | Serum creatinine>3mg/dl: **Cisplatin** 75%; creatinine clearance <80ml/min: discontinue **Cisplatin**; see Dose Modification Table |
| **Filgrastim Dosage:** | *Before planned leukapheresis 5µg/kg body weight (>70kg:480µg, <70kg 300µg); if no planned leukapheresis, give a standard dose of 300µg absolute |
| **Max. Cum. Dose :** | **Epirubicin**: Danger of cardiotoxicity; maximum cumulative dose is 1000mg/m² |
| **Efficacy Assess.** | Not applicable |
| **References:** | Adapted from: Waller CF et al, BMT 24(1);19-24, 1999; Pujol PJ et al, JCO 15(5):2082-9, 1997; Bamberga M et al, Tumori: 78(5):333-7, 1992 |

**VIP-E**

**Indication:** **PBSC Mobilization**
**(NHL, Lung Cancer, Breast Cancer, etc.)**

**13.1.2**

*This chemotherapy may cause life-threatening toxicity! It should only be administered under the supervision of an experienced medical oncologist! The protocol must first be reviewed and considered in relationship to the clinical situation of the patient.*

## Chemotherapy

| Week | Day | Compounds (generic names) in chronological order | Dosage | Diluent | Route | Duration of Infusion | Comments |
|------|-----|------|------|------|------|------|------|
| | 1 | Epirubicin | 50mg/m² | undiluted | i.v. | bolus 15min | |
| | 1 | Etoposide Phosphate | 500mg/m² | 500ml Saline 0.9% | i.v. | 1h | dose expressed in terms of Etoposide base |
| | 1 | Cisplatin | 50mg/m² | 250ml Saline 0.9% | i.v. | 1h | |
| | 1 | Ifosfamide | 4000mg/m² | 500ml Saline 0.9% | i.v. | 18h | |

| | Cycle Diagram | d1 w1 | d8 w2 | d15 w3 | d22 w4 |
|------|------|------|------|------|------|
| | Epirubicin | | | | N.C. |
| | Etop. Phos. | | | | |
| | Cisplatin | | | | |
| | Ifosfamide | | | | |

**Cautions**

Etoposide Phosphate and Sodium Bicarbonate must not be administered concomitantly through the same infusion site!
After day 1 protocol for prophylaxis of delayed emesis
Granisetron: increase dose to 3mg with emesis
Anthracycline: Danger of cardiotoxicity - monitor cardiac function

## Obligatory Pre- and Concurrent Medication

| Week | Day | Sequence and Timing | Compounds (generic names) | Dose | Diluent | Route | Duration of Infusion | Comments |
|------|-----|------|------|------|------|------|------|------|
| | 0 | prehydration | Saline 0.9% | | 1000ml | i.v. | 12h | |
| | 0,1 | before & with chemotherapy | Magnesium | 6.3 mmol/day | in Saline 0.9% | i.v. | | in saline infusion |
| | 0-3 | before chemotherapy | Sodium Bicarbonate | 2g every 6 hours | | oral | | |
| | 1 | continuously | Saline 0.9% | | 3000ml | i.v. | 24h | |
| | 1 | 30' before Cisplatin | Granisetron | 1mg | | i.v. | bolus | |
| | 1 | 30' before and after Cisplatin | Mannitol 10% | | 250ml | i.v. | 15min | |
| | 1,2 | 15' before, 0h,18h after Ifosfamide | Mesna | 800/4000/2000mg/m² | | i.v. | 18h | |
| | 1, 2, 3 | -1h before chemo/d2+3 in the morning | Aprepitant | * | | oral | | * d1: 125mg, d2+3: 80mg |
| | 1-4 | d1-15min, d2-4 in the morning | Dexamethasone | * | | i.v./oral | | * d1: 12mg/d2-4: 8mg |
| | 7-11 | mornings | Filgrastim | 300µg absolute | | s.c. | | |

| | | | | | |
|------|------|------|------|------|------|
| **Medicines As Required** | Metoclopramide, Dexamethasone, Granisetron, Heparin 15000 units on days 1 and 2, Sodium Bicarbonate oral or i.v., Famotidine, Sucralfate | | | | |
| **Routine Tests:** | **Anthracycline:** see cautions above; FBC, U&Es esp. Ca²⁺ and Mg²⁺, LFTs, serum creatinine, creatinine clearance, diuresis, ototoxicity, neurotoxicity | | | | |
| **Dose Reduction:** | Creatinine clearance <60ml/min is absolute contraindication; see Dose Modification Table | | | | |
| **Filgrastim Dosage:** | Before planned leukapheresis 5µg/kg body weight (>70kg:480µg,<70kg:300µg) | | | | |
| **Max. Cum. Dose :** | **Epirubicin:** Danger of cardiotoxicity; maximum cumulative dose is 1000mg/m² | | | | |
| **Next Cycle (N.C.):** | Day 22 | | | | |
| **References:** | Neidhart JA et al., J Clin Oncol, 1990;8:1728-38 | | | | |

# Cyclo-Mob-1d

**Indication: PBSC Mobilization**
**(Medulloblastoma, PNET, Multiple Myeloma)**

13.1.3

*This chemotherapy may cause life-threatening toxicity! It should only be administered under the supervision of an experienced medical oncologist! The protocol must first be reviewed and considered in relationship to the clinical situation of the patient.*

## Chemotherapy

| Week | Day | Compounds (generic names) in chronological order | Dosage | Diluent | Route | Duration of Infusion | Comments |
|---|---|---|---|---|---|---|---|
| | 1 | **Cyclophosphamide** | 4000mg/m² | 1000ml Saline 0.9% | i.v. | 1h | |
| | | | | | | | |
| | | | | | | | |
| | | | | | | | |

**Cautions**

After day 1 protocol for prophylaxis of delayed emesis

| Cycle Diagram | d1 w1 | d8 w2 | d15 w3 | d22 w4 |
|---|---|---|---|---|
| Cyclophos. | | | | |

## Obligatory Pre- and Concurrent Medication

| Week | Day | Sequence and Timing | Compounds (generic names) | Dose | Diluent | Route | Duration of Infusion | Comments |
|---|---|---|---|---|---|---|---|---|
| | 0 | prehydration | Saline 0.9% | | 1000ml | i.v. | 24h | |
| | 0 | before chemotherapy | Sodium Bicarbonate | 2g every 6 hours | | oral | | |
| | 0,1 | continuously | Magnesium | 3.15 mmol | 1000ml Saline 0.9% | i.v. | | in saline infusion |
| | 1 | continuously | Saline 0.9% | | 3000ml | i.v. | 24h | |
| | 1-2 | continuously | Sodium Bicarbonate | 200ml | | i.v. | 24h | |
| | 1 | 15' before chemotherapy | Furosemide | 20mg | | i.v. | bolus | |
| | 1 | 15' before chemotherapy | Granisetron | 1mg | | i.v. | bolus | |
| | 1 | 15' before, 4h & 8h after chemo. | Dexamethasone | 8mg | | i.v. | bolus | |
| | 1-2 | 0h, 4h, 8h after chemo. | Mesna | 800mg/m² | | i.v. | 15min | |
| | from day +7 | mornings | Filgrastim | 5µg/kg | | s.c. | | till end of leukapheresis: <70kg:300µg; >70kg:480µg |
| | | | | | | | | |
| | | | | | | | | |
| | | | | | | | | |
| | | | | | | | | |

| | |
|---|---|
| **Medicines As Required** | Metoclopramide, Dexamethasone, Granisetron, Furosemide, Heparin 15000 units on days 1 and 2, Sodium Bicarbonate oral or i.v. |
| **Routine Tests:** | FBC, U&Es esp. Ca²⁺ and Mg²⁺, LFTs, serum creatinine, diuresis, interim check after 4 hours: further dose of Furosemide if necessary |
| **Dose Reduction:** | Reduce **Cyclophosphamide** with impairment of liver and renal function, see Dose Modification Table |
| **Filgrastim Dosage:** | Before planned leukapheresis 5µg/kg body weight (>70kg:480µg,<70kg 300µg): if no planned leukapheresis, give a standard dose of 300µg absolute |
| **References:** | Sheridan WP et al., Lancet, 1992:339:640-644 |

# Cyclo-Mob-2d

**Indication: PBSC Mobilization (NHL, Autoimmune Diseases, etc.)**

**13.1.4**

*This chemotherapy may cause life-threatening toxicity! It should only be administered under the supervision of an experienced medical oncologist! The protocol must first be reviewed and considered in relationship to the clinical situation of the patient.*

## Chemotherapy

| Week | Day | Compounds (generic names) in chronological order | Dosage | Diluent | Route | Duration of Infusion | Comments |
|------|-----|--------------------------------------------------|--------|---------|-------|----------------------|----------|
|      | 1,2 | **Cyclophosphamide** | 2000mg/m² | 500ml Saline 0.9% | i.v. | 1h | |
|      |     | | | | | | |
|      |     | | | | | | |
|      |     | | | | | | |
|      |     | | | | | | |

**Cautions:** After day 2 protocol for prophylaxis of delayed emesis

| Cycle Diagram | d1 w1 | d8 w2 | d15 w3 | d22 w4 |
|---------------|-------|-------|--------|--------|
| Cyclophos. | | | | |
| | | | | |
| | | | | |

## Obligatory Pre- and Concurrent Medication

| Week | Day | Sequence and Timing | Compounds (generic names) | Dose | Diluent | Route | Duration of Infusion | Comments |
|------|-----|---------------------|---------------------------|------|---------|-------|----------------------|----------|
| | 0 | prehydration | Saline 0.9% | | 1000ml | i.v. | 24h | |
| | 0 | before chemotherapy | Sodium Bicarbonate | 2g every 6 hours | | oral | | |
| | 0–2 | continuously | Magnesium | 3.15 mmol | 1000ml Saline 0.9% | i.v. | 24h | in saline infusion |
| | 1,2 | continuously | Saline 0.9% | | 3000ml | i.v. | 24h | |
| | 1–3 | continuously | Sodium Bicarbonate | 200ml | | i.v. | 24h | |
| | 1,2 | 15' before chemotherapy | Furosemide | 20mg | | i.v. | bolus | |
| | 1,2 | 15' before chemotherapy | Granisetron | 1mg | | i.v. | bolus | |
| | 1,2 | 15' before, 4h & 8h after chemo. | Dexamethasone | 8mg | | i.v. | bolus | |
| | 1,2 | 0h,4h,8h after chemo. | Mesna | 400mg/m² | | i.v. | 24h | |
| | from day +7 | mornings | Filgrastim | 5µg/kg | | s.c. | | till end of leukapheresis: <70kg:300µg; >70kg:480µg |
| | | | | | | | | |
| | | | | | | | | |
| | | | | | | | | |
| | | | | | | | | |

| | |
|---|---|
| **Medicines As Required** | Metoclopramide, Dexamethasone, Granisetron, Furosemide, Heparin 15000 units on days 1 and 2, Sodium Bicarbonate oral or i.v. |
| **Routine Tests:** | FBC, U&Es esp. Ca²⁺ and Mg²⁺, LFTs, serum creatinine, diuresis, interim check after 4 hours: further dose of Furosemide if necessary |
| **Dose Reduction:** | Reduce **Cyclophosphamide** with impairment of liver and renal function, see Dose Modification Table |
| **Filgrastim Dosage:** | Before planned leukapheresis 5µg/kg body weight (>70kg:480µg,<70kg 300µg); if no planned leukapheresis, give a standard dose of 300µg absolute |
| **References:** | Rowlings PA et al., Austral N Zeal J Med, 1992;22(6):660-664; Jutner CA, Bone Marrow Transpl, 1990;5:22-24 |

# Dexa-BEAM

## Indication: PBSC Mobilization (Lymphoma)

**13.1.5**

*This chemotherapy may cause life-threatening toxicity! It should only be administered under the supervision of an experienced medical oncologist! The protocol must first be reviewed and considered in relationship to the clinical situation of the patient.*

## Chemotherapy

| Week | Day | Compounds (generic names) in chronological order | Dosage | Diluent | Route | Duration of Infusion | Comments |
|---|---|---|---|---|---|---|---|
| | 1-10 | **Dexamethasone** | 8mg every 8 hours | undiluted | i.v. | 15min | short infusion |
| | 2 | **Carmustine (BCNU)** | 60mg/m² | 500ml Glucose 5% | i.v. | 30min | protect from light |
| | 3 | **Melphalan** | 20mg/m² | 100ml Saline 0.9% | i.v. | 5min | only via central line |
| | 4-7 | **Etoposide Phosphate** | 75mg/m² | 100ml Saline 0.9% | i.v. | 30min | dose expressed in terms of Etoposide base |
| | 4-7 | **Cytarabine** | 100mg/m² twice a day | 250ml Saline 0.9% | i.v. | 30min | twice a day: 8:00 and 20:00 |

| Cycle Diagram | d1 w1 | d8 w2 | d15 w3 | d22 w4 | |
|---|---|---|---|---|---|
| Dexameth. | | | | | |
| Carmustine | | | | | |
| Melphalan | | | | | |
| Etop. Phos. | | | | | |
| Cytarabine | | | | | |

**Cautions** — Etoposide Phosphate and Sodium Bicarbonate must not be administered concomitantly through the same infusion site!

## Obligatory Pre- and Concurrent Medication

| Week | Day | Compounds (generic names) | Sequence and Timing | Dose | Diluent | Route | Duration of Infusion | Comments |
|---|---|---|---|---|---|---|---|---|
| | from day 1 | Saline 0.9% | continuously | | 2000ml | i.v. | 24h | |
| | from day 1 | Heparin | continuously | 15000 units | | i.v. | 24h | reduce dose if platelets < 30,000/µl |
| | 2-7 | Granisetron | 15' before chemotherapy | 1mg | | i.v. | bolus | increase dose to 3mg with emesis |
| | regularly | Co-trimoxazole | 1 - 0 - 1 (2x/week) | 960mg | | oral | | |
| | regularly | Amphotericin B | 1 - 1 - 1 - 1 | 100mg (1ml) | | oral | | as suspension |
| | from day 11 | Filgrastim | mornings | 5µg/kg | | s.c. | | till end of leukapheresis; <70kg:300µg; >70kg:480µg |

| | |
|---|---|
| **Medicines As Required** | Metoclopramide oral or i.v., Granisetron i.v., Allopurinol 300mg, Sucralfate |
| **Routine Tests** | FBC, U&Es, blood glucose, LFTs, serum creatinine, creatinine clearance, diuresis, pulmonary function, neurotoxicity |
| **Dose Increase:** | Etoposide phosphate 75mg/m² may be given twice a day on days 4-7 if necessary |
| **Dose Reduction:** | With bone marrow failure, reduce **BCNU** and **Etoposide**; with renal failure, reduce **BCNU** and **Melphalan**; with cerebellar symptoms, exanthema, bilirubin >3.0mg/dl, raised AST (SGOT) or ALP: stop **Cytarabine**, with cytopenia withhold therapy (no dose reduction); see Dose Modification Table |
| **Max. Cum. Dose :** | **BCNU** >1000mg/m²: Danger of pulmonary toxicity |
| **References:** | Dreger P et al., Br J Cancer, 1993, 68: 950-57 |

| IEV < 60 years | | Indication: PBSC Mobilization (Multiple Myeloma) | | | | 13.1.6 |

**Chemotherapy**

*This chemotherapy may cause life-threatening toxicity! It should only be administered under the supervision of an experienced medical oncologist! The protocol must first be reviewed and considered in relationship to the clinical situation of the patient.*

| Week | Day | Compounds (generic names) in chronological order | Dosage | Diluent | Route | Duration of Infusion | Comments |
|---|---|---|---|---|---|---|---|
| | 1 | **Epirubicin** | 100mg/m² | 100ml Saline 0.9% | i.v. | 1h | via central line |
| | 1-3 | **Etoposide Phosphate** | 150mg/m² | 100ml Saline 0.9% (from 200mg in 250ml) | i.v. | 1h | dose expressed in terms of Etoposide base |
| | 1-3 | **Ifosfamide** | 2500mg/m² | 500ml Saline 0.9% | i.v. | 18h | |

| | | | |
|---|---|---|---|
| | Cycle Diagram | d1 w1 | d8 w2 | d15 w3 | d22 w4 |
| | Epirubicin | | | | N.C. (outside the study) |
| | Etop. Phos. | | | | |
| | Ifosfamide | | | | |

**Cautions**

Etoposide Phosphate and Sodium Bicarbonate must not be administered concomitantly through the same infusion site!
Incompatibilities: Epirubicin<>alkaline solutions, Epirubicin<>Mesna, Epirubicin<>Ifosfamide, Etoposide Phos.<>alkaline solutions
Anthracycline: Danger of cardiotoxicity - monitor cardiac function
With renal insufficiency or previous Ifosfamide toxicity: EVC 980000_12
(replace Ifosfamide with Cyclophosphamide 500mg/m² on days 1-3)

**Obligatory Pre- and Concurrent Medication**

| Week | Day | Compounds (generic names) | Dose | Diluent | Route | Duration of Infusion | Comments |
|---|---|---|---|---|---|---|---|
| | 0 | Saline 0.9% | | 1000ml | i.v. | 12h | |
| | 0,1,2,3 | Magnesium | 6.3 mmol/day | in Saline 0.9% | i.v. | | |
| | 0-5 | Sodium Bicarbonate | 2g every 6 hours | | oral | | |
| | 1-3 | Saline 0.9% | | 2000ml | i.v. | 24h | |
| | 1-3 | Granisetron | 1mg | | i.v. | bolus | increase dose to 3mg with emesis |
| | 1-3 | Dexamethasone | 8mg | | i.v. | bolus | |
| | 1-4 | Mesna | 500/2500/1250mg/m² | | i.v. | 15min/18h/6h | |
| | from day 5 | Filgrastim | 5µg/kg | | s.c. | | till end of apheresis |

| | |
|---|---|
| Medicines As Required | Metoclopramide, Dexamethasone, Granisetron, Sodium Bicarbonate oral or i.v., Allopurinol |
| Routine Tests: | **Anthracycline:** see **cautions** above.; FBC, U&Es esp. Ca²⁺ and Mg²⁺, LFTs, serum creatinine, urinary pH, creatinine clearance, diuresis, neurotoxicity |
| Dose Reduction: | See Dose Modification Table |
| Max. Cum. Dose : | **Epirubicin:** Danger of cardiotoxicity; maximum cumulative dose is 1000mg/m² |
| Filgrastim Dosage: | Before planned leukapheresis 5µg/kg body weight (>70kg:480µg, <70kg:300µg) till the end of apheresis |
| Next Cycle (N.C.): | IEV for one or two cycles, starting on day 22 of cycle 1, if clinically indicated |
| Efficacy Assess. | Before next therapy |
| References: | Analogous to Holowiecki J et al., Transplant Proc., 2000; 32(6): 1412-5 |

**EVC < 60 years (instead of IEV)**

**Indication: Multiple Myeloma with Renal Failure**
**(also Mobilization Therapy)**    13.1.7

*This chemotherapy may cause life-threatening toxicity! It should only be administered under the supervision of an experienced medical oncologist! The protocol must first be reviewed and considered in relationship to the clinical situation of the patient.*

## Chemotherapy

| Week | Day | Compounds (generic names) in chronological order | Dosage | Diluent | Route | Duration of Infusion | Comments |
|---|---|---|---|---|---|---|---|
| | 1 | **Epirubicin** | 100mg/m² | 100ml Saline 0.9% | i.v. | 1h | via central line |
| | 1-3 | **Etoposide Phosphate** | 150mg/m² | 100ml Saline 0.9% (from 200mg in 250ml) | i.v. | 1h | dose expressed in terms of Etoposide base |
| | 1-3 | **Cyclophosphamide** | 500mg/m² | 500ml Saline 0.9% | i.v. | 1h | |

**Cautions**

Etoposide Phosphate and Sodium Bicarbonate must not be administered concomitantly through the same infusion site!
Incompatibilities: Epirubicin<>alkaline solutions, Epirubicin<>Mesna, Etoposide Phosphate<>alkaline solutions
Anthracycline: Danger of cardiotoxicity - monitor cardiac function

| Cycle Diagram | d1 w1 | d8 w2 | d15 w3 | d22 w4 | d2 |
|---|---|---|---|---|---|
| Epirubicin | | | | N.C. | |
| Etop. Phos. | | | | | |
| Cyclophos. | | | | | |

## Obligatory Pre- and Concurrent Medication

| Week | Day | Sequence and Timing | Compounds (generic names) | Dose | Diluent | Route | Duration of Infusion | Comments |
|---|---|---|---|---|---|---|---|---|
| | 0 | prehydration | Saline 0.9% | | 1000ml | i.v. | 12h | |
| | 0,1,2,3 | before & with chemotherapy | Magnesium | 6.3 mmol/day | in Saline 0.9% | i.v. | | |
| | 0-5 | before chemotherapy | Sodium Bicarbonate | 2g every 6 hours | | oral | | |
| | 1-3 | continuously | Saline 0.9% | | 2000ml | i.v. | 24h | |
| | 1-3 | 30' before chemotherapy | Granisetron | 1mg | | i.v. | bolus | increase dose to 3mg with emesis |
| | 1-3 | 30' before, 4h & 8h after chemo. | Dexamethasone | 8mg | | i.v. | bolus | |
| | 1-3 | 0h, 4h & 8h after Cyclophos. | Mesna | 400mg | | i.v. | bolus | |
| | from day 5 | evenings | Filgrastim | 5µg/kg | | s.c. | | till end of apheresis |

| | |
|---|---|
| **Medicines As Required** | Metoclopramide, Dexamethasone, Granisetron, Sodium Bicarbonate oral or i.v., Allopurinol |
| **Routine Tests:** | **Anthracycline**: see **cautions** above; FBC, U&Es esp. Ca²⁺ and Mg²⁺ urinary pH, LFTs, serum creatinine, creatinine clearance, diuresis, neurotoxicity |
| **Dose Reduction:** | See Dose Modification Table |
| **Max. Cum. Dose :** | **Epirubicin**: Danger of cardiotoxicity; maximum cumulative dose is 1000mg/m² |
| **Filgrastim Dosage:** | Before planned leukapheresis 5µg/kg body weight (>70kg:480µg, <70kg:300µg) till the end of apheresis |
| **Next Cycle (N.C.):** | Cycle 2 after 21 days if clinically indicated |
| **Efficacy Assess.** | Before next therapy |
| **References:** | Analogous to Holowiecki J et al., Transplant Proc., 2000; 32(6): 1412-5 |

# BEAM (≤ 65 years) — Indication: High-Dose Protocol (Lymphoma) — 14.1

*This chemotherapy may cause life-threatening toxicity! It should only be administered under the supervision of an experienced medical oncologist! The protocol must first be reviewed and considered in relationship to the clinical situation of the patient.*

## Chemotherapy

| Week | Day | Compounds (generic names) in chronological order | Dosage | Diluent | Route | Duration of Infusion | Comments |
|---|---|---|---|---|---|---|---|
| | -7 | **Carmustine (BCNU)** | 300mg/m² | 500ml Glucose 5% | i.v. | 1h | protect from light |
| | -6 to -3 | **Cytarabine** | 200mg/m² twice a day | 250ml Saline 0.9% | i.v. | 1h | twice a day: 8.00 and 18.00 |
| | -6 to -3 | **Etoposide Phosphate** | 100mg/m² twice a day | 100ml Saline 0.9% | i.v. | 30min | twice a day: 9.00 and 19.00 |
| | -2 | **Melphalan** | 140mg/m² | 500ml Saline 0.9% | i.v. | 30min | only via a central line |
| | -1 | **Therapy-free Interval** of at least 30 hours | | | | | |
| | 0 | **Peripheral Blood Stem Cell Transplantation** | | | | | |

| Cycle Diagram | d-7 w-1 | d1 w1 | d8 w2 | d15 w3 | d |
|---|---|---|---|---|---|
| Carmustine | | | | | |
| Cytarabine | | | | | |
| Etop. Phos. | | | | | |
| Melphalan | | | | | |
| No Therapy | | | | | |
| PBSCT | | | | | |

**Cautions**

Etoposide Phosphate and Sodium Bicarbonate must not be administered concomitantly through the same infusion site!

Dosage of all chemotherapy for the overweight refers to ideal body weight (IBW), calculate body surface area using IBW:

Men: IBW = 50kg + 2.3 x ((height in cm/2.53) - 60)

Women: IBW = 45.5kg + 2.3 x ((height in cm/2.53) - 60)

If IBW is more than 15kg below actual body weight, use adjusted body weight: Calculated IBW + 0.4 x (actual BW - calculated IBW )

## Obligatory Pre- and Concurrent Medication

| Week | Day | Compounds (generic names) | Sequence and Timing | Dose | Diluent | Route | Duration of Infusion | Comments |
|---|---|---|---|---|---|---|---|---|
| | -7 to -2 | Granisetron | 15' before chemotherapy | 3mg | | i.v. | bolus | |
| | -7 | Dexamethasone | 15' before Carmustine | 20mg | 100ml Saline 0.9% | i.v. | 15min | |
| | -6 to -2 | Dexamethasone | before every Cyt., Eto. & Melph. | 8mg | | i.v. | bolus | |
| | from day -7 | Saline 0.9% | continuously | | 2000ml | i.v. | 24h | |
| | from admission until day -2 | Co-trimoxazole | 1 - 0 - 1 (2x/week) | 960mg | | oral | | |
| | from admission until day -2 | Folic Acid | 1 - 0 - 0 | 5mg | | oral | | |
| | -1 | Levofloxacin | 1 - 0 - 0 | 500mg | | oral | | until possibility of i.v. antibiotics or engraftment |
| | from day -7 | Heparin | continuously | 15000 units | | i.v. | 24h | reduce dose if platelets < 30,000/µl |
| | from day 7 | Filgrastim | mornings | 5µg/kg | | s.c. | | till stable engraftment: WBC >1000/µl |
| | with stable engraftment | Co-trimoxazole | 1 - 0 - 1 (2x/week) | 960mg | | oral | | |
| | with stable engraftment | Folic Acid | 1 - 0 - 0 | 5mg | | oral | | |

**Medicines As Required** Metoclopramide, Dimenhydrinate, Allopurinol 300mg, Lynestrenol 5mg every 12 hours, Famotidine, Sucralfate

**Routine Tests** FBC, U&Es, LFTs, serum creatinine, creatinine clearance, diuresis, cardiac function, pulmonary function

**Dose Reduction:** If bilirubin >3.0mg/dl or GFR <60ml/min do not give high-dose therapy; see Dose Modification Table

**References:** Chopra R et al., Blood, 1993 ;5:1137-45; Diehl V et al., Lancet, 2002; 359(9323); 2065-71

| Melphalan 200 | Indication: Multiple Myeloma | 14.2 |
|---|---|---|

*This chemotherapy may cause life-threatening toxicity! It should only be administered under the supervision of an experienced medical oncologist! The protocol must first be reviewed and considered in relationship to the clinical situation of the patient.*

## Chemotherapy

| Week | Day | Compounds (generic names) in chronological order | Dosage | Diluent | Route | Duration of Infusion | Comments |
|---|---|---|---|---|---|---|---|
| | -3,-2 | **Melphalan** (only via central line) | 100mg/m² | 500ml Saline 0.9% | i.v. | 1h | **incompatible with glucose** |
| | -1 | **Therapy-free Interval** of at least 30 hours! | | | | | |
| | 0 | **Peripheral Blood Stem Cell Transplantation** | CD34⁺>2x10⁶/kg | | | | |

With patients >60years: Melphalan 100mg/m² for 2 days as indicated above
With patients >70years or with renal insufficiency or with Karnofsky Index <70%: Therapy according to Melphalan 140 protocol
Dosage of all chemotherapy for the overweight refers to ideal body weight (IBW), calculate body surface area using IBW:
Men: IBW = 50kg + 2.3 x ((height in cm/2.53) - 60)
Women: IBW = 45.5kg + 2.3 x ((height in cm/2.53) - 60)
If IBW is more than 15kg below actual body weight, use adjusted body weight: Calculated IBW + 0.4 x (actual BW - calculated IBW)

Cautions

| Cycle Diagram | d-7 w-1 | d1 w1 | d8 w2 | d15 w3 |
|---|---|---|---|---|
| Melphalan | | | | |
| No Therapy | | | | |
| PBSCT | | | | |

## Obligatory Pre- and Concurrent Medication

| Week | Day | Compounds (generic names) | Sequence and Timing | Dose | Diluent | Route | Duration of Infusion | Comments |
|---|---|---|---|---|---|---|---|---|
| | from day -3 | Saline 0.9% + Gluc.5% alternately | continuously | | 1000ml + 1000ml | i.v. | 24h | Start in the evening of day -3 |
| | | +Potassium Chloride | | 20ml/1000ml in hydration infusion | | | | check serum potassium |
| | | +Sodium Bicarbonate | | 100mmol | | i.v. | 24h | venous gases, pH measurement |
| | from day -3 | Heparin | continuously | 15000 units | | i.v. | 22h | reduce dose if platelets < 30,000/μl |
| | from day -3, -2 | Allopurinol | 1 - 0 - 1 | 300mg | | oral | | |
| | on days -3,-2, | Granisetron | 30' before chemotherapy | 3mg | | i.v. | bolus | |
| | on days -3,-2, | Aprepitant | 60' before chemotherapy | 125mg | | oral | | |
| | on days -3,-2 | Dexamethasone | 30' before chemotherapy | 20mg | | i.v. | bolus 15min | |
| | from admission until day -2 | Co-trimoxazole | 1 - 0 - 1 (2x/week) | 960mg | | oral | | |
| | -1 | Levofloxacin | 1 - 0 - 0 | 500mg | | oral | | until possibility of i.v. antibiotics or engraftment |
| | from admission until day -2 | Folic Acid | 1 - 0 - 0 | 5mg | | oral | | |
| | from day +7 | Filgrastim | mornings | 300μg absolute | | s.c. | | till stable engraftment: WBC >1000/μl for 2 days |
| | regularly | Aciclovir | 1 - 1 - 1 - 1 | 400mg | | oral | | daily till start of engraftment |
| | with stable engraftment | Co-trimoxazole | 1 - 0 - 1 (2x/week) | 960mg | | oral | | |
| | with stable engraftment | Folic Acid | 1 - 0 - 0 | 5mg | | oral | | |

| | |
|---|---|
| Medicines As Required | Metoclopramide, Dexamethasone 4mg every 8 hours, Dimenhydrinate, Pantoprazole 40mg, Sucralfate, Lynestrenol 5mg every 12 hours |
| Routine Tests: | FBC, U&Es, LFTs, serum creatinine, creatinine clearance, cardiac function, diuresis, pulmonary function |
| Dose Reduction: | See Dose Modification Table |
| Efficacy Assess. | **Check for remission 4-8 weeks after 1st high-dose therapy** |
| References: | Adapted from Goldschmidt et al., Ann Oncol, 1997, 8(3):243-6; Harousseau JL, Leukemia, 2002;16(9):1838-43; Child JA et al., N Engl J Med, 20 03; 348(19):1875-83; Haas P et al., AOH 2005 |

# Melphalan 140 — Indication: Multiple Myeloma

**Patients >70 years or with renal failure or with Karnofsky Index<70%**  **14.3**

*This chemotherapy may cause life-threatening toxicity! It should only be administered under the supervision of an experienced medical oncologist! The protocol must first be reviewed and considered in relationship to the clinical situation of the patient.*

## Chemotherapy

| Week | Day | Compounds (generic names) in chronological order | Dosage | Diluent | Route | Duration of Infusion | Comments |
|---|---|---|---|---|---|---|---|
| | -2 | **Melphalan** (via central line) | 140mg/m² | 500ml Saline 0.9% | i.v. | 1h | **incompatible with glucose** |
| | -1 | **Therapy-free Interval** of at least 30 hours | | | | | |
| | 0 | **Peripheral Blood Stem Cell Transplantation** | | | | | |

**Cautions**

Aprepitant is a moderate inhibitor and inducer of CYP3A4 (see Summary of Product Characteristics - SmPC)

- additional caution with Etoposide, Vinorelbine, Docetaxel, Paclitaxel, Irinotecan and Ketoconazole
- not to be given concomitantly with Pimozide, Terfenadine, Astemizole or Cisapride
- avoid concomitant use with Rifampicin, Phenytoin, Carbamazepine or other CYP3A4 inducers
- reduce the normal dose of oral Dexamethasone to 50%
- the effectiveness of oral contraceptives may be decreased until 2 months after the last dose of Aprepitant

Dosage of all chemotherapy for the overweight refers to ideal body weight (IBW), calculate body surface area using IBW:

Men: IBW = 50kg + 2.3 x (height in cm/2.53) - 60)

Women: IBW = 45.5kg + 2.3 x ((height in cm/2.53) - 60)

If IBW is more than 15kg below actual body weight, use adjusted body weight: Calculated IBW + 0.4 x (actual BW - calculated IBW)

**Cycle Diagram**

| | d-7 w-1 | d1 w1 | d8 w2 | weeks 4-16 |
|---|---|---|---|---|
| Melphalan | | | | <---N.C.---> |
| No Therapy | | | | |
| PBSCT | | | | |

## Obligatory Pre- and Concurrent Medication

| Week | Day | Sequence and Timing | Compounds (generic names) | Dose | Diluent | Route | Duration of Infusion | Comments |
|---|---|---|---|---|---|---|---|---|
| | from day -2 | continuously | Saline 0.9% | | 2000ml | i.v. | 22h | |
| | from day -2 | continuously | Heparin | 15000 units | | i.v. | 22h | reduce dose if platelets < 30,000/µl |
| | from admission until day -2 | 1 - 0 - 1 (2x week) | Co-trimoxazole | 960mg | | oral | | |
| | -1 | 1 - 0 - 0 | Levofloxacin | 500mg | | oral | | until possibility of i.v. antibiotics or engraftment |
| | from admission until day -2 | 1 - 0 - 0 | Folic Acid | 5mg | | oral | | |
| | from day -2 | 1 - 1 - 1 - 1 | Amphotericin B (as suspension) | 100mg | | oral | | |
| | day -2 | 1h before chemotherapy | Aprepitant | 125mg | | oral | | |
| | day -2 | 30' before chemotherapy | Granisetron | 1mg | | i.v. | bolus | |
| | day -2 | 30' before chemotherapy | Dexamethasone | 12mg | | oral | | |
| | on days -1, 0 | mornings | Aprepitant | 80mg | | oral | | see **Cautions** above |
| | days -1 to +1 | mornings | Dexamethasone | 8mg | | oral | | |
| | from day +7 | mornings | Filgrastim | 300µg absolute | | s.c. | | till stable engraftment: WBC >1000/µl for 2 days |
| | with stable engraftment | 1 - 0 - 1 | Co-trimoxazole | 960mg | | oral | | |
| | with stable engraftment | 1 - 0 - 0 | Folic Acid | 5mg | | oral | | |

| | |
|---|---|
| **Medicines As Required:** | Metoclopramide, Dimenhydrinate, Allopurinol 300mg, Lynestrenol 5mg every 12 hours, Famotidine, Sucralfate, |
| **Routine Tests:** | FBC, U&Es, LFTs, serum creatinine, creatinine clearance, diuresis, cardiac function, pulmonary function |
| **Dose Reduction:** | According to GFR if renal function impaired (see Dose Modification Table) |
| **Next Cycle (N.C.):** | In line with tandem transplantation, 2 cycles with an interval of about 4-16 weeks may be given |
| **Efficacy Assess.** | 1, 3, 6 months after transplantation; normal multiple myeloma remission criteria |
| **References:** | Goldschmidt et al., Ann of Oncol 8(3):243-6, 1997; Harousseau JL, Leuk mia 2002 Sep;16(9): 1838-43; Child JA et al., N Engl J Med 2003 May 8;348(19):1875-83; **Aprepitant:** SmPC, Bokemeyer C. Arzneimitteltherapie, MASCC Antiemetic guidelines 2004 www.mascc.org,Navari RM. Cancer Invest. 2004;22(4):569-76 . |

# Busulfan/Cyclophosphamide    Indication: High-Dose Protocol (Hematologic Neoplasia)    14.4

*This chemotherapy may cause life-threatening toxicity! It should only be administered under the supervision of an experienced medical oncologist! The protocol must first be reviewed and considered in relationship to the clinical situation of the patient.*

## Chemotherapy

| Week | Day | Compounds (generic names) in chronological order | Dosage | Diluent | Route | Duration of Infusion | Comments |
|---|---|---|---|---|---|---|---|
| | -7 to -4 | **Busulfan** | 4mg/kg/day | | oral | | 1 mg/kg at 6:00, 12:00, 18:00, 24:00 respectively |
| | -3 to -2 | **Cyclophosphamide** | 60mg/kg | 1000ml Saline 0.9% | i.v. | 1h | start Cyclophosphamide when urine pH >8 |
| | -1 | **Therapy-free Interval**  of at least 30 hours! | | | | | |
| | 0 | **Transplantation** | | | | | |

**Cautions**

After day 2 protocol for prophylaxis of delayed emesis

Dosage of all chemotherapy for the overweight refers to ideal body weight (IBW), calculate body surface area using IBW:

Men: IBW = 50kg + 2.3 x ((height in cm/2.53) - 60)

Women: IBW = 45.5kg + 2.3 x ((height in cm/2.53) - 60)

If IBW is more than 15kg below actual body weight, use adjusted body weight: Calculated IBW + 0.4 x (actual BW - calculated IBW )

| Cycle Diagram | d-7 w-1 | d1 w1 | d8 w2 | d15 w3 |
|---|---|---|---|---|
| Busulfan | | | | |
| Cyclophos. | | | | |
| No Therapy | | | | |
| Transplantation | | | | |

## Obligatory Pre- and Concurrent Medication

| Week | Day | Sequence and Timing | Compounds (generic names) | Dose | Diluent | Route | Duration of Infusion | Comments |
|---|---|---|---|---|---|---|---|---|
| | regularly | 1 - 0 - 0 | Fluconazole | 200mg | | oral | | |
| from admission until day -2 | 1 - 0 - 1 (2x/week) | Co-trimoxazole | 960mg | | oral | | until possibility of i.v. antibiotics or engraftment |
| | -1 | 1 - 0 - 0 | Levofloxacin | 500mg | | oral | | |
| from admission until day -2 | 1 - 0 - 0 | Folic Acid | 5mg | | oral | | |
| | -8 to -5 | 1 - 1 - 1 - 1 | Phenytoin | 100mg | | oral | | |
| | -4 to -3 | 1 - 1 - 1 | Phenytoin | 100mg | | oral | | |
| | -2 | 1 - 0 - 1 | Phenytoin | 100mg | | oral | | |
| | -1 | 1 - 0 - 0 | Phenytoin | 100mg | | oral | | |
| | -7 to -2 | 1 - 0 - 1 - 0; 30' before chemo. | Granisetron | 2mg/3mg | | oral/i.v. | | |
| | -7 to -2 | 0 - 1 - 0 - 1; 30' before chemo. | Dexamethasone | 8mg | | oral/i.v. | | |
| | -4 | 0 - 0 - 1 - 1 | Sodium Bicarbonate | 4g | | oral | | |
| | -3 to -1 | 1 - 1 - 1 - 1 | Sodium Bicarbonate | 4g | | oral | | |
| | -4 | prehydration | Saline 0.9% | | 1000ml | i.v. | 24h | +60 ml NaHCO₃ + KCl |
| | -3 to -2 | with Cyclophosphamide | Saline 0.9% + Gluc.5% alternately | | 2000ml + 2000ml | i.v. | 24h | +60 ml NaHCO₃ per liter + KCl |
| | -3 to -2 | before Cyclophosphamide | Saline 0.9% | | 500ml | i.v. | 30min | +60 ml NaHCO₃ |
| | -1 to 0 | | Saline 0.9% + Gluc.5% alternately | | 2000ml + 1000ml | i.v. | 24h | +60 ml NaHCO₃ per liter + KCl |
| | from -8 cont. | till day +30 (VOD prophylaxis) | Heparin | 15000 units | | i.v. | 24h | reduce to 5000 units/24h if platelets <30,000/µl |
| | from -3 cont. | continuously | Dopamine | 200mg | | i.v. | 24h | |
| | -3 to -2 | before Cyclophosphamide | Furosemide | 20mg | | i.v. | bolus | |
| | -3 to -1 | parallel to, and after Cyclophos. | Mesna | 100mg/kg | | i.v. | 24h | continue for 24 hours after Cyclophos. |
| | from day +7 | mornings | Filgrastim | 300µg absolute | | s.c. | | til stable engraftment: WBC >1000/µl for 2 days |
| with stable engraftment | 1 - 0 - 1 | Co-trimoxazole | 960mg | | oral | | |
| with stable engraftment | 1 - 0 - 0 | Folic Acid | 5mg | | oral | | |

**Medicines As Required** Lynestrenol 5mg every 12 hours or Goserelin s.c. 1/month, Famotidine, Sucralfate, Aciclovir 200mg orally every 6 hours, 250mg i.v. every 8 hours if HSV positive.

No medication that might lower seizure threshold should be given during **Busulfan** therapy (e.g. Metronidazole)

**Routine Tests** FBC, U&Es, LFTs, serum creatinine, diuresis, blood gases, clotting studies, pulmonary function, serum Phenytoin on day -6.

**References:** Tutschka PJ et al., Exp Hematol. 1987;15:601; Bertz H, Finke J, B Marro Transpl 1997 Jun;19(12):1169-73; Deeg et al., Blood 2002 Aug 15;100(<9):1201-7

# Busulfan monotherapy  Indication: AML  14.5

*This chemotherapy may cause life-threatening toxicity! It should only be administered under the supervision of an experienced medical oncologist! The protocol must first be reviewed and considered in relationship to the clinical situation of the patient.*

## Chemotherapy

| Week | Day | Compounds (generic names) in chronological order | Dosage | Diluent | Route | Duration of Infusion | Comments |
|---|---|---|---|---|---|---|---|
| | -6 to -3 | **Busulfan** | 4mg/kg/day | | oral | | 1mg/kg at 6:00, 12:00, 18:00, 24:00 respectively |
| | -2 to -1 | **Therapy-free Interval >48 hours** | | | | | |
| | 0 | **Transplantation** | | | | | |

**Cautions**

Dosage of all chemotherapy for the overweight refers to ideal body weight (IBW), calculate body surface area using IBW:

Men: $IBW = 50\text{kg} + 2.3 \times ((\text{height in cm}/2.53) - 60)$

Women: $IBW = 45.5\text{kg} + 2.3 \times ((\text{height in cm}/2.53) - 60)$

If IBW is more than 15kg under actual body weight, use adjusted body weight: Calculated IBW + 0.4 x (actual BW - calculated IBW )

| Cycle Diagram | d-7 w-1 | d1 w1 | d8 w2 | d15 w3 |
|---|---|---|---|---|
| Busulfan | ▓ | | | |
| No Therapy | | | | |
| Transplantation | | ■ | | |

## Obligatory Pre- and Concurrent Medication

| Week | Day | Compounds (generic names) | Sequence and Timing | Dose | Diluent | Route | Duration of Infusion | Comments |
|---|---|---|---|---|---|---|---|---|
| | from admission until day -2 | Co-trimoxazole | 1-0-1 (2x/week) | 960mg | | oral | | discontinue if i.v. antibiotics necessary |
| | -1 | Levofloxacin | 1-0-0 | 500mg | | oral | | until possibility of i.v. antibiotics or engraftment |
| | from admission until day -2 | Folic Acid | 1-0-0 | 5mg | | oral | | |
| | regularly | Aciclovir | 1-1-1-1 | 200mg | | oral | | only if HSV serology positive |
| | -8 to -5 | Phenytoin | 1-1-1-1 | 100mg | | oral | | check serum Phenytoin level on day -6 |
| | -4 to -3 | Phenytoin | 1-1-1 | 100mg | | oral | | |
| | -2 | Phenytoin | 1-0-1 | 100mg | | oral | | |
| | -1 | Phenytoin | 1-0-0 | 100mg | | oral | | |
| | -6 to -3 | Granisetron | 1-0-1-0; 30' before chemo. | 2mg | | oral | | |
| | -6 to -3 | Dexamethasone | 0-1-0-1; 30' before chemo. | 8mg | | oral | | |
| | -7 to +2 | Allopurinol | 1-0-0 | 300mg | | oral | | |
| | from -6 cont. | Heparin | till day +30 (VOD prophylaxis) | 15000 units | | i.v. | 24h | reduce to 5000 units/24h if platelets < 30,000 |
| | from day +7 | Filgrastim | mornings | 300µg absolute | | s.c. | | till stable engraftment: WBC >1000/µl |
| | with stable engraftment | Co-trimoxazole | 1-0-1 | 960mg | | oral | | |
| | with stable engraftment | Folic Acid | 1-0-0 | 5mg | | oral | | |

**Medicines As Required:** Lynestrenol 5mg every 12 hours, Famotidine

**Routine Tests:** FBC, U&Es, LFTs, serum creatinine, diuresis, blood gases, clotting studies, pulmonary function. No medication that might lower seizure threshold during **Busulfan** therapy

**References:** Study protocol CML Study IIIa 10/97; Bertz H, Finke J, B Marrow Transpl. 1997;19(12):1169-73; Deeg HJ, Appelbaum FR et al. Blood, 2002;100(4):1201-7

| VIC | Indication: High-Dose Protocol (Solid Tumors) | 14.6 |
|---|---|---|

*This chemotherapy may cause life-threatening toxicity! It should only be administered under the supervision of an experienced medical oncologist! The protocol must first be reviewed and considered in relationship to the clinical situation of the patient.*

## Chemotherapy

| Week | Day | Compounds (generic names) in chronological order | Dosage | Diluent | Route | Duration of Infusion | Comments |
|---|---|---|---|---|---|---|---|
| | -4 to -2 | **Etoposide Phosphate** | 500mg/m² | 500ml Saline 0.9% | i.v. | 1h | dose expressed in terms of Etoposide base |
| | -4 to -2 | **Carboplatin** | #AUC 6mg/mlxmin | 500ml Glucose 5% | i.v. | 18h | #dose (mg) = AUC (mg/ml x min) x [GFR (ml/min)+25] |
| | -4 to -2 | **Ifosfamide** | 4000mg/m² | 500ml Saline 0.9% | i.v. | 18h | parallel to Carboplatin |
| | -1 | **Therapy-free Interval** of at least 24 hours! | | | | | |
| | 0 | **Peripheral Blood Stem Cell Transplantation** | | | | | |

**Cautions**

Etoposide Phosphate and Sodium Bicarbonate must not be administered concomitantly through the same infusion site!
After day 2 protocol for prophylaxis of delayed emesis
Incompatibilities: Carboplatin<>Mesna, Carboplatin<>NaHCO₃, Etoposide Phosphate<>alkaline solutions
Dosage of all chemotherapy for the overweight refers to ideal body weight (IBW), calculate body surface area using IBW:
Men: IBW = 50kg + 2.3 x ((height in cm/2.53) - 60)
Women: IBW = 45.5kg + 2.3 x ((height in cm/2.53) - 60)
If IBW is more than 15kg below actual body weight, use adjusted body weight: Calculated IBW + 0.4 x (actual BW - calculated IBW)

| Cycle Diagram | d-7 w-1 | d1 w1 | d8 w2 | d15 w3 | d |
|---|---|---|---|---|---|
| Etop. Phos. | | | | | |
| Carboplatin | | | | | |
| Ifosfamide | | | | | |
| No Therapy | | | | | |
| PBSCT | | | | | |

## Obligatory Pre- and Concurrent Medication

| Week | Day | Compounds (generic names) | Dose | Diluent | Route | Duration of Infusion | Comments |
|---|---|---|---|---|---|---|---|
| | -5 | Saline 0.9% | 1000ml | | i.v. | 12h | continue infusion after chemotherapy |
| | -4 to +4 | Saline 0.9% | 3000ml | | i.v. | 24h | |
| | -5 to -2 | Magnesium | 6.3 mmol/day | Saline 0.9% | i.v. | | in saline infusion |
| from admission until day -2 | 1 - 0 - 1 | Co-trimoxazole | 960mg | | oral | | |
| | -1 | 1 - 0 - 0 | Levofloxacin | 500mg | | oral | | until possibility of i.v. antibiotics or engraftment |
| from admission until day -2 | 1 - 0 - 0 | Folic Acid | 5mg | | oral | | |
| | -4 to -2 | 15' before and 8h after chemo. | Granisetron | 3mg | | i.v. | bolus | |
| | -4 to -2 | 15' before, 4h & 8h after chemo. | Dexamethasone | 8mg | 100ml Saline 0.9% | i.v. | 15min | |
| | -4 to -1 | 15' before,4h ,8h after Ifosfamide | Mesna | 800/4000/2000mg/m² | | i.v. | B/18h/6h | |
| | from day -4 | continuously | Heparin | 15000 units | | i.v. | 24h | reduce dose if platelets < 30,000/µl |
| | -4 to -1 | continuously | Sodium Bicarbonate | 100mmol | | i.v. | 24h | |
| | -4 to +2 | continuously | Dopamine | 200mg | | i.v. | 24h | |
| | from day +7 | mornings | Filgrastim | 300µg absolute | | s.c. | | till stable engraftment: WBC >1000/µl for 2 days |
| | with stable engraftment | 1 - 0 - 1 (2x/ week) | Co-trimoxazole | 960mg | | oral | | |
| | with stable engraftment | 1 - 0 - 0 | Folic Acid | 5mg | | oral | | |

| Medicines As Required | Metoclopramide, Famotidine, Lynestrenol 5mg every 12 hours, Sucralfate |
|---|---|
| Routine Tests | FBC, U&Es esp. Ca²⁺, Mg²⁺, LFTs, serum creatinine, creatinine clearance, fluid balance, ototoxicity, neurotoxicity |
| Dose Reduction: | With renal insufficiency: reduce **Carboplatin**; with impairment of renal and liver function: reduce **Ifosfamide**; see Dose Modification Table |
| References: | According to Brugger W et al., J Clin Oncol. 1992;9:1452-9; Hartmann JT et al., Br J Cancer 2001;84(3):313-20 |

# Bu-Mel  EURO - E.W.I.N.G. 99  Indication: High-Dose Protocol Ewing's Sarcoma  14.7

*This chemotherapy may cause life-threatening toxicity! It should only be administered under the supervision of an experienced medical oncologist! The protocol must first be reviewed and considered in relationship to the clinical situation of the patient.*

## Chemotherapy

| Week | Day | Compounds (generic names) in chronological order | Dosage | Diluent | Route | Duration of Infusion | Comments |
|---|---|---|---|---|---|---|---|
| | -6 to -3 | **Busulfan** | 4mg/kg/day | | oral | | 1mg/kg at 6:00, 12:00, 18:00, 24:00 respectively |
| | - 2 | **Melphalan** | 140mg/m² | 500ml Saline 0.9% | i.v. | 30min. | incompatible with glucose |
| | -1 | **Therapy-free Interval** | | | | | via central line |
| | 0 | **Peripheral Blood Stem Cell Transplantation** | CD34⁺ 4x10⁶/kg | | | | |

**Cautions**

Dosage of all chemotherapy for the overweight refers to ideal body weight (IBW), calculate body surface area using IBW:

Men: IBW = 50kg + 2.3 x ((height in cm/2.53) - 60)

Women: IBW = 45.5kg + 2.3 x ((height in cm/2.53) - 60)

If IBW is more than 15kg under actual body weight, use adjusted body weight: Calculated IBW + 0.4 x (actual BW - calculated IBW)

| Cycle Diagram | d-7 w-1 | d1 w1 | d8 w2 | d15 w3 |
|---|---|---|---|---|
| Busulfan | | | | |
| Melphalan | | | | |
| No Therapy | | | | |
| PBSCT | | | | |

## Obligatory Pre- and Concurrent Medication

| Week | Day | Sequence and Timing | Compounds (generic names) | Dose | Diluent | Route | Duration of Infusion | Comments |
|---|---|---|---|---|---|---|---|---|
| | from admission until day -2 | 1 - 0 - 1 (2x/week) | Co-trimoxazole | 960mg | | oral | | until possibility of i.v. antibiotics or engraftment |
| | -1 | 1 - 0 - 0 | Levofloxacin | 500mg | | oral | | discontinue if i.v. antibiotics required |
| | from admission until day -2 | 1 - 0 - 0 | Folic Acid | 5mg | | oral | | |
| | from day +1 | 1 - 1 - 1 - 1 | Aciclovir | 200mg | | oral | | only if HSV serology positive |
| | -7 to -5 | 1 - 1 - 1 - 1 | Phenytoin | 100mg | | oral | | check serum Phenytoin level on day -6 |
| | -4 to -3 | 1 - 1 - 1 | Phenytoin | 100mg | | oral | | |
| | -2 | 1 - 0 - 1 | Phenytoin | 100mg | | oral | | |
| | -1 | 1 - 0 - 0 | Phenytoin | 100mg | | oral | | |
| | -6 to -3 | 1 - 0 - 0 before chemo. admin. | Granisetron | 2mg | | oral | | |
| | -2 | 15' before chemotherapy | Granisetron | 3mg | | i.v. | | |
| | -2 to -1 | 1 - 1 - 1 | Dexamethasone | 4mg | | i.v. | | |
| | from -6 cont. | till day +30 (VOD prophylaxis) | Heparin | 15000 units | | i.v. | 24h | platelets<30,000 reduce to 5000 units/24h |
| | from -6 cont. | 1 - 0 - 0 | Allopurinol | 300mg | | oral | | |
| | from day +7 | mornings | Filgrastim | 300 µg absolute | | s.c. | | till stable engraftment: WBC >1000/µl |
| | with stable engraftment | 1 - 0 - 1 | Co-trimoxazole | 960mg | | oral | | |
| | with stable engraftment | 1 - 0 - 0 | Folic Acid | 5mg | | oral | | |

**Medicines As Required** Goserelin acetate 1x/month s.c., Lynestrenol 5mg/month s.c., Lynestrenol 5mg every 12 hours, Pantoprazole 40mg, Sucralfate

**Routine Tests:** FBC, U&Es, LFTs, serum creatinine, creatinine clearance, diuresis, bloo gases, clotting studies (PTT<37"), cardiac function, pulmonary function

**Dose Reduction:** Leukocytes <2000/µl or neutrophils <1000/µl, platelets <80,000/µl  see study protocol

**Next Cycle (N.C.):** High-dose protocol

**References:** Reiffers J, Bone Marrow Transpl 1995 Jul;16(1):69-70; analogous to Murata M, Br J Haematol 1999 Jun;105(3):799-802

983

# CNS - NHL High-Dose Methotrexate

## Indication: CNS - NHL

**14.8**

*This chemotherapy may cause life-threatening toxicity! It should only be administered under the supervision of an experienced medical oncologist! The protocol must first be reviewed and considered in relationship to the clinical situation of the patient.*

## Chemotherapy

| Week | Day | Compounds (generic names) in chronological order | Dosage | Diluent | Route | Duration of Infusion | Comments |
|---|---|---|---|---|---|---|---|
| | **Prephase:** | **Dexamethasone** | 4mg every 6 hours | | oral/i.v. | | withdraw gradually over 6 days beginning with start of Methotrexate |
| | | diagnostic L.P. if intracranial pressure normal; with CSF involvement: assessment on day 20 after i.v. Methotrexate dose | | | | | |
| | 1, 11, 21, 31 | **Methotrexate** | 8000mg/m² | | i.v. | 4h | |
| | 2-6, 12-16, 22-26 | **Calcium Folinate (Leucovorin)** | 15 mg/m² | | i.v./oral | | every 6 hours, **1st dose i.v.**; commence 24h after start of Methotrexate |
| | 32-36 | | | | | | see Rescue Protocol |

**Note:** with delayed Methotrexate elimination: extension and dose increase of Leucovorin rescue in accordance with the Methotrexate Document in the COSS Database (chapter 3.5)

**Days 16-20** 1st staging: if **PR/CR**, repeat therapy (cycle 2)
if **PD/SD**, start AraC/Thiotepa therapy

| Cycle Diagram | d1 w1 | d8 w2 | d15 w3 | d22 w4 | d29 w5 | d36 w6 | d43 w7 | d50 w8 | d57 w9 |
|---|---|---|---|---|---|---|---|---|---|
| Dexameth. | | | | | | | | | |
| Methotrexate | | | PR/CR staging | | staging | | | | continue therapy with AraC/Thiotepa, starting on day 41 |
| | | | PD/SD =>CNS-NHL HD, continue therapy with AraC/TT | | | | | | |
| Leucovorin | | | | | | | | | |

Cautions

## Obligatory Pre- and Concurrent Medication

| Week | Day | Compounds (generic names) | Sequence and Timing | Dose | Diluent | Route | Duration of Infusion | Comments |
|---|---|---|---|---|---|---|---|---|
| | -5 till end of Dex. | Sucralfate | 1-1-1-1 | 1g | | oral | | during Dexamethasone therapy |
| | 0, 10, 20, 30 | Sodium Bicarbonate | 1-1-1-1 | 4g | | oral | | |
| | 1, 11, 21, 31 | Saline 0.9% | 3h before chemotherapy | | 1000ml | i.v. | 3h | urine pH must remain >7.4! |
| | | Sodium Bicarbonate | | 60ml/m² | in infusion fluid | | | |
| | 1-2,11-12,21-22,31-32 | Saline 0.9% + Gluc.5% alternately | 15min before chemotherapy | | 2000ml + 1000ml | i.v. | 24h | urine target pH = 8 |
| | 1-2,11-12,21-22,31-32 | Sodium Bicarbonate | continuously | 200mmol | | i.v. | 24h | |
| | 1, 11, 21,31 | Dexamethasone | 15min before chemotherapy | 8mg | | i.v. | 15min | |
| | 1, 11, 21,31 | Granisetron | 15min before chemotherapy | 1mg | | i.v. | bolus | |
| | 1, 11, 21,31 | Furosemide | 6h after Methotrexate | 40mg | | i.v. | bolus | |

| | |
|---|---|
| **Medicines As Required** | Potassium orally, NaHCO₃ infusion 50ml/2 hours, Famotidine, Furosemide 40mg |
| **Routine Tests:** | FBC, U&Es, LFTs, serum creatinine, creatinine clearance, fluid balance, exclude third space fluid accumulation, urine pH >7.4, serum Methotrexate level; normal values according to Rescue Sheets |
| **Dose Reduction:** | Contraindication: if GFR < 50ml/min or serum creatinine > 1.5mg% as well as serum bilirubin >2mg/dl |
| **Max. Cum. Dose :** | Unknown |
| **Next Cycle (N.C.):** | With **PR/CR**, continue therapy with next cycle starting on day 21 (cycle2) |
| **Efficacy Assess.** | Days 16-20 |
| **References:** | Freiburg protocol: therapy for primary cerebral NHL (Dr. G. Illerhaus/Prof. Dr. J. Finke). |

984

# CNS - NHL High-Dose AraC/Thiotepa

**Indication: CNS - NHL**

**14.9**

*This chemotherapy may cause life-threatening toxicity! It should only be administered under the supervision of an experienced medical oncologist! The protocol must first be reviewed and considered in relationship to the clinical situation of the patient.*

## Chemotherapy

| Week | Day | Compounds (generic names) in chronological order | Dosage | Diluent | Route | Duration of Infusion | Comments |
|---|---|---|---|---|---|---|---|
| | 1, 2, 22, 23 | **Cytarabine (AraC)** | 3000 mg/m² | | i.v. | 3h | |
| | 2, 23 | **Thiotepa** | 40mg/m² | | i.v. | 1h | |
| | 10 | **Harvest** | | | | | |
| | | | | | | | |
| | | | | | | | |
| | | | | | | | |

| Cycle Diagram | d1 w1 | d8 w2 | d15 w3 | d22 w4 | d29 w5 | d36 w6 | d43 w7 | d50 w8 |
|---|---|---|---|---|---|---|---|---|
| Cytarabine | | | | | | | | |
| Thiotepa | | | | | | | | |
| Filgrastim | | | <--> | | | | | |
| Harvest | | | | | | | | |
| Staging | | | | | | <--> | | |
| BCNU | | | | | | | | |
| PBSCT | | | | | | | | <--> |

**Cautions**

PBSCT to be carried out not less than 3 days after the last dose of Thiotepa

Thiotepa is secreted in sweat! In order to avoid a toxic induced erythroderma especially in the axillary and inguinal regions, frequent washing with a wet flannel is recommended.

## Obligatory Pre- and Concurrent Medication

| Week | Day | Sequence and Timing | Compounds (generic names) | Dose | Diluent | Route | Duration of Infusion | Comments |
|---|---|---|---|---|---|---|---|---|
| | 1, 2, 22, 23 | 30min before chemotherapy | Saline 0.9% | | 2000ml | i.v. | 24h | |
| | 1, 2, 22, 23 | 30min before chemotherapy | Dexamethasone | 8mg | | i.v. | 15min | |
| | 1, 2, 22, 23 | 30min before chemotherapy | Granisetron | 1mg | | i.v. | bolus | |
| | 1-3, 21, 22, 23 | every 6 hours | Dexamethasone eye drops (1mg/ml) | 2 drops | | each eye | | |
| | 4-8, 25-29 | every 6 hours | Dexpanthenol eye drops (50mg/ml) | 1 drop | | each eye | | |
| | 6-10, 27-31 | mornings | Filgrastim | 300μg absolute | | s.c. | | |
| | | | | | | | | |
| | | | | | | | | |
| | | | | | | | | |

| | |
|---|---|
| **Medicines As Required** | Famotidine |
| **Routine Tests:** | FBC, U&Es, LFTs, serum creatinine |
| **Dose Reduction:** | GFR < 10ml/min is a relative contraindication |
| **Max. Cum. Dose :** | Unknown |
| **Next Cycle (N.C.):** | None |
| **Efficacy Assess.** | 3rd staging between days 18 and 20, 4th staging between days 38 and 40 |
| **References:** | Freiburg protocol; therapy for primary cerebral NHL (Dr. G. Illerhaus/Prof. Dr. J. Finke). |

| CNS - NHL High-Dose BCNU/Thiotepa | Indication: CNS - NHL |
|---|---|

**14.10**

*This chemotherapy may cause life-threatening toxicity! It should only be administered under the supervision of an experienced medical oncologist! The protocol must first be reviewed and considered in relationship to the clinical situation of the patient.*

## Chemotherapy

| Week | Day | Compounds (generic names) in chronological order | Dosage | Route | Duration of Infusion | Comments |
|---|---|---|---|---|---|---|
| | 43 (-6) | **Carmustine (BCNU)** | 400 mg/m² | i.v. | 1h | |
| | 44 & 45 (-5 & -4) | **Thiotepa** | 5mg/kg twice a day | i.v. | 2h | at 12 hourly intervals |
| | 49 (0) | **Peripheral Blood Stem Cell Transplantation** | | | | |

| Cycle Diagram | d1 w1 | d8 w2 | d15 w3 | d22 w4 | d29 w5 | d36 w6 | d43 w7 | d50 w8 |
|---|---|---|---|---|---|---|---|---|
| Cytarabine | | | | | | | | |
| Thiotepa | | | | | | | | |
| Filgrastim | | | | | | | | |
| Harvest | | | | | | | | |
| Staging | | | <--> | | | | <--> | <--> |
| BCNU | | | | | | | | |
| PBSCT | | | | | | | | |

**Cautions**

PBSCT to be carried out not less than 3 days after the last dose of Thiotepa

Thiotepa is secreted in sweat! In order to avoid a toxic induced erythroderma especially in the axillary and inguinal regions, frequent washing with a wet flannel is recommended.

## Obligatory Pre- and Concurrent Medication

| Week | Day | Compounds (generic names) | Sequence and Timing | Dose | Diluent | Route | Duration of Infusion | Comments |
|---|---|---|---|---|---|---|---|---|
| | 43 | Saline 0.9% | 30min before chemotherapy | | 2000ml | i.v. | 24h | |
| | 44, 45 | Saline 0.9% | 30min before chemotherapy | | 3000ml | i.v. | 24h | |
| | 43, 44, 45 | Heparin | 30min before chemotherapy | 15000 units | | i.v. | 24h | |
| | 43, 44, 45 | Granisetron | 30min before chemotherapy | 1mg | | i.v. | bolus | |
| | 43, 44, 45 | Dexamethasone | 30min before chemotherapy | 8mg | | i.v. | 15min | |
| | 43, 44, 45 | Dexamethasone | +4h, +8h | 8mg | | i.v. | 15min | |
| | from day 53 (+5) | Filgrastim | mornings | 300µg absolute | | s.c. | | |
| | regularly | Amphotericin B | 1 - 1 - 1 - 1 | 100mg (1ml) | | oral | | as suspension |
| | regularly | Co-trimoxazole | 1 - 0 - 1 (2x/week) | 960mg | | oral | | |

| | |
|---|---|
| Medicines As Required | Metoclopramide, Famotidine |
| Routine Tests: | FBC, U&Es, LFTs, serum creatinine, pulmonary function tests including carbon monoxide diffusion capacity, echocardiogram |
| Dose Reduction: | GFR < 10ml/min, bilirubin >2mg/dl are relative contraindications |
| Max. Cum. Dose : | **Carmustine**: increased risk pulmonary toxicity when total cumulative dose >1000 mg/m² |
| Next Cycle (N.C.): | None |
| Efficacy Assess. | Day 30 |
| References: | Freiburg protocol; therapy for primary cerebral NHL (Dr. G. Illerhaus/Prof. Dr. J. Finke). |

## Prophylaxis of Delayed Emesis

## Indication: Cytostatic-induced Emesis

**14.11**

*This chemotherapy may cause life-threatening toxicity! It should only be administered under the supervision of an experienced medical oncologist! The protocol must first be reviewed and considered in relationship to the clinical situation of the patient.*

### Chemotherapy

| Time | Day | Compounds (generic names) in chronological order | Dosage | Diluent | Route | Duration of Infusion | Comments |
|------|-----|------|------|------|------|------|------|
| 6:00 and 18:00 | 1-3 days after end of chemo. | **Dexamethasone** | 8mg | | oral | | may also be given intravenously |
| 6:00 hours then 6 hourly | 1-3 days after end of chemo. | **Metoclopramide** | 30mg | | oral | | may also be given intravenously |

| Cycle Diagram (days) | 1-3 |
|------|------|
| Dexamethasone | > |
| Metoclopramide | > |

**Advice regarding the administration of a 5-HT3 antagonist as an alternative antiemetic:**

General:
- the **most effective single drug** for the prophylaxis of delayed emesis is **Dexamethasone**
- the combination of Dexamethasone with either **Metoclopramide** or a **5-HT3 antagonist is equipotent**

Indication:
- only with the occurrence of emesis or with Metoclopramide incompatibility; in **combination** with Dexamethasone
- with a contraindication to Dexamethasone e.g. uncontrolled diabetes mellitus or after stimulatory immunotherapies (e.g. Legha protocol); as a **single medication**

Administration: - orally in the mornings 1x/day in equivalent dosages (Tropisetron 5mg; Granisetron 2mg; Ondansetron 8mg (in this case, 2x/day))

Note:
- the indications concerning the prophylaxis of delayed emesis are mentioned in the relevant risk protocols
- prophylaxis may also be given at the discretion of the treating physician after non-risk protocols where there is an increased individual risk as well as episodes of acute emesis in the current cycle and a well-known history of prolonged vomiting
- with persistent vomiting in the current cycle, maximum rescue therapy according to current antiemetic regimens should continue until vomiting has ceased
- the **use of Dexamethasone**, particularly with hematological neoplasias, should only be undertaken with reference to the administration of Corticosteroids in the relevant therapy protocols and possible complications from long-term administration evaluated after **individual assessment** by the treating physician/consultant

**Cautions**

### Obligatory Pre- and Concurrent Medication

| Week | Day | Compounds (generic names) | Sequence and Timing | Dose | Diluent | Route | Duration of Infusion | Comments |
|------|-----|------|------|------|------|------|------|------|
| | | | | | | | | |
| | | | | | | | | |
| | | | | | | | | |
| | | | | | | | | |
| | | | | | | | | |
| | | | | | | | | |

Medicines As Required: With dyskinesia from Metoclopramide, give Biperiden 2.5-5mg (replace with 5-HT3 Antagonists in next cycle)

Repeat Therapy: Repeat therapy after end of next cycle if there is an existing risk profile

References: Gralla RJ et al, J Clin Oncol, 1999;17:2971-94; Koeller JM, Support Care Cancer, 2002;10:519-22; ESMO Recommendations 4/2002, Chapter13

# Amphotericin B

**Indication: PUO, Organ Mycoses**                    **14.12**

*This chemotherapy may cause life-threatening toxicity! It should only be administered under the supervision of an experienced medical oncologist! The protocol must first be reviewed and considered in relationship to the clinical situation of the patient.*

## Chemotherapy

| Week | Day | Compounds (generic names) in chronological order | Dosage | Diluent | Route | Duration of Infusion | Comments |
|---|---|---|---|---|---|---|---|
| | 1–n | **Amphotericin B** | 1mg/kg max. | 250ml Glucose 5% | i.v. | 6–12h | Test dose with first administration: |
| | | | | | | | 1mg over 30min, then the rest of the |
| | | | | | | | infusion over 6–12 hours. |
| | | | | | | | **A lipid diluent is contraindicated!** |

Cycle Diagram — day 1 ————————————————→ day n
Amphotericin | | etc.

**Cautions**

<u>Note:</u> No simultaneous administration of blood products

A time interval of 8 hours bone marrow transplantation, PBSCT or leukocyte transfusion

Close monitoring of blood pressure, pulse, respiration and temperature both during and after Amphotericin B infusion

Procedure for chills: Pethidine 25–50mg i.v.; possibly stop the infusion

Incompatibility: Amphotericin B<>Saline 0.9%

## Obligatory Pre- and Concurrent Medication

| Week | Day | Sequence and Timing | Compounds (generic names) | Dose | Diluent | Route | Duration of Infusion | Comments |
|---|---|---|---|---|---|---|---|---|
| | 1–n | –1h, +6h to +12h | Saline 0.9% | | 1000ml | i.v. | 1h | |
| | 1–n | –30min | Clemastine | 2.68mg | | i.v. | bolus | |
| | 1–n | –30min | Paracetamol | 500mg | | oral | | |
| | | as required | Dexamethasone | 4mg | | i.v. | bolus | by slow bolus infusion |

| | |
|---|---|
| **Indications:** | Organ and disseminated mycoses particularly Candidiasis, Cryptococcosis, Aspergillosis, Coccidiomycosis, Histoplasmosis |
| **Contraindications:** | Severe impairment of liver and renal function; pregnancy, lactation |
| **Dosage:** | Dosage individually adjusted for each patient; start with test dose: 1mg over 30 min, with cardiovascular stability and good tolerance: 0.3mg/kg over 6 hours; with cardiovascular impairment or poor tolerance: lower the dose e.g. 0.1mg/kg. Daily dose: 0.1–0.7mg/kg. Maximum dose:1mg/kg/day |
| **Stop Therapy:** | Serum creatinine > 3mg/dl |
| **Routine Tests** | U&Es (keep potassium and magnesium towards higher end of normal range), serum creatinine, FBC, LFTs, pulmonary function |
| **Side Effects:** | Disturbances of renal function with hypokalemia, hypomagnesemia, uremia, hyposthenuria, anemia; thrombophlebitis; fever, vomiting, diarrhea |
| **Comments:** | Increases the nephrotoxic effects of Cisplatin, amino glycosides, Cyclosporin, Foscarnet, Ganciclovir |
| **References:** | Eriksson U et al, BML, 2001:322:579–82; Cornely OA et al, Blood, 2003;101:3365–72 |

988

# Leucovorin Rescue

| Surname: | Protocol: Methotrexate Rescue | Diagnosis: | 14.13 |
|---|---|---|---|
| First Name: | Height(cm): | Cycle: | Date: |
| Date of Birth: | Weight (kg): | Day: | Doctor's Signature: |
| | SA (m²): | | |

## Leucovorin Administration

| Hours after start of MTX | Date | Time | Serum MTX level | LV dose given |
|---|---|---|---|---|
| 0 hours - start of MTX infusion | | | | |
| +4 hours - end of MTX infusion | | | | |
| +24 hours: 1st LV dose due | | | | |
| 24h | | | | |
| 30h | | | | |
| 36h | | | | |
| 42h | | | | |
| 48h | | | | |
| 54h | | | | |
| 60h | | | | |
| 66h | | | | |
| 72h | | | | |
| 78h | | | | |
| 84h | | | | |
| 90h | | | | |
| 96h | | | | |
| 102h | | | | |
| 108h | | | | |
| 114h | | | | |
| 120h | | | | |

## Serum MTX Level / Leucovorin Dosage According to Serum MTX Level

| Hours after start of MTX | Date | Time | Serum MTX level (µmol/l) | If serum MTX (µmol/l) | Leucovorin dose [mg/m²] | Leucovorin absolute dose (mg) | Duration of Leucovorin Rescue |
|---|---|---|---|---|---|---|---|
| 4h | | | | - | - | - | peak level |
| 24h | | | | <8.5 | 15 | | until day 6 |
| | | | | 8.5-12 | 90 | | |
| | | | | 12.1-18 | 150 | | |
| | | | | >18 | 300 | | |
| 42h | | | | <3.0 | 15 | | until day 6 |
| | | | | 3.0-11 | 90 | | |
| | | | | 11.1-21 | 150 | | |
| | | | | >21 | 300 | | |
| 48h | | | | <0.3 | 15 | | until day 6 |
| | | | | 0.4-1.8 | 15 | | |
| | | | | 1.9-2.8 | 30 | | |
| | | | | 2.9-8.5 | 90 | | |
| | | | | 8.6-18 | 150 | | |
| | | | | >18 | 300 | | |
| 72h | | | | <0.4 | 15 | | until day 6 |
| | | | | 0.4-1.8 | 15 | | |
| | | | | 1.9-2.8 | 30 | | |
| | | | | 2.9-9.8 | 90 | | |
| | | | | 9.9-19 | 150 | | |
| | | | | >19 | 300 | | |
| 96h | | | | proceed as for 72 hours | | | |

further serum MTX levels may be done at 120, 140, 168 hours

## Comments

**1.**
**Boxes with white background:** serum MTX level in normal range
**Boxes with grey background:** caution: serum MTX level outside normal range

**2.**
**All times and dates are with reference to the start of MTX infusion.**
**LV Rescue is commenced:**
- **24h after start of MTX, if** serum level within normal range
- **immediately, if** there are clinical signs of toxicity (even if serum MTX levels are within normal range e.g. with infections or severe inflammatory conditions) or serum MTX level>1000 µmol/l after end of MTX infusion; **LV dose must also be increased 2-4 fold**

**3.**
**Leucovorin dose every 6 hours** throughout entire Rescue (4x/day)

**4.**
**With markedly raised serum MTX:** Carboxypeptidase G2 may be given as antidote.

**5.**
**For LV Doses> 20 mg/kg BW:** dose in 250ml Saline 0.9% over 1h

**6.**
**Urinary alkalinization:** keep urine pH >7.4; check with each voiding

# Subject Index